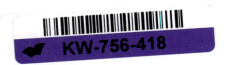

British Pharmacopoeia 2014

Volume IV

British Pharmacopoeia 2014

Volume IV

The British Pharmacopoeia Commission has caused this British Pharmacopoeia 2014 to be prepared under regulation 317(1) of the Human Medicines Regulations 2012 and, in accordance with regulation 317(4), the Ministers have arranged for it to be published. It has been notified in draft to the European Commission in accordance with Directive 98/34/EEC.

The monographs of the Seventh Edition of the European Pharmacopoeia (2010), as amended by Supplements 7.1 to 7.8, published by the Council of Europe are reproduced either in this edition of the British Pharmacopoeia or in the associated edition of the British Pharmacopoeia (Veterinary).

See General Notices

Effective date: 1 January 2014

see Notices

London: The Stationery Office

In respect of Great Britain:

THE DEPARTMENT OF HEALTH

In respect of Northern Ireland:

THE DEPARTMENT OF HEALTH, SOCIAL SERVICES AND
PUBLIC SAFETY

© Crown Copyright 2013

Published by The Stationery Office on behalf of the Medicines and
Healthcare products Regulatory Agency (MHRA) except that:

European Pharmacopoeia monographs are reproduced with the permission
of the Council of Europe and are not Crown Copyright. These are
identified in the publication by a chaplet of stars.

This publication is a 'value added' product. If you wish to re-use the
Crown Copyright material from this publication, applications must be made
in writing, clearly stating the material requested for re-use, and the purpose
for which it is required. Applications should be sent to: Dr S Atkinson,
MHRA, 5th Floor, 151 Buckingham Palace Road, London SW1W 9SZ.

First Published 2013

ISBN 978 011 3229 352

British Pharmacopoeia Commission Office:
MHRA
151 Buckingham Palace Road,
London SW1W 9SZ
Telephone: +44 (0)20 3080 6561
E-mail: bpcom@mhra.gsi.gov.uk
Web site: http://www.pharmacopoeia.com

Laboratory:
British Pharmacopoeia Commission Laboratory
Queen's Road
Teddington
Middlesex TW11 0LY
Telephone: +44 (0)20 8943 8960
Fax: +44 (0)20 8943 8962
E-mail: bpcrs@mhra.gsi.gov.uk
Web site: http://www.pharmacopoeia.com

Contents

Contents of Volume IV

Contents of Volume V

Notices

Monographs of the European Pharmacopoeia are distinguished by a chaplet of stars against the title. The term European Pharmacopoeia, used without qualification, means the seventh edition of the European Pharmacopoeia comprising, unless otherwise stated, the main volume, published in 2010, as amended by any subsequent supplements and revisions.

Patents In this Pharmacopoeia certain drugs and preparations have been included notwithstanding the existence of actual or potential patent rights. In so far as such substances are protected by Letters Patent their inclusion in this Pharmacopoeia neither conveys, nor implies, licence to manufacture.

Effective dates New and revised monographs of national origin enter into force on 1 January 2014. The monographs are brought into effect under regulation 320(2) of the Human Medicines Regulations 2012.

Monographs of the European Pharmacopoeia have previously been published by the European Directorate for the Quality of Medicines & HealthCare in accordance with the Convention on the Elaboration of a European Pharmacopoeia and have been brought into effect under European Directives 2001/82/EC, 2001/83/EC and 2003/63/EC, as amended, on medicines for human and veterinary use.

General Notices

CONTENTS OF THE GENERAL NOTICES

General Notices

Part I

The British Pharmacopoeia comprises the entire text within this publication.
The word 'official' is used in the Pharmacopoeia to signify 'of the Pharmacopoeia'.
It applies to any title, substance, preparation, method or statement included in the
general notices, monographs and appendices of the Pharmacopoeia.
The abbreviation for British Pharmacopoeia is BP.

European
Pharmacopoeia

Monographs of the European Pharmacopoeia are reproduced in this edition of the British Pharmacopoeia by incorporation of the text published under the direction of the Council of Europe (Partial Agreement) in accordance with the Convention on the Elaboration of a European Pharmacopoeia (Treaty Series No. 32 (1974) CMND 5763) as amended by the Protocol to the Convention (Treaty Series No. MISC16 (1990) CMND 1133). They are included for the convenience of users of the British Pharmacopoeia. In cases of doubt or dispute reference should be made to the Council of Europe text.

Monographs of the European Pharmacopoeia are distinguished by a chaplet of stars against the title and by reference to the European Pharmacopoeia monograph number included immediately below the title in italics. The beginning and end of text from the European Pharmacopoeia are denoted by means of horizontal lines with the symbol '*Ph Eur*' ranged left and right, respectively.

The general provisions of the European Pharmacopoeia relating to different types of dosage form are included in the appropriate general monograph in that section of the British Pharmacopoeia entitled Monographs: Formulated Preparations. These general provisions apply to all dosage forms of the type defined, whether an individual monograph is included in the British Pharmacopoeia or not.

Texts of the European Pharmacopoeia are governed by the General Notices of the European Pharmacopoeia. These are reproduced as Part III of these notices.

Part II

The following general notices apply to the statements made in the monographs of the British Pharmacopoeia other than those reproduced from the European Pharmacopoeia and to the statements made in the Appendices of the British Pharmacopoeia other than when a method, test or other matter described in an appendix is invoked in a monograph reproduced from the European Pharmacopoeia.

Official Standards The requirements stated in the monographs of the Pharmacopoeia apply to articles that are intended for medicinal use but not necessarily to articles that may be sold under the same name for other purposes. An article intended for medicinal use that is described by means of an official title must comply with the requirements of the relevant monograph. A formulated preparation must comply throughout its assigned shelf-life (period of validity). The subject of any other monograph must comply throughout its period of use.

A monograph is to be construed in accordance with any general monograph or notice or any appendix, note or other explanatory material that is contained in this edition and that is applicable to that monograph. All statements contained in the monographs, except where a specific general notice indicates otherwise and with the exceptions given below, constitute standards for the official articles. An article is not of pharmacopoeial quality unless it complies with all of the requirements stated. This does not imply that a manufacturer is obliged to perform all the tests in a monograph in order to assess compliance with the Pharmacopoeia before release of a product. The manufacturer may assure himself that a product is of pharmacopoeial quality by other means, for example, from data derived from validation studies of the manufacturing process, from in-process controls or from a combination of the two. Parametric release in appropriate circumstances is thus not precluded by the need to comply with the Pharmacopoeia. The general notice on Assays and Tests indicates that analytical methods other than those described in the Pharmacopoeia may be employed for routine purposes.

Requirements in monographs have been framed to provide appropriate limitation of potential impurities rather than to provide against all possible impurities. Material found to contain an impurity not detectable by means of the prescribed tests is not of pharmacopoeial quality if the nature or amount of the impurity found is incompatible with good pharmaceutical practice.

The status of any statement given under the headings Definition, Production, Characteristics, Storage, Labelling or Action and use is defined within the general notice relating to the relevant heading. In addition to any exceptions indicated by one of the general notices referred to above, the following parts of a monograph do not constitute standards: (a) a graphic or molecular formula given at the beginning of a monograph; (b) a molecular weight; (c) a Chemical Abstracts Service Registry Number; (d) any information given at the end of a monograph concerning impurities known to be limited by that monograph; (e) information in any annex to a monograph. Any statement containing the word 'should' constitutes non-mandatory advice or recommendation.

The expression 'unless otherwise justified and authorised' means that the requirement in question has to be met, unless a competent authority authorises a modification or exemption where justified in a particular case. The term 'competent authority' means the national, supranational or international body or organisation vested with the authority for making decisions concerning the issue in question. It may, for example, be a licensing authority or an official control laboratory. For a formulated preparation that is the subject of monograph in the British Pharmacopoeia any justified and authorised modification to, or exemption from, the requirements of the relevant general monograph of the European Pharmacopoeia is stated in the individual monograph. For example, the general monograph for Tablets requires that Uncoated Tablets, except for chewable tablets, disintegrate within 15 minutes; for Calcium Lactate Tablets a time of 30 minutes is permitted.

Many of the general monographs for formulated preparations include statements and requirements additional to those of the European Pharmacopoeia that are applicable to the individual monographs of the British Pharmacopoeia. Such statements and requirements apply to all monographs for that dosage form included in the Pharmacopoeia unless otherwise indicated in the individual monograph.

Where a monograph on a biological substance or preparation refers to a strain, a test, a method, a substance, etc., using the qualifications 'suitable' or 'appropriate' without further definition in the text, the choice of such strain, test, method, substance, etc., is made in accordance with any international agreements or national regulations affecting the subject concerned.

Definition of Terms

Where the term 'about' is included in a monograph or test it should be taken to mean approximately (fairly correct or accurate; near to the actual value).

Where the term 'corresponds' is included in a monograph or test it should be taken to mean similar or equivalent in character or quantity.

Where the term 'similar' is included in a monograph or test it should be taken to mean alike though not necessarily identical.

Further qualifiers (such as numerical acceptance criteria) for the above terms are not included in the BP. The acceptance criteria for any individual case is set based on the range of results obtained from known reference samples, the level of precision of the equipment or apparatus used and the level of accuracy required for the particular application. The user should determine the variability seen in his/her own laboratory and set in-house acceptance criteria that he/she judges to be appropriate based on the local operating conditions.

Expression of Standards

Where the standard for the content of a substance described in a monograph is expressed in terms of the chemical formula for that substance an upper limit exceeding 100% may be stated. Such an upper limit applies to the result of the assay calculated in terms of the equivalent content of the specified chemical formula. For example, the statement 'contains not less than 99.0% and not more than 101.0% of $C_{20}H_{24}N_2O_2,HCl$' implies that the result of the assay is not less than 99.0% and not more than 101.0%, calculated in terms of the equivalent content of $C_{20}H_{24}N_2O_2,HCl$.

Where the result of an assay or test is required to be calculated with reference to the dried, anhydrous or ignited substance, the substance free from a specified solvent or to the peptide content, the determination of loss on drying, water content, loss on ignition, content of the specified solvent or peptide content is carried out by the method prescribed in the relevant test in the monograph.

Temperature The Celsius thermometric scale is used in expressing temperatures.

Weights and Measures The metric system of weights and measures is employed; SI Units have generally been adopted. Metric measures are required to have been graduated at 20° and all measurements involved in the analytical operations of the Pharmacopoeia are intended, unless otherwise stated, to be made at that temperature. Graduated glass apparatus used in analytical operations should comply with Class A requirements of the appropriate International Standard issued by the International Organization for Standardization. The abbreviation for litre is 'L' throughout the Pharmacopoeia. In line with European Directive 80/181/EEC, the abbreviation 'l' is also permitted for use.

Atomic Weights The atomic weights adopted are the values given in the Table of Relative Atomic Weights 2001 published by the International Union of Pure and Applied Chemistry (Appendix XXV).

Constant Weight The term 'constant weight', used in relation to the process of drying or the process of ignition, means that two consecutive weighings do not differ by more than 0.5 mg, the second weighing being made after an additional period of drying or ignition under the specified conditions appropriate to the nature and quantity of the residue (1 hour is usually suitable).

Expression of Concentrations The term 'per cent' or more usually the symbol '%' is used with one of four different meanings in the expression of concentrations according to circumstances. In order that the meaning to be attached to the expression in each instance is clear, the following notation is used:

Per cent w/w (% w/w) (percentage weight in weight) expresses the number of grams of solute in 100 g of product.

Per cent w/v (% w/v) (percentage weight in volume) expresses the number of grams of solute in 100 mL of product.

Per cent v/v (% v/v) (percentage volume in volume) expresses the number of millilitres of solute in 100 mL of product.

Per cent v/w (% v/w) (percentage volume in weight) expresses the number of millilitres of solute in 100 g of product.

Usually the strength of solutions of solids in liquids is expressed as percentage weight in volume, of liquids in liquids as percentage volume in volume and of gases in liquids as percentage weight in weight.

When the concentration of a solution is expressed as parts per million (ppm), it means weight in weight, unless otherwise specified.

When the concentration of a solution is expressed as parts of dissolved substance in parts of the solution, it means parts by weight (g) of a solid in parts by volume (mL) of the final solution; or parts by volume (mL) of a liquid in parts by volume (mL) of the final solution; or parts by weight (g) of a gas in parts by weight (g) of the final solution.

When the concentration of a solution is expressed in molarity designated by the symbol M preceded by a number, it denotes the number of moles of the stated solute contained in sufficient Purified Water (unless otherwise stated) to produce 1 litre of solution.

Water Bath The term 'water bath' means a bath of boiling water, unless water at some other temperature is indicated in the text. An alternative form of heating may be employed providing that the required temperature is approximately maintained but not exceeded.

Reagents The reagents required for the assays and tests of the Pharmacopoeia are defined in appendices. The descriptions set out in the appendices do not imply that the materials are suitable for use in medicine.

Indicators Indicators, the colours of which change over approximately the same range of pH, may be substituted for one another but in the event of doubt or dispute as to the equivalence of indicators for a particular purpose, the indicator specified in the text is alone authoritative.

The quantity of an indicator solution appropriate for use in acid-base titrations described in assays or tests is 0.1 mL unless otherwise stated in the text.

Any solvent required in an assay or test in which an indicator is specified is previously neutralised to the indicator, unless a blank test is prescribed.

Caution Statements A number of materials described in the monographs and some of the reagents specified for use in the assays and tests of the Pharmacopoeia may be injurious to health unless adequate precautions are taken. The principles of good laboratory practice and the provisions of any appropriate regulations such as those issued in the United Kingdom in accordance with the Health and Safety at Work *etc.* Act 1974 should be observed at all times in carrying out the assays and tests of the Pharmacopoeia.

Attention is drawn to particular hazards in certain monographs by means of an italicised statement; the absence of such a statement should not however be taken to mean that no hazard exists.

Titles Subsidiary titles, where included, have the same significance as the main titles. An abbreviated title constructed in accordance with the directions given in Appendix XXI A has the same significance as the main title.

Titles that are derived by the suitable inversion of words of a main or subsidiary title, with the addition of a preposition if appropriate, are also official titles. Thus, the following are all official titles: Aspirin Tablets, Tablets of Aspirin; Atropine Injection, Injection of Atropine.

A title of a formulated preparation that includes the full nonproprietary name of the active ingredient or ingredients, where this is not included in the title of the monograph, is also an official title. For example, the title Promethazine Hydrochloride Oral Solution has the same significance as Promethazine Oral Solution and the title Brompheniramine Maleate Tablets has the same significance as Brompheniramine Tablets.

Where the English title at the head of a monograph in the European Pharmacopoeia is different from that at the head of the text incorporated into the British Pharmacopoeia, an Approved Synonym has been created on the recommendation of the British Pharmacopoeia Commission. Approved Synonyms have the same significance as the main title and are thus official titles. A cumulative list of such Approved Synonyms is provided in Appendix XXI B.

Where the names of pharmacopoeial substances, preparations and other materials occur in the text they are printed with capital initial letters and this indicates that materials of Pharmacopoeial quality must be used. Words in the text that name a reagent or other material, a physical characteristic or a process that is described or defined in an appendix are printed in italic type, for example, *methanol*, *absorbance*, *gas chromatography*, and these imply compliance with the requirements specified in the appropriate appendix.

Chemical Formulae
When the chemical composition of an official substance is known or generally accepted, the graphic and molecular formulae, the molecular weight and the Chemical Abstracts Service Registry Number are normally given at the beginning of the monograph for information. This information refers to the chemically pure substance and is not to be regarded as an indication of the purity of the official material. Elsewhere, in statements of standards of purity and strength and in descriptions of processes of assay, it is evident from the context that the formulae denote the chemically pure substances.

Where the absolute stereochemical configuration is specified, the International Union of Pure and Applied Chemistry (IUPAC) *R/S* and *E/Z* systems of designation have been used. If the substance is an enantiomer of unknown absolute stereochemistry the sign of the optical rotation, as determined in the solvent and under the conditions specified in the monograph, has been attached to the systematic name. An indication of sign of rotation has also been given where this is incorporated in a trivial name that appears on an IUPAC preferred list.

All amino acids, except glycine, have the L-configuration unless otherwise indicated. The three-letter and one-letter symbols used for amino acids in peptide and protein sequences are those recommended by the Joint Commission on Biochemical Nomenclature of the International Union of Pure and Applied Chemistry and the International Union of Biochemistry and Molecular Biology.

In the graphic formulae the following abbreviations are used:

Me	$-CH_3$	Bu^s	$-CH(CH_3)CH_2CH_3$
Et	$-CH_2CH_3$	Bu^n	$-CH_2CH_2CH_2CH_3$
Pr^i	$-CH(CH_3)_2$	Bu^t	$-C(CH_3)_3$
Pr^n	$-CH_2CH_2CH_3$	Ph	$-C_6H_5$
Bu^i	$-CH_2CH(CH_3)_2$	Ac	$-COCH_3$

Definition
Statements given under the heading Definition constitute an official definition of the substance, preparation or other article that is the subject of the monograph. They constitute instructions or requirements and are mandatory in nature.

Certain medicinal or pharmaceutical substances and other articles are defined by reference to a particular method of manufacture. A statement that a substance or article *is* prepared or obtained by a certain method constitutes part of the official definition and implies that other methods are not permitted. A statement that a substance *may be* prepared or obtained by a certain method, however, indicates that this is one possible method and does not imply that other methods are proscribed.

Additional statements concerning the definition of formulated preparations are given in the general notice on Manufacture of Formulated Preparations.

Production Statements given under the heading Production draw attention to particular aspects of the manufacturing process but are not necessarily comprehensive. They constitute mandatory instructions to manufacturers. They may relate, for example, to source materials, to the manufacturing process itself and its validation and control, to in-process testing or to testing that is to be carried out by the manufacturer on the final product (bulk material or dosage form) either on selected batches or on each batch prior to release. These statements cannot necessarily be verified on a sample of the final product by an independent analyst. The competent authority may establish that the instructions have been followed, for example, by examination of data received from the manufacturer, by inspection or by testing appropriate samples.

The absence of a section on Production does not imply that attention to features such as those referred to above is not required. A substance, preparation or article described in a monograph of the Pharmacopoeia is to be manufactured in accordance with the principles of good manufacturing practice and in accordance with relevant international agreements and supranational and national regulations governing medicinal products.

Where in the section under the heading Production a monograph on a vaccine defines the characteristics of the vaccine strain to be used, any test methods given for confirming these characteristics are provided as examples of suitable methods. The use of these methods is not mandatory.

Additional statements concerning the production of formulated preparations are given in the general notice on Manufacture of Formulated Preparations.

Manufacture of Formulated Preparations Attention is drawn to the need to observe adequate hygienic precautions in the preparation and dispensing of pharmaceutical formulations. The principles of good pharmaceutical manufacturing practice should be observed.

The Definition in certain monographs for pharmaceutical preparations is given in terms of the principal ingredients only. Any ingredient, other than those included in the Definition, must comply with the general notice on Excipients and the product must conform with the Pharmacopoeial requirements.

The Definition in other monographs for pharmaceutical preparations is presented as a full formula. No deviation from the stated formula is permitted except those allowed by the general notices on Colouring Agents and Antimicrobial Preservatives. Where additionally directions are given under the heading Extemporaneous Preparation these are intended for the extemporaneous preparation of relatively small quantities for short-term supply and use. When so prepared, no deviation from the stated directions is permitted. If, however, such a pharmaceutical preparation is manufactured on a larger scale with the intention that it may be stored, deviations from the stated directions are permitted provided that the final product meets the following criteria:

(1) compliance with all of the requirements stated in the monograph;

(2) retention of the essential characteristics of the preparation made strictly in accordance with the directions of the Pharmacopoeia.

Monographs for yet other pharmaceutical preparations include both a Definition in terms of the principal ingredients and, under the side-heading Extemporaneous Preparation, a full formula together with, in some cases, directions for their preparation. Such full formulae and directions are intended for the extemporaneous preparation of relatively small quantities for short-term supply and use. When so prepared, no deviation from the stated formula and directions is permitted. If, however, such a pharmaceutical preparation is manufactured on a larger scale with the intention that it may be stored, deviations from the formula and directions stated under the heading Extemporaneous Preparation are permitted provided that any ingredient, other than those included in the Definition, complies with the general notice on Excipients and that the final product meets the following criteria:

(1) accordance with the Definition stated in the monograph;

(2) compliance with all of the requirements stated in the monograph;

(3) retention of the essential characteristics of the preparation made strictly in accordance with the formula and directions of the Pharmacopoeia.

In the manufacture of any official preparation on a large scale with the intention that it should be stored, in addition to following any instruction under the heading Production, it is necessary to ascertain that the product is satisfactory with respect to its physical and chemical stability and its state of preservation over the claimed shelf-life. This applies irrespective of whether the formula of the Pharmacopoeia and any instructions given under the heading Extemporaneous Preparation are followed precisely or modified. Provided that the preparation has been shown to be stable in other respects, deterioration due to microbial contamination may be inhibited by the incorporation of a suitable antimicrobial preservative. In such circumstances the label states appropriate storage conditions, the date after which the product should not be used and the identity and concentration of the antimicrobial preservative.

Freshly and Recently Prepared The direction, given under the heading Extemporaneous Preparation, that a preparation must be freshly prepared indicates that it must be made not more than 24 hours before it is issued for use. The direction that a preparation should be recently prepared indicates that deterioration is likely if the preparation is stored for longer than about 4 weeks at 15° to 25°.

Methods of Sterilisation The methods of sterilisation used in preparing the sterile materials described in the Pharmacopoeia are given in Appendix XVIII. For aqueous preparations, steam sterilisation (heating in an autoclave) is the method of choice wherever it is known to be suitable. Any method of sterilisation must be validated with respect to both the assurance of sterility and the integrity of the product and to ensure that the final product complies with the requirements of the monograph.

Water The term water used without qualification in formulae for formulated preparations means either potable water freshly drawn direct from the public supply and suitable for drinking or freshly boiled and cooled Purified

Water. The latter should be used if the public supply is from a local storage tank or if the potable water is unsuitable for a particular preparation.

Excipients   Where an excipient for which there is a pharmacopoeial monograph is used in preparing an official preparation it shall comply with that monograph. Any substance added in preparing an official preparation shall be innocuous, shall have no adverse influence on the therapeutic efficacy of the active ingredients and shall not interfere with the assays and tests of the Pharmacopoeia. Particular care should be taken to ensure that such substances are free from harmful organisms.

Colouring Agents   If in a monograph for a formulated preparation defined by means of a full formula a specific colouring agent or agents is prescribed, suitable alternatives approved in the country concerned may be substituted.

Antimicrobial Preservatives   When the term 'suitable antimicrobial preservative' is used it is implied that the preparation concerned will be effectively preserved according to the appropriate criteria applied and interpreted as described in the test for *efficacy of antimicrobial preservation* (Appendix XVI C). In certain monographs for formulated preparations defined by means of a full formula, a specific antimicrobial agent or agents may be prescribed; suitable alternatives may be substituted provided that their identity and concentration are stated on the label.

Characteristics   Statements given under the heading Characteristics are not to be interpreted in a strict sense and are not to be regarded as official requirements. Statements on taste are provided only in cases where this property is a guide to the acceptability of the material (for example, a material used primarily for flavouring). The status of statements on solubility is given in the general notice on Solubility.

   Solubility   Statements on solubility given under the heading Characteristics are intended as information on the approximate solubility at a temperature between 15° and 25°, unless otherwise stated, and are not to be considered as official requirements.

   Statements given under headings such as Solubility in ethanol express exact requirements and constitute part of the standards for the substances under which they occur.

   The following table indicates the meanings of the terms used in statements of approximate solubilities.

Descriptive term	Approximate volume of solvent in millilitres per gram of solute
very soluble	less than 1
freely soluble	from 1 to 10
soluble	from 10 to 30
sparingly soluble	from 30 to 100
slightly soluble	from 100 to 1000
very slightly soluble	from 1000 to 10,000
practically insoluble	more than 10,000

   The term 'partly soluble' is used to describe a mixture of which only some of the components dissolve.

Identification   The tests described or referred to under the heading Identification are not necessarily sufficient to establish absolute proof of identity. They provide a means of verifying that the identity of the material being examined is in accordance with the label on the container.

Unless otherwise prescribed, identification tests are carried out at a temperature between 15° and 25°.

Reference spectra Where a monograph refers to an infrared reference spectrum, this spectrum is provided in a separate section of the Pharmacopoeia. A sample spectrum is considered to be concordant with a reference spectrum if the transmission minima (absorption maxima) of the principal bands in the sample correspond in position, relative intensities and shape to those of the reference. Instrumentation software may be used to calculate concordance with a previously recorded reference spectrum.

When tests for infrared absorption are applied to material extracted from formulated preparations, strict concordance with the specified reference spectrum may not always be possible, but nevertheless a close resemblance between the spectrum of the extracted material and the specified reference spectrum should be achieved.

Assays and Tests   The assays and tests described are the official methods upon which the standards of the Pharmacopoeia depend. The analyst is not precluded from employing alternative methods, including methods of micro-analysis, in any assay or test if it is known that the method used will give a result of equivalent accuracy. Local reference materials may be used for routine analysis, provided that these are calibrated against the official reference materials. In the event of doubt or dispute, the methods of analysis, the reference materials and the reference spectra of the Pharmacopoeia are alone authoritative.

Where the solvent used for a solution is not named, the solvent is Purified Water.

Unless otherwise prescribed, the assays and tests are carried out at a temperature between 15° and 25°.

A temperature in a test for Loss on drying, where no temperature range is given, implies a range of $\pm 2°$ about the stated value.

Visual comparative tests, unless otherwise prescribed, are carried out using identical tubes of colourless, transparent, neutral glass with a flat base. The volumes of liquid prescribed are for use with tubes 16 mm in internal diameter; tubes with a larger internal diameter may be used but the volume of liquid examined must be increased so that the depth of liquid in the tubes is not less than that obtained when the prescribed volume of liquid and tubes 16 mm in internal diameter are used. Equal volumes of the liquids to be compared are examined down the vertical axis of the tubes against a white background or, if necessary, against a black background. The examination is carried out in diffuse light.

Where a direction is given that an analytical operation is to be carried out 'in subdued light', precautions should be taken to avoid exposure to direct sunlight or other strong light. Where a direction is given that an analytical operation is to be carried out 'protected from light', precautions should be taken to exclude actinic light by the use of low-actinic glassware, working in a dark room or similar procedures.

For preparations other than those of fixed strength, the quantity to be taken for an assay or test is usually expressed in terms of the active ingredient. This means that the quantity of the active ingredient expected to be present and the quantity of the preparation to be taken are calculated from the strength stated on the label.

In assays the approximate quantity to be taken for examination is indicated but the quantity actually used must not deviate by more than 10% from that stated. The quantity taken is accurately weighed or measured and the result of the assay is calculated from this exact quantity. Reagents are measured and the procedures are carried out with an accuracy commensurate with the degree of precision implied by the standard stated for the assay.

In tests the stated quantity to be taken for examination must be used unless any divergence can be taken into account in conducting the test and calculating the result. The quantity taken is accurately weighed or measured with the degree of precision implied by the standard or, where the standard is not stated numerically (for example, in tests for Clarity and colour of solution), with the degree of precision implied by the number of significant figures stated. Reagents are measured and the procedures are carried out with an accuracy commensurate with this degree of precision.

The limits stated in monographs are based on data obtained in normal analytical practice; they take account of normal analytical errors, of acceptable variations in manufacture and of deterioration to an extent considered acceptable. No further tolerances are to be applied to the limits prescribed to determine whether the article being examined complies with the requirements of the monograph.

In determining compliance with a numerical limit, the calculated result of a test or assay is first rounded to the number of significant figures stated, unless otherwise prescribed. The last figure is increased by 1 when the part rejected is equal to or exceeds one half-unit, whereas it is not modified when the part rejected is less than a half-unit.

In certain tests, the concentration of impurity is given in parentheses either as a percentage or in parts per million by weight (ppm). In chromatographic tests such concentrations are stated as a percentage irrespective of the limit. In other tests they are usually stated in ppm unless the limit exceeds 500 ppm. In those chromatographic tests in which a secondary spot or peak in a chromatogram obtained with a solution of the substance being examined is described as corresponding to a named impurity and is compared with a spot or peak in a chromatogram obtained with a reference solution of the same impurity, the percentage given in parentheses indicates the limit for that impurity. In those chromatographic tests in which a spot or peak in a chromatogram obtained with a solution of the substance being examined is described in terms other than as corresponding to a named impurity (commonly, for example, as any (other) *secondary spot* or *peak*) but is compared with a spot or peak in a chromatogram obtained with a reference solution of a named impurity, the percentage given in parentheses indicates an impurity limit expressed in terms of a nominal concentration of the named impurity. In chromatographic tests in which a comparison is made between spots or peaks in chromatograms obtained with solutions of different concentrations of the substance being examined, the percentage given in parentheses indicates an impurity limit expressed in terms of a nominal concentration of the medicinal substance itself. In some monographs, in particular those for certain formulated preparations, the impurity limit is expressed in terms of a nominal concentration of the active moiety rather than of the medicinal substance itself. Where necessary for clarification the terms in which the limit is expressed are stated within the monograph.

In all cases where an impurity limit is given in parentheses, the figures given are approximations for information only; conformity with the requirements is determined on the basis of compliance or otherwise with the stated test.

The use of a proprietary designation to identify a material used in an assay or test does not imply that another equally suitable material may not be used.

Biological Assays and Tests

Methods of assay described as Suggested methods are not obligatory, but when another method is used its precision must be not less than that required for the Suggested method.

For those antibiotics for which the monograph specifies a microbiological assay the potency requirement is expressed in the monograph in International Units (IU) per milligram. The material is not of pharmacopoeial quality if the upper fiducial limit of error is less than the stated potency. For such antibiotics the required precision of the assay is stated in the monograph in terms of the fiducial limits of error about the estimated potency.

For other substances and preparations for which the monograph specifies a biological assay, unless otherwise stated, the precision of the assay is such that the fiducial limits of error, expressed as a percentage of the estimated potency, are within a range not wider than that obtained by multiplying by a factor of 10 the square roots of the limits given in the monograph for the fiducial limits of error about the stated potency.

In all cases fiducial limits of error are based on a probability of 95% ($P = 0.95$).

Where the biological assay is being used to ascertain the purity of the material, the stated potency means the potency stated on the label in terms of International Units (IU) or other Units per gram, per milligram or per millilitre. When no such statement appears on the label, the stated potency means the fixed or minimum potency required in the monograph. This interpretation of stated potency applies in all cases except where the monograph specifically directs otherwise.

Where the biological assay is being used to determine the total activity in the container, the stated potency means the total number of International Units (IU) or other Units stated on the label or, if no such statement appears, the total activity calculated in accordance with the instructions in the monograph.

Wherever possible the primary standard used in an assay or test is the respective International Standard or Reference Preparation established by the World Health Organization for international use and the biological activity is expressed in International Units (IU).

In other cases, where Units are referred to in an assay or test, the Unit for a particular substance or preparation is, for the United Kingdom, the specific biological activity contained in such an amount of the respective primary standard as the appropriate international or national organisation indicates. The necessary information is provided with the primary standard.

Unless otherwise directed, animals used in an assay or a test are healthy animals, drawn from a uniform stock, that have not previously been treated with any material that will interfere with the assay or test. Unless otherwise stated, guinea-pigs weigh not less than 250 g or, when used in systemic toxicity tests, not less than 350 g. When used in skin tests they are white or light coloured. Unless otherwise stated, mice weigh not less than 17 g and not more than 22 g.

Certain of the biological assays and tests of the Pharmacopoeia are such that in the United Kingdom they may be carried out only in accordance with the Animals (Scientific Procedures) Act 1986. Instructions included in such assays and tests in the Pharmacopoeia, with respect to the handling of animals, are therefore confined to those concerned with the accuracy and reproducibility of the assay or test.

Reference Substances and Reference Preparations

Certain monographs require the use of a reference substance, a reference preparation or a reference spectrum. These are chosen with regard to their intended use as prescribed in the monographs of the Pharmacopoeia and are not necessarily suitable in other circumstances.

Any information necessary for proper use of the reference substance or reference preparation is given on the label or in the accompanying leaflet or brochure. Where no drying conditions are stated in the leaflet or on the label, the substance is to be used as received. No certificate of analysis or other data not relevant to the prescribed use of the product are provided. The products are guaranteed to be suitable for use for a period of three months from dispatch when stored under the appropriate conditions. The stability of the contents of opened containers cannot be guaranteed. The current lot is listed in the BP Laboratory website catalogue. Additional information is provided in Supplementary Chapter III E.

Chemical Reference Substances The abbreviation BPCRS indicates a Chemical Reference Substance established by the British Pharmacopoeia Commission. The abbreviation CRS or EPCRS indicates a Chemical Reference Substance established by the European Pharmacopoeia Commission. Some Chemical Reference Substances are used for the microbiological assay of antibiotics and their activity is stated, in International Units, on the label or on the accompanying leaflet and defined in the same manner as for Biological Reference Preparations.

Biological Reference Preparations The majority of the primary biological reference preparations referred to are the appropriate International Standards and Reference Preparations established by the World Health Organisation. Because these reference materials are usually available only in limited quantities, the European Pharmacopoeia has established Biological Reference Preparations (indicated by the abbreviation BRP or EPBRP) where appropriate. Where applicable, the potency of the Biological Reference Preparations is expressed in International Units. For some Biological Reference Preparations, where an international standard or reference preparation does not exist, the potency is expressed in European Pharmacopoeia Units.

Storage

Statements under the side-heading Storage constitute non-mandatory advice. The substances and preparations described in the Pharmacopoeia are to be stored under conditions that prevent contamination and, as far as possible, deterioration. Unless otherwise stated in the monograph, the substances and preparations described in the Pharmacopoeia are kept in well-closed containers and stored at a temperature not exceeding 25°. Precautions that should be taken in relation to the effects of the atmosphere, moisture, heat and light are indicated, where appropriate, in the monographs. Further precautions may be necessary when some materials are stored in tropical climates or under other severe conditions.

The expression 'protected from moisture' means that the product is to be stored in an airtight container. Care is to be taken when the container is opened in a damp atmosphere. A low moisture content may be maintained, if necessary, by the use of a desiccant in the container provided that direct contact with the product is avoided.

The expression 'protected from light' means that the product is to be stored either in a container made of a material that absorbs actinic light sufficiently to protect the contents from change induced by such light or in a container enclosed in an outer cover that provides such protection or stored in a place from which all such light is excluded.

The expression 'tamper-evident container' means a closed container fitted with a device that reveals irreversibly whether the container has been opened, whereas, the expression 'tamper-proof container' means a closed container in which access to the contents is prevented under normal conditions of use. The two terms are considered to be synonymous by the European Pharmacopoeia Commission.

Labelling The labelling requirements of the Pharmacopoeia are not comprehensive, and the provisions of regulations issued in accordance with the requirements of the territory in which the medicinal product is to be used should be met.

Licensed medicines intended for use within the United Kingdom must comply with the requirements of The Human Medicines Regulations 2012 and European Directive 2001/83/EC, Title V (as amended) in respect of their labelling and package leaflets, together with those regulations for the labelling of hazardous materials.

Best practice guidance on the labelling and packaging of medicines for use in the United Kingdom advises that certain items of information are deemed critical for the safe use of the medicine (see "Best Practice Guidance on the Labelling and Packaging of Medicines" issued by the MHRA, 2012). Further information and guidance on the labelling of medicinal products can be found in Supplementary Chapter I G.

Such matters as the exact form of wording to be used and whether a particular item of information should appear on the primary label and additionally, or alternatively, on the package or exceptionally in a leaflet are, in general, outside the scope of the Pharmacopoeia. When the term 'label' is used in Labelling statements of the Pharmacopoeia, decisions as to where the particular statement should appear should therefore be made in accordance with relevant legislation.

The label of every official formulated preparation other than those of fixed strength also states the content of the active ingredient or ingredients expressed in the terms required by the monograph. Where the content of active ingredient is required to be expressed in terms other than the weight of the official medicinal substance used in making the formulation, this is specifically stated under the heading Labelling. Unless otherwise stated in the monograph, the content of the active ingredient is expressed in terms of the official medicinal substance used in making the formulation.

These requirements do not necessarily apply to unlicensed preparations supplied in accordance with a prescription. For requirements for unlicensed medicines see the general monograph on Unlicensed Medicines.

Action and Use The statements given under this heading in monographs are intended only as information on the principal pharmacological actions or the uses of the materials in medicine or pharmacy. It should not be assumed that the substance has no other action or use. The statements are not intended to be binding on prescribers or to limit their discretion.

Crude Drugs; Traditional Herbal and Complementary Medicines *Herbal and complementary medicines are classed as medicines under European Directive 2001/83/EC as amended. It is emphasised that, although requirements for the quality of the material are provided in the monograph to assist the registration scheme by the UK Licensing Authority, the British Pharmacopoeia Commission has not assessed the safety or efficacy of the material in traditional use.*

Monograph Title For traditional herbal medicines, the monograph title is a combination of the binomial name together with a description of use. Monographs for the material that has not been processed (the herbal drug) and the processed material (the herbal drug preparation) are published where possible. To distinguish between the two, the word 'Processed' is included in the relevant monograph title.

Definition Under the heading Definition, the botanical name together with any synonym is given. Where appropriate, for material that has not been processed, information on the collection/harvesting and/or treatment/drying of the whole herbal drug may be given. For processed materials, the method of processing, where appropriate, will normally be given in a separate section.

Characteristics References to odour are included only where this is highly characteristic. References to taste are not included.

Control methods Where applicable, the control methods to be used in monographs are:

(a) macroscopical and microscopical descriptions and chemical/chromatographic tests for identification

(b) tests for absence of any related species

(c) microbial test to assure microbial quality

(d) tests for inorganic impurities and non-specific purity tests, including extractive tests, Sulfated ash and Heavy metals where appropriate

(e) test for Loss on drying or Water

(f) wherever possible, a method for assaying the active constituent(s) or suitable marker constituent(s).

The macroscopical characteristics include those features that can be seen by the unaided eye or by the use of a hand lens. When two species/subspecies of the same plant are included in the Definition, individual differences between the two are indicated where possible.

The description of the microscopical characteristics of the powdered drug includes information on the dominant or the most specific characters. Where it is considered to be an aid to identification, illustrations of the powdered drug may be provided.

The following aspects are controlled by the general monograph for Herbal Drugs: they are required to be free from moulds, insects, decay, animal matter and animal excreta. Unless otherwise prescribed the amount of foreign matter is not more than 2% w/w. Microbial contamination should be minimal.

In determining the content of the active constituents or the suitable marker substances measurements are made with reference to the dried or anhydrous herbal drug. In the tests for Acid-insoluble ash, Ash, Extractive soluble in ethanol, Loss on drying, Sulfated ash, Water, Water-soluble ash and Water-soluble extractive of herbal drugs, the calculations are made with reference to the herbal drug that has not been specifically dried unless otherwise prescribed in the monograph.

Homoeopathic Medicines

Homoeopathic medicines are classed as medicines under European Directive 2001/83/EC as amended. It is emphasised that, although requirements for the quality of the material are provided in the relevant monograph in order to assist the simplified registration scheme by the UK Licensing Authority, the British Pharmacopoeia Commission has not assessed the safety or efficacy of the material in use.

All materials used for the production of homoeopathic medicines, including excipients, must comply with European Pharmacopoeia or British Pharmacopoeia monographs for those materials. Where such European Pharmacopoeia or British Pharmacopoeia monographs do not exist, each material used for the production of homoeopathic medicines must comply with an official national pharmacopoeia of a Member State.

British Pharmacopoeia monographs for homoeopathic medicines apply to homoeopathic stocks and mother tinctures only, but may be prefaced by a section which details the quality requirements applicable to the principle component where there is no European Pharmacopoeia or British Pharmacopoeia monograph for the material. These monographs also include either general statements on the methods of preparation or refer to specific methods of preparation given in the European Pharmacopoeia. Homoeopathic stocks and mother tinctures undergo the further process referred to as potentisation. Potentisation is a term specific to homoeopathic medicine and is a process of dilution of stocks and mother tinctures to produce the final product.

Identification tests are established for the components in homoeopathic stocks and usually relate to those applied to the materials used in the production of the homoeopathic stocks. An assay is included for the principal component(s) where possible. For mother tinctures, an identification test, usually chromatographic, is established and, where applicable, an assay for the principle component(s); where appropriate, other tests, related to the solvent, dry matter or known adulterants, are included.

Specifications have not been set for final homoeopathic products due to the high dilution used in their preparation and the subsequent difficulty in applying analytical methodology.

Statements under Crude Drugs; Traditional Herbal and Complementary Medicines also apply to homoeopathic stocks and mother tinctures, when appropriate.

Unlicensed Medicines

The General Monograph for Unlicensed Medicines applies to those formulations used in human medicine that are prepared under a Manufacturer's 'Specials' Licence or prepared extemporaneously under the supervision of a pharmacist, whether or not there is a published monograph for the specific dosage form.

An article intended for medicinal use that is described by means of an official title must comply with the requirements of the relevant monograph.

A formulated preparation must comply throughout its assigned shelf-life (period of validity). The subject of any other monograph must comply throughout its period of use.

Unlicensed medicines that are prepared under a Manufacturer's 'Specials' Licence comply with the requirements of the general monograph and, where applicable, the requirements of the individual monograph for the specific dosage form.

Unlicensed medicines prepared extemporaneously under the supervision of a pharmacist comply with the requirements of the general monograph and, where applicable, the requirements of the individual monograph for the specific dosage form. While it is expected that extemporaneous preparations will demonstrate pharmacopoeial compliance when tested, it is recognised that it might not be practicable to carry out the pharmacopoeial tests routinely on such formulations. In the event of doubt or dispute, the methods of analysis, the reference materials and the reference spectra of the Pharmacopoeia are alone authoritative.

Part III

Monographs and other texts of the European Pharmacopoeia that are incorporated in this edition of the British Pharmacopoeia are governed by the general notices of the European Pharmacopoeia; these are reproduced below.

GENERAL NOTICES OF THE EUROPEAN PHARMACOPOEIA

1.1. GENERAL STATEMENTS

The General Notices apply to all monographs and other texts of the European Pharmacopoeia.

The official texts of the European Pharmacopoeia are published in English and French. Translations in other languages may be prepared by the signatory States of the European Pharmacopoeia Convention. In case of doubt or dispute, the English and French versions are alone authoritative.

In the texts of the European Pharmacopoeia, the word 'Pharmacopoeia' without qualification means the European Pharmacopoeia. The official abbreviation Ph. Eur. may be used to indicate the European Pharmacopoeia.

The use of the title or the subtitle of a monograph implies that the article complies with the requirements of the relevant monograph. Such references to monographs in the texts of the Pharmacopoeia are shown using the monograph title and reference number in *italics*.

A preparation must comply throughout its period of validity; a distinct period of validity and/or specifications for opened or broached containers may be decided by the competent authority. The subject of any other monograph must comply throughout its period of use. The period of validity that is assigned to any given article and the time from which that period is to be calculated are decided by the competent authority in light of experimental results of stability studies.

Unless otherwise indicated in the General Notices or in the monographs, statements in monographs constitute mandatory requirements. General chapters become mandatory when referred to in a monograph, unless such reference is made in a way that indicates that it is not the intention to make the text referred to mandatory but rather to cite it for information.

The active substances, excipients, pharmaceutical preparations and other articles described in the monographs are intended for human and veterinary use (unless explicitly restricted to one of these uses). An article is not of Pharmacopoeia quality unless it complies with all the requirements stated in the monograph. This does not imply that performance of all the tests in a monograph is necessarily a prerequisite for a manufacturer in assessing compliance with the Pharmacopoeia before release of a product. The manufacturer may obtain assurance that a product is of Pharmacopoeia quality from data derived, for example, from validation studies of the manufacturing process and from in-process controls. Parametric release in circumstances deemed appropriate by the competent authority is thus not precluded by the need to comply with the Pharmacopoeia.

The tests and assays described are the official methods upon which the standards of the Pharmacopoeia are based. With the agreement of the competent authority, alternative methods of analysis may be used for control purposes, provided that the methods used enable an unequivocal decision to be made as to whether compliance with the standards of the monographs would be achieved if the official methods were used. In the event of doubt or dispute, the methods of analysis of the Pharmacopoeia are alone authoritative.

Certain materials that are the subject of a pharmacopoeial monograph may exist in different grades suitable for different purposes. Unless otherwise indicated in the monograph, the requirements apply to all grades of the material. In some monographs, particularly those on excipients, a list of functionality-related characteristics that are relevant to the use of the substance may be appended to the monograph for information. Test methods for determination of one or more of these characteristics may be given, also for information.

Quality systems The quality standards represented by monographs are valid only where the articles in question are produced within the framework of a suitable quality system.

General monographs Substances and preparations that are the subject of an individual monograph are also required to comply with relevant, applicable general monographs. Cross-references to applicable general monographs are not normally given in individual monographs.

General monographs apply to all substances and preparations within the scope of the Definition section of the general monograph, except where a preamble limits the application, for example to substances and preparations that are the subject of a monograph of the Pharmacopoeia.

General monographs on dosage forms apply to all preparations of the type defined. The requirements are not necessarily comprehensive for a given specific preparation and requirements additional to those prescribed in the general monograph may be imposed by the competent authority.

General monographs and individual monographs are complementary. If the provisions of a general monograph do not apply to a particular product, this is expressly stated in the individual monograph.

Validation of pharmacopoeial methods The test methods given in monographs and general chapters have been validated in accordance with accepted scientific practice and current recommendations on analytical validation. Unless otherwise stated in the monograph or general chapter, validation of the test methods by the analyst is not required.

Implementation of pharmacopoeial methods When implementing a pharmacopoeial method, the user must assess whether and to what extent the suitability of the method under the actual conditions of use needs to be demonstrated according to relevant monographs, general chapters and quality systems.

Conventional terms The term 'competent authority' means the national, supranational or international body or organisation vested with the authority for making decisions concerning the issue in question. It may, for example, be a national pharmacopoeia authority, a licensing authority or an official control laboratory.

The expression 'unless otherwise justified and authorised' means that the requirements have to be met, unless the competent authority authorises a modification or an exemption where justified in a particular case.

Statements containing the word 'should' are informative or advisory.

In certain monographs or other texts, the terms 'suitable' and 'appropriate' are used to describe a reagent, micro-organism, test method etc.; if criteria for suitability are not described in the monograph, suitability is demonstrated to the satisfaction of the competent authority.

Medicinal product (a) Any substance or combination of substances presented as having properties for treating or preventing disease in human beings and/or animals; or (b) any substance or combination of substances that may be used in or administered to human beings and/or animals with a view either to restoring, correcting or modifying physiological functions by exerting a pharmacological, immunological or metabolic action, or to making a medical diagnosis.

Herbal medicinal product Any medicinal product, exclusively containing as active ingredients one or more herbal drugs or one or more herbal drug preparations, or one or more such herbal drugs in combination with one or more such herbal drug preparations.

Active substance Any substance intended to be used in the manufacture of a medicinal product and that, when so used, becomes an active ingredient of the medicinal product. Such substances are intended to furnish a pharmacological activity or other direct effect in the diagnosis, cure, mitigation, treatment or prevention of disease, or to affect the structure and function of the body.

Excipient (auxiliary substance) Any constituent of a medicinal product that is not an active substance. Adjuvants, stabilisers, antimicrobial preservatives, diluents, antioxidants, for example, are excipients.

Interchangeable methods Certain general chapters contain a statement that the text in question is harmonised with the corresponding text of the Japanese Pharmacopoeia and/or the United States Pharmacopeia and that these texts are interchangeable. This implies that if a substance or preparation is found to comply with a requirement using an interchangeable method from one of these pharmacopoeias it complies with the requirements of the European Pharmacopoeia. In the event of doubt or dispute, the text of the European Pharmacopoeia is alone authoritative.

References to regulatory documents Monographs and general chapters may contain references to documents issued by regulatory authorities for medicines, for example directives and notes for guidance of the European Union. These references are provided for information for users for the Pharmacopoeia. Inclusion of such a reference does not modify the status of the documents referred to, which may be mandatory or for guidance.

1.2. OTHER PROVISIONS APPLYING TO GENERAL CHAPTERS AND MONOGRAPHS

Quantities In tests with numerical limits and assays, the quantity stated to be taken for examination is approximate. The amount actually used, which may deviate by not more than 10 per cent from that stated, is accurately weighed or measured and the result is calculated from this exact quantity. In tests where the limit is not numerical, but usually depends upon comparison with the behaviour of a reference substance in the same conditions, the stated quantity is taken for examination. Reagents are used in the prescribed amounts.

Quantities are weighed or measured with an accuracy commensurate with the indicated degree of precision. For weighings, the precision corresponds to plus or minus 5 units after the last figure stated (for example, 0.25 g is to be interpreted as 0.245 g to 0.255 g). For the measurement of volumes, if the figure after the decimal point is a zero or ends in a zero (for example, 10.0 mL or 0.50 mL), the volume is measured using a pipette, a volumetric flask or a burette, as appropriate; otherwise, a graduated measuring cylinder or a graduated pipette may be used. Volumes stated in microlitres are measured using a micropipette or microsyringe.

It is recognised, however, that in certain cases the precision with which quantities are stated does not correspond to the number of significant figures stated in a specified numerical limit. The weighings and measurements are then carried out with a sufficiently improved accuracy.

Apparatus and procedures Volumetric glassware complies with Class A requirements of the appropriate International Standard issued by the International Organisation for Standardisation.

Unless otherwise prescribed, analytical procedures are carried out at a temperature between 15 °C and 25 °C.

Unless otherwise prescribed, comparative tests are carried out using identical tubes of colourless, transparent, neutral glass with a flat base; the volumes of liquid prescribed are for use with tubes having an internal diameter of 16 mm, but tubes with a larger internal diameter may be used provided the volume of liquid used is adjusted *(2.1.5)*. Equal volumes of the liquids to be compared are examined down the vertical axis of the tubes against a white background, or if necessary against a black background. The examination is carried out in diffuse light.

Any solvent required in a test or assay in which an indicator is to be used is previously neutralised to the indicator, unless a blank test is prescribed.

Water-bath The term 'water-bath' means a bath of boiling water unless water at another temperature is indicated. Other methods of heating may be substituted provided the temperature is near to but not higher than 100 °C or the indicated temperature.

Drying and ignition to constant mass The terms 'dried to constant mass' and 'ignited to constant mass' mean that 2 consecutive weighings do not differ by more than 0.5 mg, the 2nd weighing following an additional period of drying or of ignition respectively appropriate to the nature and quantity of the residue.

Where drying is prescribed using one of the expressions 'in a desiccator' or '*in vacuo*', it is carried out using the conditions described in chapter *2.2.32. Loss on drying*.

Reagents The proper conduct of the analytical procedures described in the Pharmacopoeia and the reliability of the results depend, in part, upon the quality of the reagents used. The reagents are described in general chapter *4*. It is assumed that reagents of analytical grade are used; for some reagents, tests to determine suitability are included in the specifications.

Solvents Where the name of the solvent is not stated, the term 'solution' implies a solution in water.

Where the use of water is specified or implied in the analytical procedures described in the Pharmacopoeia or for the preparation of reagents, water complying with the requirements of the monograph *Purified water (0008)* is used, except that for many purposes the requirements for bacterial endotoxins (*Purified water in bulk*) and microbial contamination (*Purified water in containers*) are not relevant. The term 'distilled water' indicates purified water prepared by distillation.

The term 'ethanol' without qualification means anhydrous ethanol. The term 'alcohol' without qualification means ethanol (96 per cent). Other dilutions of ethanol are indicated by the term 'ethanol' or 'alcohol' followed by a statement of the percentage by volume of ethanol (C_2H_6O) required.

Expression of content

In defining content, the expression 'per cent' is used according to circumstances with one of 2 meanings:

— per cent *m/m* (percentage, mass in mass) expresses the number of grams of substance in 100 grams of final product;

— per cent *V/V* (percentage, volume in volume) expresses the number of millilitres of substance in 100 mL of final product.

The expression 'parts per million' (or ppm) refers to mass in mass, unless otherwise specified.

Temperature

Where an analytical procedure describes temperature without a figure, the general terms used have the following meaning:

— in a deep-freeze: below −15 °C;

— in a refrigerator: 2 °C to 8 °C;

— cold or cool: 8 °C to 15 °C;

— room temperature: 15 °C to 25 °C.

1.3. GENERAL CHAPTERS

Containers

Materials used for containers are described in general chapter *3.1*. General names used for materials, particularly plastic materials, each cover a range of products varying not only in the properties of the principal constituent but also in the additives used. The test methods and limits for materials depend on the formulation and are therefore applicable only for materials whose formulation is covered by the preamble to the specification. The use of materials with different formulations, and the test methods and limits applied to them, are subject to agreement by the competent authority.

The specifications for containers in general chapter *3.2* have been developed for general application to containers of the stated category, but in view of the wide variety of containers available and possible new developments, the publication of a specification does not exclude the use, in justified circumstances, of containers that comply with other specifications, subject to agreement by the competent authority.

Reference may be made within the monographs of the Pharmacopoeia to the definitions and specifications for containers provided in chapter *3.2. Containers*. The general monographs for pharmaceutical dosage forms may, under the heading Definition/Production, require the use of certain types of container; certain other monographs may, under the heading Storage, indicate the type of container that is recommended for use.

1.4. MONOGRAPHS

Titles   Monograph titles are in English and French in the respective versions and there is a Latin subtitle.

Relative Atomic and Molecular Masses   The relative atomic mass (A_r) or the relative molecular mass (M_r) is shown, as and where appropriate, at the beginning of each monograph. The relative atomic and molecular masses and the molecular and graphic formulae do not constitute analytical standards for the substances described.

Chemical Abstracts Service (CAS) Registry Number   CAS registry numbers are included for information in monographs, where applicable, to provide convenient access to useful information for users. CAS Registry Number[®] is a Registered Trademark of the American Chemical Society.

Definition   Statements under the heading Definition constitute an official definition of the substance, preparation or other article that is the subject of the monograph.

Limits of content Where limits of content are prescribed, they are those determined by the method described under Assay.

Herbal drugs In monographs on herbal drugs, the definition indicates whether the subject of the monograph is, for example, the whole drug or the drug in powdered form. Where a monograph applies to the drug in several states, for example both to the whole drug and the drug in powdered form, the definition states this.

Production   Statements under the heading Production draw attention to particular aspects of the manufacturing process but are not necessarily comprehensive. They constitute mandatory requirements for manufacturers, unless otherwise stated. They may relate, for example, to source materials; to the manufacturing process itself and its validation and control; to in-process testing; or to testing that is to be carried out by the manufacturer on the final article, either on selected batches or on each batch prior to release. These statements cannot necessarily be verified on a sample of the final article by an independent analyst. The competent authority may establish that the instructions have been followed, for example, by examination of data received from the manufacturer, by inspection of manufacture or by testing appropriate samples.

The absence of a Production section does not imply that attention to features such as those referred to above is not required.

Choice of vaccine strain, Choice of vaccine composition The Production section of a monograph may define the characteristics of a vaccine strain or vaccine composition. Unless otherwise stated, test methods given for verification of these characteristics are provided for information as examples of suitable methods. Subject to approval by the competent authority, other test methods may be used without validation against the method shown in the monograph.

Potential Adulteration   Due to the increasing number of fraudulent activities and cases of adulteration, information may be made available to Ph. Eur. users to help detect adulterated materials (i.e. active substances, excipients, intermediate products, bulk products and finished products).

To this purpose, a method for the detection of potential adulterants and relevant limits, together with a reminder that all stages of production and sourcing are subjected to a suitable quality system, may be included in this section of monographs on substances for which an incident has occurred or that present a risk of deliberate contamination. The frequency of testing by manufacturers or by users (e.g. manufacturers of intermediate products, bulk products and finished products, where relevant) depends on a risk assessment, taking into account the level of knowledge of the whole supply chain and national requirements.

This section constitutes requirements for the whole supply chain, from manufacturers to users (e.g. manufacturers of intermediate products, bulk products and finished products, where relevant). The absence of this section does not imply that attention to features such as those referred to above is not required.

Characters

The statements under the heading Characters are not to be interpreted in a strict sense and are not requirements.

Solubility In statements of solubility in the Characters section, the terms used have the following significance, referred to a temperature between 15 °C and 25 °C.

Descriptive term	Approximate volume of solvent in millilitres per gram of solute		
Very soluble	less than	1	
Freely soluble	from	1	to 10
Soluble	from	10	to 30
Sparingly soluble	from	30	to 100
Slightly soluble	from	100	to 1000
Very slightly soluble	from	1000	to 10 000
Practically insoluble	more than		10 000

The term 'partly soluble' is used to describe a mixture where only some of the components dissolve. The term 'miscible' is used to describe a liquid that is miscible in all proportions with the stated solvent.

Identification

Scope The tests given in the Identification section are not designed to give a full confirmation of the chemical structure or composition of the product; they are intended to give confirmation, with an acceptable degree of assurance, that the article conforms to the description on the label.

First and second identifications Certain monographs have subdivisions entitled 'First identification' and 'Second identification'. The test or tests that constitute the 'First identification' may be used in all circumstances. The test or tests that constitute the 'Second identification' may be used in pharmacies provided it can be demonstrated that the substance or preparation is fully traceable to a batch certified to comply with all the other requirements of the monograph.

Certain monographs give two or more sets of tests for the purpose of the first identification, which are equivalent and may be used independently. One or more of these sets usually contain a cross-reference to a test prescribed in the Tests section of the monograph. It may be used to simplify the work of the analyst carrying out the identification and the prescribed tests. For example, one identification set cross-refers to a test for enantiomeric purity while the other set gives a test for specific optical rotation: the intended purpose of the two is the same, that is, verification that the correct enantiomer is present.

Powdered herbal drugs Monographs on herbal drugs may contain schematic drawings of the powdered drug. These drawings complement the description given in the relevant identification test.

Tests and Assays   *Scope* The requirements are not framed to take account of all possible impurities. It is not to be presumed, for example, that an impurity that is not detectable by means of the prescribed tests is tolerated if common sense and good pharmaceutical practice require that it be absent. See also below under Impurities.

Calculation Where the result of a test or assay is required to be calculated with reference to the dried or anhydrous substance or on some other specified basis, the determination of loss on drying, water content or other property is carried out by the method prescribed in the relevant test in the monograph. The words 'dried substance' or 'anhydrous substance' etc. appear in parentheses after the result.

Where a quantitative determination of a residual solvent is carried out and a test for loss on drying is not carried out, the content of residual solvent is taken into account for the calculation of the assay content of the substance, the specific optical rotation and the specific absorbance. No further indication is given in the specific monograph.

Limits The limits prescribed are based on data obtained in normal analytical practice; they take account of normal analytical errors, of acceptable variations in manufacture and compounding and of deterioration to an extent considered acceptable. No further tolerances are to be applied to the limits prescribed to determine whether the article being examined complies with the requirements of the monograph.

In determining compliance with a numerical limit, the calculated result of a test or assay is first rounded to the number of significant figures stated, unless otherwise prescribed. The limits, regardless of whether the values are expressed as percentages or as absolute values, are considered significant to the last digit shown (for example 140 indicates 3 significant figures). The last figure of the result is increased by one when the part rejected is equal to or exceeds one half-unit, whereas it is not modified when the part rejected is less than a half-unit.

Indication of permitted limit of impurities The acceptance criteria for related substances are expressed in monographs either in terms of comparison of peak areas (comparative tests) or as numerical values. For comparative tests, the approximate content of impurity tolerated, or the sum of impurities, may be indicated in brackets for information only. Acceptance or rejection is determined on the basis of compliance or non-compliance with the stated test. If the use of a reference substance for the named impurity is not prescribed, this content may be expressed as a nominal concentration of the substance used to prepare the reference solution specified in the monograph, unless otherwise described.

Herbal drugs For herbal drugs, the sulfated ash, total ash, water-soluble matter, alcohol-soluble matter, water content, content of essential oil and content of active principle are calculated with reference to the drug that has not been specially dried, unless otherwise prescribed in the monograph.

Equivalents Where an equivalent is given, for the purposes of the Pharmacopoeia only the figures shown are to be used in applying the requirements of the monograph.

Culture media The culture media described in monographs and general chapters have been found to be satisfactory for the intended purpose. However, the components of media, particularly those of biological origin, are of variable quality, and it may be necessary for optimal performance to modulate the concentration of some ingredients, notably:

— peptones and meat or yeast extracts, with respect to their nutritive properties;
— buffering substances;
— bile salts, bile extract, deoxycholate, and colouring matter, depending on their selective properties;
— antibiotics, with respect to their activity.

Storage The information and recommendations given under the heading Storage do not constitute a pharmacopoeial requirement but the competent authority may specify particular storage conditions that must be met.

The articles described in the Pharmacopoeia are stored in such a way as to prevent contamination and, as far as possible, deterioration. Where special conditions of storage are recommended, including the type of container (see section 1.3. General chapters) and limits of temperature, they are stated in the monograph.

The following expressions are used in monographs under Storage with the meaning shown.

In an airtight container means that the product is stored in an airtight container *(3.2)*. Care is to be taken when the container is opened in a damp atmosphere. A low moisture content may be maintained, if necessary, by the use of a desiccant in the container provided that direct contact with the product is avoided.

Protected from light means that the product is stored either in a container made of a material that absorbs actinic light sufficiently to protect the contents from change induced by such light, or in a container enclosed in an outer cover that provides such protection, or is stored in a place from which all such light is excluded.

Labelling In general, labelling of medicines is subject to supranational and national regulation and to international agreements. The statements under the heading Labelling are not therefore comprehensive and, moreover, for the purposes of the Pharmacopoeia only those statements that are necessary to demonstrate compliance or non-compliance with the monograph are mandatory. Any other labelling statements are included as recommendations. When the term 'label' is used in the Pharmacopoeia, the labelling statements may appear on the container, the package, a leaflet accompanying the package, or a certificate of analysis accompanying the article, as decided by the competent authority.

Warnings Materials described in monographs and reagents specified for use in the Pharmacopoeia may be injurious to health unless adequate precautions are taken. The principles of good quality control laboratory practice and the provisions of any appropriate regulations are to be observed at all times. Attention is drawn to particular hazards in certain monographs by means of a warning statement; absence of such a statement is not to be taken to mean that no hazard exists.

Impurities A list of all known and potential impurities that have been shown to be detected by the tests in a monograph may be given. See also chapter *5.10. Control of impurities in substances for pharmaceutical use.* The impurities are designated by a letter or letters of the alphabet. Where a letter appears to be missing, the impurity designated by this letter has been deleted from the list during monograph development prior to publication or during monograph revision.

Functionality-Related Characteristics of Excipients Monographs on excipients may have a section on functionality-related characteristics. The characteristics, any test methods for determination and any tolerances are not mandatory requirements; they may nevertheless be relevant for use of the excipient and are given for information (see also section 1.1. General statements).

Reference Standards Certain monographs require the use of reference standards (chemical reference substances, herbal reference standards, biological reference preparations, reference spectra). See also chapter *5.12. Reference standards.* The European Pharmacopoeia Commission establishes the official reference standards, which are alone authoritative in case of arbitration. These reference standards are available from the European Directorate for the Quality of Medicines & HealthCare (EDQM). Information on the available reference standards and a batch validity statement can be obtained via the EDQM website.

1.5. ABBREVIATIONS AND SYMBOLS

A	Absorbance		mp	Melting point
$A_{1\,cm}^{1\,per\,cent}$	Specific absorbance		n_D^{20}	Refractive index
A_r	Relative atomic mass		Ph. Eur. U.	European Pharmacopoeia Unit
$[\alpha]_D^{20}$	Specific optical rotation		ppb	Parts per billion (micrograms per kilogram)
bp	Boiling point		ppm	Parts per million (milligrams per kilogram)
BRP	Biological Reference Preparation		R	Substance or solution defined under
CRS	Chemical Reference Substance			*4. Reagents*
d_{20}^{20}	Relative density		R_F	Retardation factor (see chapter *2.2.46*)
λ	Wavelength		R_{st}	Used in chromatography to indicate the ratio of the distance travelled by a substance to the distance travelled by a reference substance
HRS	Herbal reference standard			
IU	International Unit		RV	Substance used as a primary standard in volumetric analysis (chapter *4.2.1*)
M	Molarity			
M_r	Relative molecular mass			

Abbreviations used in the monographs on immunoglobulins, immunosera and vaccines

LD_{50}	The statistically determined quantity of a substance that, when administered by the specified route, may be expected to cause the death of 50 per cent of the test animals within a given period		Lo/10 dose	The largest quantity of a toxin that, in the conditions of the test, when mixed with 0.1 IU of antitoxin and administered by the specified route, does not cause symptoms of toxicity in the test animals within a given period
MLD	Minimum lethal dose		Lf dose	The quantity of toxin or toxoid that flocculates in the shortest time with 1 IU of antitoxin
L+/10 dose	The smallest quantity of a toxin that, in the conditions of the test, when mixed with 0.1 IU of antitoxin and administered by the specified route, causes the death of the test animals within a given period		$CCID_{50}$	The statistically determined quantity of virus that may be expected to infect 50 per cent of the cell cultures to which it is added
L+ dose	The smallest quantity of a toxin that, in the conditions of the test, when mixed with 1 IU of antitoxin and administered by the specified route, causes the death of the test animals within a given period		EID_{50}	The statistically determined quantity of virus that may be expected to infect 50 per cent of fertilised eggs into which it is inoculated
lr/100 dose	The smallest quantity of a toxin that, in the conditions of the test, when mixed with 0.01 IU of antitoxin and injected intracutaneously causes a characteristic reaction at the site of injection within a given period		ID_{50}	The statistically determined quantity of a virus that may be expected to infect 50 per cent of the animals into which it is inoculated
			PD_{50}	The statistically determined dose of a vaccine that, in the conditions of the test, may be expected to protect 50 per cent of the animals against a challenge dose of the micro-organisms or toxins against which it is active
Lp/10 dose	The smallest quantity of toxin that, in the conditions of the test, when mixed with 0.1 IU of antitoxin and administered by the specified route, causes paralysis in the test animals within a given period		ED_{50}	The statistically determined dose of a vaccine that, in the conditions of the test, may be expected to induce specific antibodies in 50 per cent of the animals for the relevant vaccine antigens
			PFU	Pock-forming units or plaque-forming units
			SPF	Specified-pathogen-free.

Collections of micro-organisms

ATCC	American Type Culture Collection 10801 University Boulevard Manassas, Virginia 20110-2209, USA	NCTC	National Collection of Type Cultures Central Public Health Laboratory Colindale Avenue London NW9 5HT, Great Britain
C.I.P.	Collection de Bactéries de l'Institut Pasteur B.P. 52, 25 rue du Docteur Roux 75724 Paris Cedex 15, France	NCYC	National Collection of Yeast Cultures AFRC Food Research Institute Colney Lane Norwich NR4 7UA, Great Britain
IMI	International Mycological Institute Bakeham Lane Surrey TW20 9TY, Great Britain	NITE	Biological Resource Center Department of Biotechnology National Institute of Technology and Evaluation 2-5-8 Kazusakamatari, Kisarazu-shi, Chiba, 292-0818 Japan
I.P.	Collection Nationale de Culture de Microorganismes (C.N.C.M.) Institut Pasteur 25, rue du Docteur Roux 75724 Paris Cedex 15, France		
NCIMB	National Collection of Industrial and Marine Bacteria Ltd 23 St Machar Drive Aberdeen AB2 1RY, Great Britain	S.S.I.	Statens Serum Institut 80 Amager Boulevard, Copenhagen, Denmark
NCPF	National Collection of Pathogenic Fungi London School of Hygiene and Tropical Medicine Keppel Street London WC1E 7HT, Great Britain		

1.6. UNITS OF THE INTERNATIONAL SYSTEM (SI) USED IN THE PHARMACOPOEIA AND EQUIVALENCE WITH OTHER UNITS

International System Of Units (SI)

The International System of Units comprises 3 classes of units, namely base units, derived units and supplementary units[1]. The base units and their definitions are set out in Table 1.6-1.

The derived units may be formed by combining the base units according to the algebraic relationships linking the corresponding quantities. Some of these derived units have special names and symbols. The SI units used in the Pharmacopoeia are shown in Table 1.6-2.

Some important and widely used units outside the International System are shown in Table 1.6-3.

The prefixes shown in Table 1.6-4 are used to form the names and symbols of the decimal multiples and submultiples of SI units.

---

[1] The definitions of the units used in the International System are given in the booklet "Le Système International d'Unités (SI)" published by the Bureau International des Poids et Mesures, Pavillion de Breteuil, F-92310 Sèvres.

Notes   1.   In the Pharmacopoeia, the Celsius temperature is used (symbol t). This is defined by the following equation:

$$t = T - T_0$$

where $T_0 = 273.15$ K by definition. The Celsius or centigrade temperature is expressed in degree Celsius (symbol °C). The unit 'degree Celsius' is equal to the unit 'kelvin'.

2.   The practical expressions of concentrations used in the Pharmacopoeia are defined in the General Notices.

3.   The radian is the plane angle between two radii of a circle that cut off on the circumference an arc equal in length to the radius.

4.   In the Pharmacopoeia, conditions of centrifugation are defined by reference to the acceleration due to gravity (g):

$$g = 9.806\,65\ m \cdot s^{-2}$$

5.   Certain quantities without dimensions are used in the Pharmacopoeia: relative density *(2.2.5)*, absorbance *(2.2.25)*, specific absorbance *(2.2.25)* and refractive index *(2.2.6)*.

6.   The microkatal is defined as the enzymic activity that, under defined conditions, produces the transformation (e.g. hydrolysis) of 1 micromole of the substrate per second.

Table 1.6.-1. – *SI base units*

Quantity		Unit		Definition
Name	**Symbol**	**Name**	**Symbol**	
Length	l	metre	m	The metre is the length of the path travelled by light in a vacuum during a time interval of 1/299 792 458 of a second.
Mass	m	kilogram	kg	The kilogram is equal to the mass of the international prototype of the kilogram.
Time	t	second	s	The second is the duration of 9 192 631 770 periods of the radiation corresponding to the transition between the two hyperfine levels of the ground state of the caesium-133 atom.
Electric current	I	ampere	A	The ampere is that constant current which, maintained in two straight parallel conductors of infinite length, of negligible circular cross-section and placed 1 metre apart in vacuum would produce between these conductors a force equal to 2×10^{-7} newton per metre of length.
Thermodynamic temperature	T	kelvin	K	The kelvin is the fraction 1/273.16 of the thermodynamic temperature of the triple point of water.
Amount of substance	n	mole	mol	The mole is the amount of substance of a system containing as many elementary entities as there are atoms in 0.012 kilogram of carbon-12[*].
Luminous intensity	I_v	candela	cd	The candela is the luminous intensity in a given direction of a source emitting monochromatic radiation with a frequency of 540×10^{12} hertz and whose energy intensity in that direction is 1/683 watt per steradian.

[*] When the mole is used, the elementary entities must be specified and may be atoms, molecules, ions, electrons, other particles or specified groups of such particles.

Table 1.6.-2. – *SI units used in the European Pharmacopoeia and equivalence with other units*

Quantity		Unit				Conversion of other units into SI units
Name	**Symbol**	**Name**	**Symbol**	**Expression in SI base units**	**Expression in other SI units**	
Wave number	ν	one per metre	1/m	m^{-1}		
Wavelength	λ	micrometre	µm	$10^{-6}m$		
		nanometre	nm	$10^{-9}m$		
Area	A, S	square metre	m^2	m^2		
Volume	V	cubic metre	m^3	m^3		$1\ mL = 1\ cm^3 = 10^{-6}\ m^3$
Frequency	ν	hertz	Hz	s^{-1}		
Density	ρ	kilogram per cubic metre	kg/m^3	$kg \cdot m^{-3}$		$1\ g/mL = 1\ g/cm^3 = 10^3\ kg \cdot m^{-3}$
Velocity	v	metre per second	m/s	$m \cdot s^{-1}$		
Force	F	newton	N	$m \cdot kg \cdot s^{-2}$		$1\ dyne = 1\ g \cdot cm \cdot s^{-2} = 10^{-5}\ N$ $1\ kp = 9.806\ 65\ N$
Pressure	p	pascal	Pa	$m^{-1} \cdot kg \cdot s^{-2}$	$N \cdot m^{-2}$	$1\ dyne/cm^2 = 10^{-1}\ Pa = 10^{-1}\ N \cdot m^{-2}$ $1\ atm = 101\ 325\ Pa = 101.325\ kPa$ $1\ bar = 10^5\ Pa = 0.1\ MPa$ $1\ mm\ Hg = 133.322\ 387\ Pa$ $1\ Torr = 133.322\ 368\ Pa$ $1\ psi = 6.894\ 757\ kPa$
Dynamic viscosity	η	pascal second	Pa·s	$m^{-1} \cdot kg \cdot s^{-1}$	$N \cdot s \cdot m^{-2}$	$1\ P = 10^{-1}\ Pa \cdot s = 10^{-1}\ N \cdot s \cdot m^{-2}$ $1\ cP = 1\ mPa \cdot s$
Kinematic viscosity	ν	square metre per second	m^2/s	$m^2 \cdot s^{-1}$	$Pa \cdot s \cdot m^3 \cdot kg^{-1}$ $N \cdot m \cdot s \cdot kg^{-1}$	$1\ St = 1\ cm^2 \cdot s^{-1} = 10^{-4}\ m^2 \cdot s^{-1}$
Energy	W	joule	J	$m^2 \cdot kg \cdot s^{-2}$	$N \cdot m$	$1\ erg = 1\ cm^2 \cdot g \cdot s^{-2} = 1\ dyne \cdot cm = 10^{-7}\ J$ $1\ cal = 4.1868\ J$
Power Radiant flux	P	watt	W	$m^2 \cdot kg \cdot s^{-3}$	$N \cdot m \cdot s^{-1}$ $J \cdot s^{-1}$	$1\ erg/s = 1\ dyne \cdot cm \cdot s^{-1} =$ $10^{-7}\ W = 10^{-7}\ N \cdot m \cdot s^{-1} = 10^{-7}\ J \cdot s^{-1}$
Absorbed dose (of radiant energy)	D	gray	Gy	$m^2 \cdot s^{-2}$	$J \cdot kg^{-1}$	$1\ rad = 10^{-2}\ Gy$
Electric potential, electromotive force	U	volt	V	$m^2 \cdot kg \cdot s^{-3} \cdot A^{-1}$	$W \cdot A^{-1}$	
Electric resistance	R	ohm	Ω	$m^2 \cdot kg \cdot s^{-3} \cdot A^{-2}$	$V \cdot A^{-1}$	
Quantity of electricity	Q	coulomb	C	$A \cdot s$		
Activity of a radionuclide	A	becquerel	Bq	s^{-1}		$1\ Ci = 37 \cdot 10^9\ Bq = 37 \cdot 10^9\ s^{-1}$
Concentration (of amount of substance), molar concentration	c	mole per cubic metre	mol/m^3	$mol \cdot m^{-3}$		$1\ mol/L = 1\ M = 1\ mol/dm^3 = 10^3\ mol \cdot m^{-3}$
Mass concentration	ρ	kilogram per cubic metre	kg/m^3	$kg \cdot m^{-3}$		$1\ g/L = 1\ g/dm^3 = 1\ kg \cdot m^{-3}$

Table 1.6.-3. – *Units used with the International System*

Quantity	Unit		Value in SI units
	Name	**Symbol**	
Time	minute	min	1 min = 60 s
	hour	h	1 h = 60 min = 3600 s
	day	d	1 d = 24 h = 86 400 s
Plane angle	degree	°	1° = (π/180) rad
Volume	litre	L	$1 \text{ L} = 1 \text{ dm}^3 = 10^{-3} \text{ m}^3$
Mass	tonne	t	$1 \text{ t} = 10^3 \text{ kg}$
Rotational frequency	revolution per minute	r/min	$1 \text{ r/min} = (1/60) \text{ s}^{-1}$

Table 1.6.-4. – *Decimal multiples and sub-multiples of units*

Factor	Prefix	Symbol	Factor	Prefix	Symbol
10^{18}	exa	E	10^{-1}	deci	d
10^{15}	peta	P	10^{-2}	centi	c
10^{12}	tera	T	10^{-3}	milli	m
10^{9}	giga	G	10^{-6}	micro	μ
10^{6}	mega	M	10^{-9}	nano	n
10^{3}	kilo	k	10^{-12}	pico	p
10^{2}	hecto	h	10^{-15}	femto	f
10^{1}	deca	da	10^{-18}	atto	a

Monographs

Formulated Preparations: General Monographs

FORMULATED PREPARATIONS: GENERAL MONOGRAPHS

Pharmaceutical Preparations

(*Ph Eur monograph 2619*)

Ph Eur

INTRODUCTION

This monograph is intended to be a reference source of standards in the European Pharmacopoeia on active substances, excipients and dosage forms, which are to be applied in the manufacture/preparation of pharmaceuticals, but not a guide on how to manufacture as there is specific guidance available covering methods of manufacture and associated controls.

It does not cover investigational medicinal products, but competent authorities may refer to pharmacopoeial standards when authorising clinical trials using investigational medicinal products.

DEFINITION

Pharmaceutical preparations are medicinal products generally consisting of active substances that may be combined with excipients, formulated into a dosage form suitable for the intended use, where necessary after reconstitution, presented in a suitable and appropriately labelled container.

Pharmaceutical preparations may be licensed by the competent authority, or unlicensed and made to the specific needs of patients according to legislation. There are 2 categories of unlicensed pharmaceutical preparations:
— extemporaneous preparations, i.e. pharmaceutical preparations individually prepared for a specific patient or patient group, supplied after preparation;
— stock preparations, i.e. pharmaceutical preparations prepared in advance and stored until a request for a supply is received.

In addition to this monograph, pharmaceutical preparations also comply with the General Notices and with the relevant general chapters of the Pharmacopoeia. General chapters are normally given for information and become mandatory when referred to in a general or specific monograph, unless such reference is made in a way that indicates that it is not the intention to make the text referred to mandatory but rather to cite it for information.

Where relevant, pharmaceutical preparations also comply with the dosage form monographs (e.g. *Capsules (0016)*, *Tablets (0478)*) and general monographs relating to pharmaceutical preparations (e.g. *Allergen products (1063)*, *Herbal teas (1435)*, *Homoeopathic preparations (1038)*, *Immunosera for human use, animal (0084)*, *Immunosera for veterinary use (0030)*, *Monoclonal antibodies for human use (2031)*, *Radiopharmaceutical preparations (0125)*, *Vaccines for human use (0153)*, *Vaccines for veterinary use (0062))*.

Where pharmaceutical preparations are manufactured/prepared using materials of human or animal origin, the general requirements of general chapters *5.1.7. Viral safety*, *5.2.6. Evaluation of safety of veterinary vaccines and immunosera* and *5.2.8. Minimising the risk of transmitting animal spongiform encephalophathy agents via human and veterinary medicinal products* apply, where appropriate.

ETHICAL CONSIDERATIONS AND GUIDANCE IN THE PREPARATION OF UNLICENSED PHARMACEUTICAL PREPARATIONS

The underlying principle of legislation for pharmaceutical preparations is that, subject to specific exemptions, no pharmaceutical preparation may be placed on the market without an appropriate marketing authorisation.

The exemptions from the formal licensing requirement allow the supply of unlicensed products to meet the special needs of individual patients. However, when deciding to use an unlicensed preparation all health professionals involved (e.g. the prescribing practitioners and/or the preparing pharmacists) have, within their area of responsibilities, a duty of care to the patient receiving the pharmaceutical preparation.

In considering the preparation of an unlicensed pharmaceutical preparation, a suitable level of risk assessment is undertaken.

The risk assessment identifies:
— the criticality of different parameters (e.g. quality of active substances, excipients and containers; design of the preparation process; extent and significance of testing; stability of the preparation) to the quality of the preparation; and
— the risk that the preparation may present to a particular patient group.

Based on the risk assessment, the person responsible for the preparation must ensure, with a suitable level of assurance, that the pharmaceutical preparation is, throughout its shelf-life, of an appropriate quality and suitable and fit for its purpose. For stock preparations, storage conditions and shelf-life have to be justified on the basis of, for example, analytical data or professional judgement, which may be based on literature references.

PRODUCTION

Manufacture/preparation must take place within the framework of a suitable quality system and be compliant with the standards relevant to the type of product being made. Licensed products must comply with the requirements of their licence. For unlicensed products a risk assessment as outlined in the section 'Ethical considerations and guidance in the preparation of unlicensed pharmaceutical preparations' is of special importance, as these products are not previously assessed by the competent authority.

Formulation

During pharmaceutical development or prior to manufacture/preparation, suitable ingredients, processes, tests and specifications are identified and justified in order to ensure the suitability of the product for the intended purpose. This includes consideration of the properties required in order to identify whether specific ingredient properties or process steps are critical to the required quality of the pharmaceutical preparation.

Active substances and excipients

Active substances and excipients used in the formulation of pharmaceutical preparations comply with the requirements of the relevant general monographs, e.g. *Substances for pharmaceutical use (2034)*, *Essential oils (2098)*, *Extracts (0765)*, *Herbal drugs (1433)*, *Herbal drug preparations (1434)*, *Herbal drugs for homoeopathic preparations (2045)*, *Mother tinctures for homoeopathic preparations (2029)*, *Methods of preparation of homoeopathic stocks and potentisation (2371)*, *Products of fermentation (1468)*, *Products with risk of transmitting agents of animal spongiform encephalopathies (1483)*,

Products of recombinant DNA technology (0784), Vegetable fatty oils (1579).

In addition, where specific monographs exist, the quality of the active substances and excipients used complies with the corresponding monographs.

Where no specific monographs exist, the required quality must be defined, taking into account the intended use and the involved risk.

When physicochemical characteristics of active substances and functionality-related characteristics (FRCs) of excipients (e.g. particle-size distribution, viscosity, polymorphism) are critical in relation to their role in the manufacturing process and quality attributes of the pharmaceutical preparation, they must be identified and controlled.

Detailed information on FRCs is given in general chapter *5.15. Functionality-related characteristics of excipients.*

Microbiological quality

The formulation of the pharmaceutical preparation and its container must ensure that the microbiological quality is suitable for the intended use.

During development, it shall be demonstrated that the antimicrobial activity of the preparation as such or, if necessary, with the addition of a suitable preservative or preservatives, or by the selection of an appropriate container, provides adequate protection from adverse effects that may arise from microbial contamination or proliferation during the storage and use of the preparation. A suitable test method together with criteria for evaluating the preservative properties of the formulation are provided in general chapter *5.1.3. Efficacy of antimicrobial preservation.*

If preparations do not have adequate antimicrobial efficacy and do not contain antimicrobial preservatives they are supplied in single-dose containers, or in multidose containers that prevent microbial contamination of the contents after opening.

In the manufacture/preparation of non-sterile pharmaceutical preparations, suitable measures are taken to ensure their microbial quality; recommendations on this aspect are provided in general chapters *5.1.4. Microbiological quality of non-sterile pharmaceutical preparations and substances for pharmaceutical use* and *5.1.8. Microbiological quality of herbal medicinal products for oral use.*

Sterile preparations are manufactured/prepared using materials and methods designed to ensure sterility and to avoid the introduction of contaminants and the growth of micro-organisms; recommendations on this aspect are provided in general chapter *5.1.1. Methods of preparation of sterile products.*

Containers

A suitable container is selected. Consideration is given to the intended use of the preparation, the properties of the container, the required shelf-life, and product/container incompatibilities. Where applicable, containers for pharmaceutical preparations comply with the requirements for containers (*3.2* and subsections) and materials used for the manufacture of containers (*3.1* and subsections).

Stability

Stability requirements of pharmaceutical preparations are dependent on their intended use and on the desired storage time.

Where applicable, the probability and criticality of possible degradation products of the active substance(s) and/or reaction products of the active substance(s) with an excipient and/or the immediate container must be assessed. Depending on the result of this assessment, limits of degradation and/or reaction products are set and monitored in the pharmaceutical preparation. Licensed products require a stability exercise.

Methods used for the purpose of stability testing for all relevant characteristics of the preparation are validated as stability indicating, i.e. the methods allow the quantification of the relevant degradation products and physical characteristic changes.

TESTS

Relevant tests to apply in order to ensure the appropriate quality of a particular dosage form are described in the specific dosage form monographs.

Where it is not practical, for unlicensed pharmaceutical preparations, to carry out the tests (e.g. batch size, time restraints), other suitable methods are implemented to ensure that the appropriate quality is achieved in accordance with the risk assessment carried out and any local guidance or legal requirements.

Stock preparations are normally tested to a greater extent than extemporaneous preparations.

The following tests are applicable to many preparations and are therefore listed here.

Appearance

The appearance (e.g. size, shape and colour) of the pharmaceutical preparation is controlled.

Identity and purity tests

Where applicable, the following tests are carried out on the pharmaceutical preparation:
— identification of the active substance(s);
— identification of specific excipient(s), such as preservatives;
— purity tests (e.g. investigation of degradation products, residual solvents (*2.4.24*) or other related impurities, sterility (*2.6.1*));
— safety tests (e.g. safety tests for biological products).

Uniformity (*2.9.40* or *2.9.5/2.9.6*)

Pharmaceutical preparations presented in single-dose units comply with the test(s) as prescribed in the relevant specific dosage form monograph. If justified and authorised, general chapter *2.9.40* can be applicable only at the time of release.

Special uniformity requirements apply in the following cases:
— for herbal drugs and herbal drug preparations, compliance with general chapter *2.9.40* is not required;
— for homoeopathic preparations, the provisions of general chapters *2.9.6* and *2.9.40* are normally not appropriate, however in certain circumstances compliance with these chapters may be required by the competent authority;
— for single- and multivitamin and trace-element preparations, compliance with general chapters *2.9.6* and *2.9.40* (content uniformity only) is not required;
— in justified and authorised circumstances, for other preparations, compliance with general chapters *2.9.6* and *2.9.40* may not be required by the competent authority.

Reference standards

Reference standards may be needed at various stages for quality control of pharmaceutical preparations. They are established and monitored taking due account of general chapter *5.12. Reference standards.*

ASSAY

Unless otherwise justified and authorised, contents of active substances and specific excipients such as preservatives are determined in pharmaceutical preparations. Limits must be defined and justified.

Suitable and validated methods are used. If assay methods prescribed in the respective active substance monographs are used, it must be demonstrated that they are not affected by the presence of the excipients and/or by the formulation.

Reference standards

See Tests.

LABELLING AND STORAGE

The relevant labelling requirements given in the general dosage form monographs apply. In addition, relevant European Union or other applicable regulations apply.

GLOSSARY

Formulation

The designing of an appropriate formula (including materials, processes, etc.) that will ensure that the patient receives the suitable pharmaceutical preparation in an appropriate form that has the required quality and that will be stable and effective for the required length of time.

Licensed pharmaceutical preparation

A medicinal product that has been granted a marketing authorisation by a competent authority. Synonym: authorised pharmaceutical preparation.

Manufacture

All operations of purchase of materials and products, Production, Quality Control, release, storage, distribution of medicinal products and the related controls.

Preparation (of an unlicensed pharmaceutical preparation)

The 'manufacture' of unlicensed pharmaceutical preparations by or at the request of pharmacies or other healthcare establishments (the term 'preparation' is used instead of 'manufacture' in order clearly to distinguish it from the industrial manufacture of licensed pharmaceutical preparations).

Reconstitution

Manipulation to enable the use or application of a medicinal product with a marketing authorisation in accordance with the instructions given in the summary of product characteristics or the patient information leaflet.

Risk assessment

The identification of hazards and the analysis and evaluation of risks associated with exposure to those hazards.

Unlicensed pharmaceutical preparation

A medicinal product that is exempt from the need of having a marketing authorisation issued by a competent authority but is made for specific patients' needs according to legislation.

_____ *Ph Eur*

Monographs

Herbal Drugs, Herbal Drug Preparations and Herbal Medicinal Products

Herbal Drugs

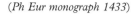

(Ph Eur monograph 1433)

Herbal Drugs comply with the requirements of the European Pharmacopoeia. These requirements are reproduced below.

Ph Eur

DEFINITION

Herbal drugs are mainly whole, fragmented, or broken plants, parts of plants, algae, fungi or lichen, in an unprocessed state, usually in dried form but sometimes fresh. Certain exudates that have not been subjected to a specific treatment are also considered to be herbal drugs. Herbal drugs are precisely defined by the botanical scientific name according to the binominal system (genus, species, variety and author).

Whole describes a herbal drug that has not been reduced in size and is presented, dried or undried, as harvested; for example: dog rose, bitter fennel or sweet fennel, Roman chamomile flower.

Fragmented describes a herbal drug that has been reduced in size after harvesting to permit ease of handling, drying and/or packaging; for example: cinchona bark, rhubarb, passion flower.

Broken describes a herbal drug in which the more-fragile parts of the plant have broken during drying, packaging or transportation; for example: belladonna leaf, matricaria flower, hop strobile.

Cut describes a herbal drug that has been reduced in size, other than by powdering, to the extent that the macroscopic description in the monograph of the herbal drug can no longer be applied. When a herbal drug is cut for a specific purpose that results in the cut herbal drug being homogeneous, for example when cut for herbal teas, it is a herbal drug preparation. Certain cut herbal drugs processed in this way may be the subject of an individual monograph.

A herbal drug that complies with its monograph and is subsequently cut for extraction shall comply in its cut form, except for its macroscopic description, with the monograph for that herbal drug, unless otherwise justified.

The term *herbal drug* is synonymous with the term *herbal substance* used in European Community legislation on herbal medicinal products.

PRODUCTION

Herbal drugs are obtained from cultivated or wild plants. Suitable collection, cultivation, harvesting, drying, fragmentation and storage conditions are essential to guarantee the quality of herbal drugs.

Herbal drugs are, as far as possible, free from impurities such as soil, dust, dirt and other contaminants such as fungal, insect and other animal contaminations. They are not rotten.

If a decontaminating treatment has been used, it is necessary to demonstrate that the constituents of the plant are not affected and that no harmful residues remain. The use of ethylene oxide is prohibited for the decontamination of herbal drugs.

IDENTIFICATION

Herbal drugs are identified using their macroscopic and microscopic descriptions and any further tests that may be required (for example, thin-layer chromatography).

TESTS

Foreign matter *(2.8.2)*
Carry out a test for foreign matter, unless otherwise prescribed or justified and authorised. The content of foreign matter is not more than 2 per cent *m/m*, unless otherwise prescribed or justified and authorised. An appropriate specific test may apply to herbal drugs liable to be adulterated. It may not be possible to perform the test for foreign matter on a herbal drug that is cut, as described under Definition, for either a specific purpose or for extraction. Under these circumstances the cut material is presumed to comply with the test for foreign matter providing that the herbal drug prior to cutting was compliant with this test.

Loss on drying *(2.2.32)*
Carry out a test for loss on drying, unless otherwise prescribed or justified and authorised.

Water *(2.2.13)*
A determination of water may be carried out instead of a test for loss on drying for herbal drugs with a high essential-oil content.

Pesticides *(2.8.13)*
Herbal drugs comply with the requirements for pesticide residues. The requirements take into account the nature of the plant, where necessary the preparation in which the plant might be used, and where available the knowledge of the complete record of treatment of the batch of the plant.

Heavy metals *(2.4.27)*
Unless otherwise stated in an individual monograph or unless otherwise justified and authorised:
— *cadmium*: maximum 1.0 ppm;
— *lead*: maximum 5.0 ppm;
— *mercury*: maximum 0.1 ppm.

Where necessary, limits for other heavy metals may be required.

Where necessary herbal drugs comply with other tests, such as the following, for example.

Total ash *(2.4.16)*.

Ash insoluble in hydrochloric acid *(2.8.1)*.

Extractable matter.

Swelling index *(2.8.4)*.

Bitterness value *(2.8.15)*.

Aflatoxin B$_1$ *(2.8.18)*
Where necessary, limits for aflatoxins may be required.

Ochratoxin A *(2.8.22)*
Where necessary, a limit for ochratoxin A may be required.

Radioactive contamination
In some specific circumstances, the risk of radioactive contamination is to be considered.

Microbial contamination
Where a herbal drug is used whole, cut or powdered as an ingredient in a medicinal product, the microbial contamination is controlled (*Microbiological quality of herbal medicinal products for oral use (5.1.8)* or *Microbiological quality of non-sterile pharmaceutical preparations and substances for pharmaceutical use (5.1.4)* (for example, for cutaneous use)).

ASSAY

Unless otherwise prescribed or justified and authorised, herbal drugs are assayed by an appropriate method.

STORAGE

Protected from light.

_____ *Ph Eur*

Processed Herbal Drugs

DEFINITION
Processed Herbal Drugs are obtained by subjecting Herbal Drugs to traditional processing methods.

Processed Herbal Drugs are defined precisely by the botanical scientific name according to the binomial system (genus, species, subspecies, variety, and author) and plant part. Monographs for Processed Herbal Drugs may refer to the relevant monograph for the unprocessed material where the binomial name is given.

PRODUCTION
Processed Herbal Drugs are obtained by subjecting Herbal Drugs to specific types of processing according to traditional processing methods. These traditional processing methods have the potential to alter the physical characteristics and/or chemical constituents of a Herbal Drug. Traditional processing methods may require the addition of processing aids to the herbal drug, for example, honey, vinegar, wine, milk and salt. The additional processing aids used should be of a suitable quality or of pharmacopoeial quality where a monograph exists. The method of traditional processing is provided under the Production section in individual monographs.

IDENTIFICATION
Processed Herbal Drugs are identified using their macroscopical and, where appropriate, microscopical descriptions and any further tests that may be required.

TESTS
A test for *foreign matter*, Appendix XI D, is carried out, unless otherwise prescribed in the individual monographs.

A specific appropriate test may be prescribed to detect potential contaminants in processed herbal drugs.

If appropriate, the Processed Herbal Drugs comply with other tests, for example, *total ash*, Appendix XI J, Method II, *ash insoluble in hydrochloric acid*, Appendix XI K, Method II, *extractable matter, swelling index*, Appendix XI C and *bitterness value*, Appendix XI N.

The test for *loss on drying*, Appendix IX D, is carried out on Processed Herbal Drugs, unless otherwise prescribed in the individual monographs. A *determination of water by distillation*, Appendix IX C, Method II, is carried out for Processed Herbal Drugs with a high essential oil content.

Processed Herbal Drugs comply with the requirements for *pesticide residues*, Appendix XI L. The requirements take into account the nature of the Processed Herbal Drugs, where necessary the preparation in which the plant might be used, and where available, the knowledge of the complete record of treatment of the batch of the Processed Herbal Drugs during cultivation, harvesting and processing. The content of pesticide residues may be determined by the method described in the annex to the general method.

The risk of contamination of Processed Herbal Drugs by heavy metals must be considered. In an individual monograph either a general limit for heavy metals or specific limits for individual heavy metal may be required.

Where necessary limits for specific toxins, for example aflatoxins or ochratoxins, may be applied.

Where processing is carried out to remove or limit specific constituents from the herbal drug a suitable limit test should be carried out.

In some specific circumstances, the risk of radioactive contamination is to be considered.

ASSAY
Unless otherwise justified and authorised Processed Herbal Drugs are assayed by an appropriate method.

Herbal Drug Preparations

(Ph Eur monograph 1434)

Herbal Drug Preparations comply with the requirements of the European Pharmacopoeia. These requirements are reproduced below.

Ph Eur

DEFINITION
Herbal drug preparations are homogeneous products obtained by subjecting herbal drugs to treatments such as extraction, distillation, expression, fractionation, purification, concentration or fermentation.

Herbal drug preparations include, for example, extracts, essential oils, expressed juices, processed exudates, and herbal drugs that have been subjected to size reduction for specific applications, for example herbal drugs cut for herbal teas or powdered for encapsulation.

Herbal teas comply with the monograph *Herbal teas (1435)*.

NOTE: the term *comminuted* used in European Community legislation on herbal medicinal products describes a herbal drug that has been either cut or powdered.

The term *herbal drug preparation* is synonymous with the term *herbal preparation* used in European Community legislation on herbal medicinal products.

Ph Eur

Essential Oils

(Ph Eur monograph 2098)

Essential Oils comply with the requirements of the European Pharmacopoeia. These requirements are reproduced below.

Ph Eur

The statements in this monograph are intended to be read in conjunction with individual monographs on essential oils in the European Pharmacopoeia. Application of the monograph to other essential oils may be decided by the competent authority.

DEFINITION
Odorous product, usually of complex composition, obtained from a botanically defined plant raw material by steam distillation, dry distillation, or a suitable mechanical process without heating. Essential oils are usually separated from the aqueous phase by a physical process that does not significantly affect their composition.

Essential oils may be subjected to a suitable subsequent treatment. Thus an essential oil may be commercially known as being deterpenated, desesquiterpenated, rectified or 'x'-free.

— A *deterpenated essential oil* is an essential oil from which monoterpene hydrocarbons have been removed, partially or totally.

— A *deterpenated and desesquiterpenated essential oil* is an essential oil from which mono- and sesquiterpene hydrocarbons have been removed, partially or totally.

— A *rectified essential oil* is an essential oil that has been subjected to fractional distillation to remove certain constituents or modify the content.
— An *'x'-free essential oil* is an essential oil that has been subjected to partial or complete removal of one or more constituents.

PRODUCTION

Depending on the monograph, the plant raw material may be fresh, wilted, dried, whole, broken or ground.

Steam distillation The essential oil is produced by the passage of steam through the plant raw material in a suitable apparatus. The steam may be introduced from an external source or generated by boiling water below the raw material or by boiling water in which the raw material is immersed. The steam and oil vapours are condensed. The water and essential oil are separated by decantation.

Dry distillation The essential oil is produced by high-temperature heating of stems or barks in a suitable apparatus without the addition of water or steam.

Mechanical process The essential oil, usually known as 'cold-pressed', is produced by a mechanical process without any heating. It is mainly applied to *Citrus* fruit and involves expression of the oil from the pericarp and subsequent separation by physical means.

In certain cases, a suitable antioxidant may be added to the essential oil.

CHARACTERS

The appearance and the odour of the essential oil is determined.

IDENTIFICATION

Essential oils are identified by their gas chromatographic profile, or failing this, by any other test that may be required (for example, a test by thin-layer chromatography).

TESTS

GENERAL TESTS
The essential oil complies with the prescribed limits for the following tests.

Relative density (*2.2.5*)

Refractive index (*2.2.6*)

Optical rotation (*2.2.7*)

Fatty oils and resinified essential oils (*2.8.7*)
SUPPLEMENTARY TESTS
If necessary, the essential oil complies with the prescribed limits for the following tests.

Freezing point (*2.2.18*)

Acid value (*2.5.1*)

Peroxide value (*2.5.5*)

Foreign esters (*2.8.6*)

Residue on evaporation (*2.8.9*)

Water (*2.8.5*)

Solubility in alcohol (*2.8.10*)

Falsification
If appropriate, a test for one or more falsifications may be carried out by thin-layer chromatography (*2.2.27*), by gas chromatography (*2.2.28*) using a chiral column if necessary, or by any other suitable method.

Chromatographic profile
Gas chromatography (*2.2.28*): use the normalisation procedure.

In addition to the system suitability test given in the specific monograph, it is necessary to check the suitability of the chromatographic system using the following test, which is to be carried out periodically within the framework of performance qualification.

The chromatogram shown in Figure 2098.-1 is given as an example.

Reference solution essential oil CRS. If necessary, the reference solution can be diluted with *heptane R*.

Column:
— *material*: fused silica;
— *size*: l = 60 m, Ø = 0.25 mm;
— *stationary phase*: macrogol 20 000 R (0.25 μm).

Carrier gas helium for chromatography R.

Flow rate 1.5 mL/min.

Split ratio 1:500. The split ratio/injection volume can be adjusted in order to fit the specific equipment used, provided that the column load stays the same.

Temperature:

	Time (min)	Temperature (°C)
Column	0 - 15	70
	15 - 100	70 → 240
	100 - 105	240
Injection port		250
Detector		270

Detection Flame ionisation.

Injection 1 μL.

Identification of components Use the chromatogram supplied with *essential oil CRS*.

System suitability Reference solution:
— *resolution*: minimum 1.5 between the peaks due to linalol and linalyl acetate;
— *signal-to-noise ratio*: minimum 100 for the peak due to decanal;
— *limits*: the percentage content of each of the 9 components is within the limits stated on the leaflet provided with *essential oil CRS*.

STORAGE

In a well-filled, airtight container, protected from light.

LABELLING

The label states:
— the scientific name of the plant raw material used;
— where applicable, the type and/or the chemotype of the essential oil;
— where applicable, the method of production;
— where applicable, the name and concentration of any added antioxidant;
— where applicable, additional processing steps that are not specified under Definition.

_____ *Ph Eur*

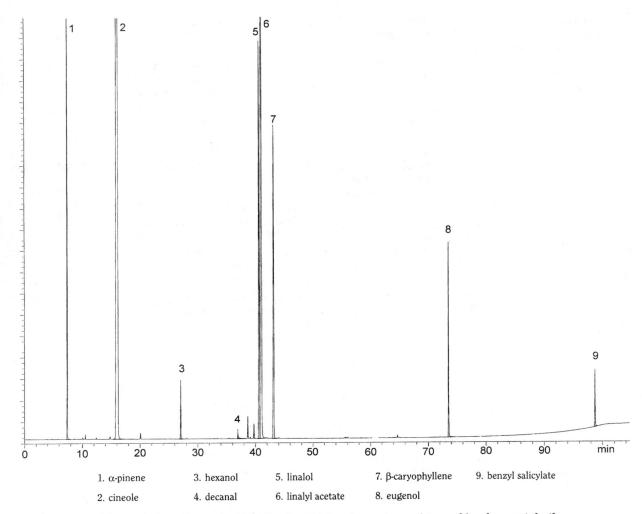

1. α-pinene   3. hexanol   5. linalol   7. β-caryophyllene   9. benzyl salicylate

2. cineole   4. decanal   6. linalyl acetate   8. eugenol

Figure 2098.-1. – *Chromatogram for the test for chromatographic profile of essential oils*

EXTRACTS

(Ph Eur monograph 0765)

Extracts comply with the requirements of the European Pharmacopoeia. These requirements are reproduced below.

Ph Eur _____

DEFINITION

Extracts are preparations of liquid (liquid extracts and tinctures), semi-solid (soft extracts and oleoresins) or solid (dry extracts) consistency, obtained from herbal drugs or animal matter, which are usually in a dry state.

Where medicinal products are manufactured using extracts of animal origin, the requirements of chapter *5.1.7. Viral safety* apply.

Different types of extract may be distinguished. Standardised extracts are adjusted within an acceptable tolerance to a given content of constituents with known therapeutic activity; standardisation is achieved by adjustment of the extract with inert material or by blending batches of extracts. Quantified extracts are adjusted to a defined range of constituents; adjustments are made by blending batches of extracts. Other extracts are essentially defined by their production process (state of the herbal drug or animal matter to be extracted, solvent, extraction conditions) and their specifications.

PRODUCTION

Extracts are prepared by suitable methods using ethanol or other suitable solvents. Different batches of the herbal drug or animal matter may be blended prior to extraction. The herbal drug or animal matter to be extracted may undergo a preliminary treatment, for example, inactivation of enzymes, grinding or defatting. In addition, unwanted matter may be removed after extraction.

Herbal drugs, animal matter and organic solvents used for the preparation of extracts comply with any relevant monograph of the Pharmacopoeia. For soft and dry extracts where the organic solvent is removed by evaporation, recovered or recycled solvent may be used, provided that the recovery procedures are controlled and monitored to ensure that solvents meet appropriate standards before re-use or admixture with other approved materials. Water used for the preparation of extracts is of a suitable quality. Except for the test for bacterial endotoxins, water complying with the section on Purified water in bulk in the monograph on *Purified water (0008)* is suitable. Potable water may be suitable if it complies with a defined specification that allows the consistent production of a suitable extract.

Where applicable, concentration to the intended consistency is carried out using suitable methods, usually under reduced pressure and at a temperature at which deterioration of the constituents is reduced to a minimum. Essential oils that have been separated during processing may be restored to the extracts at an appropriate stage in the manufacturing process. Suitable excipients may be added at various stages of the manufacturing process, for example to improve technological qualities such as homogeneity or consistency. Suitable stabilisers and antimicrobial preservatives may also be added.

Extraction with a given solvent leads to typical proportions of characterised constituents in the extractable matter; during production of standardised and quantified extracts, purification procedures may be applied that increase these proportions with respect to the expected values; such extracts are referred to as 'refined'.

IDENTIFICATION

Extracts are identified using a suitable method.

TESTS

Where applicable, as a result of analysis of the herbal drug or animal matter used for production and in view of the production process, tests for microbiological quality (*5.1.4*), heavy metals, aflatoxins and pesticide residues (*2.8.13*) in the extracts may be necessary.

ASSAY

Wherever possible, extracts are assayed by a suitable method.

LABELLING

The label states:
— the herbal drug or animal matter used;
— whether the extract is liquid, soft or dry, or whether it is a tincture;
— for standardised extracts, the content of constituents with known therapeutic activity;
— for quantified extracts, the content of constituents (markers) used for quantification;
— the ratio of the starting material to the genuine extract (extract without excipients) (DER);
— the solvent or solvents used for extraction;
— where applicable, that a fresh herbal drug or fresh animal matter has been used;
— where applicable, that the extract is 'refined';
— the name and amount of any excipient used including stabilisers and antimicrobial preservatives;
— where applicable, the percentage of dry residue.

LIQUID EXTRACTS

DEFINITION

Liquid extracts are liquid preparations of which, in general, 1 part by mass or volume is equivalent to 1 part by mass of the dried herbal drug or animal matter. These preparations are adjusted, if necessary, so that they satisfy the requirements for content of solvent, and, where applicable, for constituents.

PRODUCTION

Liquid extracts are prepared by using ethanol of a suitable concentration or water to extract the herbal drug or animal matter, or by dissolving a soft or dry extract (which has been produced using the same strength of extraction solvent as is used in preparing the liquid extract by direct extraction) of the herbal drug or animal matter in either ethanol of a suitable concentration or water. Liquid extracts may be filtered, if necessary.

A slight sediment may form on standing, which is acceptable as long as the composition of the liquid extract is not changed significantly.

TESTS

Relative density (*2.2.5*)
Where applicable, the liquid extract complies with the limits prescribed in the monograph.

Ethanol (*2.9.10*)
For alcoholic liquid extracts, carry out the determination of ethanol content. The ethanol content complies with that prescribed.

Methanol and 2-propanol (*2.9.11*)
Maximum 0.05 per cent *V/V* of methanol and maximum 0.05 per cent *V/V* of 2-propanol for alcoholic liquid extracts, unless otherwise prescribed.

Dry residue (*2.8.16*)
Where applicable, the liquid extract complies with the limits prescribed in the monograph, corrected if necessary, taking into account any excipient used.

STORAGE

Protected from light.

LABELLING

The label states in addition to the requirements listed above:
— where applicable, the ethanol content in per cent *V/V* in the final extract.

TINCTURES

DEFINITION

Tinctures are liquid preparations that are usually obtained using either 1 part of herbal drug or animal matter and 10 parts of extraction solvent, or 1 part of herbal drug or animal matter and 5 parts of extraction solvent.

PRODUCTION

Tinctures are prepared by maceration or percolation (outline methodology is given below) using only ethanol of a suitable concentration for extraction of the herbal drug or animal matter, or by dissolving a soft or dry extract (which has been produced using the same strength of extraction solvent as is used in preparing the tincture by direct extraction) of the herbal drug or animal matter in ethanol of a suitable concentration. Tinctures are filtered, if necessary.

Tinctures are usually clear. A slight sediment may form on standing, which is acceptable as long as the composition of the tincture is not changed significantly.

Production by maceration
Unless otherwise prescribed, reduce the herbal drug or animal matter to be extracted to pieces of suitable size, mix thoroughly with the prescribed extraction solvent and allow to stand in a closed container for an appropriate time. The residue is separated from the extraction solvent and, if necessary, pressed out. In the latter case, the 2 liquids obtained are combined.

Production by percolation
If necessary, reduce the herbal drug or animal matter to be extracted to pieces of suitable size. Mix thoroughly with a portion of the prescribed extraction solvent and allow to stand for an appropriate time. Transfer to a percolator and allow the percolate to flow at room temperature slowly making sure that the herbal drug or animal matter to be extracted is always covered with the remaining extraction solvent. The residue may be pressed out and the expressed liquid combined with the percolate.

TESTS

Relative density (*2.2.5*)
Where applicable, the tincture complies with the limits prescribed in the monograph.

Ethanol (*2.9.10*)
The ethanol content complies with that prescribed.

Methanol and 2-propanol (*2.9.11*)
Maximum 0.05 per cent *V/V* of methanol and maximum 0.05 per cent *V/V* of 2-propanol, unless otherwise prescribed.

Dry residue (*2.8.16*)
Where applicable, the tincture complies with the limits prescribed in the monograph, corrected if necessary, taking into account any excipient used.

STORAGE
Protected from light.

LABELLING
The label states in addition to the requirements listed above:
— for tinctures other than standardised and quantified tinctures, the ratio of starting material to extraction liquid or of starting material to final tincture;
— the ethanol content in per cent *V/V* in the final tincture.

SOFT EXTRACTS

DEFINITION
Soft extracts are semi-solid preparations obtained by evaporation or partial evaporation of the solvent used for extraction.

TESTS

Dry residue (*2.8.16*)
The soft extract complies with the limits prescribed in the monograph.

Solvents
Residual solvents are controlled as described in chapter *5.4*, unless otherwise prescribed or justified and authorised.

STORAGE
Protected from light.

OLEORESINS

DEFINITION
Oleoresins are semi-solid extracts composed of a resin in solution in an essential and/or fatty oil and are obtained by evaporation of the solvent(s) used for their production.

This monograph applies to oleoresins produced by extraction and not to natural oleoresins.

TESTS

Water (*2.2.13*)
The oleoresin complies with the limits prescribed in the monograph.

Solvents
Residual solvents are controlled as described in chapter *5.4*, unless otherwise prescribed or justified and authorised.

STORAGE
In an airtight container, protected from light.

DRY EXTRACTS

DEFINITION
Dry extracts are solid preparations obtained by evaporation of the solvent used for their production. Dry extracts have a loss on drying of not greater than 5 per cent *m/m*, unless a loss on drying with a different limit or a test on water is prescribed in the monograph.

TESTS

Water (*2.2.13*)
Where applicable, the dry extract complies with the limits prescribed in the monograph.

Loss on drying (*2.8.17*)
Where applicable, the dry extract complies with the limits prescribed in the monograph.

Solvents
Residual solvents are controlled as described in chapter *5.4*, unless otherwise prescribed or justified and authorised.

STORAGE
In an airtight container, protected from light.

_____ *Ph Eur*

Tinctures of the British Pharmacopoeia

In addition to the requirements for Tinctures of the European Pharmacopoeia (stated under Extracts), the following statements apply to those tinctures that are the subject of an individual monograph in the British Pharmacopoeia.

DEFINITION
Certain preparations of the British Pharmacopoeia entitled Tinctures do not conform strictly to the definition of the European Pharmacopoeia and consequently application of some of the above requirements is inappropriate.
Any necessary exceptions are stated in the relevant individual monographs.

Herbal Teas

(*Ph Eur monograph 1435*)

Herbal Teas comply with the requirements of the European Pharmacopoeia. These requirements are reproduced below.

Ph Eur _____

DEFINITION
Herbal teas consist exclusively of one or more herbal drugs intended for oral aqueous preparations by means of decoction, infusion or maceration. The preparation is prepared immediately before use.

Herbal teas are usually supplied in bulk form or in bags for single use.

The herbal drugs used comply with the appropriate individual European Pharmacopoeia monographs or in their absence with the general monograph *Herbal drugs (1433)*.

IDENTIFICATION
The identity of herbal drugs present in herbal teas is checked by suitable methods such as botanical examinations and/or chromatographic profiles.

TESTS
Recommendations on the microbiological quality of herbal teas (*5.1.8.*) take into account the prescribed preparation method (use of boiling or non-boiling water).

The proportion of herbal drugs present in herbal teas is checked by appropriate methods.

Herbal teas in bags comply with the following test:

Uniformity of mass

Determine the individual and the average mass of the contents of 20 randomly chosen units as follows: weigh a single full bag of herbal tea, open it without losing any fragments. Empty it completely using a brush. Weigh the empty bag and calculate the mass of the contents by subtraction. Repeat the operation on the 19 remaining bags and calculate the average mass of the contents of the 20 units. Unless otherwise justified, not more than 2 of the 20 individual masses deviate from the average mass by more than the percentage deviation shown in the table below and none deviates by more than twice that percentage.

Average mass	Percentage deviation
less than 1.5 g	15 per cent
1.5 g to 2.0 g included	10 per cent
more than 2.0 g	7.5 per cent

STORAGE

Protected from light.

Ph Eur

Instant Herbal Teas

(*Ph Eur monograph 2620*)

Ph Eur

DEFINITION

Instant herbal teas consist of 1 or more herbal drug preparations (primarily extracts with or without added essential oils), and are intended for the preparation of an oral solution immediately before use.

Instant herbal teas may also contain, in addition to herbal drug preparations, suitable excipients such as maltodextrin and added flavourings.

Instant herbal teas are presented as a powder or granules and are usually supplied in bulk form or in sachets.

The herbal drug preparations used comply with the appropriate individual European Pharmacopoeia monographs or, in the absence of such individual monographs, with the general monograph *Herbal drug preparations (1434)* and with other appropriate general monographs, for example *Extracts (0765)* or *Essential oils (2098)*.

IDENTIFICATION

The identity of herbal drug preparations present in instant herbal teas is checked by suitable methods.

TESTS

General chapter *5.1.8* contains recommendations on the microbiological quality of extract-containing herbal medicinal products such as instant herbal teas.

The proportion of herbal drug preparations present in instant herbal teas is checked by suitable methods.

Instant herbal teas in sachets comply with the following test.

Uniformity of mass

Determine the individual and the average mass of the contents of 20 randomly chosen units as follows: weigh a single full sachet of instant herbal tea, open it without losing any fragments. Empty it completely using a brush. Weigh the empty sachet and calculate the mass of the contents by subtraction. Repeat the operation on the 19 remaining sachets and calculate the average mass of the contents of the 20 units. Unless otherwise justified, not more than 2 of the individual masses deviate from the average mass by more than the percentage deviation shown in the table below and none deviates by more than twice that percentage.

Average mass	Percentage deviation
less than 1.5 g	15 per cent
1.5 g to 2.0 g included	10 per cent
more than 2.0 g	7.5 per cent

STORAGE

Protected from light.

Ph Eur

Acanthopanax Bark

(*Ph Eur monograph 2432*)

Ph Eur

DEFINITION

Dried root bark of *Eleutherococcus gracilistylus* (W.W.Sm.) S.Y.Hu var. *nodiflorus* (Dunn) H.Ohashi (*Acanthopanax gracilistylus* W.W.Sm.) collected in summer and autumn.

IDENTIFICATION

A. The bark occurs in irregular quills, 5-15 cm long, 0.4-1.4 cm in diameter, about 2 mm thick. The outer surface is greyish-brown, with slightly twisted longitudinal wrinkles and transverse lenticel-like scars. The inner surface is pale yellow or greyish-yellow, with fine longitudinal striations. The texture is light, fragile, easily broken. The fracture is irregular, greyish-white.

B. Microscopic examination (*2.8.23*). The powder is greyish-white. Examine under a microscope using *chloral hydrate solution R*. The powder shows the following diagnostic characters: cluster crystals of calcium oxalate, 8-64 µm in diameter, sometimes included in crystal cells arranged in rows; cork cells, rectangular or polygonal, thin-walled, sometimes walls of cork cells of older barks unevenly thickened, slightly pitted; fragments of secretory canals containing colourless or pale yellow secretions. Examine under a microscope using a 50 per cent *V/V* solution of *glycerol R*. The powder shows abundant starch granules, simple, polygonal or subspherical, 2-8 µm in diameter, or compound with 2-10 components.

C. Examine the chromatogram obtained in the test for *Periploca sepium*.

Results See below the sequence of zones present in the chromatograms obtained with the reference solution and the test solution. Furthermore, other faint zones may be present in the chromatogram obtained with the test solution.

TESTS

Periploca sepium

Thin-layer chromatography (*2.2.27*).

Test solution To 0.3 g of the powdered herbal drug (355) (*2.9.12*) add 3 mL of *methanol R*, heat in a water-bath at 60 °C for 1 min and filter.

Reference solution Dissolve 5 mg of *thymol R* and 8 mg of *borneol R* in 5 mL of *methanol R*.

Top of the plate	
Thymol: an orange zone	
Borneol: a brown zone	
	A broad pink zone
Reference solution	**Test solution**

Plate TLC silica gel plate R (5-40 μm) [or *TLC silica gel plate R* (2-10 μm)].

Mobile phase ethyl acetate R, methylene chloride R (2:98 V/V).

Application 20 μL [or 1 μL] as bands of 10 mm [or 8 mm].

Development Over a path of 10 cm [or 6 cm].

Drying In air.

Detection Treat with *anisaldehyde solution R*, heat at 105 °C for 5 min and examine in daylight.

Results The chromatogram obtained with the test solution shows no intense coloured zones above the zone due to borneol in the chromatogram obtained with the reference solution.

Acanthopanax giraldii
The outer surface of the root bark must not be covered with scaly covering trichomes.

Loss on drying (*2.2.32*)
Maximum 12.0 per cent, determined on 1.000 g of the powdered herbal drug (355) (*2.9.12*) by drying in an oven at 105 °C for 2 h.

Total ash (*2.4.16*)
Maximum 12.0 per cent.

Ash insoluble in hydrochloric acid (*2.8.1*)
Maximum 2.0 per cent.

Extractable matter
Minimum 16.0 per cent.

To 2.00 g of the powdered herbal drug (250) (*2.9.12*) add a mixture of 8 g of *water R* and 12 g of *ethanol (96 per cent) R* and allow to macerate for 2 h, shaking frequently. Filter, evaporate the filtrate to dryness on a water-bath *in vacuo* and dry in an oven at 100-105 °C for 2 h. The residue weighs a minimum of 320 mg.

_____ *Ph Eur*

Agnus Castus Fruit

(*Ph Eur monograph 2147*)

Ph Eur _____

DEFINITION

Whole, ripe, dried fruit of *Vitex agnus-castus* L.

Content

Minimum 0.08 per cent of casticin ($C_{19}H_{18}O_8$; M_r 374.3) (dried drug).

IDENTIFICATION

A. Agnus castus fruit is oval or almost globular, with a diameter of up to 5 mm. The persistent calyx is greenish-grey, finely pubescent, ends in 4-5 short teeth and envelops 2/3 to 3/4 of the surface of the fruit. The blackish-brown fruit consists of a pericarp that becomes progressively sclerous up to the endocarp. The style scar is often visible.

Some of the fruits may retain a stalk, about 1 mm long. A transverse section of the fruit shows 4 locules, each containing an elongated seed.

B. Reduce to a powder (355) (*2.9.12*). Examine under a microscope using *chloral hydrate solution R*. The powder shows the following diagnostic characters: fragments of the outer epidermis of the calyx composed of polygonal cells densely covered with short, bent or undulate, uni-, bi- or tri-cellular uniseriate covering trichomes; cells of the epicarp with thick walls and well-marked, large pits; isolated glandular trichomes with a unicellular stalk and a uni- or multi-cellular head; layers of parenchyma from the outer part of the mesocarp, some containing brown pigment, others extending into septa; fragments from the inner part of the mesocarp composed of thin-walled, pitted, sclerenchymatous cells and of typical isodiametric sclerous cells with very thick, deeply grooved walls and a narrow, stellate lumen; small brown cells of the endocarp; fragments of the testa containing areas of fairly large, thin-walled lignified cells with reticulate bands of thickening; numerous fragments of the endosperm composed of thin-walled parenchymatous cells containing aleurone grains and oil droplets.

C. Thin-layer chromatography (*2.2.27*).

Test solution To 1.0 g of the powdered drug (355) (*2.9.12*) add 10 mL of *methanol R*. Heat in a water-bath at 60 °C for 10 min. Allow to cool and filter.

Reference solution Dissolve 0.5 mg of *aucubin R* and 1 mg of *agnuside R* in *methanol R* and dilute to 1.0 mL with the same solvent.

Plate TLC silica gel F_{254} plate R (5-40 μm) [or *TLC silica gel F_{254} plate R* (2-10 μm)].

Mobile phase water R, methanol R, ethyl acetate R (8:15:77 V/V/V).

Application 10 μL [or 8 μL] as bands.

Development Over a path of 8 cm [or 5 cm].

Drying In air.

Detection Spray with *formic acid R* and heat at 120 °C for 10 min; examine in daylight.

Results See below the sequence of zones present in the chromatograms obtained with the reference solution and the test solution. Furthermore, other zones may be present in the chromatogram obtained with the test solution.

Top of the plate	
Agnuside: a blue zone	A blue zone (agnuside)
Aucubin: a blue zone	A blue zone (aucubin)
Reference solution	**Test solution**

TESTS

Foreign matter (*2.8.2*)
Maximum 3.0 per cent.

Other species of *Vitex*, in particular *Vitex negundo*
No fruit of other species with a much greater diameter is present.

Total ash (*2.4.16*)
Maximum 5.0 per cent.

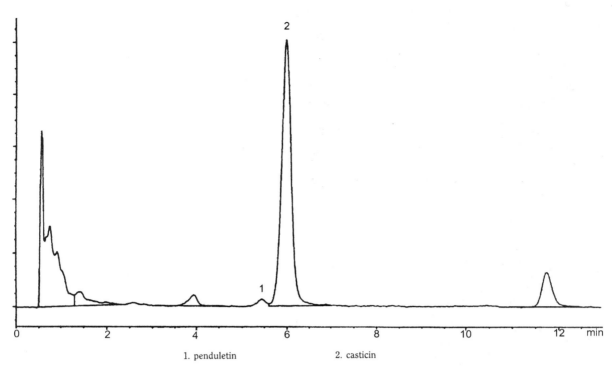

1. penduletin   2. casticin

Figure 2147.-1. – *Chromatogram for the assay of casticin in Agnus castus fruit: test solution*

Loss on drying (*2.2.32*)
Maximum 10.0 per cent, determined on 1.000 g of the powdered drug (355) (*2.9.12*) by drying in an oven at 105 °C for 2 h.

ASSAY
Liquid chromatography (*2.2.29*).

Test solution   Extract 1.000 g of the powdered drug (355) (*2.9.12*) with 40 mL of *methanol R* for 2 min using a suitable-speed homogeniser. Collect the supernatant liquid and filter into a 250 mL flask. Repeat the extraction with a further 40 mL of *methanol R*, collecting the supernatant liquid and filtering as before. Rinse the residue carefully with a small quantity of *methanol R*. Combine the methanol extracts and rinsings and evaporate to dryness *in vacuo* in a water-bath at not more than 30 °C. With the aid of ultrasound, dissolve the residue obtained in *methanol R* and dilute to 20.0 mL with the same solvent. Filter the solution through a membrane filter (nominal pore size 0.45 μm). Dilute 1.0 mL to 10.0 mL with *methanol R*.

Reference solution   Dissolve 100.0 mg of *agnus castus fruit standardised dry extract CRS* in 20.0 mL of *methanol R* with the aid of ultrasound for 20 min, then dilute to 25.0 mL with the same solvent. Filter the solution through a membrane filter (nominal pore size 0.45 μm).

Column:
— *size*: l = 0.125 m, Ø = 3.0 mm;
— *stationary phase*: octadecylsilyl silica gel for chromatography R (3 μm);
— *temperature*: 25 °C.

Mobile phase:
— *mobile phase A*: 5.88 g/L solution of *phosphoric acid R*;
— *mobile phase B*: *methanol R*;

Time (min)	Mobile phase A (per cent *V/V*)	Mobile phase B (per cent *V/V*)
0 - 13	50 → 35	50 → 65
13 - 18	35 → 0	65 → 100
18 - 23	0 → 50	100 → 50

Flow rate   1.0 mL/min.

Detection   Spectrophotometer at 348 nm.

Injection   10 μL.

System suitability   Test solution:
— *resolution*: minimum 1.5 between the peaks due to penduletin and casticin (see Figure 2147.-1).

Calculate the percentage content of casticin using the following expression:

$$\frac{F_1 \times m_2 \times p_1 \times 8}{F_2 \times m_1}$$

F_1 = area of the peak due to casticin in the chromatogram obtained with the test solution;
F_2 = area of the peak due to casticin in the chromatogram obtained with the reference solution;
m_1 = mass of the drug used to prepare the test solution, in grams;
m_2 = mass of *agnus castus fruit standardised dry extract CRS* used to prepare the reference solution, in grams;
p_1 = percentage content of casticin in *agnus castus fruit standardised dry extract CRS*.

Ph Eur

Agrimony

(*Ph Eur monograph 1587*)

Ph Eur

DEFINITION

Dried flowering tops of *Agrimonia eupatoria* L.

Content

Minimum 2.0 per cent of tannins, expressed as pyrogallol
($C_6H_6O_3$; M_r 126.1) (dried drug).

IDENTIFICATION

A. The stem is green or, more usually, reddish, cylindrical
and infrequently branched. It is covered with long, erect or
tangled hairs. The leaves are compound imparipennate with
3 or 6 opposite pairs of leaflets, with 2 or 3 smaller leaflets
between. The leaflets are deeply dentate to serrate, dark
green on the upper surface, greyish and densely tomentose
on the lower face. The flowers are small and form a terminal
spike. They are pentamerous and borne in the axils of hairy
bracts, the calyces closely surrounded by numerous terminal
hooked spires, which occur on the rim of the hairy
receptacle. The petals are free, yellow and deciduous. Fruit-
bearing obconical receptacles, with deep furrows and hooked
bristles, are usually present at the base of the inflorescence.

B. Reduce to a powder (355) (*2.9.12*). The powder is
yellowish-green or grey. Examine under a microscope using
chloral hydrate solution R. The powder shows the following
diagnostic characters (Figure 1587.-1): numerous straight or
bent, unicellular, long, thick-walled (about 500 μm) covering
trichomes [Ab, Ca, F], finely warty, and sometimes spirally
marked, often fragmented (F); fragments of the epidermis of
the stems [A] with stomata [Aa], covering trichomes (Ab)
and glandular trichomes [Ac]; fragments of upper leaf
epidermis in surface view [C] with straight walls bearing
covering trichomes (Ca), accompanied by palisade
parenchyma [Cb], with some of the cells containing calcium
oxalate prisms [Cc]; fragments of lower leaf epidermis in
surface view [J] with sinuous walls and abundant stomata
[Ja], mostly anomocytic (*2.8.3*) but occasionally anisocytic,
and glandular trichomes [Jb]; ovoid to subspherical pollen
grains, with 3 pores and a smooth exine [D]; glandular
trichomes with a multicellular, uniseriate stalk and a
unicellular to quadricellular head [B, Jb]; fragments of the
stems [H] with groups of fibres [Ha] and parenchymatous
cells, some of which contain cluster crystals of calcium
oxalate [Hb]; small spiral vessels from the leaflets [G];
fragments of large, spiral or bordered-pitted vessels from the
stem [E].

C. Thin-layer chromatography (*2.2.27*).

Test solution To 2.0 g of the powdered drug (355) (*2.9.12*)
add 20 mL of *methanol R*. Heat with shaking at 40 °C for
10 min. Filter.

Reference solution Dissolve 1.0 mg of *isoquercitroside R* and
1.0 mg of *rutin R* in 2 mL of *methanol R*.

Plate TLC silica gel plate *R*.

Mobile phase anhydrous formic acid *R*, water *R*, ethyl acetate *R*
(10:10:80 *V/V/V*).

Application 10 μL as bands.

Development Over a path of 12 cm.

Drying At 100-105 °C.

Detection Spray the still-warm plate with a 10 g/L solution
of *diphenylboric acid aminoethyl ester R* in *methanol R* and then
with a 50 g/L solution of *macrogol 400 R* in *methanol R*; allow

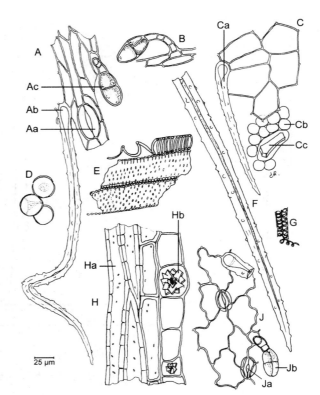

Figure 1587.-1.– *Illustration for identification test B of
powdered herbal drug of agrimony*

the plate to dry in air for 30 min and examine in ultraviolet
light at 365 nm.

Results See below the sequence of zones present in the
chromatograms obtained with the reference solution and the
test solution.

Top of the plate	
	An orange fluorescent zone may be present (quercitroside)
Isoquercitroside: an orange fluorescent zone	An orange fluorescent zone (isoquercitroside)
	An orange fluorescent zone (hyperoside)
Rutin: an orange fluorescent zone	An orange fluorescent zone (rutin)
Reference solution	**Test solution**

TESTS

Loss on drying (*2.2.32*)

Maximum 10.0 per cent, determined on 1.000 g of the
powdered drug (355) (*2.9.12*) by drying in an oven at
105 °C for 2 h.

Total ash (*2.4.16*)

Maximum 10.0 per cent.

ASSAY

Carry out the determination of tannins in herbal drugs
(*2.8.14*). Use 1.000 g of powdered drug (180) (*2.9.12*).

Ph Eur

Alchemilla

(*Ph Eur monograph 1387*)

Ph Eur _____

DEFINITION

Whole or cut, dried, flowering, aerial parts of *Alchemilla vulgaris* L. *sensu latiore*.

Content

Minimum 6.0 per cent of tannins, expressed as pyrogallol ($C_6H_6O_3$; M_r 126.1) (dried drug).

IDENTIFICATION

A. The greyish-green, partly brownish-green, radical leaves which are the main part of the drug are reniform or slightly semicircular with a diameter generally up to 8 cm, seldom up to 11 cm and have 7 to 9, or 11 lobes and a long petiole. The smaller, cauline leaves, which have a pair of large stipules at the base, have 5-9 lobes and a shorter petiole or they are sessile. The leaves are densely pubescent especially on the lower surface and have a coarsely serrated margin. Young leaves are folded with a whitish-silvery pubescence; older leaves are slightly pubescent and have a finely meshed venation, prominent on the lower surface. The greyish-green or yellowish-green petiole is pubescent, about 1 mm in diameter, with an adaxial groove. The apetalous flowers are yellowish-green or light green and about 3 mm in diameter. The calyx is double with 4 small segments of the epicalyx alternating with 4 larger sepals, subacute or triangular. They are 4 short stamens and a single carpel with a capitate stigma. The greyish-green or yellowish-green stem is pubescent, more or less longitudinally wrinkled and hollow.

B. Reduce to a powder (355) (*2.9.12*). The powder is greyish-green. Examine under a microscope using *chloral hydrate solution R*. The powder shows the following diagnostic characters: unicellular, narrow trichomes up to 1 mm long partly tortuous, acuminate, and bluntly pointed at the apex, with thick lignified walls, somewhat enlarged and pitted at the base; fragments of leaves with 2 layers of palisade parenchyma, the upper layer of which is 2-3 times longer than the lower layer and with spongy parenchyma, containing scattered cluster crystals of calcium oxalate, up to 25 μm in diameter; leaf fragments in surface view with sinuous or wavy epidermal cells, the anticlinal walls unevenly thickened and beaded, anomocytic stomata (*2.8.3*); groups of vascular tissue and lignified fibres from the petioles and stems, the vessels spirally thickened or with bordered pits; occasional thin-walled conical trichomes, about 300 μm long; thin-walled parenchyma containing cluster crystals of calcium oxalate; spherical pollen grains, about 15 μm in diameter, with 3 distinct pores and a granular exine; occasional fragments of the ovary wall with cells containing a single crystal of calcium oxalate.

C. Thin-layer chromatography (*2.2.27*).

Test solution To 0.5 g of the powdered drug (355) (*2.9.12*) add 5 mL of *methanol R* and heat in a water-bath at 70 °C under a reflux condenser for 5 min. Cool and filter.

Reference solution Dissolve 1.0 mg of *caffeic acid R* and 1.0 mg of *chlorogenic acid R* in 10 mL of *methanol R*.

Plate *TLC silica gel plate R*.

Mobile phase *anhydrous formic acid R*, *water R*, *ethyl acetate R* (8:8:84 *V/V/V*).

Application 20 μL of the test solution and 10 μL of the reference solution, as bands.

Development Over a path of 10 cm.

Drying At 100-105 °C for 5 min.

Detection Spray with a 10 g/L solution of *diphenylboric acid aminoethyl ester R* in *methanol R*. Subsequently spray with a 50 g/L solution of *macrogol 400 R* in *methanol R*. Allow to dry in air for about 30 min. Examine in ultraviolet light at 365 nm.

Results See below the sequence of the zones present in the chromatograms obtained with the reference solution and the test solution. Furthermore, other fluorescent zones may be present in the chromatogram obtained with the test solution.

Top of the plate	
	2 red fluorescent zones (chlorophyll)
Caffeic acid: a light blue florescent zone	1 or 2 intense light blue fluorescent zones
	One or several intense green or greenish-yellow fluorescent zones
————	————
Chlorogenic acid: a light blue fluorescent zone	An intense yellow or orange fluorescent zone
————	————
Reference solution	**Test solution**

TESTS

Loss on drying (*2.2.32*)
Maximum 10.0 per cent, determined on 1.000 g of powdered drug (355) (*2.9.12*) by drying in an oven at 105 °C for 2 h.

Total ash (*2.4.16*)
Maximum 12.0 per cent.

ASSAY

Carry out the determination of tannins in herbal drugs (*2.8.14*). Use 0.50 g of the powdered drug (355) (*2.9.12*).

_____ *Ph Eur*

Barbados Aloes

Curaçao Aloes

(*Ph Eur monograph 0257*)

Preparation
Standardised Aloes Dry Extract

Ph Eur _____

DEFINITION

Concentrated and dried juice of the leaves of *Aloe barbadensis* Miller.

Content

Minimum 28.0 per cent of hydroxyanthracene derivatives, expressed as barbaloin ($C_{21}H_{22}O_9$; M_r 418.4) (dried drug).

CHARACTERS

Appearance
Dark brown masses, slightly shiny or opaque with a conchoidal fracture, or brown powder.

Solubility
Partly soluble in boiling water, soluble in hot ethanol (96 per cent).

IDENTIFICATION

A. Thin-layer chromatography (2.2.27).

Test solution To 0.25 g of the powdered drug add 20 mL of *methanol R* and heat to boiling in a water-bath. Shake for a few minutes and decant the solution. Store at about 4 °C and use within 24 h.

Reference solution Dissolve 25 mg of *barbaloin R* in *methanol R* and dilute to 10 mL with the same solvent.

Plate TLC silica gel G plate R.

Mobile phase water R, methanol R, ethyl acetate R (13:17:100 *V/V/V*).

Application 10 μL, as bands of 20 mm by maximum 3 mm.

Development Over a path of 10 cm.

Drying In air.

Detection A Spray with a 100 g/L solution of *potassium hydroxide R* in *methanol R* and examine in ultraviolet light at 365 nm.

Results A The chromatogram obtained with the test solution shows in the central part a yellow fluorescent zone (barbaloin) similar in position to the zone due to barbaloin in the chromatogram obtained with the reference solution and in the lower part a light blue fluorescent zone (aloesine).

Detection B Heat at 110 °C for 5 min.

Results B In the chromatogram obtained with the test solution, a violet fluorescent zone appears just below the zone due to barbaloin.

B. Shake 1 g of the powdered drug with 100 mL of boiling *water R*. Cool, add 1 g of *talc R* and filter. To 10 mL of the filtrate add 0.25 g of *disodium tetraborate R* and heat to dissolve. Pour 2 mL of this solution into 20 mL of *water R*. Yellowish-green fluorescence appears which is particularly marked in ultraviolet light at 365 nm.

C. To 5 mL of the filtrate obtained in identification test B add 1 mL of freshly prepared *bromine water R*. A brownish-yellow precipitate is formed and the supernatant liquid is violet.

TESTS

Loss on drying (2.2.32)

Maximum 12.0 per cent, determined on 1.000 g of the powdered drug by drying in an oven at 105 °C.

Total ash (2.4.16)

Maximum 2.0 per cent.

ASSAY

Carry out the assay protected from bright light.

Introduce 0.300 g of powdered drug (180) (2.9.12) into a 250 mL conical flask. Moisten with 2 mL of *methanol R*, add 5 mL of *water R* warmed to about 60 °C, mix, then add a further 75 mL of *water R* at about 60 °C and shake for 30 min. Cool, filter into a volumetric flask, rinse the conical flask and filter with 20 mL of *water R*, add the rinsings to the volumetric flask and dilute to 1000.0 mL with *water R*. Transfer 10.0 mL of this solution to a 100 mL round-bottomed flask containing 1 mL of a 600 g/L solution of *ferric chloride R* and 6 mL of *hydrochloric acid R*. Heat in a water-bath under a reflux condenser for 4 h, with the water level above that of the liquid in the flask. Allow to cool, transfer the solution to a separating funnel, rinse the flask successively with 4 mL of *water R*, 4 mL of *1 M sodium hydroxide* and 4 mL of *water R* and add the rinsings to the separating funnel. Shake the contents of the separating funnel with 3 quantities, each of 20 mL, of *ether R*. Wash the combined ether layers with 2 quantities, each of 10 mL, of

water R. Discard the washings and dilute the organic phase to 100.0 mL with *ether R*. Evaporate 20.0 mL of the solution carefully to dryness on a water-bath and dissolve the residue in 10.0 mL of a 5 g/L solution of *magnesium acetate R* in *methanol R*. Measure the absorbance (2.2.25) at 512 nm using *methanol R* as the compensation liquid.

Calculate the percentage content of hydroxyanthracene derivatives, as barbaloin, from the following expression:

$$\frac{A \times 19.6}{m}$$

i.e. taking the specific absorbance of barbaloin to be 255.

A = absorbance at 512 nm,

m = mass of the substance to be examined, in grams.

STORAGE

In an airtight container.

_____ Ph Eur

Cape Aloes

(Ph Eur monograph 0258)

Preparation

Standardised Aloes Dry Extract

Ph Eur _____

DEFINITION

Concentrated and dried juice of the leaves of various species of *Aloe*, mainly *Aloe ferox* Miller and its hybrids.

Content

Minimum 18.0 per cent of hydroxyanthracene derivatives, expressed as barbaloin ($C_{21}H_{22}O_9$; M_r 418.4) (dried drug).

CHARACTERS

Appearance

Dark brown masses tinged with green and having a shiny conchoidal fracture, or greenish-brown powder.

Solubility

Partly soluble in boiling water, soluble in hot ethanol (96 per cent).

IDENTIFICATION

A. Examine the chromatograms obtained in the test for Barbados aloes.

Results The chromatogram obtained with the test solution shows in the central part a yellow fluorescent zone (barbaloin) similar in position to the zone due to barbaloin in the chromatogram obtained with the reference solution and in the lower part 2 yellow fluorescent zones (aloinosides A and B) and 1 blue fluorescent zone (aloesine).

B. Shake 1 g of the powdered drug with 100 mL of boiling *water R*. Cool, add 1 g of *talc R* and filter. To 10 mL of the filtrate add 0.25 g of *disodium tetraborate R* and heat to dissolve. Pour 2 mL of the solution into 20 mL of *water R*. A yellowish-green fluorescence appears which is particularly marked in ultraviolet light at 365 nm.

C. To 5 mL of the filtrate obtained in identification test B add 1 mL of freshly prepared *bromine water R*. A yellow precipitate is formed. The supernatant liquid is not violet.

TESTS

Barbados aloes

Thin-layer chromatography (2.2.27).

Test solution   To 0.25 g of the powdered drug add 20 mL of *methanol R* and heat to boiling in a water-bath. Shake for a few minutes and decant the solution. Store at about 4 °C and use within 24 h.

Reference solution   Dissolve 25 mg of *barbaloin R* in *methanol R* and dilute to 10 mL with the same solvent.

Plate   TLC silica gel G plate R.

Mobile phase   water R, methanol R, ethyl acetate R (13:17:100 V/V/V).

Application   10 µL, as bands of 20 mm by maximum 3 mm.

Development   Over a path of 10 cm.

Drying   In air.

Detection   Spray with a 100 g/L solution of *potassium hydroxide R* in *methanol R*. Heat at 110 °C for 5 min and examine in ultraviolet light at 365 nm.

Results   The chromatogram obtained with the test solution shows no violet fluorescent zone just below the zone due to barbaloin.

Loss on drying (*2.2.32*)
Maximum 10.0 per cent, determined on 1.000 g of the powdered drug by drying in an oven at 105 °C.

Total ash (*2.4.16*)
Maximum 2.0 per cent.

ASSAY
Carry out the assay protected from bright light.

Introduce 0.400 g of powdered drug (180) (*2.9.12*) into a 250 mL conical flask. Moisten with 2 mL of *methanol R*, add 5 mL of *water R* warmed to about 60 °C, mix, then add a further 75 mL of *water R* at about 60 °C and shake for 30 min. Cool, filter into a volumetric flask, rinse the conical flask and filter with 20 mL of *water R*, add the rinsings to the volumetric flask and dilute to 1000.0 mL with *water R*. Transfer 10.0 mL of this solution to a 100 mL round-bottomed flask containing 1 mL of a 600 g/L solution of *ferric chloride R* and 6 mL of *hydrochloric acid R*. Heat in a water-bath under a reflux condenser for 4 h, with the water level above that of the liquid in the flask. Allow to cool, transfer the solution to a separating funnel, rinse the flask successively with 4 mL of *water R*, 4 mL of *1 M sodium hydroxide* and 4 mL of *water R* and add the rinsings to the separating funnel. Shake the contents of the separating funnel with 3 quantities, each of 20 mL, of *ether R*. Wash the combined ether layers with 2 quantities, each of 10 mL, of *water R*. Discard the washings and dilute the organic phase to 100.0 mL with *ether R*. Evaporate 20.0 mL of the solution carefully to dryness on a water-bath and dissolve the residue in 10.0 mL of a 5 g/L solution of *magnesium acetate R* in *methanol R*. Measure the absorbance (*2.2.25*) at 512 nm using *methanol R* as the compensation liquid.

Calculate the percentage content of barbaloin from the following expression:

$$\frac{A \times 19.6}{m}$$

i.e. taking the specific absorbance of hydroxyanthracene derivatives, as barbaloin, to be 255.

A = absorbance at 512 nm,
m = mass of the substance to be examined in grams.

STORAGE
In an airtight container.

Standardised Aloes Dry Extract

(Ph Eur monograph 0259)

Ph Eur _____

DEFINITION
Standardised dry extract prepared from Barbados aloes or Cape aloes, or a mixture of both.

Content
19.0 per cent to 21.0 per cent of hydroxyanthracene derivatives, expressed as barbaloin ($C_{21}H_{22}O_9$; M_r 418.4) adjusted, if necessary (dried extract).

PRODUCTION
The extract is produced from the herbal drug by a suitable procedure using boiling water.

CHARACTERS
Appearance
Brown or yellowish-brown powder.

Solubility
Sparingly soluble in boiling water.

IDENTIFICATION
A. Thin-layer chromatography (*2.2.27*).

Test solution   To 0.25 g of the extract to be examined add 20 mL of *methanol R* and heat to boiling in a water-bath. Shake for a few minutes and decant the solution. Store at about 4 °C and use within 24 h.

Reference solution   Dissolve 25 mg of *barbaloin R* in *methanol R* and dilute to 10 mL with the same solvent.

Plate   TLC silica gel G plate R.

Mobile phase   water R, methanol R, ethyl acetate R (13:17:100 V/V/V).

Application   10 µL as bands of 20 mm by not more than 3 mm.

Development   Over a path of 10 cm.

Drying   In air.

Detection   Spray with a 100 g/L solution of *potassium hydroxide R* in *methanol R* and examine in ultraviolet light at 365 nm.

Results   The chromatogram obtained with the test solution shows, in the central part, a zone of yellow fluorescence (barbaloin) similar in position to the zone due to barbaloin in the chromatogram obtained with the reference solution and in the lower part, a zone of light blue fluorescence (aloesine). In the lower part of the chromatogram obtained with the test solution 2 zones of yellow fluorescence (aloinosides A and B) (Cape aloes) and a zone of violet fluorescence just below the zone due to barbaloin (Barbados aloes) may be present.

B. Shake 1 g with 100 mL of boiling *water R*. Cool, add 1 g of *talc R* and filter. To 10 mL of the filtrate add 0.25 g of *disodium tetraborate R* and heat to dissolve. Pour 2 mL of this solution into 20 mL of *water R*. A yellowish-green fluorescence appears which is particularly marked in ultraviolet light at 365 nm.

TESTS
Loss on drying (*2.8.17*)
Maximum 4.0 per cent *m/m*.

Total ash (*2.4.16*)
Maximum 2.0 per cent.

ASSAY

Carry out the assay protected from bright light.

Introduce 0.400 g into a 250 mL conical flask. Moisten with 2 mL of *methanol R*, add 5 mL of *water R* warmed to about 60 °C, mix, add a further 75 mL of *water R* at about 60 °C and shake for 30 min. Cool, filter into a volumetric flask, rinse the conical flask and the filter with 20 mL of *water R*, add the rinsings to the volumetric flask and dilute to 1000.0 mL with *water R*. Transfer 10.0 mL of this solution to a 100 mL round-bottomed flask containing 1 mL of a 600 g/L solution of *ferric chloride R* and 6 mL of *hydrochloric acid R*. Heat in a water-bath under a reflux condenser for 4 h, with the water level above that of the liquid in the flask. Allow to cool, transfer the solution to a separating funnel, rinse the flask successively with 4 mL of *water R*, 4 mL of *1 M sodium hydroxide* and 4 mL of *water R*, and add the rinsings to the separating funnel. Shake the contents of the separating funnel with 3 quantities, each of 20 mL, of *ether R*. Wash the combined ether layers with 2 quantities, each of 10 mL, of *water R*. Discard the washings and dilute the organic layer to 100.0 mL with *ether R*. Evaporate 20.0 mL carefully to dryness on a water-bath and dissolve the residue in 10.0 mL of a 5 g/L solution of *magnesium acetate R* in *methanol R*. Measure the absorbance (*2.2.25*) at 512 nm using *methanol R* as the compensation liquid.

Calculate the percentage content of hydroxyanthracene derivatives, expressed as barbaloin, using the following expression:

$$\frac{A \times 19.6}{m}$$

i.e. taking the specific absorbance of barbaloin to be 255.
A = absorbance at 512 nm;
m = mass of the substance to be examined, in grams.

Ph Eur

Anethum Graveolens Sowa Fruit

DEFINITION

Anethum Graveolens Sowa Fruit is the dried ripe fruit of *Anethum graveolens* L. Sowa Group.

Content

It contains not less than 3.0% v/w of essential oil calculated with reference to the anhydrous drug.

IDENTIFICATION

A. The dried fruits usually occur as separate mericarps, pedicels normally absent; broadly oval, highly compressed dorsally, about 4 mm long, 2 to 3 mm broad, with 5 dorsal ridges, each mericarp exhibiting 3 pale brown dorsal ridges, the two lateral ridges elongated into characteristic membranous wings; surface glabrous; remnants of the stylopod at the apex; commissural surface flat, often with attached, paler brown carpophore; vittae visible as two darker, arc-shaped, longitudinal bands.

B. Reduce to a powder (355). The powder is pale brown. Examine under a microscope using *chloral hydrate solution*. The powder contains numerous fragments of the epicarp, with cuticular striations and infrequent anomocytic stomata; parquetry layer of endocarp in surface view; endosperm of oval to rectangular thick-walled cells containing oil globules and aleurone grains with embedded microrosette crystals of calcium oxalate; fragments of yellowish-brown septate vittae;

parenchyma of mesocarp consisting of elongated, lignified, reticulately thickened cells; sclereids of mesocarp thick-walled with few pits.

C. Carry out the method for *thin-layer chromatography*, Appendix III A, using the following solutions.

(1) Add 10mL of *methanol (70%)* to 0.5 g of the powdered drug (355), mix and place in an ultrasonic bath for 30 minutes. Filter (a 0.45-μm PTFE is suitable) into a 10 mL volumetric flask and dilute to 10 mL with *methanol (70%)*.

(2) 0.05% w/v each of *carvone* and *dillapiole* in *methanol (70%)*.

CHROMATOGRAPHIC CONDITIONS

(a) Use high-performance *silica gel 60 F_{254}* plates (Merck silica gel 60 F_{254} HPTLC plates are suitable).

(b) Use the mobile phase as described below.

(c) Apply 10 μL of each solution as 6 mm bands.

(d) Develop the plate to 8 cm.

(e) After removal of the plate, dry in air, spray with *vanillin reagent*, heat the plate at 110° until the coloured bands appear and examine in daylight.

MOBILE PHASE

2 volumes of *acetic acid*, 10 volumes of *ethyl acetate* and 88 volumes of *toluene*.

SYSTEM SUITABILITY

The test is not valid unless the chromatogram obtained with solution (3) shows two clearly separated bands.

CONFIRMATION

The chromatogram obtained with solution (1) shows a purple band corresponding in position and colour to the band due to carvone in the chromatogram obtained with solution (2); a brown band corresponding in position and colour to the band due to dillapiole and other bands as shown in the table. Other bands may be present.

Top of the plate		
A faint brown band		
A brown band (dillapiole)		A brown band (dillapiole)
A purple band (carvone)	A purple band (carvone)	A purple band (carvone)
A grey band		
Solution (1)	**Solution (2)**	**Solution (3)**

TESTS
Apiole

Carry out the method for *gas chromatography*, Appendix III B, using the following solutions.

(1) Use the oil retained in the Assay of Essential oil.

(2) 1.0% w/v of *apiole* in *toluene*.

(3) 0.05% v/v of *β-myrcene* and 0.8% v/v of *limonene* in *toluene*.

CHROMATOGRAPHIC CONDITIONS

(a) Use a fused silica capillary column (30 m × 0.53 mm) bonded with a 1 μm film thickness, *polyethylene glycol 20,000* (DB-Wax is suitable).

(b) Use *helium* as the carrier gas at 1.5 mL per minute.

(c) Use the gradient conditions described in the table.

(d) Use a flame ionisation detector maintained at a temperature of 260°.

(e) Inject 1 μL of each solution at a temperature of 250°.

Time (min)	Temperature	Comment
0 → 5	60	isothermal
5 → 68	60 → 250	linear gradient
68 → 75	250	isothermal

SYSTEM SUITABILITY

The test is not valid unless, in the chromatogram obtained with solution (3), the *resolution factor* between the peaks due to β-myrcene and limonene, is at least 4.5.

In the chromatogram obtained with solution (3), the substances elute in the following order: β-myrcene and limonene.

CONFIRMATION

In the chromatogram obtained with solution (1), there is no peak corresponding to the peak due to apiole obtained with solution (2).

Water

Not more than 10.0% v/w, Appendix IX C, method II using 30 g of powdered drug (*1400*).

Total Ash

Not more than 8.0%, Appendix XI J, Method II.

Chromatographic profile

Carry out the method for *gas chromatography*, Appendix III B, using the following solutions.

(1) Use the oil retained in the Assay of Essential oil.

(2) 0.4% w/v each of *limonene, dihydrocarvone, carvone* and *dillapiole* in *toluene*.

(3) 0.05% v/v of *β-myrcene* and 0.8% v/v of *limonene* in *toluene*

CHROMATOGRAPHIC CONDITIONS

The chromatographic procedure described under the test for Apiole may be used.

SYSTEM SUITABILITY

The test is not valid unless, in the chromatogram obtained with solution (3), the *resolution factor* between the peaks due to β-myrcene and limonene is at least 4.5.

In the chromatogram obtained with solution (2), the substances elute in the following order: limonene, dihydrocarvone isomer 1, dihydrocarvone isomer 2, carvone and dillapiole.

In the chromatogram obtained with solution (3), the substances elute in the following order: β-myrcene and limonene.

Calculate the content of limonene, dihydrocarvone, carvone and dillapiole by normalisation. Disregard the peak due to toluene.

Limits:

— limonene: 15.0 to 28.0%,
— sum of dihydrocarvone isomers 1 and 2: 5.0 to 30.0%,
— carvone: 20.0 to 45.0%,
— dillapiole: 15.0 to 35.0%.

Disregard any peak with an area less than 0.025 times the area of the peak due to carvone in the chromatogram obtained with solution (2).

ASSAY

Essential oil

Carry out the method for *Essential Oils in Herbal Drugs*, Appendix XI E using 18 g of freshly prepared powdered drug (*1400*) with 250 mL of *water* as the distillation liquid. Distil at a rate of 2 to 3 mL per minute for 2 hours using 0.50 mL of *toluene* in the graduated tube. Measure the quantity of essential oil distilled and use in the tests for Apiole and Chromatographic profile.

Angelica Archangelica Root

(*Ph Eur monograph 1857*)

Ph Eur ⎯⎯⎯⎯⎯⎯⎯⎯⎯⎯⎯⎯⎯⎯⎯⎯⎯⎯⎯⎯⎯⎯

DEFINITION

Whole or cut, carefully dried rhizome and root of *Angelica archangelica* L. (syn. *A. officinalis* Hoffm.).

Content

Minimum 2.0 mL/kg of essential oil (dried drug).

CHARACTERS

Bitter taste.

IDENTIFICATION

A. The rhizome is greyish-brown or reddish-brown, with transversely annulated thickenings. The base bears greyish-brown or reddish-brown, cylindrical, longitudinally furrowed, occasionally branched roots often with incompletely encircling, transverse ridges. The apex sometimes shows remnants of stem and leaf bases. The fracture is uneven. The transversely cut surface shows a greyish-white, spongy, distinctly radiate bark, in which the secretory channels are visible as brown spots, and a bright yellow or greyish-yellow wood which, in the rhizome, surrounds the greyish or brownish-white pith.

B. Microscopic examination (*2.8.23*). The powder is brownish-white. Examine under a microscope using *chloral hydrate solution R*. The powder shows the following diagnostic characters (Figure 1857.-1): fragments of cork consisting of several layers of thin-walled, greyish-brown or reddish-brown cells, in surface view [C] or in transverse section [E]; large, yellowish-brown secretory channels, whole or fragmented, in transverse section [A] or in longitudinal section [F]; fragments of medullary rays, 2 or 4 cells wide [G]; fragments of xylem [B] consisting of lignified vessels with reticulate thickening [Ba] occurring singly or in small groups, and unlignified parenchyma in which some of the cells associated with the vessels are collenchymatously thickened. Examine under a microscope using a 50 per cent *V/V* solution of *glycerol R*. The powder shows numerous, simple starch granules 2-4 μm in diameter, free or included in parenchyma cells [D].

C. Examine the chromatograms obtained in the test for other species of *Angelica, Levisticum* and *Ligusticum* described in the European Pharmacopoeia.

Results A See below the sequence of zones present in the chromatograms obtained with the reference solution and the test solution. Furthermore, other faint fluorescent zones may be present in the chromatogram obtained with the test solution.

Herbal Drugs

Top of the plate	
(Z)-Ligustilide: a bluish-white fluorescent zone	
	———
Osthole: a blue fluorescent zone	A blue fluorescent zone
Imperatorin: a whitish fluorescent zone	A whitish fluorescent zone
	A blue fluorescent zone
———	———
	3 blue fluorescent zones
Reference solution	**Test solution**

Results B See below the sequence of zones present in the chromatograms obtained with the reference solution and the test solution. Furthermore, other faint quenching zones may be present in the chromatogram obtained with the test solution.

Top of the plate	
(Z)-Ligustilide: a blue fluorescent zone	
———	———
Osthole: a quenching zone	A quenching zone
Imperatorin: a quenching zone	A quenching zone
	A quenching zone
———	———
	Several quenching zones
Reference solution	**Test solution**

TESTS

Other species of *Angelica, Levisticum* and *Ligusticum* described in the European Pharmacopoeia
Thin-layer chromatography (*2.2.27*).

Test solution To 1 g of the freshly powdered herbal drug (355) (*2.9.12*) add 4 mL of *heptane R*, close and sonicate for 5 min. Centrifuge the mixture and use the supernatant.

Reference solution Dissolve 1 mg of *imperatorin R*, 1 mg of (*Z*)-*ligustilide R* and 1 mg of *osthole R* in 10 mL of *methanol R*.

Plate TLC silica gel F_{254} *plate R* (2-10 μm).

Mobile phase glacial acetic acid R, ethyl acetate R, toluene R (1:10:90 *V/V/V*).

Application 4 μL as bands of 8 mm.

Development Over a path of 6 cm.

Drying In air.

Detection A Examine in ultraviolet light at 365 nm.

Results A The chromatogram obtained with the test solution shows no zone at the position of (*Z*)-ligustilide in the chromatogram obtained with the reference solution.

Detection B Examine in ultraviolet light at 254 nm.

Results B The chromatogram obtained with the test solution shows no zone at or just below the position of (*Z*)-ligustilide in the chromatogram obtained with the reference solution.

Foreign matter (*2.8.2*)
Maximum 5 per cent of leaf bases and stem bases, maximum 5 per cent of discoloured pieces and maximum 1 per cent of other foreign matter.

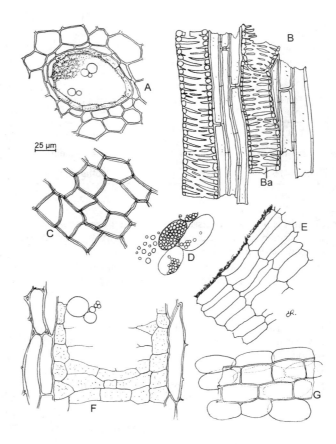

Figure 1857.-1. – *Illustration for identification test B of powdered herbal drug of angelica root*

Loss on drying (*2.2.32*)
Maximum 10.0 per cent, determined on 1.000 g of the powdered herbal drug (355) (*2.9.12*) by drying in an oven at 105 °C for 2 h.

Total ash (*2.4.16*)
Maximum 10.0 per cent.

Ash insoluble in hydrochloric acid (*2.8.1*)
Maximum 2.0 per cent.

ASSAY

Carry out the determination of essential oils in herbal drugs (*2.8.12*). Reduce the herbal drug to a powder (500) (*2.9.12*) and immediately use 40.0 g for the determination. Use a 2 L round-bottomed flask, 10 drops of *liquid paraffin R*, 500 mL of *water R* as distillation liquid and 0.50 mL of *xylene R* in the graduated tube. Distil at a rate of 2-3 mL/min for 4 h.

Ph Eur

Angelica Dahurica Root

(*Ph Eur monograph 2556*)

Ph Eur ————————————————————————

DEFINITION

Dried, whole or fragmented root, with rootlets removed, of *Angelica dahurica* (Hoffm.) Benth. & Hook. f. ex Franch. & Sav. collected in summer or autumn.

Content

Minimum 0.08 per cent of imperatorin ($C_{16}H_{14}O_4$; M_r 270.3) (dried drug).

IDENTIFICATION

A. The non-fragmented drug consists of conical roots, about 10-25 cm long and 1.5-2.5 cm in diameter. The root crown, more or less quadrangular, is obtuse and shows stem scars on prominences. It tapers to the tip. The outer surface is brownish-grey or yellowish-brown and clearly striated longitudinally, showing scars of the secondary roots and lenticel-like transverse protuberances, some of them arranged in 4 longitudinal rows. The texture is compact, hard and heavy. The fracture, white or whitish grey and mealy, is marked with concentric striations. The cambium occurs as a brown ring. Very many brown dots, corresponding to a transverse section of the secretory canals, are visible in the cortical part.

B. Microscopic examination (*2.8.23*). The powder is yellowish-white. Examine under a microscope using *chloral hydrate solution R*. The powder shows the following diagnostic characters: reticulate lignified vessels, free or in groups of 2 or 3 and accompanied by ligneous parenchyma cells with fine cellulose walls; numerous fragments of parenchyma with ovoid cells; a few orange cork fragments, consisting of several layers of superimposed cells; secretory canals, usually broken, with yellow or pale brown contents and oil droplets. Examine under a microscope using a 50 per cent *V/V* solution of *glycerol R*. The powder shows very many starch granules varying in size from 5 to 25 μm; some are simple and rounded, others consist of 2-8 elements, but most are polyhedral, either due to compound granules breaking up or to compression in the cells.

C. Examine the chromatograms obtained in the test for other officinal species of *Angelica*, *Levisticum* and *Ligusticum*.

Results A   See below the sequence of zones present in the chromatograms obtained with the reference solution and the test solution. Furthermore, other faint fluorescent zones may be present in the chromatogram obtained with the test solution.

Top of the plate	
(*Z*)-Ligustilide: a bluish-white fluorescent zone	A bluish-white fluorescent zone
	———
	A whitish fluorescent zone
Osthole: a blue fluorescent zone	A blue fluorescent zone
Imperatorin: a whitish fluorescent zone	A whitish fluorescent zone (imperatorin)
———	———
Reference solution	**Test solution**

Results B   See below the sequence of zones present in the chromatograms obtained with the reference solution and the test solution. Furthermore, other faint quenching zones may be present in the chromatogram obtained with the test solution.

Top of the plate	
(*Z*)-Ligustilide: a blue fluorescent zone	A faint quenching zone
	———
	A quenching zone
Osthole: a quenching zone	
Imperatorin: a quenching zone	A quenching zone (imperatorin)
———	———
Reference solution	**Test solution**

Results C   See below the sequence of zones present in the chromatograms obtained with the reference solution and the test solution. Furthermore, other faint zones may be present in the chromatogram obtained with the test solution.

Top of the plate	
	2 prominent reddish zones
(*Z*)-Ligustilide: a grey zone	
———	———
	A faint blue zone
Osthole: a violet zone	
Imperatorin: a grey zone	A yellow and violet double-zone
	———
	A prominent violet zone
	A yellow zone
Reference solution	**Test solution**

TESTS

Other officinal species of *Angelica*, *Levisticum* and *Ligusticum*

Thin-layer chromatography (*2.2.27*).

Test solution   To 1 g of the powdered herbal drug (355) (*2.9.12*) add 4 mL of *heptane R*, close and sonicate for 5 min. Centrifuge the mixture and use the supernatant.

Reference solution   Dissolve 1 mg of *imperatorin R*, 1 mg of (*Z*)-*ligustilide R* and 1 mg of *osthole R* in 10 mL of *methanol R*.

Plate   TLC silica gel F_{254} plate R (2-10 μm).

Mobile phase   glacial acetic acid R, ethyl acetate R, toluene R (1:10:90 *V/V/V*).

Application   4 μL as bands of 8 mm.

Development   Over a path of 6 cm.

Drying   In air.

Detection A   Examine in ultraviolet light at 365 nm.

Results A   The chromatogram obtained with the test solution shows no intense blue fluorescent zone below the position of imperatorin in the chromatogram obtained with the reference solution.

Detection B   Examine in ultraviolet light at 254 nm.

Results B   The chromatogram obtained with the test solution shows no blue fluorescent zone corresponding to the zone due to (Z)-ligustilide in the chromatogram obtained with the reference solution; the chromatogram obtained with the test solution shows no quenching zone at the position of osthole or below the position of imperatorin in the chromatogram obtained with the reference solution.

Detection C   Treat with a 10 per cent *V/V* solution of *sulfuric acid R* in *methanol R*, heat at 100 °C for 5 min and examine in daylight.

Results C   The chromatogram obtained with the test solution shows no violet zone corresponding to the zone due to osthole in the chromatogram obtained with the reference solution.

Loss on drying *(2.2.32)*

Maximum 12.0 per cent, determined on 1.000 g of the powdered herbal drug (355) *(2.9.12)* by drying in an oven at 105 °C for 2 h.

Total ash *(2.4.16)*

Maximum 6.0 per cent.

Ash insoluble in hydrochloric acid *(2.8.1)*

Maximum 1.5 per cent.

ASSAY

Liquid chromatography *(2.2.29)*.

Test solution   Disperse 0.400 g of the powdered herbal drug (355) *(2.9.12)* in 45 mL of *methanol R* and sonicate for 1 h. Cool and dilute to 50.0 mL with *methanol R*. Filter through a membrane filter (nominal pore size 0.45 µm).

Reference solution (a)   Dissolve 5.0 mg of *imperatorin CRS* in *methanol R* and dilute to 50.0 mL with the same solvent. Dilute 1.0 mL of the solution to 10.0 mL with *methanol R*.

Reference solution (b)   Disperse 80 mg of *Angelica dahurica root HRS* in 9 mL of *methanol R* and sonicate for 1 h. Cool and dilute to 10 mL with *methanol R*. Filter through a membrane filter (nominal pore size 0.45 µm).

Precolumn:
— *size: l* = 4 mm, Ø = 4.0 mm;
— *stationary phase*: *octadecylsilyl silica gel for chromatography R* (5 µm).

Column:
— *size: l* = 0.125 m, Ø = 4.0 mm;
— *stationary phase*: *octadecylsilyl silica gel for chromatography R* (5 µm).

Mobile phase:
— *mobile phase A: water R*;
— *mobile phase B: acetonitrile R1*;

Time (min)	Mobile phase A (per cent *V/V*)	Mobile phase B (per cent *V/V*)
0 - 15	45	55
15 – 33	45 → 5	55 → 95
33 - 35	5	95

Flow rate   1.0 mL/min.

Detection   Spectrophotometer at 210 nm.

Injection   20 µL.

Identification of peaks   Use the chromatogram supplied with *Angelica dahurica root HRS* and the chromatogram obtained with reference solution (b) to identify the peak due to phellopterin.

Relative retention   With reference to imperatorin (retention time = about 5 min): phellopterin = about 1.1.

System suitability   Reference solution (b):
— *resolution*: minimum 1.5 between the peaks due to imperatorin and phellopterin.

Calculate the percentage content of imperatorin using the following expression:

$$\frac{A_1 \times m_2 \times p}{A_2 \times m_1 \times 10}$$

A_1 = area of the peak due to imperatorin in the chromatogram obtained with the test solution;

A_2 = area of the peak due to imperatorin in the chromatogram obtained with reference solution (a);

m_1 = mass of the herbal drug to be examined used to prepare the test solution, in grams;

m_2 = mass of *imperatorin CRS* used to prepare reference solution (a), in grams;

p = percentage content of imperatorin in *imperatorin CRS*.

—————— Ph Eur

Angelica Pubescens Root

(Ph Eur monograph 2557)

Ph Eur _____

DEFINITION

Dried root, without rootlets, of *Angelica pubescens* Maxim. f. *biserrata* R.H.Shan et C.Q.Yuan, collected in early spring before sprouting, or in the end of autumn when stem and leaves wither.

Content

Minimum 0.50 per cent of osthole ($C_{15}H_{16}O_3$; M_r 244.3) (dried drug).

IDENTIFICATION

A. The taproot is more or less cylindrical, branching rapidly into 2-3 or more principal roots at the lower part; the whole is about 5-30 cm long. The root crown is enlarged, with transverse, annulated wrinkles and measures about 0.5-4.5 cm in diameter; it shows the remains of stems, leaves or buds. The greyish-brown or dark brown outer surface is longitudinally wrinkled and shows slightly prominent rootlet scars and transverse lenticel-like protuberances. The fracture shows greyish-yellow bark, with abundant brown dots due to secretory canals; the cambium ring is brown and the wood is greyish-yellow or yellowish-brown.

B. Microscopic examination *(2.8.23)*. The powder is yellowish-brown or brown. Examine under a microscope using *chloral hydrate solution R*. The powder shows the following diagnostic characters: fragments of lignified vessels up to 90 µm in diameter with spiral or reticulate thickenings, free or in groups of 2 or 3; fragments of phloem parenchyma with fine, sinuous fusiform cells, about 7-38 µm in diameter, with slightly thickened walls and fine, oblique criss-cross striations; orange-brown cork fragments, consisting of several layers of superimposed, somewhat polyhedral cells in surface view; secretory canals, usually broken, with yellow or pale brown contents and droplets of essential oil. Examine under a microscope using a 50 per cent *V/V* solution of *glycerol R*. The powder shows numerous small, rounded or ovoid, simple starch granules, about 10 µm in size, with a punctiform hilum that is visible on the largest granules; a few starch granules consisting of 2-10 components are also present.

C. Examine the chromatograms obtained in the test for other officinal species of *Angelica*, *Levisticum* and *Ligusticum*.

Results A   See below the sequence of zones present in the chromatograms obtained with the reference solution and the test solution. Furthermore, other faint fluorescent zones may be present in the chromatogram obtained with the test solution.

Top of the plate	
(*Z*)-Ligustilide: a bluish-white fluorescent zone	A bluish-white fluorescent zone
———	———
	A very faint whitish zone
Osthole: a blue fluorescent zone	A prominent blue fluorescent zone (osthole)
Imperatorin: a whitish fluorescent zone	A whitish fluorescent zone (may be missing)
———	———
	A blue fluorescent zone
	3 blue fluorescent zones
Reference solution	**Test solution**

Results B   See below the sequence of zones present in the chromatograms obtained with the reference solution and the test solution. Furthermore, other faint quenching zones may be present in the chromatogram obtained with the test solution.

Top of the plate	
(*Z*)-Ligustilide: a blue fluorescent zone	A faint quenching zone
———	———
Osthole: a quenching zone	A quenching zone (osthole)
	A blue fluorescent zone
Imperatorin: a quenching zone	A quenching zone (may be missing)
———	———
	2 or 3 quenching zones
Reference solution	**Test solution**

Results C   See below the sequence of zones present in the chromatograms obtained with the reference solution and the test solution. Furthermore, other faint zones may be present in the chromatogram obtained with the test solution.

Top of the plate	
	A prominent reddish zone
(*Z*)-Ligustilide: a grey zone	
———	———
Osthole: a violet zone	A violet zone (osthole)
Imperatorin: a grey zone	A violet zone (may be missing)
———	———
	A prominent violet zone
	A yellow zone
Reference solution	**Test solution**

TESTS

Other officinal species of *Angelica*, *Levisticum* and *Ligusticum*

Thin-layer chromatography (*2.2.27*).

Test solution   To 1 g of the powdered herbal drug (355) (*2.9.12*) add 4 mL of *heptane R*, close and sonicate for 5 min. Centrifuge the mixture and use the supernatant.

Reference solution   Dissolve 1 mg of *imperatorin R*, 1 mg of (*Z*)-*ligustilide R* and 1 mg of *osthole R* in 10 mL of *methanol R*.

Plate   TLC silica gel F_{254} plate *R* (2-10 μm).

Mobile phase   glacial acetic acid *R*, ethyl acetate *R*, toluene *R* (1:10:90 *V/V/V*).

Application   4 μL as bands of 8 mm.

Development   Over a path of 6 cm.

Drying   In air.

Detection A   Examine in ultraviolet light at 365 nm.

Results A   The chromatogram obtained with the test solution shows no intense whitish fluorescent zone directly above the position of osthole and no blue fluorescent zone just below the position of imperatorin in the chromatogram obtained with the reference solution.

Detection B   Examine in ultraviolet light at 254 nm.

Results B   The chromatogram obtained with the test solution shows no blue fluorescent zone corresponding to the zone due to (*Z*)-ligustilide in the chromatogram obtained with the reference solution.

Detection C   Treat with a 10 per cent *V/V* solution of *sulfuric acid R* in *methanol R*, heat at 100 °C for 5 min and examine in daylight.

Results C   The chromatogram obtained with the test solution shows no zone corresponding to the zone due to (*Z*)-ligustilide in the chromatogram obtained with the reference solution.

Loss on drying (*2.2.32*)

Maximum 10.0 per cent, determined on 1.000 g of the powdered herbal drug (355) (*2.9.12*) by drying in an oven at 105 °C for 2 h.

Total ash (*2.4.16*)

Maximum 8.0 per cent.

Ash insoluble in hydrochloric acid (*2.8.1*)

Maximum 3.0 per cent.

ASSAY

Liquid chromatography (*2.2.29*).

Test solution   Disperse 0.500 g of the powdered herbal drug (355) (*2.9.12*) in 18 mL of *methanol R* and sonicate for 30 min. Cool and dilute to 20.0 mL with *methanol R*. Mix and filter. Dilute 5.0 mL of the filtrate to 20.0 mL with *methanol R*.

Reference solution (a)   Dissolve 5.0 mg of *osthole CRS* in *methanol R* and dilute to 100.0 mL with the same solvent.

Reference solution (b)   Disperse 0.250 g of *Angelica pubescens root HRS* in 9 mL of *methanol R* and sonicate for 30 min. Cool and dilute to 10.0 mL with *methanol R*. Mix and filter. Dilute 5.0 mL of the filtrate to 20.0 mL with *methanol R*.

Column:
— *size*: l = 0.125 m, Ø = 2.0 mm;
— *stationary phase*: octadecylsilyl silica gel for chromatography *R* (4 μm).

Mobile phase   water *R*, acetonitrile *R* (40:60 *V/V*).

Flow rate   0.23 mL/min.

Detection Spectrophotometer at 322 nm.

Injection 10 μL.

Retention time Osthole = about 8 min.

System suitability Reference solution (b):

— *resolution*: minimum 1.5 between the peak due to osthole and peak 2; use the chromatogram supplied with *Angelica pubescens root HRS* to identify peak 2.

Calculate the percentage content of osthole using the following expression:

$$\frac{A_1 \times m_2 \times p \times 0.8}{A_2 \times m_1}$$

A_1 = area of the peak due to osthole in the chromatogram obtained with the test solution;

A_2 = area of the peak due to osthole in the chromatogram obtained with reference solution (a);

m_1 = mass of the herbal drug to be examined used to prepare the test solution, in grams;

m_2 = mass of *osthole CRS* used to prepare reference solution (a), in grams;

p = percentage content of osthole in *osthole CRS*.

―――――――――――――――――――――――― Ph Eur

Angelica Sinensis Root

DEFINITION

Angelica Sinensis Root is the dried whole root of *Angelica sinensis* (Oliv.) Diels. (*Angelica polymorpha* Maxim. var. *sinensis* Oliv.). The dried root consists of the top (uppermost part), main body and small lateral roots (tails).

It is collected in late autumn, removed from rootlets and dried.

It contains not less than 0.1% of *Z*-ligustilide ($C_{12}H_{14}O_2$), calculated with reference to the dried material.

IDENTIFICATION

A. The whole root is yellowish-brown to brown, up to 25 cm long, irregularly cylindrical with 3 to 5 or more branch roots arising from the lower end. The upper part is 1.5 to 5 cm in diameter, annulated on the surface and rounded at the apex which may show purple or yellowish-green remains of stems and leaves; the surface of the remainder of the main root is strongly longitudinally wrinkled and has pale, transverse lenticels; the branch roots are 0.3 to 1 cm in diameter in the upper part, twisted and tapering towards the base, the outer surface is strongly striated and has few rootlet scars.

B. Reduce to a powder (355). The powder is pale yellowish to buff. Examine under a microscope using *chloral hydrate solution*. The powder shows brown fragments of cork composed of thin-walled cells; abundant thin-walled parenchyma from the secondary cortex, phloem and medullary rays, some of the phloem cells fusiform with slightly thickened walls; lignified vessels in groups of 2 or 3 associated with small celled and pitted xylem parenchyma; the vessels are up to 80 μm in diameter and have reticulate or scalariform thickening. Examine under a microscope using 50% v/v of *glycerol*. The powder shows small groups of single starch granules, spherical to ovoid, up to about 8 μm in diameter.

C. Carry out the method for *thin-layer chromatography*, Appendix III A, using the following solutions.

(1) Add 4 mL of *heptane* to 1.0 g of the powdered drug, mix with the aid of ultrasound for 5 minutes and filter (use a 0.22 μm membrane filter).

(2) 0.1% w/v of *linoleic acid* in *methanol*.

(3) 0.1% w/v of *ferulic acid* in *methanol*.

(4) 0.1% w/v of *Z-ligustilide CRS* in *methanol*.

CHROMATOGRAPHIC CONDITIONS

(a) Use a *silica gel F_{254}* precoated plate (Merck silica gel 60 F_{254} HPTLC plates are suitable).

(b) Use the mobile phase as described below.

(c) Apply 10 μL of solution (1) and 5 μL of solutions (2) to (4), as bands.

(d) Develop the plate to 15 cm.

(e) Remove the plate, allow to dry in a stream of warm air for 5 minutes or until the solvents are completely removed. Examine under *ultraviolet light (254 nm)*. Spray the plate with *methanolic sulfuric acid (5%)*, heat at 105° for 3 minutes and examine in daylight.

MOBILE PHASE

1 volume of *formic acid*, 10 volumes of *ethyl acetate* and 90 volumes of *toluene*.

SYSTEM SUITABILITY

When examined under *ultraviolet light (254 nm)* the violet band with an Rf value of approximately 0.7 the chromatogram obtained with solution (4) corresponds in colour and position to that in the chromatogram obtained with solution (1). A band with an Rf value of approximately 0.23 in the chromatogram obtained with solution (3) corresponds in position to a band in the chromatogram obtained with solution (1). Other bands may be present in the chromatogram obtained with solution (1).

CONFIRMATION

When sprayed with *methanolic sulfuric acid (5%)* the chromatogram obtained with solution (1) shows three spots with similar Rf values to the spots in the chromatograms obtained with solutions (2), (3) and (4). Other spots may be present in the chromatogram obtained with solution (1).

TESTS

Lovage root (*Levisticum officinale*)

Carry out the method for *gas chromatography*, Appendix III B, using the following solutions.

(1) Extract approximately 20 g of the coarsely powdered drug in a 500 mL round-bottomed flask by hydrodistillation for 2 to 3 hours in 200 mL of *water*, collecting the distillate in suitable glassware. Extract the oily drops on top of the distillate with 5 mL of *toluene*.

(2) 0.2% w/v each of *coumarin* and *eugenol* in *toluene*.

(3) 0.1% w/v of *Z-ligustilide CRS* in *acetonitrile*.

(4) 0.1% w/v of *benzyl alcohol* in *toluene*.

(5) 0.1% w/v of *(-)-carvone* in *toluene*.

(6) 0.1% w/v of *octanoic acid* in *toluene*.

(7) 0.1% w/v of *3-propylidenephthalide* in *toluene*.

CHROMATOGRAPHIC CONDITIONS

(a) Use a fused silica capillary column (50 m × 0.32 mm) bonded with a film (1.05 μm) of 5% phenyl/95% dimethylpolysiloxane (HP 5 is suitable).

(b) Use *helium* as the carrier gas at 1 mL per minute.

(c) Use an oven maintained at an initial temperature of 40° increasing linearly to 220° at a rate of 5° per minute, then maintained at 220°.

(d) Use a split injection system having a split ratio of 20:1 maintained at 250°.

(e) Use a flame ionisation detector maintained at a temperature of 250°.

(f) Inject 1 μL of each solution.

(g) Record the chromatograms for a sufficient length of time to elute all the peaks in the chromatogram obtained with solution (1) (55 minutes may be suitable).

SYSTEM SUITABILITY

The test is not valid unless, in the chromatogram obtained with solution (2), the resolution between coumarin (eluting at approximately 34 minutes) and eugenol (eluting at approximately 37 minutes) is at least 3.0.

CONFIRMATION

In the chromatogram obtained with solution (1):
— there are no peaks corresponding to the principal peaks in the chromatograms obtained with solutions (4), (5), (6) and (7);
— there is a peak corresponding to the principal peak in the chromatogram obtained with solution (3).

Loss on drying
When dried at 100° to 105° for 2 hours, loses not more than 12.0% of its weight. Use 1 g.

Total ash
Not more than 7.0%, Appendix XI J, Method II.

Acid-insoluble ash
Not more than 2.0%, Appendix XI K.

Ethanol-soluble extractive
Not less than 45%, Appendix XI B1.

ASSAY
Carry out the method for *liquid chromatography*, Appendix III D, using the following solutions.

(1) Finely powder not less than 5.0 g of the drug being examined. Transfer 0.5 g of the powder into a 25 mL volumetric flask and add 20 mL of *methanol*, place in an ultrasonic bath (maintained at a low temperature by adding ice to the bath) for 100 minutes, equilibrate to ambient temperature and dilute to volume with *methanol*. Centrifuge the solution at 5000 rpm for 5 minutes or until a clear supernatant is obtained. Filter through a 0.45-μm filter.

(2) 0.025% w/v of Z-ligustilide CRS in *acetonitrile*.

CHROMATOGRAPHIC CONDITIONS

(a) Use a stainless steel column (15 cm × 4.6 mm) packed with *octadecylsilyl silica gel for chromatography* (5 μm) (Hypersil ODS is suitable).

(b) Use isocratic elution and the mobile phase described below.

(c) Use a flow rate of 1.0 mL per minute.

(d) Use a detection wavelength of 350 nm.

(e) Inject 10 μL of each solution.

MOBILE PHASE

A mixture of 8 volumes of *water* and 12 volumes of *acetonitrile*.

SYSTEM SUITABILITY

Inject solution (2) not less than five times. The test is not valid unless the relative standard deviation of the peak areas of the Z-ligustilide peak is not more than 3.0%, the relative standard deviation of the retention times of the Z-ligustilide peak is not more than 3.0%. The *column efficiency*, determined on the Z-ligustilide peak, is not less than 5000

theoretical plates. The *symmetry factor*, determined on the Z-ligustilide peak, is not more than 1.3.

Inject solution (1). The test is not valid unless the *resolution factor* between the Z-ligustilide peak and the closest peak (relative retention about 0.9 with respect to Z-ligustilide) is not less than 1.5.

DETERMINATION OF CONTENT

Using the retention time and the peak area from the chromatograms obtained with solution (2), locate and integrate the peak due to Z-ligustilide in the chromatogram obtained with solution (1).

Calculate the content of Z-ligustilide in the sample using the declared content of Z-ligustilide ($C_{12}H_{14}O_2$) in *Z-ligustilide CRS* and the following expression:

$$\frac{A_1}{A_2} \times \frac{m_2}{V_2} \times \frac{V_1}{m_1} \times p \times \frac{100}{100-d}$$

A_1 = Area of the peak due to Z-ligustilide in the chromatogram obtained with solution (1).

A_2 = Area of the peak due to Z-ligustilide in the chromatogram obtained with solution (2).

m_1 = Weight of the drug being examined in mg.

m_2 = Weight of Z-*ligustilide CRS* in mg.

V_1 = Dilution volume of solution (1) in mL.

V_2 = Dilution volume of solution (2) in mL.

p = Percentage content of $C_{12}H_{14}O_2$ in Z-*ligustilide CRS*.

d = Percentage loss on drying of the herbal drug being examined.

STORAGE
Angelica Sinensis Root should be protected from moisture.

Processed Angelica Sinensis Root

(Angelica Sinensis Root, Ph Eur monograph 2558)

Ph Eur _____

DEFINITION
Smoke-dried, whole or fragmented root, with rootlets removed, of *Angelica sinensis* (Oliv.) Diels collected in late autumn.

Content
Minimum 0.050 per cent of *trans*-ferulic acid ($C_{10}H_{10}O_4$; M_r 194.2) (dried drug).

IDENTIFICATION
A. Taproot branching rapidly into 10 or more conical principal roots; the whole is about 15-25 cm long.
The annulated root crown is about 1.5-4 cm in diameter; its blunt, rounded tip shows the yellowish-green remains of stems and petioles of leaves. The outer surface is light brownish-yellow or dark brown, lumpy, irregularly striated longitudinally and shows scars of secondary roots and transversal lenticel-like markings. The branching roots have a thick upper part (0.3-1 cm in diameter) and a thin lower part. They are frequently twisted and show few scars of secondary roots. The texture is friable. The fracture, yellowish-white or yellowish-brown, shows a thick bark with some clefts and numerous brown dots due to secretory canals. The cambium occurs as a yellowish-brown ring. The wood is light coloured.

The fragmented roots occur as long strips about 1.5-2 mm thick, 1.5-4 cm wide at the root crown and 10-15 cm long.

B. Microscopic examination (*2.8.23*). The powder is yellowish-white. Examine under a microscope using *chloral hydrate solution R*. The powder shows the following diagnostic characters: reticulate or scalariform lignified vessels up to 80 µm in diameter, free or in groups of 2 or 3 and accompanied by ligneous parenchyma cells with thick walls; numerous fragments of parenchyma with ovoid cells; orange cork fragments, consisting of several layers of superimposed cells, more or less rectangular in surface view; very small calcium oxalate prisms, visible in polarised light, in the cork; rare secretory canals, usually broken, with orange-yellow contents, up to 170 µm in diameter. Examine under a microscope using a 50 per cent *V/V* solution of *glycerol R*: the powder shows small (less than 10 µm), simple, rounded or ovoid starch granules, usually included in parenchyma cells.

C. Examine the chromatograms obtained in the test for other officinal species of *Angelica*, *Levisticum* and *Ligusticum*.

Results A See below the sequence of zones present in the chromatograms obtained with the reference solution and the test solution. Furthermore, other faint fluorescent zones may be present in the chromatogram obtained with the test solution.

Top of the plate	
(*Z*)-Ligustilide: a bluish-white fluorescent zone	A prominent bluish-white fluorescent zone ((*Z*)-ligustilide)
Osthole: a blue fluorescent zone	
Imperatorin: a whitish fluorescent zone	
Reference solution	Test solution

Results B See below the sequence of zones present in the chromatograms obtained with the reference solution and the test solution. Furthermore, other faint quenching zones may be present in the chromatogram obtained with the test solution.

Top of the plate	
(*Z*)-Ligustilide: a blue fluorescent zone	A prominent blue fluorescent zone ((*Z*)-ligustilide)
	A faint quenching zone
Osthole: a quenching zone	A faint quenching zone
Imperatorin: a quenching zone	
Reference solution	Test solution

TESTS

Other officinal species of *Angelica*, *Levisticum* and *Ligusticum*

Thin-layer chromatography (*2.2.27*).

Test solution To 1 g of the powdered herbal drug (355) (*2.9.12*) add 4 mL of *heptane R*, close and sonicate for 5 min. Centrifuge and use the supernatant.

Reference solution Dissolve 1 mg of (*Z*)-*ligustilide R*, 1 mg of *imperatorin R* and 1 mg of *osthole R* in 10 mL of *methanol R*.

Plate TLC silica gel F$_{254}$ plate R (2-10 µm).

Mobile phase Glacial acetic acid R, ethyl acetate R, toluene R (1:10:90 *V/V/V*).

Application 4 µL as bands of 8 mm.

Development Over a path of 6 cm.

Drying In air.

Detection A Examine in ultraviolet light at 365 nm.

Results A The chromatogram obtained with the test solution shows no intense blue fluorescent zone at or below the position of osthole in the chromatogram obtained with the reference solution.

Detection B Examine in ultraviolet light at 254 nm.

Results B The chromatogram obtained with the test solution shows no quenching zone at or below the position of imperatorin in the chromatogram obtained with the reference solution.

Loss on drying (*2.2.32*)
Maximum 12.0 per cent, determined on 1.000 g of the powdered herbal drug (355) (*2.9.12*) by drying in an oven at 105 °C for 2 h.

Total ash (*2.4.16*)
Maximum 7.0 per cent.

Ash insoluble in hydrochloric acid (*2.8.1*)
Maximum 2.0 per cent.

ASSAY

Liquid chromatography (*2.2.29*).

Test solution Disperse 0.200 g of the powdered herbal drug (355) (*2.9.12*) in 20.0 mL of a 70 per cent *V/V* solution of *methanol R* in a conical flask, stopper tightly and weigh. Heat under a reflux condenser for 30 min, cool and weigh again. Compensate the loss of solvent with a 70 per cent *V/V* solution of *methanol R*, mix well and allow to stand. Filter the supernatant through a membrane filter (nominal pore size 0.45 µm); use the filtrate.

Reference solution (a) In a brown-glass volumetric flask, dissolve 10.0 mg of *ferulic acid CRS* in a 70 per cent *V/V* solution of *methanol R* and dilute to 100.0 mL with the same solvent.

Reference solution (b) In order to prepare *cis*-ferulic acid *in situ*, introduce 2 mL of reference solution (a) into a transparent vial and expose to ultraviolet light at 254 nm for about 60 min.

Column:
— *size*: *l* = 0.150 m, Ø = 2.0 mm;
— *stationary phase*: octadecylsilyl silica gel for chromatography R (4 µm);
— *temperature*: 35 °C.

Mobile phase acetonitrile R, 0.085 per cent *V/V* solution of phosphoric acid R (17:83 *V/V*).

Flow rate 0.23 mL/min.

Detection Spectrophotometer at 316 nm.

Injection 10 µL.

Retention time *trans*-ferulic acid = about 13 min; *cis*-ferulic acid = about 14 min.

System suitability Reference solution (b):
— *resolution*: minimum 1.3 between the peaks due to *trans*-ferulic acid and *cis*-ferulic acid.

Calculate the percentage content of *trans*-ferulic acid using the following expression:

$$\frac{A_1 \times m_2 \times p}{A_2 \times m_1 \times 5}$$

A_1 = area of the peak due to *trans*-ferulic acid in the chromatogram obtained with the test solution;

A_2 = area of the peak due to *trans*-ferulic acid in the chromatogram obtained with reference solution (a);

m_1 = mass of the herbal drug to be examined used to prepare the test solution, in grams;

m_2 = mass of *ferulic acid CRS* used to prepare reference solution (a), in grams;

p = percentage content of *trans*-ferulic acid in *ferulic acid CRS*.

———————————————————— Ph Eur

Aniseed

Anise

(*Ph Eur monograph 0262*)

When Powdered Aniseed is prescribed or demanded, material complying with the requirements below, with the exception of Identification test A and the test for Foreign matter, shall be dispensed or supplied.

Ph Eur _____

DEFINITION

Whole, dry cremocarp of *Pimpinella anisum* L.

Content

Minimum 20 mL/kg of essential oil (anhydrous drug).

CHARACTERS

Reminiscent odour of anethole.

The fruit is a cremocarp and generally entire; a small fragment of the thin, rigid, slightly curved pedicel is frequently attached.

IDENTIFICATION

A. The cremocarp is ovoid or pyriform and slightly compressed laterally, yellowish-green or greenish-grey, 3-5 mm long and up to 3 mm wide, surmounted by a stylopod with 2 short, reflexed stylar points. The mericarps are attached by their tops to the carpophore with a plane commissural surface and a convex dorsal surface, the latter being covered with short, warty trichomes visible using a lens; each mericarp shows 5 primary ridges, running longitudinally, comprising 3 dorsal ridges and 2 lateral ridges, non-prominent, and lighter in colour.

B. Microscopic examination (*2.8.23*). The powder is greenish-yellow or brownish-green. Examine under a microscope using *chloral hydrate solution R*. The powder shows the following diagnostic characters (Figure 0262.-1): fragments of epicarp in surface view [D] with a striated cuticle, occasional anomocytic stomata (*2.8.3*) [Da], bases of covering trichomes [Dc] and whole covering trichomes [Db], mostly unicellular, sometimes curved, with a blunt apex and a warty cuticle; isolated fragments of covering trichomes [E]; fragments [H] of numerous narrow, branched vittae [Ha], often accompanied by elongated cells of the commissural surface [Hb]; fragments of testa [B] consisting of a layer of brown, polyhedral, thin-walled cells; fragments of endosperm [G] containing oil droplets [Ga], aleurone grains and small cluster crystals of calcium oxalate [Gb]; oblong sclereids from the mesocarp [C] or the commissural surface of the fruit; bundles of short sclerenchymatous fibres [A] from the

carpophore and the pedicel [Ab], accompanied by vessels with spiral or annular thickening [Aa, F].

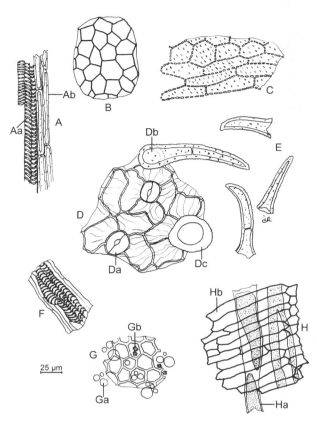

Figure 0262.-1. – *Illustration for identification test B of powdered herbal drug of aniseed*

C. Thin-layer chromatography (*2.2.27*).

Test solution Shake 0.10 g of the powdered herbal drug (1400) (*2.9.12*) with 2 mL of *methylene chloride R* for 15 min. Filter and carefully evaporate the filtrate to dryness on a water-bath at 60 °C. Dissolve the residue in 0.5 mL of *toluene R*.

Reference solution Dissolve 3 µL of *anethole R* and 40 µL of *olive oil R* in 1 mL of *toluene R*.

Plate TLC silica gel GF$_{254}$ plate R.

Mobile phase toluene R.

Application 2 µL and 3 µL of the test solution, then 1 µL, 2 µL and 3 µL of the reference solution, at 2 cm intervals.

Development Over a path of 10 cm.

Drying In air.

Detection A Examine in ultraviolet light at 254 nm.

Results A The chromatograms show a quenching zone (anethole) in the central part against a light background.

Detection B Spray with a freshly prepared 200 g/L solution of *phosphomolybdic acid R* in *ethanol (96 per cent) R*, using 10 mL for a 200 mm square plate, and heat at 120 °C for 5 min.

Results B The spots due to anethole appear blue against a yellow background. In the chromatogram obtained with 2 µL of the test solution, the spot due to anethole is intermediate in size between the corresponding spots in the chromatograms obtained with 1 µL and 3 µL of the reference solution. The chromatograms obtained with the test solution show in the lower third a blue spot (triglycerides) similar in position to the spot in the lower third of the chromatograms obtained with the reference solution (triglycerides of olive oil).

TESTS

Water (2.2.13)
Maximum 70 mL/kg, determined on 20.0 g of the powdered herbal drug.

Total ash (2.4.16)
Maximum 12.0 per cent.

Ash insoluble in hydrochloric acid (2.8.1)
Maximum 2.5 per cent.

ASSAY

Carry out the determination of essential oils in herbal drugs (2.8.12). Use 10.0 g of the herbal drug reduced to a coarse powder immediately before the determination, a 250 mL round-bottomed flask, and 100 mL of *water R* as the distillation liquid. Place 0.50 mL of *xylene R* in the graduated tube. Distil at a rate of 2.5-3.5 mL/min for 2 h.

_____ *Ph Eur*

Star Anise

(*Ph Eur monograph 1153*)

Preparation
Concentrated Anise Water

Ph Eur _____

DEFINITION

Dried composite fruit of *Illicium verum* Hooker fil.

Content:
— minimum 70 mL/kg of essential oil (anhydrous drug),
— minimum 86.0 per cent of *trans*-anethole in the essential oil.

CHARACTERS

The fruit carpels are brown.

Odour of anethole.

IDENTIFICATION

A. The fruit generally consists of 8 developed, one-seeded follicles, each 12-22 mm long and 6-12 mm high, radially arranged around a short, central, blunt-ending columella. In some fruits 1 or 2 follicles may be missing, but their position is clearly visible. Each follicle is boat-shaped or boot-shaped, with a greyish-brown dorsal surface showing rough markings and lateral surfaces bearing scars from the neighbouring follicles. One or more follicles are split open along the ventral suture, exposing a single, lenticular, shiny, reddish-brown seed about 8 mm in diameter. The markings on the dorsal surface are not visible from the ventral surface. Some of the follicles (1-3) may be imperfectly developed. Isolated follicles, pedicels and seeds may be present.

B. Reduce to a powder (355) (2.9.12). The powder is reddish-brown. Examine under a microscope using *chloral hydrate solution R*. The powder shows the following diagnostic characters: brown epicarpal cells, polygonal in surface view, with a strongly striated cuticle and occasional anomocytic stomata (2.8.3); fragments of the endocarp with long palisade-like cells; fragments of the mesocarp with large parenchymatous cells, vessels, oil-containing cells and groups of stone cells; fragments of the seed testa with palisade-like, sclerified, strongly pitted, yellow cells up to 200 μm long;

fragments of the columella and the fruit stalk with strongly and irregularly thickened, star-shaped stone cells about 400 μm long and 150 μm wide; rhomboidal or rectangular crystals of calcium oxalate.

C. Examine the chromatograms obtained in test B for *Illicium anisatum* (= *I. religiosum*) and certain other *Illicium* spp.

Results See below the sequence of the zones present in the chromatograms obtained with the reference solution and the test solution. Furthermore, other weaker zones may be present in the chromatogram obtained with the test solution.

Top of the plate	
—	—
Caffeic acid: a light blue fluorescent zone	
Quercitrin: a brownish-yellow fluorescent zone	
	A brownish-yellow fluorescent zone
	A greenish fluorescent zone
Hyperoside: a brownish-yellow fluorescent zone	A brownish-yellow fluorescent zone
Chlorogenic acid: a light blue fluorescent zone	
	A green fluorescent zone
Rutin: a brownish-yellow fluorescent zone	A brownish-yellow fluorescent zone
Reference solution	**Test solution**

TESTS

Illicium anisatum (= _I. religiosum_) and certain other _Illicium_ spp.

A. Adulteration with *Illicium anisatum* or certain other *Illicium* spp. is indicated by the presence of fruits mainly consisting of more than 8 follicles; fruits either smaller than 2.5 cm or greater than 3.5 cm; follicles with the suture edged with a thickening extending to the neighbouring follicle, or with dorsal markings visible from the ventral surface; follicles somewhat undulate and ending in a fine beak or a small, ventrally turned hook; follicles with a profile fitting into a rectangle; pedicels more than 5 cm long; seedless fruits; seeds either very flat or almost spherical.

B. Thin-layer chromatography (2.2.27).

Test solution To 2.0 g of the powdered drug (355) (2.9.12) add 10 mL of *methanol R* and heat under a reflux condenser in a water-bath at 60 °C for 5 min. Allow to cool and filter.

Reference solution Dissolve 1 mg of *caffeic acid R*, 1 mg of *chlorogenic acid R*, 2.5 mg of *quercitrin R*, 2.5 mg of *rutin R* and 2.5 mg of *hyperoside R* in 10 mL of *methanol R*.

Plate TLC silica gel plate R (2-10 μm).

Mobile phase anhydrous formic acid R, glacial acetic acid R, water R, ethyl acetate R (11:11:26:100 V/V/V/V).

Application 5 μL as bands.

Development Over a path of 6 cm.

Drying In a current of warm air.

Detection Spray with a 10 g/L solution of *diphenylboric acid aminoethyl ester R* in *methanol R* and then with a 50 g/L solution of *macrogol 400 R* in *methanol R*; after 30 min, examine in ultraviolet light at 365 nm.

Results The chromatogram obtained with the test solution shows no brownish-yellow fluorescent zone at or above the position of the zone due to quercitrin in the chromatogram obtained with the reference solution. No yellow fluorescent zone is seen at or above the position of the zone due to caffeic acid in the chromatogram obtained with the reference solution. No brownish-yellow fluorescent zone is seen directly above the zone due to hyperoside in the chromatogram obtained with the reference solution.

Water (*2.2.13*)
Maximum 100 mL/kg, determined by distillation on 20.0 g of the powdered drug (355) (*2.9.12*).

Total ash (*2.4.16*)
Maximum 4.0 per cent.

ASSAY
Essential oil
Carry out the determination of essential oils in herbal drugs (*2.8.12*). Use a 250 mL round-bottomed flask and 100 mL of *water R* as the distillation liquid. Immediately before the determination, reduce 50.0 g of the drug to a coarse powder (1400) (*2.9.12*) and mix. Further reduce about 10.0 g of this mixture to a finer powder (710) (*2.9.12*). Use 2.50 g of the powder for the determination. Introduce 0.50 mL of *xylene R* into the graduated tube. Distil at a rate of 2-3 mL/min for 2 h.

***trans*-Anethole**
Gas chromatography (*2.2.28*): use the normalisation procedure.

Test solution Dilute the mixture of essential oil and *xylene R* obtained in the assay of essential oil to 5.0 mL with *xylene R* by rinsing the apparatus.

Reference solution To 1.0 mL of *xylene R* add 20 μL of *estragole R*, 20 mg of *α-terpineol R* and 60 μL of *anethole R*.

Column:
— *material*: fused silica;
— *size*: l = 30 m, Ø = 0.25 mm;
— *stationary phase*: macrogol 20 000 R.

Carrier gas helium for chromatography R.

Flow rate 1.0 mL/min.

Split ratio 1:100.

Temperature:

	Time (min)	Temperature (°C)
Column	0 - 5	60
	5 - 80	60 → 210
	80 - 95	210
Injection port		200
Detector		220

Detection Flame ionisation.

Injection 1 μL.

Elution order Order indicated in the preparation of the reference solution.

System suitability Reference solution:
— *resolution*: minimum 5 between the peaks due to estragole and α-terpineol.

Use the retention times from the chromatogram obtained with the reference solution locate the components of the reference solution in the chromatogram obtained with the test solution.

Calculate the percentage content of *trans*-anethole. Disregard any peak due to the solvent or with an area less than

0.05 per cent of the area of the principal peak in the chromatogram obtained with the test solution.

Ph Eur

Star Anise Oil

(*Ph Eur monograph 2108*)

Ph Eur

DEFINITION
Essential oil obtained by steam distillation from the dry ripe fruits of *Illicium verum* Hook. fil.

CHARACTERS
Appearance
Clear, colourless or pale yellow liquid.

IDENTIFICATION
First identification B.
Second identification A.

A. Thin-layer chromatography (*2.2.27*).

Test solution Dissolve 1 g of the substance to be examined in *toluene R* and dilute to 10 mL with the same solvent.

Reference solution Dissolve 10 μL of *linalol R*, 30 μL of *anisaldehyde R* and 200 μL of *anethole R* and in *toluene R* and dilute to 15 mL with the same solvent. Dilute 1 mL of this solution to 5 mL with *toluene R*.

Plate TLC silica gel F_{254} plate R.

Mobile phase ethyl acetate R, toluene R (7:93 *V/V*).

Application 5 μL as bands of 10 mm (for normal TLC plates) or 2 μL as bands of 10 mm (for fine particle TLC plates).

Development Over a path of 15 cm (for normal TLC plates) or over a path of 6 cm (for fine particle size plates).

Drying In air.

Detection A Examine in ultraviolet light at 254 nm.

Results A See below the sequence of zones present in the chromatograms obtained with the reference solution and the test solution. Furthermore, other zones may be present in the chromatogram obtained with the test solution.

Top of the plate	
	A quenching zone, partly separated
Anethole: a quenching zone	A very strong quenching zone (anethole)
	———
Anisaldehyde: a quenching zone	A quenching zone (anisaldehyde)
———	
Reference solution	**Test solution**

Detection B Spray with *methyl 4-acetylbenzoate reagent R* and heat at 100-105 °C for 10 min; examine the still hot plate in daylight within 10 min.

Results B See below the sequence of zones present in the chromatograms obtained with the reference solution and the test solution. Furthermore, other zones may be present in the chromatogram obtained with the test solution.

Top of the plate	
	A violet-brown zone, not fully separated
Anethole: a brown zone	A very strong brown zone (anethole)
———	———
Anisaldehyde: a yellow zone	A yellow zone (anisaldehyde)
———	———
Linalol: a grey zone	A grey zone (linalol)
Reference solution	**Test solution**

B. Examine the chromatograms obtained in the test for chromatographic profile.

Results   The characteristic peaks in the chromatogram obtained with the test solution are similar in retention time to those in the chromatogram obtained with the reference solution.

TESTS

Relative density (*2.2.5*)
0.979 to 0.985.

Refractive index (*2.2.6*)
1.553 to 1.556.

Freezing point (*2.2.18*)
15 °C to 19 °C.

Fenchone
Gas chromatography (*2.2.28*) as described in the test for chromatographic profile with the following modifications.

Test solution   Dissolve 400 µL of the substance to be examined in 2.0 mL of *hexane R*.

Reference solution (a)   Dilute 10 µL of *fenchone R* to 1.2 g with *hexane R*.

Reference solution (b)   Dilute 100 µL of reference solution (a) to 100 mL with *hexane R*.

System suitability   Reference solution (b):
— *signal-to-noise ratio*: minimum 10 for the principal peak.
Limit:
— *fenchone*: maximum 0.01 per cent.

Pseudoisoeugenyl 2-methylbutyrate
Gas chromatography (*2.2.28*) as described in the test for chromatographic profile with the following modifications.

Test solution   The substance to be examined.

Reference solution (a)   Dilute 10 mg of the test solution to 1.000 g with *hexane R*. Dilute 0.5 mL of this solution to 100 mL with *hexane R*.

Reference solution (b)   *Pseudoisoeugenyl 2-methylbutyrate for peak identification CRS*.

System suitability:
— the chromatogram obtained with reference solution (b) is similar to the chromatogram provided with *pseudoisoeugenyl 2-methylbutyrate for peak identification CRS*.
— *signal-to-noise ratio*: minimum 10 for the principal peak in the chromatogram obtained with reference solution (a).

Limit   Locate the peak due to pseudoisoeugenyl 2-methylbutyrate by comparison with the chromatogram provided with *pseudoisoeugenyl 2-methylbutyrate for peak identification CRS*.
— *pseudoisoeugenyl 2-methylbutyrate*: maximum 0.01 per cent.

Fatty oils and resinified essential oils (*2.8.7*)
It complies with the test for fatty oils and resinified essential oils.

Chromatographic profile
Gas chromatography (*2.2.28*): use the normalisation procedure.

Test solution   Dissolve 200 µL of the substance to be examined in 1.0 mL of *hexane R*.

Reference solution   To 1.0 mL of *hexane R*, add 20 µL of *linalol R*, 20 µL of *estragole R*, 20 µL of *α-terpineol R*, 60 µL of *anethole R* and 30 µL of *anisaldehyde R*.

Column:
— *material*: fused silica,
— *size*: *l* = 30 m, Ø = 0.25 mm,
— *stationary phase*: *macrogol 20 000 R* (film thickness 0.25 µm).

Carrier gas   *helium for chromatography R*.

Flow rate   1.0 mL/min.

Split ratio   1:100.

Temperature:

	Time (min)	Temperature (°C)
Column	0 - 5	60
	5 - 80	60 → 210
	80 - 95	210
Injection port		200
Detector		220

Detection   Flame ionisation.

Injection   0.2 µL.

Elution order   Order indicated in the composition of the reference solution; record the retention times of these substances.

System suitability   Reference solution:
— *resolution*: minimum 1.5 between the peaks due to estragole and α-terpineol.

Using the retention times determined from the chromatogram obtained with the reference solution, locate the components of the reference solution in the chromatogram obtained with the test solution and locate *cis*-anethole and foeniculin using the chromatogram shown in Figure 2108.-1 (disregard any peak due to hexane).

Determine the percentage content of these components. The percentages are within the following ranges:
— *linalol*: 0.2 per cent to 2.5 per cent,
— *estragole*: 0.5 per cent to 6.0 per cent,
— *α-terpineol*: maximum 0.3 per cent,
— *cis-anethole*: 0.1 per cent to 0.5 per cent,
— *trans-anethole*: 86 per cent to 93 per cent,
— *anisaldehyde*: 0.1 per cent to 0.5 per cent,
— *foeniculin*: 0.1 per cent to 3.0 per cent.

STORAGE
At a temperature not exceeding 25 °C.

_____ *Ph Eur*

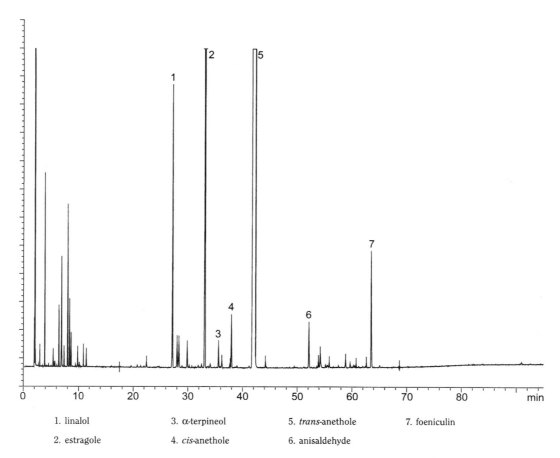

Figure 2108.-1. – *Chromatogram for the test for chromatographic profile of star anise oil*

1. linalol	3. α-terpineol	5. *trans*-anethole	7. foeniculin
2. estragole	4. *cis*-anethole	6. anisaldehyde	

Anise Oil

Aniseed Oil

(*Ph Eur monograph 0804*)

Preparation

Concentrated Anise Water

Ph Eur ___

DEFINITION

Essential oil obtained by steam distillation from the dry ripe fruits of *Pimpinella anisum* L.

CHARACTERS

Appearance

Clear, colourless or pale yellow liquid.

IDENTIFICATION

First identification   B.

Second identification   A.

A. Thin-layer chromatography (*2.2.27*).

Test solution   Dissolve 1 g of the substance to be examined in *toluene R* and dilute to 10 mL with the same solvent.

Reference solution   Dissolve 10 µL of *linalol R*, 30 µL of *anisaldehyde R* and 200 µL of *anethole R* in *toluene R* and dilute to 15 mL with the same solvent. Dilute 1 mL of this solution to 5 mL with *toluene R*.

Plate   TLC silica gel F_{254} plate R.

Mobile phase   ethyl acetate R, toluene R (7:93 *V/V*).

Application   5 µL as bands of 10 mm (for normal TLC plates) or 2 µL as bands of 10 mm (for fine particle size plates).

Development   Over a path of 15 cm (for normal TLC plates) or over a path of 6 cm (for fine particle size plates).

Drying   In air.

Detection A   Examine in ultraviolet light at 254 nm.

Results A   See below the sequence of zones present in the chromatograms obtained with the reference solution and the test solution. Furthermore, other zones may be present in the chromatogram obtained with the test solution.

Top of the plate	
Anethole: a quenching zone	A very strong quenching zone (anethole)
	A quenching zone
Anisaldehyde: a quenching zone	A quenching zone (anisaldehyde)
Reference solution	**Test solution**

Detection B   Spray with *methyl 4-acetylbenzoate reagent R* and heat at 100-105 °C for 10 min; examine the still hot plate in daylight within 5 min.

Results B   See below the sequence of zones present in the chromatograms obtained with the reference solution and the test solution. Furthermore, other zones may be present in the chromatogram obtained with the test solution.

Top of the plate	
Anethole: a brown zone	A violet-brown zone (monoterpene hydrocarbons) (solvent front)
	A very strong brown zone (anethole), distinctly separated
———	———
Anisaldehyde: a yellow zone	A grey zone
	A yellow zone (anisaldehyde)
———	———
Linalol: a grey zone	A grey zone (linalol)
	A grey zone
Reference solution	**Test solution**

B. Examine the chromatograms obtained in the test for chromatographic profile.

Results   The characteristic peaks in the chromatogram obtained with the test solution are similar in retention time to those in the chromatogram obtained with the reference solution.

TESTS
Relative density (*2.2.5*)
0.980 to 0.990.

Refractive index (*2.2.6*)
1.552 to 1.561.

Freezing point (*2.2.18*)
15 °C to 19 °C.

Fenchone
Gas chromatography (*2.2.28*) as described in the test for chromatographic profile with the following modifications.

Test solution   Dissolve 400 µL of the substance to be examined in 2.0 mL of *hexane R*.

Reference solution (a)   Dilute 10 µL of *fenchone R* to 1.2 g with *hexane R*.

Reference solution (b)   Dilute 100 µL of reference solution (a) to 100 mL with *hexane R*.

System suitability   Reference solution (b):
— *signal-to-noise ratio*: minimum 10 for the principal peak.

Limit:
— *fenchone*: maximum 0.01 per cent.

Foeniculin
Gas chromatography (*2.2.28*) as described in the test for chromatographic profile with the following modifications.

Test solution   The substance to be examined.

Reference solution (a)   Dilute 10 mg of the test solution to 1.000 g with *hexane R*. Dilute 0.5 mL of this solution to 100 mL with *hexane R*.

Reference solution (b)   *Foeniculin for peak identification CRS*.

System suitability:
— the chromatogram obtained with reference solution (b) is similar to the chromatogram provided with *foeniculin for peak identification CRS*,
— *signal-to-noise ratio*: minimum 10 for the principal peak in the chromatogram obtained with reference solution (a).

Limit   Locate the peak due to foeniculin by comparison with the chromatogram provided with *foeniculin for peak identification CRS*.

— *foeniculin*: maximum 0.01 per cent.

Fatty oils and resinified essential oils (*2.8.7*)
It complies with the test for fatty oils and resinified essential oils.

Chromatographic profile
Gas chromatography (*2.2.28*): use the normalisation procedure.

Test solution   Dissolve 200 µL of the substance to be examined in 1.0 mL of *hexane R*.

Reference solution   To 1.0 mL of *hexane R*, add 20 µL of *linalol R*, 20 µL of *estragole R*, 20 µL of α-*terpineol R*, 60 µL of *anethole R* and 30 µL of *anisaldehyde R*.

Column:
— *material*: fused silica,
— *size*: l = 30 m, Ø = 0.25 mm,
— *stationary phase*: *macrogol 20 000 R* (film thickness 0.25 µm).

Carrier gas   *helium for chromatography R*.

Flow rate   1.0 mL/min.

Split ratio   1:100.

Temperature:

	Time (min)	Temperature (°C)
Column	0 – 5	60
	5 – 80	60 → 210
	80 – 95	210
Injection port		200
Detector		220

Detection   Flame ionisation.

Injection   0.2 µL.

Elution order   Order indicated in the composition of the reference solution. Record the retention times of these substances.

System suitability   Reference solution:
— *resolution*: minimum 1.5 between the peaks due to estragole and α-terpineol.

Using the retention times determined from the chromatogram obtained with the reference solution, locate the components of the reference solution in the chromatogram obtained with the test solution and locate *cis*-anethole and pseudoisoeugenyl 2-methylbutyrate using the chromatogram shown in Figure 0804.-1 (disregard any peak due to hexane).

Determine the percentage content of these components. The percentages are within the following ranges:
— *linalol*: maximum 1.5 per cent,
— *estragole*: 0.5 per cent to 5.0 per cent,
— α-*terpineol*: maximum 1.2 per cent,
— *cis*-anethole: 0.1 per cent to 0.4 per cent,
— *trans*-anethole: 87 per cent to 94 per cent,
— *anisaldehyde*: 0.1 per cent to 1.4 per cent,
— *pseudoisoeugenyl 2-methylbutyrate*: 0.3 per cent to 2.0 per cent.

STORAGE
At a temperature not exceeding 25 °C.

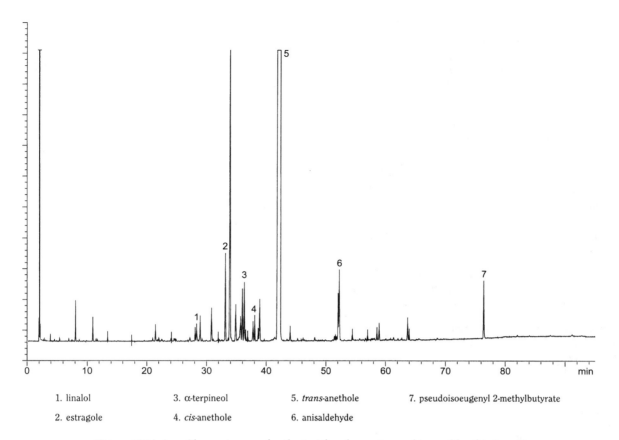

1. linalol   3. α-terpineol   5. *trans*-anethole   7. pseudoisoeugenyl 2-methylbutyrate

2. estragole   4. *cis*-anethole   6. anisaldehyde

Figure 0804.-1. – *Chromatogram for the test for chromatographic profile of anise oil*

Concentrated Anise Water

DEFINITION

Anise Oil or Star Anise Oil	20 mL
Ethanol (90 per cent)	700 mL
Water	Sufficient to produce
	1000 mL

Extemporaneous preparation

The following directions apply.

Dissolve the Anise Oil or Star Anise Oil in the Ethanol (90 per cent) and add gradually, with vigorous shaking after each addition, sufficient Water to produce 1000 mL. Add 50 g of previously sterilised Purified Talc, or other suitable filtering aid, allow to stand for a few hours, shaking occasionally, and filter.

The water complies with the requirements stated under Aromatic Waters and with the following requirements.

TESTS

Ethanol content

60 to 64% v/v, Appendix VIII F.

Weight per mL

0.898 to 0.908 g, Appendix V G.

Arnica Flower

(Ph Eur monograph 1391)

Preparation

Arnica Tincture

Ph Eur

DEFINITION

Whole or partially broken, dried flower-heads of *Arnica montana* L.

Content

Minimum 0.40 per cent *m/m* of total sesquiterpene lactones, expressed as dihydrohelenalin tiglate (dried drug).

CHARACTERS

Aromatic odour.

The capitulum, when spread out, is about 20 mm in diameter and about 15 mm deep, and has a peduncle 2-3 cm long. The involucre consists of 18-24 elongated lanceolate bracts, with acute apices, arranged in 1-2 rows: the bracts, about 8-10 mm long, are green with yellowish-green external hairs visible under a lens. The receptacle, about 6 mm in diameter, is convex, alveolate and covered with hairs. Its periphery bears about 20 ligulate florets 20-30 mm long; the disc bears a greater number of tubular florets about 15 mm long. The ovary, 4-8 mm long, is crowned by a pappus of whitish bristles 4-8 mm long. Some brown achenes, crowned or not by a pappus, may be present.

IDENTIFICATION

A. The involucre consists of elongated oval bracts with acute apices; the margin is ciliated. The ligulate floret has a reduced calyx crowned by fine, shiny, whitish bristles, bearing small coarse trichomes. The orange-yellow corolla bears 7-10 parallel veins and ends in 3 small lobes. The stamens, with free anthers, are incompletely developed. The narrow, brown ovary bears a stigma divided into 2 branches curving outwards. The tubular floret is actinomorphic. The ovary and the calyx are similar to those of the ligulate floret. The short corolla has 5 reflexed triangular lobes; the 5 fertile stamens are fused at the anthers.

B. Microscopic examination (*2.8.23*). Separate the capitulum into its different parts. Examine under a microscope using *chloral hydrate solution R*. The powder shows the following diagnostic characters (Figure 1391.-1): the epidermises of the bracts of the involucre [L, M, O, Q] have stomata [Lb, Oa, Qa] and trichomes, more abundant on the outer (abaxial) surface. There are several different types of trichomes: uniseriate multicellular covering trichomes, varying in length from 50-500 μm, particularly abundant on the margins of the bract, whole [La] or fragmented [P]; secretory trichomes with uni- or biseriate multicellular stalks and with multicellular, globular heads, about 300 μm long, abundant on the outer surface of the bract [Qb]; secretory trichomes with multicellular stalks and with multicellular, globular heads, about 80 μm long, abundant on the inner surface of the bract, in surface view [Ob] or in side view [Ma].

The epidermis of the ligulate corolla [C, G, H, J] consists of lobed or elongated cells covered by a striated cuticle [Ga], a few stomata and trichomes of different types: covering trichomes, with very sharp ends, whose length may exceed 500 μm, consisting of 1-3 proximal, thick-walled cells and 2-4 distal, thin-walled cells [C, Hb]; secretory trichomes with biseriate multicellular heads in surface view [Gb] or in side view [Ja]; secretory trichomes with multicellular stalks and multicellular globular heads [K]. The ligule ends in rounded papillose cells [Ha]. Fragments of the epidermis of the ovary [A, B, D] are covered with trichomes of 2 types: secretory trichomes with short stalks and multicellular globular heads, in surface view [Aa] or in side view [Da]; twinned covering trichomes usually consisting of 2 longitudinally united cells, with common pitted walls, in surface view [Ab] or in side view [Ba]; their ends are sharp and sometimes bifid. The epidermises of the calyx consist of elongated cells bearing short, unicellular, covering trichomes pointing towards the upper end of the bristle [E]. The pollen grains have a diameter of about 30 μm, are rounded, with a spiny exine, and have 3 germinal pores [F, N].

C. Examine the chromatograms obtained in the test for *Calendula officinalis* L. - *Heterotheca inuloides* Cass.

Results   The chromatogram obtained with the test solution shows, in the middle, a fluorescent blue zone corresponding to the zone due to chlorogenic acid in the chromatogram obtained with the reference solution; it shows, above this zone, 3 fluorescent yellowish-brown or orange-yellow zones, and above these 3 zones a fluorescent greenish-yellow zone due to astragalin; the zone located below the astragalin zone is due to isoquercitroside; the zone located just below this zone is due to luteolin-7-glucoside; it also shows a fluorescent greenish-blue zone below the zone due to caffeic acid in the chromatogram obtained with the reference solution.

TESTS

Foreign matter (*2.8.2*)
Maximum 5.0 per cent.

Calendula officinalis L. - **Heterotheca inuloides** Cass
Thin-layer chromatography (*2.2.27*).

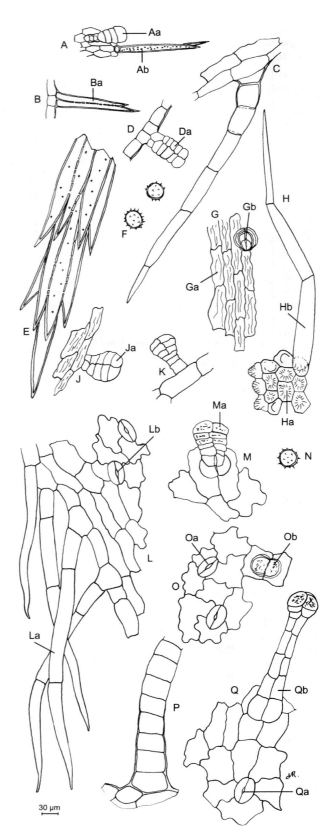

Figure 1391.-1. – *Illustration for identification test B of powdered herbal drug of arnica flower*

Test solution   To 2.00 g of the powdered herbal drug (710) (*2.9.12*) add 10 mL of *methanol R*. Heat in a water-bath at 60 °C for 5 min with shaking. Cool and filter.

Reference solution   Dissolve 2.0 mg of *caffeic acid R*, 2.0 mg of *chlorogenic acid R* and 5.0 mg of *rutin R* in *methanol R* and dilute to 30 mL with the same solvent.

Plate   TLC silica gel plate R.

Mobile phase   anhydrous formic acid R, water R, methyl ethyl ketone R, ethyl acetate R (10:10:30:50 *V/V/V/V*).

Application   15 µL as bands.

Development   Over a path of 15 cm.

Drying   In air for a few minutes.

Detection   Spray with a 10 g/L solution of *diphenylboric acid aminoethyl ester R* in *methanol R*, and then with a 50 g/L solution of *macrogol 400 R* in *methanol R*; heat at 100-105 °C for 5 min, allow to dry in air and examine in ultraviolet light at 365 nm.

Results   The chromatogram obtained with the reference solution shows in the lower part an orange-yellow fluorescent zone due to rutin, in the middle part a fluorescent zone due to chlorogenic acid and in the upper part a light bluish fluorescent zone due to caffeic acid; the chromatogram obtained with the test solution does not show a fluorescent orange-yellow zone corresponding to the zone due to rutin in the chromatogram obtained with the reference solution, nor does it show a zone below this.

Loss on drying (*2.2.32*)
Maximum 10.0 per cent, determined on 1.000 g of the powdered herbal drug (355) (*2.9.12*) by drying in an oven at 105 °C for 2 h.

Total ash (*2.4.16*)
Maximum 10.0 per cent.

ASSAY
Liquid chromatography (*2.2.29*).

Internal standard solution   Dissolve immediately before use 0.010 g of *santonin CRS*, accurately weighed, in 10.0 mL of *methanol R*.

Test solution   Introduce 1.00 g of the powdered herbal drug (355) (*2.9.12*) into a 250 mL round-bottomed flask, add 50 mL of a mixture of equal volumes of *methanol R* and *water R* and heat under a reflux condenser in a water-bath at 50-60 °C for 30 min, shaking frequently. Allow to cool and filter through a paper filter. Add the paper filter, cut into pieces, to the residue in the round-bottomed flask, add 50 mL of a mixture of equal volumes of *methanol R* and *water R* and heat under a reflux condenser in a water-bath at 50-60 °C for 30 min, shaking frequently. Repeat this procedure twice. To the combined filtrates add 3.00 mL of the internal standard solution and evaporate to 18 mL under reduced pressure. Rinse the round-bottomed flask with *water R* and dilute, with the washings, to 20.0 mL. Transfer the solution to a chromatography column about 0.15 m long and about 30 mm in internal diameter containing 15 g of *kieselguhr for chromatography R*. Allow to stand for 20 min. Elute with 200 mL of a mixture of equal volumes of *ethyl acetate R* and *methylene chloride R*. Evaporate the eluate to dryness in a 250 mL round-bottomed flask. Dissolve the residue in 10.0 mL of *methanol R* and add 10.0 mL of *water R*. Add 7.0 g of *neutral aluminium oxide R*, shake for 120 s, centrifuge at 5000 *g* for 10 min and filter through a paper filter. Evaporate 10.0 mL of the filtrate to dryness. Dissolve the residue in 3.0 mL of a mixture of equal volumes of *methanol R* and *water R* and filter.

Column:
— *size:* l = 0.12 m, Ø = 4 mm;

— stationary phase: octadecylsilyl silica gel for chromatography R (4 µm).

Mobile phase:
— mobile phase A: water R;
— mobile phase B: methanol R;

Time (min)	Mobile phase A (per cent *V/V*)	Mobile phase B (per cent *V/V*)
0 - 3	62	38
3 - 20	62 → 55	38 → 45
20 - 30	55	45
30 - 55	55 → 45	45 → 55
55 - 57	45 → 0	55 → 100
57 - 70	0	100
70 - 90	62	38

Flow rate   1.2 mL/min.

Detection   Spectrophotometer at 225 nm.

Injection   20 µL loop injector.

Calculate the percentage content of total sesquiterpene lactones, expressed as dihydrohelenalin tiglate, using the following expression:

$$\frac{S_{LS} \times C \times V \times 1.187 \times 100}{S_S \times m \times 1000}$$

S_{LS} = area of all peaks due to sesquiterpene lactones appearing after the santonin peak in the chromatogram obtained with the test solution;

S_S = area of the peak due to santonin in the chromatogram obtained with the test solution;

m = mass of the herbal drug to be examined, in grams;

C = concentration of santonin in the internal standard solution used for the test solution, in milligrams per millilitre;

V = volume of the internal standard solution used for the test solution, in millilitres;

1.187 = peak correlation factor between dihydrohelenalin tiglate and santonin.

Ph Eur

Arnica Tincture

(*Ph Eur monograph 1809*)

Ph Eur

DEFINITION
Tincture produced from *Arnica flower (1391)*.

Content
Minimum 0.04 per cent of sesquiterpene lactones expressed as dihydrohelenalin tiglate ($C_{20}H_{26}O_5$; M_r 346.42).

PRODUCTION
The tincture is produced from the herbal drug by a suitable procedure using 10 parts of ethanol (60-70 per cent *V/V*) for 1 part of drug.

CHARACTERS
Appearance
Yellowish-brown liquid.

IDENTIFICATION

Examine the chromatograms obtained in the test for *Calendula officinalis - Heterotheca inuloides*.

Chromatogram obtained with the test solution:

— in the middle, a fluorescent blue zone corresponding to the zone due to chlorogenic acid in the chromatogram obtained with the reference solution;

— above this zone, 3 fluorescent yellowish-brown to orange-yellow zones, and above these 3 zones a fluorescent greenish-yellow zone corresponding to astragalin; the zone located below the astragalin zone corresponds to isoquercitrin; the zone located just below this zone corresponds to luteolin-7-glucoside;

— a fluorescent greenish-blue zone below the zone due to caffeic acid in the chromatogram obtained with the reference solution.

TESTS

Calendula officinalis - Heterotheca inuloides

Thin-layer chromatography (*2.2.27*).

Test solution The tincture to be examined.

Reference solution Dissolve 2.0 mg of *caffeic acid R*, 2.0 mg of *chlorogenic acid R* and 5.0 mg of *rutin R* in *methanol R* and dilute to 30.0 mL with the same solvent.

Plate TLC silica gel plate R (5-40 μm) [or TLC silica gel plate R (2-10 μm)].

Mobile phase anhydrous formic acid R, water R, methyl ethyl ketone R, ethyl acetate R (10:10:30:50 V/V/V/V).

Application 30 μL [or 8 μL] as bands.

Development Over a path of 15 cm [or 8 cm].

Drying At 80-105 °C.

Detection Spray the plate whilst still hot with a 10 g/L solution of *diphenylboric acid aminoethyl ester R* in *methanol R* and then with a 50 g/L solution of *macrogol 400 R* in *methanol R*; heat 5 min at 100-105 °C, allow the plate to dry in air and examine in ultraviolet light at 365 nm.

Results The chromatogram obtained with the reference solution shows in the lower part an orange-yellow fluorescent zone (rutin), in the middle part a fluorescent zone due to chlorogenic acid and in the upper part a light bluish fluorescent zone (caffeic acid). The chromatogram obtained with the test solution does not show any fluorescent orange-yellow zone corresponding to rutin in the chromatogram obtained with the reference solution and no zone below the zone corresponding to rutin.

Ethanol (*2.9.10*)

The final ethanol concentration is not less than 90 per cent of that of the initial extraction solvent.

Methanol and 2-propanol (*2.9.11*)

Maximum 0.05 per cent *V/V* of methanol and maximum 0.05 per cent *V/V* of 2-propanol.

Dry residue (*2.8.16*)

Minimum 1.7 per cent.

ASSAY

Liquid chromatography (*2.2.29*).

Internal standard solution Dissolve immediately before use 0.010 g accurately weighed of *santonin CRS* and 0.02 g of *butyl 4-hydroxybenzoate R* in 10.0 mL of *methanol R*.

Test solution In a round-bottomed flask introduce 5.00 g of the tincture to be examined, add 2.00 mL of the internal standard solution and 3 g of *anhydrous aluminium oxide R*, shake for 120 s and filter through a filter paper. Rinse the round-bottomed flask and filter with 5 mL of a mixture of equal volumes of *methanol R* and *water R* and filter. Evaporate the filtrate to dryness. Dissolve the residue in 2.0 mL of a mixture of 20 volumes of *water R* and 80 volumes of *methanol R* and filter through a membrane filter (nominal pore size 0.45 μm).

Reference solution Dissolve 0.02 g of *methyl 4-hydroxybenzoate R* and 0.02 g of *ethyl 4-hydroxybenzoate R* in *methanol R* and dilute to 10.0 mL with the same solvent.

Column:

— *size*: l = 0.12 m, Ø = 4 mm;

— *stationary phase*: end-capped octadecylsilyl silica gel for chromatography R (5 μm);

— *temperature*: 20 °C.

Mobile phase:

— *mobile phase A*: water R;

— *mobile phase B*: methanol R;

Time (min)	Mobile phase A (per cent *V/V*)	Mobile phase B (per cent *V/V*)
0 - 3	62	38
3 - 20	62 → 55	38 → 45
20 - 30	55	45
30 - 55	55 → 45	45 → 55

Flow rate 1.2 mL/min.

Detector Spectrophotometer at 225 nm.

Injection 20 μL.

Relative retention With reference to santonin (retention time = about 9.5 min): butyl 4-hydroxybenzoate = about 4.6.

System suitability Reference solution:

— *resolution*: minimum 5 between the peaks due to methyl 4-hydroxybenzoate and ethyl 4-hydroxybenzoate.

Calculate the percentage of lactone sesquiterpenes, expressed as dihydrohelenalin tiglate, using the following expression:

$$\frac{F_1 \times C \times V \times 1.187}{F_2 \times m \times 10}$$

F_1 = area of all peaks appearing between the peaks due to santonin and butyl 4-hydroxybenzoate in the chromatogram obtained with the test solution;

F_2 = area of the peak due to santonin in the chromatogram obtained with the test solution;

m = mass of the tincture to be examined, in grams;

C = concentration of santonin in the internal standard solution used to prepare the test solution, in milligrams per millilitre;

V = volume of the internal standard solution used to prepare the test solution, in millilitres;

1.187 = peak correlation factor between dihydrohelenalin tiglate and santonin.

Ph Eur

Artichoke Leaf

(*Ph Eur monograph 1866*)

Preparation

Artichoke Leaf Dry Extract

Ph Eur _____

DEFINITION

Whole or cut, dried leaf of *Cynara cardunculus* L. (syn. *C. scolymus* L.).

Content

Minimum 0.8 per cent of chlorogenic acid ($C_{16}H_{18}O_9$; M_r 354.3) (dried drug).

IDENTIFICATION

A. The entire leaf may be up to 70 cm long and 30 cm wide. The lamina is deeply lobed in the upper part to within 1-2 cm of the petiole on either side, in the lower part the leaf becomes pinnate; all the segments have markedly dentate margins and taper at the apex. Spines are absent. The upper surface of the lamina is green with a fine covering of whitish hairs, the lower surface is pale green or white and densely tomentose with long, tangled hairs. The petiole and main veins are flat on the upper surface, prominently raised and longitudinally ridged on the lower surface, with conspicuous hairs on both surfaces.

B. Reduce to a powder (1000) (*2.9.12*). The powder is greenish-grey. Examine under a microscope using *chloral hydrate solution* R. The powder shows the following diagnostic characters (Figure 1866.-1): fragments of the epidermises of the lamina, in surface view; the upper epidermis [F] is composed of cells with straight or slightly sinuous walls [Fa], accompanied by palisade parenchyma [Fb]; the lower epidermis [C] is composed of more sinuous-walled cells; abundant anomocytic stomata (*2.8.3*) on both surfaces [D] and multicellular, uniseriate covering trichomes in felted masses, the majority fragmented [Ca] with a short stalk composed of several cells and a very long, narrow and frequently curled terminal cell, others consisting of 4-6 cylindrical cells; very occasional glandular trichomes with a short stalk and a uniseriate or biseriate head, in surface view [E] or in transverse section [Ba]; abundant fragments of covering trichomes [G]; fragments of the lamina, in transverse section [B]; abundant fragments of vascular tissue from the petiole and veins [A].

C. Thin-layer chromatography (*2.2.27*).

Test solution To 2.0 g of the powdered drug (1000) (*2.9.12*) add 20 mL of *ethanol (60 per cent V/V)* R. Allow to stand for 2 h with occasional stirring. Filter.

Reference solution Dissolve 5 mg of *luteolin-7-glucoside* R and 5 mg of *chlorogenic acid CRS* in *methanol* R and dilute to 10 mL with the same solvent.

Plate TLC silica gel plate R (5-40 µm) [or *TLC silica gel plate* R (2-10 µm)].

Mobile phase anhydrous formic acid R, glacial acetic acid R, water R, ethyl acetate R (11:11:27:100 *V/V/V/V*).

Application 10 µL [or 2 µL] as bands of 10 mm [or 8 mm].

Development Over a path of 13 cm [or 6 cm].

Drying In air.

Detection Heat at 100 °C for 5 min; spray the warm plate with a 10 g/L solution of *diphenylboric acid aminoethyl ester* R in *methanol* R followed by a 50 g/L solution of *macrogol 400* R in *methanol* R; examine in ultraviolet light at 365 nm.

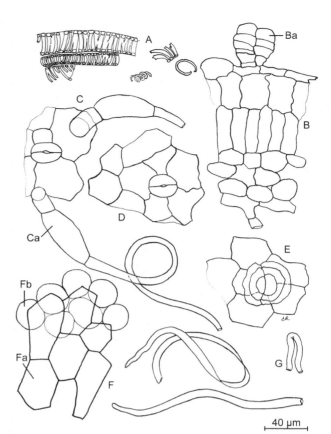

Figure 1866.-1. – *Illustration for identification test B of powdered herbal drug of artichoke leaf*

Results See below the sequence of fluorescent zones present in the chromatograms obtained with the reference solution and the test solution. Furthermore, other fluorescent zones may be present in the chromatogram obtained with the test solution.

Top of the plate	
	A light blue fluorescent zone
———	———
Luteolin-7-glucoside: a yellow or orange fluorescent zone	A yellow or orange fluorescent zone (luteolin-7-glucoside)
Chlorogenic acid: a light blue fluorescent zone	A light blue fluorescent zone (chlorogenic acid)
———	———
Reference solution	**Test solution**

TESTS

Total ash (*2.4.16*)
Maximum 20.0 per cent.

Loss on drying (*2.2.32*)
Maximum 12.0 per cent, determined on 1.000 g of the powdered drug (710) (*2.9.12*) by drying in an oven at 105 °C for 2 h.

ASSAY

Liquid chromatography (*2.2.29*).

Test solution To 0.500 g of the powdered drug (1000) (*2.9.12*) add 50.0 mL of *methanol* R and heat under a reflux condenser on a water-bath at 70 °C for 1 h. Centrifuge and

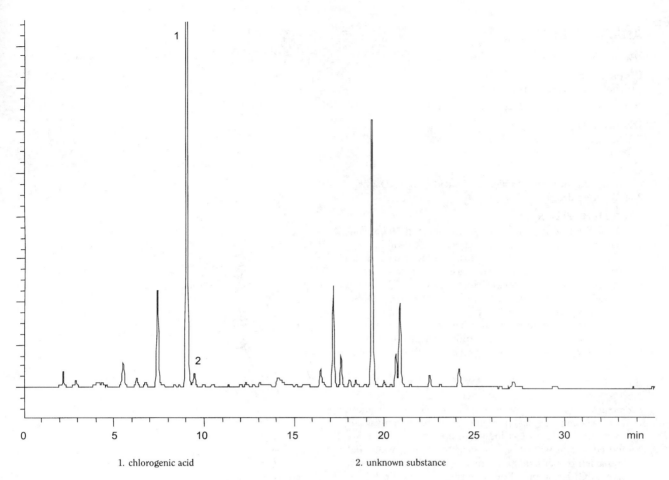

1. chlorogenic acid   2. unknown substance

Figure 1866.-2. – *Chromatogram for the assay of artichoke leaf: test solution*

transfer the supernatant to a 200 mL volumetric flask.
Repeat the procedure and dilute to 200.0 mL with *water R*.

Reference solution   Dissolve 5.0 mg of *chlorogenic acid CRS* in
50.0 mL of *methanol R*. Transfer 5.0 mL of this solution to a
volumetric flask, add 5 mL of *methanol R* and dilute to
20.0 mL with *water R*.

Column:
— *size: l* = 0.25 m, Ø = 4.6 mm;
— *stationary phase: octadecylsilyl silica gel for chromatography R*
  (5 μm);
— *temperature*: 40 °C.

Mobile phase:
— *mobile phase A: phosphoric acid R, water R* (0.5:99.5 *V/V*);
— *mobile phase B: phosphoric acid R, acetonitrile R*
  (0.5:99.5 *V/V*);

Time (min)	Mobile phase A (per cent *V/V*)	Mobile phase B (per cent *V/V*)
0 - 1	92	8
1 - 20	92 → 75	8 → 25
20 - 33	75	25
33 - 35	75 → 0	25 → 100

Flow rate   1.2 mL/min.

Detection   Spectrophotometer at 330 nm.

Injection   25 μL.

System suitability Test solution:
— the chromatogram obtained is similar to the
  chromatogram shown in Figure 1866.-2;
— *resolution*: minimum 2.0 between the peak due to
  chlorogenic acid and the subsequent peak (peak 2).

Calculate the percentage content of chlorogenic acid using
the following expression:

$$\frac{A_1 \times m_2 \times p}{A_2 \times m_1}$$

A_1 = area of the peak due to chlorogenic acid in the
chromatogram obtained with the test solution;

A_2 = area of the peak due to chlorogenic acid in the
chromatogram obtained with the reference solution;

m_1 = mass of the drug to be examined in the test
solution, in grams;

m_2 = mass of *chlorogenic acid CRS* in the reference
solution, in grams;

p = percentage content of chlorogenic acid in *chlorogenic
acid CRS*.

Ph Eur

Artichoke Leaf Dry Extract

(Ph Eur monograph 2389)

Ph Eur

DEFINITION

Dry extract produced from *Artichoke leaf (1866)*.

Content

Minimum 0.6 per cent of chlorogenic acid ($C_{16}H_{18}O_9$; M_r 354.3) (dried extract).

PRODUCTION

The extract is produced from the herbal drug by a suitable procedure using water of minimum 80 °C.

CHARACTERS

Appearance

Light brown or brown, amorphous powder.

IDENTIFICATION

Thin-layer chromatography (*2.2.27*).

Test solution   Dissolve 1.0 g of the extract to be examined in 10 mL of *ethanol (60 per cent V/V) R*. Sonicate for 5 min and filter.

Reference solution   Dissolve 5 mg of *luteolin-7-glucoside R* and 5 mg of *chlorogenic acid R* in 10 mL of *methanol R*.

Plate   *TLC silica gel plate R* (5-40 µm) [or *TLC silica gel plate R* (2-10 µm)].

Mobile phase   anhydrous formic acid R, glacial acetic acid R, water R, ethyl acetate R (11:11:27:100 V/V/V/V).

Application   10 µL [or 2 µL] as bands of 10 mm [or 8 mm].

Development   Over a path of 13 cm [or 6 cm].

Drying   In air.

Detection   Heat at 100 °C for 5 min; spray the warm plate with a 10 g/L solution of *diphenylboric acid aminoethyl ester R* in *methanol R* followed by a 50 g/L solution of *macrogol 400 R* in *methanol R*; examine in ultraviolet light at 365 nm.

Results   See below the sequence of fluorescent zones present in the chromatograms obtained with the reference solution and the test solution. Furthermore, other fluorescent zones may be present in the chromatogram obtained with the test solution.

Top of the plate	
	A light blue fluorescent zone
_____	_____
Luteolin-7-glucoside: a yellow or orange fluorescent zone	A yellow or orange fluorescent zone (luteolin-7-glucoside)
Chlorogenic acid: a light blue fluorescent zone	A light blue fluorescent zone (chlorogenic acid)
	_____
Reference solution	**Test solution**

TESTS

Loss on drying (*2.8.17*)
Maximum 6.0 per cent.

Total ash (*2.4.16*)
Maximum 30.0 per cent.

ASSAY

Liquid chromatography (*2.2.29*).

Solvent mixture   methanol R, water R (30:70 V/V).

Test solution   Dissolve 30.0 mg of the extract to be examined in the solvent mixture and dilute to 25.0 mL with the solvent mixture.

Reference solution (a)   Dissolve 5.0 mg of *chlorogenic acid CRS* in 50.0 mL of *methanol R*. Transfer 5.0 mL of this solution to a volumetric flask, add 5 mL of *methanol R* and dilute to 20.0 mL with *water R*.

Reference solution (b)   Dissolve 30 mg of the *artichoke leaf dry extract HRS* in the solvent mixture and dilute to 25.0 mL with the solvent mixture.

Column:
— *size*: l = 0.25 m, Ø = 4.6 mm;
— *stationary phase*: octadecylsilyl silica gel for chromatography R (5 µm);
— *temperature*: 40 °C.

Mobile phase:
— *mobile phase A*: phosphoric acid R, water R (0.5:99.5 V/V);
— *mobile phase B*: phosphoric acid R, acetonitrile R (0.5:99.5 V/V);

Time (min)	Mobile phase A (per cent V/V)	Mobile phase B (per cent V/V)
0 - 1	92	8
1 - 20	92 → 75	8 → 25
20 - 33	75	25
33 - 35	75 → 0	25 → 100

Flow rate   1.2 mL/min.

Detection   Spectrophotometer at 330 nm.

Injection   25 µL.

System suitability   Reference solution (b):
— *peak-to-valley ratio*: minimum 2.5, where H_p = height above the baseline of the peak immediately after the peak due to chlorogenic acid and H_v = height above the baseline of the lowest point of the curve separating this peak from the peak due to chlorogenic acid;
— the chromatogram obtained is similar to the chromatogram supplied with the *artichoke leaf dry extract HRS*.

Calculate the percentage content of chlorogenic acid using the following expression:

$$\frac{A_1 \times m_2 \times p \times 0.125}{A_2 \times m_1}$$

A_1 =   area of the peak due to chlorogenic acid in the chromatogram obtained with the test solution;

A_2 =   area of the peak due to chlorogenic acid in the chromatogram obtained with reference solution (a);

m_1 =   mass of the extract to be examined used to prepare the test solution, in milligrams;

m_2 =   mass of *chlorogenic acid CRS* used to prepare reference solution (a), in milligrams;

p =   percentage content of chlorogenic acid in *chlorogenic acid CRS*.

Ph Eur

Ash Leaf

(*Ph Eur monograph 1600*)

Ph Eur _____

DEFINITION

Dried leaf of *Fraxinus excelsior* L. or *Fraxinus angustifolia* Vahl (syn. *Fraxinus oxyphylla* M. Bieb) or of hybrids of these 2 species or of a mixture.

Content

Minimum 2.5 per cent of total hydroxycinnamic acid derivatives, expressed as chlorogenic acid ($C_{16}H_{18}O_9$; M_r 354.3) (dried drug).

IDENTIFICATION

A. The leaf consists of leaflets that are sometimes detached and separated from the rachis. The leaflet is about 6 cm long and 3 cm wide. Each leaflet is subsessile or shortly petiolate, oblong, lanceolate, somewhat unequal at the base, acuminate at the apex, with fine, acute teeth on the margins; the upper surface is dark green and the lower surface is greyish-green. The midrib and secondary veins are whitish and prominent on the lower surface.

B. Microscopic examination (*2.8.23*). The powder is greyish-green. Examine under a microscope using *chloral hydrate solution R*. The powder shows the following diagnostic characters (Figure 1600.-1): fragments of the upper epidermis of the lamina in surface view [B], with some of the cells showing cuticular striations, accompanied by underlying palisade parenchyma [Ba]; fragments of the lower epidermis in surface view [A] consisting of cells covered by fine cuticular striations [Aa], numerous anomocytic stomata (*2.8.3*) [Ab] and rare peltate glandular trichomes with a unicellular stalk and a glandular head composed of radiating cells [Ac]; fragments of lamina in transverse section [F] with 2 layers of palisade parenchyma [Fa], spongy parenchyma [Fb] and, occasionally, glandular trichomes embedded in the epidermis [Fc]; occasional multicellular, uniseriate, conical covering trichomes composed of cells with thick striated walls, either on an epidermis [C] or fragmented [D]; fragments of vascular tissue from the leaflets [E] composed of spiral vessels [Ea], short fibres [Eb] and sometimes palisade parenchyma [Ec]; fragments of vascular tissue from the veins [G] composed of fibres [Ga], sometimes accompanied by cells with thick, pitted walls from the medullary rays [Gb].

C. Examine the chromatograms obtained in the test for *Fraxinus ornus*.

Results See below the sequence of zones present in the chromatograms obtained with the reference solution and the test solution. The intensity of the zones present in the chromatogram obtained with the test solution may vary depending on the presence of *F. excelsior*, *F. angustifolia*, their hybrids or their concentration in a mixture. Furthermore, other fluorescent zones may be present in the chromatogram obtained with the test solution.

TESTS

Foreign matter (*2.8.2*)

Maximum 3.0 per cent of stems and maximum 2.0 per cent of other foreign matter.

Fraxinus ornus

Thin-layer chromatography (*2.2.27*).

Test solution To 1 g of the powdered herbal drug (355) (*2.9.12*) add 20 mL of *methanol R*. Stir with a magnetic stirrer for 10 min. Filter.

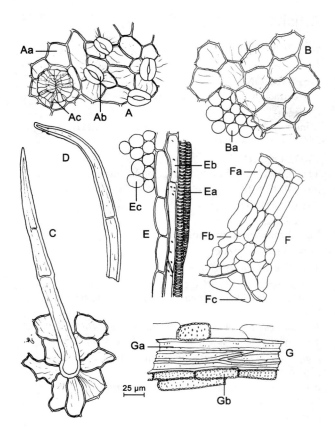

Figure 1600.-1. – *Illustration for identification test B of powdered herbal drug of ash leaf*

Reference solution Dissolve 5 mg of *rutin R* and 5 mg of *chlorogenic acid R* in 10 mL of *methanol R*.

Plate TLC silica gel plate R (5-40 µm) [or TLC silica gel plate R (2-10 µm)].

Mobile phase anhydrous formic acid R, water R, ethyl acetate R (10:10:80 *V/V/V*).

Application 10 µL [or 4 µL] as bands of 10 mm [or 8 mm].

Development Over a path of 10 cm [or 6 cm].

Drying In air.

Detection Heat at 100 °C for 3 min; treat the still-warm plate with a 10 g/L solution of *diphenylboric acid aminoethyl ester R* in *methanol R*; dry in air; treat with a 50 g/L solution of *macrogol 400 R* in *methanol R*; dry in air; examine in ultraviolet light at 365 nm.

Top of the plate	
	A light blue fluorescent zone (acteoside)
Chlorogenic acid: a light blue fluorescent zone	A light blue fluorescent zone may be present (chlorogenic acid)
	A light blue fluorescent zone
Rutin: an orange fluorescent zone	An orange fluorescent zone (rutin)
Reference solution	**Test solution**

Results   The chromatogram obtained with the test solution does not show any intense light blue fluorescent zones in the upper third of the chromatogram.

Loss on drying (*2.2.32*)
Maximum 10.0 per cent, determined on 1.000 g of the powdered herbal drug (355) (*2.9.12*) by drying in an oven at 105 °C for 2 h.

Total ash (*2.4.16*)
Maximum 12.0 per cent.

ASSAY
Test solution (a)   To 0.300 g of the powdered herbal drug (355) (*2.9.12*) add 95 mL of *ethanol (50 per cent V/V) R*. Boil in a water-bath under a reflux condenser for 30 min. Allow to cool and filter. Rinse the filter with 5 mL of *ethanol (50 per cent V/V) R*. Combine the filtrate and the rinsings in a volumetric flask and dilute to 100.0 mL with *ethanol (50 per cent V/V) R*.

Test solution (b)   To 1.0 mL of test solution (a) in a test tube, add 2 mL of *0.5 M hydrochloric acid*, 2 mL of a solution prepared by dissolving 10 g of *sodium nitrite R* and 10 g of *sodium molybdate R* in 100 mL of *water R*, then add 2 mL of *dilute sodium hydroxide solution R* and dilute to 10.0 mL with *water R*; mix.

Immediately measure the absorbance (*2.2.25*) of test solution (b) at 525 nm, using as compensation liquid a solution prepared as follows: mix 1.0 mL of test solution (a), 2 mL of *0.5 M hydrochloric acid*, 2 mL of *dilute sodium hydroxide solution R* and dilute to 10.0 mL with *water R*.

Calculate the percentage content of total hydroxycinnamic acid derivatives, expressed as chlorogenic acid, using the following expression:

$$\frac{A \times 5.3}{m}$$

taking the specific absorbance of chlorogenic acid to be 188.
A = absorbance at 525 nm;
m = mass of the herbal drug to be examined, in grams.

————————————————————————— *Ph Eur*

Astragalus Mongholicus Root

(*Ph Eur monograph 2435*)

Ph Eur ——————————————————————————

DEFINITION
Whole, dried root of *Astragalus mongholicus* var. *mongholicus* (Syn. *Astragalus membranaceus* Bunge var. *mongholicus* (Bunge) P.K. Hsiao) and *Astragalus mongholicus* var. *dahuricus* (DC.) Podlech (Syn. *Astragalus membranaceus* Bunge), freed from rootlets and rootstock, collected from spring to autumn.

Content
Minimum 0.040 per cent of astragaloside IV ($C_{41}H_{68}O_{14}$; M_r 785) (dried drug).

IDENTIFICATION
A. Cylindrical, often with branches, upper part relatively thick, 30-90 cm long and 1-3.5 cm in diameter. Externally pale brownish-yellow or pale brown, with irregular, longitudinal wrinkles or furrows. Texture hard and tenacious; uneasily broken, fracture highly fibrous and weakly (cultivated origin) or strongly starchy (wild origin), bark yellowish-white, wood pale yellow, with radiate striations and

fissures; the central region is dark brown and in older roots may be broken down to form a hollow surrounded by fragments of disintegrating tissue.

B. Reduce to a powder (355) (*2.9.12*). The powder is yellowish-white. Examine under a microscope using *chloral hydrate solution R*. The powder shows the following diagnostic characters: fibres, in bundles or scattered, 8-30 μm in diameter, thick-walled with longitudinal fissures on the surface, the primary walls often separated from the secondary walls, both ends often broken or tassel-like, or slightly truncated; colourless or orange vessels with closely arranged bordered pits; cork fragments consisting of several layers, often accompanied by collenchymatous phelloderm; stone cells occasionally visible, rounded, oblong or irregular, slightly thick-walled. Examine under a microscope using a 50 per cent *V/V* solution of *glycerol R*: the powder shows small, rounded or ovoid starch granules, usually simple or sometimes 2- or 3-compound, about 5 μm in diameter.

C. Thin-layer chromatography (*2.2.27*).

Test solution   Heat 3 g of the powdered drug (355) (*2.9.12*) with 50 mL of *methanol R* for 50 min under reflux and then filter. Evaporate the filtrate under reduced pressure to dryness and take up the residue in 1 mL of *water R*. Apply the solution to a 6 mL solid phase extraction column containing *octadecylsilyl silica gel for chromatography R* previously conditioned with 3 mL of *methanol R* and then with 3 mL of *water R*. Wash the column with 15 mL of *water R* followed by 15 mL of a 30 per cent *V/V* solution of *methanol R*. Discard the washings. Elute with 20 mL of *methanol R* and collect the eluate. Evaporate the eluate under reduced pressure to dryness and take up the residue with 2 mL of *methanol R*.

Reference solution   Dissolve 10.0 mg of *daidzin R* and 5.0 mg of *daidzein R* in 5.0 mL of *methanol R*.

Plate   TLC silica gel F_{254} *plate R* (2-10 μm).

Mobile phase   *water R*, *methanol R*, *ethyl acetate R* (10:13.5:100 *V/V/V*).

Application   3 μL as bands of 8 mm.

Development   Over a path of 7 cm.

Drying   In air.

Detection A   Examine in ultraviolet light at 254 nm.

Results A   See below the sequence of zones present in the chromatograms obtained with the reference solution and the test solution. Furthermore, other faint zones may be present in the chromatogram obtained with the test solution.

Top of the plate	
	A blue fluorescent zone
Daidzein: a quenching zone	A quenching zone
———	———
	A quenching zone
Daidzin: a quenching zone	A quenching zone
Reference solution	**Test solution**

Detection B   Treat with *anisaldehyde solution R*. Heat at 100 °C for 3 min. Examine in ultraviolet light at 366 nm.

Results B   See below the sequence of zones present in the chromatograms obtained with the reference solution and the test solution. Furthermore, other faint zones may be present in the chromatogram obtained with the test solution.

Top of the plate	
	A violet zone
Daidzein: a pale blue zone	
	A violet zone
———	———
	A violet zone
Daidzin: a pale blue zone	A brown zone
	5 brown zones
———	———
Reference solution	**Test solution**

TESTS

Foreign matter (*2.8.2*)
Maximum 5 per cent.

Loss on drying (*2.2.32*)
Maximum 10.0 per cent, determined on 1.000 g of the powdered drug (355) (*2.9.12*) by drying in an oven at 105 °C for 3 h.

Total ash (*2.4.16*)
Maximum 5.0 per cent.

Ash insoluble in hydrochloric acid (*2.8.1*)
Maximum 1.0 per cent.

ASSAY

Liquid chromatography (*2.2.29*).

Test solution   Weigh 4.0 g of the powdered drug (355) (*2.9.12*) into a Soxhlet type extractor and add 40 mL of *methanol R*. Macerate overnight. Add again 40 mL of *methanol R*. Heat under a reflux condenser for 4 h. Evaporate to dryness. Dissolve the residue in 10 mL of *water R*, heating slightly if necessary. Shake with 4 quantities, each of 40 mL, of *butanol R* saturated with *water R*. Combine the butanol extracts and wash with 2 quantities, each of 40 mL, of *ammonia R*. Discard the ammonia layers and evaporate the butanol layers to dryness. Dissolve the residue in 5 mL of *water R* and cool. Apply the solution to a solid phase extraction column containing 1 g of *octadecylsilyl silica gel for chromatography R* previously washed with 5 mL of *methanol R* and 5 mL of *water R*. Wash the column with 20 mL of *water R* and 20 mL of *ethanol (25 per cent V/V) R*. Elute with 25 mL of *ethanol (70 per cent V/V) R*. Evaporate the eluate to dryness. Dissolve the residue in 5.0 mL of *methanol R*.

Reference solution (a)   Dissolve 10.0 mg of *astragaloside IV CRS* in *methanol R* and dilute to 10.0 mL with the same solvent.

Reference solutions (b), (c), (d)   Dilute reference solution (a) to obtain 3 reference solutions of astragaloside IV, the concentrations of which span the expected value in the test solution.

Reference solution (e)   Dissolve 5.0 mg of *ginsenoside Rb1 R* in 5 mL of *methanol R* and dilute to 10.0 mL with reference solution (a).

Column:
— *size*: *l* = 0.25 m, Ø = 3.2 mm;
— *stationary phase*: *octadecylsilyl silica gel for chromatography R* (3 µm);
— *temperature*: 25 °C.

Mobile phase:
— *mobile phase A*: *water R*;
— *mobile phase B*: *acetonitrile R*;

Time (min)	Mobile phase A (per cent *V/V*)	Mobile phase B (per cent *V/V*)
0 - 5	90	10
5 - 10	90 → 80	10 → 20
10 - 20	80 → 75	20 → 25
20 - 30	75 → 67	25 → 33
30 - 40	67 → 65	33 → 35
40 - 50	65 → 40	35 → 60
50 - 55	40	60

Flow rate   0.5 mL/min.

Detection   Evaporative light-scattering detector; the following settings have been found to be suitable; if the detector has different setting parameters, adjust the detector settings so as to comply with the system suitability criterion:
— *carrier gas*: air;
— *flow rate*: 1.5 mL/min;
— *evaporator temperature*: 50 °C.

Injection   20 µL of the test solution and reference solutions (b), (c), (d) and (e).

Relative retention   With reference to ginsenoside Rb1 (retention time = about 33.6 min):
astragaloside IV = about 1.05.

System suitability:
— *resolution*: minimum 4.0 between the peaks due to astragaloside IV and ginsenoside Rb1 in the chromatogram obtained with reference solution (e).

Establish a calibration curve with the logarithm of the concentration (mg/mL) of reference solutions (b), (c) and (d) (corrected by the declared percentage content of *astragaloside IV CRS*) as the abscissa and the logarithm of the corresponding peak area as the ordinate. Calculate the percentage content of astragaloside IV using the following expression:

$$\frac{10^A \times 0.5}{m}$$

A =   logarithm of the concentration corresponding to the astragaloside IV peak in the chromatogram obtained with the test solution, determined from the calibration curve;

m =   mass of the drug to be examined used to prepare the test solution, in grams.

———————————————————— *Ph Eur*

Atractylodes Lancea Rhizome

(Ph Eur monograph 2559)

Ph Eur

DEFINITION

Dried, whole or fragmented rhizome of *Atractylodes lancea* (Thunb.) DC. (syn. *Atractylodes chinensis* (Bunge) Koidz.) with the roots removed, collected in spring and autumn.

Content

Minimum 14 mL/kg of essential oil (anhydrous drug).

IDENTIFICATION

A. The whole rhizome is curved, irregular, nodular and cylindrical, 3-10 cm long and 1-3 cm in diameter. The external surface is transversally wrinkled, dark greyish-brown or yellowish-brown; it shows numerous rounded protuberances and large circular stem scars and smaller root scars.

The fragmented rhizome occurs in slices with a highly variable diameter (1-4 cm) and a thickness of about 0.5 cm. The external surface is wrinkled, dark greyish-brown or yellowish-brown and shows numerous scars. The transverse section is pale yellow or brownish-yellow, consisting of fibrous tissues scattered with particularly abundant orange oil cavities appearing as dots.

B. Microscopic examination (*2.8.23*). The powder is brownish-yellow. Examine under a microscope using *chloral hydrate solution R*. The powder shows the following diagnostic characters: fragments of orange cork, with polyhedral cells, often accompanied by subrectangular or ovoid sclereids with very thick channelled walls from the phelloderm; isolated, ovoid or subrectangular sclereids with very thick, channelled walls and a narrow lumen, variable in shape (20-80 µm in diameter); fragments of parenchyma with polyhedral or subrectangular cells containing small needle-shaped crystals of calcium oxalate (5-30 µm) clearly visible in polarised light; fragments of fibres in bundles, with heavily thickened and slightly pitted walls (40 µm in diameter) and a narrow lumen, very often associated with xylem vessels; fragments of short, reticulate or pitted vessels, usually included in parenchyma with thin-walled cells; fragments of oil glands with thin-walled cells and granular orange-brown contents and orange oil droplets. Examine under a microscope, without heating, using *glycerol R*: the powder shows pieces of inulin, free or included in parenchyma cells.

C. Examine the chromatograms obtained in the test for *Atractylodes macrocephala*.

Results   See below the sequence of zones present in the chromatograms obtained with the reference solution and the test solution. Furthermore, other faint zones may be present in the chromatogram obtained with the test solution.

TESTS

Atractylodes macrocephala

Thin-layer chromatography (*2.2.27*).

Test solution   Introduce 0.5 g of the powdered herbal drug (355) (*2.9.12*) into a centrifuge tube, add 2 mL of *methanol R* and stopper the tube. Sonicate at 25 °C for 15 min and centrifuge.

Reference solution   Dissolve 10 mg of *β-caryophyllene R* and 10 mg of *bornyl acetate R* in 5 mL of *methanol R*.

Plate   *TLC silica gel plate R* (5-40 µm) [or *TLC silica gel plate R* (2-10 µm)].

Mobile phase   ethyl acetate *R*, heptane *R* (5:95 *V/V*).

Top of the plate	
β-Caryophyllene: a pink zone	A pink or violet zone
	An orange zone may be present
_____	
	An intense greyish-green zone
	A very faint violet zone
_____	_____
Bornyl acetate: a brown zone	A violet zone
	Several violet zones
Reference solution	**Test solution**

Application   5 µL [or 3 µL] as bands of 10 mm [or 6 mm].

Development   In an unsaturated tank, over a path of 10 cm [or 6 cm].

Drying   In air.

Detection   Treat with *anisaldehyde solution R* and heat at 105-110 °C for 5-10 min; examine in daylight.

Results   The chromatogram obtained with the test solution shows an intense greyish-green zone in the middle third. In the case of a substitution by *Atractylodes macrocephala*, no intense greyish-green zone is present in the middle third.

Water (*2.2.13*)
Maximum 100 mL/kg, determined on 20.0 g of the powdered herbal drug (355) (*2.9.12*).

Total ash (*2.4.16*)
Maximum 7.0 per cent.

Ash insoluble in hydrochloric acid (*2.8.1*)
Maximum 1.0 per cent.

ASSAY

Carry out the determination of essential oils in herbal drugs (*2.8.12*). Use 15.0 g of freshly powdered herbal drug (710) (*2.9.12*), a 500 mL round-bottomed flask, 200 mL of *water R* as the distillation liquid and 0.50 mL of *xylene R* in the graduated tube. Distil at a rate of 2-3 mL/min for 2 h.

Ph Eur

Largehead Atractylodes Rhizome

(Ph Eur monograph 2560)

Ph Eur

DEFINITION

Dried, whole or fragmented rhizome of *Atractylodes macrocephala* Koidz. with the roots removed, collected in winter when the lower leaves of the plant turn yellow and the upper leaves become fragile.

Content

Minimum 9 mL/kg of essential oil (anhydrous drug).

IDENTIFICATION

A. The whole rhizome is irregularly shaped, 3-13 cm long and 1.5-7 cm in diameter. Externally yellowish-grey or dark brown, with small knob-like protrusions, interrupted longitudinal wrinkles and grooves.

The fragmented rhizome occurs in slices with a highly variable diameter (1-7 cm) and a thickness of about 0.5 cm. The external surface is wrinkled or grooved, more or less

dark yellowish-brown with numerous root scars.
The transverse section is pale yellow, consisting of tissues with wide spaces between them and scattered with many orange oil cavities appearing as dots that are particularly abundant in the external tissues.

The fracture is hard and fibrous.

B. Microscopic examination (*2.8.23*). The powder is brownish-yellow. Examine under a microscope using *chloral hydrate solution R*. The powder shows the following diagnostic characters: fragments of orange cork, with polyhedral cells; fragments of parenchyma with polyhedral or subrectangular cells, many of which contain small needle-shaped crystals of calcium oxalate (10-32 µm) clearly visible in polarised light; sclereids, isolated or in small groups, with very thick, channelled walls, variable in shape (35-65 µm in diameter); fragments of fibres, isolated or in bundles, with moderately thickened and slightly pitted walls (40 µm in diameter); fragments of short, reticulate or pitted vessels, usually included in parenchyma with thin-walled cells; fragments of oil glands with thin-walled cells and granular orange-brown contents. Examine under a microscope, without heating, using *glycerol R*; the powder shows numerous pieces of inulin, free or included in parenchyma cells.

C. Examine the chromatograms obtained in the test for *Atractylodes lancea*.

Results See below the sequence of zones present in the chromatograms obtained with the reference solution and the test solution. Furthermore, other faint zones may be present in the chromatogram obtained with the test solution.

Top of the plate	
β-Caryophyllene: a pink zone	A pink or violet zone
	An orange zone
	A very faint violet zone
Bornyl acetate: a brown zone	
	A very faint violet zone
	Several faint violet zones
Reference solution	Test solution

D. To 0.5 g of the powdered herbal drug (355) (*2.9.12*) add 5 mL of *ethanol (96 per cent) R*, heat in a water-bath at 60 °C for 2 min and filter. To 1 mL of the filtrate add 0.25 mL of a solution freshly prepared as follows: dissolve 5 mg of *vanillin R* in 0.5 mL of *ethanol (96 per cent) R*, to this solution add 0.5 mL of *water R* and 3 mL of *hydrochloric acid R*. Shake immediately; a red or reddish-purple colour develops and persists.

TESTS

Atractylodes lancea

Thin-layer chromatography (*2.2.27*).

Test solution Introduce 0.5 g of the powdered herbal drug (355) (*2.9.12*) into a centrifuge tube, add 2 mL of *methanol R* and stopper the tube. Sonicate at 25 °C for 15 min and centrifuge.

Reference solution Dissolve 10 mg of *β-caryophyllene R* and 10 mg of *bornyl acetate R* in 5 mL of *methanol R*.

Plate *TLC silica gel plate R* (5-40 µm) [or *TLC silica gel plate R* (2-10 µm)].

Mobile phase ethyl acetate R, heptane R (5:95 *V/V*).

Application 5 µL [or 3 µL] as bands of 10 mm [or 6 mm].

Development In an unsaturated tank, over a path of 10 cm [or 6 cm].

Drying In air.

Detection Treat with *anisaldehyde solution R* and heat at 105-110 °C for 5-10 min; examine in daylight.

Results The chromatogram obtained with the test solution shows no greyish-green zone in the middle third, above the very faint violet zone.

Water (*2.2.13*)

Maximum 100 mL/kg, determined on 20.0 g of the powdered herbal drug (710) (*2.9.12*).

Total ash (*2.4.16*)

Maximum 5.0 per cent.

Ash insoluble in hydrochloric acid (*2.8.1*)

Maximum 1.0 per cent.

ASSAY

Carry out the determination of essential oils in herbal drugs (*2.8.12*). Use 15.0 g of freshly powdered herbal drug (710) (*2.9.12*), a 500 mL round-bottomed flask, 200 mL of *water R* as the distillation liquid and 0.50 mL of *xylene R* in the graduated tube. Distil at a rate of 2-3 mL/min for 2 h.

———————————————————— *Ph Eur*

Azadirachta Indica Leaf

Nimba Leaf

DEFINITION

Azadirachta Indica Leaf is the dried leaf of *Azadirachta indica* A. Juss.

It contains not less than 1.0% of tetranortriterpinoids, expressed as salannin, calculated with reference to the dried drug.

IDENTIFICATION

A. Leaflets thin and fragile, ovate to lanceolate, 3 to 10 cm long and 1 to 2.5 cm wide, curved with a serrate margin; base markedly asymmetrical, apex acuminate and terminating in a fine point; upper surface dark brownish-green, lower surface paler with distinct midrib and lateral veins running to the margins; both surfaces glabrous. Fragments of the rachis may be present; these are pale brown, slender, up to about 10 cm long, cylindrical with faint longitudinal striations and bearing alternating pairs of scars where the leaflets were attached.

B. Reduce to a powder (355). The powder is green. Examine under a microscope using *chloral hydrate solution*. The powder shows fragments of the epidermis composed of thin-walled tangentially elongated cells with abundant *anomocytic* stomata, Appendix XI H; abundant fragments of single layered palisade and thin-walled parenchymatous cells of the spongy mesophyll present, some with associated vessels; some fragments display rosette crystals of calcium oxalate often in rows.

C. Carry out the method for *thin-layer chromatography*, Appendix III A, using the following solutions.

(1) Add 30 mL of *methanol* to approximately 5 g of powdered herbal drug, mix thoroughly by hand and with the aid of ultrasound for 30 minutes. Centrifuge at 3000 rpm for 5 minutes and collect the clear supernatant liquid. Repeat the extraction twice, combine the supernatant liquid and dilute

to 100 mL with *methanol*. Filter approximately 30 mL of the solution through a 0.45-µm filter and use the filtrate.

(2) 0.025% w/v each of *azadirachtin, salannin CRS* and *β-sitosterol* in *methanol*.

CHROMATOGRAPHIC CONDITIONS

(a) Use a *silica gel 60* or high-performance *silica gel 60* precoated plate [Merck silica gel 60 HPTLC plates are suitable].

(b) Use the mobile phase as described below.

(c) Apply as bands 5 µL of each solution.

(d) Develop the plate to 15 cm [or 7 cm].

(e) After removal of the plate, spray with *vanillin reagent*, heat the plate at 100° for 3 minutes and examine in daylight.

MOBILE PHASE

3 volumes of *hexane* and 7 volumes of *ethyl acetate*.

SYSTEM SUITABILITY

The test is not valid unless the chromatogram obtained with solution (2) shows three clearly separated spots.

CONFIRMATION

In the chromatogram obtained with solution (1), a black band with an Rf value of approximately 0.15 corresponding in position to a brown band in the chromatogram for solution (2) is obtained. A black band with an Rf value of approximately 0.3 corresponding in position to the indigo band in the chromatogram for solution (2) is obtained for salannin. An indigo band with an Rf value of approximately 0.6 corresponding in position to a purple band in the chromatogram for solution (2) is obtained for β-sitosterol.

Top of the plate	
Purple band	β-sitosterol: a purple band
Black band	Salannin: an indigo band
Black band	Azadirachtin: a brown band
Solution (1)	**Solution (2)**

TESTS

Foreign matter
Not more than 2%, Appendix XI D.

Loss on drying
When dried for 2 hours at 105°, loses not more than 10.0% of its weight. Use 1 g.

Ash
Not more than 10.0%, Appendix XI J, method II.

Water-soluble extractive
Not less than 20.0%, Appendix XI B2.

ASSAY

Carry out the method for *liquid chromatography*, Appendix III D, using the following solutions.

(1) Add 30 mL of *methanol* to approximately 5 g of powdered herbal drug, mix thoroughly by hand and with the aid of ultrasound for 30 minutes. Centrifuge at 3000 rpm for 5 minutes and collect the clear supernatant liquid. Repeat the extraction twice, combine the supernatant liquid and dilute to 100 mL with *methanol*. Filter approximately 30 mL of the solution through a 0.45-µm filter and use the filtrate.

(2) 0.0025% w/v of *salannin CRS* and 0.001% w/v of *azadirachtin-A CRS* in *methanol*.

CHROMATOGRAPHIC CONDITIONS

(a) Use a stainless steel column (15 cm × 2.1 mm) packed with *octadecylsilyl silica gel for chromatography* (5 µm) (Spherisorb ODS1 is suitable).

(b) Use gradient elution and the mobile phase described below.

(c) Use a flow rate of 0.5 mL per minute.

(d) Use a column temperature of 30°.

(e) Use a detection wavelength of 217 nm.

(f) Inject 10 µL of each solution.

When the chromatograms are recorded under the prescribed conditions the retention time of the peak due to azadirachtin-A is about 15 minutes and the retention time of the peak due to salannin is about 22 minutes.

MOBILE PHASE

Mobile phase A   0.1 volume of *trifluroacetic acid* and 100 volumes of *water*.

Mobile phase B   0.1 volume of *trifluroacetic acid* and 100 volumes of *acetonitrile*.

Time (Minutes)	Mobile phase A (% v/v)	Mobile phase B (% v/v)	Comment
0-10	90→70	10→30	linear gradient
10-25	70→30	30→70	linear gradient
25-40	30	70	isocratic
40-45	30→90	70→10	linear gradient
45-50	90	10	re-equilibration

SYSTEM SUITABILITY

The test is not valid unless, in the chromatogram obtained with solution (2):

the *symmetry factor* of the peak due to azadirachtin-A is at most 1.2;

the *symmetry factor* of the peak due to salannin is at most 1.4.

DETERMINATION OF CONTENT

Calculate the total content of tetranortriterpinoids, expressed as salannin, from the sum of the areas of the peaks eluting from three minutes before to three minutes after the retention time of salannin and from the declared content of salannin in *salannin CRS* using the following expression:

$$\frac{A_1}{A_2} \times \frac{m_2}{V_2} \times \frac{V_1}{m_1} \times p \times \frac{100}{100 - d}$$

A_1 =   combined areas of the peaks in the chromatogram obtained with solution (1) with retention times from three minutes before to three minutes after the retention time of peak due to salannin in the chromatogram obtained with solution (2),

A_2 =   area of the peak due to salannin in the chromatogram obtained with solution (2),

m_1 =   weight of the drug being examined in mg,

m_2 =   weight of *salannin CRS* in mg,

V_1 =   dilution volume of solution (1),

V_2 = dilution volume of solution (2),
p = percentage content of salannin in *salannin CRS*,
d = percentage loss on drying of the herbal drug being examined.

STORAGE

Azadirachta Indica Leaf should be protected from moisture.

Bacopa Monnieri

DEFINITION

Bacopa Monnieri is the dried aerial parts of *Bacopa monnieri* (L.) Wettst.

It contains not less than 1.0% w/w of bacopa saponins, expressed as bacopaside II ($C_{47}H_{76}O_8$), calculated with reference to the dried drug.

IDENTIFICATION

A. Pieces of herb, consisting mainly of stem and leaf; buff or greenish brown, angular stems, 1 to 2 mm in diameter and 10 to 30 cm long, nodes prominent, often showing sprouting rootlets and with numerous ascending branches; greenish leaves sessile or short petioled, fleshy, glabrous on the upper surface, simple, opposite, decussate, 0.6 to 2.5 cm long and 3 to 8 mm wide, reniform, spathulate or oblanceolate, margin entire or, rarely, dentate. If present, flowers are axillary and solitary, on peduncles usually longer than the leaves; corolla up to 1 cm long, five lobed, oblong, obtuse; fruit capsule ovoid-acuminate or slightly beaked at the apex, glabrous, up to 5 mm long.

B. Reduce to a powder (355). The powder is greenish or yellowish-brown. Examine under a microscope using *chloral hydrate solution*. The powder shows fragments of the epidermis, with a thin striated cuticle, multicellular glandular trichomes, *anomocytic* stomata; numerous xylem vessels with reticulate thickening. Examine under a microscope using 50% v/v of *glycerol* in *water*. Starch granules are present, usually simple, round or ovoid, 4 to 14 µm in diameter, without a visible hilum.

C. Carry out the method for *thin-layer chromatography*, Appendix III A, using the following solutions.

(1) Add 30 mL of *methanol (70%)* to 5.0 g of the powdered herbal drug, heat on a water-bath under reflux for 30 minutes, cool, centrifuge at 3000 rpm for 5 minutes and decant the supernatant liquid. Repeat the extraction procedure with a further two 30-mL quantities of *methanol (70%)*. Combine the supernatant liquid, dilute to 100 mL with *methanol (70%)* and filter (0.45 µm PTFE is suitable).

(2) 0.05% w/v of *bacopaside II CRS* in *methanol (70%)*.

(3) 0.05% w/v each of *bacopaside I CRS* and *bacopaside II CRS* in *methanol (70%)*.

CHROMATOGRAPHIC CONDITIONS

(a) Use silica gel 60 precoated plates or high-performance *silica gel 60* (Merck silica gel 60 plates are suitable).

(b) Use the mobile phase as described below.

(c) Apply 20 µL [or 10 µL] of each solution, as bands.

(d) Develop the plate to 15 cm [or 8 cm].

(e) After removal of the plate, dip in *anisaldehyde solution R1*, heat in an oven at 105° for 5 minutes and examine in daylight.

MOBILE PHASE

10 volumes of 1% v/v of *formic acid*, 20 volumes of *methanol* and 70 volumes of *ethyl acetate*.

SYSTEM SUITABILITY

The test is not valid unless the chromatogram obtained with solution (3) shows two clearly separated bands.

CONFIRMATION

The chromatogram obtained with solution (1) shows a dark band with an Rf value of approximately 0.4 corresponding to the band obtained with bacopaside II in the chromatogram obtained with solution (3), a lighter band with an Rf value of approximately 0.3 corresponding to the band obtained with bacopaside I in the chromatogram obtained with solution (3). Bands with Rf values of approximately 0.2 and 0.8 are also present. Other bands may be present in solution (1).

Top of the plate		
unknown: dark band		
bacopaside II: dark band	bacopaside II: dark band	bacopaside II: dark band
bacopaside I: light band		bacopaside I: light band
unknown: light band		
Solution (1)	**Solution (2)**	**Solution (3)**

TESTS

Foreign matter

Not more than 1.0%, Appendix XI D.

Loss on drying

Not more than 11.0%, Appendix IX D. Use 1 g.

Ash

Not more than 13.0%, Appendix XI J, Method II.

Water-soluble extractive

Not less than 15.0%, Appendix XI B2.

ASSAY

Carry out the method for *liquid chromatography*, Appendix III D, using the following solutions.

(1) Reduce to a powder (355). To 5.0 g of the powder, add 30 mL of *methanol (70%)* and heat under reflux for 30 minutes. Allow to cool, centrifuge and collect the supernatant liquid. Repeat the extraction twice with two further 30-mL quantities of *methanol (70%)*. Combine the three supernatant liquids, dilute to 100 mL with *methanol (70%)* and filter (0.45 µm PTFE is suitable).

(2) 0.05% w/v of *bacopaside II CRS* in *methanol (70%)*.

(3) 0.05% w/v of *bacoside A CRS* in *methanol (70%)*.

CHROMATOGRAPHIC CONDITIONS

(a) Use a stainless steel column (25 cm x 4.6 mm) packed with *end-capped octadecylsilyl silica gel for chromatography* (5 µm) (Phenomenex Luna C18 is suitable).

(b) Use isocratic elution and the mobile phase described below.

(c) Use a flow rate of 1.0 mL per minute.

(d) Use a column temperature of 30°.

(e) Use a detection wavelength of 205 nm.

(f) Inject 20 µL of each solution.

(g) Record the chromatograms for 75 minutes.

MOBILE PHASE

315 volumes of *acetonitrile* and 685 volumes of 0.71% w/v *anhydrous sodium sulfate*, previously adjusted to pH 2.3 with *sulfuric acid*.

When the chromatograms are recorded under the prescribed conditions the retention time of bacopaside II is about 36 minutes. The retention times relative to bacopaside II are: bacoside A_3, about 0.9; bacopaside X, about 1.2; bacopasaponin C, about 1.3; bacopaside I, about 1.4.

SYSTEM SUITABILITY

The test is not valid unless, in the chromatogram obtained with solution (3), the *resolution factor* between the peaks due to bacoside A_3 and bacopaside II is at least 1.5 and the *resolution factor* between the peaks due to bacopaside X and bacopasaponin C is at least 2.4.

DETERMINATION OF CONTENT

Calculate the total content of bacopa saponins (bacoside A_3, bacopaside II, bacopaside X, bacopasaponin C and bacopaside I), expressed as bacopaside II from the chromatograms obtained, and using the declared content of bacopaside II in *bacopaside II CRS*.

Bearberry Leaf

Uva Ursi

(Ph Eur monograph 1054)

Ph Eur ⎯⎯⎯⎯⎯⎯⎯⎯⎯⎯⎯⎯⎯⎯⎯⎯⎯⎯⎯⎯⎯⎯

DEFINITION

Whole or fragmented, dried leaf of *Arctostaphylos uva-ursi* (L.) Spreng.

Content

Minimum 7.0 per cent of anhydrous arbutin ($C_{12}H_{16}O_7$; M_r 272.3) (dried drug).

IDENTIFICATION

A. The leaf, shiny and dark green on the adaxial surface, lighter on the abaxial surface, is generally 7-30 mm long and 5-12 mm wide. The entire leaf is obovate with smooth margins, somewhat reflexed downwards, narrowing at the base into a short petiole. The leaf is obtuse or retuse at its apex. The lamina is thick and coriaceous. The venation, pinnate and finely reticulate, is clearly visible on both surfaces. The adaxial surface is marked with sunken veinlets, giving it a characteristic grainy appearance. Only the young leaf has ciliated margins. Old leaves are glabrous.

B. Microscopic examination (*2.8.23*). The powder is green, greenish-grey or yellowish-green. Examine under a microscope using *chloral hydrate solution R*. The powder shows the following diagnostic characters (Figure 1054.-1): fragments of adaxial epidermis in surface view [A] showing thick and irregularly pitted polygonal cells [Aa] usually accompanied by palisade parenchyma [Ab]; fragments of adaxial epidermis in transverse section [G], showing straight-walled cells [Ga] covered by a thick smooth cuticle [Gb], and accompanied by palisade parenchyma [Gc] consisting of 3 or 4 layers of cells of unequal lengths, some of which contain numerous prisms of calcium oxalate [Gd]; fragments of abaxial epidermis, in surface view [B, E], showing anomocytic stomata (*2.8.3*) [Ba] surrounded by 5-11 subsidiary cells, scars of hair bases [Ea], and accompanied by spongy parenchyma [Eb]; groups of lignified fibres from the pericycle [D]; fragments of the vascular system [F] consisting of pitted vessels [Fa] and fibres [Fb] accompanied by rows of cells containing prisms of calcium oxalate [Fc]; oil droplets are present in the parenchymatous cells; occasional fragments of conical, unicellular covering trichomes [C].

C. Thin-layer chromatography (*2.2.27*).

Test solution   To 0.5 g of the powdered herbal drug (355) (*2.9.12*) add 5 mL of a mixture of equal volumes of *methanol R* and *water R*, and heat under a reflux condenser for 10 min. Filter whilst hot. Wash the flask and the filter with a mixture of equal volumes of *methanol R* and *water R* and dilute to 5 mL with the same mixture of solvents.

Reference solution   Dissolve 50 mg of *arbutin R* and 25 mg of *gallic acid R* in *methanol R* and dilute to 20.0 mL with the same solvent.

Plate   *TLC silica gel plate R* (5-40 μm) [or *TLC silica gel plate R* (2-10 μm)].

Mobile phase   *anhydrous formic acid R*, *water R*, *ethyl acetate R* (6:6:88 *V/V/V*).

Application   10 μL [or 2 μL] as bands of 15 mm [or 8 mm].

Development   Over a path of 15 cm [or 6 cm].

Drying   At 105-110 °C until the mobile phase has evaporated.

Detection   Treat with a 10 g/L solution of *dichloroquinonechlorimide R* in *methanol R*, then treat with a 20 g/L solution of *anhydrous sodium carbonate R*.

Results   See below the sequence of zones present in the chromatograms obtained with the reference solution and the test solution. Furthermore, other blue or brown zones may be present in the chromatogram obtained with the test solution.

Top of the plate	
	A brownish zone
Gallic acid: a brownish zone	
	A brown zone
Arbutin: a blue zone	An intense blue zone (arbutin)
Reference solution	**Test solution**

TESTS

Foreign matter (*2.8.2*)

Maximum 5 per cent of stems and maximum 3 per cent of other foreign matter.

Leaves of different colour

Maximum 10 per cent, determined in the same manner as foreign matter (*2.8.2*).

Loss on drying (*2.2.32*)

Maximum 10.0 per cent, determined on 1.000 g of the powdered herbal drug (355) (*2.9.12*) by drying in an oven at 105 °C for 2 h.

Total ash (*2.4.16*)

Maximum 5.0 per cent.

ASSAY

Liquid chromatography (*2.2.29*).

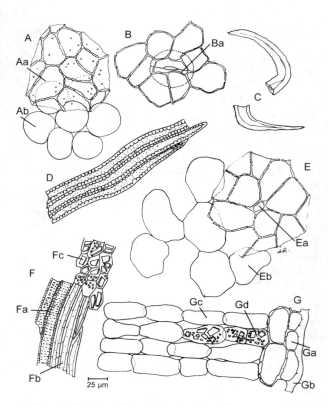

Figure 1054.-1. – *Illustration for identification test B of powdered herbal drug of bearberry leaf*

Test solution   In a 100 mL flask with a ground-glass neck, place 0.800 g of the powdered herbal drug (250) (*2.9.12*). Add 20 mL of *water R* and heat under a reflux condenser on a water-bath for 30 min. Allow to cool and filter the liquid through a plug of absorbent cotton. Add the absorbent cotton to the residue in the 100 mL flask and extract with 20 mL of *water R* under a reflux condenser on a water-bath for 30 min. Allow to cool and filter through a paper filter. Combine the filtrates and dilute to 50.0 mL with *water R*. Filter through a paper filter. Discard the first 10 mL of the filtrate.

Reference solution (a)   Dissolve 50.0 mg of *arbutin CRS* in the mobile phase and dilute to 50.0 mL with the mobile phase.

Reference solution (b)   Dissolve 2.5 mg of *hydroquinone R* in the mobile phase and dilute to 10.0 mL with the mobile phase. To 5.0 mL of the solution, add 2.5 mL of reference solution (a) and dilute to 10.0 mL with the mobile phase.

Column:
— *size*: l = 0.25 m, Ø = 4 mm;
— *stationary phase*: base-deactivated octadecylsilyl silica gel for chromatography R (5 μm).

Mobile phase   methanol R, water R (10:90 *V/V*).

Flow rate   1.2 mL/min.

Detection   Spectrophotometer at 280 nm.

Injection   20 μL.

System suitability   Reference solution (b):
— *resolution*: minimum 4.0 between the peaks due to arbutin and hydroquinone.

Calculate the percentage content of arbutin using the following expression:

$$\frac{F_1 \times m_2 \times p}{F_2 \times m_1}$$

F_1 = area of the peak due to arbutin in the chromatogram obtained with the test solution;

F_2 = area of the peak due to arbutin in the chromatogram obtained with reference solution (a);

m_1 = mass of the herbal drug to be examined used to prepare the test solution, in grams;

m_2 = mass of *arbutin CRS* used to prepare reference solution (a), in grams;

p = percentage content of arbutin in *arbutin CRS*.

Ph Eur

Belladonna Leaf

Belladonna Herb

(*Ph Eur monograph 0221*)

Preparations
Prepared Belladonna

Standardised Belladonna Leaf Dry Extract

Belladonna Tincture

When Belladonna Herb, Belladonna Leaf or Powdered Belladonna Herb is prescribed, Prepared Belladonna shall be supplied.

Ph Eur

DEFINITION
Dried leaf or dried leaf and flowering, and occasionally fruit-bearing, tops of *Atropa belladonna* L.

Content
Minimum 0.30 per cent of total alkaloids, expressed as hyoscyamine ($C_{17}H_{23}NO_3$; M_r 289.4) (dried drug).
The alkaloids consist mainly of hyoscyamine together with small quantities of hyoscine (scopolamine).

CHARACTERS
Slightly nauseous odour.

IDENTIFICATION
A. The leaves are green or brownish-green, slightly darker on the upper surface, often crumpled and rolled and partly matted together in the drug. The leaf is petiolate and the lamina is acute and decurrent. The margin is entire.
The flowering stems are flattened and bear at each node a pair of leaves unequal in size, in the axils of which occur singly the flowers or occasionally fruits. The flowers have a gamosepalous calyx and campanulate corolla. The drug may contain fruits, as globular berries, green or brownish-black and surrounded by the persistent calyx with widely spread lobes.

B. Microscopic examination (*2.8.23*). The powder is dark green. Examine under a microscope using *chloral hydrate solution R*. The powder shows the following diagnostic characters (Figure 0221.-1): fragments of the lamina showing sinuous-walled epidermal cells with striated cuticle [A, C] and part of the underlying palisade parenchyma [Aa] associated with the upper epidermis [A]; numerous stomata [Ca] more frequent on the lower epidermis [C], anisocytic and also some anomocytic (*2.8.3*); multicellular, uniseriate covering trichomes with a smooth cuticle [F], glandular trichomes with unicellular heads and multicellular, uniseriate stalks [D] or with multicellular heads and unicellular stalks [B]; parenchyma cells including rounded cells, some of which contain microsphenoidal crystals of calcium oxalate [E]; annularly and spirally thickened vessels [K]. The powdered drug may also show: fibres and reticulately thickened vessels from the stems; subspherical pollen grains, 40-50 µm in diameter, with 3 germinal pores, 3 furrows and an extensively pitted exine [H]; fragments of the corolla with a papillose epidermis [J] or bearing numerous covering or glandular trichomes of the types previously described [L]; fragments of the brownish-yellow testa consisting of irregularly sclerified cells [G].

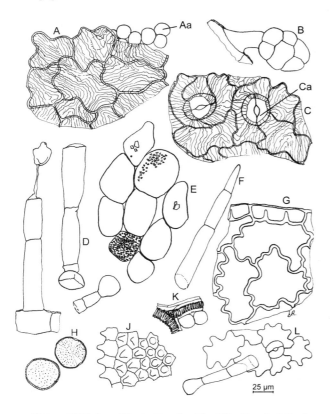

Figure 0221.-1. – Illustration for identification test B of powdered herbal drug of belladonna leaf

C. Shake 1 g of the powdered herbal drug (180) (*2.9.12*) with 10 mL of *0.05 M sulfuric acid* for 2 min. Filter and add to the filtrate 1 mL of *concentrated ammonia R* and 5 mL of *water R*. Shake cautiously with 15 mL of *ether R*, avoiding formation of an emulsion. Separate the ether layer and dry over *anhydrous sodium sulfate R*. Filter and evaporate the ether in a porcelain dish. Add 0.5 mL of *fuming nitric acid R* and evaporate to dryness on a water-bath. Add 10 mL of *acetone R* and, dropwise, a 30 g/L solution of *potassium hydroxide R* in *ethanol (96 per cent) R*. A deep violet colour develops.

D. Examine the chromatograms obtained in the chromatography test.

Results The principal zones in the chromatograms obtained with the test solution are similar in position, colour and size to the principal zones in the chromatograms obtained with the same volume of the reference solution.

TESTS
Chromatography
Thin-layer chromatography (*2.2.27*).

Test solution To 0.6 g of the powdered herbal drug (180) (*2.9.12*) add 15 mL of *0.05 M sulfuric acid*, shake for 15 min

and filter. Wash the filter with *0.05 M sulfuric acid* until 20 mL of filtrate is obtained. To the filtrate add 1 mL of *concentrated ammonia R* and shake with 2 quantities, each of 10 mL, of *peroxide-free ether R*. If necessary, separate by centrifugation. Dry the combined ether layers over *anhydrous sodium sulfate R*, filter and evaporate to dryness on a water-bath. Dissolve the residue in 0.5 mL of *methanol R*.

Reference solution Dissolve 50 mg of *hyoscyamine sulfate R* in 9 mL of *methanol R*. Dissolve 15 mg of *hyoscine hydrobromide R* in 10 mL of *methanol R*. Mix 1.8 mL of the hyoscine hydrobromide solution and 8 mL of the hyoscyamine sulfate solution.

Plate TLC silica gel G plate R.

Mobile phase concentrated ammonia R, water R, acetone R (3:7:90 V/V/V).

Application 10 µL and 20 µL, as bands of 20 mm by 3 mm, leaving 1 cm between the bands.

Development Over a path of 10 cm.

Drying At 100-105 °C for 15 min; allow to cool.

Detection A Spray with *potassium iodobismuthate solution R2*, using about 10 mL for a plate 200 mm square, until the orange or brown zones become visible against a yellow background.

Results A The zones in the chromatograms obtained with the test solution are similar in position (hyoscyamine in the lower third, hyoscine in the upper third of the chromatograms) and colour to the bands in the chromatograms obtained with the reference solution. The zones in the chromatograms obtained with the test solution are at least equal in size to the corresponding zones in the chromatogram obtained with the same volume of the reference solution. Faint secondary zones may appear, particularly in the middle of the chromatogram obtained with 20 µL of the test solution or near the starting point in the chromatogram obtained with 10 µL of the test solution.

Detection B Spray with *sodium nitrite solution R* until the coating is transparent; examine after 15 min.

Results B The zones due to hyoscyamine in the chromatograms obtained with the reference solution and the test solution change from brown to reddish-brown but not to greyish-blue (atropine) and any secondary zones disappear.

Foreign matter (*2.8.2*)
Maximum 3 per cent of stems with a diameter greater than 5 mm.

Total ash (*2.4.16*)
Maximum 16.0 per cent.

Ash insoluble in hydrochloric acid (*2.8.1*)
Maximum 4.0 per cent.

ASSAY
a) Determine the loss on drying (*2.2.32*) on 2.000 g of the powdered herbal drug (180) (*2.9.12*), by drying in an oven at 105 °C.

b) Moisten 10.00 g of the powdered herbal drug (180) (*2.9.12*) with a mixture of 5 mL of *ammonia R*, 10 mL of *ethanol (96 per cent) R* and 30 mL of *peroxide-free ether R* and mix thoroughly. Transfer the mixture to a suitable percolator, if necessary with the aid of the extracting mixture. Allow to macerate for 4 h and percolate with a mixture of 1 volume of *chloroform R* and 3 volumes of *peroxide-free ether R* until the alkaloids are completely extracted. Evaporate to dryness a few millilitres of the liquid flowing from the percolator, dissolve the residue in *0.25 M sulfuric acid* and verify the absence of alkaloids using *potassium tetraiodomercurate* solution R. Concentrate the percolate to about 50 mL by distilling on a water-bath and transfer it to a separating funnel, rinsing with *peroxide-free ether R*. Add a quantity of *peroxide-free ether R* equal to at least 2.1 times the volume of the percolate to produce a liquid of a density well below that of water. Shake the solution with no fewer than 3 quantities, each of 20 mL, of *0.25 M sulfuric acid*, separate the 2 layers by centrifugation if necessary and transfer the acid layers to a 2nd separating funnel. Make the acid layer alkaline with *ammonia R* and shake with 3 quantities, each of 30 mL, of *chloroform R*. Combine the chloroform layers, add 4 g of *anhydrous sodium sulfate R* and allow to stand for 30 min with occasional shaking. Decant the chloroform and wash the sodium sulfate with 3 quantities, each of 10 mL, of *chloroform R*. Add the washings to the chloroform extract, evaporate to dryness on a water-bath and heat in an oven at 100-105 °C for 15 min. Dissolve the residue in a few millilitres of *chloroform R*, add 20.0 mL of *0.01 M sulfuric acid* and remove the chloroform by evaporation on a water-bath. Titrate the excess of acid with *0.02 M sodium hydroxide* using *methyl red mixed solution R* as indicator.

Calculate the percentage content of total alkaloids, expressed as hyoscyamine, using the following expression:

$$\frac{57.88 \times (20 - n)}{(100 - d) \times m}$$

d = loss on drying, as a percentage;

n = volume of *0.02 M sodium hydroxide*, in millilitres;

m = mass of the powdered herbal drug, in grams.

Ph Eur

Prepared Belladonna

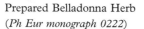

Prepared Belladonna Herb

(*Ph Eur monograph 0222*)

Ph Eur

DEFINITION
Belladonna leaf powder (180) (*2.9.12*) adjusted, if necessary, by adding powdered lactose or belladonna leaf powder with a lower alkaloidal content.

Content
0.28 per cent to 0.32 per cent of total alkaloids, expressed as hyoscyamine (M_r 289.4) (dried drug).

CHARACTERS
Slightly nauseous odour.

IDENTIFICATION
A. The powder is dark green. Examine under a microscope, using *chloral hydrate solution R*. The powder shows the following diagnostic characters: fragments of leaf lamina showing sinuous-walled epidermal cells, a striated cuticle and numerous stomata predominantly present on the lower epidermis (anisocytic and also some anomocytic) (*2.8.3*); multicellular uniseriate covering trichomes with smooth cuticle, glandular trichomes with unicellular heads and multicellular, uniseriate stalks or with multicellular heads and unicellular stalks; parenchyma cells including rounded cells containing microsphenoidal crystals of calcium oxalate; annular and spirally thickened vessels. The powdered drug may also show the following: fibres and reticulately thickened vessels from the stems; subspherical pollen grains, 40-50 μm in diameter, with 3 germinal pores, 3 furrows and an

extensively pitted exine; fragments of the corolla, with a papillose epidermis or bearing numerous covering or glandular trichomes of the types previously described; brownish-yellow seed fragments containing irregularly sclerified and pitted cells of the testa. Examined in *glycerol (85 per cent) R*, the powder may be seen to contain lactose crystals.

B. Shake 1 g with 10 mL of *0.05 M sulfuric acid* for 2 min. Filter and add to the filtrate 1 mL of *concentrated ammonia R* and 5 mL of *water R*. Shake cautiously with 15 mL of *ether R*, avoiding formation of an emulsion. Separate the ether layer and dry over *anhydrous sodium sulfate R*. Filter and evaporate the ether in a porcelain dish. Add 0.5 mL of *fuming nitric acid R* and evaporate to dryness on a water-bath. Add 10 mL of *acetone R* and, dropwise, a 30 g/L solution of *potassium hydroxide R* in *ethanol (96 per cent) R*. A deep violet colour develops.

C. Examine the chromatograms obtained in the test Chromatography.

Results The principal zones in the chromatograms obtained with the test solution are similar in position, colour and size to the principal zones in the chromatogram obtained with the same volume of the reference solution.

TESTS
Chromatography
Thin-layer chromatography (*2.2.27*).

Test solution To 0.6 g of the drug to be examined add 15 mL of *0.05 M sulfuric acid*, shake for 15 min and filter. Wash the filter with *0.05 M sulfuric acid* until 20 mL of filtrate is obtained. To the filtrate add 1 mL of *concentrated ammonia R* and shake with 2 quantities, each of 10 mL, of *peroxide-free ether R*. If necessary, separate by centrifugation. Dry the combined ether layers over *anhydrous sodium sulfate R*, filter, and evaporate to dryness on a water-bath. Dissolve the residue in 0.5 mL of *methanol R*.

Reference solution Dissolve 50 mg of *hyoscyamine sulfate R* in 9 mL of *methanol R*. Dissolve 15 mg of *hyoscine hydrobromide R* in 10 mL of *methanol R*. Mix 1.8 mL of the hyoscine hydrobromide solution and 8 mL of the hyoscyamine sulfate solution.

Plate *TLC silica gel G plate R*.

Mobile phase *concentrated ammonia R*, *water R*, *acetone R* (3:7:90 *V/V/V*).

Application 10 μL and 20 μL of each solution, as bands of 20 mm by 3 mm, leaving 1 cm between each band.

Development Over a path of 10 cm.

Drying At 100-105 °C for 15 min; allow to cool.

Detection A Spray with *potassium iodobismuthate solution R2*, using about 10 mL for a plate 200 mm square, until orange or brown zones become visible against a yellow background.

Results A The zones in the chromatograms obtained with the test solution are similar in position (hyoscyamine in the lower third, hyoscine in the upper third) and colour to those in the chromatograms obtained with the reference solution; the zones in the chromatograms obtained with the test solution are at least equal in size to the corresponding zones in the chromatogram obtained with the same volume of the reference solution; faint secondary zones may appear, particularly in the middle of the chromatogram obtained with 20 μL of the test solution or near the point of application in the chromatogram obtained with 10 μL of the test solution.

Detection B Spray with *sodium nitrite solution R* until the coating is transparent and examine after 15 min.

Results B The zones due to hyoscyamine in the chromatograms obtained with the test solution and the reference solution change from brown to reddish-brown but not to greyish-blue (atropine), and any secondary zones disappear.

Loss on drying (*2.2.32*)
Maximum 5.0 per cent, determined on 1.000 g by drying in an oven at 105 °C.

Total ash (*2.4.16*)
Maximum 16.0 per cent.

Ash insoluble in hydrochloric acid (*2.8.1*)
Maximum 4.0 per cent.

ASSAY
a) Determine the loss on drying (*2.2.32*) on 2.000 g by drying in an oven at 105 °C.

b) Moisten 10.00 g with a mixture of 5 mL of *ammonia R*, 10 mL of *ethanol (96 per cent) R* and 30 mL of *peroxide-free ether R* and mix thoroughly. Transfer the mixture to a suitable percolator, if necessary with the aid of the extracting mixture. Allow to macerate for 4 h and percolate with a mixture of 1 volume of *chloroform R* and 3 volumes of *peroxide-free ether R* until the alkaloids are completely extracted. Evaporate to dryness a few millilitres of the liquid flowing from the percolator, dissolve the residue in *0.25 M sulfuric acid* and verify the absence of alkaloids using *potassium tetraiodomercurate solution R*. Concentrate the percolate to about 50 mL by distilling on a water-bath and transfer it to a separating funnel, rinsing with *peroxide-free ether R*. Add a quantity of *peroxide-free ether R* equal to at least 2.1 times the volume of the percolate to produce a liquid of a density well below that of water. Shake the solution with no fewer than 3 quantities, each of 20 mL, of *0.25 M sulfuric acid*, separate the 2 layers by centrifugation if necessary and transfer the acid layers to a 2nd separating funnel. Make the acid layer alkaline with *ammonia R* and shake with 3 quantities, each of 30 mL, of *chloroform R*. Combine the chloroform layers, add 4 g of *anhydrous sodium sulfate R* and allow to stand for 30 min with occasional shaking. Decant the chloroform and wash the sodium sulfate with 3 quantities, each of 10 mL, of *chloroform R*. Add the washings to the chloroform extract, evaporate to dryness on a water-bath and heat in an oven at 100-105 °C for 15 min. Dissolve the residue in a few millilitres of *chloroform R*, add 20.0 mL of *0.01 M sulfuric acid* and remove the chloroform by evaporation on a water-bath. Titrate the excess of acid with *0.02 M sodium hydroxide* using *methyl red mixed solution R* as indicator.

Calculate the percentage content of total alkaloids, expressed as hyoscyamine, using the following expression:

$$\frac{57.88 \times (20 - n)}{(100 - d) \times m}$$

d = loss on drying as a percentage;
n = volume of *0.02 M sodium hydroxide* used, in millilitres;
m = mass of drug used, in grams.

STORAGE
In an airtight container.

_____ *Ph Eur*

Standardised Belladonna Leaf Dry Extract

(*Ph Eur monograph 1294*)

Ph Eur _____

DEFINITION
Standardised dry extract obtained from *Belladonna leaf (0221)*.

Content
0.95 per cent to 1.05 per cent of total alkaloids, expressed as hyoscyamine ($C_{17}H_{23}NO_3$; M_r 289.4) (dried extract).

PRODUCTION
The extract is produced from the herbal drug by a suitable procedure using ethanol (70 per cent *V/V*).

CHARACTERS
Appearance
Brown or greenish, hygroscopic powder.

IDENTIFICATION
A. Thin-layer chromatography (*2.2.27*).

Test solution To 1 g of the extract to be examined add 5.0 mL of *methanol R*. Shake for 2 min and filter.

Reference solution Dissolve 1.0 mg of *chlorogenic acid R* and 2.5 mg of *rutin R* in 10 mL of *methanol R*.

Plate TLC silica gel plate R.

Mobile phase anhydrous formic acid R, water R, methyl ethyl ketone R, ethyl acetate R (10:10:30:50 *V/V/V/V*).

Application 20 μL as bands.

Development Over a path of 15 cm.

Drying At 100-105 °C.

Detection Spray the warm plate with a 10 g/L solution of *diphenylboric acid aminoethyl ester R* in *methanol R*, then spray with a 50 g/L solution of *macrogol 400 R* in *methanol R*; allow to dry in air for 30 min and examine in ultraviolet light at 365 nm.

Results The chromatograms obtained with the reference solution and the test solution show in the central part a light blue fluorescent zone (chlorogenic acid) and in the lower part a yellowish-brown fluorescent zone (rutin); furthermore, the chromatogram obtained with the test solution shows a little above the start a yellowish-brown fluorescent zone and directly above that a yellow fluorescent zone, and a yellow or yellowish-brown fluorescent zone between the zone due to rutin and the zone due to chlorogenic acid. Further zones may be present.

B. Examine the chromatograms obtained in the test for atropine.

Results The principal zones in the chromatogram obtained with the test solution are similar in position and colour to the principal zones in the chromatogram obtained with the reference solution.

TESTS
Atropine
Thin-layer chromatography (*2.2.27*).

Test solution To 0.20 g of the extract to be examined add 10.0 mL of *0.05 M sulfuric acid*, shake for 2 min and filter. Add 1.0 mL of *concentrated ammonia R* and shake with 2 quantities, each of 10 mL, of *peroxide-free ether R*. If necessary, separate by centrifugation. Dry the combined ether layers over about 2 g of *anhydrous sodium sulfate R*, filter and evaporate to dryness on a water-bath. Dissolve the residue in 0.5 mL of *methanol R*.

HERBAL DRUGS

Reference solution   Dissolve 50 mg of *hyoscyamine sulfate R* in 9 mL of *methanol R*. Dissolve 15 mg of *hyoscine hydrobromide R* in 10 mL of *methanol R*. Mix 1.8 mL of the hyoscine hydrobromide solution and 8 mL of the hyoscyamine sulfate solution.

Plate   TLC silica gel plate R.

Mobile phase   concentrated ammonia R, water R, acetone R (3:7:90 V/V/V).

Application   20 μL as bands.

Development   Over a path of 10 cm.

Drying   At 100-105 °C for 15 min; allow to cool.

Detection A   Spray with *potassium iodobismuthate solution R2*, until orange or brown zones become visible against a yellow background.

Results A   The zones in the chromatogram obtained with the test solution are similar in position (hyoscyamine in the lower third, hyoscine in the upper third) and colour to those in the chromatogram obtained with the reference solution. Other faint zones may be present in the chromatogram obtained with the test solution.

Detection B   Spray with *sodium nitrite solution R* until the coating is transparent and examine after 15 min.

Results B   The zones due to hyoscyamine in the chromatograms obtained with the test solution and the reference solution change from orange or brown to reddish-brown but not to greyish-blue (atropine).

Loss on drying (*2.8.17*)
Maximum 5.0 per cent.

Microbial contamination
TAMC: acceptance criterion 10^4 CFU/g (*2.6.12*).
TYMC: acceptance criterion 10^2 CFU/g (*2.6.12*).
Absence of *Escherichia coli* (*2.6.13*).
Absence of *Salmonella* (*2.6.13*).

ASSAY
At each extraction stage it is necessary to check that the alkaloids have been completely extracted. If the extraction is into the organic phase this is done by evaporating to dryness a few millilitres of the last organic layer, dissolving the residue in *0.25 M sulfuric acid* and verifying the absence of alkaloids using *potassium tetraiodomercurate solution R*. If the extraction is into the acid aqueous phase, this is done by taking a few millilitres of the last acid aqueous phase and verifying the absence of alkaloids using *potassium tetraiodomercurate solution R*.

Disperse 3.00 g in a mixture of 5 mL of *ammonia R* and 15 mL of *water R*. Shake with no fewer than 3 quantities, each of 40 mL, of a mixture of 1 volume of *methylene chloride R* and 3 volumes of *peroxide-free ether R* until the alkaloids are completely extracted. Concentrate the combined organic layers to about 50 mL by distilling on a water-bath and transfer the resulting liquid to a separating funnel, rinsing with *peroxide-free ether R*. Add a quantity of *peroxide-free ether R* equal to at least 2.1 times the volume of the liquid to produce a layer having a density well below that of water. Shake the resulting solution with no fewer than 3 quantities, each of 20 mL, of *0.25 M sulfuric acid* until the alkaloids are completely extracted. Separate the layers by centrifugation, if necessary, and transfer the acid layers to a 2nd separating funnel. Make the combined acid layers alkaline with *ammonia R* and shake with no fewer than 3 quantities, each of 30 mL, of *methylene chloride R* until the alkaloids are completely extracted. Combine the organic layers, add 4 g of *anhydrous sodium sulfate R* and allow to stand for 30 min with occasional shaking. Decant the methylene chloride and wash the sodium sulfate with 3 quantities, each of 10 mL, of *methylene chloride R*. Combine the organic extracts and evaporate to dryness on a water-bath. Heat the residue in an oven at 100-105 °C for 15 min. Dissolve the residue in a few millilitres of *methylene chloride R*, evaporate to dryness on a water-bath and again heat the residue in an oven at 100-105 °C for 15 min. Dissolve the residue in a few millilitres of *methylene chloride R*, add 20.0 mL of *0.01 M sulfuric acid* and remove the methylene chloride by evaporation on a water-bath. Titrate the excess of acid with *0.02 M sodium hydroxide* using *methyl red mixed solution R* as indicator.

Calculate the percentage content of total alkaloids, expressed as hyoscyamine, using the following expression:

$$\frac{57.88 \times (20 - n)}{100 \times m}$$

n = volume of *0.02 M sodium hydroxide* used, in millilitres;
m = mass of drug used, in grams.

Ph Eur

Belladonna Tincture

(Standardised Belladonna Leaf Tincture, Ph Eur monograph 1812)

Ph Eur

DEFINITION
Tincture produced from *Belladonna leaf (0221)*.

Content
0.027 per cent to 0.033 per cent of total alkaloids, calculated as hyoscyamine ($C_{17}H_{23}NO_3$; M_r 289.4). The alkaloids consist mainly of hyoscyamine together with small quantities of hyoscine.

PRODUCTION
The tincture is produced from 1 part of the powdered drug (355) (*2.9.12*) and 10 parts of ethanol (70 per cent V/V) by a suitable procedure.

IDENTIFICATION
A. Thin-layer chromatography (*2.2.27*).

Test solution   Evaporate to dryness 10.0 mL of the tincture to be examined in a water-bath at 40 °C under reduced pressure. Dissolve the residue in 1.0 mL of *methanol R*.

Reference solution   Dissolve 1.0 mg of *chlorogenic acid R* and 2.5 mg of *rutin R* in 10 mL of *methanol R*.

Plate   TLC silica gel plate R.

Mobile phase   anhydrous formic acid R, water R, methyl ethyl ketone R, ethyl acetate R (10:10:30:50 V/V/V/V).

Application   40 μL as bands.

Development   Over a path of 15 cm.

Drying   At 100-105 °C.

Detection   Spray the warm plate with a 10 g/L solution of *diphenylboric acid aminoethyl ester R* in *methanol R*; subsequently spray the plate with a 50 g/L solution of *macrogol 400 R* in *methanol R*; allow the plate to dry in air for 30 min and examine in ultraviolet light at 365 nm.

Results   See below the sequence of zones present in the chromatograms obtained with the reference solution and the

test solution. Furthermore, other fluorescent zones may be present in the chromatogram obtained with the test solution.

Top of the plate	
Chlorogenic acid: a light blue fluorescent zone	A light blue fluorescent zone (chlorogenic acid)
	A yellow or yellowish-brown fluorescent zone
Rutin: a yellowish-brown fluorescent zone	A bluish-grey fluorescent zone
	A yellow fluorescent zone
	A yellowish-brown fluorescent zone
Reference solution	**Test solution**

B. Examine the chromatograms obtained in the test for atropine, detection A.

Results A   See below the sequence of zones present in the chromatograms obtained with the reference solution and the test solution. Faint secondary zones may appear, particularly in the middle of the chromatogram obtained with 40 µL of the test solution or near the point of application in the chromatogram obtained with 20 µL of the test solution.

Top of the plate	
Hyoscine: a brownish-orange zone	A brownish-orange zone (hyoscine)
	Faint secondary zones
Hyoscyamine: a brownish-orange zone	A brownish-orange zone (hyoscyamine)
	Faint secondary zones
Reference solution	**Test solution**

TESTS

Atropine
Thin-layer chromatography (*2.2.27*).

Test solution   To 15.0 mL of the tincture to be examined add 15 mL of *0.05 M sulfuric acid*. Filter. Add 1 mL of *concentrated ammonia R* to the filtrate and shake with 2 quantities, each of 10 mL, of *peroxide-free ether R*. Separate by centrifugation if necessary. Dry the combined ether layers over *anhydrous sodium sulfate R*. Filter and evaporate to dryness on a water-bath. Dissolve the residue in 0.5 mL of *methanol R*.

Reference solution   Dissolve 50 mg of *hyoscyamine sulfate R* in 9 mL of *methanol R*. Dissolve 15 mg of *hyoscine hydrobromide R* in 10 mL of *methanol R*. Mix 1.8 mL of the hyoscine hydrobromide solution and 8 mL of the hyoscyamine sulfate solution.

Plate   TLC silica gel plate R.

Mobile phase   concentrated ammonia R, water R, acetone R (3:7:90 *V/V/V*).

Application   20 µL and 40 µL of each solution, as bands.

Development   Over a path of 10 cm.

Drying   At 100-105 °C for 15 min.

Detection A   Spray with *potassium iodobismuthate solution R2*.

Detection B   Spray with *sodium nitrite solution R* until the plate is transparent. Examine after 15 min.

Results B   The zones due to hyoscyamine in the chromatograms obtained with the test solution and the reference solution change from brownish-orange to reddish-brown but not to greyish-blue (atropine) and any secondary zones disappear.

Ethanol (*2.9.10*)
64 per cent *V/V* to 69 per cent *V/V*.

ASSAY

Evaporate 50.0 g of the tincture to be examined to a volume of about 10 mL. Transfer quantitatively to a separating funnel, with the minimum volume of *alcohol (70 per cent V/V) R*. Add 5 mL of *ammonia R* and 15 mL of *water R*. Shake with not fewer than 3 quantities each of 40 mL of a mixture of 1 volume of *methylene chloride R* and 3 volumes of *peroxide-free ether R*, carefully to avoid emulsion, until the alkaloids are completely extracted. Combine the organic layers and concentrate the solution to a volume of about 50 mL by distilling on a water-bath. Transfer the resulting solution quantitatively to a separating funnel, rinsing with *peroxide-free ether R*. Add a quantity of *peroxide-free ether R* equal to at least 2.1 times the volume of the solution to produce a layer having a density well below that of water. Shake the resulting solution with not fewer than 3 quantities each of 20 mL of *0.25 M sulfuric acid* until the alkaloids are completely extracted. Separate the layers by centrifugation if necessary and transfer the layers to a separating funnel. Make the combined layers alkaline with *ammonia R* and shake with not fewer than 3 quantities each of 30 mL of *methylene chloride R* until the alkaloids are completely extracted. Combine the organic layers, add 4 g of *anhydrous sodium sulfate R* and allow to stand for 30 min with occasional shaking. Decant the methylene chloride and filter. Wash the sodium sulfate with 3 quantities each of 10 mL of *methylene chloride R*. Combine the organic extracts, evaporate to dryness on a water-bath. Heat the residue in an oven at 100-105 °C for 15 min. Dissolve the residue in a few millilitres of *methylene chloride R*, evaporate to dryness on a water-bath and heat the residue in an oven at 100-105 °C for 15 min again. Dissolve the residue in a few millilitres of *methylene chloride R*. Add 20.0 mL of *0.01 M sulfuric acid* and remove the methylene chloride by evaporation on a water-bath. Titrate the excess of acid with *0.02 M sodium hydroxide* using *methyl red mixed solution R* as indicator.

Calculate the percentage content of total alkaloids, expressed as hyoscyamine, using the following expression:

$$\frac{57.88 \times (20 - n)}{100 \times m}$$

n = volume of *0.02 M sodium hydroxide* used, in millilitres,
m = mass of drug used, in grams.

_____ *Ph Eur*

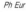

Siam Benzoin

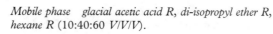

(*Ph Eur monograph 2158*)

Preparation

Siam Benzoin Tincture

Ph Eur _____

DEFINITION

Resin obtained by incising the trunk of *Styrax tonkinensis* (Pierre) Craib ex Hartwich.

Content

45.0 per cent to 55.0 per cent of total acids, calculated as benzoic acid ($C_7H_6O_2$; M_r 122.1) (dried drug).

CHARACTERS

Characteristic odour of vanillin.

IDENTIFICATION

A. Siam benzoin occurs as opaque, granular, rounded or ovoid masses (tears), varying in size from a few millimeters up to 3 cm, separated or sometimes agglomerated together by a reddish-brown, transparent resin. Individual tears are yellowish-white to reddish externally with a waxy, whitish fracture which becomes reddish on exposure to air.

B. Examine the chromatograms obtained in test B for *Styrax benzoin*.

Results See below the sequence of the zones present in the chromatograms obtained with the reference solution and the test solution. Furthermore, other faint fluorescent zones may be present in the chromatogram obtained with the test solution.

Top of the plate	
Methyl cinnamate: a very prominent quenching zone	
Benzoic acid: a quenching zone	A quenching zone (benzoic acid)
Cinnamic acid: a prominent quenching zone	
	A quenching zone
	A very prominent quenching zone
Vanillin: a quenching zone	A quenching zone (vanillin)
	Series of unresolved zones including a quenching zone
Reference solution	**Test solution**

TESTS

Styrax benzoin

A. To 0.2 g of the finely powdered drug add 10 mL of *ethanol (96 per cent) R*. Shake vigorously until almost completely dissolved and filter. Place 5 mL of the filtrate in a test-tube and add 0.5 mL of a 50 g/L solution of *ferric chloride R* in *ethanol (96 per cent) R*. A green colour is produced. No yellow colour is produced.

B. Thin-layer chromatography (*2.2.27*).

Test solution Sonicate 0.2 g of the finely powdered drug in 5 mL of *ethanol (96 per cent) R* and filter. Collect the filtrate.

Reference solution Dissolve 20 mg of *benzoic acid R*, 10 mg of *trans-cinnamic acid R*, 4 mg of *vanillin R* and 20 mg of *methyl cinnamate R* in 10 mL of *ethanol (96 per cent) R*.

Plate TLC silica gel F_{254} plate R.

Mobile phase glacial acetic acid R, di-isopropyl ether R, hexane R (10:40:60 *V/V/V*).

Application 10 µL as bands.

Development Over a path of 12 cm.

Drying In air.

Detection Examine in ultraviolet light at 254 nm.

Results The chromatogram obtained with the test solution shows no zone in the same position as the zone due to cinnamic acid in the chromatogram obtained with the reference solution.

Matter insoluble in ethanol

Maximum 5 per cent.

To 2 g of the powdered drug add 25 mL of *ethanol (90 per cent V/V) R*. Boil until almost completely dissolved. Filter through a previously tared sintered-glass filter (16) (*2.1.2*) and wash with 3 quantities, each of 5 mL, of boiling *ethanol (90 per cent V/V) R*. Heat the glass filter and its contents in an oven at 100-105 °C for 2 h. Weigh after cooling.

Loss on drying (*2.2.32*)

Maximum 5.0 per cent, determined on 2.00 g of the coarsely powdered drug by drying *in vacuo* for 4 h.

Total ash (*2.4.16*)

Maximum 2.0 per cent.

ASSAY

Place 0.750 g of the finely powdered drug in a 250 mL borosilicate glass flask and add 15.0 mL of *0.5 M alcoholic potassium hydroxide*. Boil under a reflux condenser on a water-bath for 30 min. Allow to cool and rinse the condenser with 20 mL of *ethanol (96 per cent) R*. Titrate the excess of potassium hydroxide with *0.5 M hydrochloric acid*. Determine the end-point potentiometrically (*2.2.20*). Carry out a blank titration.

1 mL of *0.5 M alcoholic potassium hydroxide* is equivalent to 61.05 mg of benzoic acid ($C_7H_6O_2$).

_____ *Ph Eur*

Siam Benzoin Tincture

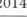

(*Ph Eur monograph 2157*

Ph Eur _____

DEFINITION

Tincture produced from *Siam benzoin (2158)*.

Content

Minimum 5.0 per cent m/m of total acids, calculated as benzoic acid ($C_7H_6O_2$; M_r 122.1).

PRODUCTION

The tincture is produced from 1 part of the drug and 5 parts of ethanol (75 per cent *V/V* to 96 per cent *V/V*) by a suitable procedure.

CHARACTERS

Appearance

Orange-yellow liquid.

It has a characteristic odour of vanillin.

IDENTIFICATION

A. Place 10 mL in a test tube; add 0.5 mL of a 50 g/L solution of *ferric chloride R* in *ethanol (96 per cent) R*. A green colour is produced.

B. Examine the chromatograms obtained in the test for Sumatra benzoin tincture.

Results   See below the sequence of the zones present in the chromatograms obtained with the reference solution and the test solution. Furthermore, other faint fluorescent zones may be present in the chromatogram obtained with the test solution.

Top of the plate	
Methyl cinnamate: a very prominent quenching zone Benzoic acid: a quenching zone Cinnamic acid: a prominent quenching zone	A quenching zone (benzoic acid)
	A quenching zone
	A very prominent quenching zone
Vanillin: a quenching zone	A quenching zone (vanillin)
	Series of unresolved zones including a quenching zone
Reference solution	**Test solution**

TESTS
Sumatra benzoin tincture
Thin-layer chromatography (*2.2.27*).

Test solution   The tincture to be examined.

Reference solution   Dissolve 20 mg of *benzoic acid R*, 10 mg of *trans-cinnamic acid R*, 4 mg of *vanillin R* and 20 mg of *methyl cinnamate R* in 20 mL of ethanol of the same concentration as that used for the production of the tincture.

Plate   TLC silica gel F_{254} *plate R* (5-40 μm) [or *TLC silica gel* F_{254} *plate R* (2-10 μm)].

Mobile phase   glacial acetic acid R, di-isopropyl ether R, hexane R (10:40:60 *V/V/V*).

Application   20 μL [or 8 μL] as bands.

Development   Over a path of 12 cm [or 6 cm].

Drying   In air.

Detection   Examine in ultraviolet light at 254 nm.

Results   The chromatogram obtained with the test solution does not show any zone in the same position as the zones due to cinnamic acid and methyl cinnamate in the chromatogram obtained with the reference solution.

Ethanol (*2.9.10*)
95 per cent to 105 per cent of the content stated on the label.

ASSAY
Place 3.50 g in a 250 mL borosilicate glass flask and add 15.0 mL of *0.5 M alcoholic potassium hydroxide*. Boil under a reflux condenser on a water-bath for 30 min. Allow to cool and rinse the condenser with 20 mL of *ethanol (96 per cent) R*. Titrate the excess of potassium hydroxide with *1 M hydrochloric acid*, determining the end-point potentiometrically (*2.2.20*). Carry out a blank titration.

1 mL of *0.5 M alcoholic potassium hydroxide* is equivalent to 61.05 mg of benzoic acid ($C_7H_6O_2$).

———————— Ph Eur

Sumatra Benzoin

(*Ph Eur monograph 1814*)

Benzoin

Preparations

Benzoin Inhalation

Compound Benzoin Tincture

Sumatra Benzoin Tincture

Ph Eur ——————————————————————

DEFINITION
Resin obtained by incising the trunk of *Styrax benzoin* Dryander.

Content
25.0 per cent to 50.0 per cent of total acids, calculated as benzoic acid ($C_7H_6O_2$; M_r 122.1) (dried drug).

IDENTIFICATION
A. Sumatra benzoin occurs as creamy white, rounded to ovoid tears, which may be embedded in a dull greyish-brown or reddish-brown matrix. It is hard and brittle and the fractured surface is dull and uneven.

B. Examine the chromatograms obtained in test B for *Styrax tonkinensis*.

Results   See below the sequence of quenching zones present in the chromatograms obtained with the reference solution and the test solution. Furthermore, other faint quenching zones may be present in the chromatogram obtained with the test solution.

Top of the plate	
	A very intense dark zone
Methyl cinnamate: a very intense dark zone Benzoic acid: a dark zone Cinnamic acid: an intense dark zone	A dark zone
	A very weak dark zone (benzoic acid)
	A very intense dark zone (cinnamic acid)
	A dark zone
	A very intense dark zone
	A dark zone
Vanillin: a dark zone	A very weak dark zone (vanillin)
	Series of unresolved zones including 2 dark zones
Reference solution	**Test solution**

TESTS
Dammar gum
Thin-layer chromatography (*2.2.27*).

Test solution   Dissolve 0.2 g of the drug to be examined with gentle heating in 10 mL of *ethanol (90 per cent V/V) R* and centrifuge.

Plate   TLC aluminium oxide G plate R.

Mobile phase   Light petroleum R4, ether R (40:60 *V/V*).

Application   5 μL.

Development   Over a path of 10 cm.

Drying   In air.

Detection Spray with *anisaldehyde solution R* and heat at 100-105 °C for 5 min.

Results The chromatogram obtained does not show any prominent spot with an RF between 0.4 and 1.0.

Styrax tonkinensis

A. To 0.2 g of the finely powdered drug add 10 mL of *ethanol (96 per cent) R*. Shake vigorously until almost completely dissolved and filter. Place 5 mL of the filtrate in a test-tube and add 0.5 mL of a 50 g/L solution of *ferric chloride R* in *ethanol (96 per cent) R*. A yellowish, slightly green colour is produced.

B. Thin-layer chromatography (2.2.27).

Test solution Sonicate 0.2 g of the finely powdered drug in 5 mL of *ethanol (96 per cent) R* and filter. Collect the filtrate.

Reference solution Dissolve 20 mg of *benzoic acid R*, 10 mg of *trans-cinnamic acid R*, 4 mg of *vanillin R* and 20 mg of *methyl cinnamate R* in 10 mL of *ethanol (96 per cent) R*.

Plate TLC silica gel F_{254} plate R (5-40 µm) [or *TLC silica gel* F_{254} plate R (2-10 µm)].

Mobile phase glacial acetic acid R, di-isopropyl ether R, hexane R (10:40:60 *V/V/V*).

Application 10 µL [or 2 µL] as bands.

Development Over a path of 12 cm [or 5 cm].

Drying In air.

Detection Examine in ultraviolet light at 254 nm.

Results The chromatogram obtained with the test solution shows 2 faint zones in the same positions as the dark zones due to benzoic acid and vanillin in the chromatogram obtained with the reference solution.

Matter insoluble in ethanol

Maximum 20.0 per cent.

To 2.0 g of the powdered drug add 25 mL of *ethanol (90 per cent V/V) R*. Boil until almost completely dissolved. Filter through a tared sintered-glass filter (16) (2.1.2) and wash with 3 quantities, each of 5 mL, of boiling *ethanol (90 per cent V/V) R*. Heat the glass filter and its contents in an oven at 100-105 °C for 2 h. Allow to cool and weigh.

Loss on drying (2.2.32)

Maximum 5.0 per cent, determined on 2.000 g of the coarsely powdered drug by drying *in vacuo* for 4 h.

Total ash (2.4.16)

Maximum 2.0 per cent.

ASSAY

Place 0.750 g of the finely powdered drug in a 250 mL borosilicate glass flask and add 15.0 mL of *0.5 M alcoholic potassium hydroxide*. Boil under a reflux condenser on a water-bath for 30 min. Allow to cool and rinse the condenser with 20 mL of *ethanol (96 per cent) R*. Titrate the excess of potassium hydroxide with *0.5 M hydrochloric acid*, determining the end-point potentiometrically (2.2.20). Carry out a blank titration.

1 mL of *0.5 M alcoholic potassium hydroxide* is equivalent to 61.05 mg of benzoic acid ($C_7H_6O_2$).

————————————————— Ph Eur

Sumatra Benzoin Tincture

(Ph Eur monograph 1813)

Ph Eur —————————————————

DEFINITION

Tincture produced from *Sumatra benzoin (1814)*.

Content

Minimum 4.0 per cent *m/m* of total acids, calculated as benzoic acid ($C_7H_6O_2$; M_r 122.1).

PRODUCTION

The tincture is produced from 1 part of the drug and 5 parts of ethanol (75 per cent *V/V* to 96 per cent *V/V*) by a suitable procedure.

CHARACTERS

Appearance

Orange-yellow liquid.

IDENTIFICATION

Examine the chromatograms obtained in the test for Siam benzoin tincture.

Results See below the sequence of quenching zones present in the chromatograms obtained with the reference solution and the test solution. Furthermore, other faint quenching zones may be present in the chromatogram obtained with the test solution.

Top of the plate	
	A very intense dark zone
_____	_____
Methyl cinnamate: a very intense dark zone	A dark zone
Benzoic acid: a dark zone	A very weak dark zone (benzoic acid)
Cinnamic acid: an intense dark zone	A very intense dark zone (cinnamic acid)
_____	_____
	A dark zone
	A very intense dark zone
	A dark zone
Vanillin: a dark zone	A very weak dark zone (vanillin)
	Series of unresolved dark zones
Reference solution	**Test solution**

TESTS

Siam benzoin tincture

Thin-layer chromatography (2.2.27).

Test solution The tincture to be examined.

Reference solution Dissolve 20 mg of *benzoic acid R*, 10 mg of *trans-cinnamic acid R*, 4 mg of *vanillin R* and 20 mg of *methyl cinnamate R* in 20 mL of ethanol of the same concentration as that used for the production of the tincture.

Plate TLC silica gel F_{254} plate R (5-40 µm) [or *TLC silica gel* F_{254} plate R (2-10 µm)].

Mobile phase glacial acetic acid R, di-isopropyl ether R, hexane R (10:40:60 *V/V/V*).

Application 20 µL [or 8 µL] as bands.

Development Over a path of 12 cm [or 6 cm].

Drying In air.

Detection Examine in ultraviolet light at 254 nm.

Results   The chromatogram obtained with the test solution does not show zones due to benzoic acid and vanillin that are more intense than the corresponding zones in the chromatogram obtained with the reference solution.

Ethanol (*2.9.10*)
95 per cent to 105 per cent of the content stated on the label.

ASSAY
Place 3.50 g in a 250 mL borosilicate glass flask and add 15.0 mL of *0.5 M alcoholic potassium hydroxide*. Boil under a reflux condenser on a water-bath for 30 min. Allow to cool and rinse the condenser with 20 mL of *ethanol (96 per cent) R*. Titrate the excess of potassium hydroxide with *1 M hydrochloric acid*, determining the end-point potentiometrically (*2.2.20*). Carry out a blank titration.

1 mL of *0.5 M alcoholic potassium hydroxide* is equivalent to 61.05 mg of benzoic acid ($C_7H_6O_2$).

_____ *Ph Eur*

Compound Benzoin Tincture
Friars' Balsam

DEFINITION

Barbados Aloes or Cape Aloes	20 g
Prepared storax of commerce	100 g
Sumatra Benzoin crushed	100 g
Ethanol (90 per cent)	Sufficient to produce 1000 mL

Extemporaneous preparation
The following directions apply.

Macerate the Barbados Aloes or Cape Aloes, the prepared storax and the Sumatra Benzoin with 800 mL of Ethanol (90 per cent) in a closed vessel for not less than 2 days, shaking occasionally, filter and pass sufficient Ethanol (90 per cent) through the filter to produce 1000 mL.

The tincture complies with the requirements for Tinctures stated under Extracts and with the following requirements.

Content of total balsamic acids
Not less than 4.5% w/v, calculated as cinnamic acid, $C_9H_8O_2$.

TESTS
Ethanol content
70 to 76% v/v, Appendix VIII F, Method III.

Dry residue
15 to 19% w/w.

Relative density
0.880 to 0.910, Appendix V G.

ASSAY
Carry out the Assay described under Benzoin Inhalation using 10 mL of the tincture. Each mL of 0.1M *sodium hydroxide VS* is equivalent to 14.82 mg of total balsamic acids, calculated as cinnamic acid, $C_9H_8O_2$.

Benzoin Inhalation
Benzoin Inhalation Vapour

DEFINITION
Benzoin Inhalation is an *inhalation vapour, solution*.

Sumatra Benzoin crushed	100 g
Prepared storax of commerce	50 g
Ethanol (96 per cent)	Sufficient to produce 1000 mL

In making Benzoin Inhalation, Ethanol (96 per cent) may be replaced by Industrial Methylated Spirit[1].

Extemporaneous preparation
The following directions apply.

Macerate the crushed Sumatra Benzoin and the prepared storax with 750 mL of Ethanol (96 per cent) for 24 hours. Filter and pass sufficient Ethanol (96 per cent) through the filter to produce 1000 mL.

The inhalation complies with the requirements stated under Preparations for Inhalation and with the following requirements.

Content of total balsamic acids
Not less than 3.0% w/v, calculated as cinnamic acid, $C_9H_8O_2$.

Total solids
9.0 to 12.0% w/v when determined by drying at 105° for 4 hours, Appendix XI A. Use 2 mL.

ASSAY
Boil 10 mL with 25 mL of 0.5M *ethanolic potassium hydroxide* under a reflux condenser for 1 hour. Evaporate the ethanol, disperse the residue in 50 mL of hot *water*, cool, add 80 mL of *water* and 1.5 g of *magnesium sulfate* dissolved in 50 mL of *water*. Mix thoroughly and allow to stand for 10 minutes. Filter, wash the residue on the filter with 20 mL of *water*, acidify the combined filtrate and washings with *hydrochloric acid* and extract with four 40-mL quantities of *ether*. Discard the aqueous solution, combine the ether extracts and extract with successive quantities of 20, 20, 10, 10 and 10 mL of *sodium hydrogen carbonate solution*, washing each aqueous extract with the same 20 mL of *ether*. Discard the ether layers, carefully acidify the combined aqueous extracts with *hydrochloric acid* and extract with successive quantities of 30, 20, 20 and 10 mL of *chloroform*, filtering each extract through *anhydrous sodium sulfate* supported on absorbent cotton. Distil the chloroform from the combined filtrates until 10 mL remains and remove the remainder in a current of air. Dissolve the residue, with the aid of gentle heat, in 10 mL of *ethanol (96%)*, previously neutralised to *phenol red solution*, cool and titrate with 0.1M *sodium hydroxide VS* using *phenol red solution* as indicator. Each mL of 0.1M *sodium hydroxide VS* is equivalent to 14.82 mg of total balsamic acids, calculated as cinnamic acid, $C_9H_8O_2$.

_____
[1] *Statutory regulations governing the use of Industrial Methylated Spirit must be observed.*

Berberis Aristata

DEFINITION

Berberis Aristata is the dried, cut stem of *Berberis aristata* DC.

It contains not less than 1.4% of berberine ($C_{20}H_{19}NO_5$), calculated with reference to the dried material.

IDENTIFICATION

A. The cut pieces of stem are subcylindrical, often branched and somewhat swollen at the nodes, from about 15-20 mm diameter and varying in length. The bark is soft, about 4-8 mm thick, with a yellowish brown outer surface, finely wrinkled longitudinally or deeply furrowed, peeling off in places and exposing the inner dark yellow wood. Fracture short in the region of the bark, hard and fibrous in the wood.

B. Reduce to a powder. The powder is yellowish brown. Examine under a microscope using *chloral hydrate solution*. The powder contains numerous fragments of xylem, the vessels reticulately and spirally thickened, some tracheids; thick-walled, short, spindle-shaped, lignified, yellowish fibres of the phloem and xylem with a wide lumen; stone cells elongated with thick, pitted walls, some containing a single calcium oxalate crystal, normally present in groups; parenchyma cells of the medullary rays, some with yellow-brown contents, single prism crystals of calcium oxalate, or simple starch granules; cork cells yellowish-brown, thin-walled; numerous scattered starch grains and calcium oxalate crystals.

C. Carry out the method for *thin-layer chromatography*, Appendix III A, using the following solutions.

(1) Add 4 mL of *methanol (80%)* to 250 mg of the powdered herbal drug (180) in a centrifuge tube. Mix with the aid of ultrasound for 10 minutes. Centrifuge at 3000 rpm for 5 minutes and collect the clear supernatant. Repeat the extraction twice with a further two 2-mL portions of *methanol (80%)*. Combine the supernatants and dilute to 20 mL with *methanol (80%)*.

(2) 0.04% w/v each of *berberine chloride BPCRS* and *palmatine chloride* in *methanol (80%)*.

CHROMATOGRAPHIC CONDITIONS

(a) Use as the coating *silica gel* F_{254}.

(b) Use the mobile phase as described below.

(c) Apply 20 µL of each solution as 6 mm bands.

(d) Develop the plate to 15 cm.

(e) After removal of the plate, dry in air and examine under *ultraviolet light (254 nm)*.

MOBILE PHASE

10 volumes of *anhydrous formic acid*, 10 volumes of *water* and 80 volumes of *ethyl acetate*.

SYSTEM SUITABILITY

The test is not valid unless the chromatogram obtained with solution (2) shows two clearly separated bands.

CONFIRMATION

The chromatogram obtained with solution (1) shows a principal yellow band corresponding in colour and position to the band obtained for berberine chloride in solution (2), a yellow band corresponding in colour and position to the band obtained for palmatine in solution (2) and several other bands as shown in the table. Other bands may be present.

Top of the plate	
Yellow band (berberine chloride)	Yellow band (berberine chloride)
Faint yellow band	
Yellow band (palmatine)	Yellow band (palmatine)
Purple band	
Solution (1)	**Solution (2)**

TESTS

D-Tetrahydropalmatine

Carry out the method for *liquid chromatography*, Appendix III D, using the following solutions.

(1) To 0.5 g of powdered sample, add 400 mL of a mixture of equal volumes of *acetonitrile* and 0.1% v/v *orthophosphoric acid*. Mix with the aid of ultrasound for 40 minutes and allow to cool. Dilute to 500 mL with the mobile phase and filter through a 0.45-µm filter.

(2) 0.01% w/v each of *palmatine chloride* and *berberine chloride BPCRS* in the mobile phase.

(3) 0.01% w/v of *D-tetrahydropalmatine hydrochloride* in the mobile phase.

CHROMATOGRAPHIC CONDITIONS

(a) Use a stainless steel column (15 cm × 4.6 mm) packed with *end-capped octadecylsilyl silica gel for chromatography* (5 µm) (Phenomenex Luna C18 is suitable).

(b) Use isocratic elution and the mobile phase described below.

(c) Use a flow rate of 1.2 mL per minute.

(d) Use an ambient column temperature.

(e) Use a detection wavelength of 235 nm.

(f) Inject 10 µL of each solution.

When the chromatograms are recorded under the prescribed conditions the retention times relative to palmatine (retention time = about 8 minutes) are berberine chloride = about 1.1; D-tetrahydropalmitine = about 1.6.

MOBILE PHASE

27 volumes of *acetonitrile* and 73 volumes of a 1.36% w/v solution of *potassium dihydrogen orthophosphate*.

SYSTEM SUITABILITY

The test is not valid unless, in the chromatogram obtained with solution (2), the *resolution factor* between the peaks due to palmatine and berberine chloride is at least 2.0.

CONFIRMATION

In the chromatogram obtained with solution (1), there are no peaks corresponding to the peak due to D-tetrahydropalmitine in the chromatogram obtained with solution (3).

Loss on drying

When dried for 2 hours at 105°, loses not more than 10.0% of its weight, Appendix IX D. Use 1 g.

Total Ash

Not more than 3.0%, Appendix XI J, Method II.

ASSAY

Carry out the method for *liquid chromatography*, Appendix III D, using the following solutions.

(1) To 0.5 g of powdered sample, add 400 mL of a mixture of equal volumes of *acetonitrile* and 0.1% v/v *orthophosphoric acid*. Mix with the aid of ultrasound for 40 minutes and allow to cool. Dilute to 500 mL with the mobile phase and filter through a 0.45-μm filter.

(2) 0.01% w/v each of *palmatine chloride* and *berberine chloride BPCRS* in the mobile phase.

CHROMATOGRAPHIC CONDITIONS

The chromatographic conditions described under the test for D-tetrahydropalmatine may be used.

MOBILE PHASE

27 volumes of *acetonitrile* and 73 volumes of a 1.36% w/v solution of *potassium dihydrogen orthophosphate*.

SYSTEM SUITABILITY

The test is not valid unless, in the chromatogram obtained with solution (2), the *resolution factor* between the peaks due to palmatine and berberine chloride is at least 2.0.

DETERMINATION OF CONTENT

Using the retention time and the peak area from the chromatogram obtained with solution (2), locate and integrate the peak due to berberine chloride in the chromatogram obtained with solution (1). Calculate the content of berberine in the sample using the declared content of berberine in *berberine chloride BPCRS* and the following expression:

$$\frac{A_1}{A_2} \times \frac{m_2}{V_2} \times \frac{V_1}{m_1} \times p \times \frac{100}{100 - d}$$

A_1 = area of the peak due to berberine in the chromatogram obtained with solution (1),

A_2 = area of the peak due to berberine in the chromatogram obtained with solution (2),

m_1 = weight of the drug being examined in mg,

m_2 = weight of *berberine chloride BPCRS* in mg,

V_1 = dilution volume of solution (1) in mL,

V_2 = dilution volume of solution (2) in mL,

p = percentage content of berberine in *berberine chloride BPCRS*,

d = percentage loss on drying of the herbal drug being examined.

STORAGE

Berberis Aristata should be protected from moisture.

Dried Bilberry

(*Dried Bilberry Fruit, Ph Eur monograph 1588*)

Ph Eur

DEFINITION

Dried ripe fruit of *Vaccinium myrtillus* L.

Content

Minimum 1.0 per cent of tannins, expressed as pyrogallol ($C_6H_6O_3$; M_r 126.1) (dried drug).

CHARACTERS

Sweet and slightly astringent taste.

IDENTIFICATION

A. Dried bilberry is a dark blue, subglobular, shrunken berry about 5 mm in diameter, with a scar at the lower end and surmounted by the persistent calyx, which appears as a circular fold and the remains of the style. The deep violet, fleshy mesocarp contains numerous small, brown, ovoid seeds.

B. Reduce to a powder (355) (*2.9.12*). The powder is violet-brown. Examine under a microscope using *chloral hydrate solution R*. The powder shows: violet-pink sclereids from the endocarp and the mesocarp, usually aggregated, with thick, channelled walls; reddish-brown fragments of the epicarp consisting of polygonal cells with moderately thickened walls; brownish-yellow fragments of the outer seed testa made up of elongated cells with U-shaped thickened walls; clusters and prisms crystals of various size of calcium oxalate.

C. Thin-layer chromatography (*2.2.27*)

Test solution   To 2 g of the powdered drug (355) (*2.9.12*) add 20 mL of *methanol R*. Shake for 15 min and filter.

Reference solution   Dissolve 5 mg of *chrysanthemin R* in 10 mL of *methanol R*.

Plate   TLC silica gel plate R.

Mobile phase   anhydrous formic acid R, water R, butanol R (16:19:65 *V/V/V*).

Application   10 μL, as bands.

Development   Over a path of 10 cm.

Drying   In air.

Detection   Examine in daylight.

Results   See below the sequence of the zones present in the chromatograms obtained with the reference and test solutions.

Top of the plate	
	A violet-red zone of low intensity
Chrysanthemin: a violet-red zone	A principal violet-red zone
	A compact set of other principal zones:
	— a violet-red zone
	— several violet-blue zones
Reference solution	**Test solution**

TESTS

Loss on drying (*2.2.32*)

Maximum 12.0 per cent, determined on 1.000 g of the powdered drug by drying in an oven at 105 °C for 2 h.

Total ash (*2.4.16*)

Maximum 5.0 per cent.

ASSAY

Carry out the determination of tannins in herbal drugs (*2.8.14*). Use 1.500 g of the powdered drug (355) (*2.9.12*).

_____ *Ph Eur*

Fresh Bilberry

(*Fresh Bilberry Fruit, Ph Eur monograph 1602*)

Preparation
Fresh Bilberry Fruit Dry Extract, Refined and Standardised

Ph Eur _____

DEFINITION
Fresh or frozen, ripe fruit of *Vaccinium myrtillus L.*

Content
Minimum 0.30 per cent of anthocyanins, expressed as cyanidin 3-*O*-glucoside chloride (chrysanthemin, $C_{21}H_{21}ClO_{11}$; M_r 484.8) (dried drug).

CHARACTERS
Sweet and slightly astringent taste.

IDENTIFICATION
A. The fresh fruit is a blackish-blue globular berry about 5 mm in diameter. Its lower end shows a scar or, rarely, a fragment of the pedicel. The upper end is flattened and surmounted by the remains of the persistent style and of the calyx, which appears as a circular fold. The violet, fleshy mesocarp includes 4 to 5 locules containing numerous small, brown, ovoid seeds.

B. The crushed fresh fruit is violet-red. Examine under a microscope using *chloral hydrate solution R*. It shows violet-pink sclereids from the endocarp and the mesocarp, usually aggregated, with thick, channelled walls; reddish-brown fragments of the epicarp consisting of polygonal cells with moderately thickened walls; brownish-yellow fragments of the outer layer of the testa composed of elongated cells with U-shaped thickened walls; cluster crystals of calcium oxalate.

C. Thin-layer chromatography (*2.2.27*).

Test solution To 5 g of the freshly crushed drug, add 20 mL of *methanol R*. Stir for 15 min and filter.

Reference solution Dissolve 5 mg of *chrysanthemin R* in 10 mL of *methanol R*.

Plate TLC silica gel plate R.

Mobile phase anhydrous formic acid R, water R, butanol R (16:19:65 *V/V/V*).

Application 10 µL, as bands.

Development Over a path of 10 cm.

Drying In air.

Detection Examine in daylight.

Results See below the sequence of the zones present in the chromatograms obtained with the reference solution and the test solution.

Top of the plate	
	A violet-red zone
Chrysanthemin: a violet-red zone	A principal violet-red zone
	A compact set of other principal zones:
	– a violet-red zone
	– several violet-blue zones
Reference solution	**Test solution**

TESTS
Total ash (*2.4.16*)
Maximum 0.6 per cent.

Loss on drying (*2.2.32*)
80.0 per cent to 90.0 per cent, determined on 5.000 g of the freshly crushed drug by drying in an oven at 105 °C.

ASSAY
Crush 50 g extemporaneously. To about 5.00 g of the crushed, accurately weighed drug, add 95 mL of *methanol R*. Stir mechanically for 30 min. Filter into a 100.0 mL volumetric flask. Rinse the filter and dilute to 100.0 mL with *methanol R*. Prepare a 50-fold dilution of this solution in a 0.1 per cent *V/V* solution of *hydrochloric acid R* in *methanol R*.

Measure the absorbance (*2.2.25*) of the solution at 528 nm, using a 0.1 per cent *V/V* solution of *hydrochloric acid R* in *methanol R* as the compensation liquid.

Calculate the percentage content of anthocyanins, expressed as cyanidin 3-*O*-glucoside chloride, using the following expression:

$$\frac{A \times 5000}{718 \times m}$$

718 = specific absorbance of cyanidin 3-*O*-glucoside chloride at 528 nm
A = absorbance at 528 nm
m = mass of the substance to be examined in grams.

STORAGE
When frozen, store at or below − 18 °C.

_____ *Ph Eur*

Refined and Standardised Fresh Bilberry Fruit Dry Extract

(*Ph Eur monograph 2394*)

Ph Eur _____

DEFINITION
Refined and standardised dry extract produced from *Bilberry fruit, fresh (1602)*.

Content
32.4 per cent to 39.6 per cent of anthocyanins, expressed as cyanidin 3-*O*-glucoside chloride [chrysanthemin ($C_{21}H_{21}ClO_{11}$; M_r 484.8)] (dried extract).

PRODUCTION
The extract is produced from the herbal drug by a suitable procedure using ethanol (96 per cent *V/V*) or methanol (minimum 60 per cent *V/V*). Refinement may be performed by ion-exchange chromatography.

CHARACTERS
Appearance
Dark reddish-violet, amorphous, hygroscopic powder.

IDENTIFICATION
First identification B.
Second identification A.

A. Thin-layer chromatography (*2.2.27*).

Test solution Dissolve 0.10 g of the extract to be examined in 25 mL of *methanol R*. Stir for 15 min and filter.

Reference solution Dissolve 2 mg of *chrysanthemin R* and 2 mg of *myrtillin R* in 5 mL of *methanol R*.

Plate TLC plate coated with *cellulose for chromatography R* (5-40 µm) [or TLC plate coated with *cellulose for chromatography R* (2-10 µm)].

*Mobile phase: mobile phase A: hydrochloric acid R, acetic
acid R, water R (3:15:82 V/V/V);*

mobile phase B: water R, acetic acid R (40:60 V/V).

Application   10 µL [or 2 µL] as bands of 10 mm [or 6 mm].

Development A   Over a path of 10 cm [or 6 cm] with mobile
phase A.

Drying A   In warm air.

Development B   Over a path of 10 cm [or 6 cm] with mobile
phase B.

Drying B   In air.

Detection   Examine in daylight.

Results   See below the sequence of zones present in the
chromatograms obtained with the reference solution and the
test solution. Furthermore, other faint zones may be present
in the chromatogram obtained with the test solution.

Top of the plate		
———		———
	A violet-red zone	
Chrysanthemin: a violet-red zone	A violet-red zone (chrysanthemin)	
Myrtillin: a violet-red zone	A violet-red zone (myrtillin)	
———		———
Reference solution	**Test solution**	

B. Liquid chromatography (*2.2.29*) as described in the test
for total anthocyanidins.

The characteristic anthocyanin peaks (peaks 1-8, 10-15 and
17) in the chromatogram obtained with the test solution are
similar in their retention times to those in the chromatogram
obtained with reference solution (b).

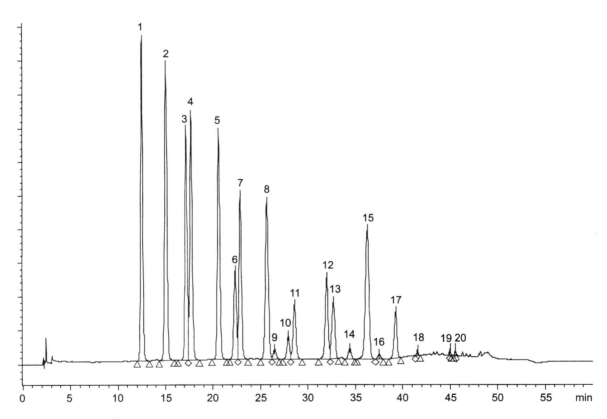

1. delphinidin 3-*O*-galactoside chloride

2. myrtillin (delphinidin 3-*O*-glucoside chloride)

3. cyanidin 3-*O*-galactoside chloride

4. delphinidin 3-*O*-arabinoside chloride

5. chrysanthemin (cyanidin 3-*O*-glucoside chloride)

6. petunidin 3-*O*-galactoside chloride

7. cyanidin 3-*O*-arabinoside chloride

8. petunidin 3-*O*-glucoside chloride

9. delphinidin chloride

10. peonidin 3-*O*-galactoside chloride

11. petunidin 3-*O*-arabinoside chloride

12. peonidin 3-*O*-glucoside chloride

13. malvidin 3-*O*-galactoside chloride

14. peonidin 3-*O*-arabinoside chloride

15. malvidin 3-*O*-glucoside chloride

16. cyanidin chloride

17. malvidin 3-*O*-arabinoside chloride

18. petunidin chloride

19. peonidin chloride

20. malvidin chloride

Figure 2394.-1. – *Chromatogram for the assay of refined and standardised fresh bilberry fruit dry extract*

TESTS

Loss on drying (*2.8.17*)
Maximum 4.5 per cent.

Total ash (*2.4.16*)
Maximum 2.0 per cent.

Total anthocyanidins

Liquid chromatography (*2.2.29*). *Maintain the solutions at 4 °C.*

Solvent mixture hydrochloric acid R, methanol R (2:98 *V/V*).

Test solution Dissolve 0.1250 g of the extract to be examined in the solvent mixture and dilute to 25.0 mL with the solvent mixture. Dilute 5.0 mL of this solution to 20.0 mL with *dilute phosphoric acid R*.

Reference solution (a) Dissolve 10.0 mg of *cyanidin chloride CRS* in the solvent mixture and dilute to 25.0 mL with the solvent mixture. Dilute 2.0 mL of this solution to 100.0 mL with *dilute phosphoric acid R*.

Reference solution (b) Dissolve 0.1250 g of *bilberry dry extract CRS* in the solvent mixture and dilute to 25.0 mL with the solvent mixture. Dilute 5.0 mL of this solution to 20.0 mL with *dilute phosphoric acid R*.

Column:
— *size*: l = 0.250 m, Ø = 4.6 mm;
— *stationary phase*: octadecylsilyl silica gel for chromatography R (5 µm);
— *temperature*: 30 °C.

Mobile phase:
— *mobile phase A*: anhydrous formic acid R, water R (8.5:91.5 *V/V*);
— *mobile phase B*: anhydrous formic acid R, acetonitrile R, methanol R, water R, (8.5:22.5:22.5:41.5 *V/V/V/V*);

Time (min)	Mobile phase A (per cent *V/V*)	Mobile phase B (per cent *V/V*)
0 - 35	93 → 75	7 → 25
35 - 45	75 → 35	25 → 65
45 - 46	35 → 0	65 → 100
46 - 50	0	100

Flow rate 1.0 mL/min.

Detection Spectrophotometer at 535 nm.

Injection 10 µL.

Identification of peaks Use the chromatogram supplied with *bilberry dry extract CRS* and the chromatograms obtained with reference solutions (a) and (b) to identify the peaks due to the anthocyanins and the anthocyanidins.

Retention times The retention times and the elution order of the peaks are similar to those shown in the chromatogram (Figure 2394.-1).

System suitability Reference solution (b):
— *peak-to-valley ratio*: minimum 2.0, where H_p = height above the baseline of the peak due to cyanidin 3-*O*-galactoside (peak 3) and H_v = height above the baseline of the lowest point of the curve separating this peak from the peak due to delphinidin 3-*O*-arabinoside (peak 4).

Calculate the percentage content of total anthocyanidins, expressed as cyanidin chloride, using the following expression:

$$\frac{A_1 \times m_2 \times 100 \times p}{m_1 \times A_2 \times 1250}$$

A_1 = sum of the areas of the peaks due to the anthocyanidins (peaks 9, 16, 18-20) in the chromatogram obtained with the test solution;

A_2 = area of the peak due to cyanidin chloride (peak 16) in the chromatogram obtained with reference solution (a);

m_1 = mass of the extract to be examined used to prepare the test solution, in grams;

m_2 = mass of *cyanidin chloride CRS* used to prepare reference solution (a), in grams;

p = percentage content of cyanidin chloride in *cyanidin chloride CRS*.

Limits Not more than 1.0 per cent of total anthocyanidins, expressed as cyanidin chloride.

ASSAY

Liquid chromatography (*2.2.29*) as described in the test for total anthocyanidins with the following modification.

Injection Test solution and reference solution (b).

Calculate the percentage content of total anthocyanins, expressed as cyanidin 3-*O*-glucoside chloride, using the following expression:

$$\frac{A_1 \times m_2 \times p}{m_1 \times A_2}$$

A_1 = sum of the areas of the peaks due to the anthocyanins (peaks 1-8, 10-15 and 17) in the chromatogram obtained with the test solution;

A_2 = area of the peak due to cyanidin 3-*O*-glucoside chloride (peak 5) in the chromatogram obtained with reference solution (b);

m_1 = mass of the extract to be examined used to prepare the test solution, in grams;

m_2 = mass of *bilberry dry extract CRS* used to prepare reference solution (b), in grams;

p = percentage content of cyanidin 3-*O*-glucoside chloride in *bilberry dry extract CRS*.

_____ *Ph Eur*

Birch Leaf

(*Ph Eur monograph 1174*)

Ph Eur _____

DEFINITION

Whole or fragmented, dried leaves of *Betula pendula* Roth and/or *Betula pubescens* Ehrh. as well as hybrids of both species.

Content: minimum 1.5 per cent of flavonoids, expressed as hyperoside ($C_{21}H_{20}O_{12}$; M_r 464.4) (dried drug).

IDENTIFICATION

A. The leaves of both species are dark green on the adaxial surface and lighter greenish-grey on the abaxial surface; they show a characteristic dense reticulate venation. The veins are light brown or almost white.

The leaves of *B. pendula* are glabrous and show closely spaced glandular pits on both surfaces. The leaves of *B. pendula* are 3-7 cm long and 2-5 cm wide; the petiole is long and the doubly dentate lamina is triangular or rhomboid and broadly cuneate or truncate at the base. The angle on each side is unrounded or slightly rounded, and the apex is long and acuminate.

The leaves of *B. pubescens* show few glandular trichomes and are slightly pubescent on both surfaces. The abaxial surface shows small bundles of yellowish-grey trichomes at the branch points of the veins. The leaves of *B. pubescens* are slightly smaller, oval or rhomboid and more rounded. They are more roughly and more regularly dentate. The apex is neither long nor acuminate.

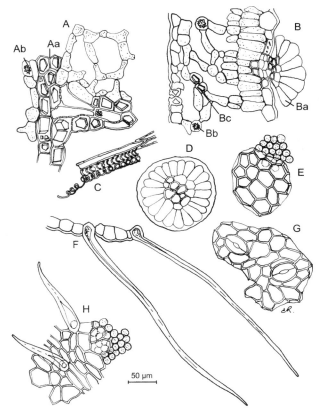

Figure 1174.-1. – *Illustration for identification test B of powdered herbal drug of birch leaf*

B. Microscopic examination (*2.8.23*). The powder is greenish-grey. Examine under a microscope using *chloral hydrate solution R*. The powder shows the following diagnostic characters (Figure 1174.-1): numerous fragments of the lamina, in surface view, with straight-walled, adaxial epidermal cells accompanied by underlying palisade parenchyma [E] and cells of the abaxial epidermis surrounding anomocytic stomata (*2.8.3*) [G]; large, free, glandular trichomes usually measuring 100-120 µm [D]; fragments of the lamina in transverse section [B], showing glandular trichomes on the epidermises [Ba], heterogeneous, asymmetrical mesophyll containing cluster crystals [Bb] and prisms [Bc] of calcium oxalate; fragments of spongy parenchyma [A] accompanied by crystal sheaths [Aa] and cells containing cluster crystals of calcium oxalate [Ab]; fragments of vessels and sclerenchyma fibres [C]. If *B. pubescens* is present, the powder also contains unicellular covering trichomes with very thick walls, about 80-600 µm long, usually 100-200 µm, numerous on the margin of the lamina [F] or on the epidermises, in surface view [H].

C. Thin-layer chromatography (*2.2.27*).

Test solution   To 1 g of the powdered herbal drug (355) (*2.9.12*) add 10 mL of *methanol R* and shake. Heat on a water-bath at 60 °C for 5 min. Cool and filter the solution.

Reference solution   Dissolve 1 mg of *chlorogenic acid R*, 1 mg of *caffeic acid R*, 2.5 mg of *hyperoside R* and 2.5 mg of *rutin R* in 10 mL of *methanol R*.

Plate   TLC *silica gel plate R*.

Mobile phase   anhydrous formic acid R, water R, methyl ethyl ketone R, ethyl acetate R (10:10:30:50 V/V/V/V).

Application   10 µL as bands.

Development   Over a path of 10 cm.

Drying   In a current of warm air.

Detection   Treat with a 10 g/L solution of *diphenylboric acid aminoethyl ester R* in *methanol R*; subsequently treat with a 50 g/L solution of *macrogol 400 R* in *methanol R*; allow to dry in air for 30 min and examine in ultraviolet light at 365 nm.

Results   The chromatogram obtained with the reference solution shows 3 zones in its lower half: in increasing order of R_F, a yellowish-brown fluorescent zone (rutin), a light blue fluorescent zone (chlorogenic acid) and a yellowish-brown fluorescent zone (hyperoside), and in its upper third, a light blue fluorescent zone (caffeic acid). The chromatogram obtained with the test solution shows 3 zones similar in position and fluorescence to the zones due to rutin, chlorogenic acid and hyperoside in the chromatogram obtained with the reference solution. The zone due to rutin is very faint and the zone due to hyperoside is intense. It also shows other yellowish-brown faint fluorescent zones between the zones due to caffeic acid and chlorogenic acid in the chromatogram obtained with the reference solution. Near the solvent front, the red fluorescent zone due to chlorophylls is visible. In the chromatogram obtained with the test solution, between this zone and the zone due to caffeic acid in the chromatogram obtained with the reference solution, there is a brownish-yellow zone due to quercetin.

TESTS

Foreign matter (*2.8.2*)

Maximum 3 per cent of fragments of female catkins and maximum 3 per cent of other foreign matter.

Loss on drying (*2.2.32*)

Maximum 10.0 per cent, determined on 1.000 g of powdered herbal drug (355) (*2.9.12*) by drying in an oven at 105 °C for 2 h.

Total ash (*2.4.16*)

Maximum 6.0 per cent.

ASSAY

Stock solution   In a 100 mL round-bottomed flask introduce 0.200 g of the powdered herbal drug (355) (*2.9.12*), 1 mL of a 5 g/L solution of *hexamethylenetetramine R*, 20 mL of *acetone R* and 2 mL of *hydrochloric acid R1*. Boil the mixture under a reflux condenser for 30 min. Filter the liquid through a plug of absorbent cotton into a 100 mL flask. Add the absorbent cotton to the residue in the round-bottomed flask and extract with 2 quantities, each of 20 mL, of *acetone R*, each time boiling under a reflux condenser for 10 min. Allow to cool to room temperature, filter the liquid through a plug of absorbent cotton then through a filter paper into the volumetric flask, and dilute to 100.0 mL with *acetone R* by rinsing the flask and filter. Introduce 20.0 mL of the solution into a separating funnel, add 20 mL of *water R* and extract the mixture with 1 quantity of 15 mL and then 3 quantities, each of 10 mL, of *ethyl acetate R*. Combine the ethyl acetate extracts in a separating funnel, wash with 2 quantities, each of 50 mL, of *water R*, and filter the extract over 10 g of *anhydrous sodium sulfate R* into a 50 mL volumetric flask and dilute to 50.0 mL with *ethyl acetate R*.

Test solution To 10.0 mL of the stock solution add 1 mL of *aluminium chloride reagent R* and dilute to 25.0 mL with a 5 per cent *V/V* solution of *glacial acetic acid R* in *methanol R*.

Compensation liquid Dilute 10.0 mL of the stock solution to 25.0 mL with a 5 per cent *V/V* solution of *glacial acetic acid R* in *methanol R*.

Measure the absorbance (*2.2.25*) of the test solution after 30 min, by comparison with the compensation liquid at 425 nm.

Calculate the percentage content of flavonoids, expressed as hyperoside, using the following expression:

$$\frac{A \times 1.25}{m}$$

i.e. taking the specific absorbance of hyperoside to be 500.

A = absorbance at 425 nm;

m = mass of the herbal drug to be examined, in grams.

——————————————————— Ph Eur

Bistort Rhizome

(*Ph Eur monograph 2384*)

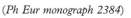

Ph Eur

DEFINITION
Whole or fragmented, dried rhizome of *Persicaria bistorta* (L.) Samp. (syn. *Polygonum bistorta* L.) without adventitious roots.

Content
Minimum 3.0 per cent of tannins, expressed as pyrogallol ($C_6H_6O_3$; M_r 126.1) (dried drug).

CHARACTERS
The whole rhizome is up to 13 cm long and 2.5 cm in diameter. The remnants of the roots are not longer than 1 cm and are about 1 mm in diameter.

IDENTIFICATION
A. The whole rhizome, reddish-brown or blackish-brown, is thick, twisted, and turned back on itself. Its outer surface shows transverse striations and blackish spots. It is flattened and somewhat depressed on the upper surface, convex on the lower surface. It shows adventitious root scars on the surface. The fracture, pinkish-beige, shows an elliptical zone of whitish pits corresponding to the vessels. The drug may also be obtained as more-or-less cylindrical fragments about 0.3 cm in diameter and up to 1 cm long, with a reddish-brown outer surface, marked by adventitious root scars and a pinkish-beige fracture.

B. Reduce to a powder (355) (*2.9.12*). The powder is reddish-brown. Examine under a microscope using *chloral hydrate solution R*. The powder shows the following diagnostic characters: fragments of parenchyma; very numerous calcium oxalate cluster crystals either free or inside parenchyma cells; a few reticulate lignified vessels; rare cork fragments. Examine under a microscope using a 50 per cent *V/V* solution of *glycerol R*. The powder shows rounded to ovoid starch granules, simple, about 10 µm in diameter.

C. Thin-layer chromatography (*2.2.27*).

Test solution To 1.0 g of the powdered drug (355) (*2.9.12*) add 10 mL of a mixture of equal volumes of *water R* and *methanol R*, heat on a water-bath at about 65 °C for 30 min and filter.

Reference solution Dissolve 5 mg of *fructose R* and 5 mg of *catechin R* in 5 mL of *methanol R*.

Plate TLC silica gel plate R (2-10 µm).

Mobile phase water R, anhydrous formic acid R, ethyl acetate R (5:10:85 *V/V/V*).

Application 2 µL as bands.

Development Over a path of 7 cm.

Drying In air.

Detection Spray with *anisaldehyde solution R* and heat at 100-105 °C for 5 min; examine in daylight.

Results See below the sequence of zones present in the chromatograms obtained with the reference solution and the test solution. Furthermore, other faint zones may be present in the chromatogram obtained with the test solution.

Top of the plate	
Catechin: a brown zone	A brown zone (catechin)
	A brown zone
	A violet zone
	A brown zone
	An orange zone
Fructose: a green zone	A green zone (fructose)
Reference solution	**Test solution**

TESTS
Paris polyphylla or *Paris quadrifolia*
Examine the powdered drug (355) (*2.9.12*) under a microscope using *chloral hydrate solution R*. The presence of raphides of calcium oxalate, free or in bundles, indicates adulteration by the rhizome of *Paris polyphylla* Smith var. *yunnanensis* (Franch.) Hand.-Mazz or *Paris polyphylla* Smith var. *chinensis* (Franch.) Hara or *Paris quadrifolia* L.

Loss on drying (*2.2.32*)
Maximum 12.0 per cent, determined on 1.000 g of the powdered drug (355) (*2.9.12*) by drying in an oven at 105 °C.

Total ash (*2.4.16*)
Maximum 9.0 per cent.

Ash insoluble in hydrochloric acid (*2.8.1*)
Maximum 1.0 per cent.

ASSAY
Carry out the determination of tannins in herbal drugs (*2.8.14*). Use 1.000 g of the powdered drug (180) (*2.9.12*).

——————————————————— Ph Eur

Black Cohosh

(Ph Eur monograph 2069)

Ph Eur

DEFINITION
Dried, whole or fragmented rhizome and root of *Actaea racemosa* L. (syn. *Cimicifuga racemosa* (L.) Nutt.).

Content
Minimum 1.0 per cent of triterpene glycosides, expressed as monoammonium glycyrrhizate ($C_{42}H_{65}NO_{16}$; M_r 840) (dried drug).

IDENTIFICATION
A. *Whole drug* The rhizome is dark brown, hard, subcylindrical and somewhat knotted; 1.5-2.5 cm in diameter and 2-15 cm long; it shows numerous closely arranged, upright or curved branches each terminating in the remains of a bud or in a circular, cup-shaped scar. The fracture is horny, the transverse section shows a thin outer bark surrounding a ring of numerous pale, narrow wedges of vascular tissue alternating with darker medullary rays and a large central pith. Roots attached to the lower surface of the rhizome are usually broken off, leaving circular scars.
The roots are dark brown, 1-3 mm in diameter, brittle, nearly cylindrical or obtusely quadrangular and longitudinally wrinkled; the fracture is short; the transverse section shows a wide outer bark, a dark brown cylinder, in which the central region is composed of 3-6 lighter wedges of vascular tissue united at the centre and separated by broad, non-lignified medullary rays.

Fragmented drug More or less angular, irregular pieces of the rhizome and cylindrical pieces of the roots. The hard, horny rhizome fragments usually show a dark brown surface corresponding to the outer surface and several frequently striated, light brown surfaces corresponding to the section. The dark brown, more or less cylindrical root fragments are wrinkled longitudinally. The lighter coloured transverse section shows a distinct cambium line separating a thick outer bark from a central region composed of 3-6 wedges of vascular tissue united at the centre and separated by broad medullary rays.

B. Microscopic examination (*2.8.23*). The powder is light brown. Examine under a microscope using *chloral hydrate solution R*. The powder shows the following diagnostic characters: numerous fragments of thin-walled parenchyma; groups of small, lignified vessels with closely-arranged bordered pits or, less frequently, with reticulate thickening; lignified thin-walled fibres and xylem parenchyma; fragments of brown, suberised cells with moderately thickened walls. Examine under a microscope using a mixture of equal volumes of *glycerol R* and *water R*. The powder shows abundant starch granules, spherical or polygonal, simple or 2 or 3 (sometimes up to 6) compound; individual granules are 3-15 μm in diameter with a central, slit-shaped hilum.

C. Examine the chromatograms obtained in the test for substitution by *Cimicifuga americana* Michx., *C. foetida* L., *C. dahurica* (Turcz.) Maxim. or *C. heracleifolia* Kom.

Results B Use the chromatograms supplied with *Actaea racemosa HRS* and the chromatogram obtained with reference solution (a) to identify the bands corresponding to *A. racemosa.*

See below the sequence of zones present in the chromatograms obtained with reference solutions (a) and (b) and the test solution. Furthermore, other faint zones may be present in the chromatograms obtained with reference solution (a) and the test solution.

Top of the plate		
_____	_____	_____
Actein: a brown zone 23-Epi-26-deoxyactein: a brown zone	Actein: a brown zone	A brown zone (actein) A brown zone (23-epi-26-deoxyactein)
_____	_____	_____
A violet zone A violet zone A brown zone		A violet zone A violet zone A brown zone
Reference solution (a)	**Reference solution (b)**	**Test solution**

TESTS
Loss on drying (*2.2.32*)
Maximum 12 per cent, determined on 1.000 g of the powdered herbal drug (355) (*2.9.12*) by drying in an oven at 105 °C for 2 h.

Foreign matter (*2.8.2*)
Maximum 5 per cent.

Total ash (*2.4.16*)
Maximum 10 per cent.

Ash insoluble in hydrochloric acid (*2.8.1*)
Maximum 5 per cent.

Substitution by *Cimicifuga americana* Michx., *C. foetida* L., *C. dahurica* (Turcz.) Maxim. or *C. heracleifolia* Kom
Thin-layer chromatography (*2.2.27*).

Test solution To 0.50 g of the powdered herbal drug (355) (*2.9.12*) add 10 mL of *ethanol (50 per cent V/V) R* and shake well. Sonicate for 10 min and centrifuge. Use the supernatant.

Reference solution (a) To 0.50 g of *Actaea racemosa HRS* add 10 mL of *ethanol (50 per cent V/V) R* and shake well. Sonicate for 10 min and centrifuge. Use the supernatant.

Reference solution (b) Dissolve 2 mg of *actein R* in *methanol R* and dilute to 10 mL with the same solvent.

Plate TLC silica gel F_{254} plate R (2-10 μm).

Mobile phase anhydrous formic acid R, ethyl formate R, toluene R (20:30:50 *V/V/V*).

Application 2 μL as bands of 8 mm (see Table 2069.-1).

Development Over a path of 6 cm.

Drying In air.

System suitability Reference solution (b):
— the R_F value of the zone due to actein is between 0.35 and 0.40 (detection B).

Detection A Examine in ultraviolet light at 254 nm.

Results A The chromatogram obtained with the test solution does not show any quenching zones more intense than those

Table 2069.-1.– *Application scheme*

Track	1	2	3	4	5	6	7
Application volume (µL)	2	2	2	-	2	2	2
Solution	Reference solution (a)	Reference solution (b)	Test solution	Blank	Reference solution (a)	Reference solution (b)	Test solution

After development, the plate is cut along track 4 (blank). Tracks 1-3 are used for detection of a substitution by *C. americana*, *C. foetida*, *C. dahurica* or *C. heracleifolia* (detection A), tracks 5-7 for identification C (detection B).

Table 2069.-2.– *Application scheme*

Track	1	2	3	4	5	6	7	8	9
Application volume (µL)	20	2	2	20	-	20	2	2	20
Solution	Reference solution (a)	Reference solution (b)	Reference solution (c)	Test solution	Blank	Reference solution (a)	Reference solution (b)	Reference solution (c)	Test solution

After development and examination for detection of *C. americana* (detection A), the plate is cut along track 5 (blank). Tracks 1-4 are used for detection of adulteration with *C. foetida* (detection B), tracks 6-9 for detection of adulteration with *C. heracleifolia* and/or *C. dahurica* (detection C).

in the chromatogram obtained with reference solution (a) between R_F value 0.2 and R_F value 0.35.

Detection B   Treat with a 10 per cent *V/V* solution of *sulfuric acid R* in *methanol R*; heat at 100 °C for 5 min; allow to cool to room temperature and examine in daylight.

Adulteration with *Cimicifuga americana* Michx., *C. foetida* L., *C. dahurica* (Turcz.) Maxim. and/or *C. heracleifolia* Kom

Thin-layer chromatography (*2.2.27*) as described in the test for substitution by *Cimicifuga americana* Michx., *C. foetida* L., *C. dahurica* (Turcz.) Maxim. or *C. heracleifolia* Kom., with the following modifications.

Reference solution (c)   Dissolve 2 mg of *cimifugin R* in *methanol R* and dilute to 10 mL with the same solvent.

Application   2 µL of reference solutions (b) and (c), 20 µL of the test solution and reference solution (a), as bands of 8 mm (see Table 2069.-2).

System suitability   Reference solution (b):
— the R_F value of the zone due to actein is between 0.35 and 0.40 (detections B and C).

Detection A   Examine in ultraviolet light at 254 nm.

Results A   Absence of more than 10 per cent of *C. americana*.

Compare the chromatogram supplied with *Actaea racemosa HRS* for *C. americana* and the chromatograms obtained with the test solution and reference solution (a).
The chromatogram obtained with the test solution does not show any quenching zone at R_F value 0.3 (zone presented in capitals in the chromatogram of *C. americana*, see below). The presence of this zone in the chromatogram obtained with the test solution indicates adulteration with *C. americana* at a level greater than 10 per cent.

Top of the plate	
———	———
A weak zone	A weak zone
2 weak zones	2 weak zones
A weak zone	A weak zone
———	———A DARK ZONE
A weak zone	A weak zone
A dark zone	A dark zone
A dark zone	A dark zone
Reference solution (a)	***C. americana* (10 per cent)**

Detection B   Dissolve 4.5 g of *boric acid R* in 150 mL of *anhydrous ethanol R* (solution A); dissolve 5 g of *oxalic acid R* in 50 mL of *anhydrous ethanol R* (solution B); combine solutions A and B and mix well; treat the plate with this freshly prepared solution and heat at 120 °C for 5 min; examine in ultraviolet light at 365 nm.

Results B   Absence of more than 5 per cent of *C. foetida*.

Compare the chromatogram supplied with *Actaea racemosa HRS* for *C. foetida* and the chromatograms obtained with the test solution and reference solutions (a), (b) and (c).
The chromatogram obtained with the test solution does not show any intense fluorescent zone between R_F value 0.03 and R_F value 0.06 or at the same position as the bright fluorescent zone in the chromatogram obtained with reference solution (c) (zones presented in capitals in the chromatogram of *C. foetida*, see below). The presence of 1 or both zones in the chromatogram obtained with the test solution indicates adulteration with *C. foetida* at a level greater than 5 per cent.

Top of the plate			
Actein: a weak whitish zone	Actein: a weak whitish zone		A weak whitish zone (actein)
A bluish zone			A bluish zone
		Cimifugin: a bright fluorescent zone	A BRIGHT FLUORESCENT ZONE (CIMIFUGIN)
A brownish zone			A brownish zone
A bluish zone			A bluish zone
			A FLUORESCENT ZONE
Reference solution (a)	**Reference solution (b)**	**Reference solution (c)**	**C. foetida (5 per cent)**

Detection C   Dissolve 8 g of *antimony trichloride R* in 200 mL of *methylene chloride R*; treat with this solution and heat at 120 °C for 10 min; examine in ultraviolet light at 365 nm.

Results C   Absence of more than 5 per cent of *C. heracleifolia* and/or *C. dahurica*.

Compare the chromatogram supplied with *Actaea racemosa HRS* for *C. heracleifolia* and *C. dahurica* and the chromatograms obtained with the test solution and reference solutions (a) and (b). The chromatogram obtained with the test solution does not show any bright fluorescent zone just above the zone due to actein (zone presented in capitals in the chromatogram of *C. heracleifolia* or *C. dahurica*, see below). The presence of this zone in the chromatogram obtained with the test solution indicates adulteration with *C. heracleifolia* and/or *C. dahurica* at a level greater than 5 per cent.

Top of the plate		
		A BRIGHT FLUORESCENT ZONE
Actein: a weak brownish zone	Actein: a weak brownish zone	A weak brownish zone (actein)
A brownish zone		A brownish zone
A bluish zone		A bluish zone
Reference solution (a)	**Reference solution (b)**	**C. heracleifolia (5 per cent) and/or C. dahurica (5 per cent)**

ASSAY

Liquid chromatography (*2.2.29*).

Test solution   Introduce 4.00 g of the powdered herbal drug (355) (*2.9.12*) into a 200 mL screw-cap bottle. Add 50.0 mL of a mixture of equal volumes of *methanol R* and *water R*. Sonicate for 45 min and shake for 15 min. Filter through a membrane filter (nominal pore size 0.45 µm).

Reference solution (a)   Dissolve 10.0 mg of *Actaea racemosa for assay CRS* (containing monoammonium glycyrrhizate) in *methanol R* with the aid of ultrasound and dilute to 10.0 mL with the same solvent.

Reference solution (b)   Dilute 5.0 mL of reference solution (a) to 10.0 mL with *methanol R*.

Reference solution (c)   Dilute 2.0 mL of reference solution (a) to 10.0 mL with *methanol R*.

Reference solution (d)   Dilute 1.0 mL of reference solution (a) to 20.0 mL with *methanol R*.

Reference solution (e)   Dissolve 500 mg of *Actaea racemosa dry extract for system suitability HRS* in *methanol R* and dilute to 10.0 mL with the same solvent; sonicate and filter through a membrane filter (nominal pore size 0.45 µm).

Column:
— *size*: l = 0.25 m, Ø = 4.6 mm;
— *stationary phase*: *octadecylsilyl silica gel for chromatography R* (5 µm).

Mobile phase:
— *mobile phase A*: 0.1 per cent *V/V* solution of *anhydrous formic acid R* in *water R*;
— *mobile phase B*: 0.1 per cent *V/V* solution of *anhydrous formic acid R* in a mixture of equal volumes of *acetonitrile R* and *methanol R*;

Time (min)	Mobile phase A (per cent V/V)	Mobile phase B (per cent V/V)
0 - 40	50 → 20	50 → 80
40 - 41	20 → 5	80 → 95
41 - 44	5	95

Flow rate   1.0 mL/min.

Detection   Evaporative light-scattering detector; the following settings have been found to be suitable; if the detector has different setting parameters, adjust the detector settings so as to comply with the system suitability criterion for the signal-to-noise ratio:
— *carrier gas*: *nitrogen R*;
— *flow rate*: 0.8 mL/min;
— *evaporator temperature*: 100 °C;
— *nebuliser temperature*: 60 °C.

Injection   10 µL.

Identification of peaks   Use the chromatogram supplied with *Actaea racemosa dry extract for system suitability HRS* and the chromatogram obtained with reference solution (e) to identify the peaks to be quantified.

System suitability:
— *signal-to-noise ratio*: minimum 4.0 for the peak due to monoammonium glycyrrhizate in the chromatogram obtained with reference solution (d);
— *peak-to-valley ratio*: minimum 3, where H_p = height above the baseline of peak 4 and H_v = height above the baseline of the lowest point of the curve separating this peak from peak 5 in the chromatogram obtained with reference solution (e).

Establish a calibration curve with the logarithm to base 10 of the concentration (in milligrams per millilitre) of reference solutions (a), (b), (c) and (d) (corrected by the assigned percentage content of monoammonium glycyrrhizate in *Actaea racemosa for assay CRS*) as the abscissa and the logarithm to base 10 of the corresponding peak area as the ordinate.

Calculate the percentage content of each peak using the following expression:

$$\frac{10^A \times 5}{m}$$

A = logarithm to base 10 of the concentration of each peak in the chromatogram obtained with the test solution, determined from the calibration curve;

m = mass of the herbal drug to be examined used to prepare the test solution, in grams.

Calculate the percentage content of triterpene glycosides by taking the sum of the percentage contents of peaks 1 to 12.

Ph Eur

Black Currant

Preparation
Black Currant Syrup

DEFINITION

Black Currant consists of the fresh ripe fruits of *Ribes nigrum* L., together with their pedicels and rachides.

CHARACTERISTICS

Odour, strong and characteristic.

Macroscopical Berries: globose, ranging in diameter from about 7 to 15 mm, occurring in pendulous racemes; epicarp shiny black externally, enclosing a yellowish green translucent pulp containing numerous flattened ovoid seeds, about 2.5 mm long, 1.25 mm wide and 1 mm thick; berry crowned with withered remains of five-cleft calyx; pedicels thin, up to about 10 mm long, attached to a rachis of variable length.

Microscopical Epicarp: glands yellow, disc-shaped, roughly circular or broadly elliptical, varying in diameter from about 140 to 240 μm, each consisting of a single layer of cells attached in the centre to the epicarp by means of a short, multiseriate stalk. Calyx: trichomes unicellular, blunt-ended with thin, crooked walls, about 10 to 14 μm wide and averaging about 350 μm in length. Seed: testa with pigment layer composed of small cells with horseshoe-shaped wall thickenings as seen in cross section, each cell containing one or two prismatic crystals of calcium oxalate; endosperm cells with irregularly thickened walls.

Black Currant Syrup

DEFINITION

Black Currant Syrup is prepared either from the clarified juice of Black Currant or from concentrated black currant juice of commerce. It contains a suitable antioxidant. Permitted food grade colours may be added.

PRODUCTION

It is prepared by dissolving 700 g of Sucrose either in 560 mL of clarified juice, previously diluted with Water to a weight per mL of 1.045 g, or in 560 mL of a solution of the same weight per mL prepared from the concentrated juice of commerce and Water, and adding to this solution sufficient Benzoic Acid to give a final concentration of not more than 800 ppm, or sufficient Sodium Metabisulfite or other suitable sulfite to give a final concentration of not more than 350 ppm of sulfur dioxide.

The syrup complies with the requirements stated under Oral Liquids and with the following requirements.

Content of ascorbic acid[1], $C_6H_8O_6$
Not less than 0.055% w/w.

TESTS
Sulfur dioxide
Not more than 350 ppm, Appendix IX B.

Weight per mL
1.27 to 1.30 g, Appendix V G.

ASSAY
Mix 5 g with 25 mL of a freshly prepared 20% w/v solution of *metaphosphoric acid*, add 20 mL of *acetone* and dilute to 100 mL with *water*. To four 3 mL quantities of this solution add 0.4, 0.5, 0.6 and 0.7 mL, respectively, of *double-strength standard 2,6-dichlorophenolindophenol solution*, mix well by agitation with a fine stream of carbon dioxide, add 3 mL of *chloroform*, agitate for a further 15 seconds, examine the solutions against a white background and select the two that are on either side of the end point (that is, one colourless and one pink). Prepare a further six solutions as directed above, but adding to the first an amount of dye solution equal to that added to the selected colourless solution, successively increasing this volume by 0.02 mL increments in the second to the fifth solutions and adding to the sixth solution a volume equal to that added to the selected pink solution. Select the solution exhibiting the faintest pink colour. Each mL of *double-strength standard 2,6-dichlorophenolindophenol solution* added to this solution is equivalent to 0.200 mg of $C_6H_8O_6$.

STORAGE
Black Currant Syrup should be kept in a well-filled container and protected from light.

Black Currant Syrup contains, in 10 mL, about 7.5 mg of ascorbic acid.

[1]The *requirement for Content of ascorbic acid does not apply when Black Currant Syrup is used as a flavouring agent for pharmaceutical purposes.*

Blackcurrant Leaf

(*Ph Eur monograph 2528*)

Ph Eur

DEFINITION
Dried leaf of *Ribes nigrum* L.

Content
Minimum 1.0 per cent of flavonoids, expressed as isoquercitroside ($C_{21}H_{20}O_{12}$; M_r 464.4) (dried drug).

IDENTIFICATION

A. The leaf is simple. The lamina may be up to 10 cm long and 12 cm wide and shows 3 (rarely 5) rounded triangular lobes, dentate or crenate on the margins, with the median lobe being the largest. The light-brown midrib and secondary veins are very visible on the lower surface, and form a characteristic network through numerous anastomoses.
The rigid, light-brown petiole shows a very distinct gutter on the upper part and its length is equal to half the length of the lamina.

B. Microscopic examination (*2.8.23*). The powder is brownish-green. Examine under a microscope using *chloral hydrate solution R*. The powder shows the following diagnostic characters (Figure 2528.-1): curved, unicellular covering trichomes, with moderately thickened, slightly verrucose walls [D]; orange-yellow, globular or ovoid glandular trichomes, lacking a visible stalk, with a multicellular head up to 200 μm in diameter, in surface view [A]; fragments of the lower epidermis, in surface view [B], composed of cells with irregularly thickened walls [Ba], numerous anomocytic stomata (*2.8.3*) [Bb] accompanied by spongy parenchyma [Bc]; fragments, in surface view [C] or in transverse section

[E], of the upper epidermis [Ca, Ea], accompanied by palisade parenchyma [Cb, Eb]; cluster crystals of calcium oxalate up to 30 µm in diameter, isolated [F] or included in parenchymatous cells [Bd, Cc, Ec].

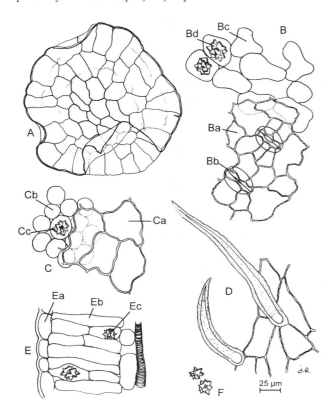

Figure 2528.-1. – *Illustration for identification test B of powdered herbal drug of blackcurrant leaf*

C. Thin-layer chromatography (*2.2.27*).

Test solution   To 1 g of the powdered herbal drug (355) (*2.9.12*) add 10 mL of *methanol R*. Heat in a water-bath at 60 °C for 10 min with occasional stirring. Allow to cool. Filter.

Reference solution   Dissolve 5 mg of *isoquercitroside R* and 5 mg of *rutin R* in 10 mL of *methanol R*.

Plate   *TLC silica gel plate R* (5-40 µm) [or *TLC silica gel plate R* (2-10 µm)].

Mobile phase   *anhydrous formic acid R*, *water R*, *ethyl acetate R* (10:10:80 *V/V/V*).

Application   10 µL [or 5 µL] as bands of 10 mm [or 8 mm].

Development   Over a path of 10 cm [or 6 cm].

Drying   At 100-105 °C for 10 min.

Detection   Treat with a 10 g/L solution of *diphenylboric acid aminoethyl ester R* in *methanol R*, then with a 50 g/L solution of *macrogol 400 R* in *methanol R*; allow to dry in air for about 30 min, then examine in ultraviolet light at 365 nm.

Results   See below the sequence of zones present in the chromatograms obtained with the reference solution and the test solution. Furthermore, other fluorescent zones may be present in the chromatogram obtained with the test solution.

TESTS

Foreign matter (*2.8.2*)
Maximum 3 per cent.

Top of the plate	
	A green zone
Isoquercitroside: an orange zone	An orange zone (mainly isoquercitroside)
	A light blue zone
Rutin: an orange-yellow zone	An orange-yellow zone (rutin)
Reference solution	**Test solution**

Loss on drying (*2.2.32*)
Maximum 10.0 per cent, determined on 1.000 g of the powdered herbal drug (355) (*2.9.12*) by drying in an oven at 105 °C for 2 h.

Total ash (*2.4.16*)
Maximum 12.0 per cent.

ASSAY

Liquid chromatography (*2.2.29*).

Test solution   Disperse 0.200 g of the powdered herbal drug (355) (*2.9.12*) in 10 mL of an 80 per cent *V/V* solution of *methanol R*. Heat under a reflux condenser in a water-bath at 60 °C for 30 min. Sonicate for 15 min. Allow to cool, dilute to 20.0 mL with an 80 per cent *V/V* solution of *methanol R*. Filter through a membrane filter (nominal pore size 0.45 µm).

Reference solution (a)   Dissolve 5.0 mg of *isoquercitroside CRS* in an 80 per cent *V/V* solution of *methanol R* and dilute to 100.0 mL with the same solution.

Reference solution (b)   Dissolve 5.0 mg of *rutin R* in *methanol R* and dilute to 100.0 mL with the same solvent.

Reference solution (c)   Dilute 10.0 mL of reference solution (a) to 20.0 mL with reference solution (b).

Reference solution (d)   Dilute 1.0 mL of reference solution (a) to 20.0 mL with an 80 per cent *V/V* solution of *methanol R*.

Column:
— *size: l* = 0.25 m, Ø = 4 mm;
— *stationary phase: end-capped octadecylsilyl silica gel for chromatography R* (5 µm);
— *temperature*: 30 °C.

Mobile phase:
— *mobile phase A*: 0.05 per cent *V/V* solution of *trifluoroacetic acid R*;
— *mobile phase B*: *acetonitrile R*;

Time (min)	Mobile phase A (per cent *V/V*)	Mobile phase B (per cent *V/V*)
0 - 45	97 → 60	3 → 40

Flow rate   1.0 mL/min.

Detection   Spectrophotometer at 350 nm.

Injection   10 µL.

Identification of peaks   Use the chromatogram obtained with reference solution (a) to identify the peak due to isoquercitroside and the chromatogram obtained with reference solution (b) to identify the peak due to rutin.

Retention time   Rutin = about 28 min; isoquercitroside = about 29 min.

System suitability   Reference solution (c):
— *resolution*: minimum 3.0 between the peaks due to rutin and isoquercitroside.

Disregard limit: the area of the principal peak in the chromatogram obtained with reference solution (d).

Calculate the percentage content of total flavonoids, expressed as isoquercitroside, using the following expression:

$$\frac{A_1 \times m_2 \times p}{A_2 \times m_1 \times 5}$$

A_1 = sum of the areas of the peak due to rutin and all peaks eluting after the peak due to rutin in the chromatogram obtained with the test solution;

A_2 = area of the peak due to isoquercitroside in the chromatogram obtained with reference solution (a);

m_1 = mass of the herbal drug to be examined used to prepare the test solution, in grams;

m_2 = mass of *isoquercitroside CRS* used to prepare reference solution (a), in grams;

p = percentage content of isoquercitroside in *isoquercitroside CRS*.

———————————————— Ph Eur

Black Horehound

(Ph Eur monograph 1858)

Ph Eur —————

DEFINITION

Dried flowering tops of *Ballota nigra* L.

Content

Minimum 1.5 per cent of total *ortho*-dihydroxycinnamic acid derivatives, expressed as acteoside ($C_{29}H_{36}O_{15}$; M_r 625) (dried drug).

IDENTIFICATION

A. The stems are conspicuously 4-angled, longitudinally striated, dark green or reddish-brown and more or less pubescent. The leaves are greyish-green, petiolate, the lamina ovate or orbicular, 2-4 cm wide, the margin irregularly crenate, and cuneate or cordate at the base; both surfaces are covered with abundant whitish hairs; the venation is pinnate, prominent on the lower surface, slightly depressed on the upper. The flowers are sessile or very shortly pedicellate, the calyx is infundibuliform, densely pubescent, with 10 prominent ribs and 5 subequal, broadly ovate teeth; the corolla, with a tube slightly shorter than the calyx tube, is purple and bilabiate, the upper lip pubescent on the outer surface and the lower lip with 3 lobes, the middle of which is notched.

B. Microscopic examination (*2.8.23*). The powder is greyish-green and slightly flocculent. Examine under a microscope using *chloral hydrate solution R*. The powder shows the following diagnostic characters (Figure 1858.-1): numerous long, uniseriate, multicellular covering trichomes consisting of 4 or more cells, thickened and swollen at the junctions, with slightly lignified and pitted walls, free [C] or on an epidermis in transverse section [Ea]; fewer glandular trichomes, usually on epidermises, in transverse section [E, F, G]: some with a unicellular or multicellular stalk and a globose, uni- or bicellular head [Ga], others with a unicellular stalk and a multicellular head in surface view [Ac] or in transverse section [Eb], others with a unicellular stalk and an 8-celled head of lamiaceous type, in surface view [Ad] or in transverse section [Fa]; fragments of the adaxial leaf epidermis [B] with cells with sinuous walls, accompanied by cells of the palisade

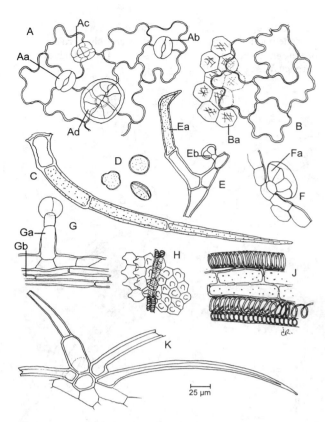

Figure 1858.-1. – *Illustration for identification test B of powdered herbal drug of black horehound*

parenchyma, most containing fine, needle-shaped crystals [Ba]; fragments of the abaxial leaf epidermis [A] bearing numerous stomata, the majority anomocytic (*2.8.3*) [Aa] but some diacytic [Ab]; fragments of the epidermis of the corolla composed of polygonal cells, those of the inner epidermis of the lips papillose [H] and those of the inner epidermis of the tube bearing uni- or bicellular covering trichomes in a stellate arrangement [K]; pollen grains subspherical with 3 pores and a smooth exine [D]; fragments from the stem (G) with groups of collenchymatous cells [Gb] and lignified vessels, with annular or spiral thickenings [J].

C. Thin-layer chromatography (*2.2.27*).

Test solution To 2 g of the powdered herbal drug (355) (*2.9.12*) add 100 mL of *methanol R*. Heat on a water-bath under a reflux condenser for 30 min. Allow to cool. Filter. Evaporate the filtrate under reduced pressure until a volume of about 10 mL is obtained.

Reference solution Dissolve 1 mg of *chlorogenic acid R* and 2.5 mg of *rutin R* in 10 mL of *methanol R*.

Plate TLC silica gel plate R.

Mobile phase anhydrous formic acid R, glacial acetic acid R, water R, ethyl acetate R (7.5:7.5:18:67 *V/V/V/V*).

Application 20 µL as bands.

Development Over a path of 15 cm.

Drying In air.

Detection spray with a solution containing 10 g/L of *diphenylboric acid aminoethyl ester R* and 50 g/L of *macrogol 400 R* in *methanol R*; allow to dry in a current of warm air; examine in ultraviolet light at 365 nm after 30 min.

Results See below the sequence of zones present in the chromatograms obtained with the reference solution and the

test solution. Furthermore, other fluorescent zones may be present in the chromatogram obtained with the test solution.

Top of the plate	
	A reddish fluorescent zone
	A faint yellow fluorescent zone
	A light blue fluorescent zone (caffeoylmalic acid)
	A greenish-blue fluorescent zone (acteoside)
	A yellowish-brown fluorescent zone (luteolin 7-lactate)
Chlorogenic acid: a light blue fluorescent zone	
	A greenish-blue fluorescent zone (forsythoside B)
Rutin: an orange-yellow fluorescent zone	2 greenish-blue fluorescent zones (arenarioside)
	A yellow fluorescent zone (luteolin 7-lactate glucoside).
	A faint greenish-blue fluorescent zone (ballotetroside).
Reference solution	Test solution

TESTS

Loss on drying (*2.2.32*)
Maximum 12.0 per cent, determined on 1.000 g of the powdered herbal drug (355) (*2.9.12*) by drying in an oven at 105 °C for 2 h.

Total ash (*2.4.16*)
Maximum 13.0 per cent.

ASSAY

Stock solution Place 1.000 g of the powdered drug (355) (*2.9.12*) in a flask. Add 90 mL of *ethanol (50 per cent V/V) R*. Heat under a reflux condenser on a water-bath for 30 min. Allow to cool and filter, collecting the filtrate in a 100 mL volumetric flask. Rinse the flask and the filter with 10 mL of *ethanol (50 per cent V/V) R*. Add the rinsings to the filtrate and dilute to 100.0 mL with *ethanol (50 per cent V/V) R*.

Test solution Into a 10 mL volumetric flask, introduce successively, with shaking after each addition, 1.0 mL of the stock solution, 2 mL of *0.5 M hydrochloric acid*, 2 mL of a solution containing 100 g/L of *sodium nitrite R* and 100 g/L of *sodium molybdate R*, and 2 mL of *dilute sodium hydroxide solution R*, and dilute to 10.0 mL with *water R*.

Compensation liquid Into a 10 mL volumetric flask, introduce 1.0 mL of the stock solution, 2 mL of *0.5 M hydrochloric acid* and 2 mL of *dilute sodium hydroxide solution R*, and dilute to 10.0 mL with *water R*.

Measure immediately the absorbance (*2.2.25*) of the test solution at 525 nm, by comparison with the compensation liquid.

Calculate the percentage content of total *ortho-*dihydroxycinnamic acid derivatives, expressed as acteoside, using the following expression:

$$\frac{A \times 1000}{185 \times m}$$

i.e. taking the specific absorbance of acteoside to be 185.
A = absorbance at 525 nm;
m = mass of the substance to be examined, in grams.

Bogbean Leaf

(*Ph Eur monograph 1605*)

Ph Eur

DEFINITION
Dried, entire or fragmented leaf of *Menyanthes trifoliata* L.

CHARACTERS
Very bitter and persistant taste.

IDENTIFICATION
A. The leaf is long-petiolated, trifoliate, with long sheaths from the base; the petiole is up to 5 mm in diameter and strongly striated longitudinally. The lamina is divided into equal leaflets, sessile, obovate up to 10 cm long and up to 5 cm wide, with an entire, occasionally sinuous margin with brownish or reddish hydathodes and a spathulate base; it is glabrous, dark green on the upper surface and paler green on the lower surface, with a wide, whitish, finely striated prominent midrib.

B. Reduce to a powder (355) (*2.9.12*). The powder is yellowish-green. Examine under a microscope using *chloral hydrate solution R*. The powder shows fragments of upper epidermis with polyhedral cells and thin wavy walls; fragments of lower epidermis with sinuous walls; anomocytic stomata (*2.8.3*), on both surfaces, with the subsidiary cells showing radiating striations; epidermal cells from the veins straight walled and papillose; fragments of mesophyll parenchyma with large intercellular spaces (aerenchyma); irregular cells with rare sclereids; fragments of spiral or annular vessels.

C. Thin-layer chromatography (*2.2.27*).

Test solution To 1.0 g of the powdered drug (355) (*2.9.12*) add 10 mL of *methanol R*. Heat, with stirring, in a water-bath at 60 °C for 5 min. Allow to cool and filter. Evaporate to dryness under reduced pressure in a water-bath at 60 °C. Dissolve the residue in 2.0 mL of *methanol R*.

Reference solution Dissolve 5 mg of *loganin R* in 15 mL of *methanol R*.

Plate TLC silica gel plate R.

Mobile phase water R, methanol R, ethyl acetate R (8:15:77 *V/V/V*).

Application 30 µL, as bands.

Development Over a path of 15 cm.

Drying In air.

Detection Spray with *vanillin reagent R*. Heat in an oven at 100-105 °C for 10 min. Examine in daylight.

Results See below the sequence of the zones present in the chromatograms obtained with the reference and test solutions. Furthermore, other zones are present in the chromatogram obtained with the test solution.

Top of the plate	
	A violet zone
	An intense blue zone
Loganine: a greyish-violet zone	A violet to greyish-violet zone
	A grey to greyish-blue zone
	A brownish zone
Reference solution	Test solution

HERBAL DRUGS

TESTS

Loss on drying (*2.2.32*)
Maximum 10.0 per cent, determined on 1.000 g of the powdered drug (355) (*2.9.12*) by drying in an oven at 105 °C for 2 h.

Total ash (*2.4.16*)
Maximum 10.0 per cent.

Bitterness value (*2.8.15*)
Minimum 3000.

—————————————————————————— *Ph Eur*

Boldo Leaf

(*Ph Eur monograph 1396*)

Preparation
Boldo Leaf Dry Extract

Ph Eur ————

DEFINITION

Whole or fragmented dried leaf of *Peumus boldus* Molina.

Content

Minimum 0.1 per cent of total alkaloids, expressed as boldine ($C_{19}H_{21}NO_4$; M_r 327.4) (anhydrous drug).

CHARACTERS

Characteristic odour, especially when rubbed.

IDENTIFICATION

A. The leaf is oval or elliptical usually 5 cm long with a short petiole, an obtuse or slightly emarginate or mucronate apex and an equal and rounded base; the margin is entire and slightly undulate and the thickened edges are more or less revolute. The lamina is greyish-green, thick, tough and brittle. The upper surface is rough with numerous prominent small protuberances and a depressed venation. The lower surface is finely pubescent, with the protuberances less well-marked, and a prominent, pinnate venation.

B. Reduce to a powder (355) (*2.9.12*). The powder is greyish-green. Examine under a microscope using *chloral hydrate solution R*. The powder shows fragments of the upper epidermis and underlying hypodermis with straight or slightly sinuous thickened and beaded walls, those of the lower epidermis with numerous stomata surrounded by 4-7 subsidiary cells; solitary, bifurcated or stellate clustered unicellular covering trichomes with more or less thickened and lignified walls; fragments of the lamina showing a two-layered palisade; debris of the spongy mesophyll including numerous large, rounded oil cells and parenchyma containing fine needle-shaped crystals; thick-walled fibres and lignified, pitted parenchymatous cells associated with vascular tissue from the veins.

C. Thin-layer chromatography (*2.2.27*).

Test solution Mix 1.5 g of the powdered drug (355) (*2.9.12*) and 5 mL of *methanol R* and sonicate for 10 min. Filter the supernatant through a 3 cm × 0.5 cm column of *cellulose for chromatography R1*. Use the first 1 mL of the eluate as the test solution.

Reference solution Dissolve 2 mg of *boldine R* and 10 mg of *hyoscine hydrobromide R* in 5 mL of *methanol R*.

Plate *TLC silica gel plate R* (5-40 µm) [or *TLC silica gel plate R* (2-10 µm)].

Mobile phase diethylamine R, methanol R, toluene R (10:10:80 *V/V/V*).

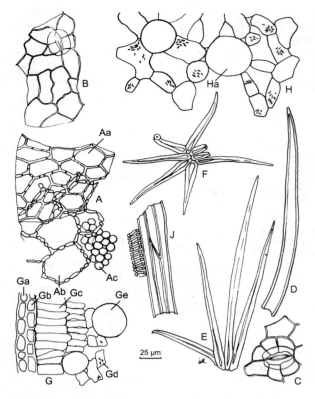

A. Fragment of the lamina, in surface view, showing the upper epidermis (Aa), hypodermis with thickened and beaded walls (Ab), and palisade parenchyma (Ac)

B and C. Lower epidermis with stomata surrounded by 4-7 subsidiary cells

D. Unicellular covering trichome, solitary

E and F. Unicellular covering trichomes, stellate clustered

G. Fragment of the lamina, in transverse section, showing the upper epidermis (Ga), hypodermis (Gb), palisade parenchyma (Gc) and spongy parenchyma (Gd) containing oil cells (Ge)

H. Spongy parenchyma containing fine needle-shaped crystals and oil cells (Ha)

J. Vascular tissue with fibres

Figure 1396.-1. – *Illustration of powdered herbal drug of boldo leaf (see Identification B)*

Application 40 µL [or 6 µL] of the test solution and 20 µL [or 2 µL] of the reference solution, as bands of 15 mm [or 8 mm].

Development Over a path of 15 cm [or 6 cm].

Drying In air.

Detection Spray with *potassium iodobismuthate solution R2*, dry for 5 min in air and spray with *sodium nitrite solution R*; examine in daylight after 30 min.

Results See below the sequence of zones present in the chromatograms obtained with the reference solution and the test solution.

TESTS

Essential oil (*2.8.12*)
Maximum 40 mL/kg (anhydrous drug).

Use 10.0 g of the freshly fragmented drug, a 1000 mL flask and 300 mL of *water R* as the distillation liquid. Distil at a rate of 2-3 mL/min for 3 h.

Foreign matter (*2.8.2*)
Maximum 4 per cent of twigs and maximum 2 per cent of other foreign matter.

Top of the plate	
	A yellowish-brown zone
Hyoscine: a pale brown zone	
	A yellow zone
	A brown zone
	A brown zone
Boldine: a brown zone	A brown zone (boldine)
	Several zones
Reference solution	Test solution

Calculate the percentage content of total alkaloids expressed as boldine using the following expression:

$$\frac{(\sum A_1) \times m_2 \times p}{A_2 \times m_1 \times 100}$$

m_1 = mass of the drug to be examined, in grams
m_2 = mass of *boldine CRS* in the reference solution, in grams
$\sum A_1$ = sum of the areas of the peaks due to the 6 alkaloids identified in the chromatogram obtained with the test solution
A_2 = of the peak due to boldine in the chromatogram obtained with the reference solution area;
p = percentage content of boldine in *boldine CRS*

—————————— Ph Eur

Water (*2.2.13*)
Maximum 100 mL/kg, determined by distillation of 20.0 g of the powdered drug (355) (*2.9.12*).

Total ash (*2.4.16*)
Maximum 13.0 per cent.

ASSAY
Alkaloids
Liquid chromatography (*2.2.29*).

Test solution   To 1.000 g of the powdered drug (355) (*2.9.12*) add 50 mL of *dilute hydrochloric acid R*. Shake in a water-bath at 80 °C for 30 min. Filter, take up the residue with 50 mL of *dilute hydrochloric acid R* and shake in a water-bath at 80 °C for 30 min. Filter and repeat the operation once on the residue obtained. Filter. Combine the cooled filtrates and shake with 100 mL of a mixture of equal volumes of *ethyl acetate R* and *hexane R*. Discard the organic layer. Adjust the aqueous layer to pH 9.5 with *dilute ammonia R1*. Shake successively with 100 mL, 50 mL and 50 mL of *methylene chloride R*. Combine the lower layers and evaporate to dryness under reduced pressure. Dissolve the residue in the mobile phase and dilute to 10.0 mL with the mobile phase.

Reference solution   Dissolve 12 mg of *boldine CRS* in the mobile phase and dilute to 100.0 mL with the mobile phase. Dilute 1.0 mL of this solution to 10.0 mL with the mobile phase.

Column:
— *size*: $l = 0.25$ m, Ø = 4.6 mm;
— *stationary phase*: *octadecylsilyl silica gel for chromatography R* (5 μm).

Solution A   Mix 0.2 mL of *diethylamine R* and 99.8 mL of *acetonitrile R*.

Solution B   Mix 0.2 mL of *diethylamine R* and 99.8 mL of *water R* and adjust to pH 3 with *anhydrous formic acid R*.

Mobile phase   Solution A, solution B (16:84 *V/V*).

Flow rate   1.5 mL/min.

Detection   Spectrophotometer at 304 nm.

Injection   20 μL.

Relative retention   With reference to boldine (retention time = about 6 min): isoboldine = about 0.9; isocorydine *N*-oxide = about 1.8; laurotetanine = about 2.2; isocorydine = about 2.8; *N*-methyllaurotetanine = about 3.2. Additional peaks may be present.

System suitability   Test solution:
— *resolution*: minimum 1 between the peaks due to isoboldine and boldine.

Boldo Leaf Dry Extract

(*Ph Eur monograph 1816*)

Ph Eur ————————————————————

DEFINITION
Extract produced from *Boldo leaf (1396)*.

Content:
— *for aqueous extracts*: minimum 0.5 per cent of total alkaloids, expressed as boldine ($C_{19}H_{21}NO_4$; M_r 327.4) (dried extract);
— *for hydroalcoholic extracts*: minimum 1.0 per cent of total alkaloids, expressed as boldine ($C_{19}H_{21}NO_4$; M_r 327.4) (dried extract).

PRODUCTION
The extract is produced from the herbal drug by a suitable procedure using either hot water at not less than 65 °C or a hydroalcoholic solvent equivalent in strength to ethanol (45-75 per cent *V/V*).

CHARACTERS
Appearance
Brown or greenish-brown, hygroscopic powder.

IDENTIFICATION
Thin-layer chromatography (*2.2.27*).

Test solution   To 0.5 g of the extract to be examined add 1 mL of *hydrochloric acid R* and 20 mL of *water R*. Sonicate for 10 min. Transfer the liquid to a separating funnel and make alkaline with 2 mL of *dilute ammonia R1*. Shake with 2 quantities, each of 20 mL, of *methylene chloride R*. Evaporate the combined organic layers to dryness. Dissolve the residue in 1 mL of *methanol R*.

Reference solution   Dissolve 2 mg of *boldine R* and 10 mg of *hyoscine hydrobromide R* in 5 mL of *methanol R*.

Plate   *TLC silica gel plate R* (5-40 μm) [or *TLC silica gel plate R* (2-10 μm)].

Mobile phase   *diethylamine R*, *methanol R*, *toluene R* (10:10:80 *V/V/V*).

Application   20 μL [or 3 μL], as bands of 15 mm [or 8 mm].

Development   Over a path of 15 cm [or 6 cm].

Drying   In air.

Detection   Spray with *potassium iodobismuthate solution R2*, allow to dry in air for 5 min and spray with *sodium nitrite solution R*; examine in daylight after 30 min.

Results   See below the sequence of zones present in the chromatograms obtained with the reference solution and the test solution. Furthermore, other faint zones may be present in the chromatogram obtained with the test solution.

Top of the plate		
———		———
	A yellowish-brown zone	
	An orange-yellow zone	
Hyoscine: a pale brown zone		
	An orange zone	
	An orange zone	
———		———
Boldine: a brown zone	A brown zone (boldine)	
	Several orange zones	
Reference solution	**Test solution**	

ASSAY

Liquid chromatography (*2.2.29*).

Test solution   To 1.000 g of the extract to be examined add 50 mL of *dilute hydrochloric acid R* and sonicate for 10 min. Transfer to a separating funnel and wash with 10 mL of a mixture of equal volumes of *ethyl acetate R* and *hexane R*. Adjust the aqueous phase to pH 9.5 with *dilute ammonia R1*. After cooling, shake successively with 100 mL, 50 mL, and a further 50 mL of *methylene chloride R*, taking care not to form an emulsion. Evaporate the combined lower layers to dryness under reduced pressure. Dissolve the residue in the mobile phase and transfer the solution to a volumetric flask. Rinse and dilute to 10.0 mL with the mobile phase.

Reference solution   Dissolve 12.0 mg of *boldine CRS* in the mobile phase and dilute to 100.0 mL with the mobile phase.

Column:
— *size*: $l = 0.25$ m, $\emptyset = 4.6$ mm;
— *stationary phase*: octadecylsilyl silica gel for chromatography R (5 μm).

Solution A   Mix 0.2 mL of *diethylamine R* with 99.8 mL of *acetonitrile R*.

Solution B   Mix 0.2 mL of *diethylamine R* with 99.8 mL of *water R* and adjust to pH 3 with *anhydrous formic acid R*.

Mobile phase   Solution A, solution B (16:84 *V/V*).

Flow rate   1.5 mL/min.

Detection   Spectrophotometer at 304 nm.

Injection   20 μL.

Relative retention   With reference to boldine (retention time = about 6 min): isoboldine = about 0.9; isocorydine *N*-oxide = about 1.8; laurotetanine = about 2.2; isocorydine = about 2.8; *N*-methyllaurotetanine = about 3.2. Additional peaks may be present.

System suitability   Test solution:
— *resolution*: minimum 1.0 between the peaks due to isoboldine and boldine.

Calculate the percentage content of total alkaloids, expressed as boldine, using the following expression:

$$\frac{\left(\sum A_1\right) \times m_2 \times p}{A_2 \times m_1 \times 10}$$

ΣA_1 = sum of the areas of the peaks due to the 6 alkaloids identified in the chromatogram obtained with the test solution

A_2 = area of the peak due to boldine in the chromatogram obtained with the reference solution

m_1 = mass of the extract to be examined used to prepare the test solution, in grams

m_2 = mass of *boldine CRS* used to prepare the reference solution, in grams

p = percentage content of boldine in *boldine CRS*.

———————————— *Ph Eur*

Buckwheat Herb

(Ph Eur monograph 2184)

Ph Eur ————————————————————

DEFINITION

Whole or fragmented aerial parts of *Fagopyrum esculentum* Moench, collected in the early flowering period prior to fruiting and dried immediately.

Content

Minimum 3.0 per cent of rutin ($C_{27}H_{30}O_{16}$; M_r 611) (dried drug).

IDENTIFICATION

A. The stem is cylindrical, hollow, finely ridged longitudinally, about 2-6 mm in diameter, brownish-green or reddish, with few branches and thickened at the internodes; the leaves are arranged spirally and have membranous, sheathing stipules; the surface is glabrous except in the region of the stipules, where short, white hairs may occur. The leaves are dark green, paler on the lower surface, up to 7 cm wide and 11 cm long, saggitate or cordate, almost pentagonal with 2 widely rounded lobes; the lower leaves are petiolate, the upper leaves sessile or amplexicaul; the lamina is glabrous and the margin finely sinuate and fringed with minute, reddish-brown projections; similar projections occur on the veins on the upper surface. The inflorescence is a cymose panicle, the individual flowers 1-2 mm long and 6 mm in diameter with 5 free, white or reddish petals.

B. Microscopic examination (*2.8.23*). The powder is dark green. Examine under a microscope using *chloral hydrate solution R*. The powder shows the following diagnostic characters (Figure 2184.-1): fragments of the epidermis of the stem, in surface view [D], composed of elongated cells showing striations on the outer walls [Da] and anomocytic stomata (*2.8.3*) [Db]; fragments of the upper epidermis of the lamina, in surface view [B], consisting of polygonal cells covered by a striated cuticle [Ba] and anomocytic stomata [Bb], often accompanied by palisade parenchyma [Bc]; fragments of the epidermis of the leaf margins [A] and of the epidermis covering the veins, often showing ovoid or rounded papilla-like projections, often reddish, with thickened and striated walls; fragments of the lower epidermis of the lamina [C] with thin-walled polygonal cells, numerous stomata [Ca] and rare glandular trichomes with a biseriate stalk and a globular head usually composed of 8 cells [Cb]; fragments of mesophyll [F] with narrow, annular or spiral vessels [Fa] and of spongy parenchyma, numerous cells of which contain cluster crystals of calcium oxalate, varying in diameter (25-100 μm) [Fb], smaller prismatic crystals of calcium oxalate [Fc], occurring scattered in the mesophyll and also in the parenchyma of the stem; fragments of lignified tissue [H] with bordered-pitted [Ha], reticulate or annular [Hb] vessels and thin-walled, pitted fibres [Hc]; occasional fragments of the corolla with a papillose epidermis [E]; spherical or ovoid pollen grains, about 50 μm in diameter, with a pitted exine and 3 furrows [G].

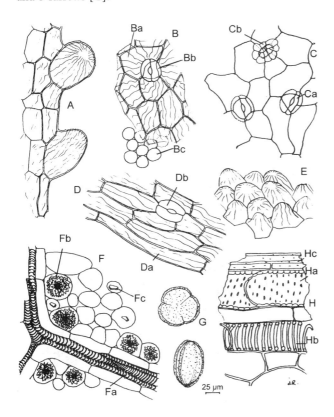

Figure 2184.-1. – *Illustration for identification test B of powdered herbal drug of buckwheat herb*

C. Thin-layer chromatography (*2.2.27*).

Test solution   To 0.5 g of the powdered herbal drug (355) (*2.9.12*) add 5.0 mL of *methanol R* and heat in a water-bath at 60 °C under a reflux condenser for 10 min. Cool and filter.

Reference solution   Dissolve 10 mg of *hyperoside R* and 10 mg of *rutin R* in 10 mL of *methanol R*.

Plate   TLC silica gel plate R (5-40 μm) [or *TLC silica gel plate R* (2-10 μm)].

Mobile phase   anhydrous formic acid R, water R, ethyl acetate R (10:10:80 *V/V/V*).

Application   20 μL [or 5 μL] as bands of 15 mm [or 8 mm].

Development   Over a path of 10 cm [or 6 cm].

Drying   At 100-105 °C.

Detection   Treat with a 10 g/L solution of *diphenylboric acid aminoethyl ester R* in *methanol R*, subsequently treat with a 50 g/L solution of *macrogol 400 R* in *methanol R*; allow to dry in air for about 30 min and examine in ultraviolet light at 365 nm.

Results   See below the sequence of zones present in the chromatograms obtained with the reference solution and the test solution. Furthermore, other fluorescent zones may be present in the chromatogram obtained with the test solution.

Top of the plate	
	2 red zones
	1-2 light blue zones
———	———
	An orange zone
	An orange zone
Hyperoside: an orange zone	2 blue zones
———	———
Rutin: an orange-yellow zone	An orange-yellow zone (rutin)
Reference solution	**Test solution**

TESTS

Loss on drying (*2.2.32*)
Maximum 10.0 per cent, determined on 1.000 g of the powdered herbal drug (355) (*2.9.12*) by drying in an oven at 105 °C for 2 h.

Total ash (*2.4.16*)
Maximum 15.0 per cent.

ASSAY
Liquid chromatography (*2.2.29*).

Test solution   To 0.500 g of the powdered herbal drug (355) (*2.9.12*), add 30 mL of an 80 per cent *V/V* solution of *methanol R*. Heat the mixture under a reflux condenser in a water-bath at 60 °C for 30 min, then extract the mixture in an ultrasonic bath for 15 min. Allow to cool, dilute to 50.0 mL with an 80 per cent *V/V* solution of *methanol R* and filter.

Reference solution (a)   Dissolve 25.0 mg of *rutoside trihydrate CRS* in an 80 per cent *V/V* solution of *methanol R* and dilute to 50.0 mL with the same solvent.

Reference solution (b)   Dissolve 20.0 mg of *troxerutin R* and 5.0 mg of *quercitrin R* in an 80 per cent *V/V* solution of *methanol R* and dilute to 50.0 mL with the same solvent.

Column:
— *size:* l = 0.125 m, Ø = 4 mm;
— *stationary phase:* octadecylsilyl silica gel for chromatography R (5 μm);
— *temperature:* 30 °C.

Mobile phase:
— *mobile phase A:* mix 50 volumes of *acetonitrile R* and 950 volumes of *water R* adjusted to pH 2 with *phosphoric acid R*;
— *mobile phase B:* mix 95 volumes of *water R* adjusted to pH 2 with *phosphoric acid R* and 905 volumes of *acetonitrile R*;

Time (min)	Mobile phase A (per cent *V/V*)	Mobile phase B (per cent *V/V*)
0 - 6	94	6
6 - 16.5	94 → 85	6 → 15
16.5 - 22	85 → 76	15 → 24
22 - 25	76 → 59	24 → 41

Flow rate   1.0 mL/min.

Detection   Spectrophotometer at 350 nm.

Injection   10 μL.

System suitability   Reference solution (b):

— *elution order*: order indicated in the composition of reference solution (b), when the chromatogram is recorded in the prescribed conditions;

— *resolution*: minimum 3 between the peaks due to troxerutin and quercitrin.

Using the retention times determined from the chromatogram obtained with reference solution (a), locate the peak due to rutin in the chromatogram obtained with the test solution.

Calculate the percentage content of rutin using the following expression:

$$\frac{A_1 \times m_2 \times p}{A_2 \times m_1}$$

A_1 = area of the peak due to rutin in the chromatogram obtained with the test solution;

A_2 = area of the peak due to rutin in the chromatogram obtained with reference solution (a);

m_1 = mass of the herbal drug to be examined used to prepare the test solution, in grams;

m_2 = mass of *rutoside trihydrate CRS* used to prepare reference solution (a), in grams;

p = percentage content of rutin in *rutoside trihydrate CRS*.

Ph Eur

Greater Burnet Root

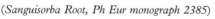

(*Sanguisorba Root, Ph Eur monograph 2385*)

Ph Eur

DEFINITION
Whole or fragmented, dried underground parts of *Sanguisorba officinalis* L. without rootlets.

Content
Minimum 5.0 per cent of tannins, expressed as pyrogallol ($C_6H_6O_3$; M_r 126.1) (dried drug).

CHARACTERS
The adventitious roots are about 5-25 cm long and up to 2 cm in diameter.

IDENTIFICATION
A. The whole drug consists of the rhizome, often ramified, thick, short, fusiform or cylindrical and the adventitious roots whose surface is reddish-brown or blackish-brown, with longitudinal striations, sometimes with transverse fissures, and showing rootlet scars.

It may also be found as more or less cylindrical fragments up to 2 cm long or elliptical or irregular discs. The fracture is light-coloured and very fibrous.

B. Reduce to a powder (355) (*2.9.12*). The powder is light yellowish-brown. Examine under a microscope using *chloral hydrate solution R*. The powder shows the following diagnostic characters: numerous, whole or fragmented phloem fibres, usually isolated, narrow, sometimes more than 500 μm long and often rough-walled; calcium oxalate cluster crystals, free or inside parenchyma cells; a few reticulate lignified vessels; rare cork fragments. Examine under a microscope using a 50 per cent *V/V* solution of *glycerol R*. The powder shows rounded or ovoid starch granules, single or in groups of 2-4; the diameter of a component granule may reach 30 μm.

Some starch granules are found in the parenchyma cells or in cells of the medullary rays.

C. Thin-layer chromatography (*2.2.27*).

Test solution To 2.0 g of the powdered drug (355) (*2.9.12*) add 50 mL of *water R* and boil under a reflux condenser for 30 min. Cool the solution and centrifuge for 10 min. Shake the supernatant with 2 quantities, each of 15 mL, of *di-isopropyl ether R* saturated with *hydrochloric acid R*. Combine the ether layers. Evaporate to dryness and dissolve the residue in 1.0 mL of *methanol R*. Filter through a polypropylene syringe filter (nominal pore size 0.45 μm).

Reference solution Dissolve 5 mg of *gallic acid R* and 20 mg of *resorcinol R* in 20 mL of *methanol R*.

Plate TLC silica gel F_{254} *plate R* (5-40 μm) [or *TLC silica gel* F_{254} *plate R* (2-10 μm)].

Mobile phase anhydrous formic acid R, ethyl acetate R, toluene R (10:30:60 *V/V/V*).

Application 10 μL [or 4 μL] as bands.

Development Over a path of 10 cm [or 6 cm].

Drying In air.

Detection A Examine in ultraviolet light at 254 nm.

Results A See below the sequence of quenching zones present in the chromatograms obtained with the reference solution and the test solution. Furthermore, other faint quenching zones may be present in the chromatogram obtained with the test solution.

Top of the plate	
	A quenching zone
Resorcinol: a quenching zone	
	A quenching zone
Gallic acid: a quenching zone	A quenching zone (gallic acid)
	A quenching zone
	A quenching zone
Reference solution	**Test solution**

Detection B Spray with a 10 g/L solution of *ferric chloride R* in *anhydrous ethanol R* and heat at 100-105 °C for 15 min; examine in daylight.

Results B See below the sequence of the zones present in the chromatograms obtained with the reference solution and the test solution. Furthermore, other faint zones may be present in the chromatogram obtained with the test solution.

Top of the plate	
Resorcinol: a brown zone	
	A blackish-blue zone
Gallic acid: a blackish-blue zone	A blackish-blue zone (gallic acid)
	A blackish-blue zone
Reference solution	**Test solution**

TESTS

Loss on drying (*2.2.32*)

Maximum 12.0 per cent, determined on 1.000 g of the powdered drug (355) (*2.9.12*) by drying in an oven at 105 °C.

Total ash (*2.4.16*)

Maximum 10.0 per cent.

Ash insoluble in hydrochloric acid (*2.8.1*)

Maximum 2.0 per cent.

ASSAY

Carry out the determination of tannins in herbal drugs (*2.8.14*). Use 0.500 g of the powdered drug (180) (*2.9.12*).

_____ *Ph Eur*

Butcher's Broom

(*Ph Eur monograph 1847*)

Ph Eur _____

DEFINITION

Dried, whole or fragmented underground parts of *Ruscus aculeatus* L.

Content

Minimum 1.0 per cent of total sapogenins, expressed as ruscogenins [mixture of neoruscogenin ($C_{27}H_{40}O_4$; M_r 428.6) and ruscogenin ($C_{27}H_{42}O_4$; M_r 430.6)] (dried drug).

IDENTIFICATION

A. The rhizome consists of yellowish, branched, articulated, somewhat knotty pieces, cylindrical or subconical, about 5-10 cm long and about 5 mm thick. The surface is marked with thin annulations about 1-3 mm wide, separated from one another; rounded scars of the aerial stems are present on the upper surface. On the lower surface numerous roots, or their scars, occur; the roots are about 2 mm in diameter and similar in colour to the rhizome. The outer layer is easily detached, revealing a yellowish-white, very hard central cylinder.

B. Reduce to a powder (355) (*2.9.12*). The powder is yellowish. Examine under a microscope using *chloral hydrate solution R*. The powder shows the following diagnostic characters (Figure 1847.-1): groups of sclereids of the rhizome, with variously-shaped cells, rounded, elongated or rectangular; the walls are moderately thickened and distinctly beaded, with large, rounded or oval pits [F, G, L, P, Q]; fragments of the endodermis composed of a single layer of irregularly thickened cells [K]; groups of rounded parenchymatous cells, thickened at the corners, with small, triangular intercellular spaces [D, E, N]; thin-walled parenchyma [J] with some cells containing raphides of calcium oxalate [C]; groups [H] of thick-walled fibres [Ha] and small vessels, up to about 50 μm in diameter, the walls showing numerous small, slit-shaped pits [A, Hb]; rare fragments of dermal tissue of the root [B]; raphides of calcium oxalate, isolated [M].

C. Thin-layer chromatography (*2.2.27*).

Test solution   Introduce 1.0 g of the powdered drug (355) (*2.9.12*) and 50 mL of *dilute hydrochloric acid R* into a 100 mL flask with a ground-glass neck. Heat on a water-bath under a reflux condenser for 40 min. Allow to cool and extract the unfiltered mixture with 3 quantities, each of 25 mL, of *methylene chloride R*. Combine the organic solutions and dry over *anhydrous sodium sulfate R*. Filter and

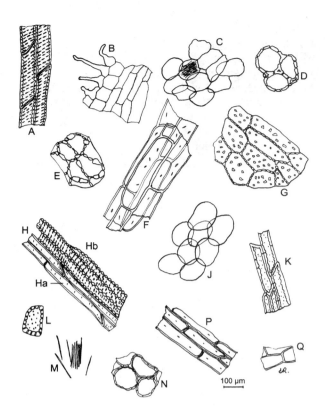

Figure 1847.-1.– *Illustration for identification test B of powdered herbal drug of butcher's broom*

evaporate to dryness. Dissolve the residue in 5 mL of *methanol R*.

Reference solution   Dissolve 1 mg of *ruscogenins CRS* and 1 mg of *stigmasterol R* in *methanol R* and dilute to 5 mL with the same solvent.

Plate   TLC *silica gel plate R* (5-40 μm) [or TLC *silica gel plate R* (2-10 μm)].

Mobile phase   methanol R, methylene chloride R (7:93 *V/V*).

Application   10 μL [or 4 μL] as bands.

Development   Over a path of 15 cm [or 6 cm].

Drying   In air.

Detection   Spray with *vanillin reagent R*, dry in an oven at 100-105 °C for 1 min and examine in daylight.

Results   See below the sequence of zones present in the chromatograms obtained with the reference solution and the test solution. Furthermore, other weak zones may be present in the chromatogram obtained with the test solution.

Top of the plate	
	Several zones of various colours
Stigmasterol: a violet zone	A violet zone
	A violet zone
Ruscogenins: a yellow zone	A yellow zone (ruscogenins)
	Several zones of various colours
Reference solution	**Test solution**

TESTS

Foreign matter (*2.8.2*)
Maximum 5 per cent.

Loss on drying (*2.2.32*)
Maximum 12.0 per cent, determined on 1.000 g of the powdered drug (355) (*2.9.12*) by drying in an oven at 105 °C for 2 h.

Total ash (*2.4.16*)
Maximum 12.0 per cent.

Ash insoluble in hydrochloric acid (*2.8.1*)
Maximum 5.0 per cent.

ASSAY

Liquid chromatography (*2.2.29*).

Test solution   To 2.000 g of the powdered drug (355) (*2.9.12*) add 60 mL of *anhydrous ethanol R*, 15 mL of *water R* and 0.2 g of *potassium hydroxide R*. Extract on a water-bath under a reflux condenser for 4 h. Allow to cool and filter into a 100 mL volumetric flask. Rinse the extraction flask and the residue in the filter with 3 quantities, each of 10 mL, of *anhydrous ethanol R* and add the rinsings to the volumetric flask. Dilute to 100.0 mL with *anhydrous ethanol R*. Introduce 25.0 mL of this solution into a round-bottomed flask fitted to a rotary evaporator and evaporate to dryness. Dissolve the residue in 10 mL of *butanol R* and add 3 mL of *hydrochloric acid R1* and 8 mL of *water R*. Heat on a water-bath under a reflux condenser for 1 h. Allow to cool and transfer to a 100 mL volumetric flask. Rinse the round-bottomed flask with 3 quantities, each of 20 mL, of *methanol R*. Add the rinsings to the volumetric flask and dilute to 100.0 mL with *methanol R*.

Reference solution   Dissolve 5.0 mg of *ruscogenins CRS* in 100 mL of *methanol R*.

Column:
— *size*: l = 0.25 m, Ø = 4.6 mm;
— *stationary phase*: octadecylsilyl silica gel for chromatography *R* (5 µm).

Mobile phase:
— *mobile phase A*: water *R*;
— *mobile phase B*: acetonitrile *R1*;

Time (min)	Mobile phase A (per cent *V/V*)	Mobile phase B (per cent *V/V*)
0 - 25	40	60
25 - 27	40 → 0	60 → 100
27 - 37	0	100

Flow rate   1.2 mL/min.

Detection   Spectrophotometer at 203 nm.

Injection   20 µL.

Identification of peaks   Use the chromatogram supplied with *ruscogenins CRS* and the chromatogram obtained with the reference solution to identify the peaks due to neoruscogenin and ruscogenin.

Relative retention   With reference to neoruscogenin (retention time = about 16 min): ruscogenin = about 1.2.

System suitability   Reference solution:
— *resolution*: minimum 1.5 between the peaks due to neoruscogenin and ruscogenin.

Calculate the percentage content of sapogenins, expressed as ruscogenins (neoruscogenin and ruscogenin), using the following expression:

$$\frac{A_1 \times m_2 \times 4 \times p_1}{A_2 \times m_1} + \frac{A_3 \times m_2 \times 4 \times p_2}{A_4 \times m_1}$$

A_1 = area of the peak due to ruscogenin in the chromatogram obtained with the test solution;

A_2 = area of the peak due to ruscogenin in the chromatogram obtained with the reference solution;

A_3 = area of the peak due to neoruscogenin in the chromatogram obtained with the test solution;

A_4 = area of the peak due to neoruscogenin in the chromatogram obtained with the reference solution;

m_1 = mass of the herbal drug to be examined used to prepare the test solution, in grams;

m_2 = mass of *ruscogenins CRS* used to prepare the reference solution, in grams;

p_1 = percentage content of ruscogenin in *ruscogenins CRS*;

p_2 = percentage content of neoruscogenin in *ruscogenins CRS*.

_____ *Ph Eur*

Calendula Flower

(*Ph Eur monograph 1297*)

Ph Eur _____

DEFINITION

Whole or cut, dried, and fully opened flowers that have been detached from the receptacle of the cultivated, double-flowered varieties of *Calendula officinalis* L.

Content

Minimum 0.4 per cent of flavonoids, expressed as hyperoside ($C_{21}H_{20}O_{12}$; M_r 464.4) (dried drug).

IDENTIFICATION

A. The ligulate florets consist of a yellow or orange-yellow ligule, about 3-5 mm wide and about 7 mm in the middle part, with a 3-toothed apex and a hairy, partly sickle-shaped, yellowish-brown or orange-brown tube with a projecting style and a bifid stigma occasionally with a partly bent yellowish-brown or orange-brown ovary. The tubular florets, about 5 mm long, are present and consist of the yellow, orange-red or reddish-violet 5-lobed corolla and the yellowish-brown or orange-brown tube, hairy in its lower part, mostly with a partly bent yellowish-brown or orange-brown ovary.

B. Reduce to a powder (355) (*2.9.12*). The powder is yellowish-brown. Examine under a microscope using *chloral hydrate solution R*. The powder shows the following diagnostic characters (Figure 1297.-1): fragments of epidermises of the corolla [C, F, K] containing light yellow oil droplets, some with fairly large anomocytic stomata (*2.8.3*) [Fa, Ka]; covering trichomes biseriate, multicellular and conical [G], usually fragmented, and glandular trichomes with a multicellular stalk [E], very abundant on the base of the corolla [D]; fragments of parenchyma of the corolla [B] containing prisms and very small cluster crystals of calcium oxalate [Ba, Da] and small vessels [Bb]; spherical pollen grains up to about 40 µm in diameter with a sharply spiny exine and 3 germinal pores [A, J]; occasional fragments of the stigmas with short, bulbous papillae [H].

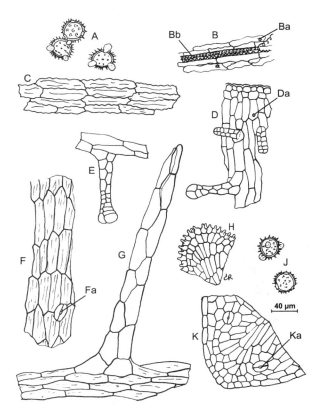

Figure 1297.-1.– Illustration for identification test B of powdered herbal drug of calendula flower

C. Thin-layer chromatography (*2.2.27*).

Test solution   Mix 1.0 g of the powdered drug (500) (*2.9.12*) and 10 mL of *methanol R* and heat on a water-bath under a reflux condenser for 10 min. Cool and filter.

Reference solution   Dissolve 1.0 mg of *caffeic acid R*, 1.0 mg of *chlorogenic acid R* and 2.5 mg of *rutin R* in 10 mL of *methanol R*.

Plate   *TLC silica gel plate R*.

Mobile phase   *anhydrous formic acid R*, *water R*, *ethyl acetate R* (10:10:80 *V/V/V*).

Application   20 µL of the test solution and 10 µL of the reference solution, as bands.

Development   Over a path of 10 cm.

Drying   At 100-105 °C.

Detection   Spray the still-warm plate with a 10 g/L solution of *diphenylboric acid aminoethyl ester R* in *methanol R* and then spray with a 50 g/L solution of *macrogol 400 R* in *methanol R*; allow to dry in air for 30 min and examine in ultraviolet light at 365 nm.

Results   The chromatogram obtained with the reference solution shows in the lower part a yellowish-brown fluorescent zone (rutin), in the middle part a light bluish fluorescent zone (chlorogenic acid) and in the upper part a light bluish fluorescent zone (caffeic acid).

The chromatogram obtained with the test solution shows a yellowish-brown fluorescent zone corresponding in position to the zone due to rutin in the chromatogram obtained with the reference solution, below and directly above it, it shows a yellowish-green fluorescent zone and a light bluish fluorescent zone corresponding to the zone due to chlorogenic acid in the chromatogram obtained with the reference solution, a yellowish-green fluorescent zone above it

and a light bluish fluorescent zone shortly below the zone due to caffeic acid in the chromatogram obtained with the reference solution. Furthermore, other zones may be present in the chromatogram obtained with the test solution.

TESTS
Foreign matter (*2.8.2*)
Maximum 5 per cent of bracts and maximum 2 per cent of other foreign matter.

Loss on drying (*2.2.32*)
Maximum 12.0 per cent, determined on 1.000 g of the powdered drug (500) (*2.9.12*) by drying in an oven at 105 °C for 2 h.

Total ash (*2.4.16*)
Maximum 10.0 per cent.

ASSAY
Stock solution   Into a 100 mL round-bottomed flask introduce 0.800 g of the powdered drug (500) (*2.9.12*), 1 mL of a 5 g/L solution of *hexamethylenetetramine R*, 7 mL of *hydrochloric acid R1* and 20 mL of *acetone R*. Boil the mixture under a reflux condenser for 30 min. Filter the liquid through a plug of absorbent cotton into a 100 mL volumetric flask. Add the absorbent cotton to the residue in the round-bottomed flask and extract with 2 quantities, each of 20 mL, of *acetone R*, each time boiling under a reflux condenser for 10 min. Allow to cool to room temperature, filter the liquid through a plug of absorbent cotton, then filter the combined acetone solution through a filter-paper into the volumetric flask, and dilute to 100.0 mL with *acetone R* by rinsing the flask and filter. Introduce 20.0 mL of this solution into a separating funnel, add 20 mL of *water R* and extract the mixture with 1 quantity of 15 mL and then with 3 quantities, each of 10 mL, of *ethyl acetate R*. Combine the ethyl acetate extracts in a separating funnel, rinse with 2 quantities, each of 50 mL, of *water R*, filter the extract over 10 g of *anhydrous sodium sulfate R* into a 50 mL volumetric flask and dilute to 50.0 mL with *ethyl acetate R*.

Test solution   To 10.0 mL of the stock solution add 1 mL of *aluminium chloride reagent R* and dilute to 25.0 mL with a 5 per cent *V/V* solution of *glacial acetic acid R* in *methanol R*.

Compensation liquid   Dilute 10.0 mL of the stock solution to 25.0 mL with a 5 per cent *V/V* solution of *glacial acetic acid R* in *methanol R*.

Measure the absorbance (*2.2.25*) of the test solution after 30 min, by comparison with the compensation liquid at 425 nm.

Calculate the percentage content of flavonoids, expressed as hyperoside, using the following expression:

$$\frac{A \times 1.25}{m}$$

i.e. taking the specific absorbance of hyperoside to be 500.
A = absorbance at 425 nm
m = mass of the drug to be examined, in grams.

Ph Eur

Capsicum

(*Ph Eur monograph 1859*)

Preparations

Refined and Quantified Capsicum Oleoresin

Standardised Capsicum Tincture

Ph Eur _____

DEFINITION

Dried ripe fruits of *Capsicum annuum* L. var. *minimum* (Miller) Heiser and small-fruited varieties of *Capsicum frutescens* L.

Content

Minimum 0.4 per cent of total capsaicinoids, expressed as capsaicin ($C_{18}H_{27}NO_3$; M_r 305.4) (dried drug).

CHARACTERS

Extremely pungent taste.

IDENTIFICATION

A. The fruit is yellowish-orange or reddish-brown, oblong conical with an obtuse apex, about 1-3 cm long and up to 1 cm in diameter at the widest part, occasionally attached to a 5-toothed inferior calyx and a straight peduncle. Pericarp somewhat shrivelled, glabrous, enclosing about 10-20 flat, reniform seeds 3-4 mm long, either loose or attached to a reddish dissepiment.

B. Reduce to a powder (355) (*2.9.12*). The powder is orange. Examine under a microscope using *chloral hydrate solution R*. The powder shows the following diagnostic characters (Figure 1859.-1): fragments of the epicarp, in surface view, with cells often arranged in rows of 5 to 7 [E], thick-walled when close to the peduncle [B] and with a cuticle uniformly striated [A]; fragments of the pericarp, in transverse section [D], showing the epicarp covered by a thick cuticle [Da] and parenchymatous cells frequently containing droplets of red oil, occasionally containing microsphenoidal crystals of calcium oxalate [Db]; fragments of endocarp [C] with characteristic island groups of sclerenchymatous cells [Ca], the groups being separated by thin-walled parenchymatous cells [Cb]; fragments of the seeds having an episperm composed of large, greenish-yellow, sinuous-walled sclereids with thin outer walls and strongly and unevenly thickened radial and inner walls which are conspicuously pitted [G]; endosperm parenchymatous cells with drops of oil and aleurone grains, 3-6 μm in diameter [H]; occasional fragments from the calyx having an outer epidermis with anisocytic stomata (*2.8.3*) [J], an inner epidermis with no stomata and many glandular trichomes with uniseriate stalks and multicellular heads [N], and a mesophyll [L] with many idioblasts containing prisms of calcium oxalate [La] or microsphenoidal crystals of calcium oxalate [Lb]; prisms [K] or clusters [M] of calcium oxalate, isolated; annularly and spirally thickened vessels [F].

C. Thin-layer chromatography (*2.2.27*).

Test solution To 0.50 g of the powdered drug (500) (*2.9.12*) add 5.0 mL of *ether R*, shake for 5 min and filter.

Reference solution Dissolve 2 mg of *capsaicin R* and 2 mg of *dihydrocapsaicin R* in 5.0 mL of *ether R*.

Plate TLC octadecylsilyl silica gel plate R.

Mobile phase water R, methanol R (20:80 *V/V*).

Application 20 μL as bands.

Development Over a path of 12 cm.

Drying In air.

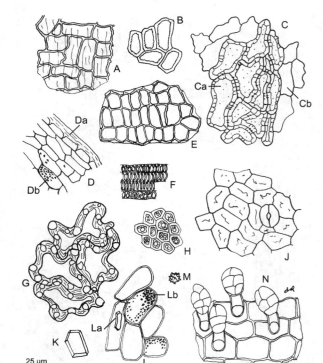

Figure 1859.-1.– *Illustration for identification test B of powdered herbal drug of capsicum*

Detection Spray with a 5 g/L solution of *dichloroquinonechlorimide R* in *methanol R*, and expose to ammonia vapour until blue zones appear; examine in daylight.

Results See below the sequence of zones present in the chromatograms obtained with the reference solution and the test solution. Furthermore, other zones may be present in the chromatogram obtained with the test solution.

Top of the plate	
———	———
Capsaicin: a blue zone	A blue zone (capsaicin)
Dihydrocapsaicin: a blue zone	A blue zone (dihydrocapsaicin)
———	———
Reference solution	**Test solution**

TESTS

Nonivamide

Liquid chromatography (*2.2.29*).

Test solution To 2.5 g of the powdered drug (500) (*2.9.12*) add 100 mL of *methanol R*. Allow to macerate for 30 min. Place in an ultrasonic bath for 15 min. Filter into a 100 mL volumetric flask, rinse the flask and filter with *methanol R*, then dilute to 100.0 mL with the same solvent.

Reference solution Dissolve 20.0 mg of *capsaicin CRS* and 4.0 mg of *nonivamide CRS* in *methanol R* and dilute to 100.0 mL with the same solvent.

Column:
— *size*: l = 0.25 m, Ø = 4.6 mm;
— *stationary phase*: *phenylsilyl silica gel for chromatography R* (5 μm);

— *temperature*: 30 °C.

Mobile phase   Mix 40 volumes of *acetonitrile R* and 60 volumes of a 1 g/L solution of *phosphoric acid R*.

Flow rate   1.0 mL/min.

Detection   Spectrophotometer at 225 nm.

Injection   10 µL.

Elution order   Nordihydrocapsaicin, nonivamide, capsaicin, dihydrocapsaicin.

System suitability   Reference solution:
— *resolution*: minimum 1.5 between the peaks due to nonivamide and capsaicin.

Calculate the percentage content of nonivamide using the following expression:

$$\frac{F_1 \times m_2 \times p_1}{F_2 \times m_1}$$

F_1 = area of the peak corresponding to nonivamide in the chromatogram obtained with the test solution;

F_2 = area of the peak corresponding to nonivamide in the chromatogram obtained with the reference solution;

m_1 = mass of the drug to be examined, in grams;

m_2 = mass of *nonivamide CRS* used to prepare the reference solution, in grams;

p_1 = percentage content of nonivamide in *nonivamide CRS*.

Limit:
— *nonivamide*: maximum 5.0 per cent of the total capsaicinoid content.

Foreign matter *(2.8.2)*

Fruits of *C. annuum* L. var. *longum* (Sendtn.) are absent.

Loss on drying *(2.2.32)*

Maximum 11.0 per cent, determined on 1.000 g of the powdered drug (500) *(2.9.12)* by drying in an oven at 105 °C for 2 h.

Total ash *(2.4.16)*

Maximum 10.0 per cent.

ASSAY

Liquid chromatography *(2.2.29)* as described in the test for nonivamide.

Calculate the percentage content of total capsaicinoids, expressed as capsaicin, using the following expression:

$$\frac{(F_3 + F_5 + F_6) \times m_4 \times p_2}{F_4 \times m_3}$$

F_3 = area of the peak corresponding to capsaicin in the chromatogram obtained with the test solution;

F_4 = area of the peak corresponding to capsaicin in the chromatogram obtained with the reference solution;

F_5 = area of the peak corresponding to dihydrocapsaicin in the chromatogram obtained with the test solution;

F_6 = area of the peak corresponding to nordihydrocapsaicin in the chromatogram obtained with the test solution;

m_3 = mass of the drug to be examined, in grams;

m_4 = mass of *capsaicin CRS* used to prepare the reference solution, in grams;

p_2 = percentage content of capsaicin in *capsaicin CRS*.

Ph Eur

Refined and Standardised Capsicum Oleoresin

(Ph Eur monograph 2336)

Ph Eur

DEFINITION

Refined and standardised oleoresin produced from *Capsicum (1859)*.

Content

12.0 per cent to 18.0 per cent *m/m* of total capsaicinoids, expressed as capsaicin ($C_{18}H_{27}NO_3$; M_r 305.4).

PRODUCTION

The oleoresin is produced from the herbal drug by an appropriate procedure, using ethanol (minimum 90 per cent *V/V*).

CHARACTERS

Appearance

Red or brown mobile extract.

IDENTIFICATION

Thin-layer chromatography *(2.2.27)*.

Test solution   Dissolve 50 mg of the oleoresin to be examined in 5 mL of *ether R*.

Reference solution   Dissolve 2 mg of *capsaicin R* and 2 mg of *dihydrocapsaicin R* in 5 mL of *ether R*.

Plate   TLC *octadecylsilyl silica gel plate R* (5-40 µm) [or TLC *octadecylsilyl silica gel plate R* (2-10 µm)].

Mobile phase   water R, methanol R (20:80 *V/V*).

Application   20 µL [or 2 µL] as bands of 15 mm [or 8 mm].

Development   Over a path of 12 cm [or 6 cm].

Drying   In air.

Detection   Treat with a 0.25 g/L solution of *dichloroquinonechlorimide R* in *ethyl acetate R*, expose to ammonia vapour until blue zones appear. Examine in daylight.

Results   See below the sequence of zones present in the chromatograms obtained with the reference solution and the test solution. Furthermore, other zones may be present in the chromatogram obtained with the test solution.

Top of the plate	
Capsaicin: a blue zone	A blue zone (capsaicin)
Dihydrocapsaicin: a blue zone	A faint blue zone (dihydrocapsaicin)
_____	_____
Reference solution	**Test solution**

TESTS

Nonivamide

Liquid chromatography *(2.2.29)*.

Test solution   Dissolve 0.300 g of the oleoresin to be examined in 60 mL of *methanol R* and dilute to 100.0 mL with the same solvent.

Reference solution   Dissolve 20.0 mg of *capsaicin CRS* and 4.0 mg of *nonivamide CRS* in 100.0 mL of *methanol R*.

Column:
— *size*: l = 0.25 m, Ø = 4.6 mm;
— *stationary phase*: phenylsilyl silica gel for chromatography R (5 µm);
— *temperature*: 30 °C.

Mobile phase   *acetonitrile R1*, 1 g/L solution of *phosphoric acid R* (40:60 *V/V*).

Flow rate   1.0 mL/min.

Detection   Spectrophotometer at 225 nm.

Injection   10 μL.

Run time   1.2 times the retention time of dihydrocapsaicin.

Elution order   Nordihydrocapsaicin, nonivamide, capsaicin, dihydrocapsaicin.

Relative retention   With reference to capsaicin (retention time = about 19 min):
nordihydrocapsaicin = about 0.9; nonivamide = about 0.95; dihydrocapsaicin = about 1.3.

System suitability   Reference solution:
— *resolution*: minimum 1.5 between the peaks due to nonivamide and capsaicin.

Calculate the percentage content of nonivamide with reference to the total capsaicinoid content, using the following expression:

$$\frac{A_1 \times m_2 \times p_1 \times 100}{A_2 \times m_1 \times C}$$

A_1 = area of the peak due to nonivamide in the chromatogram obtained with the test solution;

A_2 = area of the peak due to nonivamide in the chromatogram obtained with the reference solution;

m_1 = mass of the oleoresin to be examined used to prepare the test solution, in grams;

m_2 = mass of *nonivamide CRS* used to prepare the reference solution, in grams;

p_1 = percentage content of nonivamide in *nonivamide CRS*;

C = percentage content of total capsaicinoids, as determined in the assay.

Limit:
— *nonivamide*: maximum 5.0 per cent of the total capsaicinoid content.

Water (*2.5.12*)
Maximum 8.0 per cent, determined on 5.00 g.

ASSAY

Liquid chromatography (*2.2.29*) as described in the test for nonivamide.

Calculate the percentage content of total capsaicinoids, expressed as capsaicin, using the following expression:

$$\frac{(A_3 + A_5 + A_6) \times m_3 \times p_2}{A_4 \times m_1}$$

A_3 = area of the peak due to capsaicin in the chromatogram obtained with the test solution;

A_4 = area of the peak due to capsaicin in the chromatogram obtained with the reference solution;

A_5 = area of the peak due to dihydrocapsaicin in the chromatogram obtained with the test solution;

A_6 = area of the peak due to nordihydrocapsaicin in the chromatogram obtained with the test solution;

m_1 = mass of the oleoresin to be examined used to prepare the test solution, in grams;

m_3 = mass of *capsaicin CRS* used to prepare the reference solution, in grams;

p_2 = percentage content of capsaicin in *capsaicin CRS*.

Ph Eur

Capsicum Soft Extract, Standardised

(*Ph Eur monograph 2529*)

Ph Eur

DEFINITION

Standardised soft extract produced from *Capsicum (1859)*.

Content

2.0 per cent to 2.4 per cent of total capsaicinoids, expressed as capsaicin ($C_{18}H_{27}NO_3$; M_r 305.4).

PRODUCTION

The extract is produced from the herbal drug by a suitable procedure using ethanol (80 per cent *V/V*).

The content of total capsaicinoids in the extract is determined and adjusted, if necessary, to the value specified by adding a suitable inert excipient, for example liquid glucose.

CHARACTERS

Appearance: reddish-brown, glutinous matter.

IDENTIFICATION

Thin-layer chromatography (*2.2.27*).

Test solution   To 0.25 g of the extract to be examined add 10 mL of a mixture of *water R* and *propanol R* (40:60 *V/V*). Shake for 5 min. Filter, if necessary.

Reference solution   Dissolve 2 mg of *capsaicin R* and 1 mg of *dihydrocapsaicin R* in 5 mL of *methanol R*.

Plate   TLC octadecylsilyl silica gel plate R (5-40 μm) [or TLC octadecylsilyl silica gel plate R (2-10 μm)].

Mobile phase   *water R*, *methanol R* (20:80 *V/V*).

Application   20 μL [or 2 μL] as bands of 15 mm [or 8 mm].

Development   Over a path of 12 cm [or 6 cm].

Drying   In air.

Detection   Treat with a 0.25 g/L solution of *dichloroquinonechlorimide R* in *ethyl acetate R*, expose to ammonia vapour until blue zones appear. Examine in daylight.

Results   See below the sequence of zones present in the chromatograms obtained with the reference solution and the test solution. Furthermore, other zones may be present in the chromatogram obtained with the test solution.

Top of the plate	
Capsaicin: a blue zone	A blue zone (capsaicin)
Dihydrocapsaicin: a blue zone	A blue zone (dihydrocapsaicin)
Reference solution	**Test solution**

TESTS

Nonivamide

Liquid chromatography (*2.2.29*).

Test solution   Stir the extract to be examined until homogeneous, heating, if necessary, to not more than 60 °C. Disperse 0.350 g of the homogeneous extract in 35 mL of a mixture of *water R* and *propanol R* (40:60 *V/V*). Shake for 30 min and dilute to 50.0 mL with *propanol R*. Dilute 25.0 mL of the solution to 50.0 mL with the mobile phase and filter through a membrane filter (nominal pore size 0.45 µm).

Reference solution   Dissolve 8.0 mg of *nonivamide CRS* in the mobile phase and dilute to 100.0 mL with the mobile phase (solution A). Dissolve 8.0 mg of *capsaicin CRS* in a mixture of 5.0 mL of solution A and 45 mL of the mobile phase. Dilute to 100.0 mL with the mobile phase.

Column:
— *size: l* = 0.25 m, Ø = 4.6 mm;
— *stationary phase: phenylsilyl silica gel for chromatography R* (5 µm);
— *temperature:* 30 °C.

Mobile phase   *acetonitrile R1*, 1 g/L solution of *phosphoric acid R* (40:60 *V/V*).

Flow rate   1.0 mL/min.

Detection   spectrophotometer at 225 nm.

Injection   10 µL.

Run time   1.2 times the retention time of dihydrocapsaicin.

Elution order   nordihydrocapsaicin, nonivamide, capsaicin, dihydrocapsaicin.

Relative retention   With reference to capsaicin (retention time = about 19 min): nordihydrocapsaicin = about 0.9; nonivamide = about 0.95; dihydrocapsaicin = about 1.3.

System suitability   Reference solution:
— *resolution*: minimum 1.5 between the peaks due to nonivamide and capsaicin.

Calculate the percentage content of nonivamide with reference to the total capsaicinoid content, using the following expression:

$$\frac{A_1 \times m_2 \times p_1 \times 5}{A_2 \times m_1 \times C}$$

A_1 = area of the peak due to nonivamide in the chromatogram obtained with the test solution;
A_2 = area of the peak due to nonivamide in the chromatogram obtained with the reference solution;
m_1 = mass of the extract to be examined used to prepare the test solution, in grams;
m_2 = mass of *nonivamide CRS* used to prepare the reference solution, in grams;
p_1 = percentage content of nonivamide in *nonivamide CRS*;
C = percentage content of total capsaicinoids, as determined in the assay.

Limit:
— *nonivamide*: maximum 5.0 per cent of the total capsaicinoid content.

Dry residue *(2.8.16)*
Minimum 70.0 per cent *m/m*, determined on 2.00 g.

ASSAY
Liquid chromatography *(2.2.29)* as described in the test for nonivamide.

Calculate the percentage content of total capsaicinoids, expressed as capsaicin, using the following expression:

$$\frac{(A_3 + A_5 + A_6) \times m_3 \times p_2}{A_4 \times m_1}$$

A_3 = area of the peak due to capsaicin in the chromatogram obtained with the test solution;
A_4 = area of the peak due to capsaicin in the chromatogram obtained with the reference solution;

A_5 = area of the peak due to dihydrocapsaicin in the chromatogram obtained with the test solution;
A_6 = area of the peak due to nordihydrocapsaicin in the chromatogram obtained with the test solution;
m_1 = mass of the extract to be examined used to prepare the test solution, in grams;
m_3 = mass of *capsaicin CRS* used to prepare the reference solution, in grams;
$p2$ = percentage content of capsaicin in *capsaicin CRS*.

_____ *Ph Eur*

Standardised Capsicum Tincture

(Ph Eur monograph 2337)

Ph Eur _____

DEFINITION
Standardised tincture produced from *Capsicum (1859)* or *Refined and quantified capsicum oleoresin (2336)*.

Content
90 per cent to 110 per cent of the nominal content of total capsaicinoids, expressed as capsaicin ($C_{18}H_{27}NO_3$; M_r 305.4), stated on the label, which is between 0.020 per cent *m/m* and 0.060 per cent *m/m*.

PRODUCTION
The tincture is produced from the herbal drug or oleoresin and ethanol (70 per cent *V/V* to 85 per cent *V/V*) by an appropriate procedure.

CHARACTERS
Appearance
Yellowish-orange or reddish-orange liquid.

IDENTIFICATION
Thin-layer chromatography *(2.2.27)*.

Test solution   Shake 10 mL of the tincture to be examined with 10 mL of *hexane R*. Allow to separate and use the lower layer.

Reference solution   Dissolve 1 mg of *capsaicin R* and 1 mg of *dihydrocapsaicin R* in 5 mL of *ether R*.

Plate   TLC *octadecylsilyl silica gel plate R* (5-40 µm) [or TLC *octadecylsilyl silica gel plate R* (2-10 µm)].

Mobile phase   *water R*, *methanol R* (20:80 *V/V*).

Application   20 µL [or 2 µL] as bands of 15 mm [or 8 mm].

Development   Over a path of 12 cm [or 6 cm].

Drying   In air.

Detection   Spray with a 0.25 g/L solution of *dichloroquinonechlorimide R* in *ethyl acetate R*, expose to ammonia vapour until blue zones appear, then examine in daylight.

Results   See below the sequence of zones present in the chromatograms obtained with the reference solution and the test solution. Furthermore, other zones may be present in the chromatogram obtained with the test solution.

Top of the plate	
———	———
Capsaicin: a blue zone	A blue zone (capsaicin)
Dihydrocapsaicin: a blue zone	A faint blue zone (dihydrocapsaicin)
———	———
Reference solution	**Test solution**

TESTS

Nonivamide

Liquid chromatography (2.2.29).

Test solution Dilute 50.0 g of the tincture to be examined to 100.0 mL with *methanol R*.

Reference solution Dissolve 20.0 mg of *capsaicin CRS* and 4.0 mg of *nonivamide CRS* in 100.0 mL of *methanol R*.

Column:
— *size*: l = 0.25 m, Ø = 4.6 mm;
— *stationary phase*: phenylsilyl silica gel for chromatography R (5 μm);
— *temperature*: 30 °C.

Mobile phase acetonitrile R, 1 g/L solution of *phosphoric acid R* (40:60 *V/V*).

Flow rate 1.0 mL/min.

Detection Spectrophotometer at 225 nm.

Injection 10 μL.

Elution order Nordihydrocapsaicin, nonivamide, capsaicin, dihydrocapsaicin.

System suitability Reference solution:
— *resolution*: minimum 1.5 between the peaks due to nonivamide and capsaicin.

Calculate the percentage content of nonivamide using the following expression:

$$\frac{F_1 \times m_2 \times p_1}{F_2 \times m_1}$$

F_1 = area of the peak due to nonivamide in the chromatogram obtained with the test solution;
F_2 = area of the peak due to nonivamide in the chromatogram obtained with the reference solution;
m_1 = mass of the tincture to be examined, in grams;
m_2 = mass of *nonivamide CRS* in the reference solution, in grams;
p_1 = percentage content of nonivamide in *nonivamide CRS*.

Limit:
— *nonivamide*: maximum 5.0 per cent of the total capsaicinoid content.

Ethanol (2.9.10)

95 per cent to 105 per cent of the content stated on the label.

Methanol and 2-propanol (2.9.11)

Maximum 0.05 per cent *V/V* of methanol and maximum 0.05 per cent *V/V* of 2-propanol.

ASSAY

Liquid chromatography (2.2.29) as described in the test for nonivamide.

Calculate the percentage content of total capsaicinoids, expressed as capsaicin, using the following expression:

$$\frac{(F_3 + F_5 + F_6) \times m_4 \times p_2}{F_4 \times m_3}$$

F_3 = area of the peak due to capsaicin in the chromatogram obtained with the test solution;
F_4 = area of the peak due to capsaicin in the chromatogram obtained with the reference solution;
F_5 = area of the peak due to dihydrocapsaicin in the chromatogram obtained with the test solution;
F_6 = area of the peak due to nordihydrocapsaicin in the chromatogram obtained with the test solution;
m_3 = mass of the tincture to be examined, in grams;
m_4 = mass of *capsaicin CRS* in the reference solution, in grams;
p_2 = percentage content of capsaicin in *capsaicin CRS*.

—————————————————————— Ph Eur

Caraway

(Caraway Fruit, Ph Eur monograph 1080)

When Powdered Caraway is prescribed or demanded, material complying with the appropriate requirements below and containing not less than 2.5% v/w (25 mL/kg) of essential oil shall be dispensed or supplied.

Ph Eur ——————————————————————

DEFINITION

Whole, dry mericarp of *Carum carvi* L.

Content

Minimum 30 mL/kg of essential oil (anhydrous drug).

CHARACTERS

Odour reminiscent of carvone.

IDENTIFICATION

A. The fruit is a cremocarp of almost cylindrical shape. It is generally 3-6.5 mm long and 1-1.5 mm wide. The mericarps, usually free, are greyish-brown or brown, glabrous, mostly sickle-shaped, with both ends sharply terminated. Each bears 5 prominent narrow ridges. When cut transversely the profile shows an almost regular pentagon and 4 vittae on the dorsal surface and 2 on the commissural surface may be seen with a lens.

B. Reduce to a powder (355) (2.9.12). The powder is yellowish-brown. Examine under a microscope using *chloral hydrate solution R*. The powder shows the following diagnostic characters: fragments of the secretory cells composed of yellowish-brown or brown, thin-walled, polygonal secretory cells, frequently associated with a layer of thin-walled, transversely elongated cells, 8-12 μm wide; fragments of the epicarp with thick-walled cells and occasional anomocytic stomata (2.8.3); numerous endosperm fragments containing aleurone grains, droplets of fatty oil and microcrystals of calcium oxalate in rosette formation; spiral vessels accompanied by sclerenchymatous fibres; rarely some fibre bundles from the carpophore; groups of rectangular to sub-rectangular sclereids from the mesocarp with moderately thickened and pitted walls may be present.

C. Thin-layer chromatography (2.2.27).

Test solution Shake 0.5 g of the powdered drug (710) (2.9.12) with 5.0 mL of *ethyl acetate R* for 2-3 min. Filter over 2 g of *anhydrous sodium sulfate R*.

Reference solution Dissolve 2 μL of *carvone R* and 5 μL of *olive oil R* in 1.0 mL of *ethyl acetate R*.

Plate TLC silica gel plate R.

Mobile phase ethyl acetate R, toluene R (5:95 *V/V*).

Application   20 µL of the test solution and 10 µL of the reference solution, as bands.

Development   Over a path of 10 cm.

Drying   In air.

Detection A   Examine in ultraviolet light at 254 nm.

Results A   The chromatograms obtained with the test solution and with the reference solution show a quenching zone (carvone) in the central part against a light background.

Detection B   Spray with *anisaldehyde solution R* and, while observing, heat at 100-105 °C for 2-4 min; examine in daylight.

Results B   The zones due to carvone are dark orange-brown; the chromatogram obtained with the test solution shows above the zone due to carvone a violet zone similar in position and colour to the zone due to triglycerides of olive oil in the chromatogram obtained with the reference solution; the chromatogram obtained with the test solution shows close to the solvent front a weak violet zone due to terpene hydrocarbons and in the lower part some weak, mostly violet-greyish and brownish zones.

TESTS
Water (*2.2.13*)

Maximum 100 mL/kg, determined on 10.0 g of powdered drug.

Total ash (*2.4.16*)

Maximum 7.0 per cent.

ASSAY

Carry out the determination of essential oils in herbal drugs (*2.8.12*). Use 10.0 g of drug reduced to a powder (710) (*2.9.12*) immediately before the determination, a 500 mL round-bottomed flask, 200 mL of *water R* as the distillation liquid, and 0.50 mL of *xylene R* in the graduated tube. Distil at a rate of 2-3 mL/min for 90 min.

_____ *Ph Eur*

Caraway Oil

★ ★ ★
★   ★
★   ★
★ ★ ★

(*Ph Eur monograph 1817*)

Ph Eur _____

DEFINITION

Oil obtained by steam distillation from the dry fruits of *Carum carvi* L.

CHARACTERS

Appearance

Clear, colourless or yellow liquid.

IDENTIFICATION

First identification   B.

Second identification   A.

A. Thin-layer chromatography (*2.2.27*).

Test solution   Dissolve 40 µL of the substance to be examined in 1.0 mL of *toluene R*.

Reference solution   Dissolve 10 µL of *carvone R* and 5 µL of *carveol R* in 1.0 mL of *toluene R*.

Plate   TLC silica gel F_{254} plate R (5-40 µm) [or *TLC silica gel plate R* (2-10 µm)].

Mobile phase   ethyl acetate R, toluene R (5:95 *V/V*).

Application   10 µL [or 2 µL] as bands.

Development   Over a path of 10 cm [or 5 cm].

Drying   In air.

Detection A   Examine in ultraviolet light at 254 nm.

Results A   See below the sequence of zones present in the chromatograms obtained with the reference solution and the test solution. Furthermore, other zones may be present in the chromatogram obtained with the test solution.

Top of the plate	
———	———
Carvone: a quenching zone	A quenching zone (carvone)
———	———
Reference solution	**Test solution**

Detection B   Spray with *anisaldehyde solution R* and heat at 100-105 °C for 5-10 min. Examine immediately in daylight.

Results B   See below the sequence of zones present in the chromatograms obtained with the reference solution and the test solution. Furthermore, several zones of weak intensity are present, particularly in the lower third, in the chromatogram obtained with the test solution.

Top of the plate	
	A reddish-violet zone
———	———
	A reddish-violet zone
Carvone: a red to orange-brown zone	An intense red to orange-brown zone (carvone)
———	———
Carveol: a reddish-violet zone	A reddish-violet zone (carveol)
	A violet-blue zone
Reference solution	**Test solution**

B. Examine the chromatograms obtained in the test for chromatographic profile.

Results   The characteristic peaks in the chromatogram obtained with the test solution are similar in retention time to those in the chromatogram obtained with the reference solution.

TESTS
Relative density (*2.2.5*)

0.904 to 0.920.

Refractive index (*2.2.6*)

1.484 to 1.490.

Optical rotation (*2.2.7*)

+ 65° to + 81°.

Acid value (*2.5.1*)

Maximum 1.0, determined on 5.00 g.

Chromatographic profile

Gas chromatography (*2.2.28*): use the normalisation procedure.

Test solution   Dissolve 0.200 g of the substance to be examined in *heptane R* and dilute to 10.0 mL with the same solvent.

Reference solution (a)   Dissolve 5 µL of *β-myrcene R*, 80 µL of *limonene R*, 5 µL of *dihydrocarvone R*, 100 µL of *carvone R* and 5 µL of *carveol R* in *heptane R* and dilute to 10.0 mL with the same solvent.

Reference solution (b) Dissolve 10 μL of *carvone R* in *heptane R* and dilute to 10 mL with the same solvent. Dilute 0.1 mL of this solution to 10 mL with *heptane R*.

Column:
— *material*: fused silica,
— *size*: l = 30 m, Ø = 0.53 mm,
— *stationary phase*: macrogol 20 000 R, (film thickness 1 μm).

Carrier gas helium for chromatography R.

Flow rate 1.5 mL/min.

Split ratio 1:50.

Temperature:

	Time (min)	Temperature (°C)
Column	0 - 5	60
	5 - 68	60 → 250
	68 - 75	250
Injection port		250
Detector		260

Detection Flame ionisation.

Injection 1.0 μL.

Elution order Order indicated in the composition of reference solution (a). Record the retention times of these substances.

System suitability Reference solution (a):
— *resolution*: minimum 4.5 between the peaks due to β-myrcene and limonene.

Using the retention times determined from the chromatogram obtained with the reference solution, locate the components of the reference solution in the chromatogram obtained with the test solution.

Limits:
— *β-myrcene*: 0.1 per cent to 1.0 per cent,
— *limonene*: 30.0 per cent to 45.0 per cent,
— *trans-dihydrocarvone*: maximum 2.5 per cent,
— *carvone*: 50.0 per cent to 65.0 per cent,
— *trans-carveol*: maximum 2.5 per cent.
— *disregard limit*: the area of the peak in the chromatogram obtained with reference solution (b).

Chiral purity

Gas chromatography (*2.2.28*).

Test solution Dissolve 20 mg of the substance to be examined in *heptane R* and dilute to 10.0 mL with the same solvent.

Reference solution Dissolve 10 mg of (−)-*carvone R* and 10 mg of *carvone R1* in *heptane R* and dilute to 10.0 mL with the same solvent.

Column:
— *material*: fused silica,
— *size*: l = 30 m, Ø = 0.25 mm,
— *stationary phase*: modified β-cyclodextrine for chiral chromatography R1 (film thickness 0.25 μm).

Carrier gas helium for chromatography R.

Flow rate 2.0 mL/min.

Split ratio 1:30.

Temperature:

	Time (min)	Temperature (°C)
Column	0 - 80	50 → 170
Injection port		230
Detector		230

Detection Flame ionisation.

Injection 1 μL.

System suitability Reference solution:
— *resolution*: minimum 2.4 between the peaks due to (−)-carvone (1st peak) and *carvone R1* (2nd peak).

Calculate the percentage content of the (−)-carvone from the following expression:

$$\frac{A_1}{A_1 + A_2} \times 100$$

A_1 = area of the peak due to (−)-carvone,
A_2 = area of the peak due to carvone R1.

Limit:
— (−)-*carvone*: maximum 1 per cent.

STORAGE

At a temperature not exceeding 25 °C.

_____ *Ph Eur*

Cardamom Fruit

In making preparations of Cardamom, only the seed is used. The seed is removed from the fruit, immediately powdered or bruised and used immediately in making the preparation. Cardamom seed, after removal from the fruit, should not be stored.

DEFINITION

Cardamom Fruit consists of the dried, nearly ripe fruit of *Elettaria cardamomum* Maton var. *minuscula* Burkill.

CHARACTERISTICS

Odour and taste of the seeds, strongly aromatic.

Macroscopical Fruit: a trilocular inferior capsule, up to about 2 cm long, ovoid or oblong, dull green to pale buff, plump or slightly shrunken, obtusely triangular in cross section, nearly smooth or longitudinally striated. Seeds in each loculus in two rows, forming an adherent mass attached to the axile placenta. Seed: pale to dark reddish brown, about 4 mm long and 3 mm broad, irregularly angular, marked with six to eight transverse wrinkles, with a longitudinal channel containing the raphe, each seed enveloped by a colourless, membranous aril. Transversely cut surface of seed showing a brown testa, white starchy perisperm, grooved on one side, yellowish endosperm and a paler embryo.

Microscopical Seed: aril composed of flattened, thin-walled, parenchymatous cells. Testa composed of the following layers: (i) outer epidermis of thick-walled, narrow, axially elongated cells; (ii) a layer of collapsed parenchyma subjacent to the outer epidermis; (iii) a single layer (two or three layers near the raphe) of large, thin-walled, rectangular cells containing volatile oil; (iv) two or three layers of parenchyma; (v) layers of thin-walled, flattened cells; (vi) distinctive sclerenchymatous layer of closely packed brown, thick-walled cells, each with a bowl-shaped cavity in the upper part containing a warty silica body; (vii) inner layer consisting of flattened cells. Perisperm: cells thin-walled, packed with numerous starch granules up to 6 μm in diameter and, in a small cavity, one to seven prisms of calcium oxalate about 10 to 30 μm long. Endosperm parenchymatous, thin-walled, with a granular hyaline mass of protein in each cell. Embryo: cells small, containing aleurone grains.

TESTS

Foreign matter
Of the fruit, not more than 1.0%; of the separated seeds, not more than 3.0%, Appendix XI D.

Volatile oil
In the seeds, not less than 4.0% v/w, Appendix XI E, Method I. Use 20 g of the unground seeds and distil for 5 hours.

Acid-insoluble ash
Of the seeds, not more than 3.5%, Appendix XI K.

Ash
Of the seeds, not more than 6.0%, Appendix XI J.

Cardamom Oil

Preparations
Aromatic Cardamom Tincture
Compound Cardamom Tincture

DEFINITION
Cardamom Oil is obtained by distillation from crushed Cardamom Fruit.

CHARACTERISTICS
A clear, colourless or pale yellow liquid, visibly free from water; odour, that of Cardamom Fruit.

TESTS

Ester value
90 to 156, Appendix X C.

Optical rotation
+20° to +40°, Appendix V F.

Refractive index
1.461 to 1.467, Appendix V E.

Solubility in ethanol
Soluble, at 20°, in 6 volumes of *ethanol (70%)*, Appendix X M.

Weight per mL
0.917 to 0.940 g, Appendix V G.

STORAGE
Cardamom Oil should be kept in a well-filled container and protected from light.

Aromatic Cardamom Tincture

DEFINITION

Cardamom Oil	3 mL
Caraway Oil	10 mL
Cinnamon Oil	10 mL
Clove Oil	10 mL
Strong Ginger Tincture	60 mL
Ethanol (90 per cent)	Sufficient to produce 1000 mL

The tincture complies with the requirements for Tinctures stated under Extracts and with the following requirements.

TESTS

Ethanol content
84 to 87% v/v, Appendix VIII F, Method III.

Relative density
0.825 to 0.845, Appendix V G.

Compound Cardamom Tincture

DEFINITION

Cardamom Oil	0.450 mL
Caraway Oil	0.400 mL
Cinnamon Oil	0.225 mL
Cochineal, in *moderately coarse powder*	7 g
Glycerol	50 mL
Ethanol (60 per cent)	Sufficient to produce 1000 mL

Extemporaneous preparation
The following directions apply.

Moisten the Cochineal with a sufficient quantity of Ethanol (60 per cent) and prepare 900 mL of tincture by *percolation*, Appendix XI F. Add the Cardamom Oil, the Caraway Oil, the Cinnamon Oil and the Glycerol and sufficient Ethanol (60 per cent) to produce 1000 mL; mix. Filter, if necessary.

The tincture complies with the requirements for Tinctures stated under Extracts and with the following requirements.

TESTS

Ethanol content
52 to 57% v/v, Appendix VIII F, Method III.

Glycerol
4.5 to 5.5% v/v when determined by the following method. Dilute 20 mL to 100 mL with *water*. To 20 mL of this solution add 100 mL of *water* and 1 g of *activated charcoal* and boil under a reflux condenser for 15 minutes. Filter and wash the filter and charcoal with sufficient *water* to produce 150 mL. Add 0.25 mL of *bromocresol purple solution* and neutralise with 0.1M *sodium hydroxide* or 0.05M *sulfuric acid* to the blue colour of the indicator. Add 1.4 g of *sodium periodate* and allow to stand for 15 minutes. Add 3 mL of *propane-1,2-diol*, shake and allow to stand for 5 minutes. Add 0.25 mL of *bromocresol purple solution* and titrate with 0.1M *sodium hydroxide VS* to the same blue colour. Each mL of 0.1M *sodium hydroxide VS* is equivalent to 9.210 mg of glycerol. Calculate the percentage v/v of glycerol, taking its weight per mL to be 1.260 g.

Relative density
0.925 to 0.937, Appendix V G.

Carrageenan

(*Ph Eur monograph 2138*)

Ph Eur _____

DEFINITION
Carrageenans are polysaccharides extracted from different Rhodophyceae with boiling water or aqueous alkali solutions. Carrageenan is separated by alcohol precipitation, potassium chloride precipitation, gel pressing, drum drying or freezing. The alcohol used during separation and purification is generally 2-propanol. The main components are potassium, sodium, calcium or magnesium salts of the sulfate esters of D-galactose and 3,6-anhydro-D-galactose copolymers. They exist in different proportions depending on the biological origin of the polymer.

The prevalent copolymers are designated as κ-, ι- and λ-carrageenan.

CHARACTERS

Appearance

Yellowish, brownish, or white or almost white powder.

Solubility

Soluble in water giving a viscous or colloidal solution, insoluble in organic solvents.

IDENTIFICATION

A. Prepare a 20 g/L dispersion and heat in a water-bath at 80 °C (Solution A). Allow to cool; it becomes more viscous upon cooling and may form a gel.

To 10 mL of solution A, while still hot, add 4 drops of a 100 g/L solution of *potassium chloride R*, mix and allow to cool. A 'brittle' gel indicates a carrageenan of a predominantly κ-type; an 'elastic' gel indicates a predominantly ι-type; if the solution does not form a gel, the carrageenan is of a predominantly λ-type.

B. Dilute 1 volume of solution A with about 4 volumes of *water R* and add 2-3 drops of a 0.5 g/L solution of *methylene blue R* in *ethanol (96 per cent) R*. A blue precipitate is formed.

C. Infrared absorption spectrophotometry (2.2.24).

Preparation   Prepare a 2 g/L solution of the substance to be examined and cast films (5 μm thick when dry) on a suitable non-sticking surface.

Carrageenan has strong, broad absorption bands, typical of all polysaccharides, in the 1000-1100 cm^{-1} region. Absorption maxima are 1065 cm^{-1} and 1020 cm^{-1} for gelling and non-gelling types, respectively. Other characteristic absorption bands and their intensities relative to the absorbance at 1050 cm^{-1} are shown in Table 2138.-1.

Table 2138.-1. – *Characteristic absorption bands for carrageenan identification by infrared absorption spectrophotometry*

Wave-number (cm⁻¹)	Molecular structure	Absorbance relative to the absorbance at 1050 cm⁻¹		
		κ	ι	λ
1220 - 1260	Ester sulfate	0.7 - 1.2	1.2 - 1.6	1.4 - 2.0
928 - 933	3,6-anhydro-D-galactose	0.3 - 0.6	0.2 - 0.4	≤ 0.2
840 - 850	Galactose-4-sulfate	0.3 - 0.5	0.2 - 0.4	-
825 - 830	Galactose-2-sulfate	-	-	0.2 - 0.4
810 - 820	Galactose-6-sulfate	-	-	0.1 - 0.3
800 - 805	3,6-anhydro-D-galactose-2-sulfate	≤ 0.2	0.2 - 0.4	-

TESTS

Apparent viscosity (2.2.10)

Minimum 5 mPa·s. Heat a 15 g/L dispersion (dried substance) at 80 °C for at least 15 min to dissolve. Compensate for any loss of water by evaporation, allow to cool to 75 °C and carry out the test at this temperature.

Heavy metals (2.4.8)

Maximum 20 ppm.

Dissolve 2.0 g in 30 mL of *water R* and shake for 2 min. Allow to stand and separate the aqueous layer. 12 mL of the solution complies with test A. Prepare the reference solution using *lead standard solution (1 ppm Pb) R*.

Loss on drying (2.2.32)

Maximum 12.0 per cent, determined on 1.000 g by drying in an oven at 105 °C.

Total ash (2.4.16)

Maximum 40.0 per cent.

Ash insoluble in hydrochloric acid (2.8.1)

Maximum 2.0 per cent.

LABELLING

The label states the type of carrageenan.

FUNCTIONALITY-RELATED CHARACTERISTICS

This section provides information on characteristics that are recognised as being relevant control parameters for one or more functions of the substance when used as an excipient (see chapter 5.15). This section is a non-mandatory part of the monograph and it is not necessary to verify the characteristics to demonstrate compliance. Control of these characteristics can however contribute to the quality of a medicinal product by improving the consistency of the manufacturing process and the performance of the medicinal product during use. Where control methods are cited, they are recognised as being suitable for the purpose, but other methods can also be used. Wherever results for a particular characteristic are reported, the control method must be indicated.

The following characteristics may be relevant for carrageenan used as viscosity-increasing agent.

Gel formation

See Identification A.

Apparent viscosity

See Tests.

Ph Eur

Cascara

(*Ph Eur monograph 0105*)

Preparation

Standardised Cascara Dry Extract

When Powdered Cascara is prescribed or demanded, material complying with the requirements below with the exception of Identification test A and the test for Foreign matter shall be dispensed or supplied.

Ph Eur

DEFINITION

Dried, whole or fragmented bark of *Rhamnus purshiana* DC. (syn. *Frangula purshiana* (DC.) A.Gray).

Content

Minimum 8.0 per cent of hydroxyanthracene glycosides of which minimum 60 per cent consists of cascarosides, both expressed as cascaroside A ($C_{27}H_{32}O_{14}$; M_r 580.5) (dried drug).

IDENTIFICATION

A. The bark occurs in slightly channelled or nearly flat pieces, usually 1-5 mm in thickness, usually varying greatly in length and width. The outer surface is grey or dark greyish-brown and shows occasional lenticels that are orientated transversally. It is usually more or less completely covered by a whitish coat of lichens, epiphytic moss and foliaceous liverwort. The inner surface is yellow or reddish-brown or almost black with fine longitudinal striations; it turns red when treated with alkali. The yellow fracture is short and granular in the outer part and somewhat fibrous in the inner part.

B. Microscopic examination (2.8.23). The powder is yellowish-brown. Examine under a microscope using *chloral hydrate solution R*. The powder shows the following diagnostic characters (Figure 0105.-1): bundles [A] of partly lignified phloem fibres [Aa], accompanied by crystal sheaths containing prisms of calcium oxalate [Ab] and sometimes including medullary rays [Ac]; isolated sclereids [G] or groups of sclereids [B] accompanied by crystal sheaths [Ba]; isolated cluster crystals [C] or prisms [E] of calcium oxalate; parenchymatous cells [F, H] containing a yellow substance that becomes deep red when treated with alkali, sometimes accompanied by cells containing cluster crystals of calcium oxalate [Ha]; cork cells, in surface view [D] or in transverse section [J], associated with parenchyma, some cells of which contain cluster crystals of calcium oxalate [Ja]; frequently epiphytes [K], which may be liverworts, entire or in fragments, having a lamina 1 cell thick without a midrib and composed of isodiametric cells, or leaves of mosses, having a lamina 1 cell thick composed of elongated cells and possessing a midrib several cells thick.

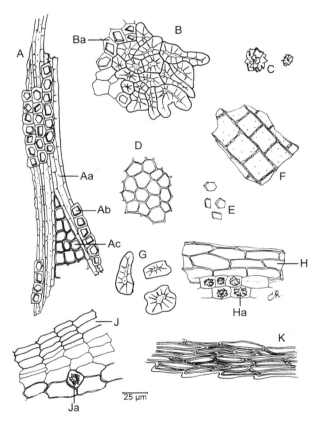

Figure 0105.-1. – *Illustration for identification test B of powdered herbal drug of cascara*

C. Examine the chromatograms obtained in test A for Other species of *Rhamnus;* anthrones.

Results   The chromatogram obtained with the test solution shows several reddish-brown zones with different intensities: there are 4 faint zones, 3 being situated at about the mid-point of the chromatogram and 1 in the lower third and there is a strong zone in the upper third of the chromatogram. Examine in ultraviolet light at 365 nm. The chromatogram obtained with the test solution shows several zones with the same fluorescence, situated above and particularly below (cascarosides) that due to barbaloin in the chromatogram obtained with the reference solution.

D. Heat 0.2 g of the powdered herbal drug (180) (*2.9.12*) with 50 mL of *water R* on a water-bath for 15 min. Allow to cool and filter. To 10 mL of the filtrate add 20 mL of *hydrochloric acid R1* and heat on a water-bath for 15 min. Allow to cool, transfer to a separating funnel and shake with 3 quantities, each of 20 mL, of *ether R*. Reserve the aqueous layer (solution A). Combine the 3 ether extracts and shake with 10 mL of *dilute ammonia R2*. The aqueous layer becomes reddish-violet. Transfer solution A to a small flask, add 5 g of *ferric chloride R* and heat on a water-bath for 30 min. Allow to cool, transfer to a separating funnel and shake with 15 mL of *ether R*. Wash the ether layer with 10 mL of *water R*, discard the aqueous layer and shake the ether layer with 5 mL of *dilute ammonia R2*. A red colour develops in the aqueous layer.

TESTS

Other species of *Rhamnus;* anthrones
Thin-layer chromatography (*2.2.27*).

Test solution   To 0.5 g of the powdered herbal drug (180) (*2.9.12*) add 5 mL of *ethanol (70 per cent V/V) R* and heat to boiling. Cool and centrifuge. Decant the supernatant immediately and use within 30 min.

Reference solution   Dissolve 20 mg of *barbaloin R* in *ethanol (70 per cent V/V) R* and dilute to 10 mL with the same solvent.

Plates   *TLC silica gel plate R* (2 plates).

Mobile phase   *water R, methanol R, ethyl acetate R* (13:17:100 *V/V/V*).

A. *Application*: 10 µL as bands.

Development   Over a path of 10 cm.

Drying   In air for 5 min.

Detection   Spray with about 10 mL of a 50 g/L solution of *potassium hydroxide R* in *ethanol (50 per cent V/V) R* and heat at 100-105 °C for 15 min; examine immediately after heating.

Results   The chromatogram obtained with the reference solution shows, in the central part, a reddish-brown zone due to barbaloin; examine in ultraviolet light at 365 nm; the zone due to barbaloin shows intense yellowish-brown fluorescence; in the chromatogram with the test solution, no zone with orange-brown fluorescence is seen between the zone due to barbaloin and the zones due to cascarosides.

B. *Application*: 10 µL of the test solution, as a band.

Development   Over a path of 10 cm.

Drying   In air for not more than 5 min.

Detection   Spray immediately with a 5 g/L solution of *nitrotetrazolium blue R* in *methanol R* and examine immediately.

Results   No violet or greyish-blue zones appear.

Foreign matter (*2.8.2*)
Maximum 1 per cent.

Loss on drying (*2.2.32*)
Maximum 10.0 per cent, determined on 1.000 g of the powdered herbal drug (180) (*2.9.12*) by drying in an oven at 105 °C for 2 h.

Total ash (*2.4.16*)
Maximum 7.0 per cent.

ASSAY
Carry out the assay in 24 h, protected from bright light.

Stir 1.00 g of the powdered herbal drug (180) (*2.9.12*) into 100 mL of boiling *water R* and continue boiling and stirring for 5 min. Allow to cool, dilute to 100.0 mL with *water R*, shake, filter and discard the first 20 mL of filtrate. Transfer 10.0 mL of the filtrate to a separating funnel, add 0.1 mL of

1 M hydrochloric acid and shake with 2 quantities, each of 20 mL, of a mixture of 1 volume of *ether R* and 3 volumes of *hexane R*. Wash the combined organic extracts with 5 mL of *water R*, discard the organic layer and return the rinsings to the aqueous layer. Shake the combined aqueous layers with 4 quantities, each of 30 mL, of *ethyl acetate R* freshly saturated with *water R* (to 150 mL of *ethyl acetate R* add 15 mL of *water R*, shake for 3 min and allow to stand) on each occasion allowing separation to take place until the organic layer is clear. Combine the ethyl acetate extracts. Use the aqueous layer for the assay for cascarosides and the organic layer for the assay for hydroxyanthracene glycosides other than cascarosides.

Hydroxyanthracene glycosides other than cascarosides
Transfer the organic layer to a suitable flask and remove the solvent by distillation, evaporating almost to dryness. Dissolve the residue in 0.3-0.5 mL of *methanol R* and transfer to a volumetric flask, rinsing the 1ˢᵗ flask with warm *water R* and adding the rinsings to the methanolic solution. Allow to cool and dilute to 50.0 mL with *water R*. Transfer 20.0 mL of this solution to a 100 mL round-bottomed flask with a ground-glass neck and containing 2 g of *ferric chloride R* and 12 mL of *hydrochloric acid R*. Attach a reflux condenser and place the flask in a water-bath so that the level of the water is above that of the liquid in the flask and heat for 4 h. Allow to cool, transfer the solution to a separating funnel and rinse the flask successively with 3-4 mL of *1 M sodium hydroxide* and 3-4 mL of *water R*, adding the rinsings to the separating funnel. Shake the contents of the separating funnel with 3 quantities, each of 30 mL, of a mixture of 1 volume of *ether R* and 3 volumes of *hexane R*. Wash the combined organic layers with 2 quantities, each of 10 mL, of *water R* and discard the rinsings. Dilute the organic layer to 100.0 mL with the mixture of ether and hexane. Take 20.0 mL, evaporate carefully to dryness on a water-bath and dissolve the residue in 10.0 mL of a 5 g/L solution of *magnesium acetate R* in *methanol R*. Measure the absorbance *(2.2.25)* at 440 nm and 515 nm using *methanol R* as the compensation liquid. If the ratio of the absorbance at 515 nm to that at 440 nm is less than 2.4, the assay is invalid.

Calculate the percentage content of hydroxyanthracene glycosides other than cascarosides, expressed as cascaroside A, using the following expression:

$$\frac{A \times 6.95}{m}$$

i.e. taking the specific absorbance to be 180.
A = absorbance at 515 nm;
m = mass of the substance to be examined, in grams.

Cascarosides
Dilute the aqueous layer to 50.0 mL with *water R*. Treat 20.0 mL of this solution as described above in the assay of hydroxyanthracene glycosides other than cascarosides. Measure the absorbance *(2.2.25)* of the test solution at 440 nm and 515 nm. If the ratio of the absorbance at 515 nm to that at 440 nm is less than 2.7, the assay is invalid.

Calculate the percentage content of cascarosides, expressed as cascaroside A, using the following expression:

$$\frac{A \times 6.95}{m}$$

i.e. taking the specific absorbance to be 180.
A = absorbance at 515 nm;
m = mass of the substance to be examined, in grams.

Ph Eur

Standardised Cascara Dry Extract

(Ph Eur monograph 1844)

Preparation
Cascara Tablets

Ph Eur

DEFINITION
Standardised dry extract obtained from *Cascara (0105)*.

Content
90 per cent to 110 per cent of the nominal content of hydroxyanthracene glycosides, expressed as cascaroside A ($C_{27}H_{32}O_{14}$; M_r 580.5), stated on the label; minimum 60 per cent of the hydroxyanthracene glycosides are cascarosides, expressed as cascaroside A. The nominal content of hydroxyanthracene glycosides is within the range 8.0 per cent to 25.0 per cent *m/m* (dried extract).

PRODUCTION
The extract is produced from the herbal drug by an appropriate procedure using either boiling water or a hydroalcoholic solvent at least equivalent in strength to ethanol (60 per cent *V/V*).

CHARACTERS
Appearance
Brown, free-flowing powder.

IDENTIFICATION
Thin-layer chromatography *(2.2.27)*.

Test solution To 0.2 g of the extract to be examined add 5 mL of *ethanol (70 per cent V/V) R* and heat to boiling. Cool and centrifuge. Decant the supernatant solution immediately and use within 30 min.

Reference solution Dissolve 20 mg of *barbaloin R* and 2 mg of *emodin R* in *ethanol (70 per cent V/V) R* and dilute to 10 mL with the same solvent.

Plate TLC silica gel plate R (5-40 µm) [or *TLC silica gel plate R* (2-10 µm)].

Mobile phase water R, methanol R, ethyl acetate R (13:17:100 *V/V/V*).

Application 10 µL [or 2 µL] as bands.

Development Over a path of 10 cm [or 6 cm].

Drying In air for 5 min.

Detection Spray with a 50 g/L solution of *potassium hydroxide R* in *ethanol (50 per cent V/V) R* and heat to 100-105 °C for 15 min; examine in ultraviolet light at 365 nm.

Results See below the sequence of zones present in the chromatograms obtained with the reference solution and the test solution. Furthermore, other zones may be present in the chromatogram obtained with the test solution.

Top of the plate	
Emodin: a red fluorescent zone	A faint red fluorescent zone
———	———
Barbaloin: a yellowish-brown fluorescent zone	A yellowish-brown fluorescent zone
	A blue fluorescent zone
———	———
	An intense yellowish-brown fluorescent zone
	3 yellowish-brown fluorescent zones
Reference solution	**Test solution**

TESTS

Loss on drying (*2.8.17*)
Maximum 5.0 per cent.

ASSAY

Carry out the assay within 24 h, protected from bright light.

To 0.500 g of the extract to be examined add 80 mL of *ethanol (70 per cent V/V) R*. Shake, and allow to stand in the dark for at least 8 h. Dilute to 100.0 mL with *ethanol (70 per cent V/V) R*. Shake and filter, discarding the first 20 mL of filtrate. Transfer 10.0 mL of the filtrate to a separating funnel, add 0.1 mL of *1 M hydrochloric acid* and shake with 2 quantities, each of 20 mL, of a mixture of 1 volume of *ether R* and 3 volumes of *hexane R*. Wash the combined organic extracts with 5 mL of *water R*. Discard the organic layer and return the rinsings to the hydroalcoholic layer. Shake with 4 quantities, each of 30 mL, of *ethyl acetate R* freshly saturated with *water R* (prepared as follows: to 150 mL of *ethyl acetate R* add 15 mL of *water R*, shake for 3 min and allow to stand), on each occasion allowing the layers to separate until the organic layer is clear. Combine the ethyl acetate extracts. Use the aqueous layer for the assay of cascarosides and the organic layer for the assay of hydroxyanthracene glycosides other than cascarosides.

Hydroxyanthracene glycosides other than cascarosides
Transfer the organic layer to a round-bottomed flask and remove the solvent by distillation, evaporating almost to dryness. Dissolve the residue in 0.5 mL of *methanol R*, add 10 mL of *water R* at 40 °C and transfer to a 50 mL volumetric flask, rinsing the round-bottomed flask with *water R* at 40 °C and adding the rinsings to the hydromethanolic solution. Allow to cool and dilute to 50.0 mL with *water R*. Transfer 20.0 mL of the solution to a 100 mL round-bottomed flask with a ground-glass neck containing 2 g of *ferric chloride R* and 12 mL of *hydrochloric acid R*. Attach a reflux condenser and place the flask in a water-bath so that the level of the water is above that of the liquid in the flask and heat for 4 h. Allow to cool, transfer the solution to a separating funnel and rinse the flask successively with 4 mL of *1 M sodium hydroxide* and 4 mL of *water R*, adding the rinsings to the separating funnel. Shake the contents of the separating funnel with 3 quantities, each of 30 mL, of a mixture of 1 volume of *ether R* and 3 volumes of *hexane R*. Wash the combined organic layers with 2 quantities, each of 10 mL, of *water R* and discard the rinsings. Dilute the organic layer to 100.0 mL with a mixture of 1 volume of *ether R* and 3 volumes of *hexane R*. Take 20.0 mL of the solution, evaporate carefully to dryness on a

water-bath and dissolve the residue in 10.0 mL of a 5 g/L solution of *magnesium acetate R* in *methanol R*. Measure the absorbance (*2.2.25*) at 440 nm and 515 nm, using *methanol R* as the compensation liquid. If the ratio of the absorbance at 515 nm to that at 440 nm is less than 2.4, the assay is invalid.

Calculate the percentage content of hydroxyanthracene glycosides other than cascarosides, expressed as cascaroside A, using the following expression:

$$\frac{A \times 6.95}{m}$$

i.e. taking the specific absorbance to be 180.
A = absorbance at 515 nm;
m = mass of the substance to be examined, in grams.

Cascarosides
Dilute the aqueous layer to 50.0 mL with *water R*. Treat 20.0 mL of this solution as described above in the assay of hydroxyanthracene glycosides other than cascarosides. Measure the absorbance (*2.2.25*) at 440 nm and 515 nm. If the ratio of the absorbance at 515 nm to that at 440 nm is less than 2.7, the assay is invalid.

Calculate the percentage content of cascarosides, expressed as cascaroside A, using the following expression:

$$\frac{A \times 6.95}{m}$$

i.e. taking the specific absorbance to be 180.
A = absorbance at 515 nm;
m = mass of the substance to be examined, in grams.

LABELLING
The label states the nominal content of hydroxyanthracene glycosides, expressed as cascaroside A.

——————————————————————————— Ph Eur

Cascara Tablets

DEFINITION
Cascara Tablets contain Standardised Cascara Dry Extract. They are coated.

The tablets comply with the requirements stated under Tablets and with the following requirements.

Content of total hydroxyanthracene derivatives
17.0 to 23.0 mg, of which not less than 60% consists of cascarosides, both expressed as cascaroside A.

IDENTIFICATION
Carry out the method for *thin-layer chromatography*, Appendix III A, using the following solutions.

(1) Boil a quantity of the powdered tablets containing the equivalent of 32 mg of total hydroxyanthracene derivatives with 5 mL of 70% v/v of *ethanol*, cool and centrifuge. Decant the supernatant liquid immediately and use within 30 minutes.

(2) Dissolve 20 mg of *barbaloin* and 2 mg of *emodin* in 70% v/v of *ethanol* and dilute to 10 mL with the same solvent.

CHROMATOGRAPHIC CONDITIONS

(a) Use *silica gel F_{254}* precoated plates or high-performance *silica gel F_{254}* (Merck *silica gel F_{254}* HPTLC plates are suitable).

(b) Use the mobile phase as described below.

(c) Apply 10 μL [or 2 μL] of each solution, as bands.

(d) Develop the plate to 10 cm [or 6 cm].

(e) After removal of the plate, dry in air, spray with a 5% w/v solution of *potassium hydroxide* in 50% v/v *ethanol*, heat at 100 to 105° for 15 minutes and examine under *ultraviolet light (365 nm)*.

MOBILE PHASE

13 volumes of *water*, 17 volumes of *methanol* and 100 volumes of *ethyl acetate*.

CONFIRMATION

The chromatogram obtained with solution (1) show yellowish-brown fluorescent bands with Rf values of between 0.2 and 0.25, an intense yellowish-brown fluorescent band with an Rf value of about 0.3, a blue fluorescent band with an Rf value of about 0.6, a yellowish-brown fluorescent band with an Rf value of about 0.7 corresponding in colour and position to the band obtained with barbaloin in solution (2) and a faint reddish fluorescent band with an Rf value of about 0.9 corresponding in position to emodin in solution (2).

Top of the plate	
A faint red fluorescent band	Emodin a red fluorescent band
A yellow-brown fluorescent band	Barbaloin: a yellow-brown fluorescent band
A blue fluorescent band	
An intense yellow-brown fluorescent band	
3 yellow-brown fluorescent bands	
Solution (1)	**Solution (2)**

TESTS

Disintegration

Comply with the requirements stated under Tablets but for sugar-coated tablets the maximum time is 120 minutes.

ASSAY

Carry out the assay within 24 hours, protected from bright light.

Add 80 mL of 70% v/v *ethanol* to a quantity of the powdered tablets containing 75 mg of total hydroxyanthracene derivatives. Shake and allow to stand in the dark for at least 8 hours. Dilute to 100.0 mL with 70% v/v of *ethanol*. Shake and filter, discarding the first 20 mL of filtrate. Transfer 10.0 mL of the filtrate to a separating funnel, add 0.1 mL of 1M *hydrochloric acid* and shake with 2-quantities, each of 20 mL, of a mixture of 1 volume of *ether* and 3 volumes of *hexane*. Wash the combined organic extracts with 5 mL of *water*. Discard the organic layer and return the rinsings to the hydroalcoholic layer. Shake with 4-quantities, each of 30 mL, of *ethyl acetate* freshly saturated with *water* prepared by shaking 150 mL of *ethyl acetate* with 15 mL of *water* for

3 minutes and allowing to stand until the layers have separated and the organic layer is clear. Combine the ethyl acetate extracts and use the aqueous layer for the assay of cascarosides and the organic layer for the assay of hydroxyanthracene glycosides other than cascarosides.

Hydroxyanthracene glycosides other than cascarosides
Transfer the organic layer to a round-bottomed flask and remove the solvent by distillation, evaporating almost to dryness. Dissolve the residue in 0.5 mL of *methanol*, add 10 mL of *water* at 40° and transfer to a 50 mL volumetric flask, rinsing the round-bottomed flask with *water* at 40° and adding the rinsings to the hydromethanolic solution. Allow to cool and dilute to 50.0 mL with *water*. Transfer 20.0 mL of the solution to a 100 mL round-bottomed flask with a ground-glass neck containing 2 g of *iron (III) chloride hexahydrate* and 12 mL of 7M *hydrochloric acid*. Attach a reflux condenser and place the flask in a water-bath so that the level of the water is above that of the liquid in the flask and heat for 4 hours. Allow to cool, transfer the solution to a separating funnel and rinse the flask successively with 4 mL of 1M *sodium hydroxide* and 4 mL of *water*, adding the rinsings to the separating funnel. Shake the contents of the separating funnel with 3-quantities, each of 30 mL, of a mixture of 1 volume of *ether* and 3 volumes of *hexane*. Wash the combined organic layers with 2-quantities, each of 10 mL, of *water* and discard the rinsings. Dilute the organic layer to 100.0 mL with a mixture of 1 volume of *ether* and 3 volumes of *hexane*. Take 20.0 mL of the solution, evaporate carefully to dryness on a water-bath and dissolve the residue in 10.0 mL of a 0.5% w/v solution of *magnesium acetate* in *methanol*. Measure the *absorbance* of the resulting solution at 440 nm and at 515 nm, *Appendix II B*, using *methanol* in the reference cell. The assay is not valid if the ratio of the absorbance at 515 nm to that at 440 nm is less than 2.4.

Calculate the percentage content of hydroxyanthracene glycosides other than cascarosides, expressed as cascaroside A, using the following expression:

$$\frac{A \times 6.95}{m}$$

i.e. taking the specific absorbance to be 180.
A = absorbance at 515 nm;
m = weight of the substance being examined, in grams.

Cascarosides
To the aqueous solution reserved from the preliminary extraction add sufficient *water* to produce 50.0 mL. Carry out the Assay for hydroxyanthracene gycosides other than cascarosides, beginning at the words, 'Transfer 20 mL …'. Measure the *absorbance* of the resulting solution at 440 nm and at 515 nm, Appendix II B, using methanol in the reference cell. The assay is not valid if the ratio of the absorbance at 515 nm to that at 440 nm is less than 2.7.

Calculate the percentage content of cascarosides, expressed as cascaroside A, using the following expression:

$$\frac{A \times 6.95}{m}$$

i.e. taking the specific absorbance to be 180.
A = absorbance at 515 nm;
m = weight of the substance being examined, in grams.

HERBAL DRUGS

LABELLING

The label states the nominal content of hydroxyanthracene glycosides, expressed as cascarosides A.

Cassia Oil

(Ph Eur monograph 1496)

8007-80-5

Ph Eur _____

DEFINITION

Essential oil obtained by steam distillation of the leaves and young branches of *Cinnamomum cassia* Blume (*C. aromaticum* Nees).

CHARACTERS

Appearance

Clear, mobile, yellow or reddish-brown liquid.

Characteristic odour reminiscent of cinnamic aldehyde.

IDENTIFICATION

First identification B.

Second identification A.

A. Thin-layer chromatography (*2.2.27*).

Test solution Dissolve 0.5 mL of the oil to be examined in *acetone R* and dilute to 10 mL with the same solvent.

Reference solution Dissolve 50 µL of *trans-cinnamic aldehyde R*, 10 µL of *eugenol R* and 50 mg of *coumarin R* in *acetone R* and dilute to 10 mL with the same solvent.

Plate TLC silica gel plate R.

Mobile phase methanol R, toluene R (10:90 *V/V*).

Application 10 µL as bands.

Development Over a path of 15 cm.

Drying In air.

Detection A Examine in ultraviolet light at 365 nm.

Results A The zone of blue fluorescence in the chromatogram obtained with the test solution is similar in position and colour to the zone in the chromatogram obtained with the reference solution (coumarin).

Detection B Spray with *anisaldehyde solution R*; examine in daylight while heating at 100-105 °C for 5-10 min.

Results B The chromatogram obtained with the reference solution shows in its upper part a violet zone (eugenol) and above this zone a greenish-blue zone (*trans*-cinnamic aldehyde). The chromatogram obtained with the test solution shows a zone similar in position and colour to the zone due to *trans*-cinnamic aldehyde in the chromatogram obtained with the reference solution and may show a very faint zone due to eugenol. Other faint zones are present.

B. Examine the chromatograms obtained in the test for chromatographic profile.

Results The principal peaks in the chromatogram obtained with the test solution are similar in retention time to those in the chromatogram obtained with the reference solution. Eugenol may be absent from the chromatogram obtained with the test solution.

TESTS

Relative density (*2.2.5*)

1.052 to 1.070.

Refractive index (*2.2.6*)

1.600 to 1.614.

Optical rotation (*2.2.7*)

− 1° to + 1°.

Chromatographic profile

Gas chromatography (*2.2.28*): use the normalisation procedure.

Test solution The oil to be examined.

Reference solution Dissolve 100 µL of *trans-cinnamic aldehyde R*, 10 µL of *cinnamyl acetate R*, 10 µL of *eugenol R*, 10 µL of *trans-2-methoxycinnamaldehyde R* and 20 mg of *coumarin R* in 1 mL of *acetone R*.

Column:

— *material*: fused silica;

— *size*: *l* = 60 m, Ø = about 0.25 mm;

— *stationary phase*: bonded macrogol 20 000 R.

Carrier gas helium for chromatography R.

Flow rate 1.5 mL/min.

Split ratio 1:100.

Temperature:

	Time (min)	Temperature (°C)
Column	0 - 10	60
	10 - 75	60 → 190
	75 - 160	190
Injection port		200
Detector		240

Detection Flame ionisation.

Injection 0.2 µL.

Elution order Order indicated in the composition of the reference solution, depending on the operating conditions and the state of the column, coumarin may elute before or after *trans*-2-methoxycinnamaldehyde; record the retention times of these substances.

System suitability Reference solution:

— *resolution*: minimum 1.5 between the peaks due to *trans*-2-methoxycinnamaldehyde and coumarin.

Identification of components Using the retention times determined from the chromatogram obtained with the reference solution, locate the components of the reference solution in the chromatogram obtained with the test solution.

Determine the percentage content of each of these components. The percentages are within the following ranges:

— *trans-cinnamic aldehyde*: 70 per cent to 90 per cent;

— *cinnamyl acetate*: 1.0 per cent to 6.0 per cent;

— *eugenol*: maximum 0.5 per cent;

— *trans-2-methoxycinnamaldehyde*: 3.0 per cent to 15 per cent;

— *coumarin*: 1.5 per cent to 4.0 per cent.

STORAGE

Protected from heat.

_____ *Ph Eur*

Greater Celandine

(*Ph Eur monograph 1861*)

Ph Eur _____

DEFINITION

Dried, whole or cut aerial parts of *Chelidonium majus* L. collected during flowering.

Content

Minimum 0.6 per cent of total alkaloids, expressed as chelidonine ($C_{20}H_{19}NO_5$; M_r 353.4) (dried drug).

IDENTIFICATION

A. The stems are rounded, ribbed, yellowish or greenish-brown, somewhat pubescent, about 3-7 mm in diameter, hollow and mostly collapsed. The leaves are thin, irregularly pinnate, the leaflets ovate to oblong with coarsely dentate margins, the terminal leaflet often 3-lobed; the adaxial surface is bluish-green and glabrous, the abaxial surface paler and pubescent, especially on the veins. The flowers have 2 deeply concavo-convex sepals, readily removed, and 4 yellow, broadly ovate, spreading petals about 8-10 mm long; the stamens are numerous, yellow, and a short style arises from a superior ovary; long, capsular, immature fruits are rarely present.

B. Microscopic examination (*2.8.23*). The powder is dark greyish-green or brownish-green. Examine under a microscope using *chloral hydrate solution R*. The powder shows the following diagnostic characters (Figure 1861.-1): numerous fragments of upper epidermis, composed of cells with sinuous walls in surface view [B], accompanied by underlying palisade parenchyma [Ba]; numerous fragments of lower epidermis in surface view [A, E] bearing anomocytic stomata (*2.8.3*) [Aa] and bases of covering trichomes [Ab], sometimes accompanied by underlying spongy parenchyma [Ea]; long, uniseriate, multicellular covering trichomes, usually fragmented, with thin-walled cells, sometimes collapsed [G]; vascular tissue from the leaves and stems consisting of pitted and spirally thickened vessels [D]; groups of fibres [C]; articulated latex tubes with yellowish-brown contents [F]; occasional fragments of the corolla [H] consisting of thin-walled cells containing numerous pale yellow droplets of oil [Ha]; spherical pollen grains about 30-40 µm in diameter with 3 pores and a finely pitted exine [J].

C. Thin-layer chromatography (*2.2.27*).

Test solution   To 0.4 g of the powdered herbal drug (710) (*2.9.12*) add 50 mL of *dilute acetic acid R*. Boil in a water-bath under a reflux condenser for 30 min. Cool and filter. To the filtrate add *concentrated ammonia R* until a strong alkaline reaction is produced. Shake with 30 mL of *methylene chloride R*. Dry the organic layer over *anhydrous sodium sulfate R*, filter and evaporate *in vacuo* to dryness. Dissolve the residue in 1.0 mL of *methanol R*.

Reference solution   Dissolve 2 mg of *methyl red R* and 2 mg of *papaverine hydrochloride R* in 10 mL of *ethanol (96 per cent) R*.

Plate   TLC *silica gel plate R*.

Mobile phase   *anhydrous formic acid R*, *water R*, *propanol R* (1:9:90 *V/V/V*).

Application   10 µL as bands.

Development   Over a path of 10 cm.

Drying   In air.

Detection   Spray with *potassium iodobismuthate solution R* and dry in air; spray with *sodium nitrite solution R* and allow to dry in air; examine in daylight.

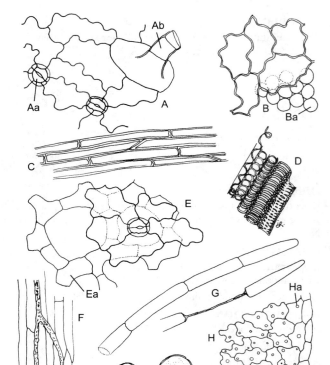

Figure 1861.-1. – *Illustration for identification test B of powdered herbal drug of greater celandine*

Results   See below the sequence of zones present in the chromatograms obtained with the reference solution and the test solution. Furthermore, other weaker zones may be present in the chromatogram obtained with the test solution.

Top of the plate	
Methyl red: a red zone	A brown zone
	A brown zone
Papaverine: a greyish-brown zone	A greyish-brown zone
___	___
	2 brown zones
Reference solution	**Test solution**

TESTS

Foreign matter (*2.8.2*)
Maximum 10.0 per cent.

Loss on drying (*2.2.32*)
Maximum 10.0 per cent, determined on 1.000 g of the powdered herbal drug (355) (*2.9.12*) by drying in an oven at 105 °C for 2 h.

Total ash (*2.4.16*)
Maximum 13.0 per cent.

ASSAY

Test solution   To 0.750 g of the powdered herbal drug (710) (*2.9.12*) add 200 mL of *dilute acetic acid R* and heat on a water-bath for 30 min, shaking frequently. Cool and dilute to 250.0 mL with *dilute acetic acid R*. Filter. Discard the first 20 mL of the filtrate. To 30.0 mL of the filtrate add 6.0 mL of *concentrated ammonia R* and 100.0 mL of *methylene chloride R*. Shake for 30 min. Separate the organic layer, place 50.0 mL in a 100 mL round-bottomed flask and evaporate to dryness *in vacuo* at a temperature not exceeding 40 °C. Dissolve the residue in about 2-3 mL of *ethanol (96 per cent) R*, warming slightly. Transfer the solution to a 25 mL volumetric flask by rinsing the round-bottomed flask with *dilute sulfuric acid R* and dilute to 25.0 mL with the same solvent. To 5.0 mL of the solution add 5.0 mL of a 10 g/L solution of *chromotropic acid, sodium salt R* in *sulfuric acid R* in a 25 mL volumetric flask, stopper the flask and mix carefully. Dilute to 25.0 mL with *sulfuric acid R* and stopper the flask.

Compensation liquid   Prepare at the same time and in the same manner as for the test solution: place in a 25 mL volumetric flask 5.0 mL of *dilute sulfuric acid R* and 5.0 mL of a 10 g/L solution of *chromotropic acid, sodium salt R* in *sulfuric acid R*, stopper the flask and mix carefully. Dilute to 25.0 mL with *sulfuric acid R* and stopper the flask.

Place both solutions on a water-bath for 10 min. Cool to about 20 °C and dilute if necessary to 25.0 mL with *sulfuric acid R*. Measure the absorbance (*2.2.25*) of the test solution at 570 nm by comparison with the compensation liquid.

Calculate the percentage content of total alkaloids, expressed as chelidonine, using the following expression:

$$\frac{A \times 2.23}{m}$$

i.e. taking the specific absorbance of chelidonine to be 933.
A = absorbance at 570 nm;
m = mass of the herbal drug to be examined, in grams.

Ph Eur

Centaury

(*Ph Eur monograph 1301*)

Ph Eur

DEFINITION
Whole or fragmented dried flowering aerial parts of *Centaurium erythraea* Rafn s. 1. including *C. majus* (H. et L.) Zeltner and *C. suffruticosum* (Griseb.) Ronn. (syn.: *Erythraea centaurium* Persoon; *C. umbellatum* Gilibert; *C. minus* Gars.).

CHARACTERS
Bitter taste.

IDENTIFICATION
A. The hollow cylindrical, light green to dark brown stem has longitudinal ridges, and is branched only in its upper part. The sessile leaves are entire, decussately arranged, and have an ovate to lanceolate lamina, up to about 3 cm long. Both surfaces are glabrous and green to brownish-green.
The inflorescence is diaxially branched. The tubular calyx is green and has 5 lanceolate, acuminate teeth. The corolla consists of a whitish tube divided into 5 elongated lanceolate pink to reddish lobes, about 5-8 mm long. 5 stamens are present attached to the top of the corolla tube. The ovary is superior and has a short style, a broad bifid stigma and numerous ovules. Cylindrical capsules, about 7-10 mm long,

with small brown markedly rough seeds are frequently present.

B. Reduce to a powder (355) (*2.9.12*). The powder is greenish-yellow or brownish. Examine under a microscope, using *chloral hydrate solution R*. The powder shows the following diagnostic characters: fragments from the stem with lignified groups of fibres associated with narrow vessels, tracheidal vessels occasional vessels with spiral thickening; pitted parenchyma of the pith and medullary rays; fragments of leaf lamina with sinuous epidermal cells and striated cuticle, especially over the margins and surrounding the stomata; numerous stomata, mainly anisocytic (*2.8.3*); fragments of the palisade mesophyll, each cell containing a single prism crystal or, less frequently, a cluster crystal of calcium oxalate; fragments of calyx and corolla, those of the calyx with straight-walled epidermal cells, those of the inner epidermis of the corolla with obtuse papillae and radially striated cuticle; parts of the endothecium with reticulate or ridge-shaped wall thickenings; triangularly rounded or elliptical, yellow pollen grains, about 30 μm in diameter, with a distinctly pitted exine and 3 germinal pores; fragments of the wall of the fruit capsule composed of crossed layers of fusiform cells; oil droplets from the seeds, fragments of the epidermis of the testa showing large, brown reticulations and a pitted surface.

C. Thin-layer chromatography (*2.2.27*).

Test solution   To 1.0 g of the powdered drug (355) (*2.9.12*) add 25 mL of *methanol R*, shake for 15 min and filter. Evaporate the filtrate to dryness under reduced pressure and at a temperature not exceeding 50 °C. Take up the residue with small quantities of *methanol R* so as to obtain 5 mL of solution, which may contain a sediment.

Reference solution   Dissolve 1 mg of *rutin R* and 1 mg of *swertiamarin R* in *methanol R* and dilute to 1 mL with the same solvent.

Plate   TLC silica gel F_{254} *plate R* (5-40 μm) [or *TLC silica gel F_{254} plate R* (2-10 μm)].

Mobile phase   *water R*, *anhydrous formic acid R*, *ethyl formate R* (4:8:88 *V/V/V*).

Application   10 μL [or 5 μL] as bands.

Development   In an unsaturated tank over a path of 12 cm [or 6 cm].

Drying   In air.

Detection A   Examine in ultraviolet light at 254 nm.

Results A   See below the sequence of the zones present in the chromatograms obtained with the reference solution and the test solution. Furthermore, other less intense quenching zones may be present in the chromatogram obtained with the test solution.

Top of the plate	
___ ___	___ ___
Swertiamarin: a quenching zone	A prominent quenching zone (swertiamarin)
Rutin: a quenching zone	
Reference solution	**Test solution**

Detection B   Spray with *anisaldehyde solution R* and heat at 100-105 °C for 5-10 min. Examine in daylight.

Results B See below the sequence of the zones present in the chromatograms obtained with the reference solution and the test solution. Furthermore, other less intense coloured zones may be present in the chromatogram obtained with the test solution.

Top of the plate	
———	———
———	———
	———
Swertiamarin: a brown zone	A brown zone (swertiamarin)
Rutin: a yellow zone	
	A brownish-grey zone
	A yellow zone
	A grey zone
Reference solution	**Test solution**

TESTS

Foreign matter (*2.8.2*)
Maximum 3 per cent.

Bitterness value (*2.8.15*)
Minimum 2000.

Loss on drying (*2.2.32*)
Maximum 10.0 per cent, determined on 1.000 g of powdered drug (355) (*2.9.12*) by drying in an oven at 105 °C for 2 h.

Total ash (*2.4.16*)
Maximum 6.0 per cent.

———————————————————————— *Ph Eur*

Centella

(*Ph Eur monograph 1498*)

Ph Eur ————————————————————————

DEFINITION
Dried, fragmented aerial parts of *Centella asiatica* (L.) Urban.

Content
Minimum 6.0 per cent of total triterpenoid derivatives, expressed as asiaticoside ($C_{48}H_{78}O_{19}$; M_r 959.15) (dried drug).

CHARACTERS
The leaves are very variable in size; the petiole is usually 5-10, sometimes 15, times longer than the lamina, which is 10-40 mm long and 20-40 mm, sometimes up to 70 mm, wide.

IDENTIFICATION
A. The leaves are alternate, sometimes grouped together at the nodes, reniform or orbicular or oblong-elliptic and have palmate nervation, usually with 7 veins, and a crenate margin. Young leaves show a few trichomes on the lower surface while adult leaves are glabrous. The inflorescence, if present, is a single umbel which usually consists of 3 flowers, rarely 2 or 4; the flowers are very small (about 2 mm) pentamerous and have an inferior ovary; the fruit, a brownish-grey, orbicular cremocarp, up to 5 mm long, is very flattened laterally and has 7-9 prominent curved ridges.

B. Reduce the drug to a powder (355) (*2.9.12*). The powder is greenish-grey. Examine under a microscope using *chloral hydrate solution R*. The powder shows the following diagnostic characters: numerous fragments of leaf epidermis with polygonal cells having an irregularly striated cuticle, and paracytic stomata (*2.8.3*) that are more numerous in the lower epidermis; fragments of petiole epidermis with elongated cells; uniseriate, long, flexuous unicellular covering trichomes, occasionally multicellular; young leaves; spiral vessels; resiniferous canals; calcium oxalate prisms and macles up to 40 μm in diameter; bundles of narrow septate fibres from the stem; fragments of the fruit: layers of wide cells in a parquetry arrangement, annular vessels, parenchyma cells containing simple or compound starch granules.

C. Thin-layer chromatography (*2.2.27*).

Test solution To 5.0 g of the powdered drug (355) (*2.9.12*) add 50 mL of *ethanol (30 per cent V/V) R*; heat to boiling under a reflux condenser and centrifuge.

Reference solution Dissolve 5 mg of *asiaticoside R* in *methanol R* and dilute to 10 mL with the same solvent.

Plate TLC silica gel G plate R.

Mobile phase acetic acid R, formic acid R, water R, ethyl acetate R (11:11:27:100 *V/V/V/V*).

Application 10 μL, as bands.

Development Over a path of 15 cm.

Drying In air.

Detection Spray with *anisaldehyde solution R* and heat at 100-105 °C; examine in daylight.

Results The chromatograms obtained with the reference solution and the test solution show in the lower third a greenish-blue zone (asiaticoside). The chromatogram obtained with the test solution shows also below this zone a violet zone (madecassoside); near the solvent front it shows a light blue zone (asiatic acid) and just below a pinkish-violet zone (madecassic acid); in the lower half it shows brown, grey and brownish-green zones between the point of application and the zone due to madecassoside, and other brownish-yellow or light yellow zones above the zone due to asiaticoside.

TESTS

Foreign matter (*2.8.2*)
Maximum 7 per cent, of which maximum 5 per cent of underground organs and maximum 2 per cent of other foreign matter.

Loss on drying (*2.2.32*)
Maximum 10.0 per cent, determined on 1.000 g of the powdered drug (355) (*2.9.12*) by drying in an oven at 105 °C for 2 h.

Total ash (*2.4.16*)
Maximum 12.0 per cent.

ASSAY
Liquid chromatography (*2.2.29*).

Test solution Place 5.0 g of the powdered drug (355) (*2.9.12*) in a cellulose fingerstall in a continuous extraction apparatus (Soxhlet type). Add 100 mL of *methanol R* and heat for 8 h. Cool and dilute the extract to 100.0 mL with *methanol R*. Filter through a 0.45 μm filter. Dilute 2.0 mL of the filtrate to 20.0 mL with *methanol R*.

Reference solution Dissolve 20.0 mg of *asiaticoside R* in *methanol R*, if necessary using sonication, and dilute to

20.0 mL with the same solvent. Dilute 2.0 mL of this solution to 100.0 mL with *methanol R*.

Column:
— *size*: $l = 0.25$ m, $\varnothing = 4$ mm;
— *stationary phase: octadecylsilyl silica gel for chromatography R* (5 μm).

Phase mobile:
— *mobile phase A: acetonitrile for chromatography R*;
— *mobile phase B*: dilute 3 mL of *phosphoric acid R* to 1000 mL with *water R*;

Time (min)	Mobile phase A (per cent *V/V*)	Mobile phase B (per cent *V/V*)
0 - 65	22	78
65 - 66	55	45
66 - 76	95	5
76 - 85	22	78

Flow rate   1.0 mL/min.

Detection   Spectrophotometer at 200 nm.

Injection   20 μL.

Relative retention   With reference to the solvent: madecassoside = about 5.8; asiaticoside = about 8.1; madecassic acid = about 17.6; Asiatic acid = about 21.7.

Calculate the response factor R_F of asiaticoside using the following expression:

$$\frac{A_1 \times V_1 \times 100}{m_1 \times HPLC_P}$$

A_1 =   area of the peak due to asiaticoside in the chromatogram obtained with the reference solution;
V_1 =   volume of the reference solution, in millilitres
m_1 =   mass of asiaticoside in the reference solution, in milligrams;
$HPLC_P$ =   purity determined for asiaticoside.

Calculate the mean response factor ($\overline{RF}$) for asiaticoside using the following expression:

$$\frac{\sum_{i=1}^{N} RF_i}{N}$$

$\sum_{i=1}^{N} RF_i$ =   sum of response factors of asiaticoside for the chromatograms obtained with the reference solution;
N =   number of injections of reference solution ($N = 4$, at least).

Calculate the percentage content of total triterpenoid derivatives, expressed as asiaticoside, using the following expression:

$$\frac{V}{m}\left[\frac{A + (B \times 1.017) + (C \times 0.526) + (D \times 0.509)}{\overline{RF}}\right]$$

V =   volume of the test solution, in millilitres;
m =   mass of the substance to be examined in the test solution, in milligrams;
A =   area of the peak due to asiaticoside in the chromatogram obtained with the test solution;

B =   area of the peak due to madecassoside in the chromatogram obtained with the test solution;
C =   area of the peak due to madecassic acid in the chromatogram obtained with the test solution;
D =   area of the peak due to asiatic acid in the chromatogram obtained with the test solution;
$\overline{RF}$ =   mean response factor of asiaticoside.

_____ *Ph Eur*

Chamomile Flowers

(*Roman Chamomile Flower, Ph Eur monograph 0380*)

Ph Eur _____

DEFINITION
Dried flower-heads of the cultivated double variety of *Chamaemelum nobile* (L.) All. (*Anthemis nobilis* L.).

Content
Minimum 7 mL/kg of essential oil (dried drug).

CHARACTERS
The flower-heads are white or yellowish-grey, composed of solitary hemispherical capitula, made up of a solid conical receptacle bearing the florets, each subtended by a transparent small palea.

Strong and characteristic odour.

IDENTIFICATION
A. The capitula have a diameter of 8-20 mm; the receptacle is solid; the base of the receptacle is surrounded by an involucre consisting of 2-3 rows of compact and imbricated bracts with scarious margins. Most florets are ligulate, but a few pale yellow tubular florets occur in the central region. Ligulate florets are white, dull, lanceolate and reflexed with a dark brown, inferior ovary, a filiform style and a bifid stigma; tubular florets have a five-toothed corolla tube, 5 syngenesious, epipetalous stamens and a gynoecium similar to that of the ligulate florets.

B. Separate the capitulum into its different parts. Examine under a microscope using *chloral hydrate solution R*. All parts of the flower-heads are covered with numerous small yellow glistening glandular trichomes. The involucral bracts and paleae have epidermal cells in longitudinal rows, sclerified at the base and they are covered with conical trichomes, about 500 μm long, each composed of 3-4 very short base cells and a long, bent, terminal cell about 20 μm wide. The corolla of the ligulate flowers consists of papillary cells with cuticular striations. The ovaries of both kinds of florets have at their base a sclerous ring consisting of a single row of cells. The receptacle and the ovaries contain small clusters of calcium oxalate. The pollen grains have a diameter of about 35 μm and are rounded or triangular with 3 germinal pores and a spiny exine.

C. Thin-layer chromatography (*2.2.27*).

Test solution   To 0.5 g of the powdered drug (710) (*2.9.12*) add 10 mL of *methanol R* and heat with shaking in a water-bath at 60 °C for 5 min. Allow to cool and filter.

Reference solution   Dissolve 2.5 mg of *apigenin R* and 2.5 mg of *apigenin 7-glucoside R* in 10 mL of *methanol R*.

Plate   TLC silica gel plate R.

Mobile phase   glacial acetic acid R, water R, butanol R (17:17:66 *V/V/V*).

Application   10 μL, as bands.

Development   Over a path of 10 cm.

Drying   At 100-105 °C for 5 min.

Detection   Spray the warm plate with a 10 g/L solution of *diphenylboric acid aminoethyl ester R* in *methanol R*, using about 10 mL for a plate 200 mm square; subsequently spray with the same volume of a 50 g/L solution of *macrogol 400 R* in *methanol R*; allow to stand for about 30 min and examine in ultraviolet light at 365 nm.

Results   The chromatogram obtained with the reference solution shows in the upper third a yellowish-green fluorescent zone (apigenin) and in the middle third a yellowish fluorescent zone (apigenin 7-glucoside). The chromatogram obtained with the test solution shows a yellowish-green fluorescent zone and a yellowish fluorescent zone similar in position and fluorescence to the zones due to apigenin and apigenin 7-glucoside in the chromatogram obtained with the reference solution; above the apigenin 7-glucoside zone there is a brownish fluorescent zone (luteolin); immediately below the apigenin 7-glucoside zone there is a light brownish fluorescent zone (apiin); immediately below the apiin zone there is a bright blue fluorescent zone and below this zone a bright blue fluorescent zone; other faint zones may be present.

TESTS

Diameter of the flower-heads

Maximum 3 per cent of flower-heads have a diameter smaller than 8 mm.

Deteriorated flower-heads

Brown or darkened flower-heads are absent.

Loss on drying (*2.2.32*)

Maximum 11.0 per cent, determined on 1.000 g of the powdered drug (355) (*2.9.12*) by drying in an oven at 105 °C for 2 h.

Total ash (*2.4.16*)

Maximum 8.0 per cent.

ASSAY

Carry out the determination of essential oils in herbal drugs (*2.8.12*). Use 20.0 g of whole drug, a 500 mL round-bottomed flask, 250 mL of *water R* as the distillation liquid and 0.50 mL of *xylene R* in the graduated tube. Distil at a rate of 3-3.5 mL/min for 3 h.

————— Ph Eur

Cinchona Bark

Cinchona; Red Cinchona Bark

(*Ph Eur monograph 0174*)

Preparation

Cinchona Liquid Extract, Standardised

When Powdered Cinchona is prescribed or demanded, material complying with the requirements below with the exception of Identification test A and the test for Foreign matter shall be dispensed or supplied.

Ph Eur _____

DEFINITION

Whole or cut, dried bark of *Cinchona pubescens* Vahl (*Cinchona succirubra* Pav.), of *Cinchona calisaya* Wedd., of *Cinchona ledgeriana* Moens ex Trimen, or of their varieties or hybrids.

Content

Minimum 6.5 per cent of total alkaloids, of which 30 per cent to 60 per cent consists of quinine-type alkaloids (dried drug).

CHARACTERS

Intense bitter, somewhat astringent taste.

IDENTIFICATION

A. The stem and branch bark is supplied in quilled or curved pieces 2-6 mm thick. The outer surface is dull brownish-grey or grey and frequently bears lichens; it is usually rough, marked with transverse fissures and longitudinally furrowed or wrinkled; exfoliation of the outer surface occurs in some varieties. The inner surface is striated and deep reddish-brown; the fracture is short in the outer part and fibrous in the inner part.

B. Reduce to a powder (355) (*2.9.12*). The powder is reddish-brown. Examine under a microscope using *chloral hydrate solution R*. The powder shows the following diagnostic characters (Figure 0174.-1): thin-walled cork cells filled with reddish-brown contents, in surface view [K] and transverse section [H]; yellow, spindle-shaped striated phloem fibres up to 90 μm in diameter and up to 1300 μm in length, very thick-walled with an uneven lumen and with conspicuous, funnel-shaped pits, whole [A] or fragmented [F, J]; parenchymatous idioblasts filled with microprisms of calcium oxalate [E, G]; clusters of thin-walled phloem parenchyma cells [L] accompanied by medullary rays in tangential section [D]. Examine under a microscope using a 50 per cent *V/V* solution of *glycerol R*. The powder shows a few starch granules 6-10 μm in diameter, mostly simple but occasionally with 2 or 3 components, free [B] or included in parenchymatous cells [C].

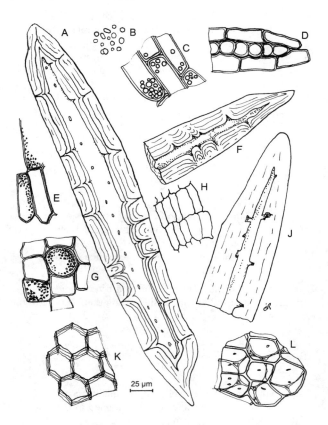

Figure 0174.-1.– *Illustration for identification test B of powdered herbal drug of cinchona bark*

C. Thin-layer chromatography (*2.2.27*).

Test solution   To 0.10 g of the powdered drug (180) (*2.9.12*) in a test-tube add 0.1 mL of *concentrated ammonia R* and 5 mL of *methylene chloride R*. Shake vigorously occasionally during 30 min and filter. Evaporate the filtrate to dryness on a water-bath and dissolve the residue in 1 mL of *anhydrous ethanol R*.

Reference solution   Dissolve 17.5 mg of *quinine R*, 2.5 mg of *quinidine R*, 10 mg of *cinchonine R* and 10 mg of *cinchonidine R* in 5 mL of *anhydrous ethanol R*.

Plate   *TLC silica gel plate R*.

Mobile phase   diethylamine R, ethyl acetate R, toluene R (10:20:70 *V/V/V*).

Application   10 μL as bands.

Development   Twice over a path of 15 cm.

Drying   At 100-105 °C, then allow to cool.

Detection A   Spray with *anhydrous formic acid R* and allow to dry in air; examine in ultraviolet light at 365 nm.

Results A   See below the sequence of zones present in the chromatograms obtained with the reference solution and the test solution. Furthermore, other fluorescent zones are present in the chromatogram obtained with the test solution.

Top of the plate	
———	———
Quinidine: a distinct blue fluorescent zone	A distinct blue fluorescent zone (quinidine)
———	———
Quinine: a distinct blue fluorescent zone	A distinct blue fluorescent zone (quinine)
Reference solution	**Test solution**

Detection B   Spray with *iodoplatinate reagent R*.

Results B   See below the sequence of zones present in the chromatograms obtained with the reference solution and the test solution. Furthermore, other zones are present in the chromatogram obtained with the test solution.

Top of the plate	
Cinchonine: a violet zone that becomes violet-grey	A violet zone that becomes violet-grey (cinchonine)
Quinidine: a violet zone that becomes violet-grey	A violet zone that becomes violet-grey (quinidine)
Cinchonidine: an intense dark blue zone	An intense dark blue zone (cinchonidine)
———	———
Quinine: a violet zone that becomes violet-grey	A violet zone that becomes violet-grey (quinine)
Reference solution	**Test solution**

TESTS

Total ash (*2.4.16*)
Maximum 6.0 per cent.

Loss on drying (*2.2.32*)
Maximum 10 per cent, determined on 1.000 g of the powdered drug (355) (*2.9.12*) by drying in an oven at 105 °C for 2 h.

ASSAY

Test solution   In a 250 mL conical flask mix 1.000 g of the powdered drug (180) (*2.9.12*) with 10 mL of *water R* and 7 mL of *dilute hydrochloric acid R*. Heat in a water-bath for 30 min, allow to cool and add 25 mL of *methylene chloride R*, 50 mL of *ether R* and 5 mL of a 200 g/L solution of *sodium hydroxide R*. Shake the mixture repeatedly for 30 min, add 3 g of *powdered tragacanth R* and shake until the mixture becomes clear. Filter through a plug of absorbent cotton and rinse the flask and the cotton with 5 quantities, each of 20 mL, of a mixture of 1 volume of *methylene chloride R* and 2 volumes of *ether R*. Combine the filtrate and washings, evaporate to dryness and dissolve the residue in 10.0 mL of *anhydrous ethanol R*. Evaporate 5.0 mL of this solution to dryness, dissolve the residue in *0.1 M hydrochloric acid* and dilute to 1000.0 mL with the same acid.

Reference solutions   Dissolve separately 30.0 mg of *quinine R* and 30.0 mg of *cinchonine R* in *0.1 M hydrochloric acid* and dilute each solution to 1000.0 mL with the same acid.

Measure the absorbances (*2.2.25*) of the 3 solutions at 316 nm and 348 nm using *0.1 M hydrochloric acid* as the compensation liquid.

Calculate the percentage content of alkaloids using the following equations:

$$x = \frac{[A_{316} \times A_{348c}] - [A_{316c} \times A_{348}]}{[A_{316q} \times A_{348c}] - [A_{316c} \times A_{348q}]} \times \frac{100}{m} \times \frac{2}{1000}$$

$$y = \frac{[A_{316} \times A_{348q}] - [A_{316q} \times A_{348}]}{[A_{316c} \times A_{348q}] - [A_{316q} \times A_{348c}]} \times \frac{100}{m} \times \frac{2}{1000}$$

m = mass of the drug used, in grams;
x = percentage content of quinine-type alkaloids;
y = percentage content of cinchonine-type alkaloids;
A_{316} = absorbance of the test solution at 316 nm;
A_{348} = absorbance of the test solution at 348 nm;
A_{316c} = absorbance of the reference solution containing cinchonine at 316 nm, corrected to a concentration of 1 mg/1000 ml;
A_{316q} = absorbance of the reference solution containing quinine at 316 nm, corrected to a concentration of 1 mg/1000 ml;
A_{348c} = absorbance of the reference solution containing cinchonine at 348 nm, corrected to a concentration of 1 mg/1000 ml;
A_{348q} = absorbance of the reference solution containing quinine at 348 nm, corrected to a concentration of 1 mg/1000 ml.

Calculate the content of total alkaloids ($x + y$), and calculate the relative content of quinine-type alkaloids using the following expression:

$$\frac{100x}{x + y}$$

——————————————— *Ph Eur*

Standardised Cinchona Liquid Extract

(Ph Eur monograph 1818)

Ph Eur ⎯⎯⎯⎯⎯⎯⎯⎯⎯⎯⎯⎯⎯⎯⎯⎯⎯⎯

DEFINITION

Liquid extract produced from *Cinchona bark (0174)*.

Content

Minimum 4.0 per cent and maximum 5.0 per cent of total alkaloids, of which 30 per cent to 60 per cent are alkaloids of the quinine type ($C_{20}H_{24}N_2O_2$; M_r 324.4).

PRODUCTION

Standardised cinchona liquid extract is produced from the herbal drug by an appropriate procedure using:

— ethanol (30 per cent *V/V* to 90 per cent *V/V*), or;
— a mixture of diluted hydrochloric acid, ethanol (96 per cent *V/V*), glycerol, water (1:2:5:20 *V/V*).

CHARACTERS

Appearance

Brownish-red liquid.

It has a bitter, astringent taste.

IDENTIFICATION

Thin-layer chromatography (*2.2.27*).

Test solution   Dilute 1 mL of the extract to be examined in 1 mL of *anhydrous ethanol R*.

Reference solution   Dissolve 2.5 mg of *quinidine R*, 10 mg of *cinchonidine R*, 10 mg of *cinchonine R* and 17.5 mg of *quinine R* in 5 mL of *anhydrous ethanol R*.

Plate   *TLC silica gel plate R* (5-40 μm) [or *TLC silica gel plate R* (2-10 μm)].

Mobile phase   *diethylamine R, ethyl acetate R, toluene R* (10:20:70 *V/V/V*).

Application   10 μL [or 2 μL] as bands.

Development   Twice over a path of 15 cm [or 6 cm].

Drying   At 100-105 °C then allow to cool.

Detection A   Spray with a 50 g/L solution of *anhydrous formic acid R* and allow to dry in air; examine in ultraviolet light at 365 nm.

Results A   See below the sequence of the zones present in the chromatograms obtained with the reference solution and the test solution. Furthermore, other fluorescent zones may be present in the chromatogram obtained with the test solution.

Top of the plate	
⎯⎯⎯	⎯⎯⎯
Quinidine: a distinct blue fluorescent zone	A distinct blue fluorescent zone (quinidine)
⎯⎯⎯	⎯⎯⎯
Quinine: a distinct blue fluorescent zone	A distinct blue fluorescent zone (quinine)
Reference solution	**Test solution**

Detection B   Spray with *iodoplatinate reagent R*.

Results B   See below the sequence of the zones present in the chromatograms obtained with the reference solution and the test solution. Furthermore, other zones may be present in the chromatogram obtained with the test solution.

Top of the plate	
Cinchonine: a violet-grey zone	A violet-grey zone (cinchonine)
Quinidine: a violet-grey zone	A violet-grey zone (quinidine)
Cinchonidine: an intense dark blue zone	An intense dark blue zone (cinchonidine)
Quinine: a violet-grey zone	A violet-grey zone (quinine)
Reference solution	**Test solution**

TESTS

Ethanol (*2.9.10*)

95 per cent to 105 per cent of the content stated on the label.

Methanol and 2-propanol (*2.9.11*)

Maximum 0.05 per cent *V/V* of methanol and maximum 0.05 per cent *V/V* of 2-propanol.

Dry residue (*2.8.16*)

Minimum 12.0 per cent for glycerol-free standardised cinchona liquid extract and minimum 30.0 per cent for glycerol-containing standardised cinchona extract, determined on 2.0 g.

ASSAY

Test solution   In a 250 mL conical flask, mix about 1.000 g of the extract to be examined with 10 mL of *water R* and 7 mL of *dilute hydrochloric acid R*. Heat in a water-bath for 30 min, allow to cool and add 25 mL of *methylene chloride R*, 50 mL of *ether R* and 5 mL of a 200 g/L solution of *sodium hydroxide R*. Shake the mixture frequently for 30 min, add 3 g of powdered *tragacanth R* and shake until the mixture becomes clear. Filter through a plug of absorbent cotton, rinse the flask and the cotton with 5 quantities, each of 20 mL, of a mixture of 1 volume of *methylene chloride R* and 2 volumes of *ether R*. Combine the filtrate and washings, evaporate to dryness and dissolve the residue in 10.0 mL of *ethanol (96 per cent) R*. Evaporate 5.0 mL of this solution to dryness, dissolve the residue in *0.1 M hydrochloric acid* and dilute to 1000.0 mL with the same acid.

Reference solution (a)   Dissolve 30.0 mg of *cinchonine R* in *0.1 M hydrochloric acid* and dilute to 1000.0 mL with the same acid.

Reference solution (b)   Dissolve 30.0 mg of *quinine R* in *0.1 M hydrochloric acid* and dilute to 1000.0 mL with the same acid.

Measure the absorbances (*2.2.25*) of the 3 solutions at 316 nm and 348 nm, using *0.1 M hydrochloric acid* as the compensation liquid.

Calculate the percentage content of alkaloids from the following equations:

$$n_1 = \frac{[A_1 \times A_{2a}] - [A_{1a} \times A_2]}{[A_{1b} \times A_{2a}] - [A_{1a} \times A_{2b}]} \times \frac{100}{m} \times \frac{2}{1000}$$

$$n_2 = \frac{[A_1 \times A_{2b}] - [A_{1b} \times A_2]}{[A_{1a} \times A_{2b}] - [A_{1b} \times A_{2a}]} \times \frac{100}{m} \times \frac{2}{1000}$$

m	=	mass of the liquid extract to be examined in grams;
n_1	=	percentage content of quinine-type alkaloids;
n_2	=	percentage content of cinchonine-type alkaloids;
A_1	=	absorbance of the test solution at 316 nm;
A_2	=	absorbance of the test solution at 348 nm;

A_{1a} = absorbance of reference solution (a) at 316 nm, corrected to a concentration of 1 mg/1000 mL;

A_{1b} = absorbance of reference solution (b) at 316 nm, corrected to a concentration of 1 mg/1000 mL;

A_{2a} = absorbance of reference solution (a) at 348 nm, corrected to a concentration of 1 mg/1000 mL;

A_{2b} = absorbance of reference solution (b) at 348 nm, corrected to a concentration of 1 mg/1000 mL.

Calculate the content of total alkaloids ($n_1 + n_2$), and the relative content of quinine-type alkaloids, from the following expression:

$$\frac{n_1 \times 100}{n_1 + n_2}$$

LABELLING

The label states the solvent composition used for the production.

———————————————— Ph Eur

Cinnamon

Cinnamon Bark; Ceylon Cinnamon

(*Ph Eur monograph 0387*)

Preparation

Cinnamon Tincture

When Powdered Cinnamon is prescribed or demanded, material complying with the requirements below with the exception of Identification test A and containing not less than 1.0% v/w (10 mL/kg) of essential oil shall be dispensed or supplied.

Ph Eur ————————————————

DEFINITION

Dried bark, freed from the outer cork and the underlying parenchyma, of the shoots grown on cut stock of *Cinnamomum verum* J.Presl.

Content

Minimum 12 mL/kg of essential oil.

CHARACTERS

Characteristic, aromatic odour.

IDENTIFICATION

A. The bark is about 0.2-0.8 mm thick and occurs in closely packed compound quills made up of single or double quills. The outer surface is smooth, yellowish-brown with faint scars marking the position of leaves and axillary buds and has fine, whitish and wavy longitudinal striations. The inner surface is slightly darker and longitudinally striated. The fracture is short and fibrous.

B. Microscopic examination (*2.8.23*). The powder is yellowish or reddish-brown. Examine under a microscope using *chloral hydrate solution R*. The powder shows the following diagnostic characters (Figure 0387.-1): rounded sclereids with pitted, channelled and moderately thickened walls, single [E, F] or in groups [C]; numerous colourless, single fibres, often whole [A], or fragmented [D], with a narrow lumen, thickened, lignified walls and few pits; small acicular crystals of calcium oxalate in parenchymatous cells [J]; very numerous oil droplets [B]. Cork fragments [G] are absent or very rare. Examine under a microscope using a 50 per cent *V/V* solution of *glycerol R*. The powder shows abundant starch granules [H].

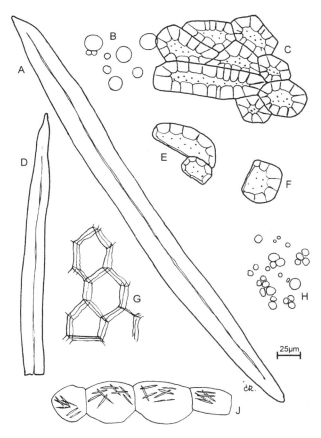

Figure 0387.-1. – *Illustration for identification test B of powdered herbal drug of cinnamon*

C. Thin-layer chromatography (*2.2.27*).

Test solution Shake 0.1 g of the powdered drug (500) (*2.9.12*) with 2 mL of *methylene chloride R* for 15 min. Filter and evaporate the filtrate carefully almost to dryness on a water-bath. Dissolve the residue in 0.4 mL of *toluene R*.

Reference solution Dissolve 50 μL of *cinnamic aldehyde R* and 10 μL of *eugenol R* in *toluene R* and dilute to 10 mL with the same solvent.

Plate TLC silica gel GF$_{254}$ plate R.

Mobile phase methylene chloride R.

Application 10 μL as bands of 20 mm by 3 mm.

Development Over a path of 10 cm.

Drying In air.

Detection A Examine in ultraviolet light at 254 nm and mark the quenching zones, then examine in ultraviolet light at 365 nm and mark the fluorescent zones.

Results A Examined in ultraviolet light at 254 nm, the chromatograms obtained with the test solution and the reference solution show a quenching zone due to cinnamaldehyde in the median part and, just above it, a weaker quenching zone due to eugenol; examined in ultraviolet light at 365 nm, the chromatogram obtained with the test solution shows a fluorescent light blue zone due to *o*-methoxycinnamaldehyde just below the zone due to cinnamaldehyde.

Detection B Spray with *phloroglucinol solution R*.

Results B The zone due to cinnamaldehyde is yellowish-brown and the zone due to *o*-methoxycinnamaldehyde is violet.

TESTS

Total ash (2.4.16)

Maximum 6.0 per cent.

ASSAY

Carry out the determination of essential oils in herbal drugs (2.8.12). Use 20.0 g of drug reduced to a powder (710) (2.9.12) immediately before the determination, a 500 mL flask, 200 mL of *0.1 M hydrochloric acid* as the distillation liquid, and 0.50 mL of *xylene R* in the graduated tube. Distil at a rate of 2.5-3.5 mL/min for 3 h.

————————————————— Ph Eur

Ceylon Cinnamon Bark Oil

Cinnamon Oil

(*Ph Eur monograph 1501*)

Preparation

Concentrated Cinnamon Water

Ph Eur ———————————————————

DEFINITION

Essential oil obtained by steam distillation of the bark of the shoots of *Cinnamomum verum* J.Presl.

CHARACTERS

Appearance

Clear, mobile, light yellow liquid becoming reddish over time.

Characteristic odour reminiscent of cinnamic aldehyde.

IDENTIFICATION

First identification   B.

Second identification   A.

A. Thin-layer chromatography (2.2.27).

Test solution   Dissolve 1 mL of the essential oil to be examined in *acetone R* and dilute to 10 mL with the same solvent.

Reference solution   Dissolve 50 µL of *trans-cinnamic aldehyde R*, 10 µL of *eugenol R*, 10 µL of *linalol R* and 10 µL of *β-caryophyllene R* in *ethanol (96 per cent) R* and dilute to 10 mL with the same solvent.

Plate   TLC silica gel plate R.

Mobile phase   methanol R, toluene R (10:90 V/V).

Application   10 µL as bands.

Development   Over a path of 15 cm.

Drying   In air.

Detection   Spray with *anisaldehyde solution R*; heat at 100-105 °C for 5-10 min and examine in daylight.

Results   The zones in the chromatogram obtained with the test solution are similar in position and colour to those in the chromatogram obtained with the reference solution.

B. Examine the chromatograms obtained in the test for chromatographic profile.

Results   The principal peaks in the chromatogram obtained with the test solution are similar in retention time to those in the chromatogram obtained with the reference solution. Safrole, coumarin and cineole may be absent from the chromatogram obtained with the test solution.

TESTS

Relative density (2.2.5)

1.000 to 1.030.

Refractive index (2.2.6)

1.572 to 1.591.

Optical rotation (2.2.7)

$- 2°$ to $+ 1°$.

Chromatographic profile

Gas chromatography (2.2.28): use the normalisation procedure.

Test solution   The essential oil to be examined.

Reference solution   Dissolve 10 µL of *cineole R*, 10 µL of *linalol R*, 10 µL of *β-caryophyllene R*, 10 µL of *safrole R*, 100 µL of *trans-cinnamic aldehyde R*, 10 µL of *eugenol R*, 20 mg of *coumarin R*, 10 µL of *trans-2-methoxycinnamaldehyde R* and 10 µL of *benzyl benzoate R* in 1 mL of *acetone R*.

Column:

— *material*: fused silica;

— *size*: $l = 60$ m, $\varnothing = 0.25$ mm;

— *stationary phase*: bonded *macrogol 20 000 R*.

Carrier gas   helium for chromatography R.

Flow rate   1.5 mL/min.

Split ratio   1:100.

Temperature:

	Time (min)	Temperature (°C)
Column	0 - 10	60
	10 - 75	60 → 190
	75 - 200	190
Injection port		200
Detector		240

Detection   Flame ionisation.

Injection   0.2 µL.

Elution order   Order indicated in the composition of the reference solution; depending on the operating conditions and the state of the column, coumarin may elute before or after *trans*-2-methoxycinnamaldehyde; record the retention times of these substances.

System suitability   Reference solution:

— *resolution*: minimum 1.5 between the peaks due to linalol and β-caryophyllene.

Identification of components   Using the retention times determined from the chromatogram obtained with the reference solution, locate the components of the reference solution in the chromatogram obtained with the test solution.

Determine the percentage content of each of these components. The percentages are within the following ranges:

— *cineole*: maximum 3.0 per cent;

— *linalol*: 1.0 per cent to 6.0 per cent;

— *β-caryophyllene*: 1.0 per cent to 4.0 per cent;

— *safrole*: maximum 0.5 per cent;

— *trans-cinnamic aldehyde*: 55 per cent to 75 per cent;

— *eugenol*: maximum 7.5 per cent;

— *coumarin*: maximum 0.5 per cent;

— *trans-2-methoxycinnamaldehyde*: 0.1 per cent to 1.0 per cent;

— *benzyl benzoate*: maximum 1.0 per cent.

STORAGE

Protected from heat.

————————————————— Ph Eur

Cinnamon Tincture

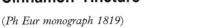

(*Ph Eur monograph 1819*)

Ph Eur _____

DEFINITION

Tincture produced from *Cinnamon (0387)*.

PRODUCTION

The tincture is produced from 1 part of the drug and 5 parts of ethanol (70 per cent *V/V*) by an appropriate procedure.

CHARACTERS

Appearance

Clear, brownish-red liquid, with a characteristic odour.

IDENTIFICATION

Thin-layer chromatography (*2.2.27*).

Test solution   Place 10 mL of the tincture to be examined, 10 mL of *saturated sodium chloride solution R* and 5 mL of *toluene R* in a ground glass-stoppered tube. Shake for 2 min and centrifuge for 10 min. Use the organic layer.

Reference solution   Dissolve 5 μL of *eugenol R*, 25 μL of *trans-cinnamic aldehyde R* and 5 μL of *trans-2-methoxycinnamaldehyde R* in *toluene R* and dilute to 10 mL with the same solvent.

Plate   TLC *silica gel G plate R*.

Mobile phase   *methylene chloride R*.

Application   20 μL, as bands.

Development   Over a path of 10 cm.

Drying   In air.

Detection A   Examine in ultraviolet light at 365 nm.

Results A   See below the sequence of the zones present in the chromatograms obtained with the reference solution and the test solution.

Top of the plate	
Trans-2-methoxycinnamaldehyde: a light blue fluorescent zone	A light blue fluorescent zone (*trans-2-* methoxycinnamaldehyde)
	A greenish fluorescent zone (above the line of application)
Reference solution	Test solution

Detection B   Spray with a 200 g/L solution of *phosphomolybdic acid R* in *ethanol R*. Examine in daylight while heating at 100-105 °C for 5-10 min.

Results B   See below the sequence of the zones present in the chromatograms obtained with the reference solution and the test solution. Furthermore, other zones may be present in the chromatogram obtained with the test solution.

Top of the plate	
	1 blue zone (terpenhydrocarbons)
Eugenol: a blue zone	A blue zone (eugenol)
Trans-cinnamic aldehyde: a blue zone	A blue zone (*trans*-cinnamic aldehyde)
Trans-2-methoxycinnamaldehyde: an orange-brown zone (the colour fades away)	A weak orange-brown zone (*trans*-2-methoxycinnamaldehyde)
	2 or 3 blue zones above the line of application
Reference solution	Test solution

TESTS

Ethanol (*2.9.10*)
64 per cent *V/V* to 70 per cent *V/V*.

Methanol and 2-propanol (*2.9.11*)
Maximum 0.05 per cent *V/V* of methanol and maximum 0.05 per cent *V/V* of 2-propanol.

Dry residue (*2.8.16*)
Minimum 1.5 per cent *m/m*, determined on 5.0 g.

_____ *Ph Eur*

Concentrated Cinnamon Water

DEFINITION

Cinnamon Oil	20 mL
Ethanol (90 per cent)	600 mL
Water	Sufficient to produce 1000 mL

Extemporaneous preparation
The following directions apply.

Dissolve the Cinnamon Oil in the Ethanol (90 per cent) and add gradually, with vigorous shaking after each addition, sufficient Water to produce 1000 mL. Add 50 g of previously sterilised Purified Talc, or other suitable filtering aid, allow to stand for a few hours, shaking occasionally, and filter.

The water complies with the requirements stated under Aromatic Waters and with the following requirements.

TESTS

Ethanol content
52 to 56% v/v, Appendix VIII F.

Weight per mL
0.914 to 0.922 g, Appendix V G.

Ceylon Cinnamon Leaf Oil

(*Ph Eur monograph 1608*)

Ph Eur _____

DEFINITION

Oil obtained by steam distillation of the leaves of *Cinnamomum verum* J.S. Presl.

CHARACTERS

Appearance

Clear, mobile, reddish-brown or dark brown liquid.

Characteristic odour reminiscent of eugenol.

IDENTIFICATION

First identification B.

Second identification A.

A. Thin-layer chromatography (*2.2.27*).

Test solution Dilute 1 mL of the substance to be examined in *acetone R* and dilute to 10 mL with the same solvent.

Reference solution Dilute about 50 µL of *trans-cinnamic aldehyde R*, 10 µL of *eugenol R*, 10 µL of *linalol R* and 10 µL of *β-caryophyllene R* in *alcohol R* and dilute to 10 mL with the same solvent.

Plate TLC silica gel plate R.

Mobile phase methanol R, toluene R (10:90 V/V).

Application 10 µL, as bands.

Development Over a path of 15 cm.

Drying In air.

Detection Spray with *anisaldehyde solution R*. Examine in day light while heating at 100-105 °C for 5-10 min.

Results The zones in the chromatogram obtained with the test solution are similar in position and colour to those in the chromatogram obtained with the reference solution. The zone due to *trans*-cinnamic aldehyde may be very faint or absent.

B. Examine the chromatogram obtained in the test for chromatographic profile.

Results The characteristic peaks in the chromatogram obtained with the test solution are similar in retention time to those in the chromatogram obtained with the reference solution. The peaks corresponding to cineole, safrole, *trans*-cinnamic aldehyde, cinnamyl acetate and coumarin may be absent in the chromatogram obtained with the test solution.

TESTS

Relative density (*2.2.5*)
1.030 to 1.059.

Refractive index (*2.2.6*)
1.527 to 1.540.

Optical rotation (*2.2.7*)
− 2.5° to + 2.0°.

Chromatographic profile
Gas chromatography (*2.2.28*): use the normalisation procedure.

Test solution The substance to be examined.

Reference solution Dissolve 10 µL of *cineole R*, 10 µL of *linalol R*, 10 µL of *β-caryophyllene R*, 10 µL of *safrole R*, 10 µL of *trans-cinnamic aldehyde R*, 10 µL of *cinnamyl acetate R*, 100 µL of *eugenol R* and 10 mg of *coumarin R* in 1 mL of *acetone R*.

Column:
— *material*: fused silica,
— *size*: l = 60 m, Ø = 0.25 mm,
— *stationary phase*: macrogol 20 000 R.

Carrier gas helium for chromatography R.

Flow rate 1.5 mL/min.

Split ratio 1/100.

Temperature:

	Time (min)	Temperature (°C)
Column	0 - 10	45
	10 - 78	45 → 180
	78 - 88	180
Injection port		200
Detector		240

Detection Flame ionisation.

Injection 0.2 µL.

Elution order The order indicated in the composition of the reference solution. Record the retention times of these substances.

System suitability Reference solution:
— *resolution*: minimum of 1.5 between the peaks due to linalol and β-caryophyllene.

Using the retention times determined from the chromatogram obtained with the reference solution, locate the components of the reference solution in the chromatogram obtained with the test solution.

Determine the percentage content of these components.

The percentages are within the following ranges:
— *cineole*: maximum 1.0 per cent,
— *linalol*: 1.5 per cent to 3.5 per cent,
— *β-caryophyllene*: 1.5 per cent to 7.0 per cent,
— *safrole*: maximum 3.0 per cent,
— *trans-cinnamic aldehyde*: maximum 3.0 per cent,
— *cinnamyl acetate*: maximum 2.0 per cent,
— *eugenol*: 70 per cent to 85 per cent,
— *coumarin*: maximum 1.0 per cent.

STORAGE
Protected from heat.

—————————————————— Ph Eur

Citronella Oil

(Ph Eur monograph 1609)

Ph Eur ————————————————————————

DEFINITION
Oil obtained by steam distillation from the fresh or partially dried aerial parts of *Cymbopogon winterianus* Jowitt.

CHARACTERS
Appearance
Pale yellow or brown-yellow liquid.
Very strong odour of citronellal.

IDENTIFICATION
First identification B.

Second identification A.

A. Thin-layer chromatography (*2.2.27*).

Test solution Dilute 0.1 g of citronella oil in 10.0 mL of *alcohol R*.

Reference solution Dilute 20 µL of *citronellal R* in 10.0 mL of *alcohol R*.

Plate TLC silica gel plate R.

Mobile phase ethyl acetate R, toluene R (10:90 V/V).

Application 5 µL, as bands.

Development Over a path of 15 cm.

Drying In air.

Detection Spray with *anisaldehyde solution R* and heat at 100-105 °C for 10 min. Examine in ultraviolet light at 365 nm.

Result See below the sequence of the zones present in the chromatograms obtained with the reference and test solutions. Furthermore, other zones are present in the chromatogram obtained with the test solution.

Top of the plate	
Citronellal: a violet zone	A zone similar in colour to the citronellal zone
	An orange zone (citronellol-geraniol)
Reference solution	**Test solution**

B. Examine the chromatograms obtained in the test for chromatographic profile.

Results The characteristic peaks in the chromatogram obtained with the test solution are similar in retention time to those in the chromatogram obtained with the reference solution. Neral and geranial may be absent in the chromatogram obtained with the test solution.

TESTS

Relative density *(2.2.5)*
0.881 to 0.895.

Refractive index *(2.2.6)*
1.463 to 1.475.

Optical rotation *(2.2.7)*
− 4° to + 1.5°.

Chromatographic profile
Gas chromatography *(2.2.28)*: use the normalisation procedure.

Test solution The substance to be examined.

Reference solution Dilute 25 µL of *limonene R*, 100 µL of *citronellal R*, 25 µL of *citronellyl acetate R*, 25 µL of *citral R*, 25 µL of *geranyl acetate R*, 25 µL of *citronellol R* and 100 µL of *geraniol R* in 5 mL of *hexane R*.

Column:
— *material*: fused silica,
— *size*: l = 60 m, Ø = 0.25 mm,
— *stationary phase*: *macrogol 20 000 R* (0.2 µm).

Carrier gas   *helium for chromatography R*.

Flow rate   1.0 mL/min.

Split ratio   1:100.

Temperature:

	Time (min)	Temperature (°C)
Column	0 - 2	80
	2 - 26	80 → 150
	26 - 42	150 → 185
	42 - 49	185 → 250
Injection port		260
Detector		260

Detection   Flame ionisation.

Injection   1 µL of the reference solution, 0.2 µL of the test solution.

Elution order   The order indicated in the composition of the reference solution. Record the retention times of these substances.

System suitability   Reference solution:
— *resolution*: minimum of 1.2 between the peaks due to geranyl acetate and citronellol.

Using the retention times determined from the chromatogram obtained with the reference solution, locate the components of the reference solution in the chromatogram obtained with the test solution. Determine the percentage content of each of these components.

The percentages are within the following values:
— *limonene*: 1.0 per cent to 5.0 per cent,
— *citronellal*: 30.0 per cent to 45.0 per cent,
— *citronellyl acetate*: 2.0 per cent to 4.0 per cent,
— *neral*: maximum 2.0 per cent,
— *geranial*: maximum 2.0 per cent,
— *geranyl acetate*: 3.0 per cent to 8.0 per cent,
— *citronellol*: 9.0 per cent to 15.0 per cent,
— *geraniol*: 20.0 per cent to 25.0 per cent.

_____ Ph Eur

Clematis Armandii Stem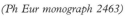

(Ph Eur monograph 2463)

Ph Eur _____

DEFINITION
Whole or fragmented, dried stem of *Clematis armandii* Franch., with cork removed, collected in spring or autumn.

Content
Minimum 0.30 per cent of oleanolic acid ($C_{30}H_{48}O_3$; M_r 456.7) (dried drug).

IDENTIFICATION
A. The whole stem is long and cylindrical, slightly twisted on itself, about 1-6.5 cm in diameter. It shows nodes, usually swollen, with leaf and branch scars. The outer surface is brownish-yellow or dull brownish-yellow, showing longitudinal grooves and striations corresponding to the ends of the medullary rays. Rare cork remnants are easily removed as longitudinal strips. The texture is hard. The fracture is difficult.

The fragmented stem occurs in thick slices, about 2-5 mm thick, with uneven margins; most of the transverse section consists of the pale yellow or slightly brownish-yellow wood and shows numerous radial striations and cracks corresponding to the medullary rays; the vessels are clearly visible in transverse section. The pale yellow or whitish pith, sometimes replaced by a hollow, is reduced.

B. Microscopic examination *(2.8.23)*. The powder is brownish-yellow. Examine under a microscope using *chloral hydrate solution R*. The powder shows the following diagnostic characters: very numerous fragments of vessels, up to 250 µm in diameter, with pitted walls, isolated or associated with elongated tracheids about 15-25 µm in diameter with lignified, thickened and pitted walls; fibres 25-30 µm in diameter, with narrow lumen and thick and partly, slightly pitted walls; parenchymatous cells of the secondary phloem and outer parts of the medullary rays, thin-walled, from the secondary xylem, inner parts of the medullary rays and pith, with slightly thickened, pitted and lignified cell walls; sub-rectangular or fusiform sclereids, about 100 µm long and 35 µm wide, with thick and pitted walls; rare orange-brown cork fragments. Examine under a microscope using a 50 per cent *V/V* solution of *glycerol R*. The powder shows rare starch granules, simple or 2-3 compound, spherical or ovate, individual granules up to 17 μm in diameter, with a punctiform or slit-shaped hilum.

C. Thin-layer chromatography (2.2.27).

Test solution   To 1 g of the powdered herbal drug (1400) (2.9.12) add 5 mL of *methanol R* and heat on a water-bath at 60 °C for 5 min. Filter.

Reference solution   Dissolve 4 mg of *hederagenin R* and 4 mg of *oleanolic acid R* in 10 mL of *methanol R*.

Plate   TLC silica gel F_{254} plate R (5-40 μm) [or TLC silica gel F_{254} plate R (2-10 μm)].

Mobile phase   acetic acid R, acetone R, toluene R (2:8:32 V/V/V).

Application   40 μL [or 10 μL] as bands of 10 mm [or 8 mm].

Development   Over a path of 13 cm [or 6 cm].

Drying   In air.

Detection   Treat with *vanillin reagent R*, heat at 100 °C for 5 min and examine in daylight.

Results   See below the sequence of zones present in the chromatograms obtained with the reference solution and the test solution. Furthermore, other mainly grey zones may be present in the chromatogram obtained with the test solution.

Top of the plate	
	A bluish-violet zone
	A reddish-violet zone
	A weak light blue or grey zone
Oleanolic acid: a reddish-violet zone	
Hederagenin: a greenish-brown zone	
	An orange zone
Reference solution	Test solution

TESTS

Aristolochia manshuriensis Kom. and other species of Aristolochia

Examine the powdered herbal drug (355) (2.9.12) under a microscope using *chloral hydrate solution R*; no cluster crystals are visible.

Aristolochic acids (2.8.21, Method A)

It complies with the test.

Loss on drying (2.2.32)

Maximum 12.0 per cent, determined on 1.000 g of the powdered herbal drug (1400) (2.9.12) by drying in an oven at 105 °C for 2 h.

Total ash (2.4.16)

Maximum 3.0 per cent.

ASSAY

Liquid chromatography (2.2.29).

Test solution   Disperse 1.00 g of the powdered herbal drug (355) (2.9.12) in *methanol R*, add 3 mL of *6 M hydrochloric acid R* and dilute to 30.0 mL with *methanol R*. Shake for 2 h. Filter, add to the filtrate 10 mL of *water R* by rinsing the flask and the filter, and extract with 3 quantities, each of 30 mL, of *methylene chloride R*. Combine the methylene chloride extracts and evaporate to dryness. Dissolve the

residue in 10.0 mL of *methanol R*, shake and filter through a membrane filter (nominal pore size 0.45 μm).

Reference solution (a)   Dissolve 10.0 mg of *oleanolic acid CRS* in *methanol R* and dilute to 20.0 mL with the same solvent.

Reference solution (b)   Dissolve 5.0 mg of *ursolic acid R* in reference solution (a) and dilute to 10.0 mL with the same solution.

Column:
— *size: l* = 0.25 m, Ø = 4.6 mm;
— *stationary phase: end-capped octadecylsilyl silica gel for chromatography R* (5 μm);
— *temperature*: 30 °C.

Mobile phase   0.4 per cent V/V solution of *acetic acid R*, *methanol R* (15:85 V/V).

Flow rate   1.0 mL/min.

Detection   Spectrophotometer at 210 nm.

Injection   20 μL.

Run time   1.2 times the retention time of ursolic acid.

Retention time   Oleanolic acid = about 21 min; ursolic acid = about 22 min.

System suitability   Reference solution (b):
— *resolution*: minimum 1.3 between the peaks due to oleanolic acid and ursolic acid.

Calculate the percentage content of oleanolic acid using the following expression:

$$\frac{A_1 \times m_2 \times p}{A_2 \times m_1 \times 2}$$

A_1 = area of the peak due to oleanolic acid in the chromatogram obtained with the test solution;

A_2 = area of the peak due to oleanolic acid in the chromatogram obtained with reference solution (a);

m_1 = mass of the herbal drug to be examined used to prepare the test solution, in grams;

m_2 = mass of *oleanolic acid CRS* used to prepare reference solution (a), in grams;

p = percentage content of oleanolic acid in *oleanolic acid CRS*.

_____ Ph Eur

Clove

(*Ph Eur monograph 0376*)

When Powdered Clove is prescribed or demanded, material complying with the requirements below with the exception of Identification test A and the test for Foreign matter and containing not less than 12.0% v/w (120 mL/kg) of essential oil shall be dispensed or supplied.

Ph Eur _____

DEFINITION

Whole flower buds of *Syzygium aromaticum* (L.) Merr. et L.M.Perry (syn. *Eugenia caryophyllus* (Spreng.) Bullock et S.G.Harrison) dried until they become reddish-brown.

Content

Minimum 150 mL/kg of essential oil.

CHARACTERS

Characteristic, aromatic odour.

IDENTIFICATION

A. The flower bud is reddish-brown and consists of a quadrangular stalked portion, the hypanthium, 10-12 mm long and 2-3 mm in diameter, surmounted by 4 divergent lobes of sepals which surround a globular head 4-6 mm in diameter. A bilocular ovary containing numerous ovules is situated in the upper part of the hypanthium. The head is globular and dome-shaped, composed of 4 imbricated petals that enclose numerous incurved stamens and a short, erect style with a nectary disc at the base. The hypanthium exudes essential oil when indented with the finger-nail.

B. Reduce to a powder (355) (*2.9.12*). The powder is dark brown and has the odour and taste of the unground drug. Examine under a microscope using *chloral hydrate solution R*. The powder shows the following diagnostic characters: fragments of the hypanthium showing the epidermis and underlying parenchyma containing large oil glands; short fibres occurring singly or in small groups, with thickened, lignified walls and few pits; abundant fragments of parenchyma containing cluster crystals of calcium oxalate; numerous triangular pollen grains about 15 μm in diameter with 3 pores in the angles. Starch granules are absent.

C. Thin-layer chromatography (*2.2.27*).

Test solution   Shake 0.1 g of the powdered drug (500) (*2.9.12*) with 2 mL of *methylene chloride R* for 15 min. Filter and carefully evaporate the filtrate to dryness on a water-bath. Dissolve the residue in 2 mL of *toluene R*.

Reference solution   Dissolve 20 μL of *eugenol R* in 2 mL of *toluene R*.

Plate   *TLC silica gel GF$_{254}$ plate R*.

Mobile phase   *toluene R*.

Application   10 μL of the reference solution and 20 μL of the test solution, as bands of 20 mm by 3 mm.

Development   Twice, in an unsaturated tank over a path of 10 cm; allow the plate to stand for 5 min between the 2 developments.

Drying   In air.

Detection A   Examine in ultraviolet light at 254 nm and mark the quenching zones.

Results A   In the chromatogram obtained with the test solution there is in the median part a quenching zone due to eugenol similar in position to the quenching zone in the chromatogram obtained with the reference solution and there may be a weak quenching zone due to acetyleugenol just below the zone due to eugenol.

Detection B   Spray with *anisaldehyde solution R* using 10 mL for a plate 200 mm square and heat at 100-105 °C for 5-10 min. Examine in daylight.

Results B   The zones due to eugenol in the chromatograms obtained with the test and reference solutions are strong brownish-violet and the zone due to acetyleugenol in the chromatogram obtained with the test solution is faint violet-blue. In the chromatogram obtained with the test solution there are other coloured zones, particularly a faint red zone in the lower part and a reddish-violet zone due to caryophyllene in the upper part.

TESTS

Foreign matter (*2.8.2*)

Maximum 6 per cent of peduncles, petioles and fruits, maximum 2 per cent of deteriorated cloves and maximum 0.5 per cent of other foreign matter.

Total ash (*2.4.16*)

Maximum 7.0 per cent.

ASSAY

Carry out the determination of essential oils in herbal drugs (*2.8.12*). Use a 250 mL flask, 100 mL of *water R* as the

distillation liquid and 0.50 mL of *xylene R* in the graduated tube. Grind 5.0 g of the drug with 5.0 g of *diatomaceous earth R* to form a fine, homogeneous powder and proceed immediately with the determination using 4.0 g of the mixture. Distil at a rate of 2.5-3.5 mL/min for 2 h.

Ph Eur

Clove Oil

(*Ph Eur monograph 1091*)

Ph Eur

DEFINITION

Essential oil obtained by steam distillation from the dried flower buds of *Syzygium aromaticum* (L.) Merr. et L.M.Perry (syn. *Eugenia caryophyllus* (Spreng.) Bullock et S.G.Harrison).

CHARACTERS

Appearance

Clear, yellow liquid, which becomes brown when exposed to air.

Solubility

Miscible with methylene chloride, with toluene and with fatty oils.

IDENTIFICATION

First identification   B.

Second identification   A.

A. Thin-layer chromatography (*2.2.27*).

Test solution   Dissolve 20 μL of the substance to be examined in 2.0 mL of *toluene R*.

Reference solution   Dissolve 15 μL of *eugenol R* and 15 μL of *acetyleugenol R* in 2.0 mL of *toluene R*.

Plate   *TLC silica gel F$_{254}$ plate R*.

Mobile phase   *toluene R*.

Application   20 μL of the test solution and 15 μL of the reference solution, as bands.

Development   Twice in an unsaturated tank over a path of 10 cm; allow to stand for 5 min between the 2 developments.

Drying   In air.

Detection A   Examine in ultraviolet light at 254 nm and mark the quenching zones.

Results A   The chromatogram obtained with the test solution shows in the middle part a quenching zone (eugenol) that is similar in position to the quenching zone in the chromatogram obtained with the reference solution; just below, there is a weak quenching zone (acetyleugenol) that is similar in position to the zone of acetyleugenol in the chromatogram obtained with the reference solution.

Detection B   Spray with *anisaldehyde solution R* and examine in daylight while heating at 100-105 °C for 5-10 min.

Results B   The zone due to eugenol in the chromatograms obtained with the test and reference solutions is strong brownish-violet and the zone due to acetyleugenol in the chromatogram obtained with the test solution is faint violet-blue; in the chromatogram obtained with the test solution there are other coloured zones, particularly a faint red zone in the lower part and a reddish-violet zone (β-caryophyllene) in the upper part.

B. Examine the chromatograms obtained in the test for chromatographic profile.

Results   The 3 principal peaks in chromatogram obtained with the test solution are similar in retention time to the

3 principal peaks in the chromatogram obtained with the reference solution.

TESTS

Relative density (*2.2.5*)
1.030 to 1.063.

Refractive index (*2.2.6*)
1.528 to 1.537.

Optical rotation (*2.2.7*)
−2° to 0°.

Fatty oils and resinified essential oils (*2.8.7*)
It complies with the test.

Solubility in alcohol (*2.8.10*)
1.0 mL is soluble in 2.0 mL and more of *ethanol (70 per cent V/V) R*.

Chromatographic profile
Gas chromatography (*2.2.28*): use the normalisation procedure.

Test solution   Dissolve 0.2 g of the substance to be examined in 10 g of *hexane R*.

Reference solution   Dissolve 7 mg of *β-caryophyllene R*, 80 mg of *eugenol R* and 4 mg of *acetyleugenol R* in 10 g of *hexane R*.

Column:
— *material*: fused silica;
— *size*: *l* = 60 m, Ø = about 0.25 mm;
— *stationary phase*: macrogol 20 000 R.

Carrier gas   helium for chromatography R.

Flow rate   1.5 mL/min.

Split ratio   1:100.

Temperature:

	Time (min)	Temperature (°C)
Column	0 - 8	60
	8 - 48	60 → 180
	48 - 53	180
Injection port		270
Detector		270

Detection   Flame ionisation.

Injection   1.0 µL.

Elution order   Order indicated in the composition of the reference solution. Record the retention times of these substances.

System suitability   Reference solution:
— *resolution*: minimum 1.5 between the peaks due to eugenol and acetyleugenol;
— *number of theoretical plates*: minimum 30 000, calculated for the peak due to β-caryophyllene at 110 °C.

Identification of components   Using the retention times determined from the chromatogram obtained with the reference solution, locate the components of the reference solution on the chromatogram obtained with the test solution.

Determine the percentage content of each of these components. The limits are within the following ranges:
— *β-caryophyllene*: 5.0 per cent to 14.0 per cent;
— *eugenol*: 75.0 per cent to 88.0 per cent;
— *acetyleugenol*: 4.0 per cent to 15.0 per cent.

STORAGE

Protected from heat.

Coix Seed

(*Ph Eur monograph 2454*)

Ph Eur ⎯⎯⎯⎯⎯⎯⎯⎯⎯⎯⎯⎯⎯⎯⎯⎯⎯⎯⎯⎯

DEFINITION

Dried, ripe, caryopsis, freed from the shell, of *Coix lacryma-jobi* L. subsp. *ma-yuen* (Rom. Caill.) T.Koyama.

Content
Minimum 0.50 per cent of triolein ($C_{57}H_{104}O_6$; M_r 885) (dried drug).

IDENTIFICATION

A. The white or pale yellow caryopsis freed from the shell is roughly ovoid or elongated-elliptical, about 4-8 mm long and 3-6 mm wide. The dorsal surface is rounded, milky white and smooth; the ventral surface shows a deep longitudinal furrow; yellowish-brown remnants of the membranous floral parts may be present. One end is obtusely rounded, the other end is relatively flat and slightly dented with an indistinct, pale brown hilum.

B. Microscopic examination (*2.8.23*). The powder is light grey or light brown. Examine under a microscope using *chloral hydrate solution R*. The powder shows the following diagnostic characters: fragments of endosperm with polygonal cells arranged in a network; fragments of epicarp with elongated, slightly sinuous cells; cells of the middle layer of the pericarp are yellowish-brown, irregularly tube-like, slightly curved and are irregularly crossed. Examine under a microscope using a 50 per cent *V/V* solution of *glycerol R*. The powder shows very numerous starch granules, simple or 2-3 compound, spherical or slightly polyhedral, 3-20 µm in diameter, with a stellate, Y-shaped, cleft-like or point-like hilum.

C. Thin-layer chromatography (*2.2.27*).

Test solution   To 1 g of the powdered herbal drug (710) (*2.9.12*) add 10 mL of *light petroleum R1* and sonicate for 30 min. Filter and reduce *in vacuo* to 1 mL.

Reference solution   Dissolve 2 mg of *oleic acid R* and 2 mg of *triolein R* in *methanol R* and dilute to 1 mL with the same solvent.

Plate   TLC octadecylsilyl silica gel plate R (5-40 µm) [or TLC octadecylsilyl silica gel plate R (2-10 µm)].

Mobile phase   methylene chloride R, glacial acetic acid R, acetone R (20:40:50 *V/V/V*).

Application   10 µL [or 2 µL] as bands of 10 mm [or 8 mm].

Development   Over a path of 7 cm.

Drying   In air.

Detection   Treat with a 100 g/L solution of *phosphomolybdic acid R* in *ethanol (96 per cent) R*, heat at 120 °C for about 3 min and examine in daylight.

Results   See below the sequence of zones present in the chromatograms obtained with the reference solution and the test solution. Furthermore, other faint zones may be present in the chromatogram obtained with the test solution.

Top of the plate	
	A purple zone
Oleic acid: a purple zone	A purple zone (oleic acid)
———	———
	A faint purple zone
	A purple zone
	A purple zone
———	———
Triolein: a purple zone	A purple zone (triolein)
Reference solution	**Test solution**

TESTS

Loss on drying (*2.2.32*)
Maximum 12.0 per cent, determined on 1.000 g of the powdered herbal drug (710) (*2.9.12*) by drying in an oven at 105 °C for 2 h.

Total ash (*2.4.16*)
Maximum 3.0 per cent.

ASSAY

Liquid chromatography (*2.2.29*).

Test solution   To 0.600 g of the powdered herbal drug (355) (*2.9.12*) add 50 mL of the mobile phase and stir with a magnetic stirrer for 2 h. Sonicate for 30 min. Allow to cool, dilute to 50.0 mL with the mobile phase and filter.

Reference solution (a)   Dissolve 10.0 mg of *triolein CRS* in the mobile phase and dilute to 50.0 mL with the mobile phase.

Reference solution (b)   To 0.600 g of *coix seed HRS* add 50 mL of the mobile phase and stir with a magnetic stirrer for 2 h. Sonicate for 30 min. Allow to cool, dilute to 50.0 mL with the mobile phase and filter.

Reference solutions (c), (d), (e), (f), (g), (h)   Dilute reference solution (a) to obtain 6 reference solutions of triolein, the concentrations of which span the expected value in the test solution.

Column:
— *size*: $l = 0.25$ m, $\varnothing = 4.6$ mm;
— *stationary phase*: end-capped octadecylsilyl silica gel for chromatography R (5 μm).

Mobile phase   methylene chloride R, acetonitrile R (35:65 *V/V*).

Flow rate   2.0 mL/min.

Detection   Evaporative light-scattering detector; the following settings have been found to be suitable; if the detector has different setting parameters, adjust the detector settings so as to comply with the system suitability criterion for signal-to-noise ratio:
— *carrier gas*: nitrogen R;
— *flow rate*: 0.8 mL/min;
— *evaporator temperature*: 100 °C.

Injection   10 μL.

Run time   35 min.

Retention time   Triolein = about 18 min.

System suitability:
— *resolution*: minimum 1.5 between the peak due to triolein and peak 2 in the chromatogram obtained with reference

solution (b); use the chromatogram supplied with *coix seed HRS* to identify peak 2;
— *signal-to-noise ratio*: minimum 30 for the peak due to triolein in the chromatogram obtained with reference solution (a).

Establish a calibration curve with the logarithm of the mass of triolein (in milligrams) per 50 mL of reference solutions (c), (d), (e), (f), (g) and (h) (corrected by the assigned percentage content of *triolein CRS*) as the abscissa and the logarithm of the corresponding peak area as the ordinate.

Calculate the percentage content of triolein using the following expression:

$$\frac{10^{A}}{m \times 10}$$

A = logarithm of the mass of triolein in the test solution, determined from the calibration curve and the area of the corresponding peak in the chromatogram obtained with the test solution;

m = mass of the herbal drug to be examined used to prepare the test solution, in grams.

Ph Eur

Cola

(*Ph Eur monograph 1504*)

Ph Eur

DEFINITION

Whole or fragmented dried seeds, freed from the testa, of *Cola nitida* (Vent.) Schott et Endl. (*C. vera* K. Schum.) and its varieties, as well as of *Cola acuminata* (P. Beauv.) Schott et Endl. (*Sterculia acuminata* P. Beauv.).

Content
Minimum 1.5 per cent of caffeine (M_r 194.2) (dried drug).

IDENTIFICATION

A. The kernels have an oblong, somewhat obtuse, sub-tetragonal shape, with deformations resulting from mutual pressure inside the fruit; they vary in size and mass, ranging from 5-15 g; the outside is hard, smooth and very dark brown, the inside is more reddish-brown. In C. *nitida* and its varieties, the kernels are divided in 2 parts, almost plano-convex, corresponding to the cotyledons and usually occurring separated in the commercial drug; the cotyledons are 3-4 cm long, 2-2.5 cm wide and 1-2 cm thick. In C. *acuminata*, the cotyledons are smaller and divided into 4-6 irregular parts.

B. Reduce to a powder (355) (*2.9.12*). The powder is reddish-brown. Examine under a microscope using a 50 per cent *V/V* solution of *glycerol R*. The powder shows the following diagnostic characters: numerous ovoid or reniform starch granules, 5-25 μm in size, with concentric striations and a stellate, slightly eccentric hilum; fragments of cotyledon tissue showing large, thick-walled, reddish polygonal cells filled with starch granules; occasional fragments of the external epidermis of the cotyledons.

C. Thin-layer chromatography (*2.2.27*).

Test solution   To 1.0 g of the powdered drug (355) (*2.9.12*) add 5 mL of *ethanol (60 per cent V/V) R*. Shake mechanically at 40 °C for 30 min and filter.

Reference solution (a) Dissolve 25 mg of *caffeine R* in 10 mL of *ethanol (60 per cent V/V) R*.

Reference solution (b) Dissolve 50 mg of *theobromine R* in 10 mL of the mobile phase. Filter.

Plate TLC *silica gel F$_{254}$ plate R*.

Mobile phase *water R, methanol R, ethyl acetate R* (10:13:77 *V/V/V*).

Application 20 µL, as bands.

Development Over a path of 10 cm.

Drying In air for 5 min.

Detection A Examine in ultraviolet light at 254 nm.

Results A The chromatogram obtained with the test solution shows 2 principal quenching zones which are similar in position to the zones in the chromatograms obtained with reference solutions (a) and (b).

Detection B Spray with a mixture of equal volumes of *ethanol (96 per cent) R* and *hydrochloric acid R* and then with a solution prepared immediately before use by dissolving 1 g of *iodine R* and 1 g of *potassium iodide R* in 100 mL of *ethanol (96 per cent) R*.

Results B The chromatogram obtained with the test solution shows a reddish-brown principal zone similar in position and colour to the zone in the chromatogram obtained with reference solution (a).

TESTS

Loss on drying *(2.2.32)*
Maximum 12.0 per cent, determined on 2.00 g of the powdered drug (355) *(2.9.12)* by drying in an oven at 105 °C for 2 h.

Total ash *(2.4.16)*
Maximum 9.0 per cent.

ASSAY

Liquid chromatography *(2.2.29)*.

Test solution To 1.00 g (m_1) of the powdered drug (355) *(2.9.12)*, add 50 mL of *methanol R*. Heat under a reflux condenser on a water-bath for 30 min. Allow to cool and filter. Rinse the filter with 10 mL of *methanol R*. Take up the residue with 50 mL of *methanol R*. Proceed as before. Combine the filtrates and the washings in a 200.0 mL volumetric flask and dilute to 200.0 mL with *methanol R*. Transfer 20.0 mL of this solution into a round-bottomed flask and evaporate to dryness under reduced pressure. Take up the residue with the mobile phase, transfer to a 50.0 mL volumetric flask and dilute to 50.0 mL with the mobile phase.

Reference solution In a 100.0 mL volumetric flask, dissolve 30.0 mg (m_2) of *caffeine CRS* and 15.0 mg of *theobromine R* in the mobile phase and dilute to 100.0 mL with the mobile phase. Transfer 10.0 mL of this solution to a 100.0 mL volumetric flask and dilute to 100.0 mL with the mobile phase.

Column:
— *size*: $l = 0.25$ m, $\emptyset = 4.6$ mm;
— *stationary phase*: *octadecylsilyl silica gel for chromatography R* (5 µm).

Mobile phase *methanol R, water R* (25:75 *V/V*).

Flow rate 1 mL/min.

Detection Spectrophotometer at 272 nm.

Injection The chosen volume of each solution; loop injector.

System suitability Reference solution:

— *resolution*: minimum 2.5 between the peaks due to caffeine and theobromine. If necessary, adjust the volume of *water R* in the mobile phase.

Calculate the caffeine content using the following expression:

$$\frac{m_2 \times A_1 \times 50}{m_1 \times A_2}$$

A_1 = area of the peak due to caffeine in the chromatogram obtained with the test solution,

A_2 = area of the peak due to caffeine in the chromatogram obtained with the reference solution,

m_1 = mass of the drug to be examined in the test solution, in grams,

m_2 = mass of *caffeine CRS* in the reference solution, in grams.

———————————————————————— *Ph Eur*

Colophony

(Ph Eur monograph 1862)

Preparation
Flexible Collodion

Ph Eur ————————————————————————

DEFINITION

Residue remaining after distillation of the volatile oil from the oleoresin obtained from various species of *Pinus*.

IDENTIFICATION

A. Translucent, pale yellow to brownish-yellow, angular, irregularly-shaped, brittle, glassy pieces of different sizes the surfaces of which bear conchoidal markings.

B. Thin-layer chromatography *(2.2.27)*.

Test solution Dissolve 1 g in 10 mL of *methanol R* by gently warming.

Reference solution Dissolve 10 mg of *thymol R* and 10 mg of *linalol R* in 10 mL of *methanol R*.

Plate TLC *silica gel plate R*.

Mobile phase *methylene chloride R*.

Application 10 µL, as bands.

Development Over a path of 15 cm.

Drying In air.

Detection Spray with *anisaldehyde solution R* and heat at 100-105 °C for 10 min; examine in daylight.

Top of the plate		
		A purple band
		A purple band
—		—
		2 purple bands
Thymol: an orange band		
—		—
Linalol: a purple band		Sequence of narrow purple bands
		Purple extended baseline band
Reference solution		**Test solution**

Results See below the sequence of the zones present in the chromatograms obtained with the reference solution and the test solution. Furthermore, other coloured zones are present in the chromatogram obtained with the test solution.

TESTS

Acid value (*2.5.1*)
145 to 180, determined on 1.0 g.

Total ash (*2.4.16*)
Maximum 0.2 per cent.

STORAGE

Do not reduce to a powder.

———————————————————————— Ph Eur

Coriander

(*Ph Eur monograph 1304*)

When Powdered Coriander is prescribed or demanded, material complying with the appropriate requirements below but containing not less than 0.2% v/w of essential oil shall be dispensed or supplied.

Ph Eur _____

DEFINITION

Dried cremocarp of *Coriandrum sativum* L.

Content
Minimum 3 mL/kg of essential oil (dried drug).

IDENTIFICATION

A. The fruit is brown or light brown, more or less spherical, about 1.5-5 mm in diameter, or oval and 2-6 mm long.
It consists of the entire cremocarp, with the mericarps usually tightly connected. The fruit is glabrous and has 10 wavy, slightly raised primary ridges and 8 straight, more prominent secondary ridges. The mericarps are concave on the internal surface. The stylopod crowns the apex and a small fragment of the pedicel may be present.

B. Microscopic examination (*2.8.23*). The powder is brown. Examine under a microscope using *chloral hydrate solution R*. The powder shows the following diagnostic characters (Figure 1304.-1): numerous oil droplets [B]; fragments of endosperm [A] with small, thick-walled, regular cells containing microrosettes [Aa] and microcrystals of calcium oxalate and oil droplets [Ab]; fragments of endocarp, in surface view [C, J] or in transverse section [H], with very narrow cells having a parquetry arrangement [Ca, Ha] and usually associated with a layer of thin-walled [Cb, Hb] or thicker-walled [Ja] rectangular sclereids of the mesocarp; fragments from the sclerenchymatous layer of the mesocarp [G] with short, strongly thickened, pitted, fusiform cells occurring in layers with the cells of adjacent layers approximately at right angles to one another; fragments of parenchyma of the mesocarp in transverse section [E] with small cells with slightly thickened walls [Ea], the remains of secretory canals [Eb] and sclereids [Ec]; fragments of epicarp, in surface view [F], with thin-walled polyhedral cells, some of which contain small prisms of calcium oxalate [Fa]; rare fragments of secretory canals with brown cells, in surface view [D]; occasional fragments of vascular bundles [K].

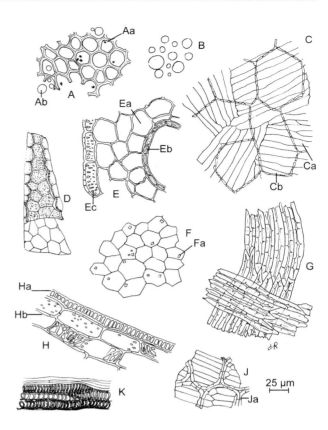

Figure 1304.-1. – *Illustration for identification test B of powdered herbal drug of coriander*

C. Thin-layer chromatography (*2.2.27*).

Test solution Shake 0.5 g of the freshly powdered herbal drug (355) (*2.9.12*) with 5 mL of *hexane R* for 2-3 min and filter over 2 g of *anhydrous sodium sulfate R*.

Reference solution Dissolve 15 µL of *linalol R* and 25 µL of *olive oil R* in 5 mL of *hexane R* immediately before use.

Plate TLC silica gel plate R.

Mobile phase ethyl acetate R, toluene R (5:95 *V/V*).

Application 20 µL of the test solution and 10 µL of the reference solution, as bands.

Development Twice over a path of 10 cm.

Drying In air.

Detection Spray with *anisaldehyde solution R* and examine in daylight while heating at 100-105 °C for 5-10 min.

Results The chromatogram obtained with the reference solution shows in the lower half a violet or greyish-violet zone (linalol) and in the upper half a bluish-violet zone (triglycerides); the chromatogram obtained with the test solution shows zones similar in position and colour to the zones in the chromatogram obtained with the reference solution; several violet-grey or brownish zones, including the zone due to geraniol, are shown between the point of application and the zone due to linalol in the chromatogram obtained with the reference solution; several faint violet-grey zones may also be shown between the zone due to triglycerides and that due to linalol in the chromatogram obtained with the reference solution.

TESTS

Foreign matter (*2.8.2*)
It complies with the test. None of the cremocarps show perforations due to insects.

Loss on drying (2.2.32)

Maximum 10.0 per cent, determined on 1.000 g of the powdered herbal drug (355) (2.9.12) by drying in an oven at 105 °C for 2 h.

Total ash (2.4.16)

Maximum 8.0 per cent.

ASSAY

Carry out the determination of essential oils in herbal drugs (2.8.12). Use a 500 mL round-bottomed flask, 200 mL of *water R* as the distillation liquid and 0.5 mL of *xylene R* in the graduated tube. Reduce the drug to a coarse powder and immediately use 30.0 g for the determination. Distil at a rate of 2-3 mL/min for 2 h.

———————————————————— *Ph Eur*

Coriander Oil

(*Ph Eur monograph 1820*)

Ph Eur ————————————————————————

DEFINITION

Essential oil obtained by steam distillation from the fruits of *Coriandrum sativum* L.

CHARACTERS

Appearance

Clear, colourless or pale yellow liquid.

Characteristic spicy odour.

IDENTIFICATION

First identification   B.

Second identification   A.

A. Examine by thin-layer chromatography (2.2.27).

Test solution   Dissolve 10 µL of the substance to be examined in 1.0 mL of *toluene R*.

Reference solution   Dissolve 10 µL *linalol R* and 2 µL of *geranyl acetate R* in 1.0 mL of *toluene R*.

Plate   TLC silica gel plate R.

Mobile phase   ethyl acetate R, toluene R (5:95 V/V).

Application   10 µL as bands.

Development   Over a path of 10 cm.

Drying   In air.

Detection   Spray with *anisaldehyde solution R* and heat at 100-105 °C for 10-15 min. Examine immediately in daylight.

Results   See below the sequence of the zones present in the chromatograms obtained with the reference solution and the test solution.

Top of the plate	
Geranyl acetate: a violet-blue zone	A violet-blue zone (geranyl acetate)
Linalol: an intense violet zone	An intense violet zone (linalol)
	A violet-blue zone (geraniol)
Reference solution	**Test solution**

B. Examine the chromatograms obtained in the test for chromatographic profile.

Results   The characteristic peaks in the chromatogram obtained with the test solution are similar in retention time to those in the chromatogram obtained with the reference solution.

TESTS

Relative density (2.2.5)

0.860 to 0.880.

Refractive index (2.2.6)

1.462 to 1.470.

Optical rotation (2.2.7)

+ 7° to + 13°.

Acid value (2.5.1)

Maximum 3.0, determined on 5.00 g of the substance to be examined.

Chromatographic profile

Gas chromatography (2.2.28): use the normalisation procedure.

Test solution   The substance to be examined.

Reference solution (a)   Dissolve 10 µL of α-pinene R, 10 µL of limonene R, 10 µL of γ-terpinene R, 10 µL of p-cymene R, 10 mg of camphor R, 20 µL of linalol R, 10 µL of α-terpineol R, 10 µL of geranyl acetate R and 10 µL of geraniol R in 1 mL of hexane R.

Reference solution (b)   Dissolve 5 µL of geraniol R in hexane R and dilute to 10 mL with the same solvent.

Column:

— *material*: fused silica,

— *size*: l = 60 m, Ø = 0.25 mm,

— *stationary phase*: macrogol 20 000 R (film thickness 0.25 µm).

Carrier gas   helium for chromatography R.

Flow rate   1 mL/min.

Split ratio   1:65.

Temperature:

	Time (min)	Temperature (°C)
Column	0 - 10	60
	10 - 75	60 → 190
	75 - 120	190
Injection port		220
Detector		240

Detection   Flame ionisation.

Injection   0.2 µL.

Elution order   Order indicated in the composition of reference solution (a). Record the retention times of these substances.

System suitability   Reference solution (a):

— *resolution*: minimum 1.5 between the peaks due to linalol and camphor.

Using the retention times determined from the chromatogram obtained with reference solution (a), locate the components of reference solution (a) in the chromatogram obtained with the test solution.

Determine the percentage content of each of these components. The percentages are within the following ranges:

— *α-pinene*: 3.0 per cent to 7.0 per cent,

— *limonene*: 1.5 per cent to 5.0 per cent,

— *γ-terpinene*: 1.5 per cent to 8.0 per cent,

— *p-cymene*: 0.5 per cent to 4.0 per cent,

— *camphor*: 3.0 per cent to 6.0 per cent,

— *linalol*: 65.0 per cent to 78.0 per cent,
— *α-terpineol*: 0.1 per cent to 1.5 per cent,
— *geranyl acetate*: 0.5 per cent to 4.0 per cent,
— *geraniol*: 0.5 per cent to 3.0 per cent,
— *disregard limit*: area of the peak in the chromatogram obtained with reference solution (b) (0.05 per cent).

Chiral purity

Gas chromatography (*2.2.28*).

Test solution   Dissolve 0.02 g of the substance to be examined in *pentane R* and dilute to 10 mL with the same solvent.

Reference solution   Dissolve 10 µL of *linalol R* and 5 mg of *borneol R* in *pentane R* and dilute to 10 mL with the same solvent.

Column:
— *material*: fused silica,
— *size*: *l* = 25 m, Ø = 0.25 mm,
— *stationary phase*: *modified β-cyclodextrin for chiral chromatography R* (film thickness 0.25 µm).

Carrier gas   *helium for chromatography R*.

Flow rate   1.3 mL/min.

Split ratio   1:30.

Temperature:

	Time (min)	Temperature (°C)
Column	0 - 65	50 → 180
Injection port		230
Detector		230

Detection   Flame ionisation.

Injection   1 µL.

System suitability   Reference solution:
— *resolution*: minimum 5.5 between the peaks due to (*R*)-linalol (1st peak) and (*S*)-linalol (2nd peak) and minimum 2.9 between the peaks due to (*S*)-linalol and borneol (3rd peak).

Limit   Calculate the percentage content of (*R*)-linalol from the expression:

$$\frac{A_R}{A_S + A_R} \times 100$$

A_S = area of the peak due to (*S*)-linalol,
A_R = area of the peak due to (*R*)-linalol.

— (*R*)-*linalol*: maximum 14 per cent.

STORAGE

At a temperature not exceeding 25 °C.

_____ *Ph Eur*

Couch Grass Rhizome

(*Ph Eur monograph 1306*)

Ph Eur _____

DEFINITION

Whole or cut, washed and dried rhizome of *Agropyron repens* (L.) P.Beauv. (*Elymus repens* (L.) Gould); the adventitious roots are removed.

IDENTIFICATION

A. The shiny yellowish, light brown or yellowish-brown pieces of the rhizome are 2-3 mm thick and longitudinally furrowed. At the nodes are the remains of very thin, more or less branched roots and whitish or brownish scale-like leaves; the internodes, up to 6 cm long, are furrowed and hollow inside. The transverse section of the nodes shows a yellowish medulla.

B. Microscopic examination (*2.8.23*). The powder is whitish-yellow. Examine under a microscope using *chloral hydrate solution R*. The powder shows the following diagnostic characters (Figure 1306.-1): fragments of the epidermis in surface view [A] covered with a thick cuticle and composed of rectangular and elongated, thick-walled cells with pitted, slightly wavy walls, which usually alternate with small, thin-walled, rounded or almost square twin cells; fragments in transverse section [B] showing the epidermis [Ba] associated with thick-walled cells of the hypodermis; fragments in transverse section [F] consisting of endodermic cells with U-shaped thickening of the walls [Fa] accompanied by pericyclic fibres [Fb]; numerous fragments of moderately thickened fibres [C]; groups of vessels [D, G] with slit-shaped pits [Da] or with spiral and annular thickening [Ga], accompanied by fibres [Db, Gb]; numerous fragments of the

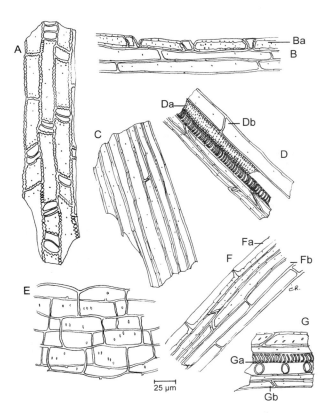

Figure 1306.-1. – *Illustration for identification test B of powdered herbal drug of couch grass rhizome*

cortical parenchyma and the pith with slightly thickened and pitted cells [E].

TESTS

Cynodon dactylon, Imperata cylindrical
Examine under a microscope using *iodine solution R1*.
No blue starch grains are visible.

Foreign matter (*2.8.2*)
Maximum 15 per cent of blackish-grey pieces of rhizome in the cut herbal drug.

Water-soluble extractive
Minimum 25 per cent.

To 5.0 g of the powdered herbal drug (355) (*2.9.12*) add 200 mL of boiling *water R*. Allow to stand for 10 min, shaking occasionally. Allow to cool, dilute to 200.0 mL with *water R* and filter. Evaporate 20.0 mL of the filtrate to dryness on a water-bath. Dry the residue in an oven at 100-105 °C. The residue weighs a minimum of 0.125 g.

Loss on drying (*2.2.32*)
Maximum 12.0 per cent, determined on 1.000 g of the powdered herbal drug (355) (*2.9.12*) by drying in an oven at 105 °C for 2 h.

Total ash (*2.4.16*)
Maximum 5.0 per cent.

Ash insoluble in hydrochloric acid (*2.8.1*)
Maximum 1.5 per cent.

———————————————————— *Ph Eur*

Dandelion Herb with Root

(*Ph Eur monograph 1851*)

Ph Eur ————————————————————

DEFINITION
Mixture of whole or fragmented, dried aerial and underground parts of *Taraxacum officinale* F.H. Wigg.

CHARACTERS
Bitter taste.

IDENTIFICATION
A. The underground parts consist of dark brown or blackish fragments 2-3 cm long, deeply wrinkled longitudinally on the outer surface. The thickened crown shows many scars left by the rosette of leaves. The fracture is short. A transverse section shows a greyish-white or brownish cortex containing concentric layers of brownish laticiferous vessels and a porous, pale yellow, non-radiate wood. Leaf fragments are green, glabrous or densely pilose. They are crumpled and usually show a clearly visible midrib on the inner surface. The lamina, with deeply dentate margins, is crumpled. The solitary flower heads, on hollow stems, consist of an involucre of green, foliaceous bracts surrounding the yellow florets, all of which are ligulate; a few achenes bearing a white, silky, outspread pappus may be present.

B. Microscopic examination (*2.8.23*). The powder is yellowish-brown. Examine under a microscope using *chloral hydrate solution R*. The powder shows the following diagnostic characters (Figure 1851.-1): fragments of cork [G] with flattened, thin-walled cells; reticulate lignified vessels [H] from the roots; fragments of parenchyma containing branched laticiferous vessels [F]; fragments of leaves, in surface view, showing upper (E) and lower [C] epidermises consisting of interlocking lobed cells and anomocytic stomata

(*2.8.3*) [Ca, Ea]; elongated, multicellular covering trichomes with constrictions, which are more or less abundant depending on the variety or sub-variety [B, D]; fragments of the upper (E) epidermis usually accompanied by underlying palisade parenchyma [Eb] and fragments of the lower (C) epidermis accompanied by underlying spongy parenchyma [Cb]; lignified, spirally or annularly thickened vessels; fragments of flower-stem epidermis with stomata and rigid-walled, elongated cells [A]; pollen grains with a pitted exine [J]. Examine under a microscope using *glycerol R*.
The powder shows angular, irregular inulin fragments, free or included in the parenchyma cells.

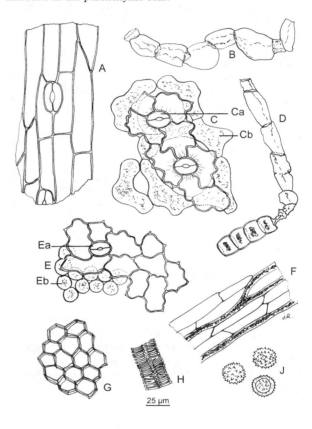

Figure 1851.-1 – *Illustration for identification test B of powdered herbal drug of dandelion herb with root*

C. Thin-layer chromatography (*2.2.27*).

Test solution To 2.0 g of the powdered herbal drug (355) (*2.9.12*) add 10 mL of *methanol R*. Heat in a water-bath at 60 °C or sonicate for 10 min. Cool and filter.

Reference solution Dissolve 2 mg of *chlorogenic acid R* and 2 mg of *rutin R* in *methanol R* and dilute to 20 mL with the same solvent.

Plate TLC silica gel plate R (5-40 μm) [or TLC silica gel plate R (2-10 μm)].

Mobile phase anhydrous formic acid R, water R, ethyl acetate R (10:10:80 *V/V/V*).

Application 20 μL [or 5 μL] as bands of 10 mm [or 8 mm].

Development Over a path of 12 cm [or 7 cm].

Drying In air.

Detection Heat at 100 °C for 5 min; spray with or dip briefly into a 10 g/L solution of *diphenylboric acid aminoethyl ester R* in *methanol R* and dry at 100 °C for 5 min; spray with or dip briefly into a 50 g/L solution of *macrogol 400 R* in methanol R; heat at 100 °C for 5 min and examine in ultraviolet light at 365 nm.

Results   See below the sequence of zones present in the chromatograms obtained with the reference solution and the test solution. Furthermore, other faint zones may be present in the chromatogram obtained with the test solution.

Top of the plate	
	A faint red zone
	A faint yellow zone
Chlorogenic acid: a blue zone	2 light blue zones
Rutin: a yellowish-brown zone	
	A light blue zone
Reference solution	**Test solution**

TESTS

Loss on drying (*2.2.32*)
Maximum 10.0 per cent, determined on 1.000 g of the powdered herbal drug (355) (*2.9.12*) by drying in an oven at 105 °C for 2 h.

Total ash (*2.4.16*)
Maximum 17.0 per cent.

Ash insoluble in hydrochloric acid (*2.8.1*)
Maximum 5.0 per cent.

Extractable matter
Minimum 30.0 per cent.

To 2.000 g of the powdered herbal drug (250) (*2.9.12*) add 40 g of *water R*. Stir for 1 h and filter. Evaporate 10 g of the filtrate to dryness on a water-bath and dry in an oven at 100-105 °C for 2 h. The residue weighs a minimum of 0.15 g.

Bitterness value (*2.8.15*)
Minimum 100.

———————————————————————— *Ph Eur*

Dandelion Root

(*Ph Eur monograph 1852*)

Ph Eur ——————————————————————————

DEFINITION

Whole or cut, dried underground parts of *Taraxacum officinale* F.H.Wigg.

CHARACTERS

Bitter taste.

IDENTIFICATION

A. The dark brown or blackish taproot shows little branching and is deeply wrinkled longitudinally on the outer surface. The thickened crown shows many scars left by the rosette of leaves. The fracture is short. A transverse section shows a greyish-white or brownish cortex containing concentric layers of brownish laticiferous vessels and a porous, pale yellow, non-radiate wood.

B. Reduce to a powder (355) (*2.9.12*). The powder is yellowish-brown. Examine under a microscope using *chloral*

hydrate solution R. The powder shows the following diagnostic characters (Figure 1852.-1): fragments of brown or reddish-brown cork, in surface view [G] and transverse section [C] with flattened, thin-walled cells [Ca], sometimes accompanied by parenchyma [Cb]; reticulate lignified vessels [E, J, M]; fragments of parenchyma [A, D, K, L], some containing branched laticiferous vessels, in longitudinal section [Ka] and transverse section [Da]; granular contents of laticiferous vessels [B, H]. Examine under a microscope using *glycerol R*. The powder shows numerous irregular, angular inulin fragments, free [F] or included in the parenchyma cells [La].

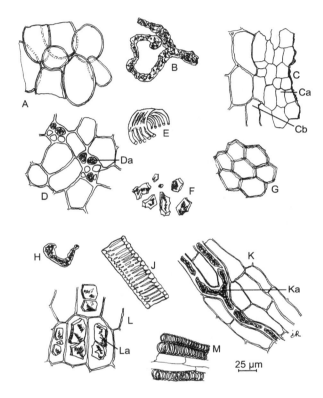

Figure 1852.-1.– Illustration for identification test B of powdered herbal drug of dandelion root

C. Thin-layer chromatography (*2.2.27*).

Test solution   To 2.0 g of the powdered herbal drug (355) (*2.9.12*) add 10 mL of *methanol R*. Heat in a water-bath at 60 °C or sonicate for 10 min. Cool and filter.

Reference solution   Dissolve 2 mg of *chlorogenic acid R* and 2 mg of *rutin R* in *methanol R* and dilute to 20 mL with the same solvent.

Plate   TLC silica gel F_{254} plate R (5-40 µm) [or *TLC silica gel* F_{254} *plate R* (2-10 µm)].

Mobile phase   anhydrous formic acid R, water R, ethyl acetate R (10:10:80 *V/V/V*).

Application   20 µL [or 5 µL] as bands of 10 mm [or 8 mm].

Development   Over a path of 12 cm [or 7 cm].

Drying   In air.

Detection   Heat at 100 °C for 5 min; spray with or dip briefly into a 10 g/L solution of *diphenylboric acid aminoethyl ester R* in *methanol R* and dry at 100 °C for 5 min; spray with or dip briefly into a 50 g/L solution of *macrogol 400 R* in *methanol R*; heat at 100 °C for 5 min and examine in ultraviolet light at 365 nm.

Results See below the sequence of zones present in the chromatograms obtained with the reference solution and the test solution. Furthermore, other faint zones may be present in the chromatogram obtained with the test solution.

Top of the plate	
	A light blue zone
———	———
Chlorogenic acid: a blue zone	A blue zone (chlorogenic acid)
———	———
Rutin: a yellowish-brown zone	
Reference solution	**Test solution**

TESTS

Loss on drying (*2.2.32*)
Maximum 10.0 per cent, determined on 1.000 g of the powdered drug (355) (*2.9.12*) by drying in an oven at 105 °C for 2 h.

Total ash (*2.4.16*)
Maximum 10.0 per cent.

Ash insoluble in hydrochloric acid (*2.8.1*)
Maximum 3.0 per cent.

Extractable matter
Minimum 20.0 per cent.

To 2.000 g of the powdered herbal drug (250) (*2.9.12*) add 40 g of *water R*. Stir for 1 h and filter. Evaporate 10 g of the filtrate to dryness on a water-bath and dry in an oven at 100-105 °C for 2 h. The residue weighs a minimum of 0.10 g.

Bitterness value (*2.8.15*)
Minimum 100.

——— Ph Eur

Devil's Claw

Harpagophytum

(*Devil's Claw Root, Ph Eur monograph 1095*)

Preparation
Devil's Claw Dry Extract

Ph Eur ———

DEFINITION

Cut and dried, tuberous secondary roots of *Harpagophytum procumbens* DC. and/or *Harpagophytum zeyheri* Decne.

Content

Minimum 1.2 per cent of harpagoside ($C_{24}H_{30}O_{11}$; M_r 494.5) (dried drug).

CHARACTERS

The root is greyish-brown or dark brown.

IDENTIFICATION

A. It consists of thick, fan-shaped or rounded slices or of roughly crushed discs. The darker outer surface is traversed by tortuous longitudinal wrinkles. The paler cut surface shows a dark cambial zone and xylem bundles distinctly aligned in radial rows. The central cylinder shows fine concentric striations. Seen under a lens, the cut surface presents yellow or brownish-red granules.

B. Reduce to a powder (355) (*2.9.12*). The powder is brownish-yellow. Examine under a microscope using *chloral hydrate solution R*. The powder shows the following diagnostic characters (Figure 1095.-1): fragments of cork consisting of yellowish-brown, thin-walled cells, in surface view [B] and in transverse section [C]; fragments of cortical parenchyma consisting of large, thin-walled cells [E, K, N, P], sometimes containing reddish-brown granular inclusions and isolated yellow droplets (P); fragments of reticulately thickened or pitted vessels [D, F, G, M] and fragments of lignified parenchyma [L], sometimes associated with vessels, from the central cylinder; prism crystals [A] and rare small needles of calcium oxalate in the parenchyma. The powder may also show rectangular or polygonal sclereids with dark reddish-brown contents [H, J]. With a solution of phloroglucinol in hydrochloric acid, the parenchyma turns green.

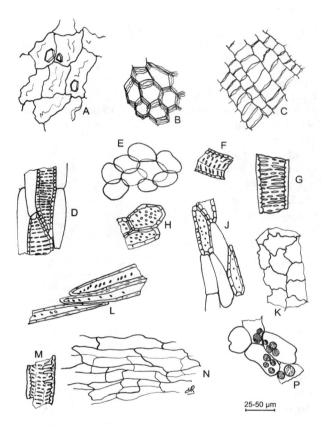

Figure 1095.-1.– *Illustration for identification test B of powdered herbal drug of devil's claw root*

C. Thin-layer chromatography (*2.2.27*).

Test solution Heat 1.0 g of the powdered drug (355) (*2.9.12*) with 10 mL of *methanol R* on a water-bath at 60 °C for 10 min. Filter and reduce the filtrate to about 2 mL under reduced pressure at a temperature not exceeding 40 °C.

Reference solution Dissolve 1 mg of *harpagoside R* and 2.5 mg of *fructose R* in 1 mL of *methanol R*.

Plate TLC silica gel plate R (5-40 µm) [or *TLC silica gel plate R* (2-10 µm)].

Mobile phase water R, methanol R, ethyl acetate R (8:15:77 *V/V/V*).

Application 20 µL [or 5 µL] as bands.

Development Over a path of 10 cm [or 7.5 cm].

Drying   In a current of warm air.

Detection A   Examine in ultraviolet light at 254 nm.

Results A   See below the sequence of zones present in the chromatograms obtained with the reference solution and the test solution; the chromatogram obtained with the test solution shows other distinct zones, mainly above the zone due to harpagoside. Furthermore, other faint zones may be present in the chromatogram obtained with the test solution.

Top of the plate	
Harpagoside: a quenching zone	A quenching zone: harpagoside
———	———
Reference solution	**Test solution**

Detection B   Spray with a 10 g/L solution of *phloroglucinol R* in *ethanol (96 per cent) R* and then with *hydrochloric acid R*; heat at 80 °C for 5-10 min and examine in daylight.

Results B   See below the sequence of zones present in the chromatograms obtained with the reference solution and the test solution; the chromatogram obtained with the test solution also shows several yellow or brown zones above the zone due to harpagoside. Furthermore, other faint zones may be present in the chromatogram obtained with the test solution.

Top of the plate	
———	———
Harpagoside: a green zone	A green zone (harpagoside)
———	———
	A yellow zone
	A light green zone
Fructose: a yellowish-grey zone	A yellowish-grey zone may be present (fructose)
	A brown zone
Reference solution	**Test solution**

TESTS

Starch

Examine the powdered drug (355) *(2.9.12)* under a microscope using *water R*. Add *iodine solution R1*. No blue colour develops.

Loss on drying *(2.2.32)*

Maximum 12.0 per cent, determined on 1.000 g of the powdered drug (355) *(2.9.12)* by drying in an oven at 105 °C.

Total ash *(2.4.16)*

Maximum 10.0 per cent.

ASSAY

Liquid chromatography *(2.2.29)*.

Test solution   To 0.500 g of the powdered drug (355) *(2.9.12)* add 100.0 mL of *methanol R*. Shake for 4 h and filter through a membrane filter (nominal pore size 0.45 µm).

Reference solution   Dissolve the contents of a vial of *harpagoside CRS* in *methanol R* and dilute to 10.0 mL with the same solvent.

Column:

— *size*: l = 0.10 m, Ø = 4.0 mm;

— *stationary phase*: octadecylsilyl silica gel for chromatography *R* (5 µm).

Mobile phase   methanol *R*, water *R* (50:50 *V/V*).

Flow rate   1.5 mL/min.

Detection   Spectrophotometer at 278 nm.

Injection   10 µL.

Run time   3 times the retention time of harpagoside.

Retention time   Harpagoside = about 7 min.

Calculate the percentage content of harpagoside using the following expression:

$$\frac{m_2 \times A_1 \times 1000}{A_2 \times m_1}$$

A_1 = area of the peak due to harpagoside in the chromatogram obtained with the test solution;

A_2 = area of the peak due to harpagoside in the chromatogram obtained with the reference solution;

m_1 = mass of the drug to be examined used to prepare the test solution, in grams;

m_2 = mass of *harpagoside CRS* in the reference solution, in grams.

————————————— Ph Eur

Devil's Claw Dry Extract

(Ph Eur monograph 1871)

Ph Eur ————————————————————

DEFINITION

Dry extract obtained from *Devil's claw root (1095)*.

Content

Minimum 1.5 per cent of harpagoside ($C_{24}H_{30}O_{11}$; M_r 494.5) (dried extract).

PRODUCTION

The extract is produced from the herbal drug by an appropriate procedure using either water or a hydroalcoholic solvent that is at most equivalent in strength to ethanol (95 per cent *V/V*).

CHARACTERS

Appearance

Light brown powder.

IDENTIFICATION

Thin-layer chromatography *(2.2.27)*.

Test solution   To 1.0 g of the extract to be examined add 10 mL of *methanol R* and heat in a water-bath at 60 °C for 10 min. Cool and filter.

Reference solution   Dissolve 1.0 mg of *harpagoside R* and 2.5 mg of *fructose R* in 1.0 mL of *methanol R*.

Plate   TLC silica gel plate *R*.

Mobile phase   water *R*, methanol *R*, ethyl acetate *R* (8:15:77 *V/V/V*).

Application   20 µL as bands.

Development   Over a path of 10 cm.

Drying   In a current of warm air.

Detection   Spray with a 10 g/L solution of *phloroglucinol R* in *ethanol (96 per cent) R* and then with *hydrochloric acid R*; heat at 80 °C for 5-10 min and examine in daylight.

Results See below the sequence of zones present in the chromatograms obtained with the reference solution and the test solution. Furthermore, other faint zones may be present in the chromatogram obtained with the test solution.

Top of the plate	
Harpagoside: a green zone	A green zone (harpagoside)
	A yellow zone
	A light green zone
Fructose: a yellowish-grey zone	A yellowish-grey zone may be present (fructose)
	A brown zone
Reference solution	**Test solution**

ASSAY

Liquid chromatography (*2.2.29*).

Test solution Introduce 0.350 g of the extract to be examined into a 100 mL volumetric flask, add 90 mL of *methanol R* and sonicate for 20 min. Cool to room temperature, dilute to 100.0 mL with *methanol R* and filter through a membrane filter (nominal pore size 0.2 μm).

Reference solution Dissolve the contents of 1 vial of *harpagoside CRS* in *methanol R* and dilute to 10.0 mL with the same solvent.

Column:
— *size: l* = 0.10 m, Ø = 4.0 mm;
— *stationary phase: octadecylsilyl silica gel for chromatography R* (5 μm).

Mobile phase *methanol R, water R* (50:50 *V/V*).

Flow rate 1.5 mL/min.

Detection Spectrophotometer at 278 nm.

Injection 10 μL.

Run time 3 times the retention time of harpagoside.

Retention time Harpagoside = about 7 min.

Calculate the percentage content of harpagoside using the following expression:

$$\frac{A_1 \times m_2 \times 1000}{A_2 \times m_1}$$

A_1 = area of the peak due to harpagoside in the chromatogram obtained with the test solution;

A_2 = area of the peak due to harpagoside in the chromatogram obtained with the reference solution;

m_1 = mass of the extract to be examined used to prepare the test solution, in grams;

m_2 = mass of harpagoside contained in 1 vial of *harpagoside CRS*, in grams.

_____ *Ph Eur*

Digitalis Leaf

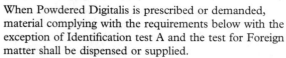

(Ph Eur monograph 0117)

When Powdered Digitalis is prescribed or demanded, material complying with the requirements below with the exception of Identification test A and the test for Foreign matter shall be dispensed or supplied.

Ph Eur _____

DEFINITION

Dried leaf of *Digitalis purpurea* L.

Content

Minimum 0.3 per cent of cardenolic glycosides, expressed as digitoxin (M_r 765) (dried drug).

CHARACTERS

Faint but characteristic odour.

The whole leaf is about 10-40 cm long and 4-15 cm wide. The lamina is ovate lanceolate or broadly ovate. The winged petiole is from 1/4 as long as to equal in length to the lamina.

IDENTIFICATION

A. The leaf is brittle and often occurs broken. The upper surface is green and the lower surface is greyish-green. The apex is subacute and the margin is irregularly crenate, dentate or serrate. The base is decurrent. The venation is pinnate, the lateral veins being prominent especially on the lower surface, leaving the midrib at about 45° and anastomosing near the margin; a veinlet terminates in each tooth of the margin and the lower veins run down the winged petiole. The upper surface is rugose and pubescent; the lower surface shows a network of raised veinlets and is densely pubescent.

B. Microscopic examination (*2.8.23*). Examine under a microscope using *chloral hydrate solution R*. The powder shows the following diagnostic characters (Figure 0117.-1): fragments of the upper epidermis, in surface view [K, L], with cells with a smooth cuticle and anticlinal walls that are slightly thickened, are straight or slightly sinuous, and may show slight beading and pitting [La] and sometimes scars of covering trichomes [Ka], accompanied by underlying palisade parenchyma [Lb]; fragments of the lower epidermis, in surface view [G], with markedly sinuous cells and anomocytic stomata (*2.8.3*) [Ga]; trichomes are of 2 types: a) uniseriate covering trichomes with blunt apex, usually consisting of 3-5 cells [H, J], often with 1 or more collapsed cells [Ja], walls mostly finely warty or faintly striated; b) glandular trichomes usually with a unicellular [C, D], sometimes a multicellular, uniseriate [A, B, E] stalk and a unicellular head [A, B, C, E] or bicellular head, in side view [D] and in surface view [F] or exceptionally a tetracellular head.

C. Thin-layer chromatography (*2.2.27*).

Test solution To 1.0 g of the powdered herbal drug (180) (*2.9.12*) add a mixture of 20 mL of *ethanol (50 per cent V/V) R* and 10 mL of *lead acetate solution R*. Boil for 2 min, allow to cool and centrifuge. Shake the supernatant solution with 2 quantities, each of 15 mL, of *chloroform R*; separate the 2 layers by centrifugation if necessary. Dry the chloroform layers over *anhydrous sodium sulfate R* and filter. Evaporate 10 mL of the solution to dryness on a water-bath and dissolve the residue in 1 mL of a mixture of equal volumes of *chloroform R* and *methanol R*.

Reference solution Dissolve 5 mg of *purpureaglycoside A CRS*, 2 mg of *purpureaglycoside B CRS*, 5 mg of *digitoxin R* and

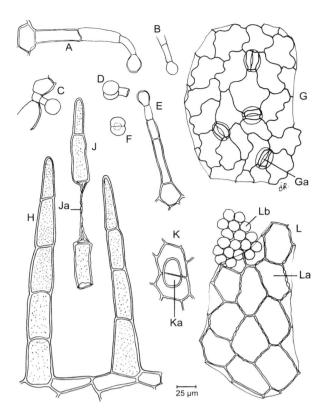

Figure 0117.-1. – *Illustration for identification test B of powdered herbal drug of digitalis leaf*

2 mg of *gitoxin R* in a mixture of equal volumes of *chloroform R* and *methanol R*, then dilute to 10 mL with the same mixture of solvents.

Plate   TLC silica gel G plate R.

Mobile phase   water R, methanol R, ethyl acetate R (7.5:10:75 *V/V/V*).

Application   20 µL as bands of 2 cm by 0.3 cm.

Development   Over a path of 10 cm.

Drying   Until the solvents have evaporated.

Detection   Treat with a mixture of 2 volumes of a 10 g/L solution of *chloramine R* and 8 volumes of a 250 g/L solution of *trichloroacetic acid R* in *ethanol (96 per cent) R*, then heat at 100-105 °C for 10 min; examine in ultraviolet light at 365 nm.

Results   The chromatogram obtained with the reference solution shows a zone of light blue fluorescence in the lower part of the chromatogram, due to purpureaglycoside B, and, just above it, a zone of brownish-yellow fluorescence due to purpureaglycoside A; a zone of light blue fluorescence, due to gitoxin, appears in the middle of the chromatogram and above it a zone of brownish-yellow fluorescence, due to digitoxin; the zones in the chromatogram obtained with the test solution are similar in position, colour and size to the zones in the chromatogram obtained with the reference solution. Other zones of fluorescence may also appear in the chromatogram obtained with the test solution.

D. Evaporate 5 mL of the chloroformic solution obtained in identification test C to dryness on a water-bath. To the residue add 2 mL of *dinitrobenzoic acid solution R* and 1 mL of *1 M sodium hydroxide*. A reddish-violet colour develops within 5 min.

E. Evaporate 5 mL of the chloroformic solution obtained in identification test C to dryness on a water-bath. To the residue add 3 mL of *xanthydrol solution R* and heat on a water-bath for 3 min. A red colour develops.

TESTS

Digitalis lanata Ehrh

The presence of leaves with few or no trichomes and with parallel venation or the presence of cells of the abaxial epidermis with beaded anticlinal walls and of cells of the adaxial epidermis with numerous stomata indicates adulteration by *Digitalis lanata* Ehrh.

Loss on drying (*2.2.32*)
Maximum 6.0 per cent, determined on 1.000 g of the powdered herbal drug (355) (*2.9.12*) by drying in an oven at 105 °C.

Total ash (*2.4.16*)
Maximum 12.0 per cent.

Ash insoluble in hydrochloric acid (2.8.1)
Maximum 5.0 per cent.

ASSAY

Shake 0.250 g of the powdered herbal drug (180) (*2.9.12*) with 50.0 mL of *water R* for 1 h. Add 5.0 mL of a 150 g/L solution of *lead acetate R*, shake, and after a few minutes add 7.5 mL of a 40 g/L solution of *disodium hydrogen phosphate R*. Filter through a pleated paper filter. Heat 50.0 mL of the filtrate with 5 mL of hydrochloric acid (150 g/L HCl) under a reflux condenser on a water-bath for 1 h. Transfer to a separating funnel, rinse the flask with 2 quantities, each of 5 mL, of *water R* and shake with 3 quantities, each of 25 mL, of *chloroform R*. Dry the combined chloroform layers over *anhydrous sodium sulfate R* and dilute to 100.0 mL with *chloroform R*. Evaporate 40.0 mL of the chloroformic solution to dryness, dissolve the residue in 7 mL of ethanol (50 per cent *V/V*) *R*, add 2 mL of *dinitrobenzoic acid solution R* and 1 mL of *1 M sodium hydroxide*. At the same time prepare a reference solution as follows. Dissolve 50.0 mg of *digitoxin CRS* in *ethanol (96 per cent) R* and dilute to 50.0 mL with the same solvent. Dilute 5.0 mL of the solution to 50.0 mL with *ethanol (96 per cent) R*. To 5.0 mL of the resulting solution add 25 mL of *water R* and 3 mL of hydrochloric acid (150 g/L HCl). Heat the solution under a reflux condenser on a water-bath for 1 h and complete the preparation as described above. Measure the absorbance (*2.2.25*) of the 2 solutions at 540 nm several times during the first 12 min until the maximum is reached, using as the compensation liquid a mixture of 7 mL of *ethanol (50 per cent V/V) R*, 2 mL of *dinitrobenzoic acid solution R* and 1 mL of *1 M sodium hydroxide*.

From the absorbances measured and the concentrations of the solutions, calculate the content of cardenolic glycosides, expressed as digitoxin.

STORAGE

Protected from moisture.

Ph Eur

Dill Oil

DEFINITION
Dill Oil is obtained by distillation from the dried ripe fruits of *Anethum graveolens* L.

CHARACTERISTICS
A clear, colourless or pale yellow liquid, visibly free from water; odour, characteristic of the crushed fruit.

TESTS
Optical rotation
+70° to +80°, Appendix V F.

Refractive index
1.481 to 1.492, Appendix V E.

Solubility in ethanol
Soluble, at 20°, in 1 volume or more of *ethanol (90%)* and in 10 volumes or more of *ethanol (80%)*, Appendix X M.

Weight per mL
0.895 to 0.910 g, Appendix V G.

Content of carvone
43.0 to 63.0% w/w when determined by the following method. To 1.5 g in a glass-stoppered tube (approximately 150 mm × 25 mm) add 10 mL of a solution prepared in the following manner. Dissolve 7.0 g of *hydroxylamine hydrochloride* in 90 mL of *ethanol (90%)*, warming gently if necessary, add 1.6 mL of *dimethyl yellow solution* and sufficient 1M *potassium hydroxide* in *ethanol (90%)* to produce a pure yellow colour and dilute to 100 mL with *ethanol (90%)*. Titrate with 1M *potassium hydroxide in ethanol (90%)* VS until the red colour changes to yellow. Place the tube in a water bath at 75° to 80° and, at 5-minute intervals, neutralise with 1M *potassium hydroxide in ethanol (90%)* VS; after 40 minutes complete the titration to the full yellow colour of the indicator. This procedure gives an approximate value for the carvone content of the oil. Repeat the procedure, using as the colour standard for the end point of the titration the titrated liquid of the first determination with the addition of 0.5 mL of 1M *potassium hydroxide in ethanol (90%)* VS. Calculate the content of carvone from the second determination. Each mL of 1M *potassium hydroxide in ethanol (90%)* VS is equivalent to 151.4 mg of carvone, $C_{10}H_{14}O$.

STORAGE
Dill Oil should be kept in a well-filled container and protected from light. It darkens in colour on storage.

Dog Rose

(*Ph Eur monograph 1510*)

Ph Eur

DEFINITION
Rose hips made up by the receptacle and the remains of the dried sepals of *Rosa canina* L., *R. pendulina* L. and other *Rosa* species, with the achenes removed.

Content
Minimum 0.3 per cent of ascorbic acid ($C_6H_8O_6$; M_r 176.1) (dried drug).

IDENTIFICATION
A. It consists of fragments of the fleshy, hollow, urceolate receptacle, bearing the remains of the reduced sepals, light pink or orange-pink, the convex outer surface shiny and strongly wrinkled; bearing on its lighter inner surface abundant bristle-like hairs.

B. Reduce to a powder (355) (*2.9.12*). The powder is orange-yellow. Examine under a microscope using *chloral hydrate solution R*. The powder shows the following diagnostic characters: numerous fragments of receptacle, the outer epidermis with orange-yellow contents and a thick cuticle, the inner epidermis composed of thin-walled cells containing cluster crystals and occasional prisms of calcium oxalate; scattered lignified cells, isodiametric, with thickened and pitted walls forming the trichome bases; abundant unicellar trichomes, up to 2 mm long and 30-45 μm thick, tapering towards each end, walls heavily thickened and with a waxy cuticle which may show fissures in a spiral arrangement; numerous oily orange-yellow globules.

C. Thin-layer chromatography (*2.2.27*).

Test solution To 5 g of the powdered drug (355) (*2.9.12*) add 25 mL of *ethanol (96 per cent) R*, shake for 30 min and filter.

Reference solution Dissolve 10 mg of *ascorbic acid R* in 5.0 mL of *ethanol (60 per cent V/V) R*.

Plate TLC *silica gel F254 plate R*.

Mobile phase *acetone R*, *glacial acetic acid R*, *methanol R*, *toluene R* (5:5:20:70 *V/V/V/V*).

Application 20 μL of the test solution and 2 μL of the reference solution.

Development Over a path of 15 cm.

Drying In air.

Detection A Examine in ultraviolet light at 254 nm.

Results A The chromatogram obtained with the test solution shows a quenching zone similar in position to the principal zone in the chromatogram obtained with the reference solution.

Detection B Spray with a 0.2 g/L solution of *dichlorophenolindophenol, sodium salt R* in *ethanol (96 per cent) R*. Examine in daylight.

Results B The chromatogram obtained with the test solution shows a white zone on a pink background (ascorbic acid) similar in position and colour to the principal zone in the chromatogram obtained with the reference solution. The chromatogram also shows an intense orange-yellow zone near the solvent front and a yellow zone in the upper third (carotenoids).

TESTS
Foreign matter (*2.8.2*)
Maximum 1 per cent.

Loss on drying (*2.2.32*)
Maximum 10.0 per cent, determined on 1.000 g of the powdered drug (355) (*2.9.12*) by drying in an oven at 105 °C.

Total ash (*2.4.16*)
Maximum 7.0 per cent.

ASSAY
Test solution In a round-bottomed flask, weigh 0.500 g of the freshly powdered drug (710) (*2.9.12*). Add a solution of 1.0 g of *oxalic acid R* in 50.0 mL of *methanol R*. Boil under a reflux condenser for 10 min, and cool in iced water until the temperature reaches 15-20 °C. Filter. Transfer 2.0 mL of the filtrate to a 50 mL conical flask. Add successively, with gentle shaking after each addition, 2.0 mL of *dichlorophenolindophenol standard solution R* and then, exactly 60 s later, 0.5 mL of a 100 g/L solution of *thiourea R* in

ethanol (50 per cent V/V) R and 0.7 mL of dinitrophenylhydrazine-sulfuric acid solution R. Heat under a reflux condenser at 50 °C for 75 min, and place immediately in iced water for 5 min. Add dropwise 5.0 mL of a mixture of 12 mL of water R and 50 mL of sulfuric acid R, taking care to carry out the addition over a period of minimum 90 s and maximum 120 s while maintaining vigorous stirring in iced water. Allow to stand for 30 min at room temperature and measure the absorbance (2.2.25) at 520 nm using solution A as compensation liquid.

Solution A   Treat 2.0 mL of the filtrate obtained during the preparation of the test solution as described but adding the dinitrophenylhydrazine-sulfuric acid solution R just before the absorbance is measured.

Reference solution   Dissolve 40.0 mg of ascorbic acid R in a freshly prepared 20 g/L solution of oxalic acid R in methanol R and dilute to 100.0 mL with the same solvent. Dilute 5.0 mL of this solution to 100.0 mL with a freshly prepared 20 g/L solution of oxalic acid R in methanol R. Treat 2.0 mL of the solution as described above for the filtrate obtained during the preparation of the test solution. Measure the absorbance (2.2.25) at 520 nm using solution B as the compensation liquid.

Solution B   Treat 2.0 mL of the reference solution as described above for solution A.

Calculate the percentage content of ascorbic acid from the following expression:

$$\frac{2.5 \times A_1 \times m_2}{A_2 \times m_1}$$

A_1 = absorbance of the test solution;
A_2 = absorbance of the reference solution;
m_1 = mass of the substance to be examined, in grams;
m_2 = mass of ascorbic acid used, in grams.

_____ Ph Eur

Drynaria Rhizome

(Ph Eur monograph 2563)

Ph Eur _____

DEFINITION
Dried rhizome of *Drynaria fortunei* (Kunze) J. Sm. The ramenta may be removed.

Content
Minimum 0.5 per cent of naringin ($C_{27}H_{32}O_{14}$; M_r 580.5) (dried drug).

IDENTIFICATION
A. Long, flattened, slat-shaped rhizome, often curved and branched, 5-15 cm long and 1-1.5 cm thick. The surface is either completely covered in scaly, dark brown hairs (rhizome with ramenta) or glabrous with dark brown dots (rhizome without ramenta). The upper surface and both sides show circular frond scars, rarely the frond bases. The lower surface shows scars or the remains of fibrous roots. The texture is light, fragile, easily broken. The section is reddish-brown; the steles form a ring of small yellow dots.

B. Microscopic examination (2.8.23). The powder is reddish-brown. Examine under a microscope using *chloral hydrate solution R*. The powder shows the following diagnostic characters: numerous parenchyma fragments, consisting of polyhedral cells with slightly and regularly thickened and

pitted walls; scalariform lignified vessels of variable diameter up to 60 µm; fragments of scaly hairs forming a tissue consisting of many reddish-brown cells forming expansions on the margins (rhizome with ramenta).

C. Thin-layer chromatography (2.2.27).

Test solution   To 0.5 g of the powdered herbal drug (355) (2.9.12) add 5 mL of *methanol R* and sonicate for 10 min. Cool, centrifuge and use the supernatant.

Reference solution   Dissolve 1 mg of *naringin R* and 1 mg of *hyperoside R* in 2 mL of *methanol R*.

Plate   *TLC silica gel plate R* (2-10 µm).

Mobile phase   acetic acid R, anhydrous formic acid R, water R, ethyl acetate R (11:11:26:100 V/V/V/V).

Application   10 µL as bands of 8 mm.

Development   Over a path of 6 cm.

Drying   In air.

Detection   Treat with *aluminium chloride reagent R*; examine in ultraviolet light at 365 nm.

Results   See below the sequence of zones present in the chromatograms obtained with the reference solution and the test solution. Furthermore, other faint zones may be present in the chromatogram obtained with the test solution.

Top of the plate	
_____	_____
Hyperoside: a yellow zone	
Naringin: a bluish-white zone	A bluish-white zone (naringin)
	A bluish-white zone
_____	_____
Reference solution	**Test solution**

TESTS
Loss on drying (2.2.32)
Maximum 13.0 per cent, determined on 1.000 g of the powdered herbal drug (355) (2.9.12) by drying in an oven at 105 °C for 2 h.

Total ash (2.4.16)
Maximum 7.0 per cent.

Ash insoluble in hydrochloric acid (2.8.1)
Maximum 2.0 per cent.

ASSAY
Liquid chromatography (2.2.29).

Test solution   Disperse 0.100 g of the powdered herbal drug (355) (2.9.12) in a 50 per cent V/V solution of *methanol R* and dilute to 10.0 mL with the same solvent. Weigh, sonicate for 45 min. Allow to cool, weigh and compensate the loss of solvent with a 50 per cent V/V solution of *methanol R*, shake well. Filter through a membrane filter (nominal pore size 0.45 µm).

Reference solution (a)   Dissolve 10.0 mg of *naringin CRS* in methanol R and dilute to 20.0 mL with the same solvent.

Reference solution (b)   Dissolve 5.0 mg of *neohesperidin R* in reference solution (a) and dilute to 10.0 mL with reference solution (a).

Reference solution (c)   Dilute 1.0 mL of reference solution (a) to 10.0 mL with *methanol R*.

Column:
— *size:* $l = 0.15$ m, $\emptyset = 4.6$ mm;
— *stationary phase*: *octadecylsilyl silica gel for chromatography R* (5 μm).

Mobile phase   *acetonitrile R*, 0.4 per cent *V/V* solution of *acetic acid R* (18:82 *V/V*).

Flow rate   1.0 mL/min.

Detection   Spectrophotometer at 283 nm.

Injection   20 μL of the test solution and reference solutions (b) and (c).

Run time   Twice the retention time of naringin.

Retention time   Naringin = about 9 min; neohesperidin = about 12 min.

System suitability   Reference solution (b):
— *resolution*: minimum 5.0 between the peaks due to naringin and neohesperidin.

Calculate the percentage content of naringin using the following expression:

$$\frac{A_1 \times m_2 \times p}{A_2 \times m_1 \times 20}$$

A_1 = area of the peak due to naringin in the chromatogram obtained with the test solution;

A_2 = area of the peak due to naringin in the chromatogram obtained with reference solution (c);

m_1 = mass of the herbal drug to be examined used to prepare the test solution, in grams;

m_2 = mass of *naringin CRS* used to prepare reference solution (a), in grams;

p = percentage content of naringin in *naringin CRS*.

Ph Eur

Echinacea Angustifolia Root

(Narrow-leaved Coneflower Root, Ph Eur monograph 1821)

Ph Eur

DEFINITION

Dried, whole or cut underground parts of *Echinacea angustifolia* (D.C.).

Content

Minimum 0.5 per cent of echinacoside ($C_{35}H_{46}O_{20}$; M_r 786.5) (dried drug).

IDENTIFICATION

First identification   A, B, C.

Second identification   A, B, D.

A. The root crown is up to about 30 mm in diameter and shows only a few stem bases. The roots are not very numerous, up to about 15 mm in diameter, cylindrical or slightly tapering and sometimes spirally twisted, the outer surface is pale brown to yellowish-brown. The fracture is short, dark brown with a radiate structure.

B. Reduce to a powder (355) (*2.9.12*). The powder is greyish-brown. Examine under a microscope using *chloral hydrate solution R*. The powder shows the following diagnostic characters: narrow lignified fibres (up to about 800 μm in length and 50 μm in diameter) joined together in long bundles surrounded by phytomelanin deposits; lignified reticulately or scalariformly thickened vessels (up to about 60 μm in diameter); abundant sclereids occuring singly or, more usually, in groups of 2 to 10, mostly elongated to rectangular, (up to about 150 μm in length and 40 μm wide), with intercellular spaces filled with phytomelanin deposit; fragments of oleoresin canal (80-150 μm in diameter) with yellowish-orange to reddish-brown content; groups of squarish to rectangular cells, about 30-45 μm from the outer layers of the roots; abundant fine-walled pitted parenchyma with sphaerocrystalline masses of inulin.

C. Examine the chromatograms obtained in the test for *Echinacea purpurea.*

Results   See below the sequence of zones present in the chromatograms obtained with the reference solution and the test solution. Furthermore, other faint dark blue fluorescent zones may be present between the zones of echinacoside and cynarin in the chromatogram obtained with the test solution.

Top of the plate	
Caffeic acid: a strong blue fluorescent zone	
Cynarin: a strong greenish fluorescent zone	A greenish fluorescent zone (cynarin)
Echinacoside: a strong greenish fluorescent zone	A strong greenish fluorescent zone (echinacoside)
Reference solution	**Test solution**

D. Examine the chromatograms obtained in the assay.

Results   The chromatogram obtained with the test solution shows 1 major peak due to echinacoside and a minor peak due to cynarin. Peaks due to caffeic acid, caftaric acid and chlorogenic acid are minor peaks or may be absent.

Figure 1821.-1. – Chromatogram for the assay of echinacoside in narrow-leaved coneflower root

TESTS

Foreign matter (*2.8.2*)
Maximum 3 per cent.

Echinacea purpurea

Thin layer chromatography (*2.2.27*).

Test solution   To 1.0 g of the powdered drug (355) (*2.9.12*) add 10 mL of *methanol R*, treat in an ultrasonic bath for 5 min. Centrifuge and use the supernatant solution.

Reference solution   Dissolve 1 mg of *echinacoside R*, 1 mg of *cynarin R* and 0.5 mg of *caffeic acid R* in 5.0 mL of *methanol R*.

Plate   *TLC silica gel F$_{254}$ plate R* (5-40 μm) [or *TLC silica gel F$_{254}$ plate R* (2-10 μm)].

Mobile phase   *anhydrous formic acid R*, *water R*, *methyl ethyl ketone R*, *ethyl acetate R* (3:3:9:15 *V/V/V/V*).

Application   25 μL [or 5 μL] of the test solution and 10 μL [or 2 μL] of the reference solution as bands.

Development   Over a path of 15 cm [or 5 cm].

Drying   In a stream of cold air for about 10 min followed by 2 min at 100-105 °C.

Detection   Treat the hot plate using a 5 g/L solution of *diphenylboric acid aminoethyl ester R* in *ethyl acetate R*; examine in ultraviolet light at 365 nm after 30 min.

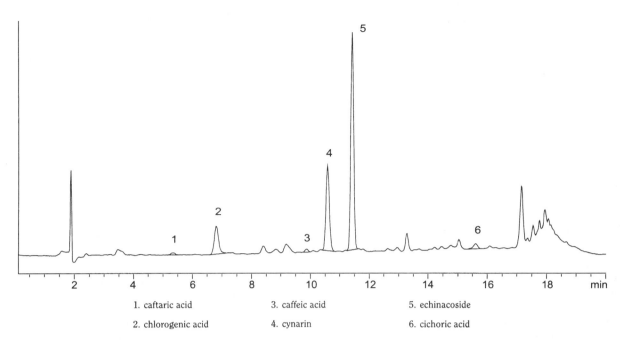

Figure 1821.-1. – *Chromatogram for the assay of echinacoside in narrow-leaved coneflower root*

| 1. caftaric acid | 3. caffeic acid | 5. echinacoside |
| 2. chlorogenic acid | 4. cynarin | 6. cichoric acid |

Results   The chromatogram obtained with the test solution shows no greenish fluorescent zone just below the zone due to caffeic acid in the chromatogram obtained with the reference solution and no greenish fluorescent zone below the zone due to cynarin in the chromatogram obtained with the reference solution. In the chromatogram obtained with the test solution no zones apart from faint dark blue fluorescent zones are visible between the zones due to echinacoside and cynarin.

Loss on drying (*2.2.32*)
Maximum 12.0 per cent, determined on 1.000 g of the powdered drug (355) (*2.9.12*) by drying in an oven at 105 °C for 2 h.

Total ash (*2.4.16*)
Maximum 9.0 per cent.

Ash insoluble in hydrochloric acid (*2.8.1*)
Maximum 3.0 per cent.

ASSAY
Liquid chromatography (*2.2.29*).

Test solution   In a 100 mL volumetric flask place 0.500 g of powdered drug (355) (*2.9.12*) and add 80 mL of *ethanol (70 per cent V/V) R*. Treat in an ultrasonic bath for 15 min and dilute to 100.0 mL with *ethanol (70 per cent V/V) R*. Mix the suspension and allow to stand for a few minutes so that visible solids settle. Filter a suitable proportion of the solution through a membrane filter (nominal pore size 0.45 μm) before injection.

Reference solution   Dissolve 10.0 mg of *chlorogenic acid CRS* and 10.0 mg of *caffeic acid R* in *ethanol (70 per cent V/V) R*, sonicate for 15 min and dilute to 10.0 mL with the same solvent. Dilute 4.0 mL of this solution to 100.0 mL with *ethanol (70 per cent V/V) R*.

Column:
— *size*: l = 0.25 m, Ø = 4.6 mm;
— *stationary phase*: *octadecylsilyl silica gel for chromatography R* (5 μm);
— *temperature*: 35 °C.

Mobile phase:
— *mobile phase A*: *phosphoric acid R, water R* (1:999 *V/V*);
— *mobile phase B*: *acetonitrile R*;

Time (min)	Mobile phase A (per cent *V/V*)	Mobile phase B (per cent *V/V*)
0	90	10
0 - 13	90 → 78	10 → 22
13 - 14	78 → 60	22 → 40
14 - 14.5	60	40

Flow rate   1.5 mL/min.

Detection   Spectrophotometer at 330 nm.

Injection   10 μL.

Relative retention   With reference to chlorogenic acid: caftaric acid = about 0.8; caffeic acid = about 1.5; cynarin = about 1.6; echinacoside = about 1.7; cichoric acid = about 2.3.

System suitability   Reference solution:
— *resolution*: minimum 10 between the peaks due to caffeic acid and chlorogenic acid.

Locate the peaks due to caffeic acid and chlorogenic acid using the chromatogram obtained with the reference solution. Locate the peaks due to echinacoside and cynarin using the chromatogram in Figure 1821.-1.

Calculate the percentage content of echinacoside from the following expression:

$$\frac{A_1 \times C_2 \times 100 \times 2.221}{A_2 \times C_1}$$

A_1 = area of the peak due to echinacoside in the chromatogram obtained with the test solution;

A_2 = area of the peak due to chlorogenic acid in the chromatogram obtained with the reference solution;

C_1 = concentration of the test solution, in milligrams per millilitre;

C_2 = concentration of chlorogenic acid in the reference solution, in milligrams per millilitre;

2.221 = peak correlation factor between chlorogenic acid and echinacoside.

STORAGE

Store uncomminuted.

_____ *Ph Eur*

Top of the plate	
	A greenish-brown to brown zone
	A yellow zone
	A violet zone
β-Sitosterol: a violet to pink zone	A violet to pink zone (β-sitosterol)
N-Isobutyldodecatetraenamide: a greyish-blue zone	
	A dark grey-blue zone
Reference solution	Test solution

Echinacea Pallida Root

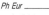

(*Pale Coneflower Root, Ph Eur monograph 1822*)

Ph Eur _____

DEFINITION

Dried, whole or cut underground parts of *Echinacea pallida* Nutt.

Content

Minimum 0.2 per cent of echinacoside ($C_{35}H_{46}O_{20}$; M_r 786.5) (dried drug).

IDENTIFICATION

A. The rhizome and roots are 4-20 mm in diameter, cylindrical and sometimes spirally twisted, longitudinally wrinkled or deeply furrowed; the outer surface is reddish-brown to greyish-brown.

B. Reduce to a powder (355) (*2.9.12*). The powder is greyish-brown to light yellow. Examine under a microscope using *chloral hydrate solution R*. The powder shows the following diagnostic characters: short lignified fibres (100-300 µm in length, up to about 80 µm in diameter) occurring singly or joined together in long bundles, sometimes with phytomelanin deposits; lignified reticulately or scalariformly thickened vessels (up to about 70 µm in diameter); abundant sclereids, occurring singly or in small groups of less than 10, varying considerably in shape from rounded to rectangular or irregular, sometimes much elongated and fibre-like and measuring up to 400 µm in length; all the sclereids have associated black, phytomelanin deposits; fragments of oleoresin canals (up to 240 µm in diameter) with yellowish-orange content; groups of squarish to rectangular cells of the outer layers (about 40 × 80 µm); abundant thin-walled pitted parenchyma with sphaerocrystalline masses of inulin.

C. Examine the chromatograms obtained in the test for other *Echinacea* species and *Parthenium integrifolium*.

Results See below the sequence of zones present in the chromatograms obtained with the reference solution and the test solution. The chromatogram obtained with the test solution may also show a weak zone close to the solvent front.

D. Examine the chromatograms obtained in the assay.

Results The major peak in the chromatogram obtained with the test solution is due to echinacoside. Peaks due to caftaric acid, caffeic acid, cynarin, chlorogenic acid and cichoric acid are minor peaks or may be absent.

TESTS

Foreign matter (*2.8.2*)

Maximum 3 per cent.

Other *Echinacea* species and *Parthenium integrifolium*

Thin-layer chromatography (*2.2.27*).

Test solution To 1.0 g of the powdered drug (355) (*2.9.12*) add 10 mL of *methylene chloride R* and sonicate for 5 min. Centrifuge and use the supernatant solution.

Reference solution Dissolve 1 mg of *β-sitosterol R* and a volume of *N-isobutyldodecatetraenamide solution R* corresponding to 1 mg of *N-isobutyldodecatetraenamide R* in *methanol R* and dilute to 5.0 mL with the same solvent.

Plate *TLC silica gel F_{254} plate R* (5-40 µm) [or *TLC silica gel F_{254} plate R* (2-10 µm)].

Mobile phase *anhydrous formic acid R, cyclohexane R, ethyl acetate R, toluene R* (0.9:3:6:24 *V/V/V/V*).

Application 25 µL [or 5 µL] of the test solution and 10 µL [or 4 µL] of the reference solution as bands.

Development Over a path of 15 cm [or 5 cm].

Drying In a stream of cold air for about 10 min.

Detection Treat the plate using *anisaldehyde solution R* and heat at 105 °C for 3 min; examine in daylight.

Results The chromatogram obtained with the test solution shows no greyish-blue zone at the position of *N*-isobutyldodecatetraenamide in the chromatogram obtained with the reference solution, and no blue zone at the position of the violet zone due to *β*-sitosterol in the chromatogram obtained with the reference solution.

Loss on drying (*2.2.32*)

Maximum 12.0 per cent, determined on 1.000 g of the powdered drug (355) (*2.9.12*) by drying in an oven at 105 °C for 2 h.

Total ash (*2.4.16*)

Maximum 7.0 per cent.

Ash insoluble in hydrochloric acid (*2.8.1*)

Maximum 2.0 per cent.

ASSAY

Liquid chromatography (*2.2.29*).

Test solution In a 100 mL volumetric flask place 0.500 g of the powdered drug (355) (*2.9.12*) and add 80 mL of *ethanol (70 per cent V/V) R*. Sonicate for 15 min and dilute to 100.0 mL with *ethanol (70 per cent V/V) R*. Mix the suspension and allow to stand for a few minutes to allow visible solids to settle. Filter a suitable proportion of the solution through a membrane filter (nominal pore size 0.45 µm) before injection.

Reference solution Dissolve 10.0 mg of *chlorogenic acid CRS* and 10.0 mg of *caffeic acid R* in *ethanol (70 per cent V/V) R*, sonicate for 15 min and dilute to 10.0 mL with the same

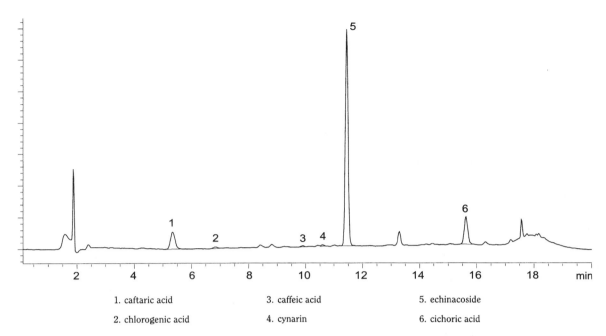

1. caftaric acid

3. caffeic acid

5. echinacoside

2. chlorogenic acid

4. cynarin

6. cichoric acid

Figure 1822.-1. – *Chromatogram for the assay of echinacoside in pale coneflower root*

solvent. Dilute 4.0 mL of this solution to 100.0 mL with *ethanol (70 per cent V/V) R*.

Column:
— *size*: l = 0.25 m, Ø = 4.6 mm;
— *stationary phase*: *octadecylsilyl silica gel for chromatography R* (5 μm);
— *temperature*: 35 °C.

Mobile phase:
— *mobile phase A*: *phosphoric acid R, water R* (1:999 *V/V*);
— *mobile phase B*: *acetonitrile R*;

Time (min)	Mobile phase A (per cent *V/V*)	Mobile phase B (per cent *V/V*)
0	90	10
0 - 13	90 → 78	10 → 22
13 - 14	78 → 60	22 → 40
14 - 20	60	40

Flow rate 1.5 mL/min.

Detection Spectrophotometer at 330 nm.

Injection 10 μL.

Relative retention With reference to chlorogenic acid (retention time = about 7 min): caftaric acid = about 0.8; caffeic acid = about 1.5; cynarin = about 1.6; echinacoside = about 1.7; cichoric acid = about 2.3.

System suitability Reference solution:
— *resolution*: minimum 10 between the peaks due to caffeic acid and chlorogenic acid.

Locate the peaks due to caffeic acid and chlorogenic acid using the chromatogram obtained with the reference solution. Locate the peaks due to echinacoside, caftaric acid and cichoric acid using the chromatogram in Figure 1822.-1.

Calculate the percentage content of echinacoside using the following expression:

$$\frac{A_1 \times C_2 \times 100 \times 2.221}{A_2 \times C_1}$$

A_1 = area of the peak due to echinacoside in the chromatogram obtained with the test solution;

A_2 = area of the peak due to chlorogenic acid in the chromatogram obtained with the reference solution;

C_1 = concentration of the test solution, in milligrams per millilitre;

C_2 = concentration of chlorogenic acid in the reference solution, in milligrams per millilitre;

2.221 = peak correlation factor between chlorogenic acid and echinacoside.

STORAGE

Uncomminuted.

_____ *Ph Eur*

Echinacea Purpurea Herb

(Purple Coneflower Herb, Ph Eur monograph 1823)

Ph Eur _____

DEFINITION

Dried, whole or cut flowering aerial parts of *Echinacea purpurea* (L.) Moench.

Content

Minimum 0.1 per cent for the sum of caftaric acid ($C_{13}H_{12}O_9$; M_r 312.2) and cichoric acid ($C_{22}H_{18}O_{12}$; M_r 474.3) (dried drug).

IDENTIFICATION

First identification A, B, C.

Second identification A, B, D.

A. The herbaceous perennial plant is 60-150 cm, rarely up to 180 cm high. The stem is green to red, upright and slightly branched. The leaves are alternate, ovate to ovate-lanceolate, irregularly serrate, rugose on both surfaces, dark green with prominent light green veins; the lamina is thick and shiny.

The involucral bracts of the large capitulum are arranged in 2 or 3 rows. The solid receptacle is slightly convex. Each of the outer violet ligulate florets (4-6 cm) and of the inner violet-pink tubular florets is attached to a reddish acute and coriaceous bract, which overtops the tubular florets.
The calyx is reduced to a very short crown, one of the sepals is up to 1 mm long.

B. Reduce to a powder (355) (2.9.12). The powder is green. Examine under a microscope using *chloral hydrate solution R*. The powder shows the following diagnostic characters: whitish-green groups of fibres, 150-200 µm in length, 10-15 µm in diameter, sometimes with black deposits; fragments of leaves in surface view showing anomocytic or anisocytic stomata (2.8.3) (about 35-40 µm in length); uniseriate covering trichomes or fragments thereof consisting mainly of 3 or 4 thick-walled cells of which the apical cell is markedly longer than the others; fragments of leaves with rosette-like arranged epidermal cells around the base of the covering trichomes; uniseriate glandular trichomes composed of very thin-walled cells; pitted parenchymatous cells from the pith of the stem as well as pitted elongated cells from the mesocarp of the achenes; fragments of parenchyma from the seeds with oil droplets; fragments of the epidermis of ligulate florets composed of red to violet papillous cells; spheroidal pollen grains, 30-40 µm in diameter, with a spiny exine.

C. Thin-layer chromatography (2.2.27).

Test solution   To 1.0 g of the powdered drug (355) (2.9.12) add 10 mL of *methanol R* and sonicate for 5 min. Centrifuge and use the supernatant solution.

Reference solution   Dissolve 0.5 mg of *caffeic acid R* and 0.5 mg of *chlorogenic acid R* in 5.0 mL of *methanol R*.

Plate   *TLC silica gel plate R* (5-40 µm) [or *TLC silica gel plate R* (2-10 µm)].

Mobile phase   *anhydrous formic acid R, water R, methyl ethyl ketone R, ethyl acetate R* (3:3:9:15 V/V/V/V).

Application   25 µL [or 5 µL] of the test solution and 10 µL [or 2 µL] of the reference solution, as bands.

Development   Over a path of 15 cm [or 5 cm].

Drying   In a stream of cold air for about 10 min, then at 100 °C for 2 min.

Detection   Spray the still-warm plate with a 5 g/L solution of *diphenylboric acid aminoethyl ester R* in *ethyl acetate R*; after 30 min, examine in ultraviolet light at 365 nm.

Results   See below the sequence of zones present in the chromatograms obtained with the reference solution and the test solution. Furthermore, other faint blue fluorescent zones may be present in the chromatogram obtained with the test solution.

D. Examine the chromatograms obtained in the assay.
The principal peak in the chromatogram obtained with the test solution is due to cichoric acid and a smaller peak is due to caftaric acid. Peaks due to caffeic acid and chlorogenic acid are minor or may be absent.

TESTS
Loss on drying (2.2.32)
Maximum 10.0 per cent, determined on 1.000 g of the powdered drug (355) (2.9.12) by drying in an oven at 105 °C for 2 h.

Total ash (2.4.16)
Maximum 12.0 per cent.

ASSAY
Liquid chromatography (2.2.29).

Top of the plate	
	An intense red fluorescent zone
Caffeic acid: a strong blue fluorescent zone	A blue fluorescent zone
———	———
	A blue fluorescent zone
Chlorogenic acid: a strong blue fluorescent zone	A faint yellow-orange fluorescent zone
———	———
Reference solution	**Test solution**

Test solution   In a 100 mL volumetric flask place 0.500 g of the powdered drug (355) (2.9.12) and add 80 mL of *ethanol (70 per cent V/V) R*. Sonicate for 15 min and dilute to 100.0 mL with *ethanol (70 per cent V/V) R*. Mix the suspension and allow to stand for a few minutes to allow visible solids to settle.

Reference solution   Dissolve 10.0 mg of *chlorogenic acid CRS* and 10.0 mg of *caffeic acid R* in *ethanol (70 per cent V/V) R*, sonicate for 15 min and dilute to 10.0 mL with the same solvent. Dilute 4.0 mL of this solution to 100.0 mL with *ethanol (70 per cent V/V) R*.

Column:
— *size*: *l* = 0.25 m, Ø = 4.6 mm;
— *stationary phase*: *octadecylsilyl silica gel for chromatography R* (5 µm);
— *temperature*: 35 °C.

Mobile phase:
— *mobile phase A*: *phosphoric acid R, water R* (1:999 V/V);
— *mobile phase B*: *acetonitrile R*;

Time (min)	Mobile phase A (per cent V/V)	Mobile phase B (per cent V/V)
0	90	10
0 - 13	90 → 78	10 → 22
13 - 14	78 → 60	22 → 40
14 - 20	60	40

Flow rate   1.5 mL/min.

Detection   Spectrophotometer at 330 nm.

Injection   10 µL.

Relative retention   With reference to chlorogenic acid (retention time = about 7 min): caftaric acid = about 0.8; caffeic acid = about 1.5; cynarin = about 1.6; echinacoside = about 1.7; cichoric acid = about 2.3.

System suitability   Reference solution:
— *resolution*: minimum 5 between the peaks due to caffeic acid and chlorogenic acid.

Locate the peaks due to caffeic acid and chlorogenic acid using the chromatogram obtained with the reference solution. Locate the peaks due to caftaric acid and cichoric acid using the chromatogram in Figure 1823.-1.

Calculate the percentage content of caftaric acid using the following expression:

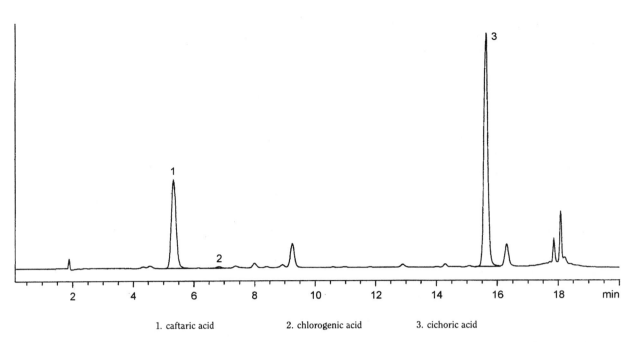

1. caftaric acid   2. chlorogenic acid   3. cichoric acid

Figure 1823.-1. – *Chromatogram for the assay of caftaric acid and cichoric acid in purple coneflower herb*

$$\frac{A_1 \times C_2 \times 100 \times 0.881}{A_2 \times C_1}$$

Calculate the percentage content of cichoric acid using the following expression:

$$\frac{A_3 \times C_2 \times 100 \times 0.695}{A_2 \times C_1}$$

A_1 = area of the peak due to caftaric acid in the chromatogram obtained with the test solution;

A_2 = area of the peak due to chlorogenic acid in the chromatogram obtained with the reference solution;

A_3 = area of the peak due to cichoric acid in the chromatogram obtained with the test solution;

C_1 = concentration of the test solution, in milligrams per millilitre;

C_2 = concentration of chlorogenic acid in the reference solution, in milligrams per millilitre;

0.695 = peak correlation factor based upon the liquid chromatography response observed;

0.881 = peak correlation factor between caftaric acid and chlorogenic acid.

STORAGE
Uncomminuted.

_____ *Ph Eur*

Echinacea Purpurea Root

(*Purple Coneflower Root, Ph Eur monograph 1824*)

Ph Eur _____

DEFINITION
Dried, whole or cut underground parts of *Echinacea purpurea* (L.) Moench.

Content
Minimum 0.5 per cent for the sum of caftaric acid ($C_{13}H_{12}O_9$; M_r 312.2) and cichoric acid ($C_{22}H_{18}O_{12}$; M_r 474.3) (dried drug).

IDENTIFICATION
First identification   A, B, C, E.

Second identification   A, B, D, E.

A. The rhizome is up to 15 cm long, branched, reddish-brown to dark brown on the surface and carries many stem bases; the inside is fibrous and white. The numerous roots are spirally twisted, light to dark brown and show a fine cross structuring on the surface.

B. Reduce to a powder (355) (*2.9.12*). The powder is light yellow to pinkish-beige. Examine under a microscope using *chloral hydrate solution R*. The powder shows the following diagnostic characters: numerous light-brown spindle-shaped fibres that are joined together in long bundles without black deposits; rare sclereids from the rhizomes and roots, usually occuring singly, those from the rhizomes being isodiametric, about 60 µm in diameter, with black deposits, those from the roots being 50-120 µm in length with no black deposits; secretory cavities up to 180 µm in diameter with yellow oil droplets; squarish to rectangular cells of the outer layers, some with reddish walls; bordered-pitted vessels from the rhizome, 30-40 µm in diameter.

C. Examine the chromatogram obtained in the test for other *Echinacea* species and *Parthenium integrifolium*.

Results   See below the sequence of zones present in the chromatograms obtained with the reference solution and the

test solution. Furthermore, faint greenish fluorescent zones may be present just below the zone situated in the middle of the chromatogram obtained with the test solution.

Top of the plate	
Caffeic acid: a strong blue fluorescent zone	A strong blue fluorescent zone
———	———
Cynarin: a strong greenish fluorescent zone	
	A blue fluorescent zone
———	———
Echinacoside: a strong greenish fluorescent zone	
Reference solution	**Test solution**

D. Examine the chromatograms obtained in the assay. The principal peak in the chromatogram obtained with the test solution is due to cichoric acid and a smaller peak is due to caftaric acid. Peaks due to caffeic acid and chlorogenic acid are minor or may be absent.

E. Thin-layer chromatography (*2.2.27*).

Test solution   To 1.0 g of the powdered drug (355) (*2.9.12*) add 10 mL of *methylene chloride R* and sonicate for 5 min. Centrifuge and use the supernatant solution.

Reference solution   Dissolve 1 mg of *β-sitosterol R* and a volume of *N-isobutyldodecatetraenamide solution R* corresponding to 1 mg of *N-isobutyldodecatetraenamide R* in 5.0 mL of *methanol R*.

Plate   TLC silica gel plate R (5-40 μm) [or *TLC silica gel plate R* (2-10 μm)].

Mobile phase   anhydrous formic acid R, cyclohexane R, ethyl acetate R, toluene R (0.9:3:6:24 *V/V/V/V*).

Application   25 μL [or 5 μL], as bands.

Development   Over a path of about 15 cm [or 5 cm].

Drying   In a stream of cold air for about 10 min.

Detection   Dip the plate into *anisaldehyde solution R* for 1 s and heat at 100-105 °C for 3 min; examine in daylight.

Results   See below the sequence of zones present in the chromatograms obtained with the reference solution and the test solution. Furthermore, other faint zones may be present in the chromatogram obtained with the test solution.

Top of the plate	
———	———
	A bluish-violet zone
	A violet or pink zone (β-sitosterol)
β-Sitosterol: a violet or pink zone	
N-Isobutyldodecatetraenamide: a greyish-blue zone	A greyish-blue zone (N-isobutyldodecatetraenamide)
———	———
	A dark greyish-blue zone
Reference solution	**Test solution**

TESTS

Other *Echinacea* species and *Parthenium integrifolium*
Thin-layer chromatography (*2.2.27*).

Test solution   To 1.0 g of the powdered drug (355) (*2.9.12*) add 10 mL of *methanol R* and sonicate for 5 min. Centrifuge and use the supernatant solution.

Reference solution   Dissolve 1 mg of *echinacoside R*, 1 mg of *cynarin R* and 0.5 mg of *caffeic acid R* in 5.0 mL of *methanol R*.

Plate   TLC silica gel plate R (5-40 μm) [or *TLC silica gel plate R* (2-10 μm)].

Mobile phase   anhydrous formic acid R, water R, methyl ethyl ketone R, ethyl acetate R (3:3:9:15 *V/V/V/V*).

Application   10 μL [or 5 μL] of the test solution and 5 μL [or 2 μL] of the reference solution, as bands.

Development   Over a path of 10 cm [or 5 cm].

Drying   In a stream of cold air for about 10 min, then at 105 °C for 2 min.

Detection   Spray the still-warm plate with a 5 g/L solution of *diphenylboric acid aminoethyl ester R* in *ethyl acetate R*; after 30 min, examine in ultraviolet light at 365 nm.

Results   The chromatogram obtained with the test solution shows no greenish fluorescent zone corresponding to the zone due to echinacoside in the chromatogram obtained with the reference solution, and no greenish fluorescent zone corresponding to the zone due to cynarin in the chromatogram obtained with the reference solution. No other zones apart from very faint dark blue fluorescent zones are seen in the lower half of the chromatogram of the test solution.

Foreign matter (*2.8.2*)
Maximum 3 per cent.

Loss on drying (*2.2.32*)
Maximum 10.0 per cent, determined on 1.000 g of the powdered drug (355) (*2.9.12*) by drying in an oven at 105 °C for 2 h.

Total ash (*2.4.16*)
Maximum 9.0 per cent.

Ash insoluble in hydrochloric acid (*2.8.1*)
Maximum 2.0 per cent.

ASSAY

Liquid chromatography (*2.2.29*).

Test solution   In a 100 mL volumetric flask place 0.500 g of the powdered drug (355) (*2.9.12*) and add 80 mL of *ethanol (70 per cent V/V) R*. Sonicate for 15 min and dilute to 100.0 mL with *ethanol (70 per cent V/V) R*. Mix the suspension and allow to stand for a few minutes to allow visible solids to settle.

Reference solution   Dissolve 10.0 mg of *chlorogenic acid CRS* and 10.0 mg of *caffeic acid R* in *ethanol (70 per cent V/V) R*, sonicate for 15 min and dilute to 10.0 mL with the same solvent. Dilute 4.0 mL of this solution to 100.0 mL with *ethanol (70 per cent V/V) R*.

Column:
— *size*: l = 0.25 m, Ø = 4.6 mm;
— *stationary phase*: octadecylsilyl silica gel for chromatography R (5 μm);
— *temperature*: 35 °C.

Mobile phase:
— *mobile phase A*: phosphoric acid R, water R (1:999 *V/V*);
— *mobile phase B*: acetonitrile R;

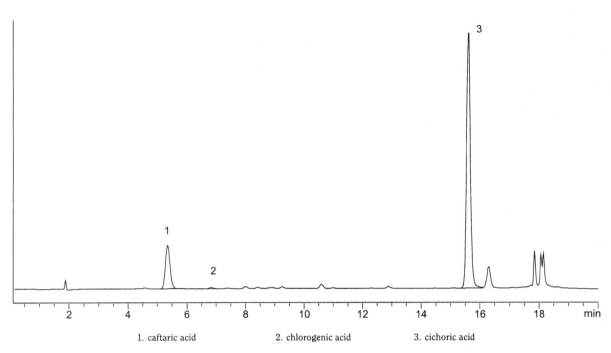

Figure 1824.-1. – *Chromatogram for the assay of caftaric acid and cichoric acid in purple coneflower root*

Time (min)	Mobile phase A (per cent V/V)	Mobile phase B (per cent V/V)
0	90	10
0 - 13	90 → 78	10 → 22
13 - 14	78 → 60	22 → 40
14 - 20	60	40

Flow rate 1.5 mL/min.

Detection Spectrophotometer at 330 nm.

Injection 10 μL.

Relative retention With reference to chlorogenic acid (retention time = about 7 min): caftaric acid = about 0.8; caffeic acid = about 1.5; cynarin = about 1.6; echinacoside = about 1.7; cichoric acid = about 2.3.

System suitability Reference solution:
— *resolution*: minimum 5 between the peaks due to caffeic acid and chlorogenic acid.

Locate the peaks due to caffeic acid and chlorogenic acid using the chromatogram obtained with the reference solution. Locate the peaks due to caftaric acid and cichoric acid using the chromatogram in Figure 1824.-1.

Calculate the percentage content of caftaric acid using the following expression:

$$\frac{A_1 \times C_2 \times 100 \times 0.881}{A_2 \times C_1}$$

Calculate the percentage content of cichoric acid using the following expression:

$$\frac{A_3 \times C_2 \times 100 \times 0.695}{A_2 \times C_1}$$

A_1 = area of the peak due to caftaric acid in the chromatogram obtained with the test solution;

A_2 = area of the peak due to chlorogenic acid in the chromatogram obtained with the reference solution;

A_3 = area of the peak due to cichoric acid in the chromatogram obtained with the test solution;

C_1 = concentration of the dried drug in the test solution, in milligrams per millilitre;

C_2 = concentration of chlorogenic acid in the reference solution, in milligrams per millilitre;

0.695 = peak correlation factor based upon the liquid chromatography response observed;

0.881 = peak correlation factor between caftaric acid and chlorogenic acid.

STORAGE

Uncomminuted.

_____ *Ph Eur*

Eclipta Prostrata Whole Plant

DEFINITION

Eclipta Prostrata Whole Plant is the dried whole plant, either entire or fragmented, of *Eclipta prostrata* (L.) L.

It contains not less than 0.04% of wedelolactone ($C_{16}H_{10}O_7$), calculated with reference to the dried material.

IDENTIFICATION

A. Stems cylindrical, four sided or flattened, 2 to 5 mm in diameter, greyish, with appressed, whitish hairs pointing towards the tip, longitudinally striated, occasionally branching and nodes distinct. Leaves dark green, sessile or subsessile, opposite, lanceolate, 2 to 8.5 cm long and 1 to 2.5 cm wide with an entire or slightly dentate margin and appressed trichomes on both surfaces. Flowerheads 2 to 6 mm in diameter, greenish-brown, solitary or in pairs on unequal axillary peduncles, up to 8 involucral bracts, ovate, with appressed hairs; ray florets spreading, no longer than the bracts, not toothed; disc florets with 4-toothed corolla, pappus usually absent or reduced to minute teeth; 5 stamens, filaments epipetalous and anthers united into a tube; pistil bicarpellary, ovary inferior, unilocular with one basal ovule. Fruits 2 to 3 mm long, pappi persistent and coroniform; unfertilised achenes pale yellow, flattened and smooth; fertilised achenes pale to dark brown, 3 to 4 angled, tuberculate and bulbous. Root, if present, cylindrical, greyish, main root up to about 7 mm in diameter, with secondary branching.

B. Reduce to a powder (355). The powder is greenish brown. Examine under a microscope using *chloral hydrate solution*. The main diagnostic characters include numerous free, whole or broken, large covering trichomes, with warty or spiny walls, up to 700 µm long, uniseriate, usually tricellular, with a broad basal cell, a long median cell and a short, pointed sub-triangular apical cell; less frequently, smaller, unicellular, pointed covering trichomes from the midrib and stem. Fragments of leaf show sinuous walled epidermal cells, underlying palisade, anomocytic stomata, cuticular striations and covering trichomes on both surfaces. Stem fragments with unicellular and multicellular trichomes, epidermis of elongated cells, or in mature stem, poorly developed rectangular cork cells; secondary cortex of parenchyma with numerous air-spaces, pericyclic fibres thick-walled, lignified, simple pitted; secretory canals may be visible; xylem vessels usually simple pitted or spirally thickened, xylem parenchyma lignified and pitted. Fragments of root, if present, show poorly developed cork, consisting of 3-5 rows of thin-walled elongated cells, a secondary cortex of parenchyma, with scattered stone cells and fibres either singly or in groups, xylem vessels and tracheids, and fibres with peg-like projections. Pollen grains with spiny exine and 3 pores.

C. Carry out the method for *thin-layer chromatography*, Appendix III A, using the following solutions.

(1) Reduce to a powder (355). To 2.0 g of powdered sample add 40 mL of *methanol*. Mix with the aid of ultrasound for 2 hours at 50° with occasional shaking and allow to cool. Dilute to 50 mL with *methanol* and filter.

(2) 0.05% w/v each of *wedelolactone EPCRS* and *rosmarinic acid* in *methanol*.

CHROMATOGRAPHIC CONDITIONS

(a) Use as the coating *silica gel F₂₅₄* (Merck silica gel HPTLC plates are suitable).

(b) Use the mobile phase as described below.

(c) Apply 10 µL of each solution as 8 mm bands.

(d) Develop the plate to 6 cm.

(e) After removal of the plate, dry in air, heat at 100° for 5 minutes, treat the plate whilst still hot with a 0.5% v/v solution of *diphenylboric acid aminoethyl ester* in *ethyl acetate* and examine under *ultraviolet light (365 nm)*.

MOBILE PHASE

1 volume of *anhydrous formic acid*, 6 volumes of *acetone* and 11 volumes of *toluene*.

SYSTEM SUITABILITY

The test is not valid unless the chromatogram obtained with solution (2) shows two clearly separated spots.

CONFIRMATION

The chromatogram obtained with solution (1) shows a fluorescent band corresponding to wedelolactone and several other fluorescent bands as shown in the table. Other fluorescent bands may be present.

Top of the plate	
A red zone A diffuse pale blue zone A greenish-white zone	
A pale blue zone	
A blue-white zone (wedelolactone) A blue-white zone	A blue-white zone (wedelolactone)
	Rosmarinic acid: A blue-white zone
A blue-white zone	
Solution (1)	**Solution (2)**

TESTS

Loss on drying
When dried at 100° to 105° for 2 hours, loses not more than 11.0% of its weight. Use 1 g.

Total Ash
Not more than 22.0%, Appendix XI J, Method II.

Acid-insoluble Ash
Not more than 11.0%, Appendix XI K.

ASSAY

Carry out the method for *liquid chromatography*, Appendix III D, using the following solutions.

(1) Reduce to a powder (355). To 2.0 g of powdered sample add 40 mL of *methanol*. Mix with the aid of ultrasound for 2 hours at 50° with occasional shaking and allow to cool. Dilute to 50 mL with *methanol* and filter.

(2) 0.005% w/v each of *wedelolactone EPCRS* and *coumestrol* in *methanol*.

CHROMATOGRAPHIC CONDITIONS

(a) Use a stainless steel column (15 cm × 4.6 mm) packed with *octadecylsilyl silica gel for chromatography* (5µm) (Waters Symmetry C18 is suitable).

(b) Use isocratic elution and the mobile phase described below.

(c) Use a flow rate of 1.0 mL per minute.

(d) Use an ambient column temperature.

(e) Use a detection wavelength of 249 nm.

(f) Inject 10 µL of each solution.

MOBILE PHASE

24 volumes of *acetonitrile* and 76 volumes of a 0.2% v/v solution of *orthophosphoric acid*.

SYSTEM SUITABILITY

The assay is not valid unless, in the chromatogram obtained with solution (2):

the *symmetry factor* of the peak due to *wedelolactone* is less than 1.2;

the *symmetry factor* of the peak due to *coumestrol* is less than 1.1.

DETERMINATION OF CONTENT

Calculate the content of wedelolactone in the sample using the declared content of wedelolactone ($C_{16}H_{10}O_7$) in *wedelolactone EPCRS* and the following expression:

$$\frac{A_1}{A_2} \times \frac{m_2}{V_2} \times \frac{V_1}{m_1} \times p \times \frac{100}{100 - d}$$

A_1 = area of the peak due to wedelolactone in the chromatogram obtained with solution (1);

A_2 = area of the peak due to wedelolactone in the chromatogram obtained with solution (2);

m_1 = weight of the herbal drug being examined in mg;

m_2 = weight of *wedelolactone EPCRS* in mg;

V_1 = dilution volume of solution (1) in mL;

V_2 = dilution volume of solution (2) in mL;

p = percentage content of wedelolactone ($C_{16}H_{10}O_7$) in *wedelolactone EPCRS*;

d = percentage loss on drying of the herbal drug being examined.

Elder Flower

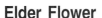

(*Ph Eur monograph 1217*)

Ph Eur

DEFINITION

Dried flowers of *Sambucus nigra* L.

Content

Minimum 0.80 per cent of flavonoids, expressed as isoquercitroside ($C_{21}H_{20}O_{12}$; M_r 464.4) (dried drug).

IDENTIFICATION

A. The flower, about 5 mm in diameter, has 3 small bracts, visible under a lens, and may have a peduncle.
The 5-toothed calyx is small; the corolla is light yellow, with 5 broadly oval petals fused at their bases into a tube.
The filaments of the 5 yellow stamens alternate with the petals. The corolla is often isolated or attached to the stamens, to which it is fused at the base. The ovary is inferior and it bears a short style with 3 obtuse stigmata.

B. Microscopic examination (*2.8.23*). The powder is greenish-yellow. Examine under a microscope using *chloral hydrate solution R*. The powder shows the following diagnostic characters (Figure 1217.-1): numerous spherical, sometimes ellipsoidal, pollen grains about 30 µm in diameter, with 3 germinal pores and very finely pitted exine [G]; cells of the lower epidermis of the sepals often containing oil globules and covered by a striated cuticle in surface view [A]; rare fragments of the rim of the sepals showing unicellular marginal teeth, in transverse section [E]; petal fragments with numerous small globules of essential oil [H]; fragments of upper epidermis of the sepals [B] or petals [F], in surface view, with slightly and irregularly thickened walls [Ba, Fa], anomocytic stomata (*2.8.3*) [Bb, Fb] and a striated cuticle; mesophyll cells of petals and sepals with idioblasts containing numerous microsphenoid crystals of calcium oxalate [Bc]; fragments of anthers in transverse section [C] and in surface view [D], showing the outer layer [Ca] and the cells of the fibrous layer [Cb, Cc, D].

C. Thin-layer chromatography (*2.2.27*).

Test solution To 0.5 g of the powdered herbal drug (355) (*2.9.12*) add 5 mL of *methanol R* and sonicate for 10 min. Centrifuge for 5 min.

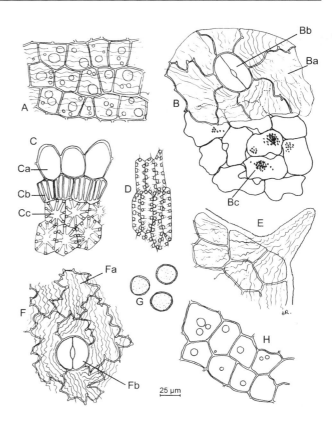

Figure 1217.-1. – *Illustration for identification B of powdered herbal drug of elder flower*

Reference solution Dissolve 1 mg of *caffeic acid R*, 1 mg of *chlorogenic acid R*, 2.5 mg of *hyperoside R* and 2.5 mg of *rutin R* in 10 mL of *methanol R*.

Plate TLC silica gel plate R (2-10 µm).

Mobile phase anhydrous formic acid R, water R, methyl ethyl ketone R, ethyl acetate R (10:10:30:50 *V/V/V/V*).

Application 4 µL as bands of 8 mm.

Development Over a path of 6 cm.

Drying In air.

Detection Heat the plate for 5 min at 100 °C and treat with a 1 g/L solution of *diphenylboric acid aminoethyl ester R* in *ethyl acetate R*, then treat with a 5 g/L solution of *macrogol 400 R* in *methylene chloride R*; allow to dry in air for 30 min. Examine in daylight (results A) and in ultraviolet light at 365 nm (results B).

Results A See below the sequence of zones present in the chromatograms obtained with the reference solution and the test solution. Furthermore, other faint zones may be present in the chromatogram obtained with the test solution.

Results B See below the sequence of zones present in the chromatograms obtained with the reference solution and the test solution. Furthermore, other faint zones may be present in the chromatogram obtained with the test solution.

TESTS

Foreign matter (*2.8.2*)

Maximum 8 per cent of fragments of coarse pedicels and other foreign matter and maximum 15 per cent of discoloured, brown flowers. Carry out the determination on 10 g.

Sambucus ebulus L

Examine the chromatograms obtained in identification C.

Top of the plate	
_____	_____
	An orange zone
Hyperoside: a dark yellow zone	
_____	_____
Rutin: a dark yellow zone	A dark yellow zone
Reference solution	Test solution

Top of the plate	
Caffeic acid: a blue fluorescent zone	
	An intense, light blue fluorescent zone
	2 light blue fluorescent zones
_____	_____
	An orange fluorescent zone
Hyperoside: an orange fluorescent zone	
Chlorogenic acid: a light blue fluorescent zone	An intense, light blue fluorescent zone
_____	_____
Rutin: an orange fluorescent zone	An orange fluorescent zone
Reference solution	Test solution

Results B The chromatogram obtained with the test solution does not show a greenish-white zone above the zone due to caffeic acid in the chromatogram obtained with the reference solution; in the chromatogram obtained with the test solution, no green fluorescent zone is seen just below the orange fluorescent zone due to rutin in the chromatogram obtained with the reference solution.

Loss on drying (*2.2.32*)
Maximum 10.0 per cent, determined on 1.000 g of the powdered herbal drug (355) (*2.9.12*) by drying in an oven at 105 °C for 2 h.

Total ash (*2.4.16*)
Maximum 10.0 per cent.

ASSAY

Stock solution In a 100 mL round-bottomed flask, introduce 0.600 g of the powdered herbal drug (355) (*2.9.12*), add 1 mL of a 5 g/L solution of *hexamethylenetetramine R*, 20 mL of *acetone R* and 2 mL of *hydrochloric acid R1*. Boil the mixture under a reflux condenser for 30 min. Filter the mixture through a plug of absorbent cotton into a flask. Add the absorbent cotton to the residue in the round-bottomed flask and extract with 2 quantities, each of 20 mL, of *acetone R*, each time boiling under a reflux condenser for 10 min. Allow to cool, filter each extract through the plug of

absorbent cotton into the flask. After cooling, filter the combined acetone extracts through a filter paper into a volumetric flask and dilute to 100.0 mL with *acetone R* by rinsing the flask and the filter paper. Introduce 20.0 mL of this solution into a separating funnel, add 20 mL of *water R* and shake the mixture with 1 quantity of 15 mL and then 3 quantities, each of 10 mL, of *ethyl acetate R*. Combine the ethyl acetate extracts in a separating funnel, wash with 2 quantities, each of 50 mL, of *water R*, and filter the extracts over 10 g of *anhydrous sodium sulfate R* into a volumetric flask and dilute to 50.0 mL with *ethyl acetate R*.

Test solution To 10.0 mL of the stock solution add 1 mL of *aluminium chloride reagent R* and dilute to 25.0 mL with a 5 per cent *V/V* solution of *glacial acetic acid R* in *methanol R*.

Compensation liquid Dilute 10.0 mL of the stock solution to 25.0 mL with a 5 per cent *V/V* solution of *glacial acetic acid R* in *methanol R*.

After 30 min, measure the absorbance (*2.2.25*) of the test solution at 425 nm, by comparison with the compensation liquid.

Calculate the percentage content of flavonoids, expressed as isoquercitroside, using the following expression:

$$\frac{A \times 1.25}{m}$$

i.e. taking the specific absorbance of isoquercitroside to be 500.
A = absorbance at 425 nm;
m = mass of the herbal drug to be examined, in grams.

Ph Eur

Eleutherococcus

Siberian Ginseng

(*Ph Eur monograph 1419*)

Ph Eur

DEFINITION

Dried, whole or cut underground organs of *Eleutherococcus senticosus* (Rupr. et Maxim.) Maxim.

Content: minimum 0.08 per cent for the sum of eleutheroside B (M_r 372.4) and eleutheroside E (M_r 742.7).

IDENTIFICATION

A. The rhizome is knotty, of irregular cylindrical shape, 1.5 cm to 4.0 cm in diameter; the surface is rugged, longitudinally wrinkled and greyish-brown to blackish-brown; the bark, about 2 mm thick, closely adheres to the xylem; the heartwood is light brown and the sapwood is pale yellow; the fracture shows short thin fibres in the bark and is coarsely fibrous, especially in the internal part of the xylem.
The lower surface bears numerous cylindrical and knotty roots, 3.5 cm to 15 cm long and 0.3 cm to 1.5 cm in diameter; with a smooth, greyish-brown to blackish-brown surface; the bark is about 0.5 mm thick, closely adhering to the pale yellow xylem; the fracture is slightly fibrous; in places where the outer layer has been removed, the outer surface is yellowish-brown.

B. Reduce to a powder (355) (*2.9.12*). The powder is yellowish-brown. Examine under a microscope, using *chloral hydrate solution R*. The powder shows numerous groups of thick-walled, lignified fibres; fragments of reticulate and bordered pitted vessels with a wide lumen; groups of secretory canals, up to 20 μm in diameter with brown contents; parenchymatous cells containing cluster crystals of calcium oxalate 10 μm to 50 μm in diameter. Examine under a microscope, using a 50 per cent *V/V* solution of *glycerol R*. The powder shows small starch granules, rounded to slightly angular in outline, single compounds or with 2 or 3 components.

C. Thin-layer chromatography (*2.2.27*).

Test solution   To 1.0 g of the powdered drug (355) (*2.9.12*) add 10 mL of *alcohol (50 per cent V/V) R* and boil under reflux for 1 h. Cool and filter. Evaporate the filtrate to dryness on a water-bath. Dissolve the residue in 2.5 mL of a mixture of 5 volumes of *water R* and 20 volumes of *alcohol (50 per cent V/V) R* and filter.

Reference solution   Dissolve 2.0 mg of *esculin R* and 2.0 mg of *catalpol R* in 20 mL of a mixture of 2 volumes of *water R* and 8 volumes of *alcohol (50 per cent V/V) R*.

Plate   *TLC silica gel plate R*.

Mobile phase   *water R, methanol R, methylene chloride R* (4:30:70 *V/V/V*).

Application   20 μL, as bands.

Development   Over a path of 10 cm.

Drying   In air.

Detection A   Examine in ultraviolet light at 365 nm.

Results A   The chromatogram obtained with the reference solution shows in the upper half a blue fluorescent zone (esculin).

Detection B   Spray with *anisaldehyde solution R* and examine in daylight while heating at 100-105 °C for 5-10 min.

Results B   See below the sequence of the zones present in the chromatograms obtained with the reference solution and the test solution. Furthermore, other faint zones are present in the chromatogram obtained with the test solution.

Top of the plate	
	A brown zone (eleutheroside B)
Esculin: a blue fluorescent zone (marked at 365 nm)	
	A reddish-brown zone (eleutheroside E)
———	———
Catalpol: a violet-brown zone	
———	———
	2 brown zones
Reference solution	**Test solution**

TESTS

Foreign matter (*2.8.2*)
Maximum 3 per cent.

Loss on drying (*2.2.32*)
Maximum 10.0 per cent, determined on 1.000 g of the powdered drug (355) (*2.9.12*) by drying in an oven at 105 °C for 2 h.

Total ash (*2.4.16*)
Maximum 8.0 per cent.

ASSAY

Liquid chromatography (*2.2.29*).

Test solution   To 0.500 g of the powdered drug (355) (*2.9.12*) in a 100 mL round-bottomed flask, add 30 mL of a mixture of equal volumes of *alcohol R* and *water R*. Heat in a

water-bath at 60 °C for 30 min. Allow to cool and filter through a sintered-glass filter (*2.1.2*). Collect the liquid in a 250 mL round-bottomed flask. Repeat this operation twice, using the residue obtained in the filtration step instead of the powdered drug. Add both fractions of supernatant liquid to the 250 mL round-bottomed flask. Evaporate under reduced pressure until about 10 mL of supernatant liquid is left in the flask. Transfer the supernatant liquid quantitatively to a 20.0 mL volumetric flask and dilute to 20.0 mL with a mixture of equal volumes of *alcohol R* and *water R*. Filter through a nylon filter (pore size 0.45 μm).

Reference solution (a)   Dissolve 10 mg of *ferulic acid R* in a mixture of equal volumes of *methanol R* and *water R* and dilute to 20.0 mL with the same mixture of solvents.

Reference solution (b)   Dissolve 10 mg of *caffeic acid R* in a mixture of equal volumes of *methanol R* and *water R* and dilute to 20.0 mL with the same mixture of solvents.

Reference solution (c)   Transfer 1 mL of reference solution (a) to a 25 mL volumetric flask and dilute to 25.0 mL with a mixture of equal volumes of *methanol R* and *water R*. Filter through a nylon filter (pore size 0.45 μm).

Reference solution (d)   Transfer 1 mL of reference solution (a) and 1 mL of reference solution (b) in a mixture of equal volumes of *methanol R* and *water R* and dilute to 25.0 mL with the same mixture of solvents. Filter through a nylon filter (pore size 0.45 μm).

Precolumn:
— *size: l* = 4 mm, Ø = 4.6 mm,
— *stationary phase: octadecylsilyl silica gel for chromatography R* (5 μm).

Column:
— *size: l* = 0.25 m, Ø = 4.6 mm,
— *stationary phase: octadecylsilyl silica gel for chromatography R* (5 μm).

Mobile phase:
— *mobile phase A: phosphoric acid R, water R* (0.5:99.5 *V/V*),
— *mobile phase B: acetonitrile for chromatography R*,

Time (min)	Mobile phase A (per cent *V/V*)	Mobile phase B (per cent *V/V*)
0 - 5	90	10
5 - 27	90 → 80	10 → 20
27 - 30	80 → 50	20 → 50
30 - 35	50	50

Flow rate   1.0 mL/min.

Detection   Spectrophotometer at 220 nm.

Injection   20 μL of the test solution and reference solutions (c) and (d).

Retention time   Eleutheroside B = about 10 min; eleutheroside E = about 22 min.

Locate the peaks due to eleutheroside B and eleutheroside E using the UV spectra shown in Figures 1419.-1 and 1419.-2.

System suitability   Reference solution (d):
— *resolution*: minimum 15 between the peaks due to caffeic acid and ferulic acid.

Calculate the total percentage content of eleutheroside B and eleutheroside E from the expression:

$$\frac{(A_B \times C \times 0.73 \times 2)}{(A_R \times m)} + \frac{(A_E \times C \times 1.90 \times 2)}{(A_R \times m)}$$

A_B = area of the peak due to eleutheroside B in the chromatogram obtained with the test solution,

A_E = area of the peak due to eleutheroside E in the chromatogram obtained with the test solution,

A_R = area of the peak due to ferulic acid in the chromatogram obtained with reference solution (c),

C = concentration of ferulic acid in reference solution (c), in micrograms per millilitre,

m = mass of the drug to be examined, in milligrams.

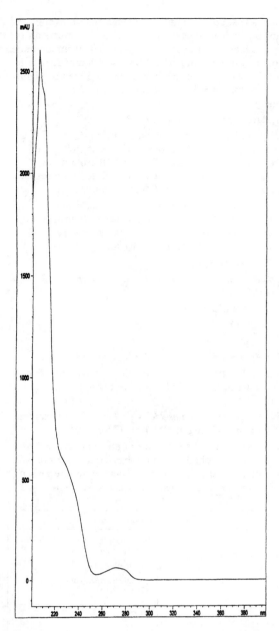

Figure 1419.-2. – *UV spectrum of eleutheroside E for the assay of eleutherococcus*

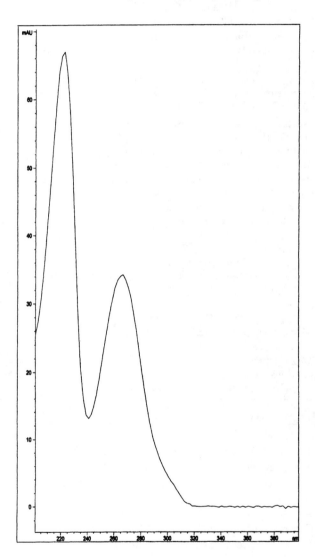

Figure 1419.-1. – *UV spectrum of eleutheroside B for the assay of eleutherococcus*

Ephedra Herb

(Ph Eur monograph 2451)

Ph Eur _____

Top of the plate	
_____ 2-Indanamine: a purple spot	 A purple spot may be present _____
_____ Ephedrine: a purple spot at the border between the middle and lower thirds	A purple spot (ephedrine) at the border between the middle and lower thirds
Reference solution	**Test solution**

DEFINITION

Dried herbaceous stem of *Ephedra sinica* Stapf, *Ephedra intermedia* Schrenk et C.A.Mey. or *Ephedra equisetina* Bunge.

Content

Minimum 1.0 per cent of ephedrine ($C_{10}H_{15}NO$; M_r 165.2) (dried drug).

IDENTIFICATION

A. Thin cylindrical pale green or yellowish-green stems up to 30 cm long and 1-3 mm in diameter; longitudinally striated and slightly rough; internodes varying in length between 1 cm and 6 cm; opposite and decussate leaves reduced to sheaths surrounding the stem, carrying diminutive laminae 1.5-4 mm long with 2 lobes (rarely 3), acutely triangular, apex greyish-white, base tubular and reddish-brown or blackish-brown. Fracture slightly fibrous.

B. Reduce to a powder (355) *(2.9.12)*. The powder is greenish-yellow. Examine under a microscope using *chloral hydrate solution R*. The powder shows the following diagnostic characters: fragments of the epidermis, in surface view, composed of rectangular cells and numerous stomata with a small depression at each end, the guard cells large and broadly elliptical; epidermal fragments, in transverse section, showing a thick cuticle and some of the cells extended to form projections; fibres in groups or single, with thick, usually lignified walls; fragments of lignified tissue composed of small, bordered-pitted tracheids, vessels with spiral thickening and groups of sclereids; groups of parenchyma, some with thickened and pitted walls; scattered prism crystals of calcium oxalate.

C. Thin-layer chromatography *(2.2.27)*.

Test solution   To 0.2 g of the powdered drug (355) *(2.9.12)* add 0.5 mL of *concentrated ammonia R* and 10 mL of *methylene chloride R*. Boil in a water-bath under a reflux condenser for 1 h. Allow to cool, filter and evaporate the filtrate to dryness; dissolve the residue in 2 mL of *methanol R*.

Reference solution   Dissolve 1 mg of *ephedrine hydrochloride CRS* and 1 mg of *2-indanamine hydrochloride R* in 2 mL of *methanol R*.

Plate   *TLC silica gel plate R* (5-40 µm) [or *TLC silica gel plate R* (2-10 µm)].

Mobile phase   concentrated ammonia R, methanol R, methylene chloride R (0.5:5:20 *V/V/V*).

Application   10 µL [or 1 µL] as spots with a diameter of 5 mm [or 2 mm].

Development   Over a path of 10 cm [or 6 cm].

Drying   In air.

Detection   Spray with a 2 g/L solution of *ninhydrin R* in *ethanol (96 per cent) R*; heat at 110 °C for 10 min and examine immediately in daylight.

Results   See below the sequence of spots present in the chromatograms obtained with the reference solution and the test solution. Furthermore, other faint spots may be present in the chromatogram obtained with the test solution.

TESTS

Loss on drying *(2.2.32)*

Maximum 10.0 per cent, determined on 1.000 g of the powdered drug (355) *(2.9.12)* by drying in an oven at 105 °C for 2 h.

Total ash *(2.4.16)*

Maximum 9.0 per cent.

ASSAY

Liquid chromatography *(2.2.29)*.

Test solution   To 0.200 g of the powdered drug (355) *(2.9.12)* add 25.0 mL of *methanol R*, weigh and sonicate for 45 min. Allow to cool, weigh and adjust to the original mass with *methanol R*, shake well and filter. Transfer 1.0 mL of the filtrate to a small column (1 cm in diameter) packed with 1.50 g of *neutral aluminium oxide R* (60-210 µm). Elute with a mixture of equal volumes of *methanol R* and *water R*. Collect about 9 mL of the eluate, add 0.5 mL of *phosphoric acid R* and dilute to 10.0 mL with a mixture of equal volumes of *methanol R* and *water R*.

Reference solution (a)   Dissolve 10.0 mg of *ephedrine hydrochloride CRS* in *methanol R* and dilute to 100.0 mL with the same solvent. Dilute 2.0 mL of the solution to 25.0 mL with the mobile phase.

Reference solution (b)   Dissolve 1 mg of *ephedrine hydrochloride CRS* and 1 mg of *terbutaline sulfate CRS* in *methanol R* and dilute to 10 mL with the same solvent. Dilute 2 mL of the solution to 25 mL with the mobile phase.

Column:
— *size: l* = 0.25 m, Ø = 4.6 mm;
— *stationary phase: octadecylsilyl silica gel for chromatography R* (5 µm).

Mobile phase   acetonitrile R1, 0.1 per cent *V/V* solution of *phosphoric acid R* (15:85 *V/V*).

Flow rate   2.0 mL/min.

Detection   Spectrophotometer at 207 nm.

Injection   10 µL.

Run time   3 times the retention time of ephedrine.

System suitability   Reference solution (b):
— *resolution*: minimum 3.5 between the peaks due to terbutaline and ephedrine.

Calculate the percentage content of ephedrine using the following expression:

$$\frac{A_1 \times m_2 \times p \times 165.2}{A_2 \times m_1 \times 5 \times 201.7}$$

A_1 = area of the peak due to ephedrine in the chromatogram obtained with the test solution;

A_2 = area of the peak due to ephedrine in the chromatogram obtained with reference solution (a);

m_1 = mass of the drug to be examined used to prepare the test solution, in grams;

m_2 = mass of *ephedrine hydrochloride CRS* used to prepare reference solution (a), in grams;

p = percentage content of ephedrine hydrochloride in *ephedrine hydrochloride CRS*.

——————— *Ph Eur*

Eucalyptus Leaf

(*Ph Eur monograph 1320*)

Ph Eur —————————————————————

DEFINITION

Whole or cut dried leaves of older branches of *Eucalyptus globulus* Labill.

Content

Minimum 20 mL/kg of essential oil for the whole drug (anhydrous drug) and minimum 15 mL/kg of essential oil for the cut drug (anhydrous drug).

CHARACTERS

Aromatic odour of cineole.

IDENTIFICATION

A. The leaves which are mainly greyish-green and relatively thick are elongated, elliptical and slightly sickle-shaped and usually up to 25 cm in length, and up to 5 cm in width. The petiole is twisted, strongly wrinkled and is 2-3 cm, rarely 5 cm, in length. The coriaceous, stiff leaves are entire and glabrous and have a yellowish-green mid rib. Lateral veins anastomose near the margin to a continuous line. The margin is even and somewhat thickened. On both surfaces are minute, irregularly distributed, warty dark brown spots. Small oil glands may be seen in transmitted light.

B. Reduce to a powder (355) (*2.9.12*). The powder is greyish-green. Examine under a microscope, using *chloral hydrate solution R*. The powder shows the following diagnostic characters: fragments of glabrous lamina with small thick-walled epidermal cells bearing a thick cuticle, numerous anomocytic stomata (*2.8.3*) of more than 80 μm in diameter and occasionally groups of brown cork cells, 300 μm in diameter and brownish-black in their centre; fragments of isobilateral mesophyll with 2-3 layers of palisade parenchyma on each side and in the centre several layers of spongy mesophyll with elongated cells with the same orientation as the palisade cells and containing prisms and cluster crystals of calcium oxalate; fragments of mesophyll containing large schizogenous oil glands.

C. Thin-layer chromatography (*2.2.27*).

Test solution   Shake 0.5 g of the freshly powdered drug (355) (*2.9.12*) with 5 mL of *toluene R* for 2-3 min and filter over about 2 g of *anhydrous sodium sulfate R*.

Reference solution   Dissolve 50 μL of *cineole R* in *toluene R* and dilute to 5 mL with the same solvent.

Plate   TLC silica gel plate R.

Mobile phase   ethyl acetate R, toluene R (10:90 *V/V*).

Application   10 μL, as bands.

Development   Over a path of 15 cm.

Drying   In air.

Detection   Spray with *anisaldehyde solution R*. Examine in daylight while heating at 100-105 °C for 5-10 min.

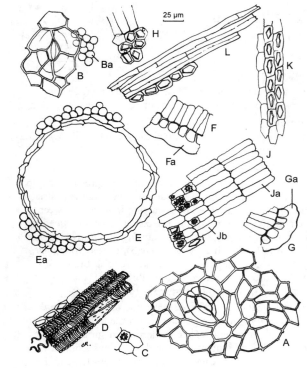

A. Thick-walled epidermal cells and anomocytic stomata, in surface view

B. Thick-walled epidermal cells and anomocytic stomata, with attached palisade parenchyma (Ba), in surface view

C. Parenchyma cells with cluster crystal of calcium oxalate

D. Vascular tissue

E. Schizogenous oil gland with attached palisade parenchyma (Ea)

F and G. Epidermis covered by a thick cuticle (Fa and Ga), in transverse section

H and J. Palisade parenchyma (Ja) with attached spongy mesophyll (Jb) containing prisms and cluster crystals of calcium oxalate

K. Cells containing prisms of calcium oxalate

L. Fibres

Figure 1320.-1. – *Illustration of powdered herbal drug of eucalyptus leaf (see Identification B)*

Results   The chromatogram obtained with the reference solution shows in the middle a zone due to cineole.

The main zone in the chromatogram obtained with the test solution is similar in position and colour to the zone due to cineole in the chromatogram obtained with the reference solution, it also shows an intense violet zone (hydrocarbons) near the solvent front and there may also be other fainter zones.

TESTS

Foreign matter (*2.8.2*)

Maximum 3 per cent of dark and brown leaves, maximum 5 per cent of stems and maximum 2 per cent of other foreign matter. Cordate or ovate sessile leaves of young branches, with numerous glands on both sides, visible as points in transmitted light, are not present. Determine by using 30 g of the drug to be examined.

Water (*2.2.13*)

Maximum 100 mL/kg, determined on 20.0 g of powdered drug (355) (*2.9.12*).

Total ash (*2.4.16*)

Maximum 6.0 per cent.

ASSAY

Carry out the determination of essential oil in herbal drugs (*2.8.12*). Use 10.0 g of the drug, cut immediately before determination, a 500 mL round-bottomed flask, 200 mL of *water R* and 100 mL of *glycerol R* as the distillation liquid and 0.5 mL of *xylene R* in the graduated tube. Distil at a rate of 2-3 mL/min for 2 h.

—————————————————— Ph Eur

Eucalyptus Oil

(Ph Eur monograph 0390)

Ph Eur _____

DEFINITION
Essential oil obtained by steam distillation and rectification from the fresh leaves or the fresh terminal branchlets of various species of *Eucalyptus* rich in 1,8-cineole. The species mainly used are *Eucalyptus globulus* Labill., *Eucalyptus polybractea* R.T.Baker and *Eucalyptus smithii* R.T.Baker.

CHARACTERS
Appearance
Colourless or pale yellow liquid.

Odour
Reminiscent of 1,8-cineole.

IDENTIFICATION
First identification   B.

Second identification   A.

A. Thin-layer chromatography (*2.2.27*).

Test solution   Dissolve 0.1 g of the oil to be examined in *toluene R* and dilute to 10 mL with the same solvent.

Reference solution   Dissolve 20 µL of α-*terpineol R* and 50 µL of *cineole R* in *toluene R* and dilute to 5 mL with the same solvent.

Plate   *TLC silica gel plate R* (5-40 µm) [or *TLC silica gel plate R* (2-10 µm)].

Mobile phase   ethyl acetate R, toluene R (10:90 V/V).

Application   10 µL [or 2 µL] as bands of 10 mm [or 6 mm].

Development   Over a path of 15 cm [or 6 cm].

Drying   In air.

Detection   Spray with *anisaldehyde solution R* and heat at 100-105 °C for 5-10 min; examine in daylight.

Results   See below the sequence of zones present in the chromatograms obtained with the reference solution and the test solution. Furthermore, other faint zones may be present in the chromatogram obtained with the test solution, near the solvent front and at the level of α-terpineol.

Top of the plate	
—	—
1,8-Cineole: a violet-brown zone	An intense violet-brown zone (1,8-cineole)
—	—
α-Terpineol: a violet-brown zone	
Reference solution	**Test solution**

B. Examine the chromatograms obtained in the test for chromatographic profile.

Results   The characteristic peaks due to α-pinene, β-pinene, α-phellandrene, limonene and 1,8-cineole in the chromatogram obtained with the test solution are similar in retention time to those in the chromatogram obtained with

reference solution (a). Sabinene and camphor may be present in the chromatogram obtained with the test solution.

TESTS
Relative density (*2.2.5*)
0.906 to 0.927.

Refractive index (*2.2.6*)
1.458 to 1.470.

Optical rotation (*2.2.7*)
0° to + 10°.

Solubility in alcohol (*2.8.10*)
It is soluble in 5 volumes of *ethanol (70 per cent V/V) R*.

Aldehydes
To 10 mL in a ground-glass-stoppered tube 25 mm in diameter and 150 mm long, add 5 mL of *toluene R* and 4 mL of *alcoholic hydroxylamine solution R*. Shake vigorously and titrate immediately with *0.5 M potassium hydroxide* in alcohol (60 per cent V/V) until the red colour changes to yellow. Continue the titration with shaking; the end-point is reached when the pure yellow colour of the indicator is permanent in the lower layer after shaking vigorously for 2 min and allowing separation to take place. The reaction is complete in about 15 min. Repeat the titration using a further 10 mL of the substance to be examined and, as a reference solution for the end-point, the titrated liquid from the 1st determination to which has been added 0.5 mL of *0.5 M potassium hydroxide* in alcohol (60 per cent V/V). Not more than 2.0 mL of *0.5 M potassium hydroxide* in *alcohol (60 per cent V/V)* is required in the 2nd titration.

Chromatographic profile
Gas chromatography (*2.2.28*): use the normalisation procedure.

Test solution   Dissolve 200 µL of the oil to be examined in *heptane R* and dilute to 10.0 mL with the same solvent.

Reference solution (a)   Dissolve 10 µL of α-*pinene R*, 5 µL of β-*pinene R*, 5 µL of *sabinene R*, 5 µL of α-*phellandrene R*, 10 µL of *limonene R*, 50 µL of *cineole R* and 5 mg of *camphor R* in *heptane R* and dilute to 10 mL with the same solvent.

Reference solution (b)   Dissolve 5 µL of *limonene R* in *heptane R* and dilute to 50.0 mL with the same solvent. Dilute 0.5 mL of the solution to 5.0 mL with *heptane R*.

Column:
— *material*: fused silica;
— *size*: l = 60 m, Ø = about 0.25 mm;
— *stationary phase*: macrogol 20 000 R (film thickness 0.25 µm).

Carrier gas   helium for chromatography R.

Flow rate   1.5 mL/min.

Split ratio   1:50.

Temperature:

	Time (min)	Temperature (°C)
Column	0 - 5	60
	5 - 33	60 → 200
	33 - 38	200
Injection port		220
Detector		220

Detection   Flame ionisation.

Injection   1 µL.

Elution order   Order indicated in the composition of reference solution (a). Record the retention times of these substances.

System suitability   Reference solution (a):
— *resolution*: minimum 1.5 between the peaks due to limonene and cineole.

Identification of components   Using the retention times determined from the chromatogram obtained with reference solution (a), locate the components of reference solution (a) in the chromatogram obtained with the test solution.

Determine the percentage content of each of these components. The percentages are within the following ranges:
— *α-pinene*: 0.05 per cent to 10.0 per cent;
— *β-pinene*: 0.05 per cent to 1.5 per cent;
— *sabinene*: maximum 0.3 per cent;
— *α-phellandrene*: 0.05 per cent to 1.5 per cent;
— *limonene*: 0.05 per cent to 15.0 per cent;
— *1,8-cineole*: minimum 70.0 per cent;
— *camphor*: maximum 0.1 per cent;
— *disregard limit*: the area of the principal peak in the chromatogram obtained with reference solution (b) (0.05 per cent).

STORAGE

At a temperature not exceeding 25 °C.

———————————————————————— *Ph Eur*

Bitter Fennel

(Ph Eur monograph 0824)

Ph Eur ————————————————————————

DEFINITION

Dry cremocarps and mericarps of *Foeniculum vulgare* Mill. ssp. *vulgare* var. *vulgare*.

Content:
— *essential oil*: minimum 40 mL/kg (anhydrous drug);
— *anethole*: minimum 60.0 per cent in the essential oil;
— *fenchone*: minimum 15.0 per cent in the essential oil.

CHARACTERS

Bitter fennel is greenish-brown, brown or green.

IDENTIFICATION

A. The fruit of bitter fennel is a cremocarp, of almost cylindrical shape with a rounded base and a narrower summit crowned with a large stylopod. It is generally 3-12 mm long and 3-4 mm wide. The mericarps, usually free, are glabrous. Each bears 5 prominent, slightly carenated ridges. When cut transversely, 4 vittae on the dorsal surface and 2 on the commissural surface may be seen with a lens.

B. Microscopic examination (2.8.23). The powder is greyish-brown or greyish-yellow. Examine under a microscope using *chloral hydrate solution R*. The powder shows the following diagnostic characters (Figure 0824.-1): yellow fragments of wide secretory canals, often made up of yellowish-brown-walled polygonal secretory cells [D, H]; reticulate parenchyma of the mesocarp [B]; numerous fibre bundles [G] from the ridges [Ga], often accompanied by narrow spiral vessels [Gb]; very numerous endosperm fragments [F] containing aleurone grains [Fb] and very small cluster crystals of calcium oxalate [Fa]; some fibre bundles from the carpophore [E]; fragments of the endocarp, in surface view [A, K], consisting of thin-walled, transversely elongated cells,

2-9 μm wide, having a parquetry arrangement, sometimes accompanied by the inner layer of the mesocarp [Aa]; fragments of the epicarp with stomata accompanied by oil droplets [C]; very numerous oil droplets [J].

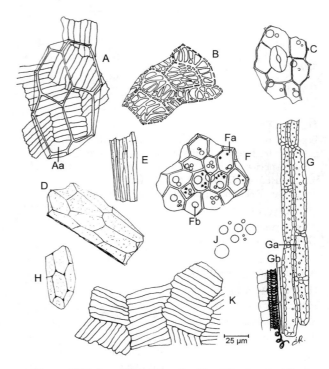

Figure 0824.-1. – *Illustration for identification test B of powdered herbal drug of bitter fennel*

C. Thin-layer chromatography (2.2.27).

Test solution   Shake 0.3 g of the freshly powdered herbal drug (1400) (2.9.12) with 5.0 mL of *methylene chloride R* for 15 min. Filter and carefully evaporate the filtrate to dryness on a water-bath at 60 °C. Dissolve the residue in 0.5 mL of *toluene R*.

Reference solution   Dissolve 50 μL of *anethole R* and 10 μL of *fenchone R* in 5.0 mL of *hexane R*.

Plate   TLC silica gel GF_{254} plate R.

Mobile phase   hexane R, toluene R (20:80 V/V).

Application   10 μL as bands of 20 mm by 3 mm.

Development   Over a path of 10 cm.

Drying   In air.

Detection A   Examine in ultraviolet light at 254 nm.

Results A   The chromatograms show in the central part a quenching zone due to anethole.

Detection B   Treat with *sulfuric acid R* and heat at 140 °C for 5-10 min until a yellow zone due to fenchone appears in the lower third of the chromatograms.

Results B   Anethole appears as a violet band in the central part; the chromatogram obtained with the test solution also shows a reddish-brown zone in its upper third (terpenes).

TESTS
Estragole
Gas chromatography (2.2.28): use the normalisation procedure.

Test solution   Dilute the mixture of essential oil and *xylene R* obtained in the determination of essential oil to 5.0 mL with *xylene R*, by rinsing the apparatus.

Reference solution   Dissolve 5 mg of *estragole R* in 0.5 mL of *xylene R*.

Column:
— *size: l* = 30-60 m, Ø = 0.3 mm;
— *stationary phase: macrogol 20 000 R.*

Carrier gas   *nitrogen for chromatography R.*

Flow rate   0.40 mL/min.

Split ratio   1:200.

Temperature:

	Time (min)	Temperature (°C)
Column	0 - 4	60
	4 - 26	60 → 170
	26 - 41	170
Injection port		220
Detector		270

Detection   Flame ionisation.

Injection   1 µL.

Limit:
— *estragole*: maximum 5.0 per cent in the essential oil obtained in the assay.

Foreign matter (*2.8.2*)
Maximum 1.5 per cent of peduncles and maximum 1.5 per cent of other foreign matter.

Water (*2.2.13*)
Maximum 100 mL/kg, determined on 20.0 g of the powdered herbal drug (710) (*2.9.12*).

Total ash (*2.4.16*)
Maximum 10.0 per cent.

ASSAY

Essential oil
Carry out the determination of essential oils in herbal drugs (*2.8.12*). Use a 500 mL round-bottomed flask and 200 mL of *water R* as the distillation liquid. Reduce the herbal drug to a coarse powder (1400) (*2.9.12*) and immediately use 5.0 g for the determination. Introduce 0.50 mL of *xylene R* in the graduated tube. Distil at a rate of 2-3 mL/min for 2 h.

Anethole and fenchone
Gas chromatography (*2.2.28*) as described in the test for estragole with the following modifications.

Reference solution   Dissolve 5 mg of *fenchone R* and 5 mg of *anethole R* in 0.5 mL of *xylene R.*

Elution order   The order indicated in the composition of the reference solution; record the retention times of these substances.

STORAGE

Protected from moisture.

_____ *Ph Eur*

Bitter-Fennel Fruit Oil

(*Ph Eur monograph 1826*)

Ph Eur ____

DEFINITION
Essential oil obtained by steam distillation from the ripe fruits of *Foeniculum vulgare* Miller, ssp. *vulgare* var. *vulgare.*

Content:
— *fenchone*: 12.0 per cent to 25.0 per cent,
— *trans*-anethole: 55.0 per cent to 75.0 per cent.

CHARACTERS

Appearance
Clear, colourless or pale yellow liquid.

Characteristic odour.

IDENTIFICATION

First identification   B.

Second identification   A.

A. Thin-layer chromatography (*2.2.27*).

Test solution   Dissolve 0.1 mL of the oil to be examined in 5 mL of *toluene R.*

Reference solution   Dissolve 10 µL of *fenchone R* and 80 µL of *anethole R* in 5 mL of *toluene R.*

Plate   TLC silica gel plate R.

Mobile phase   ethyl acetate R, toluene R (5:95 *V/V*).

Application   10 µL as bands.

Development   Over a path of 15 cm.

Drying   In air.

Detection   Spray with a freshly prepared 200 g/L solution of *phosphomolybdic acid R* in *ethanol (96 per cent) R* and heat at 150 °C for 15 min; examine in daylight.

Results   See below the sequence of the zones present in the chromatograms obtained with the reference solution and the test solution. Furthermore, other zones may be present in the chromatogram obtained with the test solution.

Top of the plate	
Anethole: a dark blue to dark violet zone	A dark blue to dark violet zone (anethole)
_____	_____
Fenchone: a blue or bluish-grey zone	A blue or bluish-grey zone (fenchone)
_____	_____
Reference solution	**Test solution**

B. Examine the chromatograms obtained in the test for chromatographic profile.

Results   The characteristic peaks in the chromatogram obtained with the test solution are similar in retention time to those in the chromatogram obtained with the reference solution.

TESTS

Relative density (*2.2.5*)
0.961 to 0.975.

Refractive index (*2.2.6*)
1.528 to 1.539.

Optical rotation (*2.2.7*)
+ 10.0° to + 24.0°.

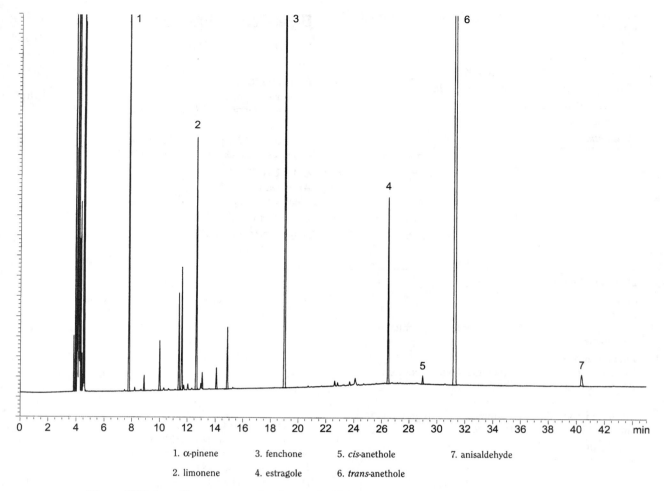

1. α-pinene   3. fenchone   5. *cis*-anethole   7. anisaldehyde

2. limonene   4. estragole   6. *trans*-anethole

Figure 1826.-1. – *Chromatogram for the test for chromatographic profile of bitter-fennel fruit oil*

Chromatographic profile

Gas chromatography (*2.2.28*): use the normalisation procedure.

Test solution   Dissolve 0.20 mL of the oil to be examined in *heptane R* and dilute to 10.0 mL with the same solvent.

Reference solution   Dissolve 20 μL of *α-pinene R*, 20 μL of *limonene R*, 50 μL of *fenchone R*, 20 μL of *estragole R*, 100 μL of *anethole R* and 20 μL of *anisaldehyde R* in *heptane R* and dilute to 10.0 mL with the same solvent.

Column:
— *material*: fused silica,
— *size*: *l* = 60 m, Ø = 0.25 mm,
— *stationary phase*: *macrogol 20 000 R* (film thickness 0.25 μm).

Carrier gas   *helium for chromatography R*.

Flow rate   1 mL/min.

Split ratio   1:200.

Detection   Flame ionisation.

Injection   1.0 μL.

Elution order   Order indicated in the composition of the reference solution. Record the retention times of these substances.

System suitability   Reference solution:
— *resolution*: minimum 5.0 between the peaks due to estragole and trans-anethole.

Temperature:

	Time (min)	Temperature (°C)
Column	0 – 4	60
	4 – 26	60 → 170
	26 – 41	170
Injection port		220
Detector		270

Using the retention times determined from the chromatogram obtained with the reference solution, locate the components of the reference solution on the chromatogram obtained with the test solution and locate *cis*-anethole using Figure 1826.-1. (Disregard the peak due to heptane).

Determine the percentage content of each of these components. The percentages are within the following ranges:
— *α-pinene*: 1.0 per cent to 10.0 per cent,
— *limonene*: 0.9 per cent to 5.0 per cent,
— *fenchone*: 12.0 per cent to 25.0 per cent,
— *estragole*: maximum 6.0 per cent,
— *cis-anethole*: maximum 0.5 per cent,
— *trans-anethole*: 55.0 per cent to 75.0 per cent,
— *anisaldehyde*: maximum 2.0 per cent.

The ratio of α-pinene content to limonene content is greater than 1.0.

STORAGE

At a temperature not exceeding 25 °C.

Ph Eur

Bitter-Fennel Herb Oil

(Ph Eur monograph 2380)

Ph Eur

DEFINITION

Essential oil obtained by steam distillation of the aerial parts of *Foeniculum vulgare* Mill. ssp. *vulgare*, var. *vulgare* collected during fruiting.

CHARACTERS

Appearance

Clear, pale or intense yellow liquid.

Anise-like odour.

IDENTIFICATION

First identification B.

Second identification A.

A. Thin-layer chromatography (*2.2.27*).

Test solution Dissolve 0.1 mL of the oil to be examined in 5 mL of *toluene R*.

Reference solution Dissolve 10 μL of *fenchone R* and 40 μL of *anethole R* in 5 mL of *toluene R*.

Plate TLC silica gel plate R (5-40 μm) [or *TLC silica gel plate R* (2-10 μm)].

Mobile phase ethyl acetate R, toluene R (5:95 V/V).

Application 10 μL [or 3 μL] as bands of 10 mm [or 8 mm].

Development Over a path of 8 cm [or 6 cm].

Drying In air.

Detection Spray with a freshly prepared 200 g/L solution of *phosphomolybdic acid R* in *ethanol (96 per cent) R* and heat at 150 °C for 15 min; examine in daylight.

Results See below the sequence of zones present in the chromatograms obtained with the reference solution and the test solution. Furthermore, other faint zones may be present in the chromatogram obtained with the test solution.

Top of the plate	
Anethole: a dark blue or dark violet zone	A dark blue or dark violet zone (anethole)
_____	_____
Fenchone: a blue or bluish-grey zone	A sometimes faint blue or bluish-grey zone (fenchone)
_____	_____
Reference solution	**Test solution**

B. Examine the chromatograms obtained in the test for chromatographic profile.

Results:

— *Spanish type*: the characteristic peaks due to α-pinene, β-pinene, β-myrcene, α-phellandrene, limonene, fenchone, estragole and *trans*-anethole in the chromatogram obtained with the test solution are similar in retention time to those in the chromatogram obtained with reference solution (a);

— *Tasmanian type*: the characteristic peaks due to α-pinene, α-phellandrene, limonene, fenchone, estragole and *trans*-anethole in the chromatogram obtained with the test solution are similar in retention time to those in the chromatogram obtained with reference solution (a).

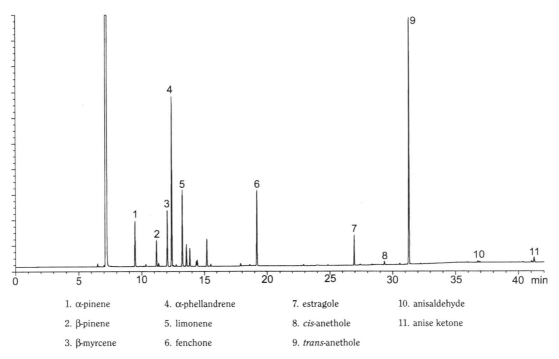

1. α-pinene
2. β-pinene
3. β-myrcene
4. α-phellandrene
5. limonene
6. fenchone
7. estragole
8. *cis*-anethole
9. *trans*-anethole
10. anisaldehyde
11. anise ketone

Figure 2380.-1. – *Chromatogram for the test for chromatographic profile of Spanish-type bitter-fennel herb oil*

TESTS

Relative density (*2.2.5*):
— *Spanish type*: 0.877 to 0.921;
— *Tasmanian type*: 0.940 to 0.973.

Refractive index (*2.2.6*):
— *Spanish type*: 1.487 to 1.501;
— *Tasmanian type*: 1.512 to 1.538.

Optical rotation (*2.2.7*):
— *Spanish type*: + 42° to + 68°;
— *Tasmanian type* + 11° to + 35°.

Solubility in alcohol (*2.8.10*):
— *Spanish type*: 1 volume is soluble in 2 volumes and more of *ethanol (90 per cent V/V) R*;
— *Tasmanian type*: 1 volume is soluble in 10 volumes and more of *ethanol (85 per cent V/V) R*.

Chromatographic profile

Gas chromatography (*2.2.28*): use the normalisation procedure.

Test solution Dissolve 0.20 mL of the oil to be examined in *acetone R* and dilute to 10.0 mL with the same solvent.

Reference solution (a) Dissolve 20 µL of *α-pinene R*, 10 µL of *β-pinene R*, 20 µL of *β-myrcene R*, 20 µL of *α-phellandrene R*, 20 µL of *limonene R*, 40 µL of *fenchone R*, 10 µL of *estragole R*, 40 µL of *anethole R*, 10 µL of *anisaldehyde R* and 10 µL of *anise ketone R* in *acetone R* and dilute to 10.0 mL with the same solvent.

Reference solution (b) Dissolve 5 µL of *anethole R* in 25.0 mL of *acetone R*. Dilute 0.5 mL of this solution to 20.0 mL with *acetone R*.

Column:
— *material*: fused silica;
— *size*: l = 60 m, Ø = 0.25 mm;
— *stationary phase*: *macrogol 20 000 R* (film thickness 0.25 µm).

Carrier gas *helium for chromatography R*.

Flow rate 1 mL/min.

Split ratio 1:50.

Temperature:

	Time (min)	Temperature (°C)
Column	0 - 35	70 → 210
	35 - 42	210
Injection port		250
Detector		270

Detection Flame ionisation.

Injection 1 µL.

Elution order Order indicated in the composition of the reference solution; record the retention times of these substances.

System suitability Reference solution (a):
— *resolution*: minimum 1.5 between the peaks due to β-myrcene and α-phellandrene.

Using the chromatogram obtained with the reference solution, locate the relevant components for the type of the essential oil to be examined in the chromatogram obtained with the test solution, and locate *cis*-anethole using Figures 2380.-1 and 2380.-2.

Determine the percentage content of each of these components.

For Spanish-type bitter-fennel herb oil, the percentages are within the following ranges:
— *α-pinene*: 2.0 to 8.0 per cent;
— *β-pinene*: 1.0 to 4.0 per cent;
— *β-myrcene*: 1.0 to 12.0 per cent;
— *α-phellandrene*: 1.0 to 25.0 per cent;
— *limonene*: 8.0 to 30.0 per cent;
— *fenchone*: 7.0 to 16.0 per cent;

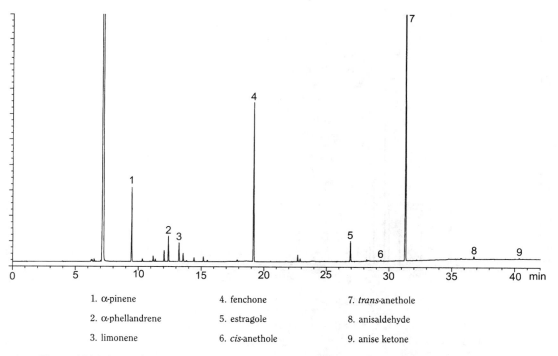

1. α-pinene
2. α-phellandrene
3. limonene
4. fenchone
5. estragole
6. *cis*-anethole
7. *trans*-anethole
8. anisaldehyde
9. anise ketone

Figure 2380.-2. – Chromatogram for the test for chromatographic profile of Tasmanian-type bitter-fennel herb oil

— *estragole*: 2.0 to 7.0 per cent;
— *cis-anethole*: maximum 0.5 per cent;
— *trans-anethole*: 15.0 to 40.0 per cent;
— *anisaldehyde*: maximum 1.0 per cent;
— *anise ketone*: maximum 0.05 per cent;
— *disregard limit*: the area of the principal peak in the chromatogram obtained with reference solution (b) (0.025 per cent).

For Tasmanian-type bitter-fennel herb oil, the percentages are within the following ranges:
— α-*pinene*: 2.0 to 11.0 per cent;
— α-*phellandrene*: 1.0 to 8.5 per cent;
— *limonene*: 1.0 to 6.0 per cent;
— *fenchone*: 10.0 to 25.0 per cent;
— *estragole*: 1.5 to 6.0 per cent;
— *cis-anethole*: maximum 0.5 per cent;
— *trans-anethole*: 45.0 to 78.0 per cent;
— *anisaldehyde*: maximum 1.0 per cent;
— *anise ketone*: maximum 0.05 per cent;
— *disregard limit*: the area of the principal peak in the chromatogram obtained with reference solution (b) (0.025 per cent).

STORAGE
At a temperature not exceeding 25 °C.

LABELLING
The label states that the content is Spanish-type or Tasmanian-type.

——————————————————————— *Ph Eur*

Sweet Fennel

(Ph Eur monograph 0825)

Ph Eur ————

DEFINITION
Dry cremocarps and mericarps of *Foeniculum vulgare* Mill. subsp. *vulgare* var. *dulce* (Mill.) Batt. & Trab.

Content:
— *essential oil*: minimum 20 mL/kg (anhydrous drug);
— *anethole*: minimum 80.0 per cent in the essential oil.

CHARACTERS
Sweet fennel is pale green or pale yellowish-brown.

IDENTIFICATION
A. The fruit of sweet fennel is a cremocarp of almost cylindrical shape with a rounded base and a narrowed summit crowned with a large stylopod. It is generally 3-12 mm long and 3-4 mm wide. The mericarps, usually free, are glabrous. Each bears 5 prominent, slightly carenated ridges. When cut transversely, 4 vittae on the dorsal surface and 2 on the commissural surface may be seen with a lens.

B. Microscopic examination (*2.8.23*). The powder is greyish-brown or greyish-yellow. Examine under a microscope using *chloral hydrate solution R*. The powder shows the following diagnostic characters (Figure 0825.-1.): yellow fragments of wide secretory canals, often made up of yellowish-brown-walled polygonal secretory cells [D, H]; reticulate parenchyma of the mesocarp [B]; numerous fibre bundles [G] from the ridges [Ga], often accompanied by narrow spiral vessels [Gb]; very numerous endosperm fragments [F] containing aleurone grains [Fb] and very small calcium oxalate cluster crystals [Fa]; some fibre bundles from the carpophore [E]; fragments of the endocarp, in surface view

[K, A], consisting of thin-walled, transversely elongated cells 2-9 μm wide, having a parquetry arrangement, sometimes accompanied by the inner layer of the mesocarp [Aa]; fragments of the epicarp with stomata accompanied by oil droplets [C]; very numerous oil droplets [J].

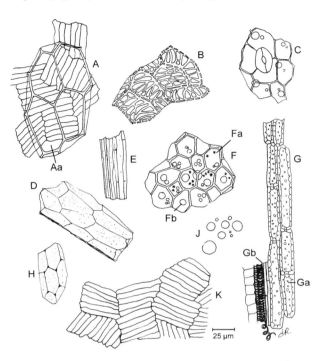

Figure 0825.-1. – *Illustration for identification test B of powdered herbal drug of sweet fennel*

C. Thin-layer chromatography (*2.2.27*).

Test solution   Shake 0.3 g of the freshly powdered herbal drug (1400) (*2.9.12*) with 5.0 mL of *methylene chloride R* for 15 min. Filter and carefully evaporate the filtrate to dryness on a water-bath at 60 °C. Dissolve the residue in 0.5 mL of *toluene R*.

Reference solution   Dissolve 60 μL of *anethole R* in 5.0 mL of *hexane R*.

Plate   TLC silica gel GF$_{254}$ plate R.

Mobile phase   hexane R, toluene R (20:80 *V/V*).

Application   10 μL as bands of 20 mm by 3 mm.

Development   Over a path of 10 cm.

Drying   In air.

Detection A   Examine in ultraviolet light at 254 nm.

Results A   The chromatograms show in the central part a quenching zone due to anethole.

Detection B   Spray with *sulfuric acid R* and heat at 140 °C for 5 min; examine in daylight.

Results B   The chromatograms show in the central part a violet band due to anethole; the chromatogram obtained with the test solution also shows a reddish-brown zone in the upper third (terpenes).

TESTS
Estragole and fenchone
Gas chromatography (*2.2.28*): use the normalisation procedure.

Test solution   Dilute the mixture of essential oil and *xylene R* obtained in the assay of essential oil to 5.0 mL with *xylene R*, by rinsing the apparatus.

Reference solution Dissolve 5 mg of *estragole R* and 5 mg of *fenchone R* in 0.5 mL of *xylene R*.

Column:
— *size: l* = 30-60 m, Ø = 0.3 mm;
— *stationary phase:* macrogol 20 000 R.

Carrier gas nitrogen for chromatography R.

Flow rate 0.40 mL/min.

Split ratio 1:200.

	Time (min)	Temperature (°C)
Column	0 - 4	60
	4 - 26	60 → 170
	26 - 41	170
Injection port		220
Detector		270

Detection Flame ionisation.

Injection 1 µL.

Limits:
— *estragole*: maximum 10.0 per cent in the essential oil;
— *fenchone*: maximum 7.5 per cent in the essential oil.

Foreign matter (*2.8.2*)
Maximum 1.5 per cent of peduncles and maximum 1.5 per cent of other foreign matter.

Water (*2.2.13*)
Maximum 80 mL/kg, determined on 20.0 g of the powdered herbal drug (710) (*2.9.12*).

Total ash (*2.4.16*)
Maximum 10.0 per cent.

ASSAY

Essential oil (*2.8.12*)
Use 10.0 g of the herbal drug reduced to a coarse powder (1400) (*2.9.12*) immediately before the assay, a 500 mL round-bottomed flask, 200 mL of *water R* as the distillation liquid, and 0.50 mL of *xylene R* in the graduated tube. Distil at a rate of 2-3 mL/min for 2 h.

Anethole
Gas chromatography (*2.2.28*) as described in the test for estragole and fenchone with the following modification.

Reference solution Dissolve 5 mg of *anethole R* in 0.5 mL of *xylene R*.

STORAGE
Protected from moisture.

———————— *Ph Eur*

Fenugreek

(*Ph Eur monograph 1323*)

Ph Eur ————————

DEFINITION
Dried, ripe seeds of *Trigonella foenum-graecum* L.

CHARACTERS
Strong characteristic aromatic odour.

IDENTIFICATION
A. The seed is hard, flattened, brown or reddish-brown and more or less rhomboidal with rounded edges. It is 3-5 mm long, 2-3 mm wide and 1.5-2 mm thick. The widest surfaces are marked by a groove that divides the seed into 2 unequal parts. The smaller part contains the radicle; the larger part contains the cotyledons.

B. Reduce to a powder (355) (*2.9.12*). The powder is yellowish-brown. Examine under a microscope using *chloral hydrate solution R*. The powder shows the following diagnostic characters: fragments of the testa in sectional view with thick cuticle covering lageniform epidermal cells, with an underlying hypodermis of large cells, narrower at the upper end and constricted in the middle, with bar-like thickenings of the radial walls; yellowish-brown fragments of the epidermis in surface view, composed of small, polygonal cells with thickened and pitted walls, frequently associated with the hypodermal cells, circular in outline with thickened and closely beaded walls; fragments of the hypodermis viewed from below, composed of polygonal cells whose bar-like thickenings extend to the upper and lower walls; parenchyma of the testa with elongated, rectangular cells with slightly thickened and beaded walls; fragments of endosperm with irregularly thickened, sometimes elongated cells, containing mucilage.

C. Thin-layer chromatography (*2.2.27*).

Test solution Place 1.0 g of the powdered drug (710) (*2.9.12*) in a 25 mL conical flask and add 5.0 mL of *methanol R*. Heat in a water-bath at 65 °C for 5 min. Cool and filter.

Reference solution Dissolve 3.0 mg of *trigonelline hydrochloride R* in 1.0 mL of *methanol R*.

Plate TLC silica gel F254 plate R.

Mobile phase water R, methanol R (30:70 *V/V*).

Application 20 µL of the test solution and 10 µL of the reference solution, as bands.

Development Over a path of 10 cm.

Drying In air.

Detection A Examine in ultraviolet light at 254 nm.

Results A The chromatogram obtained with the test solution shows in its lower half a quenching zone similar in position and fluorescence to the zone in the chromatogram obtained with the reference solution.

Detection B Spray with *potassium iodobismuthate solution R2*.

Results B The chromatogram obtained with the test solution shows an intense orange-red zone similar in position and colour to the zone in the chromatogram obtained with the reference solution. It also shows in its upper half, a broad light brownish-yellow zone (triglycerides).

TESTS

Loss on drying (*2.2.32*)
Maximum 12.0 per cent, determined on 1.000 g of the powdered drug by drying in an oven at 105 °C for 2 h.

Total ash (*2.4.16*)
Maximum 5.0 per cent.

Swelling index (*2.8.4*)
Minimum 6, determined on the powdered drug (710) (*2.9.12*).

———————— *Ph Eur*

Feverfew

(Ph Eur monograph 1516)

Ph Eur _____

DEFINITION

Dried, whole or fragmented aerial parts of *Tanacetum parthenium* (L) Schultz Bip.

Content

Minimum 0.20 per cent of parthenolide ($C_{15}H_{20}O_3$; M_r 248.3) (dried drug).

CHARACTERS

Camphoraceous odour.

IDENTIFICATION

A. The leafy, more or less branched stem has a diameter of up to 5 mm; it is almost quadrangular, channelled longitudinally and slightly pubescent. The leaves are ovate, 2-5 cm long, sometimes up to 10 cm, yellowish-green, petiolate and alternate. They are pinnate or bipinnate, deeply divided into 5-9 segments, each with a coarsely crenate margin and an obtuse apex. Both surfaces are somewhat pubescent and the midrib is prominent on the lower surface. When present, the flowering heads are 12-22 mm in diameter with long pedicels; they are clustered into broad corymbs consisting of 5-30 flower-heads. The hemispherical involucre is 6-8 mm wide and consists of many overlapping bracts, which are rather narrow, obtuse and scarious and have membranous margins. The central flowers are yellow, hermaphrodite, tube-shaped with 5 teeth and have 5 stamens inserted in the corolla; the filaments of the stamens are separate from each other but the anthers are fused into a tube through which passes the style, bearing 2 stigmatic branches. The peripheral flowers are female and have a white, three-toothed ligule, 2-7 mm long. The fruit is an achene, 1.2-1.5 mm long, brown when ripe, with 5-10 white longitudinal ribs. It is glandular and bears a short, crenate, membranous crown.

B. Reduce to a powder (355) (*2.9.12*). The powder is yellowish-green. Examine under a microscope using *chloral hydrate solution R*. The powder shows the following diagnostic characters: numerous large, multicellular, uniseriate covering trichomes consisting of a rhomboidal basal cell, 3-5 smaller, thick-walled rectangular cells and a very long, flat, slender terminal cell, often curved at a right angle to the axis of the basal cell; glandular trichomes with a short, biseriate, 2-4 celled stalk and a biseriate head of 4 cells around which the cuticle forms a bladder-like covering; epidermal cells with very sinuous, anticlinal walls, a striated cuticle and anomocytic stomata (*2.8.3*); numerous spirally and annularly thickened vessels; stratified parenchyma and collenchyma. Fragments of disc florets containing pale yellow amorphous masses and small rosette crystals of calcium oxalate may be present; spherical pollen grains about 25 μm in diameter, with 3 pores and a spiny exine may be present.

C. Thin-layer chromatography (*2.2.27*).

Test solution   To 1 g of the powdered drug (355) (*2.9.12*) add 20 mL of *methanol R*. Heat in a water-bath at 60 °C for 15 min. Allow to cool and filter. Evaporate to dryness under reduced pressure and dissolve the residue in 2 mL of *methanol R*.

Reference solution   Dissolve 5 mg of *parthenolide R* in *methanol R* and dilute to 5 mL with the same solvent.

Plate   TLC silica gel plate R.

Mobile phase   acetone R, toluene R (15:85 *V/V*).

Application   20 μL, as bands.

Development   Over a path of 10 cm.

Drying   In air.

Detection   Spray with a 5 g/L solution of *vanillin R* in a mixture of 20 volumes of *anhydrous ethanol R* and 80 volumes of *sulfuric acid R*. Examine in daylight after 5 min.

Results   The chromatogram obtained with the test solution shows in its central part a blue principal zone that is similar in position, colour and size to the principal zone in the chromatogram obtained with the reference solution, and somewhat below the principal zone a 2nd blue zone may be present; 1 or 2 blue zones are also present in its lower third; other violet zones may be present.

TESTS

Foreign matter (*2.8.2*)

Maximum 10.0 per cent of stem with a diameter greater than 5 mm and maximum 2.0 per cent of other foreign matter.

Loss on drying (*2.2.32*)

Maximum 10.0 per cent, determined on 1.000 g of the powdered drug (355) (*2.9.12*) by drying in an oven at 105 °C for 2 h.

Total ash (*2.4.16*)

Maximum 12.0 per cent.

ASSAY

Liquid chromatography (*2.2.29*).

Test solution   Completely reduce about 50 g of the drug to be examined to a powder (355) (*2.9.12*). After homogenisation, introduce 1.00 g of the powdered drug into a flask and add 40 mL of *methanol R*. Heat in a water-bath at 60 °C for 10 min. Allow to cool and filter. Rinse the filter with 15 mL of *methanol R*. Take up the residue with 40 mL of *methanol R*. Repeat the operation. Collect the filtrates and rinsings and evaporate to dryness under reduced pressure. Take up the residue with *methanol R* and dilute to 20.0 mL with the same solvent. Dilute 10.0 mL of this solution to 50.0 mL with the mobile phase. Filter (0.45 μm).

Reference solution   Dissolve 5.0 mg of *parthenolide R* in *methanol R* and dilute to 10.0 mL with the same solvent. Dilute 2.0 mL of this solution to 50.0 mL with the mobile phase.

Column:
— *size*: l = 0.25 m, Ø = 4.6 mm;
— *stationary phase*: octadecylsilyl silica gel for chromatography R (5 μm).

Mobile phase   acetonitrile R, water R (40:60 *V/V*).

Flow rate   1 mL/min.

Detection   Spectrophotometer at 220 nm.

Injection   20 μL.

Retention time   Parthenolide = about 11.5 min.

Calculate the percentage content of parthenolide using the following expression:

$$\frac{A_1 \times m_2 \times 40}{A_2 \times m_1}$$

A_1 = area of the peak due to parthenolide in the chromatogram obtained with the test solution;

A_2 = area of the peak due to parthenolide in the chromatogram obtained with the reference solution;

m_1 = mass of the drug to be examined in the test solution, in grams;

m_2 = mass of parthenolide in the reference solution, in grams.

_____ *Ph Eur*

Fig

DEFINITION

The sun-dried succulent fruit of *Ficus carica* L.

CHARACTERISTICS

Odour, pleasantly fruity; taste, sweet.

Macroscopical Fruit compound: soft, fleshy, brown or yellowish brown, sometimes covered with a saccharine efflorescence; at the summit a small opening surrounded by scales and at the base a short, stalk-like prolongation; fruit up to about 5 cm in length and breadth, consisting of a hollow receptacle bearing on the inner surface numerous drupelets, each containing a stone about 1.5 to 2.0 mm long; seed containing endosperm and a curved embryo.

Microscopical Receptacle: epidermal cells polyhedral, stomata raised, trichomes unicellular, thick walled, of varying length up to about 300 µm; hypodermis composed of rounded polyhedral cells, some containing small rosette crystals of calcium oxalate; parenchyma made up of large, irregular cells, forming the greater part of the receptacle, containing large rosette crystals of calcium oxalate and interspersed with numerous latex tubes, about 30 to 50 µm wide, and slender vascular bundles. Pericarp: epicarp consisting of radially elongated cells with mucilaginous outer walls; mesocarp of delicate, often disorganised cells; endocarp of radially elongated sclereids with pitted walls. Endosperm and embryo: small cells containing aleurone grains and fixed oil; starch absent.

Water-soluble extractive

Not less than 60.0% when determined by the following method. To 25 g, minced, add 500 mL of *water*, boil under a reflux condenser for 1 hour, cool and filter. To 20 mL of the filtrate add 20 g of washed and ignited sand, evaporate to dryness in a tared, flat bottomed shallow dish and dry the residue to constant weight at 100°. Calculate the water-soluble extractive by subtracting the weight of sand from the weight of the residue obtained.

STORAGE

Figs should be stored in a dry place.

Frangula Bark

(*Ph Eur monograph 0025*)

Preparation

Standardised Frangula Bark Dry Extract

When Powdered Frangula Bark is prescribed or demanded, material complying with the requirements below, with the exception of Identification test A and the test for Foreign matter, shall be dispensed or supplied.

Ph Eur _____

DEFINITION

Dried, whole or fragmented bark of the stems and branches of *Rhamnus frangula* L. (*Frangula alnus* Miller).

Content

Minimum 7.0 per cent of glucofrangulins, expressed as glucofrangulin A ($C_{27}H_{30}O_{14}$; M_r 578.5) (dried drug).

IDENTIFICATION

A. The bark occurs in curved, almost flat or rolled fragments or in single or double quilled pieces usually 0.5-2 mm thick and variable in length and width. The greyish-brown or dark brown outer surface is wrinkled longitudinally and covered with numerous greyish, transversely elongated lenticels; when the outer layers are removed, a dark red layer is exposed. The orange-brown or reddish-brown inner surface is smooth and bears fine longitudinal striations; it becomes red when treated with alkali. The fracture is short, fibrous in the inner part.

B. Microscopic examination (*2.8.23*). The powder is yellowish or reddish-brown. Examine under a microscope using *chloral hydrate solution R*. The powder shows the following diagnostic characters (Figure 0025.-1): numerous phloem fibres, in tangential section [D] or in longitudinal section [K], partially lignified, in groups [Da, Ka] with crystal sheaths containing calcium oxalate prisms [Db, Kb], sometimes including medullary rays [Dc]; reddish-brown fragments of cork [H]; fragments of phloem parenchyma, in longitudinal section [G] containing calcium oxalate cluster crystals [A, E] or in tangential section [C] including medullary rays [Ca] and cells containing calcium oxalate cluster crystals [Cb]; a few fragments of collenchyma [F]; isolated calcium oxalate cluster crystals [B] and prisms [J].

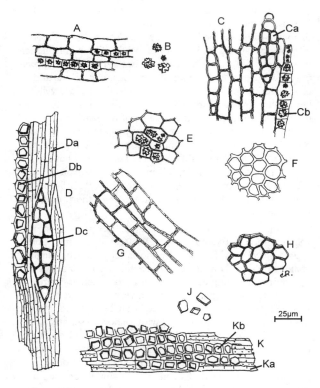

Figure 0025.-1. – *Illustration for identification test B of powdered herbal drug of frangula bark*

C. Examine the chromatogram obtained in test A for other species of *Rhamnus*; anthrones in ultraviolet light at 365 nm.

Results The chromatogram obtained with the test solution shows 2 orange-brown zones (glucofrangulins) in the lower third and 2-4 red zones (frangulins, not always clearly separated, and above them frangula-emodin) in the upper third.

D. To about 50 mg of the powdered herbal drug (180) (*2.9.12*) add 25 mL of dilute *hydrochloric acid R* and heat the mixture on a water-bath for 15 min. Allow to cool, shake with 20 mL of *ether R* and discard the aqueous layer. Shake the ether layer with 10 mL of *dilute ammonia R1*. The aqueous layer becomes reddish-violet.

TESTS

Other species of *Rhamnus*; anthrones

Thin-layer chromatography (*2.2.27*).

Test solution   To 0.5 g of the powdered herbal drug (180) (*2.9.12*) add 5 mL of *ethanol (70 per cent V/V) R* and heat to boiling. Cool and centrifuge. Decant the supernatant solution immediately and use within 30 min.

Reference solution   Dissolve 20 mg of *barbaloin R* in *ethanol (70 per cent V/V) R* and dilute to 10 mL with the same solvent.

Plates   TLC silica gel plate R (2 plates).

Mobile phase   *water R, methanol R, ethyl acetate R* (13:17:100 *V/V/V*).

A. Application: 10 μL as bands.

Development   Over a path of 10 cm.

Drying   In air for 5 min.

Detection   Spray with a 50 g/L solution of *potassium hydroxide R* in *ethanol (50 per cent V/V) R*, and heat at 100-105 °C for 15 min; examine in ultraviolet light at 365 nm.

Results   The chromatogram obtained with the reference solution shows a brownish-yellow zone due to barbaloin in the central part; the chromatogram obtained with the test solution shows no zones of intense yellow fluorescence and no zone of orange or reddish fluorescence similar in position to the zone due to barbaloin in the chromatogram obtained with the reference solution.

B. Application: 10 μL of the test solution as a band.

Development   Over a path of 10 cm.

Drying   In air for maximum 5 min.

Detection   Spray immediately with a 5 g/L solution of *nitrotetrazolium blue R* in *methanol R*; examine immediately.

Results   No violet or greyish-blue zones appear.

Foreign matter (*2.8.2*)

Maximum 1 per cent.

Loss on drying (*2.2.32*)

Maximum 10.0 per cent, determined on 1.000 g of the powdered herbal drug (355) (*2.9.12*) by drying in an oven at 105 °C for 2 h.

Total ash (*2.4.16*)

Maximum 6.0 per cent.

ASSAY

Carry out the assay protected from bright light.

In a tared, round-bottomed flask with a ground-glass neck, weigh 0.250 g of the powdered herbal drug (180) (*2.9.12*). Add 25.0 mL of a 70 per cent *V/V* solution of *methanol R*; mix and weigh. Heat in a water-bath under a reflux condenser for 15 min. Allow to cool, weigh and adjust to the original mass with a 70 per cent *V/V* solution of *methanol R*. Filter and transfer 5.0 mL of the filtrate to a separating funnel. Add 50 mL of *water R* and 0.1 mL of *hydrochloric acid R*. Shake with 5 quantities, each of 20 mL, of *light petroleum R*. Allow the layers to separate and transfer the aqueous layer to a 100 mL volumetric flask. Combine the light petroleum layers and wash with 2 quantities, each of 15 mL, of *water R*. Use this water for washing the separating funnel and add it to the aqueous solution in the volumetric flask. Add 5 mL of a 50 g/L solution of *sodium carbonate R* and dilute to 100.0 mL with *water R*. Discard the light petroleum layer. Transfer 40.0 mL of the aqueous solution to a 200 mL round-bottomed flask with a ground-glass neck. Add 20 mL of a 200 g/L solution of *ferric chloride R* and heat

under a reflux condenser for 20 min in a water-bath with the water level above that of the liquid in the flask. Add 2 mL of *hydrochloric acid R* and continue heating for 20 min, shaking frequently, until the precipitate is dissolved. Allow to cool, transfer the mixture to a separating funnel and shake with 3 quantities, each of 25 mL, of *ether R*, previously used to rinse the flask. Combine the ether extracts and wash with 2 quantities, each of 15 mL, of *water R*. Transfer the ether layer to a volumetric flask and dilute to 100.0 mL with *ether R*. Evaporate 20.0 mL carefully to dryness and dissolve the residue in 10.0 mL of a 5 g/L solution of *magnesium acetate R* in *methanol R*. Measure the absorbance (*2.2.25*) at 515 nm using *methanol R* as the compensation liquid.

Calculate the percentage content of glucofrangulins, expressed as glucofrangulin A, using the following expression:

$$\frac{A \times 3.06}{m}$$

i.e. taking the specific absorbance of glucofrangulin A to be 204.

A =   absorbance at 515 nm;

m =   mass of the substance to be examined, in grams.

Ph Eur

Standardised Frangula Bark Dry Extract

(*Ph Eur monograph 1214*)

Ph Eur

DEFINITION

Standardised dry extract obtained from *Frangula bark (0025)*.

Content

15.0 per cent to 30.0 per cent of glucofrangulins, expressed as glucofrangulin A ($C_{27}H_{30}O_{14}$; M_r 578.5) (dried extract); the measured content does not deviate from that stated on the label by more than ± 10 per cent.

PRODUCTION

The extract is produced from the herbal drug by a suitable procedure using ethanol (50-90 per cent *V/V*).

CHARACTERS

Appearance

Yellowish-brown, fine powder.

IDENTIFICATION

A. Thin-layer chromatography (*2.2.27*).

Test solution   To 0.05 g of the extract to be examined add 5 mL of *ethanol (70 per cent V/V) R* and heat to boiling. Cool and centrifuge. Decant the supernatant solution immediately and use within 30 min.

Reference solution   Dissolve 20 mg of *barbaloin R* in *ethanol (70 per cent V/V) R* and dilute to 10 mL with the same solvent.

Plate   TLC silica gel plate R.

Mobile phase   *water R, methanol R, ethyl acetate R* (13:17:100 *V/V/V*).

Application   10 μL as bands.

Development   Over a path of 10 cm.

Drying   In air for 5 min.

Detection   Spray with a 50 g/L solution of *potassium hydroxide R* in *ethanol (50 per cent V/V) R* and heat at 100-105 °C for 15 min; examine immediately after heating.

Results   The chromatogram obtained with the reference solution shows in the middle third a reddish-brown zone due to barbaloin. The chromatogram obtained with the test solution shows 2 orange-brown zones (glucofrangulins) in the lower third and 2-4 red zones (frangulins, not always clearly separated, and above them frangula-emodin) in the upper third.

B. To about 25 mg add 25 mL of *dilute hydrochloric acid R* and heat the mixture on a water-bath for 15 min. Allow to cool, shake with 20 mL of *ether R* and discard the aqueous layer. Shake the ether layer with 10 mL of *dilute ammonia R1*. The aqueous layer becomes reddish-violet.

TESTS

Loss on drying (*2.8.17*)
Maximum 5.0 per cent.

Microbial contamination
TAMC: acceptance criterion 10^4 CFU/g (*2.6.12*).
TYMC: acceptance criterion 10^2 CFU/g (*2.6.12*).
Absence of *Escherichia coli* (*2.6.13*).
Absence of *Salmonella* (*2.6.13*).

ASSAY

Carry out the assay protected from bright light.

Into a tared round-bottomed flask with a ground-glass neck, weigh 0.100 g. Add 25.0 mL of a 70 per cent *V/V* solution of *methanol R*, mix and weigh again. Heat the flask in a water-bath under a reflux condenser at 70 °C for 15 min. Allow to cool, weigh and adjust to the original mass with a 70 per cent *V/V* solution of *methanol R*. Filter and transfer 5.0 mL of the filtrate to a separating funnel. Add 50 mL of *water R* and 0.1 mL of *hydrochloric acid R*. Shake with 5 quantities, each of 20 mL, of *light petroleum R1*. Allow the layers to separate and transfer the aqueous layer to a 100 mL volumetric flask. Combine the light petroleum layers and wash with 2 quantities, each of 15 mL, of *water R*. Use this water for washing the separating funnel and add it to the aqueous solution in the volumetric flask. Add 5 mL of a 50 g/L solution of *sodium carbonate R* and dilute to 100.0 mL with *water R*. Discard the light petroleum layer. Transfer 40.0 mL of the aqueous solution to a 200 mL round-bottomed flask with a ground-glass neck. Add 20 mL of a 200 g/L solution of *ferric chloride R* and heat under a reflux condenser for 20 min in a water-bath with the water level above that of the liquid in the flask. Add 2 mL of *hydrochloric acid R* and continue heating for 20 min, shaking frequently, until the precipitate is dissolved. Allow to cool, transfer the mixture to a separating funnel and shake with 3 quantities, each of 25 mL, of *ether R*, previously used to rinse the flask. Combine the ether extracts and wash with 2 quantities, each of 15 mL, of *water R*. Transfer the ether layer to a volumetric flask and dilute to 100.0 mL with *ether R*. Evaporate 20.0 mL carefully to dryness and dissolve the residue in 10.0 mL of a 5 g/L solution of *magnesium acetate R* in *methanol R*. Measure the absorbance (*2.2.25*) at 515 nm using *methanol R* as the compensation liquid.

Calculate the percentage content of glucofrangulins, expressed as glucofrangulin A, using the following expression:

$$\frac{A \times 3.06}{m}$$

i.e. taking the specific absorbance of glucofrangulin A to be 204, calculated on the basis of the specific absorbance of barbaloin.

A = absorbance at 515 nm;
m = mass of the preparation to be examined, in grams.

LABELLING
The label states the content of glucofrangulins.

Ph Eur

Indian Frankincense

(*Ph Eur monograph 2310*)

Ph Eur

DEFINITION
Air-dried gum-resin exudate, obtained by incision in the stem or branches of *Boswellia serrata* Roxb. ex Colebr.

Content:
— *11-keto-β-boswellic acid* ($C_{30}H_{46}O_4$; M_r 470.7): minimum 1.0 per cent (dried drug);
— *acetyl-11-keto-β-boswellic acid* ($C_{32}H_{48}O_5$; M_r 512.7): minimum 1.0 per cent (dried drug).

IDENTIFICATION
A. Indian frankincense consists of translucent, roundish or irregularly shaped, variable size pieces of up to 3 cm. They are yellowish or reddish-brown. Their surface is covered with grey dust. The fracture is dull or slightly glossy.

B. Thin-layer chromatography (*2.2.27*).

Test solution   To 1.0 g of the powdered drug (355) (*2.9.12*) add 90 mL of *methanol R* and sonicate for 10 min. Shake the mixture vigorously 3 or 4 times during this procedure. Dilute to 100 mL with *methanol R*. Centrifuge and use the clear supernatant solution.

Reference solution   Dissolve 2 mg of *11-keto-β-boswellic acid R* and 2 mg of *acetyl-11-keto-β-boswellic acid R* in 20 mL of *methanol R*.

Plate   TLC silica gel F_{254} plate R (5-40 μm) [or *TLC silica gel* F_{254} *plate R* (2-10 μm)].

Mobile phase   anhydrous formic acid R, heptane R, ethyl acetate R, toluene R (3:10:20:80 *V/V/V/V*).

Application   10 μL [or 3 μL] as bands.

Development   Over a path of 8 cm [or 6 cm].

Drying   In air.

Detection   Examine in ultraviolet light at 254 nm.

Results   See below the sequence of zones present in the chromatograms obtained with the reference solution and the test solution. The zones due to 11-keto-β-boswellic acid and acetyl-11-keto-β-boswellic acid in the test solution are of approximately equivalent intensity. Furthermore, other weak quenching zones may be present in the chromatogram obtained with the test solution.

Top of the plate	
___	___
___	___
Acetyl-11-keto-β-boswellic acid: a quenching zone	A quenching zone (acetyl-11-keto-β-boswellic acid)
11-Keto-β-boswellic acid: a quenching zone	A quenching zone (11-keto-β-boswellic acid)
Reference solution	**Test solution**

TESTS

Loss on drying (*2.2.32*)

Maximum 8.0 per cent, determined on 1.000 g of powdered drug (355) (*2.9.12*) by drying in an oven at 105 °C for 3 h.

Total ash (*2.4.16*)

Maximum 10.0 per cent.

ASSAY

Liquid chromatography (*2.2.29*).

Test solution   To 1.0 g of the powdered drug (355) (*2.9.12*) add 90 mL of *methanol R* and sonicate for 10 min. Shake the mixture vigorously 3 or 4 times during this procedure. Dilute to 100.0 mL with *methanol R*. Centrifuge for 5 min. Dilute 1.0 mL of the clear solution to 10.0 mL with a mixture of 16 volumes of mobile phase A and 84 volumes of mobile phase B.

Reference solution   Dissolve 1.0 mg of *11-keto-β-boswellic acid R* and 1.0 mg of *acetyl-11-keto-β-boswellic acid R* in 20.0 mL of *methanol R*. Dilute 1.0 mL of this solution to 10.0 mL with a mixture of 16 volumes of mobile phase A and 84 volumes of mobile phase B.

Column:
— *size: l* = 0.25 m, Ø = 4.6 mm;
— *stationary phase: octadecylsilyl silica gel for chromatography R* (5 μm).

Mobile phase:
— *mobile phase A: phosphoric acid R, water R* (0.1:99.9 *V/V*);
— *mobile phase B: phosphoric acid R, acetonitrile R* (0.1:99.9 *V/V*);

Time (min)	Mobile phase A (per cent *V/V*)	Mobile phase B (per cent *V/V*)
0 - 12.5	16 → 6	84 → 94
12.5 - 13.5	6 → 0	94 → 100
13.5 - 28	0	100

Flow rate   1.0 mL/min.

Detection   Spectrophotometer at 250 nm.

Injection   20 μL.

Retention time   11-keto-β-boswellic acid = about 8 min; acetyl-11-keto-β-boswellic acid = about 12 min.

System suitability   Reference solution:
— *resolution*: minimum 6.0 between the peaks due to 11-keto-β-boswellic acid and acetyl-11-keto-β-boswellic acid.

Calculate the percentage content of 11-keto-β-boswellic acid using the following expression:

$$\frac{A_1 \times m_1 \times 5 \times p_1}{A_2 \times m}$$

A_1 =   area of the peak due to 11-keto-β-boswellic acid in the chromatogram obtained with the test solution;

A_2 =   area of the peak due to 11-keto-β-boswellic acid in the chromatogram obtained with the reference solution;

m =   mass of the substance to be examined, in grams;

m_1 =   mass of *11-keto-β-boswellic acid R* in the reference solution, in grams;

p_1 =   percentage content of *11-keto-β-boswellic acid in 11-keto-β-boswellic acid R*.

Calculate the percentage content of acetyl-11-keto-β-boswellic acid using the following expression:

$$\frac{A_3 \times m_2 \times 5 \times p_2}{A_4 \times m}$$

A_3 =   area of the peak due to acetyl-11-keto-β-boswellic acid in the chromatogram obtained with the test solution;

A_4 =   area of the peak due to acetyl-11-keto-β-boswellic acid in the chromatogram obtained with the reference solution;

m =   mass of the substance to be examined, in grams;

m_2 =   mass of *acetyl-11-keto-β-boswellic acid R* in the reference solution, in grams;

p_2 =   percentage content of acetyl-11-keto-β-boswellic acid in *acetyl-11-keto-β-boswellic acid R*.

Ph Eur

Fumitory

(*Ph Eur monograph 1869*)

Ph Eur

DEFINITION

Whole or fragmented, dried aerial parts of *Fumaria officinalis* L. harvested in full bloom.

Content

Minimum 0.40 per cent of total alkaloids, expressed as protopine ($C_{20}H_{19}NO_5$; M_r 353.4) (dried drug).

IDENTIFICATION

A. The hollow, angular stem is light green or greenish-brown. The leaves are alternate, bipinnatisect with 2 or 3 leaf segments, the ultimate lobes lanceolate or obovate; they are greenish-blue and glabrous on both surfaces. The flowers are small and occur in loose racemes; each has a short pedicel and is subtended by a leafy bract; they are pink or purplish-red, dark purple or brown at the apex; the calyx is short, composed of 2 petalloid sepals and the corolla is tubular with 4 petals, the upper petal slightly spurred; there are 6 stamens united by their filaments into 2 groups of 3. The greenish-brown, indehiscent fruits are globular or keel-shaped, truncated or slightly emarginate at the apex, and each contains a small brown seed.

B. Microscopic examination (*2.8.23*). The powder is green. Examine under a microscope using *chloral hydrate solution R*. The powder shows the following diagnostic characters (Figure 1869.-1): fragments of the leaf lamina in surface view with the upper epidermis [D] composed of irregularly polygonal cells [Da], some of which contain microcrystals of calcium oxalate [Db], and underlying palisade parenchyma [Dc]; marginal cells at the apex of the lamina elongated to form blunt papillae [Dd], and with the lower epidermis [A] composed of cells having wavier walls [Aa] and underlying spongy parenchyma [Ac]; anomocytic stomata (*2.8.3*) [Ab,

De] on both surfaces; groups [G] of lignified fibres [Ga] and spiral [Gb], reticulate or bordered-pitted [B] vessels from the stem; fragments of the epidermis of the petals [F] composed of polygonal cells with sinuous or wavy anticlinal walls and no papillae; spherical pollen grains [E], about 30 μm in diameter, with a pitted exine and 6 large pores; fragments of the fruit with polygonal cells with a thick, warty cuticle, from the epicarp [H], and sinuous sclereids with thick and channelled walls, from the endocarp [C].

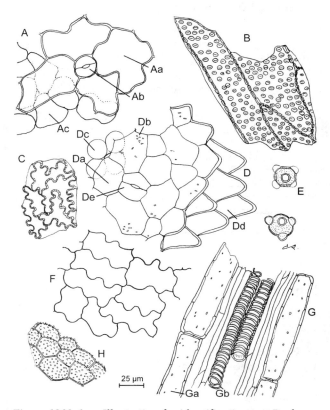

Figure 1869.-1. – *Illustration for identification test B of powdered herbal drug of fumitory*

C. Thin-layer chromatography (*2.2.27*).

Test solution   To 2 g of the powdered herbal drug (355) (*2.9.12*) add 15 mL of *0.05 M sulfuric acid* and stir for 15 min. Filter. Dilute the filtrate to 20 mL with *0.05 M sulfuric acid*. Add 1 mL of *concentrated ammonia R* and 10 mL of *ethyl acetate R*. Stir and centrifuge. Collect the upper organic layer. Repeat the extraction in the same manner. Collect the organic layers and dry over *anhydrous sodium sulfate R*. Evaporate to dryness under reduced pressure. Take up the residue with 0.5 mL of *methanol R*.

Reference solution   Dissolve 5 mg of *protopine hydrochloride R* and 5 mg of *quinine R* in 10 mL of *methanol R*.

Plate   TLC silica gel plate R.

Mobile phase   concentrated ammonia R, ethanol (96 per cent) R, acetone R, toluene R (2:6:40:52 V/V/V/V).

Application   30 μL as bands.

Development   Over a path of 15 cm.

Drying   In air.

Detection A   Examine in ultraviolet light at 365 nm.

Results A   See below the sequence of zones present in the chromatogram obtained with the reference solution and the test solution. Furthermore, other blue fluorescent zones are present in the chromatogram obtained with the test solution.

Top of the plate	
	4 blue fluorescent zones
Quinine: a blue fluorescent zone	
	A greenish-blue fluorescent zone
Reference solution	**Test solution**

Detection B   Treat with a mixture of *potassium iodobismuthate solution R2*, *acetic acid R* and *water R* (1:2:10 V/V/V) until orange zones appear against a yellow background.

Results B   See below the sequence of zones present in the chromatograms obtained with the reference solution and the test solution. Furthermore, other less intense orange zones are present in the chromatogram obtained with the test solution.

Top of the plate	
Protopine: an orange zone	An orange zone (protopine)
	2 orange zones
Quinine: an orange zone	A faint orange zone
Reference solution	**Test solution**

TESTS

Cadmium (*2.4.27*)
Maximum 1.5 ppm.

Loss on drying (*2.2.32*)
Maximum 12.0 per cent, determined on 1.000 g of the powdered herbal drug (355) (*2.9.12*) by drying in an oven at 105 °C.

Total ash (*2.4.16*)
Maximum 15.0 per cent.

ASSAY

To 5.000 g of the powdered herbal drug (355) (*2.9.12*) add 5 mL of *dilute ammonia R1* and 50 mL of *ethyl acetate R*. Shake for 15 min. Filter. Repeat the procedure in the same manner and combine the filtrates. Evaporate the filtrates to dryness under reduced pressure. Dissolve the residue by sonication for 10 min in 50 mL of *0.05 M sulfuric acid*. Filter. Dilute the filtrate to 100 mL with *0.05 M sulfuric acid*. Adjust to pH 9-10 with *concentrated ammonia R* and then add 50 mL of *ethyl acetate R*. Shake gently. Collect the upper organic layer, after centrifugation if necessary. Repeat the procedure in the same manner. Combine the organic layers and dry over *anhydrous sodium sulfate R*. Evaporate to dryness under reduced pressure. Take up the residue with 100 mL of *anhydrous acetic acid R*. Titrate with *0.02 M perchloric acid*, determining the end-point potentiometrically (*2.2.20*).

1 mL of *0.02 M perchloric acid* is equivalent to 7.068 mg of protopine.

Calculate the percentage content of total alkaloids, expressed as protopine, using the following expression:

$$\frac{n \times 706.8}{m}$$

n　=　volume of *0.02 M perchloric acid* used, in millilitres;
m　=　mass of the herbal drug to be examined, in milligrams.

———————————————— Ph Eur

Garlic Powder

(*Ph Eur monograph 1216*)

Ph Eur _____

DEFINITION
Bulbs of *Allium sativum* L., cut, freeze-dried or dried at a temperature not exceeding 65 °C and powdered.

Content
Minimum 0.45 per cent of allicin ($C_6H_{10}OS_2$; M_r 162.3) (dried drug).

CHARACTERS
Appearance
Light yellowish powder.

IDENTIFICATION
A. Examine under a microscope using *chloral hydrate solution R*. The powder shows the following diagnostic characters: numerous fragments of parenchyma and groups of spiral or annular vessels accompanied by thin-walled parenchyma.

B. Thin-layer chromatography (*2.2.27*).

Test solution　To 1.0 g of garlic powder add 5.0 mL of *methanol R*, shake for 60 s and filter.

Reference solution　Dissolve 5 mg of *alanine R* in 10 mL of *water R* and dilute to 20 mL with *methanol R*.

Plate　TLC silica gel plate R.

Mobile phase　glacial acetic acid R, propanol R, water R, anhydrous ethanol R (20:20:20:40 *V/V/V/V*).

Application　20 μL of the test solution and 10 μL of the reference solution, as bands.

Development　Over a path of 10 cm.

Drying　In air.

Detection　Spray with a 2 g/L solution of *ninhydrin R* in a mixture of 5 volumes of *glacial acetic acid R* and 95 volumes of *butanol R* and heat at 105-110 °C for 5-10 min; examine in daylight.

Results　The chromatogram obtained with the reference solution shows a violet zone (alanine) in its central third. The chromatogram obtained with the test solution shows a violet or brownish-red zone similar in position to that in the chromatogram obtained with the reference solution and corresponding to alliin; above and below this zone are other, generally fainter, violet zones.

TESTS
Starch
Examine the powdered drug under a microscope using *water R*. Add *iodine solution R1*. No blue colour develops.

Loss on drying (*2.2.32*)
Maximum 7.0 per cent, determined on 1.000 g of the powdered drug by drying in an oven at 105 °C.

Total ash (*2.4.16*)
Maximum 5.0 per cent.

ASSAY
Liquid chromatography (*2.2.29*). Carry out the assay as quickly as possible.

Internal standard solution　Dissolve 20.0 mg of *butyl parahydroxybenzoate CRS* in 100.0 mL of a mixture of equal volumes of *methanol R* and *water R*.

Test solution　To 0.800 g of garlic powder add 20.0 mL of *water R* and homogenise the mixture in an ultrasonic bath at 4 °C for 5 min. Allow to stand at room temperature for 30 min. Then centrifuge for 30 min. Dilute 10.0 mL of the supernatant to 25.0 mL with a mixture of 40 volumes of a 1 per cent *V/V* solution of *anhydrous formic acid R* and 60 volumes of *methanol R* (stock solution). Shake and centrifuge for 5 min. Place 0.50 mL of the internal standard solution in a volumetric flask and dilute to 10.0 mL with the stock solution.

Precolumn:
— *size*: l = 20 mm, Ø = 4 mm,
— *stationary phase*: *silanised octadecylsilyl silica gel for chromatography R* (5 μm).

Column:
— *size*: l = 0.25 m, Ø = 4 mm,
— *stationary phase*: *silanised octadecylsilyl silica gel for chromatography R* (5 μm).

Mobile phase　Mix 40 volumes of a 1 per cent *V/V* solution of *anhydrous formic acid R* and 60 volumes of *methanol R*.

Flow rate　0.8 mL/min.

Detection　Spectrophotometer at 254 nm.

Injection　Loop injector, 1 μL of the internal standard solution and 10 μL of the test solution.

Calculate the percentage of allicin using the following expression:

$$\frac{S_1 \times m_2 \times 22.75}{S_2 \times m_1}$$

S_1　=　area of the peak due to allicin (principal peak) in the chromatogram obtained with the test solution,
S_2　=　area of the peak due to butyl parahydroxybenzoate in the chromatogram obtained with the test solution,
m_1　=　mass of the drug to be examined, in grams,
m_2　=　mass of butyl parahydroxybenzoate in 100.0 ml of the internal standard solution, in grams. 1 mg of butylparahydroxybenzoate corresponds to 8.65 mg of allicin.

———————————————— Ph Eur

Gentian

(*Gentian Root, Ph Eur monograph 0392*)

Preparations
Compound Gentian Infusion

Gentian Tincture

When Powdered Gentian is prescribed or demanded, material complying with the requirements below with the exception of Identification test A shall be dispensed or supplied.

Ph Eur

DEFINITION

Dried, fragmented underground organs of *Gentiana lutea* L.

CHARACTERS

Characteristic odour.

Strong and persistent bitter taste.

Gentian root occurs as single or branched subcylindrical pieces of various lengths and usually 10-40 mm thick but occasionally up to 80 mm thick at the crown.

IDENTIFICATION

A. The surface is brownish-grey, and the colour of a transverse section is yellowish or reddish-yellow, but not reddish-brown. The root is longitudinally wrinkled and bears occasional rootlet scars. The branches of the rhizome frequently bear a terminal bud and are always encircled by closely arranged leaf scars. The rhizome and root are brittle when dry and break with a short fracture but they absorb moisture readily to become flexible. The smoothed, transversely cut surface shows a bark, occupying about one-third of the radius, separated by the well-marked cambium from an indistinctly radiate and mainly parenchymatous xylem.

B. Reduce to a powder (355) (*2.9.12*). The powder is light brown or yellowish-brown. Examine under a microscope using *chloral hydrate solution R*. The powder shows the following diagnostic characters: fragments of the subero-phellodermic layer, consisting of thin-walled yellowish-brown cork cells and thick-walled collenchyma (phelloderm); fragments of cortical and ligneous parenchymatous cells with moderately thickened walls containing droplets of oil and small prisms and minute needles of calcium oxalate; fragments of lignified vessels with spiral or reticulate thickening.

C. Thin-layer chromatography (*2.2.27*).

Test solution To 1.0 g of the powdered drug (355) (*2.9.12*) add 25 mL of *methanol R*, shake for 15 min and filter. Evaporate the filtrate to dryness under reduced pressure, at a temperature not exceeding 50 °C. Take up the residue with small quantities of *methanol R* so as to obtain 5 mL of a solution, which may contain a sediment.

Reference solution Dissolve 5 mg of *hyperoside R* and 5 mg of *phenazone R* in 10 mL of *methanol R*.

Plate TLC silica gel F_{254} plate R.

Mobile phase water R, anhydrous formic acid R, ethyl formate R (4:8:88 *V/V/V*).

Application 20 µL as bands.

Development In an unsaturated tank, over a path of 8 cm.

Drying In air.

Detection A Examine in ultraviolet light at 254 nm.

Results A See below the sequence of the zones present in the chromatograms obtained with the reference solution and the test solution. Furthermore, other zones may be present in the chromatogram obtained with the test solution.

Top of the plate	
Phenazone: a quenching zone	A prominent quenching zone
	A weak quenching zone (amarogentin)
_____	_____
_____	_____
Hyperoside: a quenching zone	A prominent quenching zone (gentiopicroside)
Reference solution	**Test solution**

Detection B Spray with a 100 g/L solution of *potassium hydroxide R* in *methanol R* and then with a freshly prepared 2 g/L solution of *fast blue B salt R* in a mixture of 50 volumes of *anhydrous ethanol R* and 50 volumes of *water R*. Examine in daylight.

Results B See below the sequence of the zones present in the chromatograms obtained with the reference solution and the test solution. Furthermore, other zones may be present in the chromatogram obtained with the test solution.

Top of the plate	
	A prominent dark violet zone
	A violet-red zone (amarogentin)
_____	_____
_____	_____
Hyperoside: a brownish-red zone	A weak light brown zone (gentiopicroside)
Reference solution	**Test solution**

TESTS

Other species of *Gentiana*

Examine the chromatograms obtained in identification test C, detection B.

Results The chromatogram obtained with the test solution does not show violet zones immediately above the zone due to amarogentin.

Total ash (*2.4.16*)

Maximum 6.0 per cent.

Bitterness value (*2.8.15*)

Minimum 10 000.

Water-soluble extractive

Minimum 33 per cent.

To 5.0 g of powdered drug (710) (*2.9.12*) add 200 mL of boiling *water R*. Allow to stand for 10 min, shaking occasionally. Allow to cool, dilute to 200.0 mL with *water R* and filter. Evaporate 20.0 mL of the filtrate to dryness on a water-bath. Dry the residue in an oven at 100-105 °C. The residue weighs a minimum of 0.165 g.

Ph Eur

Compound Gentian Infusion

DEFINITION

Concentrated Compound Gentian Infusion	100 ml
Water	Sufficient to produce 1000 ml

The infusion complies with the requirements stated under Infusions.

CONCENTRATED COMPOUND GENTIAN INFUSION

DEFINITION

Gentian, cut small and bruised	125 g
Dried Bitter-orange Peel, cut small	125 g
Dried Lemon Peel, cut small	125 g
Ethanol (25 per cent)	1200 ml

Extemporaneous preparation

The following directions apply.

Macerate the Gentian, the Dried Bitter-orange Peel and the Dried Lemon Peel in a covered vessel for 48 hours with 1000 ml of the Ethanol (25 per cent); express the liquid. To the pressed marc add 200 ml of the Ethanol (25 per cent), macerate for 24 hours, press and add the liquid to the product of the first pressing. Allow to stand for not less than 14 days; filter.

TESTS

Ethanol content
20 to 24% v/v, Appendix VIII F.

Total solids
Not less than 9.5% w/v, Appendix XI A.

Gentian Tincture

(Ph Eur monograph 1870)

Ph Eur ⎯⎯⎯⎯⎯⎯⎯⎯⎯⎯⎯⎯⎯⎯⎯⎯⎯⎯⎯⎯⎯⎯⎯

DEFINITION

Tincture produced from *Gentian root (0392)*.

PRODUCTION

The tincture is produced from 1 part of the comminuted drug and 5 parts of ethanol (70 per cent *V/V*) by a suitable procedure.

CHARACTERS

Appearance

Yellowish-brown or reddish-brown liquid.

It has a strong bitter taste.

IDENTIFICATION

Thin-layer chromatography (*2.2.27*).

Test solution   The tincture to be examined.

Reference solution   Dissolve 5 mg of *phenazone R* and 5 mg of *hyperoside R* in 10 mL of *methanol R*.

Plate   TLC silica gel F_{254} plate R.

Mobile phase   water R, anhydrous formic acid R, ethyl formate R (4:8:88 *V/V/V*).

Application   20 μL, as bands.

Development   Over a path of 8 cm, in an unsaturated tank.

Drying   In air.

Detection A   Examine in ultraviolet light at 254 nm.

Results A   See below the sequence of the zones present in the chromatograms obtained with the reference solution and the test solution. Furthermore, other zones may be present in the chromatogram obtained with the test solution.

Top of the plate	
	A prominent quenching zone
Phenazone: a quenching zone	A weak quenching zone (amarogentin)
⎯⎯⎯	⎯⎯⎯
⎯⎯⎯	⎯⎯⎯
Hyperoside: a quenching zone	A prominent quenching zone (gentiopicroside)
Reference solution	**Test solution**

Detection B   Spray with a 10 per cent *V/V* solution of *potassium hydroxide R* in *methanol R* and then with a freshly prepared 2 g/L solution of *fast blue B salt R* in a mixture of *ethanol R* and *water R* (50:50 *V/V*). Examine in daylight.

Results B   See below the sequence of the zones present in the chromatograms obtained with the reference solution and the test solution. Furthermore, other zones may be present in the chromatogram obtained with the test solution.

Top of the plate	
	A prominent dark violet zone
	A violet-red zone (amarogentin)
⎯⎯⎯	⎯⎯⎯
⎯⎯⎯	⎯⎯⎯
Hyperoside: a brownish-red zone	A weak light brown zone (gentiopicroside)
Reference solution	**Test solution**

TESTS

Ethanol content (*2.9.10*)
62 per cent *V/V* to 67 per cent *V/V*.

Bitterness value (*2.8.15*)
Minimum 1000.

Dry residue (*2.8.16*)
Minimum 5.0 per cent m/m, determined on 3.00 g.

⎯⎯⎯⎯⎯⎯⎯⎯⎯⎯⎯⎯⎯⎯⎯⎯⎯⎯⎯⎯⎯⎯⎯ *Ph Eur*

Acid Gentian Mixture

Acid Gentian Oral Solution

DEFINITION

Acid Gentian Mixture is an *oral solution* containing 10% v/v of Concentrated Compound Gentian Infusion and 5% v/v of Dilute Hydrochloric Acid in a suitable vehicle.

Extemporaneous preparation

It is recently prepared according to the following formula.

Concentrated Compound Gentian Infusion	100 mL
Dilute Hydrochloric Acid	50 mL
Double-strength Chloroform Water	500 mL
Water	Sufficient to produce 1000 mL

The mixture complies with the requirements stated under Oral Liquids and with the following requirements.

Content of hydrochloric acid, HCl

0.48 to 0.56% w/v.

ASSAY

To 10 mL add 10 mL of *water*, adjust the pH to between 5.0 and 6.0 with 2M *sodium hydroxide* and dilute to 25 mL with *water*. Add 75 mL of *acetate buffer pH 5.0* and titrate with 0.1M *silver nitrate VS* determining the end point potentiometrically using a silver indicator electrode and a glass reference electrode and stirring throughout the titration. Each mL of 0.1M *silver nitrate VS* is equivalent to 3.646 mg of HCl.

Alkaline Gentian Mixture

Alkaline Gentian Oral Solution

DEFINITION

Alkaline Gentian Mixture is an *oral solution* containing 10% v/v of Concentrated Compound Gentian Infusion and 5% w/v of Sodium Bicarbonate in a suitable vehicle.

Extemporaneous preparation

It is recently prepared according to the following formula.

Concentrated Compound Gentian Infusion	100 mL
Sodium Bicarbonate	50 g
Double-strength Chloroform Water	500 mL
Water	Sufficient to produce 1000 mL

The mixture complies with the requirements stated under Oral Liquids and with the following requirements.

Content of sodium bicarbonate, NaHCO₃

4.75 to 5.25% w/v.

ASSAY

To 10 mL of the mixture add 100 mL of *water* and 25 mL of 0.5M *hydrochloric acid VS*, boil for 10 minutes and titrate the excess of hydrochloric acid with 0.5M *sodium hydroxide VS* using 0.5 mL of *methyl red solution* as indicator. Each mL of 0.5M *hydrochloric acid VS* is equivalent to 42.00 mg of NaHCO₃.

Ginger

(*Ph Eur monograph 1522*)

Preparation

Strong Ginger Tincture

Ginger may be known in commerce as unbleached ginger. When Powdered Ginger is prescribed or demanded, material complying with the appropriate requirements below shall be dispensed or supplied.

Ph Eur _____

DEFINITION

Dried, whole or cut rhizome of *Zingiber officinale* Roscoe, with the cork removed, either completely or from the wide, flat surfaces only.

Content

Minimum 15 mL/kg of essential oil (anhydrous drug).

CHARACTERS

Characteristic aromatic odour.

Spicy and burning taste.

IDENTIFICATION

A. The rhizome is laterally compressed, bearing short, flattened, obovate oblique branches on the upper side, each sometimes having a depressed scar at the apex; the whole rhizomes are about 5-10 cm long, 1.5-3 cm or 4 cm wide and 1-1.5 cm thick, sometimes split longitudinally. The scraped rhizome with a light-brown external surface shows longitudinal striations and occasional loose fibres; the outer surface of the unscraped rhizome varies from pale to dark brown and is more or less covered with cork that shows conspicuous, narrow, longitudinal and transverse ridges; the cork readily exfoliates from the lateral surfaces but persists between the branches. The fracture is short and starchy with projecting fibres. The smoothed transversely cut surface exhibits a narrow cortex separated by an endodermis from a much wider stele; it shows numerous, scattered, fibrovascular bundles and abundant scattered oleoresin cells with yellow contents. The unscraped rhizome shows, in addition, an outer layer of dark brown cork.

B. Reduce to a powder (355) (*2.9.12*). The powder is pale yellow or brownish. Examine under a microscope using *chloral hydrate solution R*. The powder shows the following diagnostic characters (Figure 1522.-1): groups of large, thin-walled, septate fibres, with one wall frequently dentate [C, D, G]; fragments [K] containing vessels with reticulate thickening [Ka] often accompanied by narrow, thin-walled cells containing brown pigment [Kb] and amyliferous parenchyma [Kc]; abundant reticulate vessels, fairly large, isolated [H, L]; abundant thin-walled parenchyma of the ground tissue [J, M], some cells containing brown oleoresin [Ja]; fragments of brown cork, usually seen in surface view [F] but sometimes in transverse section [E]. Examine under a microscope using a 50 per cent *V/V* solution of *glycerol R*. The powder shows abundant starch granules, simple, flattened, oblong or oval or irregular, up to about 50 μm long and 25 μm wide, with a small point hilum situated at the narrower end; sometimes, granules show faint, transverse striations, and may be free [A], agglomerated [B] or included in parenchymatous cells (Kc).

C. Thin-layer chromatography (*2.2.27*).

Test solution   To 1.0 g of the powdered drug (710) (*2.9.12*) add 5 mL of *methanol R*. Shake for 15 min and filter.

Reference solution   Dissolve 10 μL of *citral R* and 10 mg of *resorcinol R* in 10 mL of *methanol R*. Prepare the solution immediately before use.

Plate   TLC silica gel plate R.

Mobile phase   hexane R, ether R (40:60 *V/V*).

Application   20 μL as bands.

Development   In an unsaturated tank, over a path of 15 cm.

Drying   In air.

Detection   Spray with a 10 g/L solution of *vanillin R* in *sulfuric acid R* and examine in daylight while heating at 100-105 °C for 10 min.

Results   The chromatogram obtained with the reference solution shows in the lower half an intense red zone (resorcinol) and in the upper half 2 violet zones (citral); the chromatogram obtained with the test solution shows below the zone due to resorcinol in the chromatogram obtained with the reference solution 2 intense violet zones (gingerols) and in the middle, between the zones due to

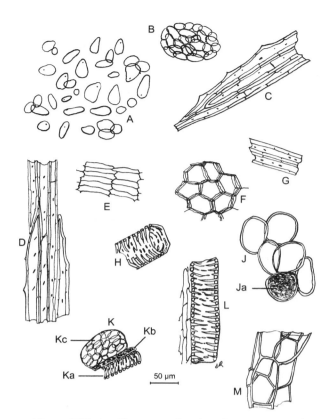

Figure 1522.-1.– *Illustration for identification test B of powdered herbal drug of ginger*

resorcinol and citral in the chromatogram obtained with the reference solution, 2 other less intense violet zones (shogaols); other zones may be present.

TESTS
Water (*2.2.13*)
Maximum 100 mL/kg, determined by distillation on 20.0 g of the powdered drug (710) (*2.9.12*).

Total ash (*2.4.16*)
Maximum 6.0 per cent.

ASSAY
Carry out the determination of essential oils in herbal drugs (*2.8.12*). Use 20.0 g of the freshly, coarsely powdered drug, a 1000 mL round-bottomed flask, 10 drops of *liquid paraffin R* or other antifoam, 500 mL of *water R* as distillation liquid and 0.5 mL of *xylene R* in the graduated tube. Distil at a rate of 2-3 mL/min for 4 h.

_____ *Ph Eur*

Strong Ginger Tincture
Ginger Essence

DEFINITION
Ginger, in moderately coarse powder	500 g
Ethanol (90 per cent)	Sufficient to produce 1000 ml

Extemporaneous preparation
The following directions apply.
Prepare by *percolation*, Appendix XI F.

The tincture complies with the requirements for Tinctures stated under Extracts and with the following requirements.

TESTS
Ethanol content
80 to 88% v/v, Appendix VIII F, Method III.

Dry residue
2.0 to 3.0% w/v.

Relative density
0.832 to 0.846, Appendix V G.

Weak Ginger Tincture

DEFINITION
Strong Ginger Tincture	200 ml
Ethanol (90 per cent)	Sufficient to produce 1000 ml

The tincture complies with the requirements for Tinctures stated under Extracts and with the following requirements.

TESTS
Ethanol content
86 to 90% v/v, Appendix VIII F, Method III.

Dry residue
Not less than 0.4% w/v. Use 10 ml.

Relative density
0.825 to 0.835, Appendix V G.

Ginkgo Leaf

(*Ph Eur monograph 1828*)

Preparation
Ginkgo Leaf Dry Extract, Refined and Quantified

Ph Eur _____

DEFINITION
Whole or fragmented, dried leaf of *Ginkgo biloba* L.

Content
Not less than 0.5 per cent of flavonoids, expressed as flavone glycosides (M_r 757) (dried drug).

IDENTIFICATION
A. The leaf is greyish or yellowish-green or yellowish-brown. The upper surface is slightly darker than the lower surface. The petioles are about 4-9 cm long. The lamina is about 4-10 cm wide, fan-shaped, usually bilobate or sometimes undivided. Both surfaces are smooth, and the venation dichotomous, the veins appearing to radiate from the base; they are equally prominent on both surfaces. The distal margin is incised, irregularly and to different degrees, and irregularly lobate or emarginate. The lateral margins are entire and taper towards the base.

B. Reduce to a powder (355) (*2.9.12*). The powder is greyish or yellowish-green or yellowish-brown. Examine under a microscope using *chloral hydrate solution R*. The powder shows the following diagnostic characters (Figure 1828.-1): irregularly-shaped fragments of the lamina [A, B, D, E], with the upper epidermis, in surface view (D) and transverse section (E), consisting of elongated cells with irregularly sinuous walls [Da], often accompanied by palisade parenchyma [Db], and the lower epidermis, in surface view (A) and transverse section (B), consisting of small cells, with a finely striated cuticle and each cell shortly papillose [Aa],

and stomata [Ab] about 60 μm, wide, deeply sunken with
6-8 subsidiary cells; fragments of vascular tissue from the
petiole and veins [C] with xylem [Ca] and parenchyma,
some cells containing abundant cluster crystals of calcium
oxalate of various sizes [Cb].

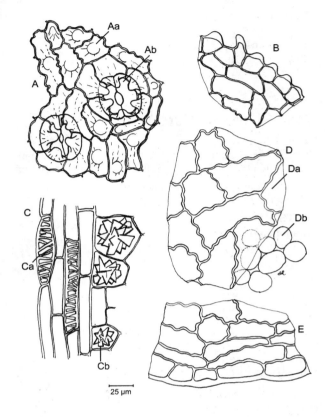

Figure 1828.-1.– *Illustration for identification test B of
powdered herbal drug of ginkgo leaf*

C. Thin-layer chromatography (*2.2.27*).

Test solution   To 2.0 g of the powdered drug (710) (*2.9.12*)
add 10 mL of *methanol R*. Heat in a water-bath at 65 °C for
10 min. Shake frequently. Allow to cool to room temperature
and filter.

Reference solution   Dissolve 1.0 mg of *chlorogenic acid R* and
3.0 mg of *rutin R* in 20 mL of *methanol R*.

Plate   *TLC silica gel plate R*.

Mobile phase   *anhydrous formic acid R, glacial acetic acid R,
water R, ethyl acetate R* (7.5:7.5:17.5:67.5 *V/V/V/V*).

Application   20 μL as bands.

Development   Over a path of 17 cm.

Drying   At 100-105 °C.

Detection   Spray the warm plate with a 10 g/L solution of
diphenylboric acid aminoethyl ester R in *methanol R*, then with
the same volume of a 50 g/L solution of *macrogol 400 R* in
methanol R; allow to dry in air for about 30 min and examine
in ultraviolet light at 365 nm.

Results   See below the sequence of zones present in the
chromatograms obtained with the reference solution and the
test solution. Furthermore, other weak fluorescent zones may
be present in the chromatogram obtained with the test
solution.

Top of the plate	
	A yellowish-brown fluorescent zone
	A green fluorescent zone
	2 yellowish-brown fluorescent zones
	An intense light blue fluorescent zone sometimes overlapped by a greenish-brown fluorescent zone
Chlorogenic acid: a light blue fluorescent zone	
	A green fluorescent zone
Rutin: a yellowish-brown fluorescent zone	2 yellowish-brown fluorescent zones
	A green fluorescent zone
	A yellowish-brown fluorescent zone
Reference solution	**Test solution**

TESTS

Foreign matter (*2.8.2*)
Maximum 5 per cent of stems and 2 per cent of other
foreign matter.

Loss on drying (*2.2.32*)
Maximum 11.0 per cent, determined on 1.000 g of the
powdered drug (355) (*2.9.12*) by drying in an oven at
105 °C for 2 h.

Total ash (*2.4.16*)
Maximum 11.0 per cent.

ASSAY
Flavonoids
Liquid chromatography (*2.2.29*).

Test solution   Heat 2.500 g of the powdered drug (710)
(*2.9.12*) in 50 mL of a 60 per cent *V/V* solution of *acetone R*
under a reflux condenser for 30 min. Filter and collect the
filtrate. Extract the drug residue a 2nd time in the same
manner, using 40 mL of a 60 per cent *V/V* solution of
acetone R and filter. Collect the filtrates and dilute to
100.0 mL with a 60 per cent *V/V* solution of *acetone R*.
Evaporate 50.0 mL of the solution to eliminate the acetone
and transfer to a 50.0 mL vial, rinsing with 30 mL of
methanol R. Add 4.4 mL of *hydrochloric acid R1*, dilute to
50.0 mL with *water R* and centrifuge. Place 10 mL of the
supernatant in a 10 mL brown-glass vial. Close with a rubber
seal and an aluminium cap and heat on a water-bath for
25 min. Allow to cool to room temperature.

Reference solution   Dissolve 10.0 mg of *quercetin dihydrate R*
in 20 mL of *methanol R*. Add 15.0 mL of *dilute hydrochloric
acid R* and 5 mL of *water R* and dilute to 50.0 mL with
methanol R.

Column:
— *size*: $l = 0.125$ m, Ø = 4 mm;
— *stationary phase*: octadecylsilyl silica gel for chromatography R
  (5 μm);
— *temperature*: 25 °C.

Mobile phase:
— *mobile phase A*: 0.3 g/L solution of *phosphoric acid R*
  adjusted to pH 2.0;
— *mobile phase B*: methanol R;

Time (min)	Mobile phase A (per cent *V/V*)	Mobile phase B (per cent *V/V*)
0 - 1	60	40
1 - 20	60 → 45	40 → 55
20 - 21	45 → 0	55 → 100
21 - 25	0	100

Flow rate 1.0 mL/min.

Detection Spectrophotometer at 370 nm.

Injection 10 µL.

Relative retention With reference to quercetin (retention time = about 12.5 min): kaempferol = about 1.4; isorhamnetin = about 1.5.

System suitability:
— *resolution*: minimum 1.5 between the peaks due to kaempferol and isorhamnetin.

Do not take into account peaks eluting before the quercetin peak or after the isorhamnetin peak in the chromatogram obtained with the test solution.

Calculate the percentage content of flavonoids, expressed as flavone glycosides, using the following expression:

$$2 \times \frac{F_1 \times m_1 \times 2.514 \times p}{F_2 \times m_2}$$

F_1 = sum of the areas of all the considered peaks in the chromatogram obtained with the test solution;

F_2 = area of the peak corresponding to quercetin in the chromatogram obtained with the reference solution;

m_1 = mass of quercetin used to prepare the reference solution, in grams;

m_2 = mass of the drug to be examined used to prepare the test solution, in grams;

p = percentage content of anhydrous quercetin in *quercetin dihydrate R*.

_____ *Ph Eur*

Refined and Quantified Ginkgo Dry Extract

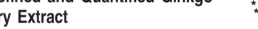

(Ph Eur monograph 1827)

Ph Eur _____

DEFINITION
Refined and quantified dry extract produced from *Ginkgo leaf (1828)*.

Content:
— *flavonoids, expressed as flavone glycosides (M_r 756.7)*: 22.0 per cent to 27.0 per cent (dried extract);
— *bilobalide*: 2.6 per cent to 3.2 per cent (dried extract);
— *ginkgolides A, B and C*: 2.8 per cent to 3.4 per cent (dried extract);
— *ginkgolic acids*: maximum 5 ppm (dried extract).

PRODUCTION
The extract is produced from the herbal drug by an appropriate procedure using organic solvents and their mixtures with water, physical separation steps as well as other suitable processes.

CHARACTERS
Appearance
Bright yellow-brown, powder or friable mass.

IDENTIFICATION
Thin-layer chromatography (2.2.27).

Test solution Dissolve 20.0 mg of the extract to be examined in 10 mL of a mixture of 2 volumes of *water R* and 8 volumes of *methanol R*.

Reference solution Dissolve 1.0 mg of *chlorogenic acid R* and 3.0 mg of *rutin R* in 20 mL of *methanol R*.

Plate TLC silica gel plate R (5-40 µm) or [TLC silica gel plate R (2-10 µm)].

Mobile phase anhydrous formic acid R, glacial acetic acid R, water R, ethyl acetate R (7.5:7.5:17.5:67.5 V/V/V/V).

Application 20 µL [or 5 µL], as bands.

Development Over a path of 17 cm [or 6 cm].

Drying At 100-105 °C.

Detection Spray the plate whilst still hot with a 10 g/L solution of *diphenylboric acid aminoethyl ester R* in *methanol R*, then spray with a 50 g/L solution of *macrogol 400 R* in *methanol R*; allow to dry in air for about 30 min and examine in ultraviolet light at 365 nm.

Results See below the sequence of zones present in the chromatograms obtained with the reference solution and the test solution. Furthermore, other, weaker fluorescent zones may be present in the chromatogram obtained with the test solution.

ASSAY
Flavonoids
Liquid chromatography (2.2.29).

Test solution Dissolve 0.200 g of the extract to be examined in 20 mL of *methanol R*. Add 15.0 mL of *dilute hydrochloric acid R* and 5 mL of *water R* and dilute to 50.0 mL with *methanol R*. Transfer 10.0 mL of this solution into a 10 mL brown-glass vial. Close the vial with a tight rubber membrane stopper and secure with an aluminium crimped cap. Heat on a water-bath for 25 min. Allow to cool to 20 °C.

Reference solution Dissolve 10.0 mg of *quercetin dihydrate CRS* in 20 mL of *methanol R*. Add 15.0 mL of *dilute hydrochloric acid R* and 5 mL of *water R* and dilute to 50.0 mL with *methanol R*.

Column:
— *size*: l = 0.125 m, Ø = 4 mm;
— *stationary phase*: octadecylsilyl silica gel for chromatography R (5 µm);
— *temperature*: 25 °C.

Mobile phase:
— *mobile phase A*: 0.3 g/L solution of *phosphoric acid R* adjusted to pH 2.0;
— *mobile phase B*: methanol R;

Time (min)	Mobile phase A (per cent *V/V*)	Mobile phase B (per cent *V/V*)
0 - 1	60	40
1 - 20	60 → 45	40 → 55
20 - 21	45 → 0	55 → 100
21 - 25	0	100

Flow rate 1.0 mL/min.

Detector Spectrophotometer at 370 nm.

Injection 10 µL.

Relative retention With reference to quercetin (retention time = about 12.5 min): kaempferol = about 1.4; isorhamnetin = about 1.5.

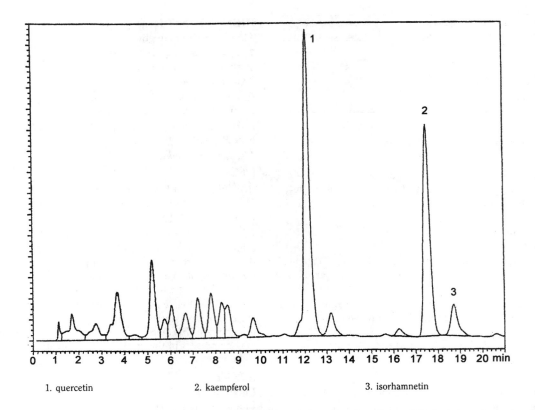

1. quercetin 2. kaempferol 3. isorhamnetin

Figure 1827.-1. – Chromatogram for the assay of flavonoids in refined and quantified ginkgo dry extract

Top of the plate		
	A blue fluorescent zone	
	Several faint coloured zones	
───────		───────
	A brown fluorescent zone	
	A green fluorescent zone	
	An intense light blue fluorescent zone sometimes overlapped by a greenish-brown fluorescent zone	
Chlorogenic acid: a light blue fluorescent zone		
	One or two green fluorescent zones	
Rutin: a yellowish-brown fluorescent zone	One or two yellowish-brown fluorescent zones	
───────		───────
	Several green and yellowish-brown fluorescent zones	
Reference solution	**Test solution**	

System suitability Test solution:
— *resolution*: minimum 1.5 between the peaks due to kaempferol and isorhamnetin.

Determine the sum of the areas including all the peaks from the peak due to quercetin to the peak due to isorhamnetin in the chromatogram obtained with the test solution (see Figure 1827.-1).

Calculate the percentage content of flavonoids, expressed as flavone glycosides, using the following expression:

$$\frac{F_1 \times m_1 \times 2.514 \times p}{F_2 \times m_2}$$

F_1 = sum of the areas of all the peaks from the peak due to quercetin to the peak due to isorhamnetin in the chromatogram obtained with the test solution

F_2 = area of the peak due to quercetin in the chromatogram obtained with the reference solution

m_1 = mass of *quercetin dihydrate CRS* in the reference solution, in grams

m_2 = mass of the extract to be examined used to prepare the test solution, in grams

p = percentage content of anhydrous quercetin in *quercetin dihydrate CRS*.

Terpene lactones
Liquid chromatography (*2.2.29*).

Test solution Place 0.120 g of the extract to be examined in a 25 mL beaker and dissolve it in 10 mL of *phosphate buffer solution pH 5.8 R* by stirring. Transfer the solution into a chromatography column, about 0.15 m long and about 30 mm in internal diameter, containing 15 g of *kieselguhr for chromatography R*. Wash the beaker with 2 quantities, each of 5 mL, of *phosphate buffer solution pH 5.8 R* and transfer the washings to the chromatography column. Allow to stand for 15 min. Elute with 100 mL of *ethyl acetate R*. Evaporate the eluate to dryness at a pressure not exceeding 4 kPa in a water-bath at 50 °C. The residue of solvent is eliminated by an air-current. Take up the residue in 2.5 mL of the mobile phase.

Reference solution (a) Dissolve 30.0 mg of *benzyl alcohol CRS* in the mobile phase and dilute to 100.0 mL with the mobile phase.

Reference solution (b)   Place 0.120 g of the *ginkgo dry extract for peak identification CRS* in a 25 mL beaker and dissolve it in 10 mL of *phosphate buffer solution pH 5.8 R* by stirring, then proceed as described for the test solution.

Column:
— *size*: $l = 0.25$ m, $\varnothing = 4$ mm;
— *stationary phase*: octylsilyl silica gel for chromatography *R* (5 µm);
— *temperature*: 25 °C.

Mobile phase   tetrahydrofuran *R*, methanol *R*, water *R* (10:20:75 *V/V/V*).

Flow rate   1.0 mL/min.

Detection   Refractometer maintained at 35 °C.

Injection   100 µL.

Identification of peaks   Use the chromatogram supplied with *ginkgo dry extract for peak identification CRS* and the chromatogram obtained with the reference solution (b) to identify the peaks due to bilobalide and ginkgolides A, B and C.

System suitability:
— the chromatogram obtained with reference solution (b) is similar to the chromatogram supplied with *ginkgo dry extract for peak identification CRS*.

Calculate the percentage content of bilobalide, using the following expression:

$$\frac{F_1 \times m_1 \times p \times 0.025 \times 1.20}{F_5 \times m_2}$$

Calculate the percentage content of ginkgolide A, using the following expression:

$$\frac{F_2 \times m_1 \times p \times 0.025 \times 1.22}{F_5 \times m_2}$$

Calculate the percentage content of ginkgolide B, using the following expression:

$$\frac{F_3 \times m_1 \times p \times 0.025 \times 1.19}{F_5 \times m_2}$$

Calculate the percentage content of ginkgolide C, using the following expression:

$$\frac{F_4 \times m_1 \times p \times 0.025 \times 1.27}{F_5 \times m_2}$$

F_1 = area of the peak due to bilobalide in the chromatogram obtained with the test solution
F_2 = area of the peak due to ginkgolide A in the chromatogram obtained with the test solution
F_3 = area of the peak due to ginkgolide B in the chromatogram obtained with the test solution
F_4 = area of the peak due to ginkgolide C in the chromatogram obtained with the test solution
F_5 = area of the peak due to benzyl alcohol in the chromatogram obtained with reference solution (a)
m_1 = mass of *benzyl alcohol CRS* in reference solution (a), in grams
m_2 = mass of the extract to be examined used to prepare the test solution, in grams
p = percentage content of benzyl alcohol in *benzyl alcohol CRS*.

Calculate the percentage content of the sum of ginkgolides A, B and C, using the following expression:

$$G_A + G_B + G_C$$

G_A = percentage content of ginkgolide A
G_B = percentage content of ginkgolide B
G_C = percentage content of ginkgolide C.

Ginkgolic acids

Liquid chromatography (*2.2.29*).

Test solution   Dissolve 0.500 g of the powdered extract to be examined in 8 mL of *methanol R*, sonicating if necessary, and dilute to 10.0 mL with the same solvent. Centrifuge if necessary.

Reference solution   Dissolve 10.0 mg of *ginkgolic acids CRS* in 8 mL of *methanol R*, sonicating if necessary, and dilute to 10.0 mL with the same solvent. Dilute 2.0 mL of this solution to 10.0 mL with *methanol R*.

Column:
— *size*: $l = 0.25$ m, $\varnothing = 4.6$ mm;
— *stationary phase*: octylsilyl silica gel for chromatography *R* (5 µm);
— *temperature*: 35 °C.

Mobile phase:
— *mobile phase A*: dilute 0.1 mL of *trifluoroacetic acid R* to 1000 mL with *water R*;
— *mobile phase B*: dilute 0.1 mL of *trifluoroacetic acid R* to 1000 mL with *acetonitrile R*;

Time (min)	Mobile phase A (per cent *V/V*)	Mobile phase B (per cent *V/V*)
0 - 30	25 → 10	75 → 90
30 - 35	10	90
35 - 36	10 → 25	90 → 75
36 - 45	25	75

Flow rate   1.0 mL/min.

Detection   Spectrophotometer at 210 nm.

Injection   50 µL.

Identification of components   Use the chromatogram supplied with *ginkgolic acids CRS* and the chromatogram obtained with the test solution to identify the peaks due to ginkgolic acids C13, C15 and C17.

System suitability   Reference solution:
— *resolution*: minimum 2.0 between the peaks due to ginkgolic acids C13 and C15;
— *symmetry factor*: 0.8 to 2.0 for the peaks due to ginkgolic acids C13, C15 and C17.

Calculate the content in parts per million of ginkgolic acids expressed as ginkgolic acid C17, using the following expression:

$$\frac{A_1 \times m_2 \times p \times 2000}{A_2 \times m_1}$$

A_1 = sum of the areas of the peaks due to the ginkgolic acids C13, C15 and C17 in the chromatogram obtained with the test solution
A_2 = area of the peak due to ginkgolic acid C17 in the chromatogram obtained with the reference solution
m_1 = mass of the extract to be examined used to prepare the test solution, in grams

Herbal Drugs

m_2 = mass of *ginkgolic acids CRS* used to prepare the reference solution, in grams

p = percentage content of ginkgolic acid C17 in *ginkgolic acids CRS*.

Ph Eur

Ginseng

(*Ph Eur monograph 1523*)

Ph Eur

DEFINITION

Whole or cut dried root, designated white ginseng; treated with steam and then dried, designated red ginseng, of *Panax ginseng* C. A. Meyer.

Content

Minimum 0.40 per cent for the sum of ginsenosides Rg1 ($C_{42}H_{72}O_{14}$,$2H_2O$; M_r 837) and Rb1 ($C_{54}H_{92}O_{23}$,$3H_2O$; M_r 1163) (dried drug).

IDENTIFICATION

A. The principal root is fusiform or cylindrical, sometimes branched, up to about 20 cm long and 2.5 cm in diameter, and may be curved or markedly re-curved. The surface is pale yellow to cream in white ginseng, brownish-red in red ginseng and shows longitudinal ridges. Stem scars may be seen at the crown. The fracture is short. The transversely-cut surface shows a wide outer zone with scattered orange-red resin canals and a finely radiate inner region. The rootlets, numerous in the lower part of white ginseng, are normally absent in red ginseng.

B. Reduce to a powder (355) (*2.9.12*). The powder is light yellow. Examine under a microscope using *chloral hydrate solution R*. The powder shows the following diagnostic characters: abundant fragments of thin-walled parenchymatous cells and fragments of large secretory canals containing yellowish-brown resin, non-lignified tracheids and partially-lignified vessels with spiral or reticulate thickening, isolated or in groups; scattered cluster crystals of calcium oxalate. Examine under a microscope using a mixture of equal volumes of *glycerol R* and *water R*. The starch granules are very abundant, simple or 2 or 3 compound, and range from 1-10 μm in diameter. In red ginseng the starch granules are often deformed and destroyed by treating with steam, or may be absent.

C. Thin-layer chromatography (*2.2.27*).

Test solution Boil 1.0 g of the powdered drug (355) (*2.9.12*) under a reflux condenser with 10 mL of a 70 per cent *V/V* solution of *methanol R* for 15 min. Filter after cooling and dilute to 10.0 mL with *methanol R*.

Reference solution Dissolve 5.0 mg of *aescin R* and 5.0 mg of *arbutin R* in 1 mL of *methanol R*.

Plate TLC silica gel plate R (5-40 μm) [or *TLC silica gel plate R* (2-10 μm)].

Mobile phase ethyl acetate R, water R, butanol R (25:50:100 *V/V/V*), allow the mixture to separate for 10 min. Use the upper layer.

Application 20 μL [or 4 μL] as bands.

Development Over 10 cm [or 5 cm] in an unsaturated tank.

Drying In air.

Detection Spray with *anisaldehyde solution R* and heat at 105-110 °C for 5-10 min. Examine in daylight.

Results See below the sequence of the zones present in the chromatograms obtained with the reference solution and the test solution.

Top of the plate	
Arbutin: a brown zone	
	A violet zone (ginsenosides Rg1 + Rg2)
	A faint violet zone (ginsenoside Rf)
	A violet zone (ginsenoside Re)
	A violet zone (ginsenoside Rd)
	A faint violet zone
	A violet zone (ginsenoside Rc)
Aescin: a grey zone	A violet zone (ginsenosides Rb1 + Rb2)
Reference solution	**Test solution**

TESTS

Panax quinquefolium

Examine the chromatograms obtained in the assay. The chromatogram obtained with the test solution shows a peak due to ginsenoside Rf (see Figure 1523.-1). In the case of a substitution by *Panax quinquefolium* no peak due to ginsenoside Rf is present.

Loss on drying (*2.2.32*)
Maximum 10.0 per cent, determined on 1.000 g of the powdered drug (355) (*2.9.12*) by drying in an oven at 105 °C.

Total ash (*2.4.16*)
Mximum 7.0 per cent.

Ash insoluble in hydrochloric acid (*2.8.1*)
Maximum 1.0 per cent.

ASSAY

Liquid chromatography (*2.2.29*).

Test solution Reduce about 50 g to a powder (355) (*2.9.12*). Place 1.00 g of the powdered drug and 70 mL of a 50 per cent *V/V* solution of *methanol R* in a 250 mL round-bottomed flask. After adding a few grains of pumice, boil on a water-bath under a reflux condenser for 1 h. After cooling, centrifuge and collect the supernatant liquid. Treat the residue as described above. Mix the collected liquids and evaporate to dryness under reduced pressure at a temperature not exceeding 60 °C. Take up the residue with 20.0 mL of a mixture of 20 volumes of *acetonitrile R* and 80 volumes of *water R*. Dilute 2.0 mL of the solution to 10.0 mL with a mixture of 20 volumes of *acetonitrile R* and 80 volumes of *water R*. Filter through a suitable membrane filter (nominal pore size 0.45 μm) before injection.

Reference solution Dissolve 3.0 mg of *ginsenoside Rg1 R*, 3.0 mg of *ginsenoside Re R*, 3.0 mg of *ginsenoside Rf R* and 3.0 mg of *ginsenoside Rb1 R* in *methanol R* and dilute to 10.0 mL with the same solvent.

Column:
— size: l = 0.125 m, Ø = 4.6 mm;
— stationary phase: *octadecylsilyl silica gel for chromatography R* (5 μm);
— temperature: 35 °C.

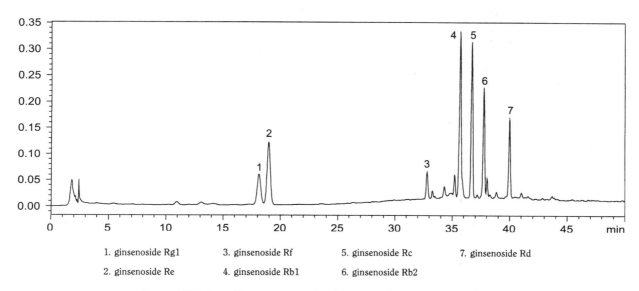

1. ginsenoside Rg1   3. ginsenoside Rf   5. ginsenoside Rc   7. ginsenoside Rd

2. ginsenoside Re   4. ginsenoside Rb1   6. ginsenoside Rb2

Figure 1523.-1. – *Chromatogram for the assay of ginseng: test solution*

Mobile phase:
— *mobile phase A: water R* adjusted to pH 2 with *phosphoric acid R*;
— *mobile phase B: acetonitrile R*;

Time (min)	Mobile phase A (per cent *V/V*)	Mobile phase B (per cent *V/V*)
0 - 8	80	20
8 - 40	80 → 60	20 → 40
40 - 45	60 → 40	40 → 60
45 - 47	40 → 0	60 → 100
47 - 52	0	100
52 - 55	0 → 80	100 → 20

Flow rate   1.0 mL/min.

Detection   Spectrophotometer at 203 nm.

Equilibration   20 min.

Injection   20 μL.

Elution order   Order indicated in the composition of the reference solution; record the retention times of these substances.

System suitability   Reference solution:
— *resolution*: minimum 1.0 between the peaks due to ginsenoside Rg1 and ginsenoside Re.

Locate the peaks due to ginsenoside Rb1 and ginsenoside Rg1 in the chromatogram obtained with the test solution.

Calculate the percentage content of ginsenosides Rb1 and Rg1 using the following expression:

$$\frac{A_1 \times m_2 \times p_1}{A_3 \times m_1 \times 100} + \frac{A_2 \times m_3 \times p_2}{A_4 \times m_1 \times 100}$$

A_1 = area of the peak due to ginsenoside Rb1 in the chromatogram obtained with the test solution,

A_2 = area of the peak due to ginsenoside Rg1 in the chromatogram obtained with the test solution,

A_3 = area of the peak due to ginsenoside Rb1 in the chromatogram obtained with the reference solution,

A_4 = area of the peak due to ginsenoside Rg1 in the chromatogram obtained with the reference solution,

m_1 = mass of the drug to be examined, in grams,

m_2 = mass of ginsenoside Rb1 in the reference solution, in milligrams,

m_3 = mass of ginsenoside Rg1 in the reference solution, in milligrams,

p_1 = percentage content of ginsenoside Rb1 in the reagent,

p_2 = percentage content of ginsenoside Rg1 in the reagent.

Ph Eur

Ginseng Dry Extract

(*Ph Eur monograph 2356*)

Ph Eur

DEFINITION

Dry extract produced from *Ginseng (1523)*.

Content

Minimum 4.0 per cent of the sum of ginsenosides Rb1, Rb2, Rc, Rd, Re, Rf, Rg1 and Rg2, expressed as ginsenoside Rb1 ($C_{54}H_{92}O_{23}$; M_r 1109) (dried extract).

PRODUCTION

The extract is produced from the herbal drug by a suitable procedure using a hydroalcoholic solvent equivalent in strength to ethanol (35-90 per cent *V/V*).

CHARACTERS

Appearance

Light brownish-yellow, hygroscopic powder or brittle mass.

IDENTIFICATION

Thin-layer chromatography (*2.2.27*).

Test solution   Dissolve 0.15 g of the extract to be examined in 10 mL of a 70 per cent *V/V* solution of *methanol R*.

Reference solution   Dissolve 0.15 g of *ginseng dry extract HRS* in 10 mL of a 70 per cent *V/V* solution of *methanol R*.

Plate   *TLC silica gel plate R* (5-40 μm) [or *TLC silica gel plate R* (2-10 μm)].

Mobile phase   *ethyl acetate R, water R, butanol R* (25:50:100 *V/V/V*); allow the phases to separate for 10 min and use the upper layer.

Application 20 μL [or 4 μL] as bands of 10 mm [or 8 mm].

Development Over a path of 10 cm [or 5 cm] in an unsaturated tank.

Drying In air.

Detection Treat with *anisaldehyde solution R* and heat at 105-110 °C for 5-10 min; examine in daylight.

Results See below the sequence of zones present in the chromatograms obtained with the reference solution and the test solution. Furthermore, other faint zones may be present in the chromatograms obtained with the test solution and the reference solution.

Top of the plate	
———	———
A violet zone (ginsenosides Rg1 + Rg2)	A violet zone (ginsenosides Rg1 + Rg2)
A faint violet zone (ginsenoside Rf)	A faint violet zone (ginsenoside Rf)
A violet zone (ginsenoside Re)	A violet zone (ginsenoside Re)
A violet zone (ginsenoside Rd)	A violet zone (ginsenoside Rd)
A faint violet zone	A faint violet zone
A violet zone (ginsenoside Rc)	A violet zone (ginsenoside Rc)
A faint violet zone	A faint violet zone
———	———
A violet zone (ginsenosides Rb1 + Rb2)	A violet zone (ginsenosides Rb1 + Rb2)
Several unresolved violet and greenish zones	Several unresolved violet and greenish zones
Reference solution	**Test solution**

TESTS

Loss on drying (*2.8.17*)
Maximum 7.0 per cent.

ASSAY

Liquid chromatography (*2.2.29*).

Buffer solution Dissolve 3.5 g of *disodium hydrogen phosphate dihydrate R* and 7.2 g of *potassium dihydrogen phosphate R* in *water R* and dilute to 1000 mL with the same solvent.

Test solution Dissolve 0.100 g of the extract to be examined in the buffer solution and dilute to 10.0 mL with the buffer solution. Prepare a ready-to-use sample-preparation cartridge containing 0.50 g of octadecylsilyl silica gel (45 μm), using 5 mL of *methanol R* followed by 20 mL of *water R*. Apply 5.0 mL of the solution to be analysed to the top of the cartridge. Wash the cartridge with 20 mL of *water R* followed by 15 mL of a 30 per cent *V/V* solution of *methanol R*. Discard the eluates after confirming that no ginsenosides are present, otherwise repeat the preparation of the solution with another brand of cartridge where no ginsenosides are eluted with a 30 per cent *V/V* solution of *methanol R*. Elute the cartridge with 20 mL of *methanol R*; collect the eluate. Under reduced pressure, evaporate the eluate to dryness. Dissolve the residue in 2.0 mL of *methanol R*. Filter through a suitable membrane filter (nominal pore size 0.45 μm).

Reference solution (a) Dissolve 0.100 g of *ginseng dry extract HRS* in the buffer solution and dilute to 10.0 mL with the buffer solution. Prepare a ready-to-use sample-preparation cartridge containing 0.50 g of octadecylsilyl silica gel (45 μm), using 5 mL of *methanol R* followed by 20 mL of

water R. Apply 5.0 mL of the solution to be analysed to the top of the cartridge. Wash the cartridge with 20 mL of *water R* followed by 15 mL of a 30 per cent *V/V* solution of *methanol R*. Discard the eluates after confirming that no ginsenosides are present, otherwise repeat the preparation of the solution with another brand of cartridge where no ginsenosides are eluted with a 30 per cent *V/V* solution of *methanol R*. Elute the cartridge with 20 mL of *methanol R*; collect the eluate. Under reduced pressure, evaporate the eluate to dryness. Dissolve the residue in 2.0 mL of *methanol R*. Filter through a suitable membrane filter (nominal pore size 0.45 μm).

Reference solution (b) Dissolve 3.0 mg of *ginsenoside Rb1 CRS* in *methanol R* and dilute to 5.0 mL with the same solvent.

Reference solution (c) Dissolve 3.0 mg of *ginsenoside Rg2 R* in *methanol R* and dilute to 5.0 mL with the same solvent.

Reference solution (d) Dilute 1.0 mL of reference solution (b) to 2.0 mL with reference solution (c).

Column:
— *size:* l = 0.125 m, Ø = 4.6 mm;
— *stationary phase: octadecylsilyl silica gel for chromatography R* (5 μm);
— *temperature:* 35 °C.

Mobile phase:
— *mobile phase A: water R* adjusted to pH 2 with *phosphoric acid R*;
— *mobile phase B: acetonitrile R1*;

Time (min)	Mobile phase A (per cent *V/V*)	Mobile phase B (per cent *V/V*)
0 - 8	80	20
8 - 40	80 → 60	20 → 40
40 - 45	60 → 40	40 → 60
45 - 47	40 → 0	60 → 100

Flow rate 1.0 mL/min.

Detection Spectrophotometer at 203 nm.

Injection 20 μL.

Elution order Ginsenoside Rg1, ginsenoside Re, ginsenoside Rf, ginsenoside Rb1, ginsenoside Rg2, ginsenoside Rc, ginsenoside Rb2, ginsenoside Rd; depending on the operating conditions and the state of the column, ginsenoside Rb1 may elute before or after ginsenoside Rg2.

Identification of peaks Use the chromatogram supplied with *ginseng dry extract HRS* and the chromatogram obtained with reference solution (a) to identify the peaks due to ginsenosides Rg1, Re, Rf, Rc, Rb2 and Rd; use the chromatogram obtained with reference solution (b) to identify the peak due to ginsenoside Rb1; use the chromatogram obtained with reference solution (c) to identify the peak due to ginsenoside Rg2.

Relative retention With reference to ginsenoside Rb1 (retention time = about 33 min):
ginsenoside Rg1 = about 0.53; ginsenoside Re = about 0.54; ginsenoside Rf = about 0.88; ginsenoside Rg2 = about 0.98; ginsenoside Rc = about 1.04; ginsenoside Rb2 = about 1.08; ginsenoside Rd = about 1.17.

System suitability Reference solution (d):
— *resolution:* minimum 1.5 between the peaks due to ginsenosides Rg2 and Rb1.

Calculate the percentage content of the sum of ginsenosides Rb1, Rb2, Rc, Rd, Re, Rf, Rg1 and Rg2, expressed as ginsenoside Rb1, using the following expression:

$$\frac{A_1 \times m_2 \times p \times 0.8}{A_2 \times m_1}$$

A_1 = sum of the areas of the peaks due to ginsenosides Rb1, Rb2, Rc, Rd, Re, Rf, Rg1 and Rg2 in the chromatogram obtained with the test solution;

A_2 = area of the peak due to ginsenoside Rb1 in the chromatogram obtained with reference solution (b);

m_1 = mass of the extract to be examined used to prepare the test solution, in grams;

m_2 = mass of *ginsenoside Rb1 CRS* used to prepare reference solution (b), in grams;

p = percentage content of ginsenoside Rb1 in *ginsenoside Rb1 CRS*.

_____ *Ph Eur*

Goldenrod

(*Ph Eur monograph 1892*)

Ph Eur _____

DEFINITION

Whole or cut, dried, flowering aerial parts of *Solidago gigantea* Ait or *Solidago canadensis* L., their varieties or hybrids and/or mixtures of these.

Content

Minimum 2.5 per cent of flavonoids, expressed as hyperoside ($C_{21}H_{20}O_{12}$; M_r 464.4) (dried drug).

IDENTIFICATION

A. The stems are greenish-yellow or greenish-brown, partly tinted reddish, roundish, more or less conspicuously grooved, glabrous and smooth in the lower part, slightly or densely pubescent in the upper part. They are solid with a whitish pith.

The leaves are green, sessile, lanceolate, with a serrate margin, 8-12 cm long and about 1-3 cm wide, the upper surface is green and more or less glabrous, the lower surface is greyish-green and pubescent, especially on the veins. The inflorescence consists of a number of unilateral, curved racemes which together form a pyramidal panicle at the end of the stems.

Each capitulum has an involucre composed of linear-lanceolate, imbricated yellowish-green bracts, surrounding a single row of yellow ligulate florets about the same length as the involucre; yellow, radially arranged tubular florets, as long as, or longer than, the ligulate florets; a brownish inferior ovary surmounted by a white pappus of silky hairs.

B. Reduce to a powder (355) (*2.9.12*). The powder is greyish-green. Examine under a microscope using *chloral hydrate solution R*. The powder shows pappus bristles and their fragments, consisting of multiseriate trichomes composed of elongated cells with the tips free from the surface and forming pointed projections over the entire length; fragments of the leaf mesophyll with vascular bundles accompanied by secretory cells; fragments of the leaf epidermis with sinuous to wavy-walled cells and stomata of the anomocytic type (*2.8.3*); uniseriate covering trichomes with up to 5 or 6 cells, some whip-like with a thicker-walled terminal cell; fragments of the style with long, slender papillae; fragments of the stem with reticulate and spiral vessels; pollen grains, with 3 germinal pores and a spiny exine; numerous whisk-shaped hairs, a few isolated twin-hairs from the ovary, absence of multicellular trichomes with a terminal cell bent at a right angle.

C. Thin-layer chromatography (*2.2.27*).

Test solution To 0.75 g of the powdered drug (355) (*2.9.12*) add 5 mL of *methanol R* and boil in a water-bath under a reflux condenser for 10 min. Cool and filter.

Reference solution Dissolve 1.0 mg of *chlorogenic acid R*, 2.5 mg of *quercitrin R* and 2.5 mg of *rutin R* in 10 mL of *methanol R*.

Plate *TLC silica gel plate R*.

Mobile phase anhydrous formic acid R, water R, methyl ethyl ketone R, ethyl acetate R (6:6:18:30 *V/V/V/V*).

Application 20 µL of the test solution and 10 µL of the reference solution as bands.

Development Over a path of 10 cm.

Drying At 100-105 °C.

Detection Spray with a 10 g/L solution of *diphenylboric acid aminoethyl ester R* in *methanol R* and then with a 50 g/L solution of *macrogol 400 R* in *methanol R*. Allow to stand for 30 min. Examine in ultraviolet light at 365 nm.

Results See below the sequence of zones present in the chromatograms obtained with the reference solution and the test solution. Furthermore, other zones may be present in the chromatogram obtained with the test solution.

Top of the plate	
	A bluish-green fluorescent zone
Quercitrin: a yellowish-brown fluorescent zone	A faint to intense yellowish-brown fluorescent zone (quercitrin)
	A more or less intense yellowish brown zone
Chlorogenic acid: a light blue fluorescent zone	A light blue zone and/or a yellow fluorescent zone (chlorogenic acid)
Rutin: an orange fluorescent zone	A faint to intense yellowish-brown fluorescent zone (rutin)
Reference solution	**Test solution**

TESTS

Foreign matter (*2.8.2*)

Maximum 5 per cent of brownish parts and maximum 2 per cent of other foreign matter.

Loss on drying (*2.2.32*)

Maximum 10 per cent, determined on 0.500 g of the powdered drug (355) (*2.9.12*) by drying in an oven at 105 °C for 2 h.

Total ash (*2.4.16*)

Maximum 7.0 per cent.

Ash insoluble in hydrochloric acid (*2.8.1*)

Maximum 1.0 per cent.

ASSAY

Stock solution In a 100 mL round-bottomed flask, introduce 0.200 g of the powdered drug (250) (*2.9.12*), add 1 mL of a 5 g/L solution of *hexamethylenetetramine R*, 20 mL of *acetone R* and 2 mL of *hydrochloric acid R1*. Boil the mixture under a reflux condenser for 30 min. Filter the liquid through a small plug of absorbent cotton into a 100 mL flask. Add the absorbent cotton to the residue in the round-bottomed flask, extract with 2 quantities, each of 20 mL of *acetone R*, each time boiling under a reflux condenser for 10 min. Allow to cool. Filter the combined acetone extracts through a filter paper into a volumetric flask. Rinse the flask and the filter paper and dilute to 100.0 mL with *acetone R*. Introduce 20.0 mL of the solution into a separating funnel, add 20 mL of *water R* and shake the mixture with 1 quantity of 15 mL and then 3 quantities, each of 10 mL, of *ethyl acetate R*. Combine the ethyl acetate extracts in a separating funnel, wash twice with 50 mL of *water R* and filter the extracts over 10 g of *anhydrous sodium sulfate R* into a volumetric flask. Dilute to 50.0 mL with *ethyl acetate R*, rinsing the separating funnel and the sodium sulfate.

Test solution To 10.0 mL of the stock solution add 1.0 mL of *aluminium chloride reagent R* and dilute to 25.0 mL with a 5 per cent *V/V* solution of *glacial acetic acid R* in *methanol R*.

Compensation solution Dilute 10.0 mL of the stock solution to 25.0 mL with a 5 per cent *V/V* solution of *glacial acetic acid R* in *methanol R*.

Measure the absorbance of the test solution (*2.2.25*) at 425 nm after 30 min by comparison with the compensation solution.

Calculate the percentage content of flavonoids, expressed as hyperoside, from the expression:

$$\frac{A \times 1.25}{m}$$

i.e. taking the value of the specific absorbance of hyperoside to be 500.

A = absorbance measured at 425 nm,
m = mass of the drug to be examined, in grams.

Ph Eur

European Goldenrod

(*Ph Eur monograph 1893*)

Ph Eur

DEFINITION
Whole or fragmented, dried, flowering aerial parts of *Solidago virgaurea* L.

Content
Minimum 0.5 per cent and maximum 1.5 per cent of flavonoids, expressed as hyperoside ($C_{21}H_{20}O_{12}$; M_r 464.4) (dried drug).

IDENTIFICATION
A. The stem is cylindrical, striated, the lower part often reddish-violet, sometimes entirely glabrous or pubescent with short, bent, apically directed hairs. The basal leaves are obovate or oblanceolate, with a serrate margin, and taper at the base into a long, winged petiole; the cauline leaves are alternate, smaller than the basal leaves and more elliptical in outline, with an entire or slightly toothed margin; they are sessile or with only a short petiole. Both surfaces of the leaves are glabrous or only slightly pubescent with a prominent reticulate venation on the lower surface. The capitula form a tightly packed panicle. At the base of the pedicels there are 2 small, linear bracts with scarious margins. The involucre consists of 2-4 rows of loosely arranged, imbricate bracts, each bract greenish-yellow with a smooth and shiny inner surface, the outer surface hairy or glabrous, with a scarious

margin. Each capitulum contains 6-12 widely separated female ray florets, about twice as long as the bracts, and about 10-30 hermaphrodite, tubular florets. All florets are yellow. The brown, inferior ovary tapers towards the base and has a ribbed surface, covered with scattered hairs; it is surmounted by a whitish pappus composed of smooth or rough, bristly hairs.

B. Microscopic examination (*2.8.23*). The powder is light green. Examine under a microscope using *chloral hydrate solution R*. The powder shows the following diagnostic characters (Figures 1893.-1 and 1893.-2): fragments of the upper epidermis of the leaf in surface view [B, H, M], covered by a distinctly striated cuticle, composed of polygonal cells with straight, beaded, thickened walls [Ba, Ma], uniseriate, multicellular covering trichomes [Ha] or rounded, thick-walled, covering trichome scars with a pitted lumen [Mb], and a few anomocytic stomata (*2.8.3*) [Bb] sometimes accompanied by underlying palisade parenchyma [Bc]; fragments of the lower epidermis of the leaf in surface view [A, K, N] covered by a slightly striated cuticle composed of cells with sinuous walls in the area of the lamina [Aa] or with more rigid walls near the veins (N), numerous anomocytic stomata (*2.8.3*) [Ab], occasional glandular trichomes with a unicellular stalk and a unicellular head [Ka, Na], covering trichomes some of which are pennant-like [Ac, F], uniseriate, multicellular, with 1-3 thin-walled basal cells [Fa], a flagella-like distal cell [Fb], and an enlarged, more or less rounded cell [Fc] between them, others are uniseriate, multicellular (up to about 10 cells), with thick, finely wrinkled walls and a rigid conical distal cell in side view [E]; rare fragments from the ovary [G] bearing paired, covering trichomes with a distinctly pitted central wall and a bifid apex in surface view [Ga] or in side view [Gb]; vascular tissue from the stems [L] composed of vessels [La] and groups of fibres [Lb]; fragments of the epidermis of the petals with a striated cuticle, through which run fine spiral vessels [S], and bearing biseriate glandular trichomes in side view [P]; spherical pollen grains, with 3 germinal pores and a spiny exine [J]; abundant pappus hairs and their fragments [C, D], multiseriate with the marginal cells overlapping outwards; fragments of parenchyma [Q], some showing cells containing small, isolated cluster crystals of calcium oxalate [Qa]; fragments of bracts [R] with a finely striated cuticle, polygonal cells [Ra], bearing pennant-like covering trichomes [Rb] and whose margin bears uniseriate, multicellular covering trichomes [Rc].

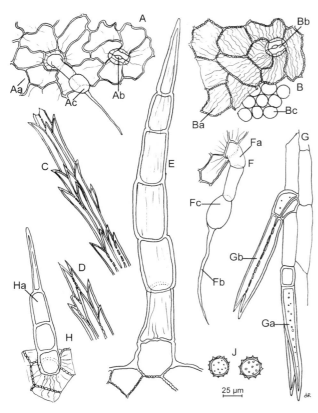

Figure 1893.-1. − *Illustration for identification test B of powdered herbal drug of European goldenrod*

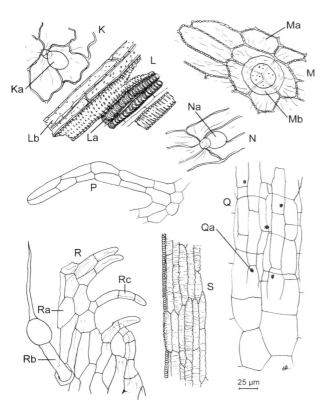

Figure 1893.-2. − *Illustration for identification test B of powdered herbal drug of European goldenrod*

C. Thin-layer chromatography (*2.2.27*) as described in the test for *Solidago gigantea* Ait. and *Solidago canadensis* L.

Results   See below the sequence of the zones present in the chromatograms obtained with the reference solution and the test solution. Furthermore, other fluorescent zones may be present in the chromatogram obtained with the test solution.

Top of the plate	
	A light blue fluorescent zone
Quercitrin: an orange fluorescent zone	
———	———
Chlorogenic acid: a light blue fluorescent zone	A light blue fluorescent zone (chlorogenic acid)
Rutin: an orange fluorescent zone	An orange fluorescent zone (rutin)
———	———
Reference solution	**Test solution**

TESTS

Foreign matter (*2.8.2*)
Maximum 5 per cent of brown coloured matter and maximum 5 per cent of other foreign matter.

***Solidago gigantea* Ait. and *Solidago canadensis* L**
Thin-layer chromatography (*2.2.27*).

Test solution   To 0.75 g of the powdered herbal drug (355) (*2.9.12*) add 5 mL of *methanol R* and heat on a water-bath under a reflux condenser for 10 min. Cool and filter.

Reference solution   Dissolve 1.0 mg of *chlorogenic acid R*, 2.5 mg of *quercitrin R* and 2.5 mg of *rutin R* in 10 mL of *methanol R*.

Plate   *TLC silica gel plate R*.

Mobile phase   anhydrous formic acid R, water R, methyl ethyl ketone R, ethyl acetate R (6:6:18:30 *V/V/V/V*).

Application   20 µL as bands.

Development   Over a path of 10 cm.

Drying   In air.

Detection   Treat the plate with a 10 g/L solution of *diphenylboric acid aminoethyl ester R* in *methanol R* and then with a 50 g/L solution of *macrogol 400 R* in *methanol R*. Examine in ultraviolet light at 365 nm after 30 min.

Results   The chromatogram obtained with the test solution shows no strong orange fluorescent zone similar in position to the zone of quercitrin in the chromatogram obtained with the reference solution.

Loss on drying (*2.2.32*)
Maximum 12.0 per cent, determined on 1.000 g of the powdered herbal drug (355) (*2.9.12*) by drying in an oven at 105 °C for 2 h.

Total ash (*2.4.16*)
Maximum 8.0 per cent.

ASSAY

Stock solution   In a 100 mL round-bottomed flask, place 0.200 g of the powdered herbal drug (355) (*2.9.12*), add 1 mL of a 5 g/L solution of *hexamethylenetetramine R*, 20 mL of *acetone R* and 2 mL of *hydrochloric acid R1*. Boil the mixture in a water-bath under a reflux condenser for 30 min. Filter the liquid through a small plug of absorbent cotton into a 100 mL flask. Add the absorbent cotton to the residue in the round-bottomed flask and extract with 2 quantities, each of 20 mL, of *acetone R*, each time boiling under a reflux condenser for 10 min. Allow to cool. Filter the combined acetone extracts through filter paper, dilute to 100.0 mL with *acetone R*, rinsing the volumetric flask and the filter paper with acetone. Introduce 20.0 mL of the solution into a suitable separating funnel, add 20 mL of *water R* and shake the mixture with 1 quantity of 15 mL and then with 3 quantities, each of 10 mL, of *ethyl acetate R*. Combine the ethyl acetate extracts in a separating funnel, wash twice with 50 mL of *water R* and filter the extracts over 10 g of *anhydrous sodium sulfate R* into a volumetric flask. Dilute to 50.0 mL with *ethyl acetate R*, rinsing the separating funnel and the sodium sulfate.

Test solution   To 10.0 mL of the stock solution add 1.0 mL of *aluminium chloride reagent R* and dilute to 25.0 mL with a 5 per cent *V/V* solution of *glacial acetic acid R* in *methanol R*.

Compensation liquid   Dilute 10.0 mL of the stock solution to 25.0 mL with a 5 per cent *V/V* solution of *glacial acetic acid R* in *methanol R*.

After 30 min, measure the absorbance (*2.2.25*) of the test solution at 425 nm by comparison with the compensation liquid.

Calculate the percentage content of flavonoids, expressed as hyperoside, using the following expression:

$$\frac{A \times 1.25}{m}$$

i.e. taking the specific absorbance of hyperoside to be 500.
A = measured absorbance at 425 nm;
m = mass of the herbal drug to be examined, in grams.

Ph Eur

Goldenseal Root

(*Goldenseal Rhizome, Ph Eur monograph 1831*)

Ph Eur

DEFINITION
Whole or cut, dried rhizome and root of *Hydrastis canadensis* L.

Content:
— *hydrastine* ($C_{21}H_{21}NO_6$; M_r 383.4): minimum 2.5 per cent (dried drug);
— *berberine* ($C_{20}H_{18}NO_4$; M_r 336.4): minimum 3.0 per cent (dried drug).

IDENTIFICATION
A. The rhizome is tortuous and knotty, about 5 cm long and 5-10 mm thick. The surface is yellowish or brownish-grey, irregularly wrinkled, and bears the remains of numerous slender, wiry roots; stem bases and scale leaves occur on the upper surface. The fracture is short and resinous.
The transversely cut surface is yellowish-brown and shows a fairly wide bark, a ring of 12-20 widely separated xylem bundles and a large, central pith.
B. Reduce to a powder (180) (*2.9.12*). The powder is greenish-yellow. Examine under a microscope using *chloral hydrate solution R*. The powder shows the following diagnostic characters (Figure 1831.-1): abundant thin-walled fragments of parenchyma [A, G, K]; occasional fragments of yellowish-brown cork from the rhizome and roots, in surface view [J] or in transverse section [F]; groups of small vessels with conspicuous perforations in the oblique end walls [L] and with simple or bordered, slit-shaped pits [B, D, E];

infrequent groups of thin-walled, pitted fibres [H], usually found associated with the vessels; numerous ovoid or spherical, orange-brown granular masses. Examine under a microscope using a 50 per cent *V/V* solution of *glycerol R*. The powder shows abundant starch granules [C], mostly simple but sometimes compound with up to 4 components; the granules are small, spherical or ovoid, up to about 10 μm in diameter, occasionally with a small, rounded or slit-shaped hilum.

C. Thin-layer chromatography (*2.2.27*).

Test solution   To 250 mg of powdered drug (180) (*2.9.12*) add 4 mL of a mixture of 20 volumes of *water R* and 80 volumes of *methanol R*. Sonicate for 10 min and filter. Wash the residue with 2 quantities, each of 2 mL, of *methanol R*. Combine the solutions and dilute to 20 mL with *methanol R*.

Reference solution   Immediately before use, dissolve 5 mg of *hydrastine hydrochloride R* and 5 mg of *berberine chloride R* in 20 mL of *methanol R*.

Plate   TLC silica gel plate R (5-40 μm) [or TLC silica gel plate R (2-10 μm)].

Mobile phase   anhydrous formic acid R, water R, ethyl acetate R (10:10:80 *V/V/V*).

Application   20 μL [or 2 μL] as bands.

Development   Over a path of 15 cm [or 6 cm].

Drying   In air.

Detection   Examine in ultraviolet light at 365 nm.

Results   See below the sequence of zones present in the chromatograms obtained with the reference solution and the test solution. Furthermore, other fluorescent zones may be present in the chromatogram obtained with the test solution.

Top of the plate	
Berberine: a bright yellow fluorescent zone	A bright yellow fluorescent zone (berberine)
Hydrastine: a deep blue fluorescent zone	A deep blue fluorescent zone (hydrastine)
	A bright light blue fluorescent zone (hydrastinine)
	A deep blue fluorescent zone
Reference solution	**Test solution**

TESTS
Loss on drying (*2.2.32*)
Maximum 10.0 per cent, determined on 1.000 g of the powdered drug (180) (*2.9.12*) by drying in an oven at 105 °C for 2 h.

Total ash (*2.4.16*)
Maximum 8.0 per cent.

Ash insoluble in hydrochloric acid (*2.8.1*)
Maximum 4.0 per cent.

ASSAY
Liquid chromatography (*2.2.29*).

Test solution   To 1.000 g of the powdered drug (355) (*2.9.12*) in a 100 mL round-bottomed flask, add 50 mL of a 1 per cent *V/V* solution of *concentrated ammonia R* in *ethanol (96 per cent) R* and boil the mixture under a reflux condenser for 30 min. Allow to cool to room temperature and filter the liquid through a plug of absorbent cotton into a flask.

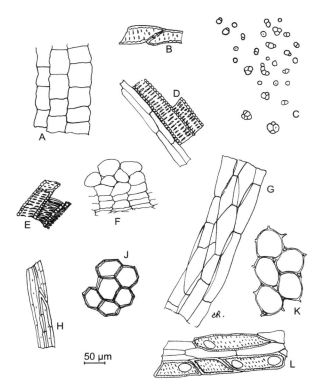

Figure 1831.-1.– *Illustration for identification test B of powdered herbal drug of goldenseal rhizome*

Using the retention times determined from the chromatogram obtained with the reference solution, locate in the chromatogram obtained with the test solution the components of the reference solution.

Calculate the percentage content of each alkaloid (hydrastine and berberine) using the following expression:

$$\frac{A_1 \times m_2 \times p}{A_2 \times m_1} \times 2.5$$

A_1 = area of the peak due to hydrastine or berberine in the chromatogram obtained with the test solution;

A_2 = area of the peak due to hydrastine or berberine in the chromatogram obtained with the reference solution;

m_1 = mass of the herbal drug to be examined used to prepare the test solution, in grams;

m_2 = mass of hydrastine hydrochloride or berberine chloride used to prepare the reference solution, in grams;

p = percentage content of hydrastine in *hydrastine hydrochloride CRS* or berberine in *berberine chloride CRS*.

Ph Eur

Add the plug of absorbent cotton to the residue in the round-bottomed flask and repeat the extraction with a further 2 quantities, each of 30 mL, of a 1 per cent *V/V* solution of *concentrated ammonia R* in *ethanol (96 per cent) R*, each time boiling under a reflux condenser for 10 min and filtering through a plug of absorbent cotton in the same flask as previously. Filter the combined filtrates through a filter paper into a 250 mL round-bottomed flask, and rinse the flask and the filter with 20 mL of a 1 per cent *V/V* solution of *concentrated ammonia R* in *ethanol (96 per cent) R*. Evaporate the filtrate to dryness *in vacuo* in a water-bath at 55 °C. Dissolve the residue in 50.0 mL of the mobile phase. Dilute 10.0 mL of this solution to 50.0 mL with the mobile phase.

Reference solution   Immediately before use, dissolve 10.0 mg of *hydrastine hydrochloride CRS* and 10.0 mg of *berberine chloride CRS* in *methanol R* and dilute to 100.0 mL with the same solvent.

Column:
— size: l = 0.125 m, Ø = 4 mm;
— stationary phase: *end-capped octadecylsilyl silica gel for chromatography R* (5 µm).

Mobile phase   Dissolve 9.93 g of *potassium dihydrogen phosphate R* in 730 mL of *water R*, add 270 mL of *acetonitrile R* and mix.

Flow rate   1.2 mL/min.

Detection   Spectrophotometer at 235 nm.

Injection   10 µL.

System suitability   Reference solution:
— elution order: order indicated in the composition of the reference solution; record the retention times of these substances;
— resolution: minimum 1.5 between the peaks due to hydrastine and berberine.

Hamamelis Leaf

(*Ph Eur* monograph 0909)

Ph Eur

DEFINITION

Whole or cut, dried leaf of *Hamamelis virginiana* L.

Content

Minimum 3 per cent of tannins, expressed as pyrogallol ($C_6H_6O_3$; M_r 126.1) (dried drug).

IDENTIFICATION

A. The leaf is green or greenish-brown, often broken, crumpled and compressed into more or less compact masses. The lamina is broadly ovate or obovate; the base is oblique and asymmetric and the apex is acute or, rarely, obtuse. The margins of the lamina are roughly crenate or dentate. The venation is pinnate and prominent on the abaxial surface. Usually, 4-6 pairs of secondary veins are attached to the main vein, emerging at an acute angle and curving gently to the marginal points where there are fine veins often at right angles to the secondary veins.

B. Reduce to a powder (355) (*2.9.12*). The powder is brownish-green. Examine under a microscope using *chloral hydrate solution R*. The powder shows the following diagnostic characters (Figure 0909.-1): fragments of adaxial epidermis with wavy anticlinal walls, in surface view [C, J], often accompanied by small, cylindrical cells of the palisade parenchyma, in surface view [Ja], or elongated, in transverse section [F]; fragments of abaxial epidermis with stomata mainly paracytic (*2.8.3*), in surface view [B], which may be accompanied by irregular-shaped cells of spongy mesophyll [K, L]; star-shaped covering trichomes, either entire or broken [A, D, M], composed of 4-12 unicellular branches that are united by their bases, elongated, conical and curved, usually up to 250 μm long, thick-walled and with a clearly visible lumen whose contents are often brown; fibres are lignified and thick-walled, isolated or in groups, and accompanied by a sheath of prismatic calcium oxalate crystals [N, P]; sclereids, frequently enlarged at 1 or both ends, 150-180 μm long, whole or fragmented [H]; fragments of annular or spiral vessels [E]; isolated prisms of calcium oxalate [G].

C. Thin-layer chromatography (*2.2.27*).

Test solution   To 1.0 g of the powdered drug (355) (*2.9.12*) add 10 mL of *ethanol (60 per cent V/V) R*, shake for 15 min and filter.

Reference solution (a)   Dissolve 30 mg of *tannic acid R* in 5 mL of *ethanol (60 per cent V/V) R*.

Reference solution (b)   Dissolve 5 mg of *gallic acid R* in 5 mL of *ethanol (60 per cent V/V) R*.

Plate   *TLC silica gel G plate R*.

Mobile phase   *anhydrous formic acid R, water R, ethyl formate R* (10:10:80 *V/V/V*).

Application   10 μL, as bands.

Development   Over a path of 10 cm.

Drying   At 100-105 °C for 10 min, then allow to cool.

Detection   Spray with *ferric chloride solution R2* until bluish-grey zones (phenolic compounds) appear.

Results   The chromatogram obtained with the test solution shows in its lower third a principal zone similar in position to the principal zone in the chromatogram obtained with reference solution (a) and, in its upper part, a narrow zone similar in position to the principal zone in the chromatogram obtained with reference solution (b); the chromatogram obtained with the test solution shows, in addition, several slightly coloured zones in the central part.

TESTS

Foreign matter (*2.8.2*)
Maximum 7 per cent of stems and maximum 2 per cent of other foreign matter, determined on 50 g.

Loss on drying (*2.2.32*)
Maximum 10.0 per cent, determined on 2.000 g of powdered drug (355) (*2.9.12*) by drying in an oven at 105 °C for 4 h.

Total ash (*2.4.16*)
Maximum 7.0 per cent.

Ash insoluble in hydrochloric acid (*2.8.1*)
Maximum 2.0 per cent.

ASSAY
Carry out the determination of tannins in herbal drugs (*2.8.14*). Use 0.750 g of the powdered drug (180) (*2.9.12*).

———————————————————————— *Ph Eur*

Hawthorn Berries

(*Ph Eur monograph 1220*)

Ph Eur ————————————————————————

DEFINITION
Dried false fruits of *Crataegus monogyna* Jacq. (Lindm.) or *C. laevigata* (Poir.) DC. (syn. *C. oxyacantha* L.) or their hybrids or a mixture of these false fruits.

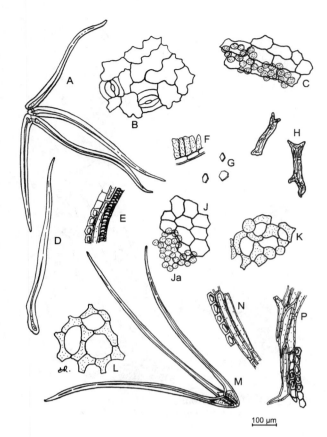

Figure 0909.-1.– *Illustration for identification test B of powdered herbal drug of hamamelis leaf*

Content
Minimum 0.06 per cent of procyanidins, expressed as cyanidin chloride ($C_{15}H_{11}ClO_6$; M_r 322.7) (dried drug).

IDENTIFICATION

A. The false fruit of *C. monogyna* is obovate or globular, generally 6-10 mm long and 4-8 mm wide, reddish-brown or dark red. The surface is pitted or, more rarely, reticulated. The upper end of the fruit is crowned by the remains of 5 reflexed sepals surrounding a small, sunken disc with a shallow, raised rim. The remains of the style occur in the centre of the disc with tufts of stiff, colourless hairs at the base. At the lower end of the fruit is a short length of pedicel or, more frequently, a small, pale, circular scar where the pedicel was attached. The receptacle is fleshy and encloses a yellowish-brown, ovoid fruit with a hard, thick wall containing a single, elongated, pale brown, smooth and shiny seed.

The false fruit of *C. laevigata* is up to 13 mm long. It contains 2-3 stony fruits, ventrally flattened, with short hairs at the top. Frequently, in the centre of the disc of the false fruit occur the remains of the 2 styles.

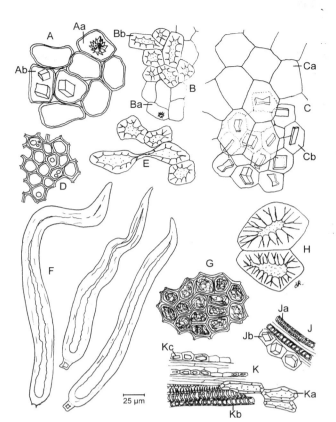

Figure 1220.-1. – *Illustration for identification test B of powdered herbal drug of hawthorn berries*

B. Microscopic examination (*2.8.23*). The powder is greyish-red. Examine under a microscope using *chloral hydrate solution R*. The powder shows the following diagnostic characters (Figure 1220.-1): covering trichomes [F] from inside the disc that are long, unicellular, frequently bent, tapering to a point, with much thickened and lignified walls; fragments of the red outer layer of the receptacle, in surface view [G]; fragments of the inner layers of the receptacle [A], some cells containing cluster crystals [Aa] or prisms [Ab] of calcium oxalate; occasional fragments [J, K] including groups of sclereids [Ka] and vascular bundles [Ja, Kb] associated with rows of cells containing prisms of calcium oxalate [Jb, Kc]; fragments of the pericarp [B] consisting of parenchyma including some cells containing cluster crystals of calcium oxalate [Ba] and groups of sclereids of various sizes with numerous pits [Bb]; thick-walled sclereids [E, H], some channelled (E), some with conspicuously branched channels (H); a few fragments of the testa [C] having an outer layer composed of hexagonal, mucilaginous cells [Ca] beneath which is a yellowish-brown pigment layer containing numerous prisms of calcium oxalate [Cb]; parenchyma of the endosperm and cotyledons consisting of cells containing aleurone grains and globules of fixed oil [D].

C. Thin-layer chromatography (*2.2.27*).

Test solution   To 1 g of the powdered herbal drug (355) (*2.9.12*) add 10 mL of *methanol R* and heat on a water bath at 65 °C for 5 min, shaking frequently. Allow to cool to room temperature and filter. Dilute the filtrate to 10 mL with *methanol R*.

Reference solution   Dissolve 2 mg of *chlorogenic acid R*, 2 mg of *caffeic acid R*, 5 mg of *hyperoside R* and 5 mg of *rutin R* in 20 mL of *methanol R*.

Plate   TLC silica gel plate R.

Mobile phase   anhydrous formic acid R, water R, methyl ethyl ketone R, ethyl acetate R (10:10:30:50 *V/V/V/V*).

Application   30 μL of the test solution and 10 μL of the reference solution, as bands.

Development   Over a path of 15 cm.

Drying   At 100-105 °C.

Detection   Spray whilst hot with a 10 g/L solution of *diphenylboric acid aminoethyl ester R* in *methanol R*; subsequently spray with a 50 g/L solution of *macrogol 400 R* in *methanol R*; allow to dry in air for 30 min and examine in ultraviolet light at 365 nm.

Results   The chromatogram obtained with the reference solution shows in the lower half, in order of increasing R_F values, a yellowish-brown fluorescent zone (rutin), a light blue fluorescent zone (chlorogenic acid) and a yellowish-brown fluorescent zone (hyperoside); in the upper third appears a light blue fluorescent zone (caffeic acid). The chromatogram obtained with the test solution shows 3 zones similar in position and fluorescence to the zones due to chlorogenic acid, hyperoside and caffeic acid in the chromatogram obtained with the reference solution, and 3 weak reddish fluorescent zones, one corresponding to the zone due to rutin in the chromatogram obtained with the reference solution and both of the others located above the zone due to hyperoside; below and above the zone due to caffeic acid some light blue zones appear.

TESTS

Foreign matter (*2.8.2*)

Maximum 5 per cent of deteriorated false fruit and maximum 2 per cent of other foreign matter. It does not contain false fruits of other *Crataegus species* (*C. nigra* Waldst. et Kit., *C. pentagyna* Waldst. et Kit. ex Willd. and *C. azarolus* L.), which are characterised by the presence of more than 3 hard stones.

Loss on drying (*2.2.32*)

Maximum 12.0 per cent, determined on 1.000 g of the powdered herbal drug (355) (*2.9.12*) by drying in an oven at 105 °C for 2 h.

Total ash (*2.4.16*)

Maximum 5.0 per cent.

ASSAY

To 2.50 g of the powdered herbal drug (355) (*2.9.12*) add 30 mL of *ethanol (70 per cent V/V) R*. Heat under a reflux condenser for 30 min and filter. Wash the residue with 10.0 mL of *ethanol (70 per cent V/V) R*. Add to the filtrate 15.0 mL of *hydrochloric acid R1* and 10.0 mL of *water R*. Heat under a reflux condenser for 80 min. Allow to cool, filter and wash the residue with *ethanol (70 per cent V/V) R* until the filtrate is colourless. Dilute the filtrate to 250.0 mL with *ethanol (70 per cent V/V) R*. Evaporate 50.0 mL of this solution in a round-bottomed flask to about 3 mL and transfer to a separating funnel. Rinse the round-bottomed flask sequentially with 10 mL and 5 mL of *water R* and transfer to the separating funnel. Shake the combined solution with 3 quantities, each of 15 mL, of *butanol R*. Combine the organic layers and dilute to 100.0 mL with *butanol R*.

Measure the absorbance (*2.2.25*) of the solution at 555 nm.

Calculate the percentage content of procyanidins, expressed as cyanidin chloride, using the following expression:

$$\frac{A \times 500}{1200 \times m}$$

i.e. taking the specific absorbance of cyanidin chloride to be 1200.

A = absorbance at 555 nm;

m = mass of the substance to be examined, in grams.

Ph Eur

Hawthorn Leaf and Flower

(*Ph Eur monograph 1432*)

Preparations

Hawthorn Leaf and Flower Dry Extract

Quantified Hawthorn Leaf and Flower Liquid Extract

Ph Eur

DEFINITION

Whole or cut, dried flower-bearing branches of *Crataegus monogyna* Jacq. (Lindm.), *C. laevigata* (Poir.) DC. (synonyms: *C. oxyacanthoides* Thuill.; *C. oxyacantha* auct.) or their hybrids or, more rarely, other European *Crataegus* species including *C. pentagyna* Waldst. et Kit. ex Willd., *C. nigra* Waldst. et Kit. and *C. azarolus* L.

Content

Minimum 1.5 per cent of total flavonoids, expressed as hyperoside ($C_{21}H_{20}O_{12}$; M_r 464.4) (dried drug).

IDENTIFICATION

A. The stems are dark brown, woody, 1-2.5 mm in diameter, bearing alternate, petiolate leaves with small, often deciduous stipules and corymbs of numerous small white flowers. The leaves are more or less deeply lobed with slightly serrate or almost entire margins; those of *C. laevigata* are pinnately lobed or pinnatifid with 3, 5 or 7 obtuse lobes, those of *C. monogyna* pinnatisect with 3 or 5 acute lobes; the adaxial surface is dark green or brownish-green, the abaxial surface is lighter greyish-green and shows a prominent, dense, reticulate venation. The leaves of *C. laevigata*, *C. monogyna* and *C. pentagyna* are glabrous or bear only isolated trichomes, those of *C. azarolus* and *C. nigra* are densely pubescent. The flowers have a brownish-green tubular calyx composed of 5 free, reflexed sepals, a corolla composed of 5 free, yellowish-white or brownish, rounded or broadly ovate and shortly unguiculate petals and numerous stamens. The ovary is fused to the calyx and consists of 1-5 carpels, each with a long style and containing a single ovule; in *C. monogyna* there is 1 carpel, in *C. laevigata* 2 or 3, in *C. azarolus* 2 or 3, or sometimes only 1, in *C. pentagyna* 5 or, rarely, 4.

B. Reduce to a powder (355) (*2.9.12*). The powder is yellowish-green. Examine under a microscope using *chloral hydrate solution R*. The powder shows the following diagnostic characters: unicellular covering trichomes, usually with a thick wall and wide lumen, almost straight or slightly curved, pitted at the base; fragments of leaf epidermis with cells which have sinuous or polygonal anticlinal walls and with large anomocytic stomata (*2.8.3*) surrounded by 4-7 subsidiary cells; parenchymatous cells of the mesophyll containing calcium oxalate clusters, usually measuring 10-20 μm, those associated with the veins containing groups of small prism crystals; fragments of petals showing rounded polygonal epidermal cells, strongly papillose, with thick walls, the cuticle of which clearly shows wavy striations; fragments of anthers showing endothecium with an arched and regularly thickened margin; fragments of stems containing collenchymatous cells, bordered pitted vessels and groups of

lignified sclerenchymatous fibres with narrow lumina; numerous spherical to elliptical or triangular pollen grains up to 45 μm in diameter, with 3 germinal pores and a faintly granular exine.

C. Thin-layer chromatography (*2.2.27*).

Test solution To 1.0 g of the powdered drug (355) (*2.9.12*) add 10 mL of *methanol R* and heat in a water-bath at 65 °C under a reflux condenser for 5 min. Cool and filter.

Reference solution Dissolve 1.0 mg of *chlorogenic acid R* and 2.5 mg of *hyperoside R* in 10 mL of *methanol R*.

Plate TLC silica gel plate R.

Mobile phase anhydrous formic acid R, water R, methyl ethyl ketone R, ethyl acetate R (10:10:30:50 *V/V/V/V*).

Application 20 μL as bands.

Development Over a path of 15 cm.

Drying At 100-105 °C.

Detection Spray the still-warm plate with a 10 g/L solution of *diphenylboric acid aminoethyl ester R* in *methanol R*, then spray with a 50 g/L solution of *macrogol 400 R* in *methanol R*; allow to dry in air for about 30 min and examine in ultraviolet light at 365 nm.

Results See below the sequence of zones present in the chromatograms obtained with the reference solution and the test solution. Furthermore, other fluorescent zones may be present in the chromatogram obtained with the test solution.

Top of the plate	
	A yellowish-green fluorescent zone (vitexin)
Hyperoside: a yellowish-orange fluorescent zone	A yellowish-orange fluorescent zone (hyperoside)
Chlorogenic acid: a light blue fluorescent zone	A light blue fluorescent zone (chlorogenic acid)
	A yellowish-green fluorescent zone (vitexin-2″-rhamnoside)
Reference solution	**Test solution**

TESTS

Foreign matter (*2.8.2*)

Maximum 8 per cent of lignified branches with a diameter greater than 2.5 mm and maximum 2 per cent of other foreign matter.

Loss on drying (*2.2.32*)

Maximum 10.0 per cent, determined on 1.000 g of powdered drug (355) (*2.9.12*) by drying in an oven at 105 °C for 2 h.

Total ash (*2.4.16*)

Maximum 10.0 per cent.

ASSAY

Stock solution Into a 200 mL flask introduce 0.400 g of the powdered drug (250) (*2.9.12*) and 40 mL of *ethanol (60 per cent V/V) R*. Heat in a water-bath at 60 °C for 10 min, shaking frequently. Allow to cool and filter through a plug of absorbent cotton into a 100 mL volumetric flask. Transfer the absorbent cotton with the drug residue back to the 200 mL flask, add 40 mL of *ethanol (60 per cent V/V) R* and heat again in a water-bath at 60 °C for 10 min, shaking frequently. Allow to cool and filter into the same 100 mL volumetric flask. Rinse the 200 mL flask with a further quantity of *ethanol (60 per cent V/V) R*, filter and transfer to the same 100 mL volumetric flask. Dilute to 100.0 mL with *ethanol (60 per cent V/V) R* and filter.

Test solution　Introduce 5.0 mL of the stock solution into a round-bottomed flask and evaporate to dryness under reduced pressure. Take up the residue with 8 mL of a mixture of 10 volumes of *methanol R* and 100 volumes of *anhydrous acetic acid R* and transfer to a 25 mL volumetric flask. Rinse the round-bottomed flask with 3 mL of a mixture of 10 volumes of *methanol R* and 100 volumes of *anhydrous acetic acid R* and transfer to the same 25 mL volumetric flask. Add 10.0 mL of a solution containing 25.0 g/L of *boric acid R* and 20.0 g/L of *oxalic acid R* in *anhydrous formic acid R* and dilute to 25.0 mL with *anhydrous acetic acid R*.

Compensation liquid　Introduce 5.0 mL of the stock solution into a round-bottomed flask and evaporate to dryness under reduced pressure. Take up the residue with 8 mL of a mixture of 10 volumes of *methanol R* and 100 volumes of *anhydrous acetic acid R* and transfer to a 25 mL volumetric flask. Rinse the round-bottomed flask with 3 mL of a mixture of 10 volumes of *methanol R* and 100 volumes of *anhydrous acetic acid R* and transfer to the same 25 mL volumetric flask. Add 10.0 mL of *anhydrous formic acid R* and dilute to 25.0 mL with *anhydrous acetic acid R*.

After 30 min, measure the absorbance (*2.2.25*) of the test solution at 410 nm, by comparison with the compensation liquid.

Calculate the percentage content of total flavonoids, expressed as hyperoside, using the following expression:

$$\frac{A \times 1.235}{m}$$

i.e. taking the specific absorbance of hyperoside to be 405.

A　=　absorbance at 410 nm;

m　=　mass of the drug to be examined, in grams.

————————————————— Ph Eur

Hawthorn Leaf and Flower Dry Extract

(*Ph Eur monograph 1865*)

Ph Eur _____

DEFINITION

Dry extract produced from *Hawthorn leaf and flower (1432)*.

Content:

— *for aqueous extracts*: minimum 2.5 per cent of total flavonoids, expressed as hyperoside ($C_{21}H_{20}O_{12}$; M_r 464.4) (dried extract);

— *for hydroalcoholic extracts*: minimum 6.0 per cent of total flavonoids, expressed as hyperoside ($C_{21}H_{20}O_{12}$; M_r 464.4) (dried extract).

PRODUCTION

The extract is produced from the herbal drug by a suitable procedure using either water or a hydroalcoholic solvent at least equivalent in strength to ethanol (45 per cent *V/V*).

CHARACTERS

Appearance

Light brown or greenish-brown powder.

IDENTIFICATION

Thin-layer chromatography (*2.2.27*).

Test solution　Suspend 0.2 g of the extract to be examined in 20 mL of *ethanol (70 per cent V/V) R* and filter.

Reference solution　Dissolve 1 mg of *chlorogenic acid R*, 2.5 mg of *hyperoside R* and 2.5 mg of *rutin R* in 10 mL of *methanol R*.

Plate　*TLC silica gel plate R.*

Mobile phase　*anhydrous formic acid R*, *water R*, *methyl ethyl ketone R*, *ethyl acetate R* (10:10:30:50 *V/V/V/V*).

Application　20 μL of the test solution and 10 μL of the reference solution, as bands.

Development　Over a path of 15 cm.

Drying　At 100-105 °C.

Detection　Spray the still-warm plate with a 10 g/L solution of *diphenylboric acid aminoethyl ester R* in *methanol R*, then spray with a 50 g/L solution of *macrogol 400 R* in *methanol R*; allow to dry in air for 30 min and examine in ultraviolet light at 365 nm.

Results　See below sequence of zones present in the chromatograms obtained with the reference solution and the test solution. Furthermore, other fluorescent zones may be present in the chromatogram obtained with the test solution.

Top of the plate	
	A light yellow fluorescent zone
Hyperoside: a yellowish-orange fluorescent zone	A yellowish-orange fluorescent zone (hyperoside)
Chlorogenic acid: a light blue fluorescent zone	A light blue fluorescent zone (chlorogenic acid)
	A yellowish-green fluorescent zone (vitexin 2″-rhamnoside)
Rutin: a yellowish-orange fluorescent zone	A yellowish-orange fluorescent zone (rutin)
Reference solution	**Test solution**

TESTS

Loss on drying (*2.2.32*)

Maximum 6.0 per cent, determined on 0.500 g of the extract to be examined by drying in an oven at 105 °C for 2 h.

ASSAY

Stock solution　Dissolve 0.100 g of the extract to be examined in *ethanol (60 per cent V/V) R* and dilute to 100.0 mL with the same solvent.

Test solution　Introduce 5.0 mL of the stock solution into a round-bottomed flask and evaporate to dryness under reduced pressure. Take up the residue in 8 mL of a mixture of 10 volumes of *methanol R* and 100 volumes of *anhydrous acetic acid R* and transfer to a 25 mL volumetric flask. Rinse the round-bottomed flask with 3 mL of a mixture of 10 volumes of *methanol R* and 100 volumes of *anhydrous acetic acid R* and transfer to the same 25 mL volumetric flask. Add 10.0 mL of a solution containing 25.0 g/L of *boric acid R* and 20.0 g/L of *oxalic acid R* in *anhydrous formic acid R* and dilute to 25.0 mL with *anhydrous acetic acid R*.

Compensation liquid　Introduce 5.0 mL of the stock solution into a round-bottomed flask and evaporate to dryness under reduced pressure. Take up the residue in 8 mL of a mixture of 10 volumes of *methanol R* and 100 volumes of *anhydrous acetic acid R* and transfer to a 25 mL volumetric flask. Rinse the round-bottomed flask with 3 mL of a mixture of 10 volumes of *methanol R* and 100 volumes of *anhydrous acetic acid R* and transfer to the same 25 mL volumetric flask. Add 10.0 mL of *anhydrous formic acid R* and dilute to 25.0 mL with *anhydrous acetic acid R*.

After 30 min, measure the absorbance (*2.2.25*) of the test solution at 410 nm, by comparison with the compensation liquid.

Calculate the percentage content of total flavonoids, expressed as hyperoside, using the following expression:

$$\frac{A \times 1.235}{m}$$

i.e. taking the specific absorbance of hyperoside to be 405.
A = absorbance at 410 nm;
m = mass of the extract to be examined, in grams.

Ph Eur

Quantified Hawthorn Leaf and Flower Liquid Extract

(*Ph Eur monograph 1864*)

Ph Eur

DEFINITION
Quantified liquid extract produced from *Hawthorn leaf with flower (1432)*.

Content
0.8 per cent to 3.0 per cent of flavonoids, expressed as hyperoside ($C_{21}H_{20}O_{12}$; M_r 464.4).

PRODUCTION
The extract is produced from the herbal drug and ethanol (30 per cent *V/V* to 70 per cent *V/V*) by an appropriate procedure.

IDENTIFICATION
Thin-layer chromatography (*2.2.27*).

Test solution Dilute 1.0 g in *methanol R* and dilute to 5 mL with the same solvent. Shake and filter.

Reference solution Dissolve 1.0 mg of *chlorogenic acid R* and 2.5 mg of *hyperoside R* in *methanol R* and dilute to 10 mL with the same solvent.

Plate *TLC silica gel plate R* (5-40 µm) [or *TLC silica gel plate R* (2-10 µm)].

Mobile phase *anhydrous formic acid R*, *water R*, *methyl ethyl ketone R*, *ethyl acetate R* (10:10:30:50 *V/V/V/V*).

Application 20 µL [or 5 µL] as bands.

Development Over a path of 15 cm [or 6 cm].

Drying At 100-105 °C.

Detection Spray with a 10 g/L solution of *diphenylboric acid aminoethyl ester R* in *methanol R*. Subsequently spray with a 50 g/L solution of *macrogol 400 R* in *methanol R*. Allow the plate to dry in air for about 30 min. Examine in ultraviolet light at 365 nm.

Results See below the sequence of zones present in the chromatograms obtained with the reference solution and the test solution. Furthermore, other fluorescent zones may be present in the chromatogram obtained with the test solution.

Top of the plate	
	A yellowish-green fluorescent zone
Hyperoside: a yellowish-orange fluorescent zone	A yellowish-orange fluorescent zone (hyperoside)
Chlorogenic acid: a light blue fluorescent zone	A light blue fluorescent zone (chlorogenic acid)
	A yellowish-green fluorescent zone
Reference solution	**Test solution**

TESTS
Ethanol (*2.9.10*): 95 per cent *V/V* to 105 per cent *V/V* of the quantity stated on the label.

ASSAY
Stock solution Dilute about 0.400 g, accurately weighed, in *ethanol (60 per cent V/V) R* and dilute to 100.0 mL with the same solvent.

Test solution Introduce 5.0 mL of the stock solution into a round-bottomed flask and evaporate to dryness under reduced pressure. Take up the residue with 8 mL of a mixture of 10 volumes of *methanol R* and 100 volumes of *glacial acetic acid R* and transfer into a 25 mL volumetric flask. Rinse the round-bottomed flask with 3 mL of a mixture of 10 volumes of *methanol R* and 100 volumes of *glacial acetic acid R* and transfer into the 25 mL volumetric flask. Add 10.0 mL of a solution containing 25.0 g/L of *boric acid R* and 20.0 g/L of *oxalic acid R* in *anhydrous formic acid R* and dilute to 25.0 mL with *anhydrous acetic acid R*.

Compensation liquid Introduce 5.0 mL of the stock solution into a round-bottomed flask and evaporate to dryness under reduced pressure. Take up the residue with 8 mL of a mixture of 10 volumes of *methanol R* and 100 volumes of *glacial acetic acid R* and transfer into a 25 mL volumetric flask. Rinse the round-bottomed flask with 3 mL of a mixture of 10 volumes of *methanol R* and 100 volumes of *glacial acetic acid R* and transfer into the 25 mL volumetric flask. Add 10.0 mL of *anhydrous formic acid R* and dilute to 25.0 mL with *anhydrous acetic acid R*.

After 30 min measure the absorbance (*2.2.25*) of the test solution at 410 nm.

Calculate the percentage content of total flavonoids, expressed as hyperoside, from the following expression:

$$\frac{A \times 1.235}{m}$$

i.e. taking the value of the specific absorbance of hyperoside to be 405.
A = absorbance at 410 nm,
m = mass of the extract to be examined, in grams.

Ph Eur

Hop Strobile

(*Ph Eur monograph 1222*)

Ph Eur

DEFINITION
Dried, generally whole, female inflorescence of *Humulus lupulus* L.

CHARACTERS

Characteristic, aromatic odour.

IDENTIFICATION

A. Hop strobiles are generally isolated and 2-5 cm long, petiolate, ovoid, made up of many oval, greenish-yellow, sessile, membranous, overlapping bracts. The external bracts are flattened and symmetrical. The internal bracts are longer and asymmetrical at the base because of a fold generally encircling an induviate fruit (achene). The ovary or rarely the fruit, the base of the bracts and especially the induvial fold, are covered with small orange-yellow glands.

B. Reduce to a powder (355) (*2.9.12*). The powder is greenish-yellow. Examine under a microscope using *chloral hydrate solution R*. The powder shows the following diagnostic characters (Figure 1222.-1): fragments of bracts and bracteoles covered by polygonal, irregular or wavy-walled epidermal cells [D, L, M]; unicellular, conical, straight or curved covering trichomes with thin, smooth walls, fragmented [E, G] or attached to an epidermis [A]; rare anomocytic stomata (*2.8.3*) [K]; glandular trichomes, usually free, with bicellular biseriate stalks and heads consisting of 8 small cells [H, N], rarely attached to an epidermis [La]; fragments of mesophyll containing small calcium oxalate cluster crystals [J]; many characteristic orange-yellow glandular trichomes with short, bicellular biseriate stalks, bearing a part widening into a cup, 150-250 μm in diameter, made up of a hemispherical layer of secretory cells with a cuticle that has been detached and distended by the accumulation of oleoresinous secretions, in surface view [B] or in side view [C]; fragments of elongated sclerenchymatous cells of the testa with thick walls showing striations and numerous pits [F].

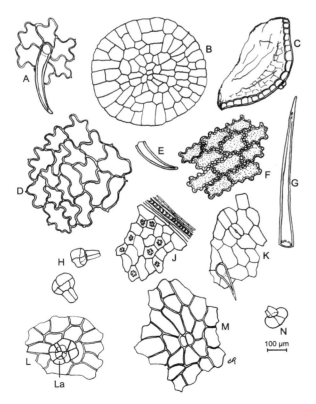

Figure 1222.-1.– *Illustration for identification test B of powdered herbal drug of hop strobile*

C. Thin-layer chromatography (*2.2.27*).

Test solution To 1.0 g of the freshly powdered drug (355) (*2.9.12*) add 10 mL of a mixture of 3 volumes of *water R* and 7 volumes of *methanol R*; shake for 15 min and filter.

Reference solution Dissolve 1.0 mg of *Sudan orange R*, 2.0 mg of *curcumin R* and 2.0 mg of *dimethylaminobenzaldehyde R* in 20 mL of *methanol R*.

Plate TLC silica gel F_{254} plate R.

Mobile phase anhydrous acetic acid R, ethyl acetate R, cyclohexane R (2:38:60 *V/V/V*).

Application 20 μL as bands.

Development Over a path of 15 cm.

Drying In air.

Detection A Examine in ultraviolet light at 254 nm.

Results A The chromatogram obtained with the reference solution shows 3 quenching zones; in the lower quarter is the faint zone due to curcumin, somewhat below the middle is the zone due to dimethylaminobenzaldehyde, and above, the zone due to Sudan orange. The chromatogram obtained with the test solution shows a number of quenching zones similar in position to the zones in the chromatogram obtained with the reference solution: at about the level of the zone due to curcumin is a faint zone due to xanthohumol, near the level of the zone due to dimethylaminobenzaldehyde are zones due to humulones, and near the level of the zone due to Sudan orange are zones due to lupulones.

Detection B Examine in ultraviolet light at 365 nm.

Results B In the chromatogram obtained with the test solution the zones due to lupulones show blue fluorescence, the zones due to humulones show brown fluorescence and the zone due to xanthohumol shows dark brown fluorescence.

Detection C Spray with *dilute phosphomolybdotungstic reagent R*; expose to ammonia vapour and examine in daylight.

Results C In the chromatogram obtained with the test solution the zones due to humulones and to lupulones are bluish-grey and the zone due to xanthohumol is greenish-grey; in the chromatogram obtained with the reference solution the zones are bluish-grey or brownish-grey.

TESTS

Matter extractable by ethanol (70 per cent *V/V*)
Minimum 25.0 per cent.

To 10.0 g of the powdered drug (355) (*2.9.12*) add 300 mL of *ethanol (70 per cent V/V) R* and heat for 10 min on a water-bath under a reflux condenser. Allow to cool, filter, and discard the first 10 mL of the filtrate. Evaporate 30.0 mL of the filtrate to dryness on a water-bath and dry in an oven at 100-105 °C for 2 h. The residue weighs a minimum of 0.250 g.

Loss on drying (*2.2.32*)
Maximum 10.0 per cent, determined on 1.000 g of the powdered drug (355) (*2.9.12*) by drying in an oven at 105 °C for 2 h.

Total ash (*2.4.16*)
Maximum 12.0 per cent.

_____ *Ph Eur*

White Horehound

(*Ph Eur monograph 1835*)

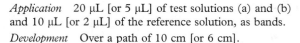

Ph Eur _____

DEFINITION

Whole or fragmented dried flowering aerial parts of
Marrubium vulgare L.

Content

Minimum 0.7 per cent of marrubiin ($C_{20}H_{28}O_4$; M_r 332.4)
(dried drug).

CHARACTERS

Bitter taste.

IDENTIFICATION

A. The stems are up to 50 cm long, quadrangular, up to
7 mm wide, young stems are densely covered with whitish
downy hairs, older stems are greenish-grey and less hairy.
The lower leaves are broadly ovate to almost orbicular, upper
leaves less broadly ovate, both petiolate; lamina 1.5-4 cm
long, 1-3.5 cm wide, apex sub-acute, base tapering or
somewhat cordate, margin dentate to crenate, petiole up to
3 cm long; venation pinnate, prominent on the lower surface,
distinctly depressed on the upper surface. Both leaf surfaces
are densely covered with fine, white, woolly hairs, older
leaves having fewer hairs on the dark greyish-green upper
surface. The flowers are small, sessile in dense axillary
clusters. The calyx is 5 mm long, persistent, with 5 long and
5 short, alternating, hooked, recurved fringing spines; throat
of calyx with an internal ring of long silky hairs; corolla
7 mm long, dull white, 4-lobed, upper lobe 2-lipped, lower-
lobe 3-lipped; 4 short stamens; style with bifid stigma.

B. Reduce to a powder (710) (*2.9.12*). The powder is
greyish-green. Examine under a microscope under *chloral
hydrate solution R*. The powder shows the following diagnostic
characters: fragments of leaves with sinuous, polygonal
epidermal cells, diacytic stomata (*2.8.3*), more numerous on
the lower surface and cells of the mesophyll with small
needles and cluster crystals of calcium oxalate; covering
trichomes very numerous, twisted or coiled, 100-200 µm
long, unicellular or multicellular and unseriate with 2-6 cells,
enlarged at the joints; stellate trichomes of 2 types, one with
15-20 branches arising from a short unicellular stalk and the
other with fewer branches arising from a sessile base; 8-celled
secretory trichomes of lamiaceous type; glandular trichomes
with 1 or 2 celled stalk and 1 to 4 celled head; the covering
trichomes on the inner surface of the calyx are up to
1000 µm long with 2 to 3 cells, strongly thickened at the
swollen joint and with the upper cell elongated; pollen grains
spherical, about 25 µm in diameter with smooth exine;
fragments of vascular tissue from the stems and veins.

C. Thin-layer chromatography (*2.2.27*).

Test solution (a)   To 1.0 g of the powdered drug (710)
(*2.9.12*) add 2 mL of *dilute hydrochloric acid R* and 8 mL of
methanol R. Heat under a reflux condenser for 30 min, cool
and filter.

Test solution (b)   To 1.0 g of the powdered drug (710)
(*2.9.12*) add 10 mL of *methanol R*. Heat under a reflux
condenser for 30 min, cool and filter.

Reference solution   Dissolve 10 mg of *cholesterol R* and 10 mg
of *guaiazulene R* in 10 mL of *methanol R*.

Plate   *TLC silica gel plate R* (5-40 µm) [or *TLC silica gel
plate R* (2-10 µm)].

Mobile phase   methanol R, toluene R (5:95 *V/V*).

Application   20 µL [or 5 µL] of test solutions (a) and (b)
and 10 µL [or 2 µL] of the reference solution, as bands.

Development   Over a path of 10 cm [or 6 cm].

Drying   In air.

Detection   Spray with a 5 g/L solution of *vanillin R* in a
mixture of 20 volumes of *ethanol (96 per cent) R* and
80 volumes of *sulfuric acid R* and examine in daylight
immediately after heating at 130 °C for 5-10 min.

Results   See below the sequence of the zones present in the
chromatograms obtained with the reference solution and test
solutions (a) and (b). Further zones in the chromatograms
obtained with test solutions (a) and (b) may be present.
The zone due to marrubiin in the chromatogram obtained
with test solution (a) is more intense than that in the
chromatogram obtained with test solution (b). During
extraction with hydrochloric acid and methanol, conversion
of pre-marrubiin to marrubiin takes place which leads to an
increase in intensity of the zone.

Top of the plate		
Guaiazulene: a reddish-violet zone	A bluish-violet zone	A bluish-violet zone
___		___
	A bluish-violet zone	A bluish-violet zone
___		___
Cholesterol: a bluish-violet zone	An intense bluish-violet zone (marrubiin)	A bluish-violet zone (marrubiin)
	A bluish-violet zone	A bluish-violet zone
	A bluish-violet zone	A bluish-violet zone
Reference solution	**Test solution (a)**	**Test solution (b)**

TESTS

Loss on drying (*2.2.32*)

Maximum 10.0 per cent, determined on 1.000 g of the
powdered drug (710) (*2.9.12*) by drying in an oven at
105 °C for 2 h.

Total ash (*2.4.16*)

Maximum 15.0 per cent.

Ash insoluble in hydrochloric acid (*2.8.1*)

Maximum 3.0 per cent.

ASSAY

Liquid chromatography (*2.2.29*).

Test solution   Reduce 50 g of the drug to a powder (250)
(*2.9.12*) and homogenise. To 1.00 g of the powdered drug in
a 50 mL round-bottomed flask add 15 mL of a mixture of
2 volumes of *dilute hydrochloric acid R* and 8 volumes of
methanol R. Heat in a water bath at 80 °C under a reflux
condenser for 30 min. Allow to cool at room temperature
and filter through a plug of adsorbent cotton into a 25 mL
volumetric flask. Dilute to 25.0 mL with *methanol R* by
rinsing the round-bottomed flask and the filter.

Reference solution   Dissolve 2.0 mg of *marrubiin R* in
10.0 mL of *methanol R*.

Column:
— size: l = 0.25 m, Ø = 4 mm,
— stationary phase: *end-capped octadecylsilyl silica gel for
   chromatography R* (5 µm).

Mobile phase:
— mobile phase A: *acetonitrile R*,
— mobile phase B: dilute 0.5 mL of *phosphoric acid R* to
   1000 mL with *water R*,

Time (min)	Mobile phase A (per cent V/V)	Mobile phase B (per cent V/V)
0 → 15	40 → 90	60 → 10
15 → 20	90 → 40	10 → 60
20 → 25	40	60

Flow rate   1.5 mL/min.

Detection   Spectrophotometer at 217 nm.

Injection   20 μL.

Locate the peak due to marrubiin by comparison with the chromatogram obtained with the reference solution.

Calculate the percentage content of marrubiin from the following expression:

$$\frac{A_1 \times m_2 \times p \times 2.5}{A_2 \times m_1}$$

A_1 = area of the peak due to marrubiin in the chromatogram obtained with the test solution,

A_2 = area of the peak due to marrubiin in the chromatogram obtained with the reference solution,

m_1 = mass of the drug to be examined, in milligrams,

m_2 = mass of *marrubiin R*, in milligrams,

p = percentage content of marrubiin in *marrubiin R*.

Ph Eur

Horsetail

(*Equisetum Stem, Ph Eur monograph 1825*)

Ph Eur

DEFINITION

Whole or cut, dried sterile aerial parts of *Equisetum arvense* L.

Content

Minimum 0.3 per cent of total flavonoids, expressed as isoquercitroside ($C_{21}H_{20}O_{12}$; M_r 464.4) (dried drug).

IDENTIFICATION

A. It consists of fragments of grooved main stems, branches with longitudinal sharp ridges and leaves in whorls, united at the base into a sheath, light green or greenish-grey. The fragments are rough to the touch, brittle and crunchy when crushed. The main stems are about 1-4.5 mm in diameter, hollow, jointed at the nodes, which occur at intervals of about 1.5-4.5 cm; distinct vertical grooves are present on the internodes, ranging in number from 4 to 14 or more. The central hollow is less than 50 per cent but more than 25 per cent of the diameter of the main stem. Verticils of widely spaced and erect branches, usually simple, each about 1 mm thick with 3-5 longitudinal, sharp ridges, occur at the nodes; at the end of each ridge is a protruding, distinct collenchymatic bundle under the epidermis. The branches are not hollow. The leaves are small, linear, verticillate at each node, concrescent at the base; they form a toothed sheath around the stem with the number of teeth corresponding to the number of grooves on the stem. Each tooth, often brown, is lanceolate-triangular. The lowest internode of each branch is longer than the sheath of the stem to which it belongs.

B. Microscopic examination (*2.8.23*). The powder is greenish-grey. Examine under a microscope using *chloral hydrate solution R*. The powder shows the following diagnostic characters (Figure 1825.-1): fragments of the epidermis in surface view [B, C] composed of rectangular cells with wavy walls and paracytic stomata (*2.8.3*) in 2-4 rows, the 2 subsidiary cells are in the same plane as the epidermis, cover the guard cells and show radial ridges; small silica pilulae are scattered on the surface of the subsidiary cells and appear more frequent at the margin forming a distinct ring surrounding the subsidiary cells (C); 2-celled papillae on the ridges, less distinct on the main stem [A] but large and rectangular on the branches, oriented longitudinally [F]; in surface view, the epidermis of the main stems consists of elongated cells [G], the epidermis of the secondary branches shows the 2-celled papillae which resemble pairs of small cells separated by a larger cell [D]; fragments of large-celled parenchyma [H] and groups of long unlignified fibres with narrow lumens; small vessels with spiral or annular thickening [E].

C. Examine the chromatograms obtained in the test for *Equisetum palustre*.

Results   See below the sequence of zones present in the chromatograms obtained with reference solution (b) and the test solution. Furthermore, other weak fluorescent zones may be present in the chromatogram obtained with the test solution.

Top of the plate	
	2 red fluorescent zones
Caffeic acid: a greenish-blue fluorescent zone	
	2 greenish-blue fluorescent zones
———	———
	An orange fluorescent zone
Hyperoside: an orange fluorescent zone	
	2 greenish-blue fluorescent zones
———	
Rutin: an orange fluorescent zone	
Reference solution (b)	**Test solution**

TESTS

Foreign matter (*2.8.2*)

Maximum 5 per cent.

Equisetum palustre

Thin-layer chromatography (*2.2.27*).

Test solution   To 1.0 g of the powdered herbal drug (355) (*2.9.12*) add 10 mL of *methanol R*. Heat in a water-bath at 60 °C for 10 min with occasional shaking. Allow to cool. Filter.

Reference solution (a)   To 100.0 mg of *Equisetum palustre HRS* add 10 mL of *methanol R*. Heat in a water-bath at 60 °C for 10 min with occasional shaking. Allow to cool. Filter.

Reference solution (b)   Dissolve 1.0 mg of *caffeic acid R*, 2.5 mg of *hyperoside R* and 2.5 mg of *rutin R* in 20 mL of *methanol R*.

Plate   TLC silica gel plate R (2-10 μm).

Mobile phase   anhydrous formic acid R, glacial acetic acid R, water R, ethyl acetate R (7.5:7.5:18:67 V/V/V/V).

Application   5 μL as bands of 8 mm.

Development   Over a path of 6 cm.

Drying   In a current of cold air for 5 min.

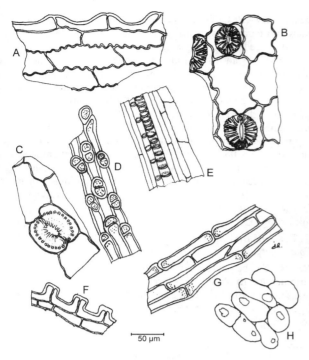

Figure 1825.-1. – *Illustration for identification test B of powdered herbal drug of equisetum stem*

Detection   Heat at 100 °C for 3 min and treat the still-warm plate with a 10 g/L solution of *diphenylboric acid aminoethyl ester R* in *methanol R*, then treat with a 50 g/L solution of *macrogol 400 R* in *methanol R*; allow to dry in a current of cold air and examine after 10 min in ultraviolet light at 365 nm.

System suitability   The chromatogram obtained with reference solution (a) shows 2 greenish fluorescent zones just above the line of application.

Results   In the chromatogram obtained with the test solution, any greenish fluorescent zones just above the line of application are not more intense than the corresponding zones (characteristic of *E. palustre* L.) in the chromatogram obtained with reference solution (a).

Loss on drying (*2.2.32*)
Maximum 10.0 per cent, determined on 1.000 g of the powdered herbal drug (355) (*2.9.12*) by drying in an oven at 105 °C for 2 h.

Ash insoluble in hydrochloric acid (*2.8.1*)
Minimum 3.0 per cent and maximum 15.0 per cent.

Total ash (*2.4.16*)
Minimum 12.0 per cent and maximum 27.0 per cent.

ASSAY
Stock solution   In a 100 mL round-bottomed flask, introduce 0.800 g of the powdered herbal drug (355) (*2.9.12*) and add 1 mL of a 5 g/L solution of *hexamethylenetetramine R*, 20 mL of *acetone R* and 2 mL of *hydrochloric acid R1*. Boil the mixture under a reflux condenser for 30 min. Filter the liquid through a plug of absorbent cotton into a flask. Add the absorbent cotton to the residue in the round-bottomed flask and extract with 2 quantities, each of 20 mL, of *acetone R*, each time boiling under a reflux condenser for 10 min. Allow to cool and filter each extract through a plug of absorbent cotton into the flask. After cooling, filter the

combined acetone extracts through a filter paper into a volumetric flask and dilute to 100.0 mL with *acetone R* by rinsing the flask and the filter paper. Introduce 20.0 mL of the solution into a separating funnel, add 20 mL of *water R* and shake the mixture with 1 quantity of 15 mL and then 3 quantities, each of 10 mL, of *ethyl acetate R*. Combine the ethyl acetate extracts in a separating funnel, wash with 2 quantities, each of 50 mL, of *water R*, and filter the extracts over 10 g of *anhydrous sodium sulfate R* into a volumetric flask. Dilute to 50.0 mL with *ethyl acetate R*.

Test solution   To 10.0 mL of the stock solution add 1 mL of *aluminium chloride reagent R* and dilute to 25.0 mL with a 5 per cent *V/V* solution of *glacial acetic acid R* in *methanol R*.

Compensation solution   Dilute 10.0 mL of the stock solution to 25.0 mL with a 5 per cent *V/V* solution of *glacial acetic acid R* in *methanol R*.

Measure the absorbance (*2.2.25*) of the test solution after 30 min, by comparison with the compensation solution at 425 nm. Calculate the percentage content of flavonoids, expressed as isoquercitroside, using the following expression:

$$\frac{A \times 1.25}{m}$$

i.e. taking the specific absorbance of isoquercitroside to be 500.
A = absorbance at 425 nm;
m = mass of the substance to be examined, in grams.

Ph Eur

Iceland Moss

(*Ph Eur monograph 1439*)

Ph Eur

DEFINITION
Whole or cut, dried thallus of *Cetraria islandica* (L) Acharius s.l.

IDENTIFICATION
A. The thallus, up to 15 cm long, is irregularly dichotomous and consists of glabrous, groove-shaped or almost flat, stiff, brittle bands, 0.3-1.5 cm wide and about 0.5 mm thick, sometimes serrated with the margin appearing ciliated (pycnidia). The upper surface is greenish or greenish-brown, the lower surface is greyish-white or light brownish and shows whitish, depressed spots (so-called respiratory cavities). On the apices of the terminal lobes, very rarely, there are brown, discoid apothecia.

B. Reduce to a powder (355) (*2.9.12*). The powder is greyish-brown. Examine under a microscope, using *chloral hydrate solution R*. The powder shows the following diagnostic characters: numerous fragments of the pseudoparenchyma consisting of narrow-lumened, thick-walled hyphae from the marginal layer and wide-lumened hyphae from the adjacent layer consisting of loosely entwined hyphae, in which, in the medullary zone, greenish or brownish algae cells up to 15 μm in diameter, are embedded; occasionally marginal fragments of the thallus with tube-like or cylindrical spermogonia, up to about 160 μm wide and up to about 400 μm long.

C. To 1.0 g of the powdered drug (355) (*2.9.12*) add 10 mL of *water R* and boil for 2-3 min. The greyish-brown solution forms a gel after cooling which gives a blue colour with *iodine solution R*.

D. Thin-layer chromatography (*2.2.27*).

Test solution   To 1.0 g of the powdered drug (355) (*2.9.12*) add 5 mL of *acetone R* and heat in a water-bath under a reflux condenser for 2-3 min. Cool and filter.

Reference solution   Dissolve 5 mg of *anethole R* and 5 mg of *caffeic acid R* in 2 mL of *acetone R*.

Plate   *TLC silica gel plate R* (5-40 μm) [or *TLC silica gel plate R* (2-10 μm)].

Mobile phase   acetone R, methanol R, anhydrous formic acid R, toluene R (5:5:10:80 *V/V/V/V*).

Application   20 μL [or 4 μL] of the test solution and 10 μL [or 2 μL] of the reference solution, as bands.

Development   Over a path of 10 cm [or 6 cm].

Drying   In air.

Detection   Spray with *anisaldehyde solution R*. Heat at 100-105 °C for 5-10 min and examine in daylight.

Results   See below the sequence of zones present in the chromatograms obtained with the reference solution and the test solution. Furthermore, other faint zones may be present in the chromatogram obtained with the test solution.

Top of the plate	
	A greyish-blue zone
Anethole: a blue or bluish-violet zone	
———	———
	2 weak greyish-blue zones
	A weak greyish-brown or grey zone
———	———
	A greyish-violet zone
Caffeic acid: a greyish-blue zone	
Reference solution	**Test solution**

TESTS

Foreign matter (*2.8.2*)
Maximum 5 per cent.

Lead (*2.4.27*)
Maximum 10.0 ppm.

Loss on drying (*2.2.32*)
Maximum 12.0 per cent, determined on 1.000 g of powdered drug (355) (*2.9.12*) by drying in an oven at 105 °C for 2 h.

Total ash (*2.4.16*)
Maximum 3.0 per cent.

Swelling value (*2.8.4*)
Minimum 4.5, determined on the powdered drug (355) (*2.9.12*).

——————————————————————— *Ph Eur*

Ipecacuanha

(*Ipecacuanha Root, Ph Eur monograph 0094*)

Preparations
Prepared Ipecacuanha
Ipecacuanha Liquid Extract
Standardised Ipecacuanha Liquid Extract
Standardised Ipecacuanha Tincture

Ph Eur ——————————————————————

DEFINITION
Fragmented and dried underground organs of *Cephaelis ipecacuanha* (Brot.) A. Rich., known as Matto Grosso ipecacuanha, or of *Cephaelis acuminata* Karsten, known as Costa Rica ipecacuanha, or of a mixture of both species. The principal alkaloids are emetine and cephaeline.

Content
Minimum 2.0 per cent of total alkaloids, expressed as emetine ($C_{29}H_{40}N_2O_4$; M_r 480.7) (dried drug).

CHARACTERS
Slight odour.

IDENTIFICATION
A. *C. ipecacuanha*. The root occurs as somewhat tortuous pieces, dark reddish-brown or very dark brown, seldom more than 15 cm long or 6 mm thick, closely annulated externally, having rounded ridges completely encircling the root; the fracture is short in the bark and splintery in the wood. The transversely cut surface shows a wide greyish bark and a small uniformly dense wood. The rhizome occurs as short lengths usually attached to roots, cylindrical, up to 2 mm in diameter, finely wrinkled longitudinally and with pith occupying approximately one-sixth of the whole diameter.

C. acuminata. The root in general resembles the root of *C. ipecacuanha*, but differs in the following particulars: it is often up to 9 mm thick; the external surface is greyish-brown or reddish-brown with transverse ridges at intervals of usually 1-3 mm, the ridges being about 0.5-1 mm wide, extending about half-way round the circumference and fading at the extremities into the general surface level.

B. Reduce to a powder (355) (*2.9.12*). The powder is light grey or yellowish-brown. Examine under a microscope, using *chloral hydrate solution R*. The powder shows the following diagnostic characters: parenchymatous cells, raphides of calcium oxalate up to 80 μm in length either in bundles or scattered throughout the powder; fragments of tracheids and vessels usually 10-20 μm in diameter, with bordered pits; larger vessels and sclereids from the rhizome. Examine under a microscope using a 50 per cent *V/V* solution of *glycerol R*. The powder shows simple or two- to eight-compound starch granules contained in parenchymatous cells, the simple granules being up to 15 μm in diameter in *C. ipecacuanha* and up to 22 μm in diameter in *C. acuminata*.

C. Thin-layer chromatography (*2.2.27*).

Test solution   To 0.1 g of the powdered drug (180) (*2.9.12*) in a test-tube add 0.05 mL of *concentrated ammonia R* and 5 mL of *ether R* and stir the mixture vigorously with a glass rod. Allow to stand for 30 min and filter.

Reference solution   Dissolve 2.5 mg of *emetine hydrochloride CRS* and 3 mg of *cephaeline hydrochloride CRS* in *methanol R* and dilute to 20 mL with the same solvent.

Plate   *TLC silica gel plate R*.

Mobile phase   concentrated ammonia R, methanol R, ethyl acetate R, toluene R (2:15:18:65 *V/V/V/V*).

Application   10 μL, as bands.

Development   Over a path of 10 cm.

Drying   In air.

Detection A   Spray with a 5 g/L solution of *iodine R* in ethanol (96 per cent) R and heat at 60 °C for 10 min. Examine in daylight.

Results A The chromatograms obtained with the test solution and with the reference solution show in the lower part a yellow zone due to emetine and below a light brown zone due to cephaeline.

Detection B Examine in ultraviolet light at 365 nm.

Results B The zone due to emetine shows an intense yellow fluorescence and that due to cephaeline a light blue fluorescence. The chromatogram obtained with the test solution shows also faint fluorescent zones.

With *C. acuminata* the principal zones in the chromatogram obtained with the test solution are similar in position, fluorescence and size to the zones in the chromatogram obtained with the reference solution.

With *C. ipecacuanha* the only difference is that the zone due to cephaeline in the chromatogram obtained with the test solution is much smaller than the corresponding zone in the chromatogram obtained with the reference solution.

TESTS

Loss on drying (*2.2.32*)
Maximum 10.0 per cent, determined on 1.000 g of powdered drug (180) (*2.9.12*) by drying in an oven at 105 °C.

Total ash (*2.4.16*)
Maximum 5.0 per cent.

Ash insoluble in hydrochloric acid (*2.8.1*)
Maximum 3.0 per cent.

ASSAY

To 7.5 g of the powdered drug (180) (*2.9.12*) in a dry flask, add 100 mL of *ether R* and shake for 5 min. Add 5 mL of *dilute ammonia R1*, shake for 1 h. Add 5 mL of *water R* and shake vigorously. Decant the ether layer into a flask through a plug of cotton. Wash the residue in the flask with 2 quantities, each of 25 mL, of *ether R*, decanting each portion through the same plug of cotton. Combine the ether solutions and eliminate the ether by distillation. Dissolve the residue in 2 mL of *ethanol (90 per cent V/V) R*, evaporate to dryness and heat at 100 °C for 5 min. Dissolve the residue in 5 mL of previously neutralised *ethanol (90 per cent V/V) R*, warming on a water-bath. Add 15.0 mL of *0.1 M hydrochloric acid* and titrate the excess acid with *0.1 M sodium hydroxide* using 0.5 mL of *methyl red mixed solution R* as indicator.

1 mL of *0.1 M hydrochloric acid* is equivalent to 24.03 mg of total alkaloids, expressed as emetine.

STORAGE

Protected from moisture.

_____ *Ph Eur*

Prepared Ipecacuanha

(*Ph Eur monograph 0093*)

Ph Eur _____

DEFINITION

Ipecacuanha root powder (180) (*2.9.12*) adjusted, if necessary, by the addition of powdered lactose or ipecacuanha root powder with a lower alkaloidal content.

Content

1.9 per cent to 2.1 per cent of total alkaloids, expressed as emetine ($C_{29}H_{40}N_2O_4$; M_r 480.7) (dried drug).

CHARACTERS

Appearance
Light grey or yellowish-brown powder.

Slight odour.

IDENTIFICATION

A. Examine under a microscope, using *chloral hydrate solution R*. The powder shows the following diagnostic characters: parenchymatous cells, raphides of calcium oxalate up to 80 μm in length either in bundles or scattered throughout the powder; fragments of tracheids and vessels usually 10-20 μm in diameter, with bordered pits; larger vessels and sclereids from the rhizome. Examine under a microscope using a 50 per cent *V/V* solution of *glycerol R*. The powder shows simple or 2-8-compound starch granules contained in parenchymatous cells, the simple granules being up to 15 μm in diameter in *Cephaelis ipecacuanha* and up to 22 μm in diameter in *C. acuminata*. Examined in *glycerol (85 per cent) R*, it may be seen to contain lactose crystals.

B. Thin-layer chromatography (*2.2.27*).

Test solution To 0.1 g of the drug to be examined in a test-tube add 0.05 mL of *concentrated ammonia R* and 5 mL of *ether R* and stir the mixture vigorously with a glass rod. Allow to stand for 30 min and filter.

Reference solution Dissolve 2.5 mg of *emetine hydrochloride CRS* and 3 mg of *cephaeline hydrochloride CRS* in *methanol R* and dilute to 20 mL with the same solvent.

Plate TLC silica gel plate R.

Mobile phase concentrated ammonia R, methanol R, ethyl acetate R, toluene R (2:15:18:65 *V/V/V/V*).

Application 10 μL, as bands.

Development Over a path of 10 cm.

Drying In air.

Detection A Spray with a 5 g/L solution of *iodine R* in *ethanol (96 per cent) R*; heat at 60 °C for 10 min and examine in daylight.

Results A The chromatograms obtained with the test solution and the reference solution show in the lower part a yellow zone due to emetine and below it a light brown zone due to cephaeline.

Detection B Examine in ultraviolet light at 365 nm.

Results B The zone due to emetine shows an intense yellow fluorescence and that due to cephaeline a light blue fluorescence. The chromatogram obtained with the test solution also shows faint fluorescent zones.

With prepared *C. acuminata*, the principal zones in the chromatogram obtained with the test solution are similar in position, fluorescence and size to the zones in the chromatogram obtained with the reference solution.

With prepared *C. ipecacuanha* , the only difference is that the zone due to cephaeline in the chromatogram obtained with the test solution is much smaller than the corresponding zone in the chromatogram obtained with the reference solution.

TESTS

Loss on drying (*2.2.32*)
Maximum 5.0 per cent, determined on 1.000 g by drying in an oven at 105 °C.

Total ash (*2.4.16*)
Maximum 5.0 per cent.

Ash insoluble in hydrochloric acid (*2.8.1*)
Maximum 3.0 per cent.

ASSAY

To 7.5 g in a dry flask, add 100 mL of *ether R* and shake for 5 min. Add 5 mL of *dilute ammonia R1*, shake for 1 h, add 5 mL of *water R* and shake vigorously. Decant the ether layer into a flask through a plug of cotton. Wash the residue in the flask with 2 quantities, each of 25 mL, of *ether R*, decanting each portion through the same plug of cotton. Combine the ether solutions and eliminate the ether by distillation. Dissolve the residue in 2 mL of *ethanol (90 per cent V/V) R*, evaporate the ethanol to dryness and heat at 100 °C for 5 min. Dissolve the residue in 5 mL of previously neutralised *ethanol (90 per cent V/V) R*, warming on a water-bath, add 15.0 mL of *0.1 M hydrochloric acid* and titrate the excess acid with *0.1 M sodium hydroxide* using 0.5 mL of *methyl red mixed solution R* as indicator.

1 mL of *0.1 M hydrochloric acid* is equivalent to 24.03 mg of total alkaloids, expressed as emetine.

STORAGE
In an airtight container.

—————————— *Ph Eur*

Ipecacuanha Liquid Extract

DEFINITION
Ipecacuanha Liquid Extract is prepared from Ipecacuanha by a method stated under the general monograph for Extracts. It contains not less than 1.90% and not more than 2.10% of total alkaloids, calculated as emetine, $C_{29}H_{40}N_2O_4$.

EXTEMPORANEOUS PREPARATION

Prepare by extracting Ipecacuanha with Ethanol (80 per cent) according to the following formula and directions.

Ipecacuanha in *fine powder*	1000 g
Ethanol (80 per cent)	A sufficient quantity

Exhaust the Ipecacuanha by *percolation*, Appendix XI F, with Ethanol (80 per cent), reserving the first 750 mL of the percolate. Remove the ethanol from the remainder of the percolate by evaporation under reduced pressure at a temperature not exceeding 60° and dissolve the residual extract in the reserved portion. Determine the proportion of alkaloids in the liquid thus obtained by the Assay described below. To the remainder of the liquid add sufficient Ethanol (80%) to produce an Ipecacuanha Liquid Extract containing 2% w/v of total alkaloids calculated as emetine. Allow to stand for not less than 24 hours; filter.

The extract complies with the requirements stated under Extracts and with the following requirements.

TESTS
Ethanol content
63 to 69% v/v, Appendix VIII F, Method III.

Relative density
0.910 to 0.960, Appendix V G.

Dry residue
The requirement for Dry residue does not apply to Ipecacuanha Liquid Extract.

ASSAY
To 5 mL in a separating funnel add 20 mL of *water*, 5 mL of 1M *sulfuric acid* and 10 mL of *chloroform* and shake well. Transfer the chloroform extract to a second separating funnel containing a mixture of 4 mL of *ethanol (96%)* and 20 mL of 0.05M *sulfuric acid*, shake, allow to separate and discard the chloroform layer. Continue the extraction of the liquid in the first separating funnel with two further 10 mL quantities of *chloroform*, transferring the chloroform solution each time to the second separating funnel and washing as before. Transfer

the acidic liquid from the second separating funnel to the first separating funnel, make distinctly alkaline with 5M *ammonia* and shake with successive quantities of *chloroform* until *complete extraction* of the alkaloids is effected, Appendix XI G, washing each chloroform solution with the same 10 mL of *water* contained in a third separating funnel. Remove the chloroform, add to the residue 2 mL of *ethanol (96%)*, evaporate to dryness and dry for 5 minutes at 80° in a current of air. Dissolve the residue in 2 mL of *ethanol (96%)*, previously neutralised to *methyl red solution*, add 10 mL of 0.05M *sulfuric acid VS* and titrate with 0.1M *sodium hydroxide VS* using *methyl red mixed solution* as indicator. Each mL of 0.05M *sulfuric acid VS* is equivalent to 24.03 mg of total alkaloids, calculated as emetine, $C_{29}H_{40}N_2O_4$.

Standardised Ipecacuanha Liquid Extract

(Ph Eur monograph 1875)

Ph Eur ——————————————————————————

DEFINITION
Standardised liquid extract produced from *Ipecacuanha root (0094)*.

Content
1.80 per cent to 2.20 per cent of total alkaloids, calculated as emetine ($C_{29}H_{40}N_2O_4$; M_r 480.7).

PRODUCTION
The extract is produced from the herbal drug and ethanol (60 to 80 per cent *V/V*) by an appropriate procedure.

CHARACTERS
Appearance
Dark brown liquid.

IDENTIFICATION
Thin-layer chromatography (*2.2.27*).

Test solution Dilute 5.0 mL of the extract to be examined to 50 mL with *ethanol (70 per cent V/V) R*. To 2.0 mL of this solution add 2 mL of *water R* and 0.1 mL of *concentrated ammonia R*. Add 10 mL of *ether R* and shake. Separate the upper layer, dry it over about 2 g of *anhydrous sodium sulfate R* and filter.

Reference solution Dissolve 2.5 mg of *emetine hydrochloride CRS* and 3 mg of *cephaeline hydrochloride CRS* in *methanol R* and dilute to 10 mL with the same solvent.

Plate   TLC silica gel plate R.

Mobile phase   concentrated ammonia R, methanol R, ethyl acetate R, toluene R (2:15:18:65 *V/V/V/V*).

Application   10 µL as bands.

Development   Over a path of 10 cm.

Drying   In air.

Detection A   Spray with a 5 g/L solution of *iodine R* in *ethanol (96 per cent) R*. Heat at 60 °C for 10 min and allow to cool for 30 min. Examine in daylight.

Results A   See below the sequence of the zones present in the chromatograms obtained with the reference solution and the test solution. Furthermore, other zones may be present in the chromatogram obtained with the test solution.

Top of the plate	
———	
	———
———	
	———
Emetine: a yellow zone	A yellow zone (emetine)
Cephaeline: a light brown zone	A light brown zone (cephaeline)
Reference solution	**Test solution**

Detection B   Examine the plate in ultraviolet light at 365 nm.

Results B   See below the sequence of the zones present in the chromatograms obtained with the reference solution and the test solution. Furthermore, other faint fluorescent zones are present in the chromatogram obtained with the test solution.

Top of the plate	
———	
	———
———	
	———
Emetine: an intense yellow fluorescent zone	An intense yellow fluorescent zone (emetine)
	A light blue fluorescent zone (cephaeline)
Reference solution	**Test solution**

With a liquid extract from *Cephaelis acuminata* root, the zones of emetine and cephaeline in the chromatogram obtained with the test solution are of similar size.

With a liquid extract from *Cephaelis ipecacuanha* root, the zone of emetine is much larger than the zone of cephaeline in the chromatogram obtained with the test solution.

TESTS

Ethanol (*2.9.10*)
95 per cent to 105 per cent of the quantity stated on the label.

ASSAY

Dilute 1.00 g of the extract to be examined to 10 mL with *ethanol (70 per cent V/V) R* and transfer to a chromatography column about 0.2 m long and about 15 mm in internal diameter, containing 8 g of *basic aluminium oxide R*, using a glass rod. After infiltration into the aluminium oxide layer, rinse the flask, glass rod and internal wall of the column with 3 quantities, each of 2 mL, of *ethanol (70 per cent V/V) R*. Elute in portions with 40 mL of *ethanol (70 per cent V/V) R*. Avoid disturbance or drying of the surface of the aluminium oxide layer. Collect the whole of the eluate. Evaporate the eluate on a water-bath to about 10 mL. Allow to cool. Add 10.0 mL of *0.02 M hydrochloric acid* and 20 mL of carbon dioxide-free *water R*. Titrate the excess acid with *0.02 M sodium hydroxide* using 0.15 mL of *methyl red mixed solution R* as indicator.

Perform a blank assay by replacing the extract to be examined with 10.0 mL of alcohol of the strength stated on the label.

1 mL of *0.02 M hydrochloric acid* is equivalent to 4.807 mg of total alkaloids, calculated as emetine.

———————————— Ph Eur

Standardised Ipecacuanha Tincture

(*Ph Eur monograph 1530*)

Ph Eur ————————————————————————

DEFINITION

Tincture produced from *Ipecacuanha root (0094)*.

Content
0.18 per cent (*m/m*) to 0.22 per cent (*m/m*) of total alkaloids, calculated as emetine ($C_{29}H_{40}N_2O_4$; M_r 480.7).

PRODUCTION

The tincture is produced from the herbal drug and ethanol (70 per cent *V/V*) by an appropriate procedure.

CHARACTERS

Appearance
Yellowish-brown liquid.

IDENTIFICATION

Thin-layer chromatography (*2.2.27*).

Test solution   To 2.0 mL of the tincture to be examined add 2 mL of *water R* and 0.1 mL of *concentrated ammonia R*. Add 10 mL of *ether R* and shake. Separate the ether layer, dry it over about 2 g of *anhydrous sodium sulfate R* and filter.

Reference solution   Dissolve 2.5 mg of *emetine hydrochloride CRS* and 3 mg of *cephaeline hydrochloride CRS* in *methanol R* and dilute to 10 mL with the same solvent.

Plate   *TLC silica gel plate R*.

Mobile phase   *concentrated ammonia R, methanol R, ethyl acetate R, toluene R* (2:15:18:65 *V/V/V/V*).

Application   10 μL as bands.

Development   Over a path of 10 cm.

Drying   In air.

Detection A   Spray with a 5 g/L solution of *iodine R* in *ethanol (96 per cent) R* and heat at 60 °C for 10 min. Examine in daylight.

Results A   See below the sequence of zones present in the chromatograms obtained with the reference solution and the test solution.

Top of the plate	
———	
	———
———	
	———
Emetine: a yellow zone	A yellow zone (emetine)
Cephaeline: a light brown zone	A light brown zone (cephaeline)
Reference solution	**Test solution**

Detection B   Examine the plate in ultraviolet light at 365 nm.

Results B   See below the sequence of zones present in the chromatograms obtained with the reference solution and the test solution. Furthermore, other faint fluorescent zones are present in the chromatogram obtained with the test solution.

Top of the plate	
_____	_____
_____	_____
	_____
Emetine: an intense yellow fluorescent zone	An intense yellow fluorescent zone (emetine)
	A light blue fluorescent zone (cephaeline)
Reference solution	**Test solution**

With a tincture from _Cephaelis acuminata_ root, the zones of emetine and cephaeline in the chromatogram obtained with the test solution are similar in size.

With a tincture from _Cephaelis ipecacuanha_ root, the zone of emetine is much larger than the zone of cephaeline in the chromatogram obtained with the test solution.

TESTS
Ethanol (_2.9.10_)
95 per cent to 105 per cent of the quantity stated on the label.

ASSAY
Transfer 10.00 g of the tincture to be examined to a chromatography column about 0.2 m long and about 15 mm in internal diameter, filled with 8 g of _basic aluminium oxide R_. After infiltration into the aluminium oxide layer rinse the internal wall of the column with 3 quantities, each of 2 mL, of _ethanol (70 per cent V/V) R_. Elute in portions, with 40 mL of _ethanol (70 per cent V/V) R_. Avoid whirling or drying of the surface of the aluminium oxide layer. Collect the whole of the eluate. Evaporate the eluate on a water-bath to about 10 mL. Allow to cool. Add 10.0 mL of _0.02 M hydrochloric acid_ and 20 mL of _carbon dioxide-free water R_. Titrate the excess acid with _0.02 M sodium hydroxide_ using 0.15 mL of _methyl red mixed solution R_ as indicator.

Perform a blank assay replacing the tincture to be examined with 10.0 mL of alcohol of the strength stated on the label.

1 mL of _0.02 M hydrochloric acid_ is equivalent to 4.807 mg of total alkaloids, calculated as emetine.

_____ _Ph Eur_

Paediatric Ipecacuanha Emetic Mixture

Paediatric Ipecacuanha Emetic; Paediatric Ipecacuanha Emetic Oral Solution

DEFINITION
Paediatric Ipecacuanha Emetic Mixture is an _oral solution_.

Ipecacuanha Liquid Extract	70 mL
Hydrochloric Acid	2.5 mL
Glycerol	100 mL
Syrup	Sufficient to produce 1000 mL

The mixture complies with the requirements stated under Oral Liquids and with the following requirements.

Content of total alkaloids
0.12 to 0.16% w/v, calculated as emetine, $C_{29}H_{40}N_2O_4$.

IDENTIFICATION
Carry out the method for _thin-layer chromatography_, Appendix III A, using the following solutions.

(1) Mix 5 mL with 10 mL of 1m _sulfuric acid_, shake with two 10 mL quantities of _chloroform_ and discard the chloroform. Add sufficient 5m _ammonia_ to make the aqueous solution distinctly alkaline to _litmus paper_, extract with four 10 mL

quantities of _chloroform_, evaporate the combined extracts to dryness, cool the residue and dissolve it in 0.5 mL of _ethanol (96%)_.

(2) 0.1% w/v of _cephaeline hydrochloride EPCRS_ in _ethanol (96%)_.

(3) 0.1% w/v of _emetine hydrochloride EPCRS_ in _ethanol (96%)_.

CHROMATOGRAPHIC CONDITIONS
(a) Use as the coating _silica gel G_.
(b) Use the mobile phase as described below.
(c) Apply 2 μL of each solution.
(d) Develop the plate to 15 cm.
(e) After removal of the plate, dry it at 105° to 110° for 30 minutes, allow to cool and spray with _dilute potassium iodobismuthate solution_.

MOBILE PHASE
10 volumes of _diethylamine_ and 90 volumes of _chloroform_.

CONFIRMATION
The principal spots in the chromatogram obtained with solution (1) correspond in colour and position to the spots in the chromatograms obtained with solutions (2) and (3). Disregard any _secondary spots_.

ASSAY
To 25 mL in a separating funnel add 20 mL of _water_ and 5 mL of 1M _sulfuric acid_, shake with three 10 mL quantities of _chloroform_ and wash each chloroform extract with a mixture of 20 mL of 0.05M _sulfuric acid_ and 4 mL of _ethanol (96%)_ contained in a second separating funnel. Transfer the acid–ethanol mixture from the second separating funnel to the first, make the combined liquids distinctly alkaline to _litmus paper_ with 5M _ammonia_ and extract with successive quantities of _chloroform_ until _complete extraction_ of the alkaloids is effected, Appendix XI G. Wash each chloroform extract with the same 10 mL of _water_, combine the chloroform extracts, evaporate the chloroform, add 2 mL of _ethanol (96%)_ to the residue, evaporate to dryness and dry the residue at 80° in a current of air for 5 minutes. Dissolve the residue in 2 mL of _ethanol (96%)_ previously neutralised to _methyl red solution_, add 10 mL of 0.01M _sulfuric acid VS_ and titrate the excess of acid with 0.02M _sodium hydroxide VS_ using _methyl red solution_ as indicator. Each mL of 0.01M _sulfuric acid VS_ is equivalent to 4.806 mg of $C_{29}H_{40}N_2O_4$.

Isatis Root

(_Ph Eur monograph 2566_)

Ph Eur _____

DEFINITION
Dried root of _Isatis tinctoria_ L. (_I. indigotica_ Fortune) collected in autumn.

Content
Minimum 1.0 per cent of arginine ($C_6H_{14}N_4O_2$; M_r 174.2) (dried drug).

IDENTIFICATION
A. The root is cylindrical, slightly tortuous, 10-20 cm long, 0.5-1 cm in diameter, externally greyish-yellow or brownish-yellow, wrinkled longitudinally and lenticellate transversally, with rootlets or rootlet scars. Root stock slightly expanded, exhibiting dark green or dark brown petiole bases arranged in

whorls, and dense tubercles. The fracture is yellowish-white, brown or dark brown in bark and yellow or brown in wood.

B. Microscopic examination (*2.8.23*). The powder is whitish-yellow or yellow. Examine under a microscope using *chloral hydrate solution R*. The powder shows the following diagnostic characters: fragments of cork consisting of 5-8 thin-walled layers; fragments of xylem with reticulate structure; thin-walled, rounded parenchyma cells. Examine under a microscope using a 50 per cent *V/V* solution of *glycerol R*. The powder shows abundant, single or compound (2, 3 or 4) starch grains. The starch grains, 1.5-3.4 μm in diameter, with spot, cleft or V-shaped hilum.

C. Thin-layer chromatography (*2.2.27*).

Test solution To 0.5 g of the powdered herbal drug (355) (*2.9.12*) add 5 mL of *ethanol (70 per cent V/V) R* and sonicate for 10 min. Centrifuge and use the supernatant.

Reference solution Dissolve 4 mg of *arginine R* and 4 mg of *cysteine hydrochloride R* in 1 mL of *ethanol (70 per cent V/V) R*.

Plate *TLC silica gel F$_{254}$ plate R* (5-40 μm) [or *TLC silica gel F$_{254}$ plate R* (2-10 μm)].

Mobile phase *anhydrous formic acid R, water R, acetonitrile R* (2:8:30 *V/V/V*).

Application 4 μL as bands of 10 mm [or 8 mm].

Development Over a path of 8.5 cm [or 6 cm].

Drying In air.

Detection Expose to *concentrated ammonia R* vapour for 5 min, treat with *ninhydrin solution R4*, then heat at 120 °C for 3 min.

Results See below the sequence of zones present in the chromatograms obtained with the reference solution and the test solution. Furthermore, other faint coloured zones may be present in the chromatogram obtained with the test solution.

Top of the plate	
___	___
	A prominent brown zone
Cysteine: a brown zone	
	A brown zone
Arginine: a brown zone	A brown zone (arginine)
	A faint brown zone
Reference solution	**Test solution**

TESTS

Loss on drying (*2.2.32*)
Maximum 9.0 per cent, determined on 1.000 g of the powdered herbal drug (355) (*2.9.12*) by drying in an oven at 105 °C for 2 h.

Total ash (*2.4.16*)
Maximum 5.0 per cent.

Ash insoluble in hydrochloric acid (*2.8.1*)
Maximum 1.0 per cent.

ASSAY

Liquid chromatography (*2.2.29*).

Test solution To 0.100 g of the powdered herbal drug (355) (*2.9.12*) add 20 mL of *ethanol (70 per cent V/V) R*, sonicate

for 20 min, filter, and evaporate the filtrate to dryness. Dissolve the residue in *ethanol (70 per cent V/V) R* and dilute to 10.0 mL with the same solvent.

Reference solution (a) Dissolve 25.0 mg of *arginine CRS* in *ethanol (70 per cent V/V) R* and dilute to 50.0 mL with the same solvent.

Reference solution (b) Dissolve 3.0 mg of *cysteine hydrochloride R* in 6.0 mL of reference solution (a) and dilute to 10.0 mL with *ethanol (70 per cent V/V) R*.

Reference solutions (c), (d), (e), (f), (g), (h) Dilute reference solution (a) to obtain 6 reference solutions of arginine, the concentrations of which span the expected value in the test solution.

Column:
— *size: l* = 0.15 m, Ø = 4.6 mm;
— *stationary phase: end-capped octadecylsilyl silica gel for chromatography R* (3 μm);
— *temperature*: 30 °C.

Mobile phase *trifluoroacetic acid R, water R* (0.2:99.8 *V/V*).

Flow rate 0.2 mL/min.

Detection Evaporative light-scattering detector; the following settings have been found to be suitable; if the detector has different setting parameters, adjust the detector settings so as to comply with the system suitability criterion for the signal-to-noise ratio:
— *carrier gas: nitrogen R*;
— *pressure*: 330 kPa;
— *evaporator temperature*: 80 °C.

Injection 10 μL.

Run time 25 min.

System suitability:
— *resolution*: minimum 1.5 between the peaks due to cysteine and arginine in the chromatogram obtained with reference solution (b);
— *signal-to-noise ratio*: minimum 50 for the peak due to arginine in the chromatogram obtained with reference solution (a).

Establish a calibration curve with the logarithm of the concentration (in milligrams per 10 mL) of reference solutions (c), (d), (e), (f), (g) and (h) (corrected by the assigned percentage content of *arginine CRS*) as the abscissa and the logarithm of the corresponding peak areas as the ordinate.

Calculate the percentage content of arginine using the following expression:

$$\frac{10^A}{m \times 10}$$

A = logarithm of the concentration of arginine in the test solution, determined from the calibration curve;

m = mass of the herbal drug to be examined used to prepare the test solution, in grams.

_____ *Ph Eur*

Ispaghula Husk

(Ph Eur monograph 1334)

Preparations
Ispaghula Husk Oral Powder
Ispaghula Husk Granules
Ispaghula Husk Effervescent Granules

Ph Eur _____

DEFINITION
Episperm and collapsed adjacent layers removed from the seeds of *Plantago ovata* Forssk. (*P. ispaghula* Roxb.).

IDENTIFICATION
A. The husk consists of pinkish-beige fragments or flakes up to about 2 mm long and 1 mm wide, some showing a light brown spot corresponding to the location of the embryo before it was removed from the seed.

B. Reduce to a powder (355) (*2.9.12*). The powder is pale yellow. Examine under a microscope using *lactic reagent R*. The powder shows the following diagnostic characters: mainly fragments of the episperm with polygonal cells filled with mucilage; fragments of the inner layers of the testa with brownish thin-walled cells often associated with the outer layers of the endosperm. Examine under a microscope using a 50 per cent *V/V* solution of *glycerol R*. The powder shows occasional starch granules, single or in groups of 2-4, measuring 3-25 µm in diameter.

C. Thin-layer chromatography (*2.2.27*).

Test solution　To 10 mg of the powdered drug (355) (*2.9.12*) in a thick-walled centrifuge tube, add 2 mL of a 230 g/L solution of *trifluoroacetic acid R* and shake vigorously. Stopper the test tube and heat at 120 °C for 1 h. Centrifuge the hydrolysate, transfer the clear supernatant liquid into a 50 mL flask, add 10 mL of *water R* and evaporate to dryness under reduced pressure. Take up the residue in 10 mL of *water R* and evaporate again to dryness under reduced pressure. Take up the residue with 2 mL of *methanol R*.

Reference solution (a)　Dissolve 10 mg of *arabinose R* in a small quantity of *water R* and dilute to 10 mL with *methanol R*.

Reference solution (b)　Dissolve 10 mg of *xylose R* in a small quantity of *water R* and dilute to 10 mL with *methanol R*.

Reference solution (c)　Dissolve 10 mg of *galactose R* in a small quantity of *water R* and dilute to 10 mL with *methanol R*.

Plate　TLC silica gel plate R.

Mobile phase　water R, acetonitrile R (15:85 *V/V*).

Application　10 µL, as bands.

Development　Over a path of 15 cm.

Detection　Spray with *aminohippuric acid reagent R* and heat at 120 °C for 5 min; examine in daylight.

Results　The chromatogram obtained with the test solution shows 2 orange-pink zones (arabinose and xylose) and a yellow zone (galactose) similar in position and colour to the zones in the chromatograms obtained with the reference solutions.

TESTS
Foreign matter (*2.8.2*)
Carry out the determination using 5.0 g.

Loss on drying (*2.2.32*)
Maximum 12.0 per cent, determined on 1.000 g of the powdered drug (355) (*2.9.12*) by drying in an oven at 105 °C for 2 h.

Total ash (*2.4.16*)
Maximum 4.0 per cent.

Swelling index (*2.8.4*)
Minimum 40, determined on 0.1 g of the powdered drug (355) (*2.9.12*).

_____ *Ph Eur*

Ispaghula Husk Granules

DEFINITION
Ispaghula Husk Granules contain Ispaghula Husk with or without suitable excipients.

The granules comply with the requirements stated under Granules and with the following requirements.

IDENTIFICATION
A. Powder the granules and examine under a microscope using *lactic reagent*. Fragments of the episperm with polygonal cells filled with mucilage and fragments of the inner layers of the testa with brownish thin-walled cells often associated with the outer layers of the endosperm are seen.

B. When mounted in *ruthenium red solution*, the particles of the powder are stained red.

TESTS
Swelling index
Not less than 40, Appendix XI C. Use a quantity of the granules containing 1.0 g of Ispaghula Husk and a 100-mL ground-glass-stoppered cylinder graduated in 1 mL divisions.

Loss on drying
When dried at 100° to 105°, loses not more than 12.0% of its weight. Use 1 g.

Ash
Not more than 5.0%, Appendix XI J, Method II.

STORAGE
Ispaghula Husk Granules should be protected from moisture.

Ispaghula Husk Effervescent Granules

DEFINITION
Ispaghula Husk Effervescent Granules contain Ispaghula Husk in a suitable, effervescent basis.

The granules comply with the requirements stated under Granules and with the following requirements.

TESTS
Disintegration
Carry out the test stated under Effervescent Granules with the following modifications. Stir the contents of the beaker occasionally to disperse the mucilage formed; evolution of gas is complete after 5 minutes.

Swelling index
Not less than 40, Appendix XI C. Use a quantity of the powdered granules containing 1.0 g of Ispaghula Husk and a 100 mL ground-glass-stoppered cylinder graduated in 1 mL divisions.

Ispaghula Husk Oral Powder

DEFINITION

Ispaghula Husk Oral Powder contains Ispaghula Husk with or without suitable excipients.

The powder complies with the requirements stated under Oral Powders and with the following requirements.

IDENTIFICATION

A. Carry out the method for *thin-layer chromatography*, Appendix III A, using the following solutions.

(1) Add 2 mL of a 23% w/v solution of *trifluoroacetic acid* to a quantity of the powder containing 10 mg of Ispaghula Husk in a thick-walled centrifuge tube, shake vigorously, close the tube and heat at 120° for 1 hour. Centrifuge the hydrolysate, transfer the clear supernatant liquid into a 50 mL flask, add 10 mL of *water* and evaporate the solution to dryness under reduced pressure. Take up the residue in 10 mL of *water*, again evaporate to dryness under reduced pressure and take up the residue in 2 mL of *methanol*.

(2) Dissolve 10 mg of *arabinose* in a small quantity of *water* and dilute to 10 mL with *methanol*.

(3) Dissolve 10 mg of *xylose* in a small quantity of *water* and dilute to 10 mL with *methanol*.

(4) Dissolve 10 mg of *galactose* in a small quantity of *water* and dilute to 10 mL with *methanol*.

CHROMATOGRAPHIC CONDITIONS

(a) Use as the coating silica gel.

(b) Use the mobile phase as described below.

(c) Apply 10 μL of each solution.

(d) Develop the plate to 15 cm.

(e) After removal of the plate, dry in air, spray with *aminohippuric acid reagent*, heat at 120° for 5 minutes and examine in daylight.

MOBILE PHASE

15 volumes of *water* and 85 volumes of *acetonitrile*.

CONFIRMATION

The chromatogram obtained with solution (1) shows two orange-pink zones (arabinose and xylose) and a yellow zone (galactose) similar in position and colour to the zones in the chromatograms obtained with solutions (2), (3) and (4).

B. When mounted in *ruthenium red solution*, the particles of the powder are stained red.

TESTS

Swelling index

Not less than 40, Appendix XI C. Use a quantity of the oral powder containing 1.0 g of Ispaghula Husk and a 100 mL ground-glass-stoppered cylinder graduated in 1 mL divisions.

Ash

Not more than 4.0%, Appendix XI J, Method II. Use a quantity of the powder containing 1 g of Ispaghula Husk.

STORAGE

Ispaghula Husk Oral Powder should be protected from moisture.

Ispaghula Seed

(Ph Eur monograph 1333)

Ph Eur

DEFINITION

Dried ripe seeds of *Plantago ovata* Forssk. (*P. ispaghula* Roxb.).

IDENTIFICATION

A. Ispaghula seed is pinkish-beige, smooth, boat-shaped and curved. It is 1.5 mm to 3.5 mm long, 1.5 mm to 2 mm wide and 1 mm to 1.5 mm thick. The concave surface shows in the centre a light coloured spot corresponding to the hilum. The convex surface shows a light brown spot corresponding to the location of the embryo and takes up about one quarter of the length of the seed.

B. Reduce to a powder (355) (*2.9.12*). The powder is pale brown. Examine under a microscope using *lactic reagent R*. The powder shows mainly fragments of the episperm with polygonal cells filled with mucilage; fragments of the inner layers of the testa with brownish thin-walled cells often associated with the outer layers of the endosperm; fragments of the endosperm with cells with thick cellulose walls containing aleurone grains and oil droplets; a few fragments of embryo with thin-walled cells. Examine under a microscope using a 50 per cent *V/V* solution of *glycerol R*. The powder shows starch granules, single or in groups of 2 to 4 and measuring 3 μm to 25 μm in diameter.

C. Thin-layer chromatography (*2.2.27*).

Test solution   To 50 mg of the powdered drug (355) (*2.9.12*) in a thick-walled centrifuge tube add 2 mL of a 230 g/L solution of *trifluoroacetic acid R*, and shake vigorously. Stopper the test tube and heat the mixture at 120 °C for 1 h. Centrifuge the hydrolysate, transfer the clear supernatant liquid into a 50 mL flask, add 10 mL of *water R* and evaporate the solution to dryness under reduced pressure. Take up the residue in 10 mL of *water R* and evaporate again to dryness under reduced pressure. Take up the residue in 2 mL of *methanol R*.

Reference solution (a)   Dissolve 10 mg of *arabinose R* in a small quantity of *water R* and dilute to 10 mL with *methanol R*.

Reference solution (b)   Dissolve 10 mg of *xylose R* in a small quantity of *water R* and dilute to 10 mL with *methanol R*.

Reference solution (c)   Dissolve 10 mg of *galactose R* in a small quantity of *water R* and dilute to 10 mL with *methanol R*.

Plate   TLC silica gel plate R

Mobile phase   water R, acetonitrile R (15:85 V/V).

Application   10 μL, as bands.

Development   Over a path of 15 cm.

Detection   Spray with *aminohippuric acid reagent R* and heat at 120 °C for 5 min. Examine in daylight.

Results   See below the sequence of the zones present in the chromatograms obtained with the reference and the test solutions.

Top of the plate	
Xylose: an orange-pink zone	An orange-pink zone (xylose)
Arabinose: an orange-pink zone	An orange-pink zone (arabinose)
Galactose: a yellow zone	A yellow zone (galactose)
Reference solution	**Test solution**

TESTS

Foreign matter (*2.8.2*)
Carry out the determination using 10.0 g.

Swelling index (*2.8.4*)
Minimum 9.

Loss on drying (*2.2.32*)
Maximum 10.0 per cent, determined on 1.000 g of the powdered drug (355) (*2.9.12*) by drying in an oven at 105 °C for 2 h.

Total ash (*2.4.16*)
Maximum 4.0 per cent.

Ph Eur

Ivy Leaf

(*Ph Eur monograph 2148*)

Ph Eur

DEFINITION

Whole or cut, dried leaves of *Hedera helix* L., collected in spring and summer.

Content

Minimum 3.0 per cent of hederacoside C ($C_{59}H_{96}O_{26}$; M_r 1221) (dried drug).

IDENTIFICATION

A. Whole leaves are coriaceous, 4-10 cm in length and width, cordate at the base. The lamina is palmately 3-5 lobed, the lobes more or less triangular with entire margins. The upper surface is dark green with a paler, radiate venation, the lower surface more greyish-green and the venation is distinctly raised. The petioles are long, cylindrical, about 2 mm in diameter and grooved longitudinally. Scattered white hairs occur on the petioles and on the surfaces of younger leaves, the older leaves are glabrous. Occasional entire, ovate-rhombic to lanceolate leaves 3-8 cm long from the flowering stems may be present.

B. Microscopic examination (*2.8.23*). The powder is green. Examine under a microscope using *chloral hydrate solution R*. The powder shows the following diagnostic characters (Figure 2148.-1): fragments of the upper epidermis, in surface view [F], showing cells with thickened, rather sinuous, finely pitted anticlinal walls [Fa] usually accompanied by underlying palisade parenchyma [Fb] including some cells containing cluster crystals of calcium oxalate [Fc]; fragments of the lower epidermis, in surface view [E], showing cells with sinuous, irregularly thickened and pitted walls [Ea], stomata that are mostly anomocytic [Eb] but occasionally anisocytic (*2.8.3*), surrounded by cells including some that show faint cuticular striations; the lower epidermis is accompanied by underlying spongy parenchyma [Ec] including some cells containing cluster crystals of calcium oxalate [Ed]; scattered stellate covering trichomes may be present, composed of 4-8 branches joined at the base on a multicellular, biseriate stalk, in surface view [B] or in

side view [A]; cluster crystals of calcium oxalate, about 40 µm in diameter, scattered [C] or occurring throughout the parenchyma (Ed, Fc); groups of lignified fibro-vascular tissue from the veins [D].

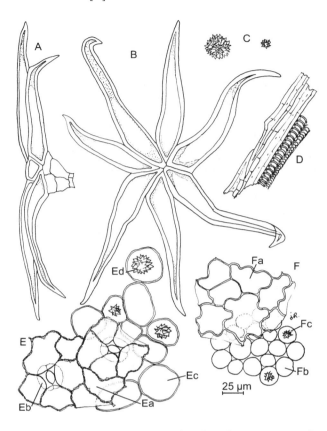

Figure 2148.-1. – *Illustration for identification test B of powdered herbal drug of ivy leaf*

C. Thin-layer chromatography (*2.2.27*).

Test solution   Extract 0.50 g of the powdered herbal drug (355) (*2.9.12*) under a reflux condenser in a water-bath at 60 °C with 5 mL of *methanol R* for 30 min. Cool and filter.

Reference solution   Dissolve 1.0 mg of *hederacoside C R* and 1.0 mg of α-*hederin R* in 1.0 mL of *methanol R*.

Plate   *TLC silica gel plate R*.

Mobile phase   *anhydrous formic acid R*, *acetone R*, *methanol R*, *ethyl acetate R* (4:20:20:30 *V/V/V/V*).

Application   20 µL as bands of 15 mm.

Development   Over a path of 12 cm.

Drying   At 100-105 °C.

Detection   Treat with *alcoholic solution of sulfuric acid R*, heat at 110 °C for 10 min and examine in daylight.

Results   See below the sequence of zones present in the chromatograms obtained with the reference solution and the test solution. Furthermore, other zones may be present in the chromatogram obtained with the test solution.

Top of the plate	
	A green zone
————	————
α-Hederin: a purple zone	A very faint purple zone (α-hederin)
	A broad yellow zone
	2-3 purple or green zones
————	————
Hederacoside C: a purple zone	A purple zone (hederacoside C)
Reference solution	**Test solution**

TESTS

Foreign matter (*2.8.2*)

Maximum 10 per cent of discoloured leaves, maximum 10 per cent of stems, and maximum 2 per cent of other foreign matter.

Loss on drying (*2.2.32*)

Maximum 10.0 per cent, determined on 1.000 g of the powdered herbal drug (355) (*2.9.12*) by drying in an oven at 105 °C for 2 h.

Total ash (*2.4.16*)

Maximum 10.0 per cent.

ASSAY

Liquid chromatography (*2.2.29*).

Solvent mixture   water R, methanol R (20:80 *V/V*).

Test solution   To 1.00 g of the powdered herbal drug (355) (*2.9.12*) in a 250 mL round-bottomed flask add 50 mL of the solvent mixture and heat under a reflux condenser in a water-bath at 80 °C for 1 h. Cool and filter through a plug of absorbent cotton into a 100 mL volumetric flask. The plug of absorbent cotton together with the residue is again extracted with 30 mL of the solvent mixture under reflux for 30 min. Filter and combine the filtrates. Rinse the round-bottomed flask and the plug of absorbent cotton with the solvent mixture and use the solvent mixture to dilute the contents of the volumetric flask to exactly 100.0 mL. Filter through a suitable membrane before use.

Reference solution   Dissolve an amount of *ivy leaf tincture HRS* corresponding to 3.0 mg of hederacoside C in *methanol R* and dilute to 5.0 mL with the same solvent.

Column:
— *size: l* = 0.125 m, Ø = 4 mm;
— *stationary phase: end-capped octadecylsilyl silica gel for chromatography R* (5 μm).

Mobile phase:
— *mobile phase A*: mix 14 volumes of *acetonitrile R* with 88 volumes of *water R* and adjust to pH 2.0 with *phosphoric acid R*;
— *mobile phase B*: *phosphoric acid R, acetonitrile R* (0.2:99.8 *V/V*);

Time (min)	Mobile phase A (per cent *V/V*)	Mobile phase B (per cent *V/V*)
0 - 5	100	0
5 - 6	100 → 94	0 → 6
6 - 40	94 → 60	6 → 40
40 - 41	60 → 0	40 → 100
41 - 55	0	100

Flow rate   1.5 mL/min.

Detection   Spectrophotometer at 205 nm.

Injection   20 μL.

System suitability   Reference solution:
— *retention time*: hederacoside C = about 20 min; if necessary, adjust the time intervals of the gradient.

Calculate the percentage content of hederacoside C with reference to the dried drug using the following expression:

$$\frac{A_1 \times m_2 \times 20 \times p}{A_2 \times m_1}$$

A_1 = area of the peak due to hederacoside C in the chromatogram obtained with the test solution;

A_2 = area of the peak due to hederacoside C in the chromatogram obtained with the reference solution;

m_1 = mass of the herbal drug to be examined used to prepare the test solution, in grams;

m_2 = mass of *ivy leaf tincture HRS* used to prepare the reference solution, in grams;

p = percentage content of hederacoside C in *ivy leaf tincture HRS*.

Ph Eur

Java Tea

(*Ph Eur monograph 1229*)

Ph Eur

DEFINITION

Fragmented, dried leaves and tops of stems of *Orthosiphon stamineus* Benth. (*O. aristatus* Miq.; *O. spicatus* Bak.).

Content

Minimum 0.05 per cent of sinensetin ($C_{20}H_{20}O_7$; M_r 372.4) (dried drug).

IDENTIFICATION

A. The leaves are friable, up to 7.5 cm in length and 2.5 cm in width. The petiole is short. The lamina is oval or lanceolate, the apex acuminate and the base cuneate. The abaxial surface of the leaves is light greyish-green and the adaxial surface is dark green or brownish-green. The venation is pinnate with few secondary veins. Examined under a lens (× 10), the secondary veins, after running parallel to the midrib, diverge at an acute angle. The margin is irregularly and roughly dentate, sometimes crenate and the abaxial surface is slightly curved. The petioles are thin, quadrangular, 4-8 mm long and, like the primary venation, usually violet-coloured. Occasionally, inflorescences in clusters of bluish-white or violet flowers, not yet opened, are found.

B. Reduce to a powder (355) (*2.9.12*). The powder is dark green. Examine under a microscope using *chloral hydrate solution R*. The powder shows the following diagnostic characters: fragments of epidermis, with cells with sinuous outlines, bearing unicellular or bicellular conical covering trichomes and articulated uniseriate trichomes up to 450 μm long, consisting of 3-8 cells with thick pitted walls; capitate trichomes with unicellular or bicellular heads; secretory trichomes with unicellular stalks and usually tetracellular heads; diacytic stomata (*2.8.3*), which are more numerous on the lower epidermis.

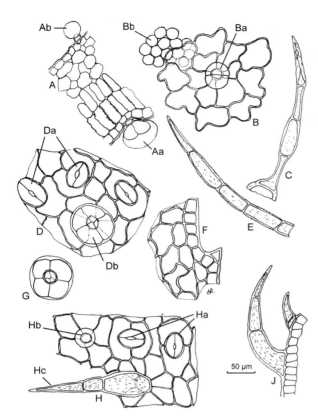

A. Lamina, in transverse section, showing a secretory trichome with a tetracellular head (Aa) and a capitate trichome with a unicellular head (Ab)

B. Upper epidermis, in surface view, showing a capitate trichome with a bicellular head (Ba) and underlying palisade parenchyma (Bb)

C. and E. Articulated covering trichomes (usually only fragments observed)

D. Lower epidermis, in surface view, with diacytic stomata (Da) and secretory trichome with a tetracellular head (Db)

F. Margin of the lamina

G. Secretory trichome

H. Lower epidermis, in surface view, with diacytic stomata (Ha), capitate trichome with a unicellular head (Hb) and multicellular covering trichome (Hc)

J. Covering trichomes on the margin of the lamina

Figure 1229.-1. – *Illustration of powdered herbal drug of Java tea (see Identification B)*

C. Thin-layer chromatography (2.2.27).

Test solution Shake 1 g of the powdered drug (710) (2.9.12) with 10 mL of *methanol R* in a water-bath at 60 °C for 5 min and filter the cooled solution.

Reference solution Dissolve 1 mg of *sinensetin R* in *methanol R* and dilute to 20 mL with the same solvent.

Plate TLC *silica gel plate R.*

Mobile phase *methanol R, ethyl acetate R, toluene R* (5:40:55 *V/V/V*).

Application 10 µL as bands.

Development Over a path of 10 cm.

Drying In air.

Detection Examine in ultraviolet light at 365 nm.

Results See below the sequence of the zones present in the chromatogram obtained with the reference solution and the test solution. Furthermore, red fluorescent zones are present in the lower third and near the solvent front of the chromatogram obtained with the test solution.

Top of the plate	
	1 or 2 more or less intense blue or violet-blue fluorescent zones
	_____
Sinensetin: an intense light blue fluorescent zone	A major blue fluorescent zone (sinensetin)
	_____
	2 bluish fluorescent zones
Reference solution	**Test solution**

TESTS

Foreign matter (2.8.2)
Maximum 5 per cent of stems with a diameter greater than 1 mm and maximum 2 per cent of other foreign matter.

Loss on drying (2.2.32)
Maximum 11.0 per cent, determined on 1.000 g of the powdered drug (355) (2.9.12) by drying in an oven at 105 °C for 2 h.

Total ash (2.4.16)
Maximum 12.5 per cent.

ASSAY

Liquid chromatography (2.2.29).

Test solution Heat 2.5 g of the powdered drug (355) (2.9.12) and 100 mL of *methylene chloride R* on a water-bath for 30 min with stirring. Filter. Collect the filtrate and repeat the operation twice, in the same manner, on the filtration residue. Combine the filtrates. Evaporate the solvent under reduced pressure. Dissolve the residue in 25.0 mL of the mobile phase, using an ultrasonic bath if necessary. Filter the solution through a nitrocellulose filter with a pore size of 0.45 µm.

Reference solution Dissolve 5 mg (m_2) of *sinensetin R* in 80 mL of the mobile phase using an ultrasonic bath if necessary and dilute to 100.0 mL with the mobile phase.

Column:
— *size*: l = 0.25 m, Ø = 4.6 mm;
— *stationary phase*: *octadecylsilyl silica gel for chromatography R* (5 µm).

Mobile phase *tetrahydrofuran R, acetic acid R, water R, methanol R* (5:8:42:45 *V/V/V/V*).

Flow rate 0.5 mL/min.

Detection Spectrophotometer at 258 nm.

Injection 20 µL.

Calculate the percentage content of sinensetin using the following expression:

$$\frac{m_2 \times F_1 \times 25}{m_1 \times F_2}$$

F_1 = area of the peak due to sinensetin in the chromatogram obtained with the test solution;
F_2 = area of the peak due to sinensetin in the chromatogram obtained with the reference solution;
m_1 = mass of the drug to be examined, in grams;
m_2 = mass of sinensetin in the reference solution, in grams.

_____ *Ph Eur*

Juniper

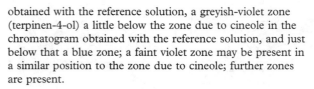

(Ph Eur monograph 1532)

Ph Eur _____

DEFINITION

Dried ripe cone berry of *Juniperus communis* L.

Content

Minimum 10 mL/kg of essential oil (anhydrous drug).

CHARACTERS

Strongly aromatic odour, especially if crushed.

IDENTIFICATION

A. The berry-shaped cone is globular, up to 10 mm in diameter, and violet-brown or blackish-brown, frequently with a bluish bloom. It consists of 3 fleshy scales. The apex has a 3-rayed closed cleft and 3 not very clearly defined projections. A remnant of peduncle is frequently attached at the base. The fleshy part is crumbly and brownish.

It contains 3 or, more rarely, 2 small, elongated, extremely hard seeds that have 3 sharp edges and are slightly rounded at the back, acuminate at the apex. The seeds are fused with the fleshy part of the cone berry in the lower part on the outside of their bases. Very large, oval oil glands containing sticky resin lie at the outer surface of the seeds.

B. Microscopic examination (*2.8.23*). The powder is brown. Examine under a microscope using *chloral hydrate solution R*. The powder shows the following diagnostic characters: fragments of epidermis of the cone berry wall containing cells with thick, pitted, colourless walls and brown glandular content, occasionnally with anomocytic stomata (*2.8.3*); fragments of the 3-rayed apical cleft of the cone berry with spaces and epidermal cells interlocked by papillous outgrowths; fragments of the hypodermis with collenchymatous thickened cells; fragments of the mesocarp consisting of large thin-walled parenchymatous cells, usually rounded, with large intercellular spaces and irregular, large, usually scarcely pitted, yellow idioblasts (barrel cells); fragments of schizogenous oil cells; fragments of the testa with thick-walled, pitted, colourless sclereids containing 1 or several prism crystals of calcium oxalate; fragments of the endosperm and embryonic tissue with thin-walled cells containing fatty oil and aleurone grains.

C. Thin-layer chromatography (*2.2.27*).

Test solution Dilute the oil-xylene mixture obtained in the assay to 5.0 mL with *hexane R*.

Reference solution Dissolve 4.0 mg of *guaiazulene R* and 50 μL of *cineole R* in 10 mL of *hexane R*.

Plate TLC silica gel plate R.

Mobile phase ethyl acetate R, toluene R (5:95 V/V).

Application 20 μL of the test solution and 10 μL of the reference solution, as bands.

Development Over a path of 15 cm.

Drying In air.

Detection Treat with *anisaldehyde solution R*, heat at 100-105 °C for 5-10 min and examine in daylight.

Results The chromatogram obtained with the reference solution shows a red zone (guaiazulene) in the upper half and a brownish-violet or greyish-violet zone (cineole) in the lower half; the chromatogram obtained with the test solution shows a strong violet zone (mono- and sesquiterpenes) similar in position to the zone due to guaiazulene in the chromatogram obtained with the reference solution, a reddish-violet zone a little above the zone due to cineole in the chromatogram

obtained with the reference solution, a greyish-violet zone (terpinen-4-ol) a little below the zone due to cineole in the chromatogram obtained with the reference solution, and just below that a blue zone; a faint violet zone may be present in a similar position to the zone due to cineole; further zones are present.

TESTS

Foreign matter (*2.8.2*)

Maximum 5 per cent of unripe or discoloured cone berries and maximum 2 per cent of other foreign matter.

Water (*2.2.13*)

Maximum 120 mL/kg, determined on 20.0 g of the crushed drug.

Total ash (*2.4.16*)

Maximum 4.0 per cent.

ASSAY

Carry out the determination of essential oils in herbal drugs (*2.8.12*). Use 20.0 g of the herbal drug reduced to a coarse powder using a suitable mill immediately before the assay, a 500 mL round-bottomed flask, 200 mL of *water R* as the distillation liquid and 0.5 mL of *xylene R* in the graduated tube. Distil at a rate of 3-4 mL/min for 90 min.

_____ *Ph Eur*

Juniper Oil

(Ph Eur monograph 1832)

Ph Eur _____

DEFINITION

Essential oil obtained by steam distillation from the ripe, non-fermented berry cones of *Juniperus communis* L. A suitable antioxidant may be added.

CHARACTERS

Appearance

Mobile, colourless or yellowish liquid.

Characteristic odour.

IDENTIFICATION

First identification B.

Second identification A.

A. Thin-layer chromatography (*2.2.27*).

Test solution Dissolve 0.2 mL of the substance to be examined in 5 mL of *heptane R*.

Reference solution Dissolve 20 mg of α-*terpineol R* and 20 μL of *terpinen-4-ol R* in 25 mL of *heptane R*.

Plate TLC silica gel plate R.

Mobile phase ethyl acetate R, toluene R (5:95 V/V).

Application 20 μL, as bands.

Development Over a path of 12 cm.

Drying In air.

Detection Treat with *anisaldehyde solution R* and heat at 100-105 °C until the zones appear; examine immediately in daylight.

Results See below the sequence of zones present in the chromatograms obtained with the reference solution and the test solution.

Top of the plate	
	An intense brownish-violet zone
	A brown zone
	A violet-pink zone
Terpinen-4-ol: a brownish-violet zone	A brownish-violet zone (terpinen-4-ol)
	A violet zone
α-Terpineol: a violet or brownish-violet zone	A violet or brownish-violet zone (α-terpineol)
Reference solution	**Test solution**

B. Examine the chromatograms obtained in the test for chromatographic profile.

Results   The characteristic peaks in the chromatogram obtained with the test solution are similar in retention time to those in the chromatogram obtained with the reference solution.

TESTS

Relative density (*2.2.5*)
0.857 to 0.876.

Refractive index (*2.2.6*)
1.471 to 1.483.

Optical rotation (*2.2.7*)
−15° to −0.5°.

Peroxide value (*2.5.5*)
Maximum 20.

Fatty oils and resinified essential oils (*2.8.7*)
It complies with the test for fatty oils and resinified essential oils.

Chromatographic profile
Gas chromatography (*2.2.28*): use the normalisation procedure.

Test solution   Dissolve 60 mg of the substance to be examined in *trimethylpentane R* and dilute to 5.0 mL with the same solvent.

Reference solution   Mix 25 μL each of *α-pinene R*, *sabinene R*, *β-pinene R*, *β-myrcene R*, *α-phellandrene R*, *limonene R*, *terpinen-4-ol R*, *bornyl acetate R* and *β-caryophyllene R* and dilute to 25.0 mL with *trimethylpentane R*.

Column:
— *material*: fused silica;
— *size: l* = 30 m (a film thickness of 1 μm may be used) to 60 m (a film thickness of 0.2 μm may be used), Ø = 0.25-0.53 mm;
— *stationary phase*: poly(dimethyl)(diphenyl)siloxane R.

Carrier gas   helium for chromatography R.

Flow rate   2.0 mL/min.

Split ratio   1:50.

Temperature:

	Time (min)	Temperature (°C)
Column	0 - 1	60
	1 - 58	60→230
Injection port		250
Detector		250

Detection   Flame ionisation.

Injection   0.5 μL.

Elution order   Order indicated in the composition of the reference solution. Record the retention times of these substances.

System suitability   Reference solution:
— *resolution*: minimum 1.5 between the peaks due to sabinene and β-pinene.

Using the retention times determined from the chromatogram obtained with the reference solution, locate the components of the reference solution in the chromatogram obtained with the test solution.

Determine the percentage content of the components. Disregard the peak due to trimethylpentane and peaks comprising less than 0.01 per cent of the total surface area. The percentages are within the following ranges:
— *α-pinene*: 20 per cent to 50 per cent;
— *sabinene*: maximum 20 per cent;
— *β-pinene*: 1.0 per cent to 12 per cent;
— *β-myrcene*: 1.0 per cent to 35 per cent;
— *α-phellandrene*: maximum 1.0 per cent;
— *limonene*: 2.0 per cent to 12 per cent;
— *terpinen-4-ol*: 0.5 per cent to 10 per cent;
— *bornyl acetate*: maximum 2.0 per cent;
— *β-caryophyllene*: maximum 7.0 per cent.

STORAGE

At a temperature not exceeding 25 °C.

_____ *Ph Eur*

Kelp

Bladderwrack; Fucus
(*Ph Eur monograph 1426*)

Ph Eur _____

DEFINITION

Fragmented dried thallus of *Fucus vesiculosus* L. or *F. serratus* L. or *Ascophyllum nodosum* Le Jolis.

Content

Minimum 0.03 per cent and maximum 0.2 per cent of total iodine (A_r 126.9) (dried drug).

CHARACTERS

Salty and mucilaginous taste.

Unpleasant marine odour.

IDENTIFICATION

A. The drug consists of fragments with a corneous consistency, blackish-brown to greenish-brown, sometimes covered with whitish efflorescence. The thallus consists of a ribbon-like blade, branching dichotomously with prominent central ribs (pseudoveins). *F. vesiculosus* typically shows a foliose blade with smooth edges and bears occasional ovoid, single or paired, air vesicles. The ends of certain branches are of ovoid shape and a little widened. They bear numerous reproductive organs (conceptacles). *F. serratus* has a foliose blade with a serrate margin and no vesicles, the branches bearing conceptacles are less swollen. The thallus of *A. nodosum* is irregularly branched, without pseudo-midrib. It shows single ovoid air vesicles; the falciform conceptacles are located at the end of small branches.

B. Reduce to a powder (355) (*2.9.12*). The powder is greenish-brown. Examine under a microscope using *chloral hydrate solution R*. The powder shows fragments of surface tissue with regular isodiametric cells with brown contents, and fragments of deep tissue with colourless, elongated cells arranged in long filaments with large mucilaginous spaces between them. Thick-walled cells in files and in closely packed groups, from the pseudovein, are sometimes visible.

C. To 1 g of the powdered drug (355) (*2.9.12*) add 20 mL of a 2 per cent *V/V* solution of *hydrochloric acid R*. Shake vigorously and filter. Wash the residue with 10 mL of *water R* and filter. To the residue add 10 mL of a 200 g/L solution of *sodium carbonate R*. Shake and centrifuge. Collect the supernatant liquid. Adjust to pH 1.5 using *sulfuric acid R*. A white, flocculent precipitate is slowly formed.

TESTS

Arsenic (*2.4.27*)
Maximum 90 ppm.

Cadmium (*2.4.27*)
Maximum 4 ppm.

Lead (*2.4.27*)
Maximum 5 ppm.

Mercury (*2.4.27*)
Maximum 0.1 ppm.

Swelling index (*2.8.4*)
Minimum 6.

Loss on drying (*2.2.32*)
Maximum 15.0 per cent, determined on 1.000 g by drying in an oven at 105 °C, for 2 h.

Total ash (*2.4.16*)
Maximum 24 per cent.

Ash insoluble in hydrochloric acid (*2.8.1*)
Maximum 3.0 per cent.

ASSAY

Total iodine
To 1.000 g of the powdered drug, in a tall silica crucible, add 5 mL of *water R* and 5 g of *potassium hydroxide R*. Stir with a magnesium rod. Heat on a water bath. Add 1 g of *potassium carbonate R*. Mix, add the tip of the magnesium rod with the residues of the drug and dry, first on a water-bath then over an open flame. Incinerate raising the temperature progressively to not more than 600 °C. Allow to cool. Add 20 mL of *water R* and heat gently to boiling, stirring with a glass rod. Filter the hot mixture through an unpleated filter, into a conical flask. Rinse the residue with 4 quantities, each of 20 mL, of hot *water R*. Rinse the filter and the crucible with 50 mL of hot *water R*. Combine the solutions. Allow to cool. Neutralise with *dilute sulfuric acid R* in the presence of *methyl orange solution R*. Add 3 mL of *dilute sulfuric acid R* and 1 mL of *bromine water R*. The solution is yellow. After 5 min add 0.6 mL of a 50 g/L solution of *phenol R*. The solution is clear. Acidify with 5 mL of *phosphoric acid R* and add 0.2 g of *potassium iodide R*. Allow to stand for 5 min protected from light. Add 1 mL of *starch solution R* and titrate with *0.01 M sodium thiosulfate*.

1 mL of *0.01 M sodium thiosulfate* is equivalent to 0.2115 mg of iodine.

LABELLING
The label states the species of kelp present.

———————————— *Ph Eur*

Knotgrass

(*Ph Eur monograph 1885*)

Ph Eur _____

DEFINITION
Whole or fragmented, dried flowering aerial parts of *Polygonum aviculare* L. *s.l.*

Content
Minimum 0.30 per cent of flavonoids, expressed as hyperoside ($C_{21}H_{20}O_{12}$; M_r 464.4) (dried drug).

IDENTIFICATION
A. The stem is 0.5-2 mm thick, branched, with nodes, cylindrical or slightly angular, and longitudinally striated. It bears sessile or shortly petiolate, glabrous, entire leaves, which differ widely in shape and size. The sheath-like stipules (ochrea) are lacerate and silvery. The small, axillary flowers have 5 greenish-white perianth segments, the tips of which are often red. The dry, indehiscent fruits are 2-4 mm, brown or black, triangular, usually punctate or striate.

B. Microscopic examination (*2.8.23*). The powder is greenish-brown. Examine under a microscope using *chloral hydrate solution R*. The powder shows the following diagnostic characters (Figure 1885.-1): fragments of lower [A] and upper [D] leaf epidermises with a striated cuticle and anisocytic stomata (*2.8.3*) [Aa, Da]; polygonal cells of the upper epidermis [D] with slightly thickened beaded walls, often associated with palisade parenchyma [Db]; cells of the lower epidermis [A], with thin, sinuous walls; fragments of the margin of the lamina of the leaf with irregular cells [J]; fragments of parenchyma [G] with numerous cells containing cluster crystals of calcium oxalate, some of which are very large [Ga], often associated with vessels [Gb]; groups of fibres [B, C] with thick walls [Ba, Cb] from the hypodermis of the stem associated either with the epidermis [Ca] or with parenchyma consisting of cells containing cluster crystals of calcium oxalate [Bb]; fragments of the ochrea [E] with elongated, thin-walled cells [Ea], along which run very elongated fibres [Eb]; globular pollen grains with a smooth exine and 3 germinal pores [H]; occasional brown fragments of the exocarp composed of cells with thick, sinuous walls [F].

C. Thin-layer chromatography (*2.2.27*).

Test solution To 1.0 g of the powdered herbal drug (355) (*2.9.12*) add 10 mL of *methanol R*. Heat the mixture in a water-bath under a reflux condenser for 10 min. Cool and filter.

Reference solution Dissolve 1 mg of *caffeic acid R*, 1 mg of *chlorogenic acid R* and 2.5 mg of *hyperoside R* in 10 mL of *methanol R*.

Plate TLC silica gel plate R.

Mobile phase anhydrous formic acid R, glacial acetic acid R, water R, ethyl acetate R (7:7:14:72 *V/V/V/V*).

Application 20 µL as bands.

Development Over a path of 10 cm.

Drying At 100-105 °C.

Detection Treat with a 10 g/L solution of *diphenylboric acid aminoethyl ester R* in *methanol R*; subsequently treat with a 50 g/L solution of *macrogol 400 R* in *methanol R*. Allow to dry in air for about 30 min. Examine in ultraviolet light at 365 nm.

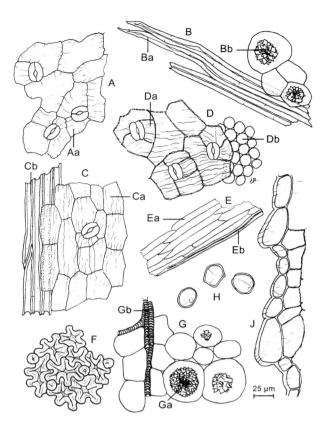

Figure 1885.-1. – *Illustration for identification test B of powdered herbal drug of knotgrass*

Loss on drying (*2.2.32*)
Maximum 10.0 per cent, determined on 1.000 g of the powdered herbal drug (710) (*2.9.12*) by drying in an oven at 105 °C for 2 h.

Total ash (*2.4.16*)
Maximum 10.0 per cent.

ASSAY

Stock solution In a 100 mL round-bottomed flask, place 0.800 g of the powdered herbal drug (355) (*2.9.12*), and add 1 mL of a 5 g/L solution of *hexamethylenetetramine R*, 20 mL of *acetone R* and 2 mL of *hydrochloric acid R1*. Boil the mixture under a reflux condenser for 30 min. Filter the liquid through a plug of absorbent cotton into a flask. Add the absorbent cotton to the residue in the round-bottomed flask and extract with 2 quantities, each of 20 mL, of *acetone R*, each time boiling under a reflux condenser for 10 min. Allow to cool, filter each extract through the plug of absorbent cotton into the flask. Filter the combined acetone extracts through a filter paper into a volumetric flask and dilute to 100.0 mL with *acetone R*, rinsing the flask and the filter paper. Introduce 20.0 mL of the solution into a separating funnel, add 20 mL of *water R* and shake the mixture with 1 quantity of 15 mL and then 3 quantities, each of 10 mL, of *ethyl acetate R*. Combine the ethyl acetate extracts in a separating funnel and wash with 2 quantities, each of 50 mL, of *water R*. Dry the extracts over 10 g of *anhydrous sodium sulfate R*, filter into a 50 mL volumetric flask and dilute to volume with *ethyl acetate R*.

Test solution To 10.0 mL of the stock solution add 1 mL of *aluminium chloride reagent R* and dilute to 25.0 mL with a 5 per cent *V/V* solution of *glacial acetic acid R* in *methanol R*.

Compensation liquid Dilute 10.0 mL of the stock solution to 25.0 mL with a 5 per cent *V/V* solution of *glacial acetic acid R* in *methanol R*.

Measure the absorbance (*2.2.25*) of the test solution after 30 min by comparison with the compensation liquid at 425 nm. Calculate the percentage content of flavonoids, calculated as hyperoside, using the following expression:

$$\frac{A \times 1.25}{m}$$

i.e. taking the specific absorbance of hyperoside to be 500.
A = absorbance at 425 nm;
m = mass of the herbal drug to be examined, in grams.

———————————— *Ph Eur*

Results See below the sequence of fluorescent zones present in the chromatograms obtained with the reference solution and the test solution. Furthermore, other fluorescent zones are present in the chromatogram obtained with the test solution.

Top of the plate	
Caffeic acid: a light blue fluorescent zone	1 or 2 blue fluorescent zones (caffeic acid)
———	———
	1 or 2 yellowish-green fluorescent zones
	A yellow fluorescent zone
Hyperoside: a yellowish-brown fluorescent zone	
	A yellowish-brown fluorescent zone
Chlorogenic acid: a light blue fluorescent zone	A light blue fluorescent zone (chlorogenic acid)
———	———
	A yellowish-brown fluorescent zone
Reference solution	**Test solution**

TESTS

Foreign matter (*2.8.2*)
Maximum 2 per cent of roots and maximum 2 per cent of other foreign matter.

Kudzuvine Root

(Ph Eur monograph 2434)

Ph Eur

DEFINITION
Fragmented, dried root of *Pueraria lobata* (Willd.) Ohwi.

Content
Minimum 6.5 per cent of total isoflavonoids, expressed as puerarin ($C_{12}H_{20}O_9$; M_r 416.4) (dried drug), of which minimum 45 per cent consists of puerarin.

IDENTIFICATION
A. Small, square pieces or thick, rectangular slices, 5-35 cm long and 0.5-1 cm thick. The outer bark is pale brown, with longitudinal wrinkles and rough; the section is yellowish-white and shows indistinct striations. The texture is strongly fibrous.

B. Microscopic examination (*2.8.23*). The powder is pale brown. Examine under a microscope using *chloral hydrate solution R*. The powder shows the following diagnostic characters: thick-walled lignified fibres, which occur in groups, surrounded by a calcium oxalate prism sheath; crystal cells with thickened walls; rare sclereids, subrounded or elliptical, about 50 μm in diameter; relatively large bordered-pitted vessels with hexagonal or elliptical pits arranged very densly. Examine under a microscope using a 50 per cent *V/V* solution of *glycerol R*. The powder shows numerous starch granules, simple or 2-20 compound; the starch granules are spheroidal, semi-rounded or polygonal with a pointed, cleft or stellate hilum, about 15 μm in diameter.

C. Thin-layer chromatography (*2.2.27*).

Test solution Sonicate 0.5 g of the powdered herbal drug (355) (*2.9.12*) with 5 mL of *methanol R*, then centrifuge; use the supernatant.

Reference solution Dissolve 5 mg of *puerarin R* and 5 mg of *daidzin R* in 5 mL of *methanol R*.

Plate TLC silica gel F_{254} plate R (2-10 μm).

Mobile phase water R, methylene chloride R, methanol R, ethyl acetate R (10:20:22:40 *V/V/V/V*); use the lower layer.

Application 7 μL as bands of 8 mm.

Development Over a path of 6 cm.

Drying In air.

Detection Examine in ultraviolet light at 254 nm.

Results See below the sequence of zones present in the chromatograms obtained with the reference solution and the test solution. Furthermore, other zones may be present in the chromatogram obtained with the test solution.

Top of the plate	
	A weak quenching zone
_____	
	A quenching zone
Daidzin: a quenching zone	A quenching zone
Puerarin: a quenching zone	A quenching zone
_____	
	At least 5 quenching zones
Reference solution	**Test solution**

TESTS
Foreign matter (*2.8.2*)
Maximum 5 per cent.

Loss on drying (*2.2.32*)
Maximum 10.0 per cent, determined on 1.000 g of the powdered herbal drug (355) (*2.9.12*) by drying in an oven at 105 °C.

Total ash (*2.4.16*)
Maximum 7.0 per cent.

Ash insoluble in hydrochloric acid (*2.8.1*)
Maximum 1.0 per cent.

ASSAY
Liquid chromatography (*2.2.29*).

Test solution Introduce 0.100 g of the powdered herbal drug (355) (*2.9.12*) into a 250 mL conical flask, add 50.0 mL of *ethanol (30 per cent V/V) R* and weigh. Heat under a reflux condenser for 30 min. Allow to cool and weigh again. Adjust to the initial mass with *ethanol (30 per cent V/V) R*, mix well and filter.

Reference solution Introduce an amount of *kudzuvine root dry extract HRS* corresponding to 3.0 mg of puerarin into a 250 mL conical flask, add 50.0 mL of *ethanol (30 per cent V/V) R* and weigh. Heat under a reflux condenser for 30 min. Allow to cool and weigh again. Adjust to the initial mass with *ethanol (30 per cent V/V) R*, mix well and filter.

Column 2 columns coupled in series:
— *size: l* = 0.10 m, Ø = 4.6 mm;
— *stationary phase: monolithic octadecylsilyl silica gel for chromatography R.*

Mobile phase:
— *mobile phase A: glacial acetic acid R, water R* (0.1:99.9 *V/V*);
— *mobile phase B: acetonitrile R*;

Time (min)	Mobile phase A (per cent *V/V*)	Mobile phase B (per cent *V/V*)
0 - 16.5	90 → 71	10 → 29

Flow rate 3.0 mL/min.

Detection Spectrophotometer at 260 nm.

Injection 10 μL.

Identification of peaks Use the chromatogram supplied with *kudzuvine root dry extract HRS* and the chromatogram obtained with the reference solution to identify the peaks due to the isoflavonoids (3-hydroxypuerarin, puerarin, 3-methoxypuerarin, 6-*O''*-D-xylosylpuerarin and daidzin).

Relative retention With reference to puerarin (retention time = about 3.4 min): 3-hydroxypuerarin = about 0.7; 3-methoxypuerarin = about 1.09; 6-*O''*-D-xylosylpuerarin = about 1.15; daidzin = about 1.4.

System suitability Reference solution:
— *peak-to-valley ratio*: minimum 10, where H_p = height above the baseline of the peak due to 3-methoxypuerarin and H_v = height above the baseline of the lowest point of the curve separating this peak from the peak due to puerarin.

Calculate the percentage content of puerarin using the following expression:

$$\frac{A_1 \times m_2 \times p}{A_2 \times m_1}$$

A_1 = area of the peak due to puerarin in the chromatogram obtained with the test solution;

A_2 = area of the peak due to puerarin in the chromatogram obtained with the reference solution;

m_1 = mass of the herbal drug to be examined used to prepare the test solution, in grams;

m_2 = mass of *kudzuvine root dry extract HRS* used to prepare the reference solution, in grams;

p = percentage content of puerarin in *kudzuvine root dry extract HRS*.

Calculate the percentage content of total isoflavonoids (3-hydroxypuerarin, puerarin, 3-methoxypuerarin, 6-O''-D-xylosylpuerarin and daidzin) using the following expression:

$$\frac{A_1 \times m_2 \times p}{A_2 \times m_1}$$

A_1 = sum of the areas of the peaks due to the isoflavonoids (3-hydroxypuerarin, puerarin, 3-methoxypuerarin, 6-O''-D-xylosylpuerarin and daidzin) in the chromatogram obtained with the test solution;

A_2 = area of the peak due to puerarin in the chromatogram obtained with the reference solution;

m_1 = mass of the herbal drug to be examined used to prepare the test solution, in grams;

$m2$ = mass of *kudzuvine root dry extract HRS* used to prepare the reference solution, in grams;

p = percentage content of puerarin in *kudzuvine root dry extract HRS*.

Ph Eur

Thomson Kudzuvine Root

(*Ph Eur monograph 2483*)

Ph Eur _____

DEFINITION

Whole or fragmented, dried root of *Pueraria thomsonii* Benth., with the outer bark removed.

Content

Minimum 0.4 per cent of total isoflavonoids, expressed as puerarin ($C_{12}H_{20}O_9$; M_r 416.4) (dried drug), of which minimum 55 per cent consists of puerarin.

IDENTIFICATION

A. Cylindrical, subfusiform or semi-cylindrical, 12-15 cm long and 4-8 cm in diameter, sometimes in longitudinally or obliquely cut thick slices, varying in size. Externally yellowish-white or pale brown. The root is heavy, texture hard and starchy, a transverse section shows pale brown concentric rings formed by fibres, a longitudinal section shows several longitudinal striations formed by fibres.

B. Microscopic examination (*2.8.23*). The powder is yellowish-white. Examine under a microscope using *chloral hydrate solution R*. The powder shows the following diagnostic characters: thick-walled lignified fibres, which occur in groups, surrounded by a calcium oxalate prism sheath; crystal cells with thickened walls; rare sclereids, subrounded or elliptical, about 50 µm in diameter; relatively large bordered-pitted vessels with hexagonal or elliptical pits, arranged very densely. Examine under a microscope using a 50 per cent *V/V* solution of *glycerol R*. The powder shows numerous starch granules, simple or 2-20 compound; the starch granules are spheroidal, semi-rounded or polygonal with a pointed, cleft or stellate hilum, about 15 µm in diameter.

C. Thin-layer chromatography (*2.2.27*).

Test solution Sonicate 0.5 g of the powdered herbal drug (355) (*2.9.12*) with 5 mL of *methanol R*, then centrifuge; use the supernatant.

Reference solution Dissolve 5 mg of *daidzin R* and 5 mg of *puerarin R* in 5 mL of *methanol R*.

Plate TLC silica gel F_{254} plate R (2-10 µm).

Mobile phase water R, methylene chloride R, methanol R, ethyl acetate R (10:20:22:40 *V/V/V/V*); use the lower layer.

Application 7 µL as bands of 8 mm.

Development Over a path of 6 cm.

Drying In air.

Detection Examine in ultraviolet light at 254 nm.

Results See below the sequence of zones present in the chromatograms obtained with the reference solution and the test solution. Furthermore, other zones may be present in the chromatogram obtained with the test solution.

Top of the plate	
	A weak quenching zone
———	———
Daidzin: a quenching zone	A weak quenching zone
Puerarin: a quenching zone	A weak quenching zone
———	———
	Several quenching zones
Reference solution	**Test solution**

TESTS

Foreign matter (*2.8.2*)
Maximum 5 per cent.

Loss on drying (*2.2.32*)
Maximum 10.0 per cent, determined on 1.000 g of the powdered herbal drug (355) (*2.9.12*) by drying in an oven at 105 °C.

Total ash (*2.4.16*)
Maximum 7.0 per cent.

Ash insoluble in hydrochloric acid (*2.8.1*)
Maximum 1.0 per cent.

ASSAY

Liquid chromatography (*2.2.29*).

Test solution Introduce 1.00 g of the powdered herbal drug (355) (*2.9.12*) into a 250 mL conical flask, add 50.0 mL of *ethanol (30 per cent V/V) R* and weigh. Heat under a reflux condenser for 30 min. Allow to cool and weigh again. Adjust to the initial mass with *ethanol (30 per cent V/V) R*, mix well and filter.

Reference solution Introduce an amount of *kudzuvine root dry extract HRS* corresponding to 3.0 mg of puerarin into a 250 mL conical flask, add 50.0 mL of *ethanol (30 per cent V/V) R* and weigh. Heat under a reflux condenser for 30 min. Allow to cool and weigh again. Adjust to the initial mass with *ethanol (30 per cent V/V) R*, mix well and filter.

Column 2 columns coupled in series:
— size: l = 0.10 m, Ø = 4.6 mm;
— stationary phase: monolithic octadecylsilyl silica gel for chromatography R.

Mobile phase:
— *mobile phase A*: glacial acetic acid R, water R
   (0.1:99.9 V/V);
— *mobile phase B*: acetonitrile R;

Time (min)	Mobile phase A (per cent V/V)	Mobile phase B (per cent V/V)
0 - 16.5	90 → 71	10 → 29

Flow rate   3.0 mL/min.

Detection   Spectrophotometer at 260 nm.

Injection   10 μL.

Identification of peaks   Use the chromatogram supplied with *kudzuvine root dry extract HRS* and the chromatogram obtained with the reference solution to identify the peaks due to the isoflavonoids (puerarin, 3-methoxypuerarin, 6-O''-D-xylosylpuerarin and daidzin).

Relative retention   With reference to puerarin (retention time = about 3.4 min): 6-O''-D-xylosylpuerarin = about 1.15; daidzin = about 1.4.

System suitability   Reference solution:
— *peak-to-valley ratio*: minimum 10, where H_p = height above the baseline of the peak due to 3-methoxypuerarin and H_v = height above the baseline of the lowest point of the curve separating this peak from the peak due to puerarin.

Calculate the percentage content of puerarin using the following expression:

$$\frac{A_1 \times m_2 \times p}{A_2 \times m_1}$$

A_1 = area of the peak due to puerarin in the chromatogram obtained with the test solution;

A_2 = area of the peak due to puerarin in the chromatogram obtained with the reference solution;

m_1 = mass of the herbal drug to be examined used to prepare the test solution, in grams;

m_2 = mass of *kudzuvine root dry extract HRS* used to prepare the reference solution, in grams;

p = percentage content of puerarin in *kudzuvine root dry extract HRS*.

Calculate the percentage content of total isoflavonoids (puerarin, 6-O''-D-xylosylpuerarin and daidzin) using the following expression:

$$\frac{A_1 \times m_2 \times p}{A_2 \times m_1}$$

A_1 = sum of the areas of the peaks due to the isoflavonoids (puerarin, 6-O''-D-xylosylpuerarin and daidzin) in the chromatogram obtained with the test solution;

A_2 = area of the peak due to puerarin in the chromatogram obtained with the reference solution;

m_1 = mass of the herbal drug to be examined used to prepare the test solution, in grams;

m_2 = mass of *kudzuvine root dry extract HRS* used to prepare the reference solution, in grams;

p = percentage content of puerarin in *kudzuvine root dry extract HRS*.

Ph Eur

Lavender Flower

(*Ph Eur monograph 1534*)

Ph Eur

DEFINITION
Dried flower of *Lavandula angustifolia* Mill. (L. *officinalis* Chaix).

Content
Minimum 13 mL/kg of essential oil (anhydrous drug).

CHARACTERS
Strongly aromatic odour.

IDENTIFICATION
First identification   A, B, D.

Second identification   A, B, C.

A. The flower has a short peduncle and consists of a bluish-grey tubular calyx divided distally into 4 very short teeth and a small rounded lobe, a blue bilabial corolla with the upper lip bifid and the lower lip trilobate and 4 didynamous stamens with ovoid anthers.

B. Microscopic examination (*2.8.23*). The powder is bluish-grey. Examine under a microscope using *chloral hydrate solution R*. The powder shows the following diagnostic characters (Figure 1534.-1): covering trichomes bifurcating at one or more levels [C, L]; secretory trichomes with short stalks and 8-celled heads of the Lamiaceae type in side view [H], in surface view [M]; glandular trichomes with unicellular [O] or multicellular [K] stalks and unicellular heads; glandular trichomes with long uneven stalks and unicellular heads, separated from the stalk by an intermediary cell with a smooth cuticle, certain trichomes show a crown of small spheroid protuberances just below the insertion point of the intermediary cell on the stalk [G]; fragments of papillose epidermis from the inner surface of the petals, in surface view [J], in side view [P]; fragments of calyx epidermis with sinuous-walled cells and containing prismatic crystals of calcium oxalate [Q]; spherical pollen grains which have a diameter of about 45 μm and an exine with 6 slit-like germinal pores and 6 ribbon-like groins radiating from the poles [A, D, E, F]; rare fragments of leaf epidermis with stomata, mostly of the diacytic type (*2.8.3*) [B]; fragments of vascular tissue with spiral vessels included in parenchyma with some cells containing small calcium oxalate cluster crystals [N].

C. Thin-layer chromatography (*2.2.27*).

Test solution   To 0.5 g of the powdered herbal drug (355) (*2.9.12*) add 5 mL of *hexane R*, shake for 5 min and filter.

Reference solution   Dissolve 10 μL of *linalol R* and 10 μL of *linalyl acetate R* in 5 mL of *hexane R*.

Plate   TLC silica gel plate R.

Mobile phase   ethyl acetate R, toluene R (5:95 V/V).

Application   10 μL as bands.

Development   Over a path of 15 cm.

Drying   In air.

Detection   Spray with *anisaldehyde solution R*. Heat at 100-105 °C for 5-10 min and examine in daylight.

Results   The chromatogram obtained with the reference solution shows in the lower third a greyish-blue zone (linalol) and in the middle third a greyish-blue zone (linalyl acetate). The chromatogram obtained with the test solution shows the zones due to linalol and linalyl acetate and in the middle, between these zones, a redish-violet zone (epoxydihydrocaryophyllene). Further zones are also present.

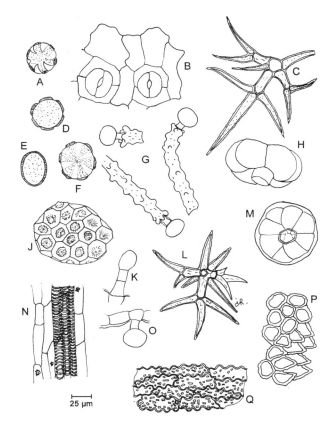

Figure 1534.-1. – *Illustration for identification test B of powdered herbal drug of lavender flower*

D. Examine the chromatograms obtained in the test for other species and varieties of lavender.

Results   The 5 principal peaks in the chromatogram obtained with the reference solution are similar in retention time to the corresponding peaks in the chromatogram obtained with the test solution. Among them are mainly linalol and linalyl acetate peaks.

TESTS

Foreign matter (*2.8.2*)
Maximum 3 per cent of stems and maximum 2 per cent of other foreign matter.

Other species and varieties of lavender
Gas chromatography (*2.2.28*): use the normalisation procedure.

Test solution   Dilute 0.2 mL of the essential oil-xylene mixture obtained in the assay to 5 mL with *hexane R*, add 1 g of *anhydrous sodium sulfate R*, shake and use the supernatant liquid.

Reference solution   Dissolve 0.1 g of *limonene R*, 0.2 g of *cineole R*, 0.05 g of *camphor R*, 0.4 g of *linalol R*, 0.6 g of *linalyl acetate R* and 0.2 g of *α-terpineol R* in 100 mL of *hexane R*.

Column:
— *material*: fused silica;
— *size*: l = 60 m, Ø = 0.25 mm;
— *stationary phase*: macrogol 20 000 R.

Carrier gas   helium for chromatography R.

Flow rate   1.5 mL/min.

Split ratio   1:100.

Temperature:

	Time (min)	Temperature (°C)
Column	0 - 15	70
	15 - 70	70 → 180
Injection port		220
Detector		220

Detection   Flame ionisation.

Injection   The same volume of each solution.

Elution order   Order indicated in the composition of the reference solution. Record the retention times of these substances.

System suitability   Reference solution:
— *resolution*: minimum 1.5 between the peaks due to limonene and cineole;
— *number of theoretical plates*: minimum 30 000, calculated for the peak due to limonene at 110 °C.

Using the retention times determined from the chromatogram obtained with the reference solution, locate the 6 components of the reference solution in the chromatogram obtained with the test solution. Disregard the peaks due to hexane and xylene.

Limit:
— *camphor*: maximum 1 per cent.

Water (*2.2.13*)
Maximum 100 mL/kg, determined on 20.0 g.

Total ash (*2.4.16*)
Maximum 9.0 per cent.

ASSAY

Carry out the determination of essential oils in herbal drugs (*2.8.12*). Use 20.0 g of the herbal drug, a 1000 mL round-bottomed flask, 500 mL of *water R* as the distillation liquid and 0.5 mL of *xylene R* in the graduated tube. Distil at a rate of 2-3 mL/min for 2 h.

_____ *Ph Eur*

Lavender Oil

(*Ph Eur monograph 1338*)

Ph Eur _____

DEFINITION

Essential oil obtained by steam distillation from the flowering tops of *Lavandula angustifolia* Mill. (*Lavandula officinalis* Chaix).

CHARACTERS

Appearance
Colourless or pale yellow, clear liquid.

Odour
Complex, reminiscent of linalyl acetate.

IDENTIFICATION

First identification   B.

Second identification   A.

A. Thin-layer chromatography (*2.2.27*).

Test solution   Dissolve 20 μL of the oil to be examined in 1 mL of *toluene R*.

Reference solution   Dissolve 10 μL of *linalol R*, 10 μL of *cineole R* and 10 μL of *linalyl acetate R* in 1 mL of *toluene R*.

Plate TLC silica gel plate R (5-40 µm) [or TLC silica gel plate R (2-10 µm)].

Mobile phase ethyl acetate R, toluene R (5:95 V/V).

Application 10 µL [or 2 µL] as bands of 10 mm [or 6 mm].

Development Over a path of 10 cm [or 8 cm].

Drying In air.

Detection Spray with *anisaldehyde solution R* and heat at 100-105 °C for 5-10 min; examine immediately in daylight.

Results See below the sequence of zones present in the chromatograms obtained with the reference solution and the test solution. Furthermore, other violet-red or greenish-brown zones are present in the chromatogram obtained with the test solution above the zone of linalyl acetate up to the solvent front.

Top of the plate	
	A violet-red or greenish-brown zone
———	———
Linalyl acetate: a violet or brown zone	A violet or brown zone (linalyl acetate)
	A violet-red zone
———	———
1,8-Cineole: a violet-brown zone	Possibly a weak violet-brown zone (1,8-cineole)
Linalol: a violet or brown zone	A violet or brown zone (linalol)
	A weak yellowish-brown zone
	Several unresolved zones
Reference solution	**Test solution**

B. Examine the chromatograms obtained in the test for chromatographic profile.

Results The characteristic peaks in the chromatogram obtained with the test solution are similar in retention time to those in the chromatogram obtained with reference solution (a).

TESTS

Relative density (*2.2.5*)
0.878 to 0.892.

Refractive index (*2.2.6*)
1.455 to 1.466.

Optical rotation (*2.2.7*)
− 12.5° to − 6.0°.

Acid value (*2.5.1*)
Maximum 1.0, determined on 5.0 g of the substance to be examined dissolved in 50 mL of the prescribed mixture of solvents.

Chromatographic profile
Gas chromatography (*2.2.28*): use the normalisation procedure.

Test solution Dissolve 200 µL of the oil to be examined in *heptane R* and dilute to 10.0 mL with the same solvent.

Reference solution (a) Dissolve 5 µL of *limonene R*, 5 µL of *cineole R*, 5 µL of *3-octanone R*, 5 mg of *camphor R*, 40 µL of *linalol R*, 50 µL of *linalyl acetate R*, 10 µL of *terpinen-4-ol R*, 5 µL of *lavandulyl acetate R*, 5 µL of *lavandulol R* and 5 mg of α-*terpineol R* in *heptane R* and dilute to 10 mL with the same solvent.

Reference solution (b) Dissolve 5 µL of *limonene R* in *heptane R* and dilute to 50.0 mL with the same solvent. Dilute 0.5 mL of the solution to 5.0 mL with *heptane R*.

Column:
— *material*: fused silica;
— *size*: l = 60 m, Ø = 0.25 mm;
— *stationary phase*: macrogol 20 000 R (film thickness 0.25 µm).

Carrier gas helium for chromatography R.

Flow rate 1.5 mL/min.

Split ratio 1:50.

Temperature:

	Time (min)	Temperature (°C)
Column	0 - 15	70
	15 - 70	70 → 180
Injection port		220
Detector		220

Detection Flame ionisation.

Injection 1 µL.

Elution order Order indicated in the composition of reference solution (a). Record the retention times of these substances.

System suitability Reference solution (a):
— *resolution*: minimum 1.4 between the peaks due to terpinen-4-ol and lavandulyl acetate.

Using the retention times determined from the chromatogram obtained with reference solution (a), locate the components of reference solution (a) in the chromatogram obtained with the test solution. Determine the percentage content of each of these components. The percentages are within the following ranges:
— *limonene*: maximum 1.0 per cent;
— *1,8-cineole*: maximum 2.5 per cent;
— *3-octanone*: 0.1 per cent to 5.0 per cent;
— *camphor*: maximum 1.2 per cent;
— *linalol*: 20.0 per cent to 45.0 per cent;
— *linalyl acetate*: 25.0 per cent to 47.0 per cent;
— *terpinen-4-ol*: 0.1 per cent to 8.0 per cent;
— *lavandulyl acetate*: minimum 0.2 per cent;
— *lavandulol*: minimum 0.1 per cent;
— α-*terpineol*: maximum 2.0 per cent;
— *disregard limit*: the area of the principal peak in the chromatogram obtained with reference solution (b) (0.05 per cent).

Chiral purity
Gas chromatography (2.2.28).

Test solution Dissolve 0.02 g of the oil to be examined in *pentane R* and dilute to 10 mL with the same solvent.

Reference solution Dissolve 10 µL of *linalol R* (mixture of (R)-linalol and (S)-linalol), add 5 mg of *borneol R* and 10 µL of *linalyl acetate R* (mixture of (R)-linalyl acetate and (S)-linalyl acetate) in *pentane R* and dilute to 10 mL with the same solvent.

Column:
— *material*: fused silica;
— *size*: l = 25 m, Ø = 0.25 mm;
— *stationary phase*: modified β-cyclodextrin for chiral chromatography R (film thickness 0.25 µm).

Carrier gas helium for chromatography R.

Flow rate   1.3 mL/min.

Split ratio   1:30.

Temperature:

	Time (min)	Temperature (°C)
Column	0 - 65	50 → 180
Injection port		230
Detector		230

Detection   Flame ionisation.

Injection   1 µL.

Elution order   (*R*)-linalol, (*S*)-linalol, borneol, (*R*)-linalyl acetate, (*S*)-linalyl acetate; depending on the operating conditions and the state of the column, borneol may elute before or after (*S*)-linalol.

System suitability   Reference solution:
— *resolution*: minimum 5.5 between the peaks due to (*R*)-linalol and (*S*)-linalol; minimum 2.9 between the peaks due to (*S*)-linalol and borneol; minimum 2.0 between the peaks due to (*R*)-linalyl acetate and (*S*)-linalyl acetate.

Calculate the percentage content of the specified (*S*)-enantiomers using the following expression:

$$\frac{A_S}{A_S + A_R} \times 100$$

A_S = area of the peak due to the corresponding (*S*)-enantiomer;

A_R = area of the peak due to the corresponding (*R*)-enantiomer.

Limits:
— *(S)-linalol*: maximum 12 per cent;
— *(S)-linalyl acetate*: maximum 1 per cent.

STORAGE

At a temperature not exceeding 25 °C.

Ph Eur

Spike Lavender Oil

(*Ph Eur monograph 2419*)

Ph Eur

DEFINITION

Essential oil obtained by steam distillation of the flowering tops of *Lavandula latifolia* Medik.

CHARACTERS

Appearance

Clear, mobile, light yellow or greenish-yellow liquid.

Odour reminiscent of cineole and camphor.

IDENTIFICATION

First identification   B.

Second identification   A.

A. Thin-layer chromatography (*2.2.27*).

Test solution   Dissolve 20 µL of the substance to be examined in 1 mL of *toluene R*.

Reference solution   Dissolve 10 µL of *cineole R*, 10 µL of *linalol R* and 10 µL of *linalyl acetate R* in 1 mL of *toluene R*.

Plate   TLC silica gel plate R (5-40 µm) [or TLC silica gel plate R (2-10 µm)].

Mobile phase   ethyl acetate R, toluene R (5:95 *V/V*).

Application   10 µL [or 2 µL], as bands of 10 mm [or 6 mm].

Development   Over a path of 10 cm [or 8 cm].

Drying   In air.

Detection   Spray with *anisaldehyde solution R* and heat at 100-105 °C for 5-10 min; examine immediately in daylight.

Results   See below the sequence of zones present in the chromatograms obtained with the reference solution and the test solution. Furthermore, other faint zones may be present in the chromatogram obtained with the test solution.

Top of the plate	
	A pink zone
Linalyl acetate: a violet or brown zone	A faint violet or brown zone may be present (linalyl acetate)
	A pink zone
Cineole: a violet-brown zone	An intense violet-brown zone (cineole)
Linalol: a violet or brown zone	An intense violet or brown zone (linalol)
	A greyish or brownish zone
	A faint violet zone
Reference solution	**Test solution**

B. Examine the chromatograms obtained in the test for chromatographic profile.

Results   The characteristic peaks in the chromatogram obtained with the test solution are similar in retention time to the peaks due to limonene, cineole, camphor, linalol, linalyl acetate, α-terpineol and *trans*-α-bisabolene in the chromatogram obtained with reference solution (a).

TESTS

Relative density (*2.2.5*)

0.894 to 0.907.

Refractive index (*2.2.6*)

1.461 to 1.468.

Optical rotation (*2.2.7*)

− 7° to + 2°.

Acid value (*2.5.1*)

Maximum 1.5, determined on 5.00 g of the substance to be examined.

Solubility in alcohol (*2.8.10*)

1.0 mL of the substance to be examined is soluble, sometimes with opalescence, in 3.0 mL of *ethanol (70 per cent V/V) R*.

Chromatographic profile

Gas chromatography (*2.2.28*): use the normalisation procedure.

Test solution   Dissolve 200 µL of the substance to be examined in *heptane R* and dilute to 10.0 mL with the same solvent.

Reference solution (a)   Dissolve 200 µL of *spike lavender oil CRS* in *heptane R* and dilute to 10.0 mL with the same solvent.

Reference solution (b)   Dissolve 5 µL of *limonene R* in 50.0 mL of *heptane R*. Dilute 0.5 mL of this solution to 5.0 mL with *heptane R*.

Column:
— *material*: fused silica;
— *size*: l = 60 m, Ø = 0.25 mm;
— *stationary phase*: *macrogol 20 000 R* (film thickness 0.25 μm).

Carrier gas *helium for chromatography R.*

Flow rate 1.5 mL/min.

Split ratio 1:50.

Temperature:

	Time (min)	Temperature (°C)
Column	0 - 15	70
	15 - 70	70 - 180
Injection port		220
Detector		220

Detection Flame ionisation.

Injection 1 μL.

Identification of peaks Use the chromatogram supplied with *spike lavender oil CRS* and the chromatogram obtained with reference solution (a) to identify the peaks due to limonene, cineole, camphor, linalol, linalyl acetate, α-terpineol and *trans*-α-bisabolene.

System suitability Reference solution (a):
— the chromatogram obtained is similar to the chromatogram supplied with *spike lavender oil CRS*;
— *resolution*: minimum 1.5 between the peaks due to limonene and cineole.

Determine the percentage content of each of these components. The percentages are within the following ranges:
— *limonene*: 0.5 per cent to 3.0 per cent;
— *cineole*: 16.0 per cent to 39.0 per cent;
— *camphor*: 8.0 per cent to 16.0 per cent;
— *linalol*: 34.0 per cent to 50.0 per cent;
— *linalyl acetate*: maximum 1.6 per cent;
— *α-terpineol*: 0.2 per cent to 2.0 per cent;
— *trans*-α-*bisabolene*: 0.4 per cent to 2.5 per cent;
— *disregard limit*: the area of the principal peak in the chromatogram obtained with reference solution (b) (0.05 per cent).

STORAGE

At a temperature not exceeding 25 °C.

——————————————————— *Ph Eur*

Lemon Balm

(Melissa Leaf, Ph Eur monograph 1447)

Preparation
Lemon Balm Dry Extract

Ph Eur ——————————————————————

DEFINITION

Dried leaf of *Melissa officinalis* L.

Content

Minimum 1.0 per cent of rosmarinic acid ($C_{18}H_{16}O_8$; M_r 360.3) (dried drug).

CHARACTERS

Odour reminiscent of lemon.

IDENTIFICATION

A. The leaves have a petiole of varying length; the lamina is broadly ovate, up to about 8 cm long and 5 cm wide, acute at the apex and rounded to cordate at the base; the margins are crenate to dentate. The upper surface is intense green, the lower surface is paler green and shows a conspicuous midrib and a raised, reticulate venation; scattered hairs occur on the upper surface and along the veins on the lower surface, which is also finely punctuate.

B. Reduce to a powder (355) (*2.9.12*). The powder is greenish. Examine under a microscope using *chloral hydrate solution R*. The powder shows the following diagnostic characters (Figure 1447.-1): fragments of the upper epidermis, in surface view, with sinuous walls [A, B, G], sometimes accompanied by palisade parenchyma [Aa]; fragments of the lower epidermis [D] with diacytic stomata (*2.8.3*) [Db]; short, straight, unicellular, conical covering trichomes with a finely striated cuticle, free [E] or attached to an epidermis [Da]; multicellular, uniseriate covering trichomes with pointed ends and thick, warty cuticles [C]; eight-celled secretory trichomes of lamiaceous type, in surface view [Ga]; secretory trichomes with unicellular to tricellular stalks and unicellular or, more rarely, bicellular heads, in surface view [Ba] or in transverse section [F].

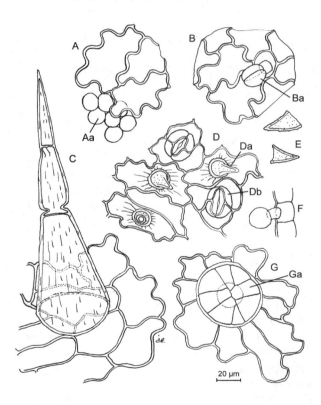

Figure 1447.-1.– *Illustration for identification test B of powdered herbal drug of melissa leaf*

C. Thin-layer chromatography (*2.2.27*).

Test solution Place 2.0 g of the powdered drug (355) (*2.9.12*) in a 250 mL round-bottomed flask and add 100 mL of *water R*. Distil for 1 h using the apparatus for the determination of essential oils in herbal drugs (*2.8.12*) and 0.5 mL of *xylene R* in the graduated tube. After distillation transfer the organic phase to a 1 mL volumetric flask, rinsing the graduated tube of the apparatus with the aid of a small portion of *xylene R*, and dilute to 1.0 mL with the same solvent.

Reference solution   Dissolve 1.0 µL of *citronellal R* and 10.0 µL of *citral R* (composed of neral and geranial) in 25 mL of *xylene R*.

Plate   TLC silica gel plate R (5-40 µm) [or *TLC silica gel plate R* (2-10 µm)].

Mobile phase   ethyl acetate R, hexane R (10:90 *V/V*).

Application   20 µL [or 4 µL] as bands.

Development   In an unsaturated tank over a path of 15 cm [or 6 cm].

Drying   In air.

Detection   Spray with *anisaldehyde solution R* and heat at 100-105 °C for 10-15 min; examine in daylight.

Results   See below the sequence of zones present in the chromatograms obtained with the reference solution and the test solution. Furthermore, other zones may be present in the chromatogram obtained with the test solution.

Top of the plate	
Citronellal: a grey or greyish-violet zone at the border between the upper and middle thirds	A grey or greyish-violet zone (citronellal) at the border between the upper and middle thirds A reddish-violet zone
Citral: 2 greyish-violet or bluish-violet zones at the border between the middle and lower thirds	2 greyish-violet or bluish-violet zones (citral) at the border between the middle and lower thirds
Reference solution	**Test solution**

TESTS

Foreign matter (*2.8.2*)
Maximum 10 per cent of stems with a diameter greater than 1 mm and maximum 2 per cent of other foreign matter, determined on 20 g.

Loss on drying (*2.2.32*)
Maximum 10.0 per cent, determined on 1.000 g of the powdered drug (355) (*2.9.12*) by drying in an oven at 105 °C for 2 h.

Total ash (*2.4.16*)
Maximum 12.0 per cent.

ASSAY

Liquid chromatography (*2.2.29*).

Test solution   Use brown-glass flasks. Disperse 0.100 g of the powdered drug (355) (*2.9.12*) in 90 mL of *ethanol (50 per cent V/V) R*. Boil in a water-bath under a reflux condenser for 30 min, cool, and filter into a 100 mL volumetric flask. Rinse the flask and the filter with 10 mL of *ethanol (50 per cent V/V) R* and dilute to 100.0 mL with the same solvent. Filter through a 0.45 µm filter.

Reference solution (a)   Dissolve 20.0 mg of *rosmarinic acid CRS* in *ethanol (50 per cent V/V) R* and dilute to 100.0 mL with the same solvent. Dilute 20.0 mL of this solution to 100.0 mL with *ethanol (50 per cent V/V) R*.

Reference solution (b)   Dissolve 5.0 mg of *ferulic acid R* in reference solution (a) and dilute to 50.0 mL with the same solution.

Column:
— *size*: *l* = 0.25 m, Ø = 4.6 mm;

— *stationary phase*: *octadecylsilyl silica gel for chromatography R* (5 µm).

Mobile phase:
— *mobile phase A*: phosphoric acid R, acetonitrile R, water R (1:19:80 *V/V/V*);
— *mobile phase B*: phosphoric acid R, methanol R, acetonitrile R (1:40:59 *V/V/V*);

Time (min)	Mobile phase A (per cent *V/V*)	Mobile phase B (per cent *V/V*)
0 - 20	100 → 55	0 → 45
20 - 25	55 → 0	45 → 100
25 - 30	0 → 100	100 → 0

Flow rate   1.2 mL/min.

Detection   Spectrophotometer at 330 nm.

Injection   20 µL.

Relative retention   With reference to rosmarinic acid (retention time = about 11 min): ferulic acid = about 0.8.

System suitability   Reference solution (b):
— *resolution*: minimum 4.0 between the peaks due to ferulic acid and rosmarinic acid.

Calculate the percentage content of rosmarinic acid using the following expression:

$$\frac{A_1 \times m_2 \times p \times 0.2}{A_2 \times m_1}$$

A_1 = area of the peak due to rosmarinic acid in the chromatogram obtained with the test solution;

A_2 = area of the peak due to rosmarinic acid in the chromatogram obtained with reference solution (a);

m_1 = mass of the drug to be examined used to prepare the test solution, in grams;

m_2 = mass of *rosmarinic acid CRS* used to prepare reference solution (a), in grams;

p = percentage content of rosmarinic acid in *rosmarinic acid CRS*.

_____ Ph Eur

Lemon Balm Dry Extract

(*Melissa Leaf Dry Extract, Ph Eur monograph 2524*)

Ph Eur _____

DEFINITION

Dry extract produced from *Melissa leaf (1447)*.

Content
Minimum 2.0 per cent of rosmarinic acid ($C_{18}H_{16}O_8$; M_r 360.3) (dried extract).

PRODUCTION

The extract is produced from the herbal drug by a suitable procedure using either hot water (not less than 70 °C) or a hydroalcoholic solvent that is at most equivalent in strength to ethanol (70 per cent *V/V*).

CHARACTERS

Appearance
Brown or greenish-brown, amorphous powder.

IDENTIFICATION

Thin-layer chromatography (*2.2.27*).

Test solution To 0.2 g of the extract to be examined add 5 mL of *methanol* R. Sonicate for 5 min and filter.

Reference solution Dissolve 1.0 mg of *hyperoside* R, 1.0 mg of *rutin* R and 5.0 mg of *rosmarinic acid* R in 10 mL of *methanol* R.

Plate TLC silica gel plate R (5-40 μm) [or *TLC silica gel plate* R (2-10 μm)].

Mobile phase anhydrous formic acid R, water R, ethyl acetate R (6:6:90 V/V/V).

Application 10 μL [or 2 μL] as bands of 15 mm [or 8 mm].

Development Over a path of 8 cm [or 6 cm].

Drying In air.

Detection Heat at 100 °C for 5 min, spray the plate whilst still hot with a 5 g/L solution of *diphenylboric acid aminoethyl ester* R in *ethyl acetate* R, and examine in ultraviolet light at 365 nm.

Results See below the sequence of fluorescent zones present in the chromatograms obtained with the reference solution and the test solution. Furthermore, other weaker fluorescent zones may be present in the chromatogram obtained with the test solution.

Top of the plate	
Rosmarinic acid: a light blue fluorescent zone	An intense light blue fluorescent zone (rosmarinic acid)
	A blue fluorescent zone
———	———
	A blue fluorescent zone
———	
Hyperoside: an orange or greenish-yellow fluorescent zone	
	A light blue fluorescent zone
Rutin: an orange or greenish-yellow fluorescent zone	
Reference solution	**Test solution**

TESTS

Loss on drying (*2.8.17*)
Maximum 6.0 per cent.

ASSAY

Liquid chromatography (*2.2.29*).

Test solution Use brown glass flasks. To 0.200 g of the extract to be examined add 50 mL of *ethanol (50 per cent V/V)* R. Sonicate for 10 min and dilute to 100.0 mL with *ethanol (50 per cent V/V)* R. Filter through a membrane filter (nominal pore size 0.45 μm).

Reference solution (a) Dissolve 20.0 mg of *rosmarinic acid CRS* in *ethanol (50 per cent V/V)* R and dilute to 100.0 mL with the same solvent. Dilute 20.0 mL of this solution to 100.0 mL with *ethanol (50 per cent V/V)* R.

Reference solution (b) Dissolve 5 mg of *ferulic acid* R in reference solution (a) and dilute to 50 mL with reference solution (a).

Column:
— *size*: l = 0.25 m, Ø = 4.6 mm;
— *stationary phase*: octadecylsilyl silica gel for chromatography R (5 μm).

Mobile phase:
— *mobile phase A*: phosphoric acid R, acetonitrile R, water R (1:19:80 V/V/V);
— *mobile phase B*: phosphoric acid R, methanol R, acetonitrile R (1:40:59 V/V/V);

Time (min)	Mobile phase A (per cent V/V)	Mobile phase B (per cent V/V)
0 - 20	100 → 55	0 → 45
20 - 25	55 → 0	45 → 100

Flow rate 1.2 mL/min.

Detection Spectrophotometer at 330 nm.

Injection 20 μL.

Relative retention With reference to rosmarinic acid (retention time = about 11 min): ferulic acid = about 0.8.

System suitability Reference solution (b):
— *resolution*: minimum 4.0 between the peaks due to ferulic acid and rosmarinic acid.

Calculate the percentage content of rosmarinic acid using the following expression:

$$\frac{A_1 \times m_2 \times p \times 0.2}{A_2 \times m_1}$$

A_1 = area of the peak due to rosmarinic acid in the chromatogram obtained with the test solution;

A_2 = area of the peak due to rosmarinic acid in the chromatogram obtained with reference solution (a);

m_1 = mass of the extract to be examined used to prepare the test solution, in grams;

m_2 = mass of *rosmarinic acid CRS* used to prepare reference solution (a), in grams;

p = percentage content of rosmarinic acid in *rosmarinic acid CRS*.

_____ *Ph Eur*

Dried Lemon Peel

DEFINITION

Dried Lemon Peel is the dried outer part of the pericarp of the ripe, or nearly ripe, fruit of *Citrus limon* (L.) Burm. f.

CHARACTERISTICS

It has the macroscopical and microscopical characters described under Identification tests A and B.

IDENTIFICATION

A. Dried Lemon Peel consists of strips or pieces, showing a marked thickening of the epicarp around the calyx. The outer surface is yellow and somewhat rough from the presence of numerous minute pits, each corresponding to an oil gland; the inner surface with only a small remnant of white, spongy pericarp. Fracture, short.

B. Prepare thin cross sections from material softened by soaking in *water* and examine under a microscope using *chloral hydrate solution*. The sections show a yellow epidermis composed of small, thin-walled cells and an underlying parenchyma with numerous large oil glands and scattered small strands of vascular tissue; prismatic crystals of calcium oxalate occur throughout the parenchyma and are particularly abundant in the layers adjacent to the epidermis.

C. Carry out the method for *thin-layer chromatography*, Appendix III A, using the following solutions.

(1) Add 1 g of freshly cut peel to 10 mL of *methanol* and heat in a water-bath at 65° for 5 minutes, shaking frequently. Allow to cool and filter.

(2) 0.01% w/v each of *caffeic acid* and *naringin* and 0.025% w/v of *rutin* in *methanol*.

CHROMATOGRAPHIC CONDITIONS

(a) Using a *TLC silica gel plate*.

(b) Use the mobile phase as described below.

(c) Apply 20 μL of each solution as bands.

(d) Develop the plate to 15 cm.

(e) After removal of the plate, dry the plate at 105° and spray the warm plate with a 1% w/v solution of *diphenylboric acid aminoethyl ester* in *methanol* and then with a 5% w/v solution of *polyethylene glycol 400* in *methanol*. Allow the plate to stand for 30 minutes and examine under *ultraviolet light (365 nm)*.

MOBILE PHASE

A mixture of 10 volumes of *anhydrous formic acid*, 10 volumes of *water*, 30 volumes of *butan-2-one* and 50 volumes of *ethyl acetate*.

CONFIRMATION

The chromatogram obtained with solution (1):

exhibits a yellowish-brown fluorescent zone corresponding in colour and position to the zone for rutin in the chromatogram obtained with solution (2);

above it an intense red fluorescent zone and further above a very weak greenish fluorescent zone corresponding in colour and position to the zone for naringin in the chromatogram obtained with solution (2);

other coloured zones are present in the chromatogram.

TESTS

Volatile oil

Not less than 2.0% v/w (1.7% w/w), Appendix XI E, using 300 mL of *water* as the distillation liquid and no xylene in the graduated tube. Use 20 g, soaked in *water* and macerated in a suitable blender, and distil for 3 hours.

Lemon Oil

(*Ph Eur monograph 0620*)

Preparation

Terpeneless Lemon Oil

Ph Eur _____

DEFINITION

Essential oil obtained by suitable mechanical means, without the aid of heat, from the fresh peel of *Citrus limon* (L.) Burman fil.

CHARACTERS

Appearance

Clear, mobile, pale yellow or greenish-yellow liquid. It may become cloudy at low temperatures.

Characteristic odour.

IDENTIFICATION

First identification   B.

Second identification   A.

A. Thin-layer chromatography (*2.2.27*).

Test solution   Mix 1 mL of the substance to be examined in 1 mL of *toluene R*.

Reference solution   Dissolve 10 mg of *citropten R* and 50 μL of *citral R* in *toluene R* and dilute to 10 mL with the same solvent.

Plate   *TLC silica gel GF₂₅₄ plate R*.

Mobile phase   *ethyl acetate R*, *toluene R* (15:85 *V/V*).

Application   10 μL, as bands.

Development   Over a path of 15 cm.

Drying   In air.

Detection A   Examine in ultraviolet light at 254 nm.

Results A   See below the sequence of the zones present in the chromatograms obtained with the reference solution and the test solution.

Top of the plate	
Citral: a quenching zone	A quenching zone (bergamotin)
	A quenching zone (citral)
Citropten: a light blue fluorescent zone	A dark blue zone (5-geranyloxy-7-methoxycoumarin)
	A light blue fluorescent zone (citropten)
	A quenching zone (psoralen derivative)
	A quenching zone (biakangelicin)
Reference solution	**Test solution**

Detection B   Examine in ultraviolet light at 365 nm.

Results B   See below the sequence of the zones present in the chromatograms obtained with the reference solution and the test solution.

Top of the plate	
Citral: a quenching zone	A yellow fluorescent zone (bergamotin)
	A quenching zone (citral)
Citropten: a bright blue fluorescent zone	A bright blue fluorescent zone (5-geranyloxy-7-methoxycoumarin)
	A bright violet-blue fluorescent zone (citropten)
	A yellow fluorescent zone (psoralen derivative)
	An orange zone (biakangelicin)
Reference solution	**Test solution**

B. Examine the chromatograms obtained in the test for chromatographic profile.

Results   The characteristic peaks in the chromatogram obtained with the test solution are similar in retention time to those in the chromatogram obtained with the reference solution.

TESTS

Relative density (*2.2.5*)

0.850 to 0.858.

Refractive index (*2.2.6*)

1.473 to 1.476.

Optical rotation (*2.2.7*)

+ 57° to + 70°.

Absorbance (*2.2.25*)

Dissolve 0.250 g of the substance to be examined in *alcohol R*, mix and dilute to 100.0 mL with the same solvent. Measure the absorbance over the range 260 nm to 400 nm. If a manual instrument is used, measure the absorbance at 5 nm intervals from 260 nm to about 12 nm before the expected absorption maximum, then at 3 nm intervals for 3 readings and at 1 nm intervals to about 5 nm beyond the maximum and finally at 10 nm intervals to 400 nm. Plot a curve representing the absorption spectrum with the absorbances as ordinates and the wavelengths as abscissae. Draw as a baseline the tangent between A and B (Figure 0620.-1). The absorption maximum C is situated at 315 $\pm$ 3 nm. From C draw a line perpendicular to the axis of abscissae and intersecting AB at D. Deduct the absorbance corresponding to point D from that corresponding to point C. The value $C - D$ is 0.20 to 0.96 and for Italian-type lemon oil it is not less than 0.45.

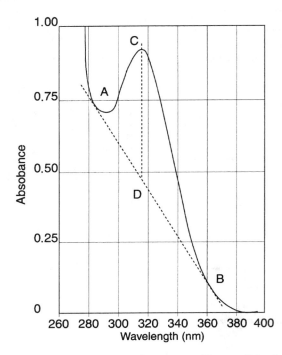

Figure 0620.-1. – *Typical spectrum of lemon oil for the test for absorbance*

Fatty oils and resinified essential oils (*2.8.7*)
It complies with the test for fatty oils and resinified essential oils.

Chromatographic profile
Gas chromatography (*2.2.28*): use the normalisation procedure.

Test solution   The substance to be examined.

Reference solution   Dissolve 20 µL of *β-pinene R*, 10 µL of *sabinene R*, 100 µL of *limonene R*, 10 µL of *γ-terpinene R*, 5 µL of *β-caryophyllene R*, 20 µL of *citral R*, 5 µL of *α-terpineol R*, 5 µL of *neryl acetate R* and 5 µL of *geranyl acetate R* in 1 mL of *acetone R*.

Column:
— *material*: fused silica,
— *size*: l = 30 m (a film thickness of 1 µm may be used) to 60 m (a film thickness of 0.2 µm may be used), Ø = 0.25-0.53 mm,
— *stationary phase*: macrogol 20 000 R.

Carrier gas   *helium for chromatography R*.

Flow rate   1.0 mL/min.

Split ratio   1:100.

Temperature:

	Time (min)	Temperature (°C)
Column	0 - 6	45
	6 - 21	45 → 90
	21 - 39	90 → 180
	39 - 55	180
Injection port		220
Detector		220

Detection   Flame ionisation.

Injection   0.5 µL of the reference solution and 0.2 µL of the test solution.

Elution order   Order indicated in the composition of the reference solution. Record the retention times of these substances.

System suitability   Reference solution:
— *resolution*: minimum 1.5 between the peaks due to β-pinene and sabinene and minimum 1.5 between the peaks due to geranial and geranyl acetate.

Using the retention times determined from the chromatogram obtained with the reference solution, locate the components of the reference solution in the chromatogram obtained with the test solution.

Determine the percentage content of these components. The percentages are within the following ranges:
— *β-pinene*: 7.0 per cent to 17.0 per cent,
— *sabinene*: 1.0 per cent to 3.0 per cent,
— *limonene*: 56.0 per cent to 78.0 per cent,
— *γ-terpinene*: 6.0 per cent to 12.0 per cent,
— *β-caryophyllene*: maximum 0.5 per cent,
— *neral*: 0.3 per cent to 1.5 per cent,
— *α-terpineol*: maximum 0.6 per cent,
— *neryl acetate*: 0.2 per cent to 0.9 per cent,
— *geranial*: 0.5 per cent to 2.3 per cent,
— *geranyl acetate*: 0.1 per cent to 0.8 per cent.

Residue on evaporation (*2.8.9*)
1.8 per cent to 3.6 per cent after heating on the water-bath for 4 h.

STORAGE
At a temperature not exceeding 25 °C.

LABELLING
The label states, where applicable, that the contents are Italian-type lemon oil.

_____ *Ph Eur*

Terpeneless Lemon Oil

Preparations
Lemon Spirit

Compound Orange Spirit

DEFINITION
Terpeneless Lemon Oil may be prepared by concentrating Lemon Oil under reduced pressure until most of the terpenes have been removed or by solvent partition. It contains not less than 40% w/w of aldehydes calculated as citral, $C_{10}H_{16}O$.

CHARACTERISTICS
A clear, colourless or pale yellow liquid, visibly free from water; odour and taste, those of lemon.

TESTS

Optical rotation
−5° to +2°, Appendix V F.

Refractive index
1.475 to 1.485, Appendix V E.

Solubility in ethanol
Soluble, at 20°, in 1 volume of *ethanol (80%)*,
Appendix X M.

Weight per mL
0.880 to 0.895 g, Appendix V G.

ASSAY

Carry out the method for *determination of aldehydes*,
Appendix X K, using 1 g, omitting the *toluene* and using a
volume, not less than 7 mL, of *alcoholic hydroxylamine solution*
that exceeds by 1 to 2 mL the volume of 0.5M *potassium*
hydroxide in ethanol (60%) VS required. Each mL of
0.5M *potassium hydroxide in ethanol (60%) VS* is equivalent to
76.73 mg of $C_{10}H_{16}O$.

STORAGE

Terpeneless Lemon Oil should be kept in a well-filled
container and protected from light.

Lemon Spirit

DEFINITION

Terpeneless Lemon Oil   100 mL
Ethanol (96 per cent)   Sufficient to produce 1000 mL

The spirit complies with the requirements stated under Spirits and
with the following requirements.

Content of aldehydes
3.45 to 4.60% w/v, calculated as citral, $C_{10}H_{16}O$.

TESTS

Ethanol content
84 to 88% v/v, Appendix VIII F.

Weight per mL
0.814 to 0.823 g, Appendix V G.

ASSAY

Carry out the method for the *determination of aldehydes*,
Appendix X K, using 10 mL, omitting the *toluene* and using
a volume, not less than 7 mL, of *alcoholic hydroxylamine*
solution that exceeds by 1 to 2 mL the volume of
0.5M *potassium hydroxide in ethanol (60%) VS* required. Each
mL of 0.5M *potassium hydroxide in ethanol (60%) VS* is
equivalent to 76.73 mg of $C_{10}H_{16}O$.

Lemon Syrup

DEFINITION

Lemon Spirit   5 mL
Citric Acid Monohydrate   25 g
Invert Syrup   100 mL
Syrup   Sufficient to produce
                                                             1000 mL

Extemporaneous preparation
The following directions apply.

Dissolve the Citric Acid Monohydrate in some of the Syrup,
add the Invert Syrup, the Lemon Spirit and sufficient Syrup
to produce 1000 mL and mix.

CHARACTERISTICS

Lemon Syrup has a weight per mL of about 1.33 g.

The syrup complies with the requirements stated under Oral
Liquids and with the following requirements.

Content of citric acid monohydrate, $C_6H_8O_7,H_2O$
2.2 to 2.6% w/v.

ASSAY

Mix 8 g with 100 mL of *water* and titrate with 0.1M *sodium*
hydroxide VS using *phenolphthalein solution R1* as indicator.
Each mL of 0.1M *sodium hydroxide VS* is equivalent to
7.005 mg of $C_6H_8O_7,H_2O$. Determine the *weight per mL*,
Appendix V G, and calculate the content of $C_6H_8O_7,H_2O$,
weight in volume.

Lemon Verbena Leaf

(*Ph Eur monograph 1834*)

Ph Eur _____

DEFINITION

Whole or fragmented, dried leaves of *Aloysia citrodora* Paláu
(syn. *Aloysia triphylla* (L'Hér.) Kuntze; *Verbena triphylla*
L'Hér.; *Lippia citriodora* Kunth).

Content:
— *acteoside* ($C_{29}H_{36}O_{15}$; Mr 625): minimum 2.5 per cent,
  expressed as ferulic acid (dried drug);
— *essential oil*: minimum 3.0 mL/kg for the whole drug and
  minimum 2.0 mL/kg for the fragmented drug (dried
  drug).

CHARACTERS

After grinding, it has a characteristic odour reminiscent of
lemon.

IDENTIFICATION

A. The leaves are simple with short petioles. They are
narrow, lanceolate, and about 4 times longer than they are
wide. The entire, slightly undulating margins are curled
towards the upper surface. The upper surface is dark green
and rough to the touch; the lower surface is paler green and
shows a prominent midrib with secondary veins running to
the margins.

B. Microscopic examination (*2.8.23*). The powder is light
green. Examine under a microscope using *chloral hydrate*
solution R. The powder shows the following diagnostic
characters (Figure 1834.-1): fragments of the upper
epidermis of the lamina in surface view [A, B, H], composed
of polygonal cells with numerous short, unicellular, thick-
walled cystolithic trichomes, each arising from a rosette of
cells at the base and containing calcium concretions (B),
glandular trichomes with a unicellular stalk and a unicellular,
globular head of variable size in surface view [Ha] and
transverse section [D, F]; these fragments are usually
accompanied by palisade parenchyma [Aa, Hb]; fragments of
the lower epidermis of the lamina in surface view [E],
covered by a striated cuticle and composed of cells more
irregular and somewhat sinuous in outline, with abundant
anomocytic stomata (*2.8.3*) [Ea] and numerous glandular
trichomes in surface view [Eb] and/or their scars [Ec];
fragments of the lamina in transverse section [G] with 2
layers of palisade parenchyma [Ga] and spongy parenchyma
[Gb]; lignified tissue from the veins [C].

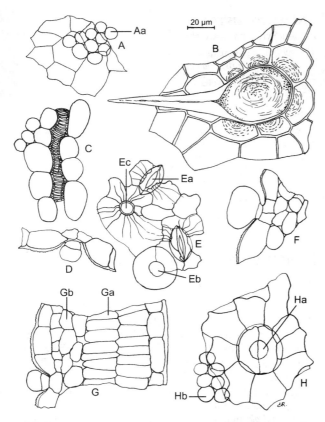

Figure 1834.-1. – *Illustration for identification test B of powdered herbal drug of lemon verbena leaf*

C. Examine the chromatograms obtained in the test for *Verbena officinalis*.

Results See below the sequence of zones present in the chromatograms obtained with the reference solution and the test solution. Furthermore, other faint zones may be present in the chromatogram obtained with the test solution. Zones may be present in the chromatogram obtained with the test solution below the zone due to rutin in the chromatogram obtained with the reference solution.

Top of the plate	
―――――	―――――
	An intense greyish-green zone
Arbutin: a blue or brown zone	
Rutin: a dark brownish-yellow zone	A blue or violet zone
―――――	―――――
Reference solution	**Test solution**

TESTS

Verbena officinalis

Thin-layer chromatography (*2.2.27*).

Test solution To 0.50 g of the powdered herbal drug (710) (*2.9.12*) add 5 mL of *methanol R*. Heat in a water-bath at 60 °C for 10 min. Cool and filter.

Reference solution Dissolve 10 mg of *arbutin R* and 10 mg of *rutin R* in *methanol R* and dilute to 10 mL with the same solvent.

Plate TLC silica gel plate R (5-40 μm) [or *TLC silica gel plate R* (2-10 μm)].

Mobile phase anhydrous formic acid R, glacial acetic acid R, water R, ethyl acetate R (11:11:27:100 *V/V/V/V*).

Application 20 μL [or 5 μL] as bands.

Development Over a path of about 12 cm [or 6 cm].

Drying In air.

Detection Spray with *anisaldehyde solution R* and dry at 100-105 °C for about 10 min; examine in daylight.

Results The chromatogram obtained with the test solution shows no brownish-grey zone at a position between that of arbutin and rutin in the chromatogram obtained with the reference solution.

Loss on drying (*2.2.32*)
Maximum 10.0 per cent, determined on 1.000 g of the powdered herbal drug (710) (*2.9.12*) by drying in an oven at 105 °C for 2 h.

Total ash (*2.4.16*)
Maximum 13.0 per cent.

Ash insoluble in hydrochloric acid (*2.8.1*)
Maximum 3.5 per cent.

ASSAY

Acteoside

Liquid chromatography (*2.2.29*).

Test solution To 1.00 g of the powdered herbal drug (710) (*2.9.12*) add 50.0 mL of the reference solution and stir for 2 h with a magnetic stirrer. Centrifuge for 15 min and pass the supernatant through a membrane filter (nominal pore size 0.45 μm).

Reference solution Dissolve 10.0 mg of *ferulic acid CRS* in ethanol (60 per cent V/V) R and dilute to 100.0 mL with the same solvent.

Precolumn:
— *size: l* = 0.01 m, Ø = 4.0 mm;
— *stationary phase*: octadecylsilyl silica gel for chromatography R (5 μm).

Column:
— *size: l* = 0.25 m, Ø = 4.0 mm;
— *stationary phase*: octadecylsilyl silica gel for chromatography R (5 μm);
— *temperature*: 20 °C.

Mobile phase:
— *mobile phase A*: 0.3 per cent *V/V* solution of *phosphoric acid R*;
— *mobile phase B*: acetonitrile R;

Time (min)	Mobile phase A (per cent *V/V*)	Mobile phase B (per cent *V/V*)
0 - 20	93 → 83	7 → 17
20 - 30	83	17
30 - 35	83 → 75	17 → 25
35 - 40	75 → 20	25 → 80
40 - 45	20 → 93	80 → 7

Flow rate 1.0 mL/min.

Detection Spectrophotometer at 330 nm.

Injection 20 μL.

System suitability Test solution:
— *resolution*: minimum 3.5 between the peaks due to ferulic acid and acteoside.

Calculate the percentage content of acteoside, expressed as ferulic acid, using the following expression:

$$\frac{A_1 \times m_2 \times p \times 0.5 \times 3.1}{A_2 \times m_1}$$

A_1 = area of the peak due to acteoside in the chromatogram obtained with the test solution;

A_2 = area of the peak due to ferulic acid in the chromatogram obtained with the reference solution;

m_1 = mass of the herbal drug in the test solution, in grams;

m_2 = mass of *ferulic acid CRS* in the reference solution, in grams;

p = percentage content of ferulic acid in *ferulic acid CRS*;

3.1 = correlation factor between acteoside and ferulic acid.

Essential oil (*2.8.12*)

Introduce 25.0 g of the freshly crushed herbal drug into a 1000 mL flask and add 500 mL of a 10 g/L solution of *sodium chloride R* as the distillation liquid. Use 0.50 mL of *xylene R* in the graduated tube. Distil at a rate of 3.0-3.5 mL/min for 3 h.

—————————————————————— *Ph Eur*

Lime Flower

(*Ph Eur monograph 0957*)

Ph Eur ————————————————————————

DEFINITION

Whole, dried inflorescence of *Tilia cordata* Miller, of *Tilia platyphyllos* Scop., of *Tilia × vulgaris* Heyne or a mixture of these.

CHARACTERS

Faint aromatic odour.

Faint, sweet and mucilaginous taste.

IDENTIFICATION

A. The inflorescence is yellowish-green. The main axis of the inflorescence bears a linguiform bract, membranous, yellowish-green, practically glabrous, the central vein of which is joined for up to about half of its length with the peduncle. The inflorescence usually consists of 2-7 flowers, occasionally up to 16. The sepals are detached easily from the perianth; they are up to 6 mm long, their abaxial surface is usually glabrous, their adaxial surface and their borders are strongly pubescent. The 5 spatulate, thin petals are yellowish-white, up to 8 mm long. They show fine venation and their borders only are sometimes covered with isolated trichomes. The numerous stamens are free and usually constitute 5 groups. The superior ovary has a pistil with a somewhat 5-lobate stigma.

B. Separate the inflorescence into its different parts. Examine under a microscope using *chloral hydrate solution R*. The adaxial epidermis of the bract shows cells with straight or slightly sinuous anticlinal walls; the abaxial epidermis shows cells with wavy-sinuous anticlinal walls and anomocytic stomata (*2.8.3*). Isolated cells in the mesophyll contain small calcium oxalate cluster crystals. The parenchyma of the sepals shows, particularly near the veins, numerous mucilaginous cells and cells containing small calcium oxalate clusters. The adaxial epidermis of sepals bears bent, thick-walled covering trichomes, unicellular or stellate with up to 5 cells. The epidermal cells of the petals show straight anticlinal walls with a striated cuticle without stomata. The parenchyma of the petals shows small calcium oxalate clusters and especially in its acuminate part mucilaginous cells. The pollen grains have a diameter of about 30-40 μm and are oval or slightly triangular with 3 germinal pores and a finely granulated exine. The ovary is glabrous or densely covered with trichomes, often very twisted, unicellular or stellate with 2-4 branches.

C. Thin-layer chromatography (*2.2.27*).

Test solution Shake 1.0 g of the powdered drug (355) (*2.9.12*) with 10 mL of *methanol R* in a water-bath at 65 °C for 5 min. Allow to cool and filter.

Reference solution Dissolve 2.0 mg of *caffeic acid R*, 5 mg of *hyperoside R* and 5 mg of *rutin R* in 10 mL of *methanol R*.

Plate TLC silica gel plate R.

Mobile phase anhydrous formic acid R, water R, methyl ethyl ketone R, ethyl acetate R (10:10:30:50 *V/V/V/V*).

Application 10 μL, as bands.

Development Over a path of 15 cm.

Drying At 100-105 °C.

Detection Spray the warm plate with a 10 g/L solution of *diphenylboric acid aminoethyl ester R* in *methanol R*. Then spray with a 50 g/L solution of *macrogol 400 R* in *methanol R*. Allow to dry for about 30 min and examine in ultraviolet light at 365 nm.

Results The chromatogram obtained with the reference solution shows in order of increasing R_F value yellowish-orange or brownish-orange fluorescent zones due to rutin and hyperoside and a greenish-blue fluorescent zone due to caffeic acid. In the chromatogram obtained with the test solution, the main zone shows brownish-yellow or orange fluorescence. This zone is situated just above the zone due to hyperoside in the chromatogram obtained with the reference solution. In daylight, this zone stands out from the other zones as the main zone. At the R_F level of rutin there is also a brownish-yellow fluorescent zone. Below this zone, 2 yellow fluorescent zones may be present. Between the zones due to rutin and hyperoside, orange and yellow fluorescent zones are visible. Between the zones due to hyperoside and caffeic acid, up to 5 yellow or orange fluorescent zones are present. Immediately below the zone due to caffeic acid is a a blue fluorescent zone.

TESTS

Foreign matter (*2.8.2*)

Maximum 2 per cent, determined on 30 g. There are no inflorescences with a bract bearing at the abaxial face stellate, five- to eight-rayed trichomes and flowers having an apparent double corolla by transformation of five stamens into petal-like staminoids and having a pistil which is not lobular nor indented. Hexamerous flowers occur only occasionally (*Tilia americana* L., *Tilia tomentosa* Moench).

Loss on drying (*2.2.32*)

Maximum 12.0 per cent, determined on 1.000 g of the powdered drug (355) (*2.9.12*) by drying in an oven at 105 °C for 2 h.

Total ash (*2.4.16*)

Maximum 8.0 per cent.

—————————————————————— *Ph Eur*

Linseed

(Ph Eur monograph 0095)

When Powdered Linseed is prescribed or demanded, material complying with the appropriate requirements below shall be dispensed or supplied.

Ph Eur _____

DEFINITION

Dried, ripe seeds of *Linum usitatissimum* L.

IDENTIFICATION

A. The seed has a flattened, elongated ovoid shape. The testa is dark reddish-brown or yellow, smooth and shiny. The seeds are 4-6 mm long, 2-3 mm wide and 1.5-2 mm thick; one end is rounded and the other end forms an oblique point near which the hilum appears as a slight depression. When viewed with a lens, the surface of the seed-coat is seen to be minutely pitted. Inside the testa a narrow, whitish endosperm and an embryo composed of 2 large, flattened, yellowish and oily cotyledons are present; the radicle points towards the hilum.

B. Microscopic examination (*2.8.23*). The powder is greasy to the touch. Examine under a microscope using *chloral hydrate solution R*. The powder shows the following diagnostic characters (Figure 0095.-1): fragments of the outer testa [A, B] with cells that are polygonal in surface view [Aa] or narrow in transverse section [Ba], and filled with mucilage [Bb]; fragments of the collenchymatously thickened sub-epidermal layer, in transverse section [Bc], or in surface view [Ab] with rounded cells with triangular intercellular spaces often attached to the sclerenchymatous layer composed of elongated cells, with thickened and pitted walls [Ca], some with strongly thickened and pitted walls [G]; fragments, in surface view [C], consisting of the hyaline layer with thin-walled cells [Cb] often remaining attached to the layer of elongated sclereids and crossing them at approximately right angles [Ca]; fragments of the inner testa, in surface view [D], composed of moderately thickened polygonal cells filled with brown-orange pigment; small polyhedral masses of pigment [H]; numerous fragments of parenchyma from the testae, with large, slightly and regularly thickened cells, in surface view [J, L]; parenchyma of the endosperm [K] and cotyledons [E] containing aleurone grains and oil droplets; very numerous isolated oil droplets [F].

TESTS

Foreign matter (*2.8.2*)
Maximum 10 per cent of seeds with a dull coat and maximum 1.5 per cent of other foreign matter.

Swelling index (*2.8.4*)
Minimum 4.

Cadmium (*2.4.27*)
Maximum 0.5 ppm.

Loss on drying (*2.2.32*)
Maximum 8.0 per cent, determined on 1.000 g of the powdered herbal drug (355) (*2.9.12*) by drying in an oven at 105 °C for 2 h.

Total ash (*2.4.16*)
Maximum 5.0 per cent.

_____ *Ph Eur*

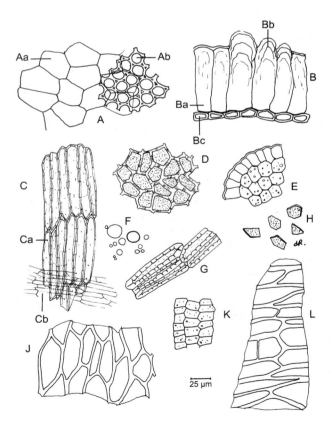

Figure 0095.-1. – *Illustration for identification test B of powdered herbal drug of linseed*

Liquorice

(Liquorice Root, Ph Eur monograph 0277)

Preparations

Liquorice Dry Extract for Flavouring Purposes

Standardised Liquorice Ethanolic Extract

Liquorice Liquid Extract

When Powdered Liquorice is prescribed or demanded, material complying with the appropriate requirements below shall be dispensed or supplied.

Ph Eur _____

DEFINITION

Dried, unpeeled or peeled, whole or cut root and stolons of *Glycyrrhiza glabra* L. and/or of *Glycyrrhiza inflata* Bat. and/or *Glycyrrhiza uralensis* Fisch.

Content

Minimum 4.0 per cent of 18β-glycyrrhizic acid ($C_{42}H_{62}O_{16}$; M_r 823) (dried drug).

IDENTIFICATION

A. The root has few branches. Its bark is brown or brownish-grey with longitudinal striations and bears traces of lateral roots. The cylindrical stolons are 1-2 cm in diameter; their external appearance is similar to that of the root but there are occasional small buds. The fracture of the root and the stolon is granular and fibrous. The cork layer is thin; the secondary phloem region is thick and light yellow with radial striations. The yellow xylem cylinder is compact, with a radiate structure. The stolon has a central pith, which is absent from the root. The external part of the bark is absent from the peeled root.

B. Microscopic examination (2.8.23). The powder is light yellow or faintly greyish. Examine under a microscope using *chloral hydrate solution R*. The powder shows the following diagnostic characters: fragments of yellow thick-walled fibres, 700-1200 μm long and 10-20 μm wide with a punctiform lumen, often accompanied by crystal sheaths containing prisms of calcium oxalate 10-35 μm long and 2-5 μm wide. The walls of the vessels are yellow, 5-10 μm thick, lignified and have numerous bordered pits with a slit-shaped aperture; fragments of cork consisting of thin-walled cells and isolated prisms of calcium oxalate occur as well as fragments of parenchymatous tissue. Fragments of cork are absent from the peeled root. Examine under a microscope using a mixture of equal volumes of *glycerol R* and *water R*. The powder shows the following diagnostic characters: simple, round or oval starch granules, 2-20 μm in diameter.

C. Thin-layer chromatography (2.2.27).

Test solution   To 0.50 g of the powdered herbal drug (180) (2.9.12) in a 50 mL round-bottomed flask add 16.0 mL of *water R* and 4.0 mL of *hydrochloric acid R1* and heat on a water-bath under a reflux condenser for 30 min. Cool and filter. Dry the filter and the round-bottomed flask at 105 °C for 60 min. Place the filter in the round-bottomed flask, add 20.0 mL of *ether R* and heat in a water-bath at 40 °C under a reflux condenser for 5 min. Cool and filter. Evaporate the filtrate to dryness. Dissolve the residue in 5.0 mL of *ether R*.

Reference solution   Dissolve 5.0 mg of *glycyrrhetic acid R* and 5.0 mg of *thymol R* in 5.0 mL of *ether R*.

Plate   TLC silica gel F_{254} plate R.

Mobile phase   concentrated ammonia R, water R, ethanol (96 per cent) R, ethyl acetate R (1:9:25:65 V/V/V/V).

Application   10 μL.

Development   Over a path of 15 cm.

Drying   In air for 5 min.

Detection A   Examine in ultraviolet light at 254 nm.

Results A   The chromatograms obtained with the test solution and the reference solution show in the lower half a quenching zone due to glycyrrhetic acid.

Detection B   Treat with *anisaldehyde solution R*, and heat at 100-105 °C for 5-10 min; examine in daylight.

Results B   The chromatogram obtained with the reference solution shows in the lower half a violet zone due to glycyrrhetic acid and in the upper third a red zone due to thymol. The chromatogram obtained with the test solution shows in the lower half a violet zone corresponding to the zone of glycyrrhetic acid in the chromatogram obtained with the reference solution and a yellow zone (isoliquiridigenine) in the upper third under the zone of thymol in the chromatogram obtained with the reference solution. Further zones may be present.

TESTS

Loss on drying (2.2.32)
Maximum 10.0 per cent, determined on 1.000 g of the powdered herbal drug (355) (2.9.12) by drying in an oven at 105 °C for 2 h.

Total ash (2.4.16)
Maximum 10.0 per cent for the unpeeled drug and maximum 6.0 per cent for the peeled drug.

Ash insoluble in hydrochloric acid (2.8.1)
Maximum 2.0 per cent for the unpeeled drug and maximum 0.5 per cent for the peeled drug.

Ochratoxin A (2.8.22)
Maximum 20 μg per kilogram of herbal drug.

ASSAY

Liquid chromatography (2.2.29).

Test solution   Place 1.000 g of the powdered herbal drug (180) (2.9.12) in a 150 mL ground-glass conical flask. Add 100.0 mL of an 8 g/L solution of *ammonia R* and treat in an ultrasonic bath for 30 min. Centrifuge a part of the solution and dilute 1.0 mL of the supernatant layer to 5.0 mL with an 8 g/L solution of *ammonia R*. Filter through a membrane filter (nominal pore size 0.45 μm); use the filtrate as the test solution.

Solution A   Dissolve 0.130 g of *monoammonium glycyrrhizate CRS* in an 8 g/L solution of *ammonia R* and dilute to 100.0 mL with the same solvent.

Reference solution (a)   Dilute 5.0 mL of solution A to 100.0 mL with an 8 g/L solution of *ammonia R*.

Reference solution (b)   Dilute 10.0 mL of solution A to 100.0 mL with an 8 g/L solution of *ammonia R*.

Reference solution (c)   Dilute 15.0 mL of solution A to 100.0 mL with an 8 g/L solution of *ammonia R*.

Column:
— size: l = 0.10 m, Ø = 4 mm;
— stationary phase: octadecylsilyl silica gel for chromatography R (5 μm).

Mobile phase   glacial acetic acid R, acetonitrile R, water R (6:30:64 V/V/V).

Flow rate   1.5 mL/min.

Detection   Spectrophotometer at 254 nm.

Injection   10 μL.

Establish a calibration curve with the mass of monoammonium glycyrrhizate in the reference solutions, in grams, as the abscissa and the corresponding peak areas as the ordinate.

Using the retention times and the peak areas determined from the chromatograms obtained with the reference solutions, locate and integrate the peak due to 18β-glycyrrhizic acid in the chromatogram obtained with the test solution.

Calculate the percentage content of 18β-glycyrrhizic acid using the following expression:

$$A \times \frac{5}{m} \times B \times \frac{823}{840}$$

A =   mass equivalent of monoammonium glycyrrhizate in the test solution, determined from the calibration curve, in grams;
B =   declared percentage content of *monoammonium glycyrrhizate CRS*;
m =   mass of the herbal drug to be examined used to prepare the test solution, in grams;
823   =   molecular mass of 18β-glycyrrhizic acid;
840   =   molecular mass of monoammonium glycyrrhizate (without any water of crystallisation).

LABELLING

The label states whether the drug is peeled or unpeeled.

_____ *Ph Eur*

Liquorice Dry Extract for Flavouring Purposes

(Ph Eur monograph 2378)

Ph Eur _____

DEFINITION
Dry extract produced from *Liquorice root (0277)*.

Content
5.0 per cent to 7.0 per cent of 18β-glycyrrhizic acid ($C_{42}H_{62}O_{16}$; M_r 823) (dried extract).

PRODUCTION
The extract is produced from the cut herbal drug by a suitable procedure using water.

CHARACTERS

Appearance
Yellowish-brown or brown powder.

Very sweet taste.

IDENTIFICATION
Thin-layer chromatography (*2.2.27*).

Solvent mixture ethyl acetate R, methanol R (50:50 *V/V*).

Test solution To 0.30 g of the extract to be examined add 30 mL of *hydrochloric acid R1* and boil on a water-bath under a reflux condenser for 60 min. After cooling, extract the mixture with 2 quantities, each of 20 mL, of *ethyl acetate R*. Combine the organic layers and filter through a filter covered with *anhydrous sodium sulfate R*. Evaporate the filtrate to dryness *in vacuo* and dissolve the residue in 2.0 mL of the solvent mixture.

Reference solution Dissolve 5.0 mg of *glycyrrhetic acid R* and 5.0 mg of *thymol R* in 5.0 mL of the solvent mixture.

Plate TLC silica gel F_{254} plate R (5-40 μm) [or *TLC silica gel F_{254} plate R* (2-10 μm)].

Mobile phase concentrated ammonia R, water R, ethanol (96 per cent) R, ethyl acetate R (1:9:25:65 *V/V/V/V*).

Application 20 μL [or 10 μL] as bands.

Development over a path of 15 cm [or 7 cm].

Drying In air for 5 min.

Detection Spray with *anisaldehyde solution R* and heat at 100-105 °C for 5-10 min; examine in daylight.

Results See below the sequence of zones present in the chromatograms obtained with the reference solution and the test solution. Furthermore, other faint zones may be present in the chromatogram obtained with the test solution.

Top of the plate	
Thymol: a red zone	
	A yellow zone
_____	_____
_____	_____
Glycyrrhetic acid: a violet zone	A violet zone (glycyrrhetic acid)
Reference solution	**Test solution**

TESTS

Loss on drying (*2.8.17*)
Maximum 7.0 per cent.

Ochratoxin A (*2.8.22*)
Maximum 80 μg per kilogram of extract.

The maximum content applies to the pure undiluted extract. Where excipients are added to reduce the strength of the extract, the maximum content should be reduced proportionally.

ASSAY
Liquid chromatography (*2.2.29*).

Solvent mixture water R, methanol R (20:80 *V/V*).

Test solution Place 0.200 g of the extract to be examined in a 150 mL ground-glass conical flask. Add 100.0 mL of the solvent mixture and sonicate for 2 min. Filter through a membrane filter (nominal pore size 0.45 μm).

Reference solution Dissolve 50.0 mg of *monoammonium glycyrrhizate CRS* in the solvent mixture and dilute to 50.0 mL with the solvent mixture. Dilute 1.0 mL of this solution to 10.0 mL with the solvent mixture.

Column:
— *size:* l = 0.10 m, Ø = 4.0 mm;
— *stationary phase*: octadecylsilyl silica gel for chromatography R (5 μm).

Mobile phase glacial acetic acid R, acetonitrile R, water R (6:30:64 *V/V/V*).

Flow rate 1.5 mL/min.

Detection Spectrophotometer at 254 nm.

Injection 10 μL.

Run time 3 times the retention time of 18β-glycyrrhizic acid.

Retention time 18β-glycyrrhizic acid = about 9 min.

Identification of peaks Use the chromatogram supplied with *monoammonium glycyrrhizate CRS* and the chromatogram obtained with the reference solution to identify the peaks due to 18β-glycyrrhizic acid and 18α-glycyrrhizic acid.

System suitability Reference solution:
— the chromatogram obtained with the reference solution is similar to the chromatogram supplied with *monoammonium glycyrrhizate CRS*;
— *resolution*: minimum 2.0 between the peaks due to 18β-glycyrrhizic acid and 18α-glycyrrhizic acid.

Calculate the percentage content of 18β-glycyrrhizic acid, using the following expression:

$$\frac{A_1 \times m_2 \times p \times 0.979}{A_2 \times m_1 \times 5}$$

A_1 = area of the peak due to 18β-glycyrrhizic acid in the chromatogram obtained with the test solution;

A_2 = area of the peak due to 18β-glycyrrhizic acid in the chromatogram obtained with the reference solution;

m_1 = mass of the extract to be examined used to prepare the test solution, in grams;

m_2 = mass of *monoammonium glycyrrhizate CRS* used to prepare the reference solution, in grams;

p = percentage content of 18β-glycyrrhizic acid in *monoammonium glycyrrhizate CRS*;

0.979 = peak correlation factor between 18β-glycyrrhizic acid and monoammonium glycyrrhizate.

_____ *Ph Eur*

Standardised Liquorice Ethanolic Liquid Extract

(Ph Eur monograph 1536)

Ph Eur —————

DEFINITION

Standardised ethanolic liquid extract produced from *Liquorice root (0277)*.

Content

3.0 per cent to 5.0 per cent of 18β-glycyrrhizic acid ($C_{42}H_{62}O_{16}$; M_r 823).

PRODUCTION

The extract is produced from the herbal drug by a suitable procedure for liquid extracts using ethanol (70 per cent *V/V*).

CHARACTERS

Appearance

Dark brown, clear liquid.

It has a faint characteristic odour and a sweet taste.

IDENTIFICATION

Thin-layer chromatography (2.2.27).

Test solution Place 1.0 g of the extract to be examined in a 50 mL round-bottomed flask, add 16.0 mL of *water R* and 4.0 mL of *hydrochloric acid R1* and heat on a water-bath under a reflux condenser for 30 min. Allow to cool and filter. Dry the filter and the round-bottomed flask at 105 °C for 60 min. Transfer the filter to the round-bottomed flask, add 20 mL of *ether R* and heat in a water-bath at 40 °C under a reflux condenser for 5 min. Allow to cool and filter. Evaporate the filtrate to dryness and dissolve the residue in 5.0 mL of *ether R*.

Reference solution Dissolve 5.0 mg of *glycyrrhetic acid R* and 5.0 mg of *thymol R* in 5 mL of *ether R*.

Plate TLC silica gel F_{254} plate R.

Mobile phase concentrated ammonia R, water R, ethanol (96 per cent) R, ethyl acetate R (1:9:25:65 *V/V/V/V*).

Application 10 µL as bands.

Development Over a path of 15 cm.

Drying In air for 5 min.

Detection A Examine in ultraviolet light at 254 nm.

Results A The chromatograms obtained with the test solution and the reference solution show in the lower half a quenching zone due to glycyrrhetic acid.

Detection B Treat with *anisaldehyde solution R*; heat at 100-105 °C for 5-10 min and examine in daylight.

Results B The chromatogram obtained with the reference solution shows in the lower half a violet zone (glycyrrhetic acid), and in the upper third a red zone (thymol); the chromatogram obtained with the test solution shows in the lower half a violet zone corresponding to glycyrrhetic acid in the chromatogram obtained with the reference solution, and in the upper third, below the zone of thymol in the chromatogram obtained with the reference solution, a yellow zone due to isoliquiritigenin; further zones are present.

TESTS

Ethanol (2.9.10)

52 per cent *V/V* to 65 per cent *V/V*.

Methanol and 2-propanol (2.9.11)

Maximum 0.05 per cent *V/V* of methanol and maximum 0.05 per cent *V/V* of 2-propanol.

Ochratoxin A (2.8.22)

Maximum 80 µg per kilogram of extract.

ASSAY

Liquid chromatography (2.2.29).

Solvent mixture dilute ammonia R1, water R (8:92 *V/V*).

Test solution Dilute 1.000 g of the extract to be examined to 100 mL with the solvent mixture and centrifuge. Dilute 2.0 mL of the supernatant to 10.0 mL with the solvent mixture.

Solution A Dissolve 0.130 g of *monoammonium glycyrrhizate CRS* in the solvent mixture and dilute to 100.0 mL with the solvent mixture.

Reference solution (a) Dilute 5.0 mL of solution A to 100.0 mL with the solvent mixture.

Reference solution (b) Dilute 10.0 mL of solution A to 100.0 mL with the solvent mixture.

Reference solution (c) Dilute 15.0 mL of solution A to 100.0 mL with the solvent mixture.

Column:
— *size: l* = 0.10 m, Ø = 4 mm;
— *stationary phase*: octadecylsilyl silica gel for chromatography R (5 µm).

Mobile phase glacial acetic acid R, acetonitrile R, water R (6:30:64 *V/V/V*).

Flow rate 1.5 mL/min.

Detection Spectrophotometer at 254 nm.

Injection 10 µL.

Establish a calibration curve with the mass of monoammonium glycyrrhizate in the reference solutions, in grams, as the abscissa and the corresponding peak areas as the ordinate.

Using the retention times and the peak areas determined from the chromatograms obtained with the reference solutions, locate and integrate the peak due to 18β-glycyrrhizic acid in the chromatogram obtained with the test solution.

Calculate the percentage content of 18β-glycyrrhizic acid using the following expression:

$$A \times \frac{5}{m} \times B \times \frac{823}{840}$$

A = mass equivalent of monoammonium glycyrrhizate in the test solution, determined from the calibration curve, in grams;

B = declared percentage content of *monoammonium glycyrrhizate CRS*;

m = mass of the extract to be examined used to prepare the test solution, in grams;

823 = molecular mass of 18β-glycyrrhizic acid;

840 = molecular mass of monoammonium glycyrrhizate (without any water of crystallisation).

————— *Ph Eur*

Liquorice Liquid Extract

DEFINITION

Liquorice Liquid Extract is prepared by extracting Liquorice with Purified Water and adding sufficient Ethanol (90 per cent) to give an ethanol content of 18% v/v in the final extract.

Extemporaneous preparation

The following formula and directions apply.

Liquorice, unpeeled, in *coarse powder*	1000 g
Purified Water	A sufficient quantity
Ethanol (90 per cent)	A sufficient quantity

Exhaust the Liquorice with Purified Water by *percolation*, Appendix XI F. Boil the percolate for 5 minutes and set aside for not less than 12 hours. Decant the clear liquid, filter the remainder, mix the two liquids and evaporate until the *weight per mL* of the liquid is 1.198 g, Appendix V G. Add to this liquid, when cold, one quarter of its volume of Ethanol (90 per cent). Allow to stand for not less than 4 weeks; filter.

The extract complies with the requirements stated under Extracts and with the following requirements.

IDENTIFICATION

Carry out the method for *thin-layer chromatography*, Appendix III A, using the following solutions.

(1) Extract 5 mL of the liquid extract with 20 mL of *chloroform*. Heat 2.5 mL of the aqueous layer with 30 mL of 0.5M *sulfuric acid* under a reflux condenser for 1 hour, cool and extract with two 20 mL quantities of *chloroform*. Dry the combined chloroform extracts over *anhydrous sodium sulfate*, filter and evaporate the filtrate to dryness; dissolve the residue in 4 mL of a mixture of equal volumes of *chloroform* and *methanol*.

(2) Dissolve 10 mg of *glycyrrhetinic acid* in 2 mL of a mixture of equal volumes of *chloroform* and *methanol*.

CHROMATOGRAPHIC CONDITIONS

(a) Use as the coating *silica gel F_{254}* (Merck 10 × 20 cm plates are suitable).

(b) Use the mobile phase as described below.

(c) Apply 10 μL of solution (1) and 5 μL of solution (2).

(d) Develop the plate to 15 cm.

(e) After removal of the plate, allow it to dry and examine under *ultraviolet light (254 nm)*.

MOBILE PHASE

5 volumes of *methanol* and 95 volumes of *chloroform*.

CONFIRMATION

The chromatogram obtained with solution (1) exhibits a dark spot corresponding to the principal spot in the chromatogram obtained with solution (2).

TESTS

Ethanol content

16 to 20% v/v, Appendix VIII F, Method III.

Ammonia

Place 5 mL in a distillation apparatus of about 500 mL capacity fitted with an efficient splash-head and a delivery tube that dips below the surface of a mixture of 10 mL of 0.05M *sulfuric acid VS* and 50 mL of *water* contained in the receiver. Add 200 mL of *water*, a little *pumice powder* and 30 mL of a solution prepared by dissolving 1.43 g of *potassium dihydrogen orthophosphate* and 9.1 g of *dipotassium hydrogen orthophosphate* in 100 mL of *water* and distil until about 175 mL of distillate has been collected. Titrate the excess of acid with 0.1M *sodium hydroxide VS* using *methyl red*

solution as indicator. Not less than 5 mL of 0.1M *sodium hydroxide VS* is required.

Dry residue

40 to 45% w/v, Appendix XIP

Relative density

1.125 to 1.140, Appendix V G.

Ochratoxin A

Not more than 40 ppb, Appendix XI S2.

Liquorice Root for use in TCM

DEFINITION

Liquorice Root for use in TCM is the dried unpeeled root and rhizome of *Glycyrrhiza uralensis* Fisch., and/or *Glycyrrhiza inflata* Bat. and/or *Glycyrrhiza glabra* L.

It is collected in spring and autumn, separated from the rootlets and dried in the sun.

It contains not less than 2.0% of glycyrrhizic acid ($C_{42}H_{62}O_{16}$), calculated with reference to the dried material.

IDENTIFICATION

A. The root has few branches. Its bark is brownish-grey or brown with longitudinal striations and bears traces of lateral roots. The cylindrical stolons are 1-2 cm in diameter; their external appearance is similar to that of the root but there are occasional small buds. The fracture of the root and the stolon is granular and fibrous. The cork layer is thin; the secondary phloem region is thick and light yellow with radial striations. The yellow xylem cylinder is compact, with a radiate structure. The stolon has a central pith, which is absent from the root.

B. Reduce to a powder. The powder is yellowish-brown. Examine under a microscope using *chloral hydrate solution*. The powder shows abundant fibres occurring in groups, each group surrounded by a calcium oxalate prism crystal sheath, the individual fibres with very thick, partially lignified walls and few small pits; lignified bordered-pitted vessels, singly or in small groups and sometimes accompanied by lignified parenchymatous cells with moderately thickened and pitted walls, some of the individual vessels are very large, with pit apertures much elongated and the borders difficult to discern; prism crystals of calcium oxalate up to about 35 μm long occur scattered and in parenchymatous tissue; fragments of cork composed of thin-walled, slightly lignified polygonal cells. Examine under a microscope using 50% w/w glycerol in water. The powder shows abundant starch granules, mostly simple, spherical to ovoid, 3 μm to 20 μm in diameter.

C. Carry out the method for *thin-layer chromatography*, Appendix III A, using the following solutions.

(1) Add 16 mL of *water* and 4 mL of *hydrochloric acid R1* to 0.5 g of the powdered drug, heat on a water-bath under reflux for 30 minutes, cool and filter. Dry the filter paper and residue in a flask at 105° for 60 minutes, add 20 mL of ether, heat on a water-bath at 40°C under reflux for 5 minutes, cool and filter. Evaporate the filtrate to dryness and dissolve the residue in 5 mL of *ether*.

(2) 0.1% w/v each of *glycyrrhetic acid* and *thymol* in *ether*.

CHROMATOGRAPHIC CONDITIONS

(a) Use as the coating substance *silica gel F_{254}* (Merck 10 × 20 cm plates are suitable).

(b) Use the mobile phase as described below.

(c) Apply 10 μL of each solution as a band.

(d) Develop the plate to 15 cm.

(e) Remove the plate and allow it to dry in air for 5 minutes. Examine under *ultraviolet light (254 nm)*. Spray the plate with *anisaldehyde solution* and heat at 100° to 105° for 10 minutes and examine in daylight.

MOBILE PHASE

1 volume of *concentrated ammonia*, 9 volumes of *water*, 25 volumes of *ethanol (96%)* and 65 volumes of *ethyl acetate*.

SYSTEM SUITABILITY

Under ultra-violet light, the chromatogram obtained with solution (2) shows in the lower half a quenching zone due to glycyrrhetic acid. When sprayed, the chromatogram obtained with solution (2) shows in the lower half the violet zone of glycyrrhetic acid and in the upper third the red zone of thymol.

CONFIRMATION

The chromatogram obtained with solution (1) shows in the lower half a violet zone corresponding to the zone of glycyrrhetic acid in the chromatogram obtained with solution (2) and a yellow zone (isoliquiridigenine) in the upper third under the zone of thymol in the chromatogram obtained with solution (2). Further zones may be present.

TESTS
Total Ash
Not more than 7.0%, Appendix XI J, Method II.

Acid-insoluble ash
Not more than 2.0%, Appendix XI K, Method II.

Loss on drying
When dried for 2 hours at 100° to 105°, loses not more than 12.0%. Use 1 g.

Ochratoxin A
Not more than 20 ppb, Appendix XI S2.

ASSAY
Carry out the method for *liquid chromatography*, Appendix III D, using the following solutions.

(1) Mix 1 g of the powdered drug with 100 mL of 0.8% w/v of *ammonia*, place in an ultrasonic bath for 30 minutes, centrifuge, dilute 1 mL of supernatant solution to 5 mL with 0.8% w/v of *ammonia* and filter through a 0.45-μm filter.

(2) 0.0065% w/v of *monoammonium glycyrrhizate EPCRS* in 0.8% w/v of *ammonia*.

(3) 0.013% w/v of *monoammonium glycyrrhizate EPCRS* in 0.8% w/v of *ammonia*.

(4) 0.0195% w/v of *monoammonium glycyrrhizate EPCRS* in 0.8% w/v of *ammonia*.

CHROMATOGRAPHIC CONDITIONS

(a) Use a stainless steel column (12.5 cm × 4 mm) packed with *octadecylsilyl silica gel for chromatography* (5 μm) (Hypersil ODS SS is suitable).

(b) Use isocratic elution and the mobile phase described below.

(c) Use a flow rate of 1.5 mL per minute.

(d) Use ambient column temperature.

(e) Use a detection wavelength of 254 nm.

(f) Inject 10 μL of each solution.

MOBILE PHASE

6 volumes of *glacial acetic acid*, 30 volumes of *acetonitrile* and 64 volumes of *water*.

SYSTEM SUITABILITY

The assay is not valid unless (a) the *column efficiency*, determined on the peak due to glycyrrhizic acid in the chromatogram obtained with solution (2), is at least 30,000 theoretical plates per metre and (b) the *symmetry factor* of the peak is not more than 1.3.

DETERMINATION OF CONTENT

Inject solution (4). Adjust the sensitivity of the system so that the height of the peaks is at least 50% of the full scale of the recorder. Inject solutions (2), (3) and (4) and determine the peak areas. Prepare a calibration curve with the concentration of the solutions (g per 100 mL) as the abscissa and the corresponding areas as the ordinate. Inject solution (1). Using the retention time and the peak area from the chromatograms obtained with solutions (2), (3) and (4), locate and integrate the peak due to glycyrrhizic acid in the chromatogram obtained with solution (1).

Calculate the percentage content of glycyrrhizic acid from the following expression:

$$A \times \frac{5}{m} \times B \times \frac{822}{840}$$

A = concentration of monoammonium glycyrrhizate in solution (1) determined from the calibration curve, in g per 100 mL,

B = declared percentage content of *monoammonium glycyrrhizate EPCRS*,

m = weight of the substance being examined in grams,

822 = molecular weight of glycyrrhizic acid,

840 = molecular weight of monoammonium glycyrrhizate (without any water of crystallisation).

STORAGE
Liquorice Root for use in TCM should be protected from moisture.

Processed Liquorice Root for use in TCM

DEFINITION
Processed Liquorice Root for use in TCM is the processed Liquorice Root for use in TCM.

It contains not less than 2.0% of glycyrrhizic acid ($C_{42}H_{62}O_{16}$) calculated with reference to the dried material.

PRODUCTION
Processed Liquorice Root for use in TCM is cleaned, softened thoroughly, sliced transversely or longitudinally to form uniform pieces and dried.

IDENTIFICATION
A. The transversely-cut pieces are 0.5 to 2.5 cm in diameter, irregularly circular to ovoid, up to about 3 mm thick. The outer surface is dark reddish-brown and longitudinally wrinkled. The transverse surface is cream to yellow and shows a thin layer of cork and a pale brown cambium line separating the radiate phloem region from the distinctly radiate xylem. In pieces cut from the rhizome there is a central, whitish pith; in those cut from the roots the radiate xylem continues to the centre.

The longitudinally-cut pieces have been sliced obliquely and usually include a small portion of the outer surface at the tapering ends; they are about 6 to 8 cm long, 1 to 1.5 cm wide and 3 mm thick. The outer surface is reddish-brown and longitudinally wrinkled with scattered transverse ridges; the smooth cut surface is cream to yellow, faintly fibrous and shows a distinct cambium; on some of the pieces the vessel cavities are visible in the central region.

B. Reduce to a powder. The powder is yellowish-brown. Examine under a microscope using chloral hydrate solution. The powder shows abundant fibres occurring in groups, each group surrounded by a calcium oxalate prism crystal sheath, the individual fibres have very thick, partially lignified walls and few small pits; lignified bordered-pitted vessels, singly or in small groups and sometimes accompanied by lignified parenchymatous cells with moderately thickened and pitted walls, some of the individual vessels are very large, with pit apertures much elongated and the borders difficult to discern; prism crystals of calcium oxalate up to about 35 μm long occur scattered and in parenchymatous tissue; fragments of cork composed of thin-walled, slightly lignified polygonal cells. Examine under a microscope using 50% w/w glycerol in water. The powder shows abundant starch granules, mostly simple, spherical to ovoid, 3 μm to 20 μm in diameter.

C. Carry out the method for *thin-layer chromatography*, Appendix III A, using the following solutions.

(1) Add 16 mL of *water* and 4 mL of *hydrochloric acid (25%)* to 0.5 g of the powdered drug, heat on a water-bath under reflux for 30 minutes, cool and filter. Dry the filter paper and residue in a flask at 105° for 60 minutes, add 20 mL of *ether*, heat on a water-bath at 40° under reflux for 5 minutes, cool and filter. Evaporate the filtrate to dryness and dissolve the residue in 5 mL of *ether*.

(2) 0.1% w/v each of *glycyrrhetic acid* and *thymol* in *ether*.

CHROMATOGRAPHIC CONDITIONS

(a) Use as the coating substance *silica gel F₂₅₄* (Merck 10 × 20 cm plates are suitable).

(b) Use the mobile phase as described below.

(c) Apply 10 μL of each solution as a band.

(d) Develop the plate to 15 cm.

(e) Remove the plate and allow it to dry in air for 5 minutes. Examine under *ultraviolet light (254 nm)*. Spray the plate with *anisaldehyde solution* and heat at 100° to 105° for 10 minutes and examine in daylight.

MOBILE PHASE

1 volume of *concentrated ammonia*, 9 volumes of *water*, 25 volumes of *ethanol (96%)* and 65 volumes of *ethyl acetate*.

SYSTEM SUITABILITY

Under ultra-violet light, the chromatogram obtained with solution (2) shows in the lower half a quenching zone due to glycyrrhetic acid. When sprayed, the chromatogram obtained with solution (2) shows in the lower half the violet zone of glycyrrhetic acid and in the upper third the red zone of thymol.

CONFIRMATION

The chromatogram obtained with solution (1) shows in the lower half of violet zone corresponding to the zone of glycyrrhetic acid in the chromatogram obtained with solution (2) and a yellow zone (isoliquiridigenine) in the upper third under the zone of thymol in the chromatogram obtained with solution (2). Further zones may be present.

TESTS
Total Ash
Not more than 5.0%, Appendix XI J, Method II.

Acid-insoluble ash
Not more than 1.0%, Appendix XI K, Method II.

Loss on drying
When dried for 2 hours at 100° to 105°, loses not more than 10.0% of its weight. Use 1 g.

Ochratoxin A
Not more than 20 ppb, Appendix XI S2.

ASSAY
Carry out the method for *liquid chromatography*, Appendix III D, using the following solutions.

(1) Mix 1 g of the powdered drug with 100 mL of 0.8% w/v of *ammonia*, place in an ultrasound bath for 30 minutes, centrifuge, dilute 1 mL of the supernatant solution to 5 mL with 0.8% w/v of *ammonia* and filter through a 0.45-μm filter.

(2) 0.0065% w/v of *monoammonium glycyrrhizate EPCRS* in 0.8% w/v of *ammonia*.

(3) 0.013% w/v of *monoammonium glycyrrhizate EPCRS* in 0.8% w/v of *ammonia*.

(4) 0.0195% w/v of *monoammonium glycyrrhizate EPCRS* in 0.8% w/v of *ammonia*.

CHROMATOGRAPHIC CONDITIONS

(a) Use a stainless steel column (12.5 cm × 4 mm) packed with *octadecylsilyl silica gel for chromatography* (5 μm) (Hypersil ODS SS is suitable).

(b) Use isocratic elution and the mobile phase described below.

(c) Use a flow rate of 1.5 mL per minute.

(d) Use ambient column temperature.

(e) Use a detection wavelength of 254 nm.

(f) Injection 10 μL of each solution.

MOBILE PHASE

6 volumes of *glacial acetic acid*, 30 volumes of *acetonitrile* and 64 volumes of *water*.

SYSTEM SUITABILITY

The assay is not valid unless (a) the *column efficiency*, determined on the peak due to glycyrrhizic acid in the chromatogram obtained with solution (2), is at least 30,000 theoretical plates per metre and (b) the *symmetry factor* of the peak is not more than 1.3.

DETERMINATION OF CONTENT

Inject solution (4). Adjust the sensitivity of the system so that the height of the peaks is at least 50% of the full scale of the recorder. Inject solutions (2), (3) and (4) and determine the peak areas. Prepare a calibration curve with the concentration of the solutions (g per 100 mL) as the abscissa and the corresponding areas as the ordinate. Inject solution (1). Using the retention time and the peak area from the chromatograms obtained with solutions (2), (3) and (4), locate and integrate the peak due to glycyrrhizic acid in the chromatogram obtained with solution (1).

Calculate the percentage content of glycyrrhizic acid from the following expression:

$$A \times \frac{5}{m} \times B \times \frac{822}{840}$$

A = concentration of monoammonium glycyrrhizate in the solution (1) determined from the calibration curve, in g per 100 mL,

B = declared percentage content of *monoammonium glycyrrhizate EPCRS*,

m = weight of the substance being examined in grams,

822 = molecular weight of glycyrrhizic acid,

840 = molecular weight of the monoammonium glycyrrhizate (without any water of crystallisation).

STORAGE

Processed Liquorice Root for use in TCM should be protected from moisture.

Long Pepper

(*Ph Eur monograph 2453*)

Ph Eur

DEFINITION

Dried, ripe or nearly ripe fruiting spikes of *Piper longum* L. or *Piper retrofractum* Vahl (syn. *P. chaba* Hunter and *P. officinarum* (Miq.) C.DC.) or a mixture of both species.

Content:

— *essential oil*: minimum 6.0 mL/kg (dried drug);

— *piperine* ($C_{17}H_{19}NO_3$; M_r 285.3): minimum 3.0 per cent (dried drug).

IDENTIFICATION

A. *P. longum*. The fruiting spikes are cylindrical or irregularly cylindrical, 1-2.5 cm long (rarely longer than 2.5 cm), 3-5 mm in diameter, blackish-brown or almost black. The spikes are quite compact, tough, composed of small fruits firmly fixed on the receptacle in regular or oblique rows. The berries are spherical, about 1 mm in diameter. The bracts are black, small, punctiform, confined to depressions between adjacent berries. The remains of the peduncle may be present at the base of the cylinder. Spikes can be easily broken; the fracture is irregular and granular.

P. retrofractum. The fruiting spikes are similar to those of *P. longum* but clearly more robust, straight and cylindrical, 2.5-4 cm long (rarely smaller than 2.5 cm), 5-8 mm in diameter, brown or reddish-brown. The berries are also firmly fixed on the receptacle but, in contrast to those of *P. longum*, arranged more obviously in spiral rows. The bracts are more prominent than those of *P. longum*.

B. Microscopic examination (*2.8.23*). The powder is greyish-beige. Examine under a microscope using *chloral hydrate solution R*. The powder shows the following diagnostic characters: fragments of the endocarp in surface view, consisting of more or less elongated sclereids about 75 μm long, which have irregularly thickened walls and wide channels and which are sometimes associated with the brown pigment layer of the testa; fragments of the endocarp, in transverse section, showing sclereids with thickened inner walls on the 3 lower sides, usually associated with the testa; fragments of the testa consisting of a layer of reddish-brown pigmented cells and a layer of very thin-walled polygonal cells constituting the 'hyaline layer'; fragments of the parenchyma of the mesocarp containing more or less polygonal sclereids, isolated or in groups, and oil cells about 50 μm in diameter; numerous thin-walled, ovoid or polygonal cells of the parenchyma of the seed; fragments of the epicarp with extremely thin-walled, reddish-brown pigmented cells associated with the outer layers of the mesocarp consisting of groups of sclereids with strongly thickened walls; rare, elongated sclereids about 400 μm long with slightly thickened walls, from the centre of the spike; a few fragments of vascular tissue with spiral or striated vessels. Examine under a microscope using a 50 per cent *V/V* solution of *glycerol R*. Rounded, compound starch granules about 20 μm in diameter made up of tiny individual granules, ovoid or polyhedral by compression, free or included in the parenchymatous cells of the seed.

C. Thin-layer chromatography (*2.2.27*).

Test solution To 0.5 g of the powdered herbal drug (355) (*2.9.12*) add 5 mL of *methanol R*. Sonicate for 10 min, centrifuge and use the supernatant.

Reference solution Dissolve 10 mg of *borneol R* and 15 mg of *piperine R* in 10 mL of *methanol R*.

Plate TLC silica gel F_{254} plate R (5-40 μm) [or *TLC silica gel F_{254} plate R* (2-10 μm)].

Mobile phase ethyl acetate R, cyclohexane R (30:50 *V/V*).

Application 10 μL [or 5 μL] as bands of 10 mm [or 8 mm].

Development Over a path of 15 cm [or 6 cm].

Drying In air.

Detection A Examine in ultraviolet light at 254 nm.

Results A See below the sequence of zones present in the chromatograms obtained with the reference solution and the test solution. Furthermore, other faint quenching zones may be present in the chromatogram obtained with the test solution.

Top of the plate	
———	———
	2 strong quenching zones
	A quenching zone
———	———
	A quenching zone
	A strong quenching zone (piperine)
Piperine: a quenching zone	
Reference solution	**Test solution**

Detection B Treat with *anisaldehyde solution R* and heat at 100 °C for 5 min; examine in daylight.

Results B See below the sequence of zones present in the chromatograms obtained with the reference solution and the test solution. Furthermore, other zones may be present in the chromatogram obtained with the test solution.

Top of the plate	
	A purple-grey zone
	———
	A purple zone
Borneol: a yellowish-brown zone	A violet zone
	A purple-grey zone
———	
Piperine: a green or brownish zone	A green or brownish zone (piperine)
Reference solution	**Test solution**

HERBAL DRUGS

TESTS

Foreign matter (*2.8.2*)
Maximum 3 per cent.

Loss on drying (*2.2.32*)
Maximum 11.0 per cent, determined on 1.000 g of the freshly powdered herbal drug (355) (*2.9.12*) by drying in an oven at 105 °C for 2 h.

Total ash (*2.4.16*)
Maximum 5.0 per cent.

ASSAY

Essential oil (*2.8.12*)
Use 25.0 g of the freshly, coarsely powdered herbal drug (1400) (*2.9.12*), a 1000 mL round-bottomed flask, 400 mL of *water R* as the distillation liquid and 0.5 mL of *xylene R* in the graduated tube. Distil at a rate of 2-3 mL/min for 3 h.

Piperine
Liquid chromatography (*2.2.29*). *Carry out the assay protected from light.*

Test solution Disperse 0.250 g of the powdered herbal drug (355) (*2.9.12*) in 40 mL of *ethanol (96 per cent) R*. Sonicate for 20 min and filter. Rinse the flask and the filter with 5 mL of *ethanol (96 per cent) R*, combine the filtrate and washings and dilute to 50.0 mL with the same solvent. Filter through a membrane filter (nominal pore size 0.45 μm).

Reference solution (a) Dissolve 15.0 mg of *piperine CRS* in *ethanol (96 per cent) R* and dilute to 100.0 mL with the same solvent.

Reference solution (b) Disperse 0.250 g of *long pepper for system suitability HRS* (355) (*2.9.12*) in 40 mL of *ethanol (96 per cent) R*. Sonicate for 20 min and filter. Rinse the flask and the filter with 5 mL of *ethanol (96 per cent) R*, combine the filtrate and washings and dilute to 50.0 mL with the same solvent. Filter through a membrane filter (nominal pore size 0.45 μm).

Column:
— *size: l* = 0.15 m, Ø = 4.6 mm;
— *stationary phase*: end-capped octadecylsilyl silica gel for chromatography R (5 μm).

Mobile phase:
— *mobile phase A: water R;*
— *mobile phase B: acetonitrile R;*

Time (min)	Mobile phase A (per cent *V/V*)	Mobile phase B (per cent *V/V*)
0 - 5	50	50
5 - 20	50 → 5	50 → 95
20 - 22	5 → 0	95 → 100

Flow rate 1.0 mL/min.

Detection Spectrophotometer at 343 nm.

Injection 10 μL.

Retention time Piperine = about 10 min.

Identification of peaks Use the chromatogram supplied with *long pepper for system suitability HRS* and the chromatogram obtained with reference solution (b) to identify the peak due to piperine and peak 2.

System suitability Reference solution (b):
— *peak-to-valley ratio*: minimum 4, where H_p = height above the baseline of peak 2 and H_v = height above the baseline of the lowest point of the curve separating the peak due to piperine from peak 2.

Calculate the percentage content of piperine using the following expression:

$$\frac{A_1 \times m_2 \times p}{A_2 \times m_1 \times 2}$$

A_1 = area of the peak due to piperine in the chromatogram obtained with the test solution;

A_2 = area of the peak due to piperine in the chromatogram obtained with reference solution (a);

m_1 = mass of the herbal drug to be examined used to prepare the test solution, in grams;

m_2 = mass of *piperine CRS* used to prepare reference solution (a), in grams;

p = percentage content of piperine in *piperine CRS*.

———————————————————————— Ph Eur

Loosestrife

(Ph Eur monograph 1537)

Ph Eur ————————————————————————

DEFINITION
Dried flowering tops, whole or cut, of *Lythrum salicaria* L.

Content
Minimum 5.0 per cent of tannins, expressed as pyrogallol ($C_6H_6O_3$; M_r 126.1) (dried drug).

IDENTIFICATION

A. The stems are rigid, 4-angled, branching at the top, brownish-green, longitudinally wrinkled and pubescent. The leaves are opposite, decussate, rarely verticillate in threes and sometimes alternate at the inflorescence which forms a long terminal spike. The leaves are sessile, lanceolate and cordate at the base, 5-15 cm long and 1-2.5 cm wide, pubescent on the lower surface; the subsidiary veins form arcs that anastomose near the leaf margin. The flowers have a pubescent, tubular, persistent gamosepalous calyx, 4-8 mm long, consisting of 6 sepals bearing 6 small, triangular teeth alternating with 6 large, acute teeth at least half as long as the tube; a polypetalous corolla consisting of 6 violet-pink petals, each expanded at the top with a wavy outline and narrowing at the base. The androecium consists of 2 verticils of 6 stamens (1 verticil with short, barely emerging stamens, the other with long stamens extending well out of the corolla). The fruit, if formed, is a small capsule included in the persistent calyx.

B. Microscopic examination (*2.8.23*). The powder is greenish-yellow. Examine under a microscope using *chloral hydrate solution R*. The powder shows the following diagnostic characters (Figure 1537.-1): unicellular [Ea] or bicellular [Aa], uniseriate, thick-walled, finely pitted covering trichomes from the epidermis of the leaf [A] and stem [E]; numerous uniseriate, unicellular [Ga] or bicellular [Gb], thin-walled, finely pitted, annularly striated covering trichomes from the calyx, in side view [G]; transparent violet-pink fragments from the petals [F] consisting of epidermal cells with sinuous walls and a grainy cuticle [Fa], covering fine spiral vessels [Fb]; fragments of parenchyma from the leaf [D] with numerous cells containing cluster crystals of calcium oxalate [Da], associated with spiral vessels [Db]; pollen grains with 3 pores and a thin and slightly granular exine [C]; fragments of the upper epidermis of the leaf [A] with large polygonal cells and sinuous walls, covered by a finely striated cuticle [Ab]; fragments of the lower epidermis of the leaf [B] with smaller polygonal cells [Ba] and anomocytic stomata [Bb] (*2.8.3*);

chlorogenic acid in the chromatogram obtained with the reference solution, a yellow fluorescent zone similar in position to the zone due to hyperoside in the chromatogram obtained with the reference solution, and a bright green fluorescent zone corresponding to the zone due to vitexin in the chromatogram obtained with the reference solution.

TESTS
Loss on drying (*2.2.32*)
Maximum 12.0 per cent, determined on 1.000 g of the powdered herbal drug (355) (*2.9.12*) by drying in an oven at 105 °C.

Total ash (*2.4.16*)
Maximum 7.0 per cent.

ASSAY
Carry out the determination of tannins in herbal drugs (*2.8.14*). Use 0.750 g of the powdered herbal drug (180) (*2.9.12*).

Ph Eur

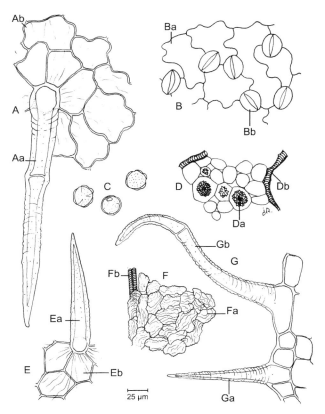

Figure 1537.-1. − *Illustration for identification test B of powdered herbal drug of loosestrife*

fragments of the stem [E] consisting of polygonal cells with straight anticlinal walls and a striated cuticle [Eb].

C. Thin-layer chromatography (*2.2.27*).

Test solution To 1.0 g of the powdered herbal drug (355) (*2.9.12*) add 10 mL of *methanol R* and heat in a water-bath at 65 °C for 5 min with frequent shaking. Cool and filter. Dilute the filtrate to 10 mL with *methanol R*.

Reference solution Dissolve 0.5 mg of *chlorogenic acid R*, 1 mg of *hyperoside R*, 1 mg of *rutin R* and 1 mg of *vitexin R* in 10 mL of *methanol R*.

Plate TLC silica gel plate R.

Mobile phase anhydrous acetic acid R, anhydrous formic acid R, water R, ethyl acetate R (7.5:7.5:18:67 V/V/V/V).

Application 10 μL as bands.

Development Over a path of 15 cm.

Drying At 100-105 °C.

Detection Treat the still-warm plate with a 10 g/L solution of *diphenylboric acid aminoethyl ester R* in *methanol R*. Subsequently treat with a 50 g/L solution of *macrogol 400 R* in *methanol R*. Allow to dry in air for 30 min and examine in ultraviolet light at 365 nm.

Results The chromatogram obtained with the reference solution shows in the lower third a yellowish-brown fluorescent zone due to rutin and in the middle third a light blue fluorescent zone due to chlorogenic acid, above it a yellowish-brown fluorescent zone due to hyperoside and a green fluorescent zone due to vitexin. The chromatogram obtained with the test solution shows a bright green fluorescent zone slightly above the zone due to rutin in the chromatogram obtained with the reference solution, a yellow fluorescent zone similar in position to the zone due to

Lovage Root

(*Ph Eur monograph 1233*)

Ph Eur

DEFINITION
Whole or cut, dried rhizome and root of *Levisticum officinale* Koch.

Content
Minimum 4.0 mL/kg of essential oil for the whole drug and minimum 3.0 mL/kg of essential oil for the cut drug (dried drug).

IDENTIFICATION
A. The rhizome and the large roots are often split longitudinally. The rhizome is short, up to 5 cm in diameter, light greyish-brown or yellowish-brown, simple or with several protuberances; the roots, showing little ramification, are the same colour as the rhizome; they are usually up to 1.5 cm thick and up to about 25 cm long; the fracture is usually smooth and shows a very wide yellowish-white bark and a narrow brownish-yellow wood.

B. Microscopic examination (*2.8.23*). The powder is brownish-yellow. Examine under a microscope using *chloral hydrate solution R*. The powder shows the following diagnostic characters: cork cells, polygonal or rounded in surface view, with brown contents; abundant parenchyma, mostly thin-walled and rounded but some with thicker walls; groups of small, reticulately thickened vessels embedded in small-celled, unlignified parenchyma; fragments of larger vessels with reticulate thickening, up to 125 μm in diameter; fragments of secretory canals up to 180 μm wide. Examine under a microscope using a 50 per cent *V/V* solution of *glycerol R*. The powder shows starch granules, simple, rounded or ovoid, up to about 12 μm, and numerous larger, compound granules, many with several components.

C. Examine the chromatograms obtained in the test for species of *Angelica* and *Ligusticum* described in the European Pharmacopoeia.

Results A See below the sequence of zones present in the chromatograms obtained with the reference solution and the test solution. Furthermore, other weak fluorescent zones may be present in the chromatogram obtained with the test solution.

Top of the plate	
(Z)-Ligustilide: a bluish-white fluorescent zone	A bluish-white fluorescent zone
———	———
Osthole: a blue fluorescent zone	
Imperatorin: a whitish fluorescent zone	A weak whitish fluorescent zone
———	———
	A weak whitish fluorescent zone
Reference solution	**Test solution**

Results B   See below the sequence of zones present in the chromatograms obtained with the reference solution and the test solution. Furthermore, other weak quenching zones may be present in the chromatogram obtained with the test solution.

Top of the plate	
(Z)-Ligustilide: a bluish fluorescent zone	A bluish fluorescent zone
———	———
Osthole: a quenching zone	A weak quenching zone
Imperatorin: a quenching zone	
———	———
Reference solution	**Test solution**

Results C   See below the sequence of zones present in the chromatograms obtained with the reference solution and the test solution. Furthermore, other faint zones may be present in the chromatogram obtained with the test solution.

Top of the plate	
	2 prominent reddish zones
(Z)-Ligustilide: a grey zone	A grey zone
———	———
Osthole: a violet zone	
Imperatorin: a grey zone	
	———
	2 purple zones
	A distinct brown zone
Reference solution	**Test solution**

TESTS

Species of *Angelica* and *Ligusticum* described in the European Pharmacopoeia
Thin-layer chromatography (*2.2.27*).

Test solution   To 1 g of the freshly powdered herbal drug (355) (*2.9.12*) add 4 mL of *heptane R* and sonicate for 5 min. Centrifuge the mixture and use the supernatant.

Reference solution   Dissolve 1 mg of *imperatorin R*, 1 mg of *(Z)-ligustilide R* and 1 mg of *osthole R* in 10 mL of *methanol R*.

Plate   TLC silica gel F_{254} plate R (2-10 µm).

Mobile phase   glacial acetic acid R, ethyl acetate R, toluene R (1:10:90 *V/V/V*).

Application   4 µL, as bands of 8 mm.

Development   Over a path of 6 cm.

Drying   In air.

Detection A   Examine in ultraviolet light at 365 nm.

Results A   The chromatogram obtained with the test solution shows no blue fluorescent zone just below or above the zone due to imperatorin in the chromatogram obtained with the reference solution.

Detection B   Examine in ultraviolet light at 254 nm.

Results B   The chromatogram obtained with the test solution shows no zone at or just below the zone due to imperatorin in the chromatogram obtained with the reference solution.

Detection C   Treat the plate with a solution of 20 mL of *sulfuric acid R* in 180 mL of ice-cooled *methanol R*; heat at 100-105 °C for 5 min and examine in daylight.

Results C   The chromatogram obtained with the test solution shows no purple zone between the 2 reddish zones at the top of the chromatogram and the zone due to (Z)-ligustilide in the chromatogram obtained with the reference solution; the chromatogram obtained with the test solution shows no purple zone between the zones due to (Z)-ligustilide and osthole in the chromatogram obtained with the reference solution.

Foreign matter (*2.8.2*)
Maximum 3 per cent, determined on 50 g.

Loss on drying (*2.2.32*)
Maximum 12.0 per cent, determined on 1.000 g of the powdered herbal drug (355) (*2.9.12*) by drying in an oven at 105 °C for 2 h.

Total ash (*2.4.16*)
Maximum 8.0 per cent.

Ash insoluble in hydrochloric acid (*2.8.1*)
Maximum 2.0 per cent.

ASSAY

Carry out the determination of essential oils in herbal drugs (*2.8.12*). Use a 2 L flask, 10 drops of *liquid paraffin R*, 500 mL of *water R* as the distillation liquid and 0.50 mL of *xylene R* in the graduated tube. Reduce the herbal drug to a powder (500) (*2.9.12*) and immediately use 40.0 g for the determination. Distil at a rate of 2-3 mL/min for 4 h.

———————————————— *Ph Eur*

Magnolia Officinalis Bark

(*Ph Eur monograph 2567*)

Ph Eur ————————————————————————

DEFINITION

Dried stem and branch bark of *Magnolia officinalis* Rehder et E.H.Wilson.

Content

Minimum 2.0 per cent of the sum of magnolol ($C_{18}H_{18}O_2$; M_r 266.3) and honokiol ($C_{18}H_{18}O_2$; M_r 266.3) (dried drug).

IDENTIFICATION

A. Fragments of stem and branch bark, quilled singly or double quilled, about 30 cm long and 2-7 mm thick. The outer surface is brownish-grey, rough, sometimes scaly, easily exfoliated, with distinct lenticels and longitudinal striations. The inner surface is reddish-brown or dark brown, smooth, with numerous fine longitudinal striations. The texture is hard and difficult to break. The fracture is granular, brownish-grey in the outer layers and reddish-brown or dark brown in the inner layers.

B. Microscopic examination (*2.8.23*). The powder is yellowish-brown. Examine under a microscope using *chloral hydrate solution R*. The powder shows the following diagnostic characters: numerous sclereids of varying shape and size, up to 100 μm long, often branched, free or in groups, with conspicuous pit canals; oval or rounded oil cells, about 60 μm in diameter, with orange-yellow contents; narrow fibres with thick walls and often in bundles; brown cork fragments.

C. Thin-layer chromatography (*2.2.27*).

Test solution Reduce to a powder (355) (*2.9.12*), avoiding heating. To 0.5 g of the powdered herbal drug add 5 mL of *methanol R*, sonicate for 5 min, centrifuge, and use the supernatant. Filter through a membrane filter (nominal pore size 0.45 μm) if necessary.

Reference solution Dissolve 1 mg of *honokiol R*, 1 mg of *magnolol R* and 2 mg of *eugenol R* in 1 mL of *methanol R*.

Plate *TLC silica gel F_{254} plate R* (5-40 μm) [or *TLC silica gel F_{254} plate R* (2-10 μm)].

Mobile phase *methanol R*, *ethyl acetate R*, *toluene R* (4:8:120 *V/V/V*).

Application 5 μL [or 2 μL] as bands of 15 mm [or 8 mm].

Development Over a path of 15 cm [or 7 cm].

Drying In air.

Detection A Examine in ultraviolet light at 254 nm.

Results A See below the sequence of zones present in the chromatograms obtained with the reference solution and the test solution. Furthermore, other faint zones may be present in the chromatogram obtained with the test solution.

Top of the plate	
———	———
Eugenol: a faint quenching zone	
Magnolol: a dark blue fluorescent zone	A dark blue fluorescent zone (magnolol)
Honokiol: a quenching zone	A quenching zone (honokiol)
———	———
Reference solution	**Test solution**

Detection B Treat with *vanillin reagent R*, heat at 100-105 °C for 5-10 min and examine in daylight.

Results B See below the sequence of zones present in the chromatograms obtained with the reference solution and the test solution. Furthermore, other faint zones of various colours may be present in the chromatogram obtained with the test solution.

TESTS

Loss on drying (*2.2.32*)
Maximum 11.0 per cent, determined on 1.000 g of the powdered herbal drug (355) (*2.9.12*) by drying in an oven at 105 °C for 2 h.

Total ash (*2.4.16*)
Maximum 5.0 per cent.

Ash insoluble in hydrochloric acid (*2.8.1*)
Maximum 3.0 per cent.

Top of the plate	
	A bluish-violet zone
	———
Eugenol: a brown zone	
Magnolol: a pinkish-violet zone	A pinkish-violet zone (magnolol)
Honokiol: a dark violet zone	A dark violet zone (honokiol)
	A bluish-violet zone
———	———
Reference solution	**Test solution**

ASSAY

Liquid chromatography (*2.2.29*).

Test solution To 0.500 g of the powdered herbal drug (355) (*2.9.12*) add 80 mL of *methanol R* and heat in a water-bath under a reflux condenser for 30 min. Cool, then dilute to 100.0 mL with *methanol R*. Filter through a membrane filter (nominal pore size 0.45 μm).

Reference solution (a) Dissolve 4.0 mg of *honokiol CRS* and 4.0 mg of *magnolol CRS* in *methanol R* and dilute to 20.0 mL with the same solvent.

Reference solution (b) Dissolve 2.0 mg of *honokiol CRS* in 2.0 mL of *acetonitrile R*. To 1.0 mL of the solution add 15 μL of *acetic anhydride R* and mix. Heat at 50 °C for 60 min. Cool. Add successively, mixing after each addition, 16 μL of *concentrated ammonia R*, 1.0 mL of *acetonitrile R* and 2.0 mL of *water R*. Filter through a membrane filter (nominal pore size 0.45 μm).

Column:
— *size: l* = 0.25 m, Ø = 4.6 mm;
— *stationary phase*: end-capped octadecylsilyl silica gel for chromatography R1 (5 μm);
— *temperature*: 30 °C.

Mobile phase 0.5 per cent *V/V* solution of *acetic acid R*, *acetonitrile for chromatography R* (40:60 *V/V*).

Flow rate 1.0 mL/min.

Detection Spectrophotometer at 290 nm.

Injection 10 μL.

Run time Twice the retention time of honokiol for the test solution and reference solution (a); 3 times the retention time of honokiol for reference solution (b).

Relative retention With reference to honokiol (retention time = about 8 min): magnolol = about 1.4; honokiol monoacetate isomer 1 = about 1.5; honokiol monoacetate isomer 2 = about 1.6; honokiol diacetate = about 2.6.

System suitability Reference solution (b):
— *resolution*: minimum 1.8 between the peaks due to honokiol monoacetate isomers 1 and 2.

Calculate the sum of the percentage contents of honokiol and magnolol using the following expression:

$$\frac{A_1 \times m_2 \times p_1 \times 5}{A_2 \times m_1} + \frac{A_3 \times m_3 \times p_2 \times 5}{A_4 \times m_1}$$

A_1 = area of the peak due to honokiol in the chromatogram obtained with the test solution;

A_2 = area of the peak due to honokiol in the chromatogram obtained with reference solution (a);

A_3 = area of the peak due to magnolol in the chromatogram obtained with the test solution;

A_4 = area of the peak due to magnolol in the chromatogram obtained with reference solution (a);

m_1 = mass of the herbal drug to be examined used to prepare the test solution, in grams;

m_2 = mass of *honokiol CRS* used to prepare reference solution (a), in grams;

m_3 = mass of *magnolol CRS* used to prepare reference solution (a), in grams;

p_1 = percentage content of honokiol in *honokiol CRS*;

p_2 = percentage content of magnolol in *magnolol CRS*.

_____ *Ph Eur*

Magnolia Officinalis Flower

(*Ph Eur monograph 2568*)

Ph Eur _____

DEFINITION
Steamed and dried, unopened flower of *Magnolia officinalis* Rehder et E.H. Wilson.

Content
Minimum 0.20 per cent of the sum of magnolol ($C_{18}H_{18}O_2$; M_r 266.3) and honokiol ($C_{18}H_{18}O_2$; M_r 266.3) (dried drug).

IDENTIFICATION
A. The greyish-yellow pedicel is short (0.5-2 cm) and densely tomentose. The brown or reddish-brown flower bud is elongated, conical, 4-7 cm long and 1.5-2.5 cm in diameter at the base; it usually consists of 12 perianth segments in several whorls. The stamens are numerous with a fine, short filament and a linear, yellowish-brown anther. The carpels are free and numerous, spirally arranged on a conical receptacle.

B. Microscopic examination (*2.8.23*). The powder is reddish-brown. Examine under a microscope using *chloral hydrate solution R*. The powder shows the following diagnostic characters: fragments of the perianth segments with polyhedral or elliptical epidermal cells, with irregularly thickened walls and anomocytic stomata (4-6 subsidiary cells) (*2.8.3*), accompanied by parenchyma that includes oval or rounded oil cells about 50 μm in diameter with orange-yellow contents; certain fragments contain epidermal cells with rounded papillae; numerous, branched sclereids, with channelled walls and a large lumen, about 15 μm in diameter; numerous elliptical pollen grains about 50 μm long and 40 μm wide, with a smooth exine.

C. Examine the chromatograms obtained in the test for other *Magnolia* species.

Detection A Examine in ultraviolet light at 254 nm.

Results A See below the sequence of zones present in the chromatograms obtained with the reference solution and the test solution. Furthermore, other faint zones may be present in the chromatogram obtained with the test solution.

Top of the plate	
Eugenol: a faint quenching zone	
Magnolol: a dark blue fluorescent zone	A dark blue fluorescent zone (magnolol)
Honokiol: a quenching zone	A quenching zone (honokiol)
Reference solution	**Test solution**

Detection B Treat with *vanillin reagent R*, heat at 100-105 °C for 5-10 min and examine in daylight.

Results B See below the sequence of zones present in the chromatograms obtained with the reference solution and the test solution. Furthermore, other faint zones of various colours may be present in the chromatogram obtained with the test solution.

Top of the plate	
	A bluish-violet zone
Eugenol: a brown zone	
Magnolol: a pinkish-violet zone	A pinkish-violet zone (magnolol)
Honokiol: a dark violet zone	A dark violet zone (honokiol)
	A bluish-violet zone
Reference solution	**Test solution**

TESTS
Other Magnolia species
Thin-layer chromatography (*2.2.27*).

Test solution Reduce the herbal drug to a powder (710) (*2.9.12*), avoiding heating. To 0.5 g of the powdered herbal drug add 2.5 mL of *methanol R*. Sonicate for 15 min at a power of 80 W and a frequency of 37 kHz (sonication time may be adapted according to the power and frequency used), then centrifuge at 1500-2000 g for 10 min and transfer the supernatant to a 5 mL flask. Add 2 mL of *methanol R* to the residue, sonicate for 15 min and centrifuge. Transfer the supernatant into the same 5 mL flask. Dilute to 5 mL with *methanol R*. Filter through a membrane filter (nominal pore size 0.45 μm) if necessary.

Reference solution Dissolve 1 mg of *honokiol R*, 1 mg of *magnolol R* and 2 mg of *eugenol R* in 4 mL of *methanol R*.

Plate TLC silica gel F_{254} plate R (2-10 μm).

Mobile phase methanol R, ethyl acetate R, toluene R (1:5:30 *V/V/V*).

Application 8 μL as bands of 8 mm.

Development Over a path of 7 cm.

Drying In air.

Detection Examine in ultraviolet light at 365 nm.

Results The chromatogram obtained with the test solution shows no blue fluorescent zone in the lower part of the plate and no green fluorescent zone in the upper part, nor any other fluorescent zone.

Loss on drying (*2.2.32*)

Maximum 11.0 per cent, determined on 1.000 g of the powdered herbal drug (710) (*2.9.12*) by drying in an oven at 105 °C.

Total ash (*2.4.16*)

Maximum 8.0 per cent.

ASSAY

Liquid chromatography (*2.2.29*).

Test solution Reduce the herbal drug to a powder (710) (*2.9.12*) using a blade grinder equipped with a double-walled grinding chamber cooled to a temperature of about 10 °C. To 0.500 g of the powdered herbal drug add 10 mL of *methanol R*. Sonicate for 1 h at a power of 80 W and a frequency of 37 kHz (sonication time may be adapted according to the power and frequency used). Change the water of the ultrasonic bath after 30 min of sonication to prevent heating. Centrifuge at 1500-2000 g for 15 min. Transfer the supernatant to a 20.0 mL flask. Add 9.5 mL of *methanol R* to the residue. Repeat the sonication for 1 h. Change the water of the ultrasonic bath after 30 min of sonication to prevent heating. Centrifuge. Transfer the supernatant to the same 20.0 mL flask. Cool, then dilute to 20.0 mL with *methanol R*. Filter through a membrane filter (nominal pore size 0.45 μm).

Reference solution (a) Dissolve 5.0 mg of *honokiol CRS* in *methanol R* and dilute to 5.0 mL with the same solvent. Dilute 1.0 mL of the solution to 25.0 mL with *methanol R*.

Reference solution (b) Dissolve 6.0 mg of *magnolol CRS* in *methanol R* and dilute to 20.0 mL with the same solvent.

Reference solution (c) Dissolve 2.0 mg of *honokiol R* in 2.0 mL of *acetonitrile R*. Add 30 μL of *acetic anhydride R* and mix. Heat at 50 °C for 60 min. Cool. Add successively, mixing after each addition, 32 μL of *concentrated ammonia R*, 2.0 mL of *acetonitrile R* and 4.0 mL of *water R*. Filter through a membrane filter (nominal pore size 0.45 μm).

Column:
— *size: l* = 0.15 m, Ø = 4.6 mm;
— *stationary phase: end-capped polar-embedded octadecylsilyl amorphous organosilica polymer R* (3.5 μm);
— *temperature*: 25 ± 2 °C.

Mobile phase:
— *mobile phase A*: anhydrous formic acid R, water R (0.1:99.9 *V/V*);
— *mobile phase B*: acetonitrile for chromatography R;

Time (min)	Mobile phase A (per cent *V/V*)	Mobile phase B (per cent *V/V*)
0 - 20	47	53
20 - 22	47 → 5	53 → 95
22 - 27	5	95

Flow rate 1.0 mL/min.

Detection Spectrophotometer at 292 nm.

Injection 20 μL.

Relative retention With reference to honokiol (retention time = about 10 min): magnolol = about 1.3; honokiol monoacetate isomer 1 = about 1.4; honokiol monoacetate isomer 2 = about 1.5; honokiol diacetate = about 1.9.

System suitability Reference solution (c):
— *resolution*: minimum 2.0 between the peaks due to honokiol monoacetate isomers 1 and 2.

If necessary, dilute the test solution to obtain peaks of honokiol and magnolol that are similar in height to the corresponding peaks in reference solutions (a) and (b).

Calculate the sum of the percentage contents of honokiol and magnolol using the following expression:

$$\frac{A_1 \times m_2 \times 0.16 \times p_1 \times d}{A_2 \times m_1} + \frac{A_3 \times m_3 \times p_2 \times d}{A_4 \times m_1}$$

A_1 = area of the peak due to honokiol in the chromatogram obtained with the test solution;

A_2 = area of the peak due to honokiol in the chromatogram obtained with reference solution (a);

A_3 = area of the peak due to magnolol in the chromatogram obtained with the test solution;

A_4 = area of the peak due to magnolol in the chromatogram obtained with reference solution (b);

m_1 = mass of the herbal drug to be examined used to prepare the test solution, in grams;

m_2 = mass of *honokiol CRS* used to prepare reference solution (a), in grams;

m_3 = mass of *magnolol CRS* used to prepare reference solution (b), in grams;

p_1 = percentage content of honokiol in *honokiol CRS*;

p_2 = percentage content of magnolol in *magnolol CRS*;

d = dilution factor of the test solution.

Ph Eur

Mallow Flower

(*Ph Eur monograph 1541*)

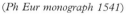

Ph Eur

DEFINITION

Whole or fragmented dried flower of *Malva sylvestris* L. or its cultivated varieties.

IDENTIFICATION

A. The flower consists of an epicalyx with 3 oblong or elliptical-lanceolate parts that are shorter than those of the calyx and situated immediately below it; a calyx with 5 pubescent triangular lobes, gamosepalous at the base; a corolla 3-4 times longer than the calyx with 5 wedge-shaped, notched petals fused to the staminal tube at their base; numerous stamens, the filaments of which fuse into a staminal tube covered by small star-shaped trichomes and occasional simple trichomes visible using a lens; numerous wrinkled carpels, glabrous or sometimes pubescent, enclosed in the staminal tube and arranged into a circle around a central style ending with numerous filiform stigmas. In cultivated varieties, the epicalyx is 3-7 partite, the calyx 5-8 partite and the corolla 5-10 partite.

B. Reduce to a powder (355) (*2.9.12*). The powder is bluish-grey. Examine under a microscope using *chloral hydrate solution R*. The powder shows the following diagnostic characters (Figure 1541.-1): unicellular, thick-walled, flexuous covering trichomes, from the calyx and the epicalyx, up to 2 mm in length, whole [L] or, most often, fragmented [Q]; fragments of the epidermis of the sepals in surface view [D, J] with anomocytic stomata (*2.8.3*) [Dc]; club-shaped glandular trichomes with multicellular heads [Db] and short unicellular covering trichomes, somewhat curved, either isolated [JJ] or in star-shaped groups of 2-6 [Da]; fragments of covering trichomes [N]; isolated glandular trichomes in surface view, [F]; or in transverse section [G]; fragments of the mesophyll of the calyx and the epicalyx whose cells contain small cluster crystals of calcium oxalate [K]; veins of the sepals [P] with vessels [Pa] accompanied by cells with cluster crystals of calcium oxalate [Pb]; fragments of petal epidermis, with elongated cells and sinuous margins, narrow in the wild plant [A], shorter and broader in the cultivated varieties [B], bearing sessile glandular trichomes with multicellular club-shaped heads [Ba, C, E]; fragments of petal mesophyll [H] consisting of large mucilage cells [Hc], sometimes cells with small cluster crystals of calcium oxalate [Hb] and spiral vessels [Ha]; spherical pollen grains, about 150 μm in diameter, with a roughly spiny exine [M].

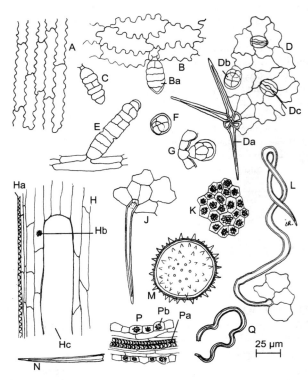

Figure 1541.-1.– *Illustration for identification test B of powdered herbal drug of mallow flower*

C. Thin-layer chromatography (*2.2.27*).

Test solution   To 1 g of the powdered drug (355) (*2.9.12*) add 10 mL of *ethanol (60 per cent V/V) R*. Stir for 15 min and filter.

Reference solution   0.5 g/L solution of *quinaldine red R* in *ethanol (96 per cent) R*.

Plate   *TLC silica gel plate R*.

Mobile phase   *glacial acetic acid R, water R, butanol R* (15:30:60 *V/V/V*).

Application   10 μL of the test solution and 5 μL of the reference solution, as bands.

Development   Over a path of 10 cm.

Drying   In air.

Detection   Examine in daylight.

Results   The chromatogram obtained with the reference solution shows an orange-red zone in the upper part of the middle third ; the chromatogram obtained with the test solution shows, below the zone in the chromatogram obtained with the reference solution, 2 violet zones in the

middle third, with the principal zone (6″-malonyl malvin) situated just below the other violet zone (malvin).

TESTS

Loss on drying (*2.2.32*)
Maximum 12.0 per cent, determined on 1.000 g of the powdered drug by drying in an oven at 105 °C.

Total ash (*2.4.16*)
Maximum 14.0 per cent.

Ash insoluble in hydrochloric acid (*2.8.1*)
Maximum 2.0 per cent.

Swelling index (*2.8.4*)
Minimum 15, determined on 0.2 g of the powdered drug (710) (*2.9.12*) moistened with 0.5 mL of *anhydrous ethanol R*

—————— *Ph Eur*

Mallow Leaf

(*Ph Eur monograph 2391*)

Ph Eur —————————————————————

DEFINITION

Whole or fragmented, dried leaf of *Malva sylvestris* L., *Malva neglecta* Wallr. or a mixture of both species.

IDENTIFICATION

A. The leaves of *M. sylvestris* are up to 12 cm long and up to 15 cm wide with 3, 5 or 7 lobes and sinuate at the base; the leaves of *M. neglecta* are up to 9 cm long and wide, round or kidney-shaped with 5-7 indistinct lobes. The leaves of both species have irregular dentate margins and are green or brownish-green. The abaxial surface of the lamina bears more hairs and shows a more prominent venation than the adaxial surface. The major veins on the upper surface of the leaves and the petioles may be violet. The petioles are as long as the leaves, up to 2 mm wide, rounded and somewhat flattened, longitudinally slightly grooved, green or brownish-green or violet. The fragmented drug consists of occasionally agglomerated, crumpled pieces of leaves showing prominent veins.

B. Microscopic examination (*2.8.23*). The powder is green or yellowish-green. Examine under a microscope using *chloral hydrate solution R*. The powder shows the following diagnostic characters (Figure 2391.-1): fragments of the lamina, in transverse section [F], consisting of the lower epidermis, in surface view [C], and the upper epidermis, in surface view [D] or in transverse section [Fb], with cells that show straight, or more or less sinuous anticlinal walls; stomata mostly anisocytic (*2.8.3*) on both surfaces [Ca, Da]; long covering trichomes with thickened walls and tapering to a point at the apex, usually unicellular, whole [A, Fa] or fragmented [Db], but in *M. Sylvestris* they may be stellate with 2-8 components [H], each strongly pitted at the base; club-shaped glandular trichomes composed of 2-6 cells [E] occur in both species; fragments of the mesophyll consisting of palisade parenchyma, in surface view [Dc] or in transverse section [Fc], and spongy mesophyll cells containing mucilage, cells containing cluster crystals of calcium oxalate, often associated with vessels [B]; occasional spherical pollen grains, 110-170 μm in diameter, with a spiny exine [G].

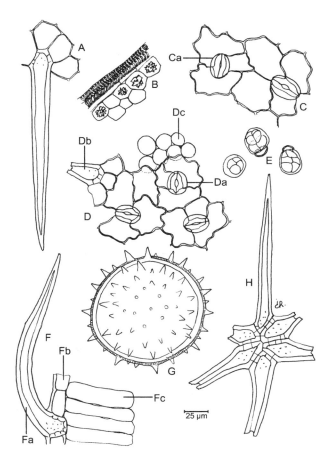

Figure 2391.-1. − *Illustration for identification test B of powdered herbal drug of mallow leaf*

Top of the plate	
	____
Hyperoside: a yellow fluorescent zone	
	A yellow fluorescent zone
	____
Rutin: a yellow fluorescent zone	
	A yellow fluorescent zone
	A light blue fluorescent zone
	An orange fluorescent zone
	An orange fluorescent zone
Reference solution	**Test solution**

C. Thin-layer chromatography (*2.2.27*).

Test solution To 2.0 g of the powdered drug (710) (*2.9.12*) add 20 mL of an 80 per cent *V/V* solution of *tetrahydrofuran R*; extract for 10 min using sonication and filter.

Reference solution Dissolve 3 mg of *hyperoside R* and 3 mg of *rutin R* in 20 mL of *methanol R*.

Plate *TLC silica gel plate R* (5-40 μm) [or *TLC silica gel plate R* (2-10 μm)].

Mobile phase *anhydrous formic acid R*, *anhydrous acetic acid R*, *water R*, *ethyl formate R*, *3-pentanone R* (4:11:14:20:50 *V/V/V/V/V*).

Application 10 μL [or 4 μL] as bands of 10 mm [or 8 mm].

Development Over a path of 10-12 cm [or 6 cm].

Drying In air.

Detection Heat at 100 °C for 10 min; spray or dip the warm plate in a 10 g/L solution of *diphenylboric acid aminoethyl ester R* in *methanol R*; remove the solvent with cold air; spray or dip the plate in a 50 g/L solution of *macrogol 400 R* in *methanol R*, dry in air and examine after 15 min in ultraviolet light at 365 nm.

Results See below the sequence of fluorescent zones present in the chromatograms obtained with the reference solution and the test solution. Furthermore, other faint fluorescent zones may be present in the chromatogram obtained with the test solution.

TESTS

Foreign matter (*2.8.2*)
Maximum 5 per cent of foreign organs, maximum 5 per cent of leaves with blisters of spores of *Puccinia malvacearum* and maximum 2 per cent of foreign elements.

Foreign organs can be flowers, fruits and parts of the stem. The blisters of spores on the leaves are mostly 1 mm wide, and red or brown. Examine under a microscope using *chloral hydrate solution R*. The spores of *Puccinia malvacearum* are oblong or oval with brownish walls and a small appendage.

Loss on drying (*2.2.32*)
Maximum 12.0 per cent, determined on 1.000 g of the powdered drug (710) (*2.9.12*) by drying in an oven at 105 °C for 2 h.

Total ash (*2.4.16*)
Maximum 17.0 per cent.

Ash insoluble in hydrochloric acid (*2.8.1*)
Maximum 3.0 per cent.

Swelling index (*2.8.4*)
Minimum 7, determined on 1.0 g of the powdered drug (710) (*2.9.12*).

Ph Eur

Mandarin Oil

(*Ph Eur monograph 2355*)

Ph Eur

DEFINITION
Essential oil obtained without heating, by suitable mechanical treatment, from the peel of the fresh fruit of *Citrus reticulata* Blanco.

CHARACTERS
Appearance
Greenish, yellow or reddish orange liquid showing blue fluorescence.

Characteristic odour.

IDENTIFICATION
First identification B.
Second identification A.

A. Thin-layer chromatography (*2.2.27*).

Test solution Dilute 0.1 mL of the substance to be examined to 1 mL with *toluene R*.

Reference solution Dissolve 2 μL of *methyl N-methylanthranilate R*, 4 mg of *guaiazulene R* and 10 mg of α-*terpineol R* in 10 mL of *toluene R*.

Plate *TLC silica gel plate R* (5-40 μm) [or *TLC silica gel plate R* (2-10 μm)].

Mobile phase ethyl acetate R, toluene R (15:85 V/V).

Application 10 μL [or 2 μL] as bands.

Development Over a path of 15 cm [or 6 cm].

Drying In air.

Detection A Examine in ultraviolet light at 365 nm.

Results A The intense blue fluorescent zone in the chromatogram obtained with the test solution is similar in position and fluorescence to the zone due to methyl N-methylanthranilate in the chromatogram obtained with the reference solution. Furthermore, other fluorescent zones may be present in the chromatogram obtained with the test solution.

Detection B Spray with a 200 g/L solution of *phosphomolybdic acid R* in *ethanol (96 per cent) R* and heat at 100 °C for 10 min; examine in daylight.

Results B See below the sequence of the zones present in the chromatograms obtained with the reference solution and the test solution. Furthermore, other zones may be present in the chromatogram obtained with the test solution.

Top of the plate	
	A blue zone
Guaiazulene: a blue zone	A blue zone
	A blue zone
————	————
	A blue zone
————	————
α-Terpineol: a blue zone	A blue zone (α-terpineol)
Reference solution	**Test solution**

B. Examine the chromatograms obtained in the test for chromatographic profile.

Results The characteristic peaks in the chromatogram obtained with the test solution are similar in retention time to those in the chromatogram obtained with the reference solution.

TESTS

Relative density (*2.2.5*)
0.848 to 0.855.

Refractive index (*2.2.6*)
1.474 to 1.478.

Optical rotation (*2.2.7*)
+ 64° to + 75°.

Fatty oils and resinified essential oils (*2.8.7*)
It complies with the test.

Chromatographic profile
Gas chromatography (*2.2.28*): use the normalisation procedure.

Test solution Dilute 0.20 g of the substance to be examined to 10.0 mL with *heptane R*.

Reference solution (a) Dilute 5 μL of α-*pinene R*, 5 μL of *sabinene R*, 5 μL of β-*pinene R*, 5 μL of β-*myrcene R*, 5 μL of *p*-cymene R, 70 μL of *limonene R*, 20 μL of γ-*terpinene R* and

5 μL of *methyl N-methylanthranilate R* to 5.0 mL with *heptane R*.

Reference solution (b) Dissolve 5 μL of *limonene R* in 50 mL of *heptane R*. Dilute 0.5 mL of this solution to 5.0 mL with *heptane R*.

Column:
— *material*: fused silica;
— *size*: $l = 60$ m, Ø = 0.25 mm;
— *stationary phase*: *poly(dimethyl)(diphenyl)siloxane R* (film thickness 0.25 μm).

Carrier gas helium for chromatography R.

Flow rate 1.4 mL/min.

Split ratio 1:70.

Temperature:

	Time (min)	Temperature (°C)
Column	0 - 90	50 → 230
Injection port		250
Detector		250

Detection Flame ionisation.

Injection 1 μL.

Elution order Order indicated in the composition of reference solution (a); record the retention times of these substances.

System suitability Reference solution (a):
— *resolution*: minimum 1.5 between the peaks due to sabinene and β-pinene and minimum 1.5 between the peaks due to *p*-cymene and limonene.

Identification of components Using the retention times determined from the chromatogram obtained with reference solution (a), locate the components of reference solution (a) in the chromatogram obtained with the test solution. Disregard the peak due to heptane.

Determine the percentage content of each of these components. The limits are within the following ranges:
— α-*pinene*: 1.6 per cent to 3.0 per cent;
— *sabinene*: maximum 0.3 per cent;
— β-*pinene*: 1.2 per cent to 2.0 per cent;
— β-*myrcene*: 1.5 per cent to 2.0 per cent;
— *p*-cymene: maximum 1.0 per cent;
— *limonene*: 65.0 per cent to 75.0 per cent;
— γ-*terpinene*: 16.0 per cent to 22.0 per cent;
— *methyl N-methylanthranilate*: 0.30 per cent to 0.60 per cent;
— *disregard limit*: area of the principal peak in the chromatogram obtained with reference solution (b).

Residue on evaporation (*2.8.9*)
1.6 per cent to 4.0 per cent, determined after heating on a water-bath for 4 h.

STORAGE
At a temperature not exceeding 25 °C.

_____ *Ph Eur*

Marshmallow Leaf

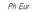

(*Ph Eur monograph 1856*)

Ph Eur _____

DEFINITION

Whole or cut, dried leaf of *Althaea officinalis* L.

IDENTIFICATION

A. The leaves have long petioles and are about 7-10 cm long; the lamina is cordate or ovate with 3-5 shallow lobes and crenate or dentate margins; the venation is palmate. The petioles and both surfaces of the lamina are greyish-green and densely pubescent. Rarely, fragments of the inflorescence or immature fruits may be present.

B. Microscopic examination (*2.8.23*). The powder is greyish-green. Examine under a microscope using *chloral hydrate solution R*. The powder shows the following diagnostic characters (Figure 1856.-1): numerous long, rigid, unicellular covering trichomes with thick walls, pointed at the apex, often fragmented [C], angular and pitted at the base where they are sometimes still united to form stellate structures with up to 8 components, in surface view [B] or in transverse section [E]; few secretory trichomes, isolated, with unicellular stalks and globular, multicellular heads [F]; fragments of the lower [A] and upper [D] leaf epidermises in surface view with anomocytic [Aa] or paracytic [Da] stomata (*2.8.3*), glandular trichomes [Ab] and basal cells of covering trichomes [Ac], often accompanied by palisade parenchyma [Db]; cluster crystals of calcium oxalate, isolated [H] or included in the parenchyma of the mesophyll [Gc, Kb]; fragments of veins [G] with small, spiral [Gb] or annular [Ga] vessels, often accompanied by sheaths containing cluster crystals of calcium oxalate [Gc]; fragments of the lamina, in transverse section [K], showing the epidermises bearing broken covering trichomes [Ka], a symmetrical, heterogeneous mesophyll with some cells containing cluster crystals of calcium oxalate [Kb]; occasional pollen grains, spherical, with a roughly spiny exine, about 150 µm in diameter [J]. Examine under a microscope using *ruthenium red solution R*. The powder shows groups of parenchyma containing mucilage, which stains orange-red.

C. Thin-layer chromatography (*2.2.27*).

Test solution   To 1 g of the powdered herbal drug (355) (*2.9.12*) add 10 mL of *methanol R*. Heat in a water-bath under a reflux condenser for 5 min. Allow to cool and filter. Distil the filtrate under reduced pressure until the total volume is about 2 mL.

Reference solution   Dissolve 2.5 mg of *chlorogenic acid R* and 2.5 mg of *quercitrin R* in 10 mL of *methanol R*.

Plate   *TLC silica gel plate R*.

Mobile phase   anhydrous formic acid R, glacial acetic acid R, water R, ethyl acetate R (11:11:27:100 *V/V/V/V*).

Application   10 µL as bands.

Development   Over a path of 15 cm.

Drying   At 100-105 °C.

Detection   Spray with a 10 g/L solution of *diphenylboric acid aminoethyl ester R* in *methanol R*, then with a 50 g/L solution of *macrogol 400 R* in *methanol R*; allow to dry in air for 30 min and examine in ultraviolet light at 365 nm.

Results   See below the sequence of zones present in the chromatograms obtained with the reference solution and the test solution. Furthermore, other fluorescent zones may be present in the chromatogram obtained with the test solution.

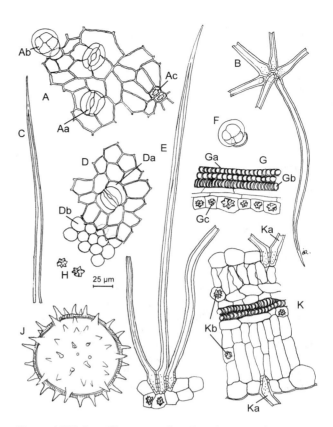

Figure 1856.-1. – *Illustration for identification test B of powdered herbal drug of marshmallow leaf*

Top of the plate	
	A blue fluorescent zone
	A yellow fluorescent zone
Quercitrin: an orange zone	
———	———
	An orange fluorescent zone
	An orange fluorescent zone
Chlorogenic acid: a blue fluorescent zone	
	A blue fluorescent zone
	An orange fluorescent zone
	An intense yellow fluorescent zone
Reference solution	**Test solution**

TESTS

Foreign matter (*2.8.2*)

Maximum 4 per cent of leaves infected by *Puccinia malvacearum*, showing red spots, and maximum 2 per cent of other foreign matter.

Loss on drying (*2.2.32*)

Maximum 10.0 per cent, determined on 1.000 g of the powdered herbal drug (355) (*2.9.12*) by drying in an oven at 105 °C for 2 h.

Total ash (*2.4.16*)

Maximum 18.0 per cent.

Herbal Drugs

Ash insoluble in hydrochloric acid (*2.8.1*)
Maximum 2.0 per cent.

Swelling index (*2.8.4*)
Minimum 12, determined on 0.2 g of the powdered herbal drug (355) (*2.9.12*).

———————————————— *Ph Eur*

Marshmallow Root

(*Ph Eur monograph 1126*)

Ph Eur ————————————————————

DEFINITION
Peeled or unpeeled, whole or cut, dried root of *Althaea officinalis* L.

IDENTIFICATION
A. The unpeeled, non-fragmented drug consists of cylindrical, slightly twisted roots, up to 2 cm thick, with deep longitudinal furrows. The outer surface is greyish-brown and bears numerous rootlet scars. The fracture is fibrous externally, rugged and granular internally. The section shows a more or less thick, whitish bark with brownish periderm, separated by the well-marked, brownish cambium from a white xylem. The stratified structure of the bark and the radiate structure of xylem become more distinct when moistened.

The peeled drug has a greyish-white, finely fibrous outer surface. Cork and external cortical parenchyma are absent.

B. Microscopic examination (*2.8.23*). The powder is greyish-brown (unpeeled root) or whitish (peeled root). Examine under a microscope using *chloral hydrate solution R*.
The powder shows the following diagnostic characters (Figure 1126.-1): fragments of colourless, mainly unlignified, thick-walled fibres [C, D, M] with split or pointed ends [D], sometimes accompanied by parenchymatous cells of the medullary rays [M], or grouped [C]; fragments of vessels, bordered-pitted or with reticulate or scalariform thickenings [G, H]; cluster crystals of calcium oxalate about 20-35 μm, mostly 25-30 μm in size, isolated [K] or included in parenchymatous cells [B]; fragments of parenchyma [E] with cells containing mucilage [Ea, F]; fragments of cork with thin-walled, tabular cells in surface view [A] and transverse section [L] (unpeeled root). Examine under a microscope using *ruthenium red solution R*. The powder shows groups of parenchyma containing mucilage, which stains orange-red.

Examine under a microscope using *water R*. The powder shows numerous starch granules [J], about 3-25 μm in size, occasionally with a longitudinal hilum. The starch granules are mostly simple [Ja], a few being 2-4 compound [Jb].

TESTS
Foreign matter (*2.8.2*)
Maximum 2 per cent of brown deteriorated drug.

Loss on drying (*2.2.32*)
Maximum 12.0 per cent, determined on 1.000 g of the powdered herbal drug (710) (*2.9.12*) by drying in an oven at 105 °C for 2 h.

Total ash (*2.4.16*)
Maximum 6.0 per cent for the peeled root and maximum 8.0 per cent for the unpeeled root.

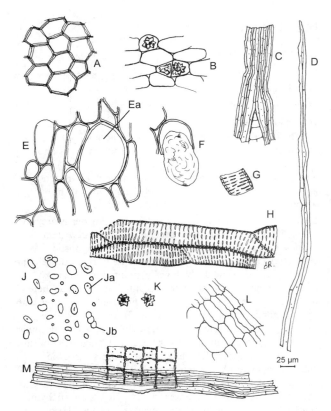

Figure 1126.-1. – *Illustration for identification test B of powdered herbal drug of marshmallow root*

Swelling index (*2.8.4*)
Minimum 10, determined on the powdered herbal drug (710) (*2.9.12*).

———————————————— *Ph Eur*

Mastic

(*Ph Eur monograph 1876*)

Ph Eur ————————————————————

DEFINITION
Dried resinous exudate obtained from stems and branches of *Pistacia lentiscus* L. var. *latifolius* Coss.

Content
Minimum 10 mL/kg of essential oil (anhydrous drug).

IDENTIFICATION
A. Small light yellow to greenish-yellow, non-uniform, spherical or pyriform, clear or opaque, hard glassy fragments.

B. Thin-layer chromatography (*2.2.27*).

Test solution   Dissolve 1 g of the substance to be examined in 10 mL of *methylene chloride R* and filter after 1-2 min.

Reference solution   Dissolve 25 mg of *eugenol R* and 25 mg of *borneol R* in 3 mL of *methylene chloride R*.

Plate   TLC silica gel plate R.

Mobile phase   light petroleum R, toluene R (5:95 V/V).

Application   1 μL, as bands.

Development   Over a path of 10 cm.

Drying   In air.

Detection   Spray with *vanillin reagent R* and heat at 100-105 °C for 5 min.

Results   See below the sequence of the zones present in the chromatograms obtained with the reference solution and the test solution. Furthermore, other zones of various colours may be present in the chromatogram obtained with the test solution.

Top of the plate	
————	A violet zone
	————
————	A pale violet zone
	A very pale violet zone
————	————
Eugenol: a brown zone	A blue zone
Borneol: a greenish-blue zone	A bluish-violet zone
	A dark violet zone
Reference solution	**Test solution**

TESTS

Acid value (*2.5.1*)
50 to 70, determined on 1.0 g.

Water (*2.2.13*)
Maximum 10 mL/kg, determined on 25.0 g of the drug reduced to a coarse powder (1400) (*2.9.12*).

Total ash (*2.4.16*)
Maximum 0.5 per cent.

ASSAY

Essential oil (*2.8.12*)
Use a 500 mL round-bottomed flask and 200 mL of *water R* as the distillation liquid. Reduce the drug to a coarse powder (1400) (*2.9.12*) and immediately use 20.0 g for the determination. Introduce 0.50 mL of *xylene R* in the graduated tube. Distil at a rate of 2-3 mL/min for 2 h.

STORAGE

Do not powder.

_____ *Ph Eur*

Matricaria Flowers

(*Matricaria Flower, Ph Eur monograph 0404*)

Preparation
Matricaria Liquid Extract

Ph Eur _____

DEFINITION

Dried capitula of *Matricaria recutita* L. (*Chamomilla recutita* (L.) Rauschert).

Content:
— *blue essential oil*: minimum 4 mL/kg (dried drug);
— *total apigenin 7-glucoside* ($C_{21}H_{20}O_{10}$): minimum 0.25 per cent (dried drug).

IDENTIFICATION

A. Capitula, when spread out, consisting of an involucre made up of many bracts arranged in 1-3 rows; an elongated-conical receptacle, occasionally hemispherical (young capitula); 12-20 marginal ligulate florets with a white ligule;

several dozen yellow central tubular florets. The involucre bracts are ovate or lanceolate, with a brownish-grey scarious margin. The receptacle is hollow, without paleae. The corolla of the ligulate florets has a brownish-yellow tube at the base extending to form a white, elongated-oval ligule. The inferior ovary is dark brown, ovoid or spherical, and has a long style and bifid stigma. The tubular florets are yellow and have a five-toothed corolla tube, 5 syngenesious, epipetalous stamens and a gynoecium similar to that of the ligulate florets.

B. Separate the capitulum into its different parts. Examine under a microscope using *chloral hydrate solution R*.
The bracts have a margin composed of thin-walled cells and a central region composed of elongated sclereids with occasional stomata (*2.8.3*). The inner epidermis of the corolla of the ligulate florets, in surface view, consisting of thin-walled, polygonal cells, slightly papillose, those of the outer epidermis markedly sinuous and strongly striated; corolla of the tubular florets with longitudinally elongated epidermal cells, and with small groups of papillae near the apex of the lobes. Glandular trichomes each consisting of a short stalk and a head of 2-3 tiers of 2 cells each occur on the outer surfaces of the bracts and on the corollas of both types of florets. The ovaries have a sclerous ring at the base and the wall is composed of vertical bands of thin-walled, longitudinally elongated cells with numerous glandular trichomes, alternating with fusiform groups of small, radially elongated cells containing mucilage. The cells at the apex of the stigmas are extended to form rounded papillae.
Numerous small, cluster crystals of calcium oxalate occur in the inner tissues of the ovaries and the anther lobes. Pollen grains spherical to triangular, about 30 μm in diameter with 3 pores and a spiny exine.

C. Thin-layer chromatography (*2.2.27*).

Test solution   Dilute 50 μL of essential oil obtained in the assay of essential oil in 1 mL of *xylene R*.

Reference solution   Dissolve 2 μL of *chamazulene R*, 5 μL of (–)-α-*bisabolol R* and 10 mg of *bornyl acetate R* in 5 mL of *toluene R*.

Plate   TLC silica gel plate R.

Mobile phase   ethyl acetate R, toluene R (5:95 *V/V*).

Application   10 μL, as bands.

Development   Over a path of 10 cm.

Drying   In air.

Detection   Spray with *anisaldehyde solution R* and heat at 100-105 °C for 5-10 min. Examine immediately in daylight.

Results   See below the sequence of zones present in the chromatograms obtained with the reference solution and the test solution. Furthermore, other zones are present in the chromatogram obtained with the test solution.

TESTS

Broken drug
Maximum 25 per cent, determined on 20.0 g, passes through a sieve (710) (*2.9.12*).

Loss on drying (*2.2.32*)
Maximum 12.0 per cent, determined on 1.000 g of the powdered drug (355) (*2.9.12*) by drying in an oven at 105 °C for 2 h.

Total ash (2.4.16)
Maximum 13.0 per cent.

Top of the plate	
	1 or 2 blue or bluish-violet zones
Chamazulene: a red or reddish-violet zone	A red or reddish-violet zone (chamazulene)
_____	_____
Bornyl acetate: a yellowish-brown zone	
	A brown zone (en-yne-dicycloether)
_____	_____
(–)-α-Bisabolol: a reddish-violet or bluish-violet zone	A reddish-violet or bluish-violet zone ((–)-α-bisabolol)
Reference solution	**Test solution**

ASSAY

Essential oil (*2.8.12*)

Use 30 g of whole drug, a 1000 mL flask, 300 mL of *water R* as distillation liquid and 0.50 mL of *xylene R* in the graduated tube. Distil at a rate of 3-4 mL/min for 4 h. Towards the end of this period, stop the flow of water to the condenser assembly but continue distilling until the blue, steam-volatile components have reached the lower end of the condenser. Immediately re-start the flow of water to the condenser assembly to avoid warming the separation space. Stop the distillation after a further 10 min.

Total apigenin 7-glucoside

Liquid chromatography (*2.2.29*).

Test solution   Reduce 40 g of the drug to a powder (500) (*2.9.12*). Place 2.00 g of the powdered drug in a 500 mL round-bottomed flask. Add 200 mL of *ethanol (96 per cent) R*. Heat the mixture under a reflux condenser on a water-bath for 15 min. Cool and filter. Rinse the filter and the residue with a few millilitres of *ethanol (96 per cent) R*. To the filtrate add 10 mL of freshly prepared *dilute sodium hydroxide solution R* and heat the mixture under a reflux condenser on a water-bath for about 1 h. Cool. Dilute to 250.0 mL with *ethanol (96 per cent) R*. To 50.0 mL of the solution add 0.5 g of *citric acid R*. Shake for 5 min and filter. Dilute 5.0 mL of this solution to 10.0 mL with the mobile phase (initial mixture).

Reference solution (a)   Dissolve 10.0 mg of *apigenin 7-glucoside R* in 100.0 mL of *methanol R*. Dilute 25.0 mL of this solution to 200.0 mL with the mobile phase (initial mixture).

Reference solution (b)   Dissolve 10.0 mg of *5,7-dihydroxy-4-methylcoumarin R* in 100.0 mL of *methanol R*. Dilute 25.0 mL of this solution to 100.0 mL of the mobile phase (initial mixture). To 4.0 mL of this solution add 4.0 mL of reference solution (a) and dilute to 10.0 mL with the mobile phase (initial mixture).

Precolumn:
— *size*: l = 8 mm, Ø = 4.6 mm;
— *stationary phase*: octadecylsilyl silica gel for chromatography R (5 µm).

Column:
— *size*: l = 0.25 m, Ø = 4.6 mm;
— *stationary phase*: octadecylsilyl silica gel for chromatography R (5 µm).

Mobile phase:
— *mobile phase A*: phosphoric acid R, water R (0.5:99.5 V/V);
— *mobile phase B*: phosphoric acid R, acetonitrile R (0.5:99.5 V/V);

Time (min)	Mobile phase A (per cent V/V)	Mobile phase B (per cent V/V)
0 - 9	75	25
9 - 19	75 → 25	25 → 75
19 - 24	25	75

Flow rate   1 mL/min.

Detection   Spectrophotometer at 340 nm.

Injection   20 µL.

System suitability   Reference solution (b):
— *resolution*: minimum 1.8 between the peaks due to apigenin 7-glucoside and 5,7-dihydroxy-4-methylcoumarin.

Calculate the percentage content of total apigenin 7-glucoside using the following expression:

$$\frac{A_1 \times m_2}{A_2 \times m_1} \times P \times 0.625$$

A_1 = area of the peak due to apigenin 7-glucoside in the chromatogram obtained with the test solution;

A_2 = area of the peak due to apigenin 7-glucoside in the chromatogram obtained with the reference solution;

m_1 = mass of the drug in the test solution, in grams;

m_2 = mass of *apigenin 7-glucoside R* in reference solution (a), in grams;

P = percentage content of apigenin 7-glucoside in the reagent.

_____ *Ph Eur*

Matricaria Oil

(*Ph Eur monograph 1836*)

Ph Eur _____

DEFINITION

Blue essential oil obtained by steam distillation from the fresh or dried flower-heads or flowering tops of *Matricaria recutita* L. (*Chamomilla recutita* L. Rauschert). There are 2 types of matricaria oil which are characterised as rich in bisabolol oxides, or rich in (−)-α-bisabolol.

CHARACTERS

Appearance

Clear, intensely blue, viscous liquid.

Intense characteristic odour.

IDENTIFICATION

First identification   B.

Second identification   A.

A. Thin-layer chromatography (*2.2.27*).

Test solution   Dissolve 20 µL of the substance to be examined in 1.0 mL of *toluene R*.

Reference solution   Dissolve 2 mg of *guaiazulene R*, 5 µL of (−)-α-bisabolol R and 10 mg of *bornyl acetate R* in 5.0 mL of *toluene R*.

Plate   TLC silica gel plate R.

Mobile phase   ethyl acetate R, toluene R (5:95 V/V).

Application   10 µL, as bands.

Development   Over a path of 10 cm.

Drying   In air.

Detection A   Examine in daylight.

Results A   See below for the sequence of the zones present in the chromatograms obtained with the reference solution and the test solution.

Top of the plate	
Guaiazulene: a blue zone	A blue zone (chamazulene)
———	———
———	———
Reference solution	**Test solution**

Detection B   Spray with *anisaldehyde solution R* and heat at 100-105 °C for 5-10 min. Examine immediately in daylight.

Results B   See below for the sequence of the zones present in the chromatograms obtained with the reference solution and the test solution. Furthermore, yellowish-brown to greenish-yellow zones (lower third), violet zones (lower third) and further weak zones may be present in the chromatogram obtained with the test solution.

B. Examine the chromatograms obtained in the test for chromatographic profile.

Results   The characteristic peaks due to (−)-α-bisabolol and chamazulene in the chromatogram obtained with the test solution are similar in retention time to those in the chromatogram obtained with the reference solution.

TESTS
Chromatographic profile

Gas chromatography (*2.2.28*): use the normalisation procedure.

Top of the plate	
	1 or 2 blue to bluish-violet zones
Guaiazulene: a red to reddish-violet zone	A red to reddish-violet zone (chamazulene)
	———
Bornyl acetate: a yellowish-brown to greyish-green zone	A brown zone (en-yne-dicycloether)
	———
(−)-α-Bisabolol: a reddish-violet to bluish-violet zone	A reddish-violet to bluish-violet zone ((−)-α-bisabolol)
	A brownish zone
Reference solution	**Test solution**

Test solution   Dissolve 20 µL of the oil to be examined in *cyclohexane R* and dilute to 5.0 mL with the same solvent.

Reference solution   Dissolve 20 µL of *(−)-α-bisabolol R*, 5 mg of *chamazulene R* and 6 mg of *guaiazulene R* in *cyclohexane R* and dilute to 5.0 mL with the same solvent.

Column:
— *material*: fused silica,
— *size*: l = 30 m (a film thickness of 1 µm may be used) to 60 m (a film thickness of 0.2 µm may be used), Ø = 0.25-0.53 mm, when using a column longer than 30 m, an adjustment of the temperature programme may be necessary,
— *stationary phase*: macrogol 20 000 R.

Carrier gas   helium for chromatography R.

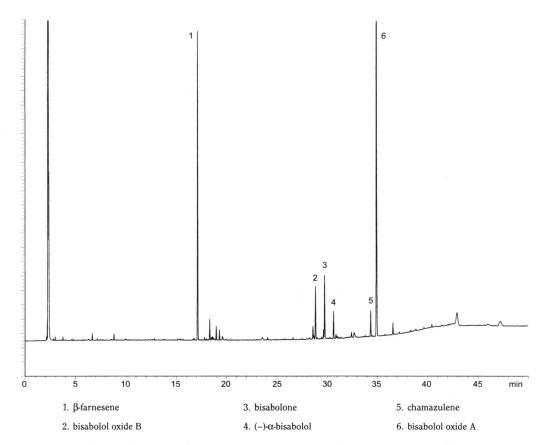

1. β-farnesene
2. bisabolol oxide B
3. bisabolone
4. (−)-α-bisabolol
5. chamazulene
6. bisabolol oxide A

Figure 1836.-1. – *Chromatogram of matricaria oil rich in bisabolol oxides*

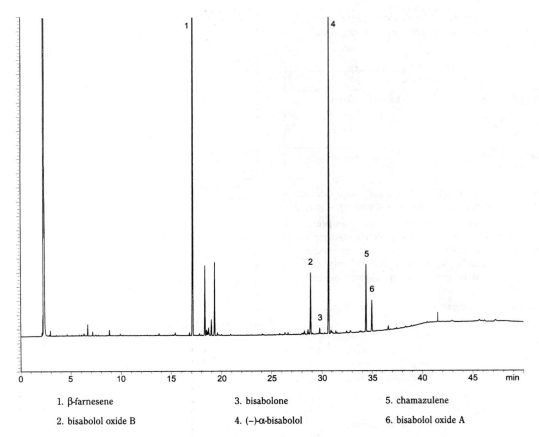

1. β-farnesene   3. bisabolone   5. chamazulene

2. bisabolol oxide B   4. (–)-α-bisabolol   6. bisabolol oxide A

Figure 1836.-2. – *Chromatogram of matricaria oil rich in (–)-α-bisabolol*

Flow rate   1-2 mL/min.

Split ratio   1:100.

Temperature:

	Time (min)	Temperature (°C)
Column	0 - 40	70 → 230
	40 - 50	230
Injection port		250
Detector		250

Detection   Flame ionisation.

Injection   1.0 μL.

Elution order   Order indicated in the composition of the reference solution. Record the retention times of these substances.

Relative retention   With reference to chamazulene (retention time = about 34.4 min): β-farnesene = about 0.5; bisabolol oxide B = about 0.8; bisabolone = about 0.87; (–)-α-bisabolol = about 0.9; bisabolol oxide A = about 1.02.

System suitability   Reference solution:

— *resolution*: minimum 1.5 between the peaks due to chamazulene and guaiazulene.

Using the retention times determined from the chromatogram obtained with the reference solution, locate (–)-α-bisabolol and chamazulene in the chromatogram obtained with the test solution; locate bisabolol oxides (bisabolol oxide B, bisabolone and bisabolol oxide A) using Figures 1836.-1 and 1836.-2 (disregard the peak due to cyclohexane). The chromatogram obtained with the test

solution does not show a peak with the retention time of guaiazulene.

Determine the percentage content of the components. The limits are within the following ranges.

	Matricaria oil rich in bisabolol oxides (per cent)	Matricaria oil rich in (–)-α-bisabolol (per cent)
Bisabolol oxides	29 - 81	
(–)-α-Bisabolol		10 - 65
Chamazulene	≥ 1.0	≥ 1.0
Total of bisabolol oxides and (–)-α-Bisabolol		≥ 20

STORAGE

At a temperature not exceeding 25 °C.

Ph Eur

Matricaria Liquid Extract

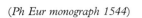

(Ph Eur monograph 1544)

Ph Eur

DEFINITION

Liquid extract produced from *Matricaria flower (0404)*.

Content

Minimum 0.30 per cent of blue residual oil.

PRODUCTION

The extract is produced from the herbal drug by a suitable procedure for liquid extracts using a mixture of 2.5 volumes of a 10 per cent *m/m* solution of ammonia (NH₃), 47.5 volumes of water and 50 volumes of ethanol (96 per cent).

CHARACTERS

Appearance

Brownish, clear liquid.

Intense characteristic odour and characteristic bitter taste.

Solubility

Miscible with water and with ethanol (96 per cent) with development of turbidity, soluble in ethanol (50 per cent *V/V*).

IDENTIFICATION

A. Thin-layer chromatography (*2.2.27*).

Test solution Place 10 mL of the extract to be examined in a separating funnel and shake with 2 quantities, each of 10 mL, of *pentane R*. Combine the pentane layers, dry over 2 g of *anhydrous sodium sulfate R* and filter. Evaporate the filtrate to dryness on a water-bath and dissolve the residue in 0.5 mL of *toluene R*.

Reference solution Dissolve 4 mg of *guaiazulene R*, 20 mg of *(-)-α-bisabolol R* and 20 mg of *bornyl acetate R* in 10 mL of *toluene R*.

Plate TLC silica gel F_{254} *plate R*.

Mobile phase ethyl acetate R, toluene R (5:95 *V/V*).

Application 10 μL as bands.

Development Over a path of 10 cm.

Drying In air.

Detection A Examine in ultraviolet light at 254 nm.

Results A The chromatogram obtained with the test solution shows several quenching zones, of which 2 main zones are in the middle third (en-yne-dicycloether).

Detection B Examine in ultraviolet light at 365 nm.

Results B The chromatogram obtained with the test solution shows in the middle part an intense blue fluorescent zone (herniarin).

Detection C Spray with *anisaldehyde solution R* and examine in daylight while heating at 100-105 °C for 5-10 min.

Results C The chromatogram obtained with the reference solution shows in the lower third a reddish-violet or bluish-violet zone ((-)-α-bisabolol), in the middle third a yellowish-brown or greyish-green zone (bornyl acetate) and in the upper third a red or reddish-violet zone (guaiazulene). The chromatogram obtained with the test solution shows in the lower third yellowish-brown or greenish-yellow and violet zones and a reddish-violet or bluish-violet zone due to (-)-α-bisabolol in the chromatogram obtained with the reference solution; a brownish zone (en-yne-dicycloether) similar in position to the zone due to bornyl acetate in the chromatogram obtained with the reference solution; a red or reddish-violet zone (chamazulene) corresponding to

guaiazulene in the chromatogram obtained with the reference solution and immediately above it 1 or 2 blue or bluish-violet zones; further weak zones may be present in the chromatogram obtained with the test solution.

B. Thin-layer chromatography (*2.2.27*).

Test solution The extract to be examined.

Reference solution Dissolve 1.0 mg of *chlorogenic acid R*, 2.5 mg of *hyperoside R* and 2.5 mg of *rutin R* in 10 mL of *methanol R*.

Plate TLC silica gel *plate R*.

Mobile phase anhydrous formic acid R, glacial acetic acid R, water R, ethyl acetate R (7.5:7.5:18:67 *V/V/V/V*).

Application 10 μL as bands.

Development Over a path of 15 cm.

Drying At 100-105 °C.

Detection Spray the warm plate with a 10 g/L solution of *diphenylboric acid aminoethyl ester R* in *methanol R*; subsequently spray with a 50 g/L solution of *macrogol 400 R* in *methanol R*; allow to dry in air for about 30 min and examine in ultraviolet light at 365 nm.

Results The chromatogram obtained with the reference solution shows in the middle part a light blue fluorescent zone (chlorogenic acid), below it a yellowish-brown fluorescent zone (rutin) and above it a yellowish-brown fluorescent zone (hyperoside). The chromatogram obtained with the test solution shows a yellowish-brown fluorescent zone corresponding to the zone of rutin in the chromatogram obtained with the reference solution, a light blue fluorescent zone corresponding to the zone of chlorogenic acid in the chromatogram obtained with the reference solution, a yellowish-brown fluorescent zone similar in position to the zone of hyperoside in the chromatogram obtained with the reference solution; it also shows above the yellowish-brown fluorescent zone a green fluorescent zone, then several bluish or greenish fluorescent zones and near the solvent front a yellowish fluorescent zone.

TESTS

Ethanol (*2.9.10*)

38 per cent *V/V* to 53 per cent *V/V*.

Dry residue (*2.8.16*)

Minimum 12.0 per cent.

ASSAY

Place 20.0 g in a 1000 mL round-bottomed flask, add 300 mL of *water R* and distil until 200 mL has been collected in a flask. Transfer the distillate into a separating funnel. Dissolve 65 g of *sodium chloride R* in the distillate and shake with 3 quantities, each of 30 mL, of *pentane R* previously used to rinse the reflux condenser and the flask. Combine the pentane layers, dry over 2 g of *anhydrous sodium sulfate R* and filter into a tared 100 mL round-bottomed flask which has been dried in a desiccator for 3 h. Rinse the anhydrous sodium sulfate and the filter with 2 quantities, each of 20 mL, of *pentane R*. Evaporate the pentane in a water-bath at 45 °C. The residue of pentane is eliminated in a current of air for 3 min. Dry the flask in a desiccator for 3 h and weigh. The residual oil is blue (chamazulene).

Ph Eur

Meadowsweet

(Ph Eur monograph 1868)

Ph Eur

DEFINITION

Whole or cut, dried flowering tops of *Filipendula ulmaria* (L.) Maxim. (syn. *Spiraea ulmaria* L.).

Content

Minimum 1 mL/kg of essential oil (dried drug).

CHARACTERS

Aromatic odour of methyl salicylate, after crushing.

IDENTIFICATION

A. The stem, up to 5 mm in diameter, is greenish-brown, stiff, angular, hollow except at the apex, and has regular, straight, longitudinal furrows. The petiolate leaf, compound imparipinnate, has 2 reddish-brown angular stipules.
It consists of 3-9 pairs of leaflets, unevenly dentate, some of which are small and fan-shaped. The leaflets are dark green and glabrous on the upper surface, tomentose and lighter, sometimes silvery on the lower surface. The terminal leaflet, the largest, is divided into 3 segments. The veins are prominent and brown on the lower surface.
The inflorescence is complex and composed of very numerous flowers arranged in irregular cymose panicles. The flowers are creamish-white and about 3-6 mm in diameter; the calyx consists of 5 dark green, reflexed and hairy sepals fused at the base to a concave receptacle; the 5 free petals, which are readily detached, are pale yellow, obovate and distinctly narrowed at the base; the stamens are numerous with rounded anthers and they extend beyond the petals; the gynoecium consists of about 4-6 carpels, each with a short style and a globular stigma; the carpels become twisted together spirally to form yellowish-brown fruits with a helicoidal twist. Unopened flower buds are frequently present. If the fruit is present, it has a helicoidal twist and contains brownish seeds.

B. Microscopic examination (*2.8.23*). The powder is green or yellowish-green. Examine under a microscope using *chloral hydrate solution R*. The powder shows the following diagnostic characters (Figure 1868.-1): fragments of the epidermises of the leaves and sepals [C, E, F] with sinuous or wavy cells [Ca, Ea, Fa], short, thick-walled, conical covering trichomes thickened at the base, in surface view [Eb] and in side view [J], unicellular covering trichomes, thin-walled, very long and flexuous, with pointed ends in surface view [Fc] and in side view [A], or their scars (flexuous trichome [Fd], conical trichome [Fe]) and occasional clavate glandular trichomes with a 1- to 3-celled ([Ed] and [G], respectively), uniseriate stalk, a multicellular head and dense brown contents; fragments of the upper epidermis often accompanied by palisade parenchyma [Cb] including some hypertrophied cells containing a cluster crystal of calcium oxalate [Cc]; fragments of the lower epidermis with anomocytic stomata (*2.8.3*) [Ec, Fb], sometimes accompanied by spongy parenchyma [Ff] with some cells containing cluster crystals of calcium oxalate [Fg]; fragments of the petals [H] with thin-walled epidermal cells, some showing rounded papillae [Ha]; numerous spherical pollen grains with 3 pores and a faintly pitted exine [Bb]; fragments of the anther [B, D] whose fibrous layer shows specific thickenings, in surface view [D] and in side view [Ba]; fragments of the ovary [K] with an epidermis bearing stomata [Ka] and with parenchyma containing prism crystals of calcium oxalate [Kb]; fragments

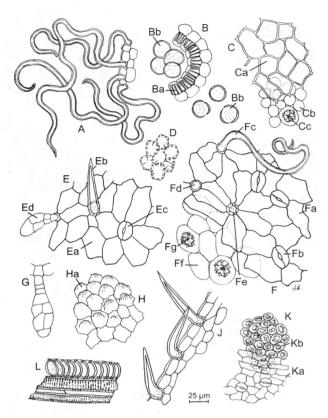

Figure 1868.-1. − *Illustration for identification test B of powdered herbal drug of meadowsweet*

of vascular tissue [L] with annular, spiral or pitted vessels from the leaves and stems.

C. Thin-layer chromatography (*2.2.27*).

Test solution   Xylene solution obtained in the assay.

Reference solution   Dissolve 0.1 mL of *methyl salicylate R* and 0.1 mL of *salicylaldehyde R* in *xylene R* and dilute to 5 mL with the same solvent.

Plate   *TLC silica gel plate R*.

Mobile phase   hexane R, toluene R (50:50 *V/V*).

Application   10 μL as bands.

Development   Over a path of 10 cm.

Drying   In air.

Detection   Treat with 3 mL of *ferric chloride solution R3* and examine in daylight.

Results   See below the sequence of zones present in the chromatograms obtained with the reference solution and the test solution. Furthermore, other zones are present in the chromatogram obtained with the test solution.

Top of the plate	
———	———
Methyl salicylate: a violet-brown zone	A violet-brown zone (methyl salicylate)
Salicylaldehyde: a violet-brown zone	A violet-brown zone (salicylaldehyde)
———	———
Reference solution	**Test solution**

TESTS

Foreign matter (*2.8.2*)

Maximum 5.0 per cent of stems with a diameter greater than 5 mm and maximum 2.0 per cent of other foreign matter.

Loss on drying (*2.2.32*)

Maximum 12.0 per cent, determined on 1.000 g of the powdered herbal drug (355) (*2.9.12*) by drying in an oven at 105 °C for 2 h.

Total ash (*2.4.16*)

Maximum 7.0 per cent.

ASSAY

Carry out the determination of essential oils in herbal drugs (*2.8.12*). Use 50.0 g of the cut herbal drug, a 1000 mL flask, 300 mL of *dilute hydrochloric acid R* as the distillation liquid, and 0.5 mL of *xylene R* in the graduated tube. Distil at a rate of 2-3 mL/min for 2 h.

Ph Eur

Melilot

(*Ph Eur monograph 2120*)

Ph Eur

DEFINITION

Whole or cut, dried aerial parts of *Melilotus officinalis* (L.) Lam.

Content

Minimum 0.3 per cent of coumarin ($C_9H_6O_2$; M_r 146.1) (dried drug).

IDENTIFICATION

A. The stem is green, cylindrical, glabrous and finely ridged. The leaves are alternate, petiolate and trifoliate with 2 lanceolate stipules; the leaflets are up to about 3 cm long and 20 mm wide, elongated or ovate with a finely dentate margin, acute at the apex and base; the upper surface is dark green and glabrous, the lower surface paler green with short, fine hairs, especially at the base. The inflorescence is racemose with numerous pale yellow flowers, about 7 mm long, each having a hairy calyx with 5 deeply-divided, unequal teeth, and a papilionate corolla. The fruit is an indehiscent pod, often persistent within the calyx, yellowish-brown, short and tapering at the apex; the surface is glabrous and transversely wrinkled.

B. Microscopic examination (*2.8.23*). The powder is yellowish-green. Examine under a microscope using *chloral hydrate solution R*. The powder shows the following diagnostic characters (Figure 2120.-1): fragments of the leaf lamina in surface view [D] showing unevenly thickened, slightly sinuous epidermal cells; numerous stomata [Db], mostly anomocytic (*2.8.3*) with 3-6 subsidiary cells [Da] and frequently, underlying palisade parenchyma [Dc]; uniseriate covering trichomes with 2 short, smooth-walled basal cells and a long terminal cell, bent at right angles, with a thick wall and a warty cuticle [A, B]; occasional glandular trichomes with a short, 2- or 3- celled stalk and ovoid, biseriate head with 4 indistinct cells [H]; fragments of the petals composed of cells with wavy walls [M]; fragments of vascular tissue from the stem [F, G], including large vessels [G], sometimes associated with unlignified septate fibres [Fa] and a sheath of parenchymatous cells containing prisms of calcium oxalate [Fb]; fragments of mesophyll [J] including some cells which may occasionally contain cluster crystals of calcium oxalate [Ja]; fragments of the stem epidermis with elongated, straight-walled cells and anomocytic (*2.8.3*) stomata [L]; fragments of the fibrous layer of the anthers in surface view [E] and in transverse section [K]; spherical or ovoid pollen grains about 25 µm long with 3 germinal pores and a smooth exine [C].

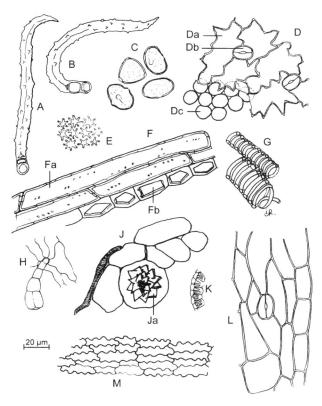

Figure 2120.-1. – *Illustration for identification test B of powdered herbal drug of melilot*

C. Thin-layer chromatography (*2.2.27*).

Test solution To 0.3 g of the powdered herbal drug (355) (*2.9.12*) add 3 mL of *methanol R*. Heat on a water-bath at 100 °C for 1 min and filter.

Reference solution Dissolve 50 mg of *coumarin CRS* and 20 mg of *o-coumaric acid R* in 50 mL of *methanol R*.

Plate TLC silica gel plate R (5-40 µm) [or *TLC silica gel plate R* (2-10 µm)].

Mobile phase *dilute acetic acid R*, *ether R*, *toluene R* (10:50:50 *V/V/V*); use the upper layer.

Application 25 µL [or 3 µL] as bands of 10 mm [or 8 mm].

Development Over a path of 12 cm [or 6 cm].

Drying In air.

Detection Spray with *2 M alcoholic potassium hydroxide R* and examine in ultraviolet light at 365 nm.

Results See below the sequence of zones present in the chromatograms obtained with the reference solution and the test solution. Furthermore, other faint zones of various colours may be present in the chromatogram obtained with the test solution.

Top of the plate	
Coumarin: a greenish-yellow fluorescent zone	A greenish-yellow fluorescent zone (coumarin)
	——
	A blue fluorescent zone
o-Coumaric acid: a greenish-yellow fluorescent zone	A greenish-yellow fluorescent zone (o-coumaric acid) may be present
——	——
Reference solution	**Test solution**

TESTS

Foreign matter (*2.8.2*)
Maximum 2 per cent of stems with a diameter greater than 3 mm and maximum 2 per cent of other foreign matter.

Loss on drying (*2.2.32*)
Maximum 12.0 per cent, determined on 1.000 g of the powdered herbal drug (355) (*2.9.12*) by drying in an oven at 105 °C for 2 h.

Total ash (*2.4.16*)
Maximum 10.0 per cent.

ASSAY

Liquid chromatography (*2.2.29*).

Test solution   Completely reduce about 50 g of the herbal drug to a powder (500) (*2.9.12*). To 5.00 g of the powdered herbal drug add 90 mL of *methanol R* and boil under a reflux condenser for 30 min. Allow to cool. Filter under vacuum through a fibre-glass filter. Take up the residue and the fragmented filter with 90 mL of *methanol R*. Treat in the same manner as before. Combine the filtrates and dilute to 250.0 mL with *methanol R*.

Reference solution   Dissolve 25.0 mg of *coumarin CRS* in *methanol R* and dilute to 250.0 mL with the same solvent.

Column:
— *size: l* = 0.25 m, Ø = 4 mm;
— *stationary phase: end-capped octadecylsilyl silica gel for chromatography R* (5 μm).

Mobile phase   acetonitrile R, 5 g/L solution of *phosphoric acid R* (22:78 *V/V*).

Flow rate   1.7 mL/min.

Detection   Spectrophotometer at 275 nm.

Injection   20 μL.

System suitability:
— *retention time*: coumarin = about 7.8 min.

Calculate the percentage content of coumarin using the following expression:

$$\frac{A_1 \times m_2 \times p}{A_2 \times m_1}$$

A_1 = area of the peak due to coumarin in the chromatogram obtained with the test solution;
A_2 = area of the peak due to coumarin in the chromatogram obtained with the reference solution;
m_1 = mass of the herbal drug to be examined used to prepare the test solution, in grams;
m_2 = mass of *coumarin CRS* used to prepare the reference solution, in grams;
p = percentage content of coumarin in *coumarin CRS*.

_____ *Ph Eur*

Menthol and Benzoin Inhalation

Menthol and Benzoin Inhalation Vapour

DEFINITION

Menthol and Benzoin Inhalation is an *inhalation vapour, solution.*

Racementhol or Levomenthol	20 g
Benzoin Inhalation	Sufficient to produce 1000 mL

Extemporaneous preparation
The following directions apply.

Dissolve the Racementhol or the Levomenthol in a portion of the Benzoin Inhalation, add sufficient Benzoin Inhalation to produce 1000 mL and mix.

The inhalation complies with the requirements stated under Preparations for Inhalation and with the following requirements.

Content of total balsamic acids
Not less than 2.8% w/v, calculated as cinnamic acid, $C_9H_8O_2$.

Total solids
9.0 to 12.0% w/v when determined by drying at 105° for 4 hours, Appendix XI A. Use 2 mL.

ASSAY
Boil 10 mL with 25 mL of 0.5M *ethanolic potassium hydroxide* under a reflux condenser for 1 hour. Evaporate the ethanol, disperse the residue in 50 mL of hot *water*, cool, add 80 mL of *water* and 1.5 g of *magnesium sulfate* dissolved in 50 mL of *water*. Mix thoroughly and allow to stand for 10 minutes. Filter, wash the residue on the filter with 20 mL of *water*, acidify the combined filtrate and washings with *hydrochloric acid* and extract with four 40 mL quantities of *ether*. Discard the aqueous solution, combine the ether extracts and extract with successive quantities of 20, 20, 10, 10 and 10 mL of *sodium hydrogen carbonate solution*, washing each aqueous extract with the same 20 mL of *ether*. Discard the ether layers, carefully acidify the combined aqueous extracts with *hydrochloric acid* and extract with successive quantities of 30, 20, 20 and 10 mL of *chloroform*, filtering each extract through *anhydrous sodium sulfate* supported on absorbent cotton. Distil the chloroform from the combined filtrates until 10 mL remains and remove the remainder in a current of air. Dissolve the residue, with the aid of gentle heat, in 10 mL of *ethanol (96%)*, previously neutralised to *phenol red solution*, cool and titrate with 0.1M *sodium hydroxide VS* using *phenol red solution* as indicator. Each mL of 0.1M *sodium hydroxide VS* is equivalent to 14.82 mg of total balsamic acids, calculated as cinnamic acid, $C_9H_8O_2$.

Milk-thistle Fruit

(Ph Eur monograph 1860)

Preparation

Refined and Standardised Milk Thistle Dry Extract

Ph Eur _____

DEFINITION

Mature fruit, devoid of the pappus, of *Silybum marianum* L. Gaertner.

Content

Minimum 1.5 per cent of silymarin, expressed as silibinin ($C_{25}H_{22}O_{10}$; M_r 482.4) (dried drug).

CHARACTERS

No rancid odour.

IDENTIFICATION

A. The achene is strongly compressed, elongate-obovate, about 6-8 mm long, 3 mm broad and 1.5 mm thick; the outer surface is smooth and shiny with a grey or pale brown ground colour variably streaked dark brown longitudinally to give an overall pale greyish or brown colour; the fruit is tapering at the base and crowned at the apex with a glistening, pale yellow extension forming a collar about 1 mm high surrounding the remains of the style.
Cut transversely, the fruit shows a narrow, brown outer area and 2 large, dense, white oily cotyledons.

B. Reduce to a powder (355) (*2.9.12*). The powder is brownish-yellow with darker specks. Examine under a microscope using *chloral hydrate solution R*. The powder shows the following diagnostic characters: fragments of the epicarp composed of colourless cells, polygonal in surface view, the lumen appearing fairly large or as a small slit, depending on the orientation; groups of parenchymatous cells from the pigment layer, some of them containing colouring matter which appears bright red; very abundant groups of large sclereids from the testa with bright yellow pitted walls and a narrow lumen; occasionally fragments of small-celled parenchyma with pitted and beaded walls; abundant thin-walled parenchymatous cells from the cotyledons containing oil globules and scattered cluster crystals of calcium oxalate; a few larger, prismatic crystals of calcium oxalate.

C. Thin-layer chromatography (*2.2.27*).

Test solution To 1.0 g of powdered drug (500) (*2.9.12*) add 10 mL of *methanol R*. Heat under reflux in a water-bath at 70 °C for 5 min. Cool and filter. Evaporate the filtrate to dryness and dissolve the residue in 1.0 mL of *methanol R*.

Reference solution Dissolve 2 mg of *silibinin R* and 5 mg of *taxifolin R* in 10 mL of *methanol R*.

Plate TLC silica gel plate R.

Mobile phase anhydrous formic acid R, acetone R, methylene chloride R (8.5:16.5:75 V/V/V).

Application 30 μL of the test solution and 10 μL of the reference solution, as bands.

Development Over a path of 10 cm.

Drying At 100-105 °C.

Detection Spray the warm plate with a 10 g/L solution of *diphenylboric acid aminoethyl ester R* in *methanol R* and subsequently spray with a 50 g/L solution of *macrogol 400 R* in *methanol R*. Allow to dry for 30 min and examine in ultraviolet light at 365 nm.

Results See below the sequence of zones present in the chromatograms obtained with the reference solution and the test solution. Furthermore, other orange and yellowish-green fluorescent zones are present between the zones of silibinin and taxifolin in the chromatogram obtained with the test solution.

Top of the plate	
Silibinin: a yellowish-green fluorescent zone	A yellowish-green fluorescent zone (silibinin)
————	————
Taxifolin: an orange fluorescent zone	An orange fluorescent zone (taxifolin)
	A yellowish-green fluorescent zone (silicristin)
————	————
	A light blue fluorescent zone (line of application)
Reference solution	**Test solution**

TESTS

Loss on drying (*2.2.32*)

Maximum 8.0 per cent, determined on 1.000 g of the powdered drug (500) (*2.9.12*) by drying in an oven at 105 °C for 2 h.

Total ash (*2.4.16*)

Maximum 8.0 per cent.

ASSAY

Liquid chromatography (*2.2.29*).

Test solution Place 5.00 g of the powdered drug (500) (*2.9.12*) in a continuous-extraction apparatus. Add 100 mL of *light petroleum R* and heat in a water-bath for 8 h. Allow the defatted drug to dry at room temperature. In a continuous-extraction apparatus, extract the latter with 100 mL of *methanol R* in a water-bath for 5 h. Evaporate the methanolic extract *in vacuo* to a volume of about 30 mL. Filter into a 50 mL volumetric flask, rinsing the extraction flask and the filter, and diluting to 50.0 mL with *methanol R*. Dilute 5.0 mL of this solution to 50.0 mL with *methanol R*.

Reference solution Dissolve a quantity of *milk thistle standardised dry extract CRS* equivalent to 5.0 mg of silibinin (m_1 g) in *methanol R* and dilute to 50.0 mL with the same solvent.

Column:
— *size*: l = 0.125 m, Ø = 4 mm;
— *stationary phase*: octadecylsilyl silica gel for chromatography R (5 μm).

Mobile phase:
— *mobile phase A*: phosphoric acid R; methanol R, water R (0.5:35:65 V/V/V);
— *mobile phase B*: phosphoric acid R; methanol R, water R (0.5:50:50 V/V/V);

Time (min)	Mobile phase A (per cent V/V)	Mobile phase B (per cent V/V)
0 - 28	100 → 0	0 → 100
28 - 35	0	100
35 - 36	0 → 100	100 → 0
36 - 51	100	0

Flow rate 0.8 mL/min.

Detection Spectrophotometer at 288 nm.

Injection 10 μL.

Retention time Silibinin B = about 30 min. If necessary, adjust the time periods of the gradient.

System suitability Reference solution:
— *resolution*: minimum 1.8 between the peaks due to silibinin A and silibinin B;
— the chromatogram obtained is similar to the chromatogram supplied with *milk thistle standardised dry extract CRS*.

Locate silicristin, silidianin, silibinin A, silibinin B, isosilibinin A and isosilibinin B by comparison with the chromatogram supplied with *milk thistle standardised dry extract CRS*. In the chromatogram obtained with the test solution the peak due to silidianin may vary in size, be absent or be present as the principal peak. Determine the area of the peaks due to silicristin, silidianin, silibinin A, silibinin B, isosilibinin A and isosilibinin B.

Calculate the percentage content of silymarin, calculated as silibinin, using the following expression:

$$\frac{(A1 + A2 + A3 + A4 + A5 + A6) \times m_1 \times p \times 1000}{(A7 + A8) \times m_2 \times (100 - d)}$$

$A1$ = area of the peak due to silicristin in the chromatogram obtained with the test solution;

$A2$ = area of the peak due to silidianin in the chromatogram obtained with the test solution;

$A3$ = area of the peak due to silibinin A in the chromatogram obtained with the test solution;

$A4$ = area of the peak due to silibinin B in the chromatogram obtained with the test solution;

$A5$ = area of the peak due to isosilibinin A in the chromatogram obtained with the test solution;

$A6$ = area of the peak due to isosilibinin B in the chromatogram obtained with the test solution;

$A7$ = area of the peak due to silibinin A in the chromatogram obtained with the reference solution;

$A8$ = area of the peak due to silibinin B in the chromatogram obtained with the reference solution;

m_1 = mass of *milk thistle standardised dry extract CRS* used to prepare the reference solution, in grams;

m_2 = mass of the drug to be examined, in grams;

p = combined percentage content of silibinin A and silibinin B in *milk thistle standardised dry extract CRS*;

d = percentage loss on drying of the drug.

Ph Eur

Refined and Standardised Milk Thistle Dry Extract

(*Ph Eur monograph 2071*)

Ph Eur

DEFINITION
Dry extract, refined and standardised, produced from *Milk-thistle fruit (1860)*.

Content
90 per cent to 110 per cent of the nominal content of silymarin, expressed as silibinin ($C_{25}H_{22}O_{10}$; M_r 482.4), stated on the label. The nominal content of silymarin is within the range 30 per cent *m/m* to 65 per cent *m/m* (dried extract).

The content of silymarin corresponds to:
— *sum of the contents of silicristin and silidianin* (both $C_{25}H_{22}O_{10}$; M_r 482.4): 20 per cent to 45 per cent, calculated with reference to total silymarin;

— *sum of the contents of silibinin A and silibinin B* (both $C_{25}H_{22}O_{10}$; M_r 482.4): 40 per cent to 65 per cent, calculated with reference to total silymarin;
— *sum of the contents of isosilibinin A and isosilibinin B* (both $C_{25}H_{22}O_{10}$; M_r 482.4): 10 per cent to 20 per cent, calculated with reference to total silymarin.

PRODUCTION
The extract is produced from the herbal drug by an appropriate procedure, using one or more of the following solvents:
— ethyl acetate;
— acetone or mixture of acetone and water;
— ethanol or mixture of ethanol and water;
— methanol or mixture of methanol and water.

CHARACTERS
Appearance
Yellowish-brown, amorphous powder.

IDENTIFICATION
Thin-layer chromatography (*2.2.27*).

Test solution Dissolve 0.250 g of the extract to be examined in 5 mL of *methanol R*.

Reference solution Dissolve 2 mg of *silibinin R* and 5 mg of *taxifolin R* in 10 mL of *methanol R*.

Plate TLC silica gel plate R (5-40 μm) [or *TLC silica gel plate R (2-10 μm)*].

Mobile phase anhydrous formic acid R, acetone R, methylene chloride R (8.5:16.5:75 *V/V/V*).

Application 10 μL [or 8 μL] of the test solution and 10 μL [or 2 μL] of the reference solution, as bands.

Development Over a path of 10 cm [or 6 cm].

Drying At 100-105 °C.

Detection Spray with a 10 g/L solution of *diphenylboric acid aminoethyl ester R* in *methanol R* and subsequently spray with a 50 g/L solution of *macrogol 400 R* in *methanol R*. Allow the plate to dry in air for about 30 min and examine in ultraviolet light at 365 nm.

Results See below the sequence of zones present in the chromatograms obtained with the reference solution and the test solution. Furthermore, other yellowish-green fluorescent zones may be present between the zones due to silibinin and taxifolin in the chromatogram obtained with the test solution.

Top of the plate	
Silibinin: a yellowish-green fluorescent zone	A yellowish-green fluorescent zone (silibinin)
———	———
Taxifolin: an orange fluorescent zone	An orange fluorescent zone (taxifolin)
	A yellowish-green fluorescent zone
———	
	A fluorescent zone (line of application)
Reference solution	**Test solution**

TESTS
Loss on drying (*2.8.17*)
Maximum 5.0 per cent.

ASSAY
Liquid chromatography (*2.2.29*).

Test solution Dissolve 60.0 mg of the extract to be examined in *methanol R* and dilute to 100.0 mL with the same solvent.

Reference solution   Dissolve a quantity of *milk thistle standardised dry extract CRS* corresponding to 10.0 mg (m_1 g) of silibinin in *methanol R* and dilute to 100.0 mL with the same solvent.

Column:
— *size: l* = 0.125 m, Ø = 4 mm;
— *stationary phase: octadecylsilyl silica gel for chromatography R* (5 μm).

Mobile phase:
— *mobile phase A: phosphoric acid R, methanol R, water R* (0.5:35:65 *V/V/V*);
— *mobile phase B: phosphoric acid R, methanol R, water R* (0.5:50:50 *V/V/V*);

Time (min)	Mobile phase A (per cent *V/V*)	Mobile phase B (per cent *V/V*)
0 - 28	100 → 0	0 → 100
28 - 35	0	100
35 - 36	0 → 100	100 → 0
36 - 51	100	0

Flow rate   0.8 mL/min.

Detection   Spectrophotometer at 288 nm.

Injection   10 μL.

Retention time   Silibinin B = about 30 min; if necessary, adjust the time periods of the gradient.

System suitability   Reference solution:
— *resolution*: minimum 1.8 between the peaks due to silibinin A and silibinin B.
— the chromatogram obtained with the reference solution is similar to the chromatogram supplied with *milk thistle standardised dry extract CRS*.

Locate the peaks due to silicristin, silidianin, silibinin A, silibinin B, isosilibinin A and isosilibinin B using the chromatogram supplied with *milk thistle standardised dry extract CRS*. In the chromatogram obtained with the test solution the peak due to silidianin may vary in size or be absent.

Calculate the percentage content of total silymarin, expressed as silibinin, using the following expression:

$$\frac{(F_1 + F_2 + F_3 + F_4 + F_5 + F_6) \times m_1}{(F_7 + F_8) \times m_2}$$

Calculate the percentage content of the sum of silicristin and silidianin, with reference to total silymarin, using the following expression:

$$\frac{(F_1 + F_2) \times 100}{F_1 + F_2 + F_3 + F_4 + F_5 + F_6}$$

Calculate the percentage content of the sum of silibinin A and silibinin B, with reference to total silymarin, using the following expression:

$$\frac{(F_3 + F_4) \times 100}{F_1 + F_2 + F_3 + F_4 + F_5 + F_6}$$

Calculate the percentage content of the sum of isosilibinin A and isosilibinin B, with reference to total silymarin, using the following expression:

$$\frac{(F_5 + F_6) \times 100}{F_1 + F_2 + F_3 + F_4 + F_5 + F_6}$$

F_1 = area of the peak due to silicristin in the chromatogram obtained with the test solution;

F_2 = area of the peak due to silidianin in the chromatogram obtained with the test solution;

F_3 = area of the peak due to silibinin A in the chromatogram obtained with the test solution;

F_4 = area of the peak due to silibinin B in the chromatogram obtained with the test solution;

F_5 = area of the peak due to isosilibinin A in the chromatogram obtained with the test solution;

F_6 = area of the peak due to isosilibinin B in the chromatogram obtained with the test solution;

F_7 = area of the peak due to silibinin A in the chromatogram obtained with the reference solution;

F_8 = area of the peak due to silibinin B in the chromatogram obtained with the reference solution;

m_1 = mass of silibinin in the reference solution, in grams;

m_2 = mass of the extract to be examined, in grams.

Ph Eur

Dementholised Mint Oil

(Partly Dementholised Mint Oil, Ph Eur monograph 1838)

Ph Eur

DEFINITION
Essential oil obtained by steam distillation from the fresh, flowering aerial parts, recently gathered from *Mentha canadensis* L. (syn. *M. arvensis* L. var. *glabrata* (Benth) Fern., *M. arvensis* var. *piperascens* Malinv. ex Holmes), followed by partial separation of menthol by crystallisation.

CHARACTERS
Appearance
Colourless, pale yellow or greenish-yellow liquid.
Characteristic odour.

IDENTIFICATION
First identification   B.

Second identification   A.

A. Thin-layer chromatography (*2.2.27*).

Test solution   Dissolve 0.1 mL of the substance to be examined in 1.0 mL of *toluene R*.

Reference solution   Dissolve 4 μL of *carvone R*, 4 μL of *pulegone R*, 10 μL of *menthyl acetate R*, 20 μL of *cineole R* and 50 mg of *menthol R* in 5 mL of *toluene R*.

Plate   TLC *silica gel F$_{254}$ plate R*.

Mobile phase   ethyl acetate *R*, toluene *R* (5:95 *V/V*).

Application   10 μL, as bands.

Development   Over a path of 15 cm.

Drying   In air.

Detection A   Examine in ultraviolet light at 254 nm.

Results A   See below the sequence of the zones present in the chromatograms obtained with the reference solution and the test solution. Furthermore, a quenching zone may be present in the upper third of the chromatogram obtained with the test solution.

Top of the plate	
Carvone and pulegone: a quenching zone	A quenching zone
	A quenching zone
Reference solution	**Test solution**

Detection B Spray with *anisaldehyde solution R* and heat at 100-105 °C for 5-10 min. Examine immediately in daylight.

Results B See below the sequence of the zones present in the chromatograms obtained with the reference solution and the test solution. Furthermore, the zone due to cineole in the reference solution is absent in the chromatogram obtained with the test solution. No yellowish-brown zone below the intense reddish-violet zone is present in the chromatogram obtained with the test solution.

Top of the plate	
	An intense reddish-violet zone (near the solvent front)
Menthyl acetate: a bluish-violet zone	A bluish-violet zone (menthyl acetate)
	A strongly greenish zone
	A greenish zone
Carvone and pulegone: a reddish zone	A reddish zone
Cineole: a violet zone	
	A distinctly violet zone
Menthol: an intense blue zone	A very intense blue zone (menthol)
Reference solution	**Test solution**

B. Examine the chromatograms obtained in the test for chromatographic profile.

Results The characteristic peaks in the chromatogram obtained with the test solution are approximately similar in retention time to those in the chromatogram obtained with the reference solution. Carvone may be absent from the chromatogram obtained with the test solution.

TESTS

Relative density (*2.2.5*)
0.888 to 0.910.

Refractive index (*2.2.6*)
1.456 to 1.470.

Optical rotation (*2.2.7*)
− 16.0° to − 34.0°.

Acid value (*2.5.1*)
Maximum 1.0, determined on 5.00 g of the substance to be examined dissolved in 50 mL of the prescribed mixture of solvents.

Chromatographic profile
Gas chromatography (*2.2.28*): use the normalisation procedure.

Test solution Dissolve 0.20 g of the substance to be examined in *hexane R* and dilute to 10.0 mL with the same solvent.

Reference solution Dissolve 10 mg of *limonene R*, 20 mg of *cineole R*, 40 mg of *menthone R*, 10 mg of *isomenthone R*, 40 mg of *menthyl acetate R*, 20 mg of *isopulegol R*, 60 mg of *menthol R*, 20 mg of *pulegone R* and 10 mg of *carvone R* in *hexane R* and dilute to 10.0 mL with the same solvent.

Column:
— *material*: fused silica,
— *size*: l = 30 m (a film thickness of 1 µm may be used) to 60 m (a film thickness of 0.2 µm may be used), Ø = 0.25-0.53 mm,
— *stationary phase*: macrogol 20 000 R.

Carrier gas helium for chromatography R.

Flow rate 1.5 mL/min.

Split ratio 1:100.

Temperature:

	Time (min)	Temperature (°C)
Column	0 - 10	60
	10 - 70	60 → 180
	70 - 75	180
Injection port		200
Detector		220

Detection Flame ionisation.

Injection 1.0 µL.

Elution order Order indicated in the composition of the reference solution. Record the retention times of these substances.

System suitability Reference solution:
— *resolution*: minimum 1.5 between the peaks due to limonene and cineole.

Using the retention times determined from the chromatogram obtained with the reference solution, locate the components of the reference solution in the chromatogram obtained with the test solution.

Determine the percentage content of these components. The percentages are within the following ranges:
— *limonene*: 1.5 per cent to 7.0 per cent,
— *cineole*: maximum 1.5 per cent,
— *menthone*: 17.0 per cent to 35.0 per cent,
— *isomenthone*: 5.0 per cent to 13.0 per cent,
— *menthyl acetate*: 1.5 per cent to 7.0 per cent,
— *isopulegol*: 1.0 per cent to 3.0 per cent,
— *menthol*: 30.0 per cent to 50.0 per cent,
— *pulegone*: maximum 2.5 per cent,
— *carvone*: maximum 2.0 per cent.

The ratio of cineole content to limonene content is less than 1.

STORAGE
At a temperature not exceeding 25 °C.

_____ *Ph Eur*

Motherwort

(Ph Eur monograph 1833)

Ph Eur

DEFINITION
Whole or cut, dried flowering aerial parts of *Leonurus cardiaca*
L.

Content
Minimum 0.2 per cent of flavonoids, expressed as hyperoside
($C_{21}H_{20}O_{12}$; M_r 464.4) (dried drug).

IDENTIFICATION
A. The stem pieces are hairy, longitudinally striated,
quadrangular, hollow, and up to about 10 mm wide; they
bear opposite and decussate, petiolate leaves and, in the axils
of the upper leaves, about 6-12 small flowers, arranged in
sessile whorls forming a long, leafy spike. The lower leaves
are ovate-orbicular, palmately 3- to 5-lobed, rarely 7-lobed,
the lobes irregularly dentate. The upper leaves are entire or
slightly trifid, lanceolate with a serrate margin and cuneate at
the base. The upper surface of the leaves is green with
scattered hairs, the lower surface is paler green, densely
pubescent and shows a prominent palmate and reticulate
venation. The flowers have a funnel-shaped calyx, 3 mm to
5 mm long with 5 stiff, recurved teeth; the corolla is
2-lipped, the upper lip pink and pubescent on the outer
surface, the lower lip white with purplish spots; stamens 4,
densely pubescent.

B. Microscopic examination (*2.8.23*). The powder is green.
Examine under a microscope using *chloral hydrate solution R*.
The powder shows the following diagnostic characters
(Figure 1833.-1): numerous covering trichomes [A], whole
[Aa] or fragmented [Ab], uniseriate, with warty walls,
composed of 2-8 cells with slight swellings at the junctions,
up to 1500 µm long; fragments of the upper epidermis, in
surface view [B], with cells with straight or sinuous anticlinal
walls [Ba], often accompanied by palisade parenchyma [Bb];
fragments of the lower epidermis, in surface view [C], with
cells with sinuous anticlinal walls [Ca], diacytic stomata
(*2.8.3*) [Cb], bearing glandular trichomes with a short
unicellular stalk and a globular head composed of 8-16 cells
[Cc], glandular trichomes with a uni- or bicellular stalk and a
bi- or tetracellular head [Cd] and sometimes covering
trichomes; fragments of the lamina, in transverse section [D],
composed of epidermises bearing glandular trichomes with a
globular head consisting of 8-16 cells [Da] or a bi- or
tetracellular head [Db], a 1-layered palisade mesophyll
extending almost halfway across the section [Dc], and a
loosely arranged spongy parenchyma [Dd]; fragments of the
calyx [G] with an epidermis consisting of polygonal cells
bearing uni- or bicellular conical covering trichomes, with
spiny walls [Ga], often associated with fusiform mesophyll
cells with thick walls and containing small prism crystals of
calcium oxalate [Gb]; isolated glandular trichomes [H],
either with a multicellular stalk and a unicellular head from
the anthers [Ha] or a uni- or multicellular stalk and bi- to
tetracellular head [Hb]; spherical pollen grains, about
25-30 µm in diameter, with 3 pores and 3 furrows and a
smooth exine [E]; thick-walled, lignified fibres [F]; fragments
from the stem with spirally and annularly thickened vessels
[K]; occasional fragments of pericarp [J] consisting of lobed
cells with thick, pitted walls, each containing a single prism
crystal of calcium oxalate [Ja].

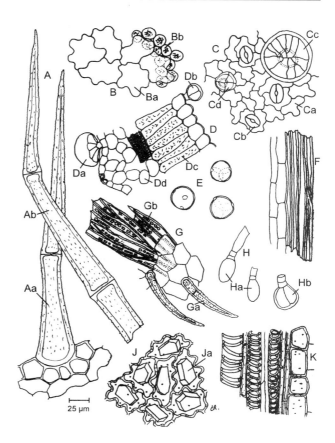

Figure 1833.-1. − *Illustration for identification test B of*
powdered herbal drug of motherwort

C. Thin-layer chromatography (*2.2.27*).

Test solution   To 0.5 g of the powdered herbal drug (355)
(*2.9.12*) add 5 mL of *methanol R*. Heat on a water-bath at
65 °C for 5 min with shaking. Cool and filter.

Reference solution   Dissolve 5 mg of *naphthol yellow S R* and
2.0 mg of *catalpol R* in 5.0 mL of *methanol R*.

Plate   *TLC silica gel plate R*.

Mobile phase   glacial acetic acid R, water R, ethyl acetate R
(20:20:60 *V/V/V*).

Application   20 µL as bands.

Development   Over a path of 10 cm.

Drying   In air.

Detection   Treat with *dimethylaminobenzaldehyde solution R2*,
using about 5 mL for a plate 200 mm square; heat at
100-105 °C for 10 min until the spots appear; examine in
daylight.

Results   See below the sequence of zones present in the
chromatograms obtained with the reference solution and the
test solution. Furthermore, other weak greyish-blue zones
may be present in the chromatogram obtained with the test
solution.

Top of the plate	
	A wide white zone
	A greyish-blue zone (iridoid)
Naphthol yellow S: an intense yellow zone	1 or 2 greyish-blue zones (iridoid)
Catalpol: a greyish-blue zone	
Reference solution	Test solution

TESTS

Foreign matter (*2.8.2*)

Maximum 2 per cent of brown or yellow leaves and maximum 2 per cent of other foreign matter.

Loss on drying (*2.2.32*)

Maximum 12.0 per cent, determined on 1.000 g of the powdered herbal drug (355) (*2.9.12*) by drying in an oven at 105 °C for 2 h.

Total ash (*2.4.16*)

Maximum 12.0 per cent.

ASSAY

Stock solution   In a 100 mL round-bottomed flask place 1.00 g of the powdered herbal drug (355) (*2.9.12*), add 1 mL of a 5 g/L solution of *hexamethylenetetramine R*, 20 mL of *acetone R* and 2 mL of *hydrochloric acid R1*. Boil the mixture under a reflux condenser for 30 min. Filter the liquid through a plug of absorbent cotton into a flask. Add the absorbent cotton to the residue in the round-bottomed flask and extract with 2 quantities, each of 20 mL, of *acetone R*, each time boiling under a reflux condenser for 10 min. Allow to cool and filter each extract through the plug of absorbent cotton into the flask. After cooling, filter the combined acetone extracts through a paper filter into a volumetric flask and dilute to 100.0 mL with *acetone R* by rinsing the flask and the paper filter. Introduce 20.0 mL of the solution into a separating funnel, add 20 mL of *water R* and shake the mixture with 1 quantity of 15 mL and then 3 quantities, each of 10 mL, of *ethyl acetate R*. Combine the ethyl acetate extracts in a separating funnel, wash with 2 quantities, each of 50 mL, of *water R*, filter the extracts over 10 g of *anhydrous sodium sulfate R* into a volumetric flask and dilute to 50.0 mL with *ethyl acetate R*.

Test solution   To 10.0 mL of the stock solution add 1 mL of *aluminium chloride reagent R* and dilute to 25.0 mL with a 5 per cent *V/V* solution of *glacial acetic acid R* in *methanol R*.

Compensation liquid   Dilute 10.0 mL of the stock solution to 25.0 mL with a 5 per cent *V/V* solution of *glacial acetic acid R* in *methanol R*.

Measure the absorbance (*2.2.25*) of the test solution after 30 min, by comparison with the compensation liquid at 425 nm. Calculate the percentage content of flavonoids, calculated as hyperoside, using the following expression:

$$\frac{A \times 1.25}{m}$$

i.e. taking the specific absorbance of hyperoside to be 500.

A = absorbance at 425 nm;

m = mass of the substance to be examined, in grams.

Mullein Flower

(*Ph Eur monograph 1853*)

Ph Eur _____

DEFINITION

Dried flower, reduced to the corolla and the androecium, of *Verbascum thapsus* L., *V. densiflorum* Bertol. (*V. thapsiforme* Schrad), and *V. phlomoides* L.

IDENTIFICATION

A. The corolla of *V. thapsus* is pale yellow, yellow or brown, funnel-shaped, about 20 mm in diameter, with 5 slightly unequal and spreading lobes. The corolla lobes are densely hairy on the outer surface, glabrous on the inner surface, with a fine network of light brown veins. There are 5 stamens, alternating with the petal lobes; 2 of these are long, with glabrous filaments, the other 3 shorter, with densely tomentose filaments. The anthers are attached transversely. In *V. phlomoides* the corolla is up to about 30 mm in diameter, bright yellow or orange, and the anthers are obliquely attached to the filaments. The corolla of *V. densiflorum*, about 30 mm in diameter, is almost flat and deeply divided into 5 slightly unequal lobes, with rounded apices.

B. Reduce to a powder (355) (*2.9.12*). The powder is yellow or yellowish-brown. Examine under a microscope using *chloral hydrate solution R*. The powder shows the following diagnostic characters (Figure 1853.-1): many covering trichomes from the corolla, whole and fragmented, pluricellular, of the candelabra type, with a central uniseriate axis from which whorls of branch cells arise at the position of the cross walls and at the apex, in side view [A, B] or in surface view [F]; the covering trichomes from the stamen filaments [G] are unicellular, long, thin-walled and tubular, have a distinctly granular or striated surface with a sharp tip [Ga] or sometimes with a club-shaped tip [Gb, Gc]; numerous pollen grains, ovoid with a finely granular exine with 3 pores [D]; fragments of the fibrous layer of the anther with thickened walls giving a characteristic star-shaped appearance [C]; yellow fragments of the petals, in surface view [E], the epidermal cells polygonal and isodiametric [Ea]; fragments of the underlying mesophyll consisting of irregular parenchymatous cells [Eb] sometimes accompanied by spiral vessels [Ec].

C. Thin-layer chromatography (*2.2.27*).

Test solution   Heat 1.0 g of the powdered drug (355) (*2.9.12*) in 10 mL of *methanol R* in a water-bath at 60 °C for 5 min, with stirring. Cool and filter.

Reference solution   Dissolve 1 mg of *caffeic acid R*, 2.5 mg of *hyperoside R* and 2.5 mg of *rutin R* in *methanol R* and dilute to 10 mL with the same solvent.

Plate   TLC silica gel plate R.

Mobile phase   anhydrous formic acid R, water R, methyl ethyl ketone R, ethyl acetate R (10:10:30:50 *V/V/V/V*).

Application   10 µL of the reference solution and 30 µL of the test solution, as bands.

Development   Over a path of 15 cm.

Drying   At 100-105 °C.

Detection   Spray the warm plate with a 10 g/L solution of *diphenylboric acid aminoethyl ester R* in *methanol R*, then with a 50 g/L solution of *macrogol 400 R* in *methanol R*; allow to dry in air for 30 min and examine in ultraviolet light at 365 nm.

Results   See below the sequence of zones present in the chromatograms obtained with the reference solution and the

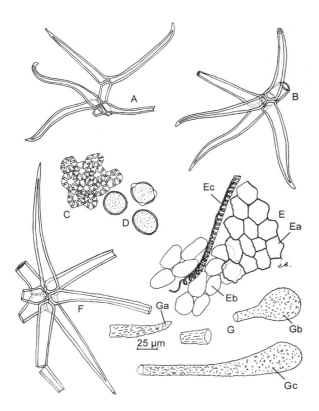

Figure 1853.-1.– *Illustration for identification test B of powdered herbal drug of mullein flower*

test solution. Furthermore, other faint zones may be present in the chromatogram obtained with the test solution.

Top of the plate	
	A yellow or yellowish-green fluorescent zone
Caffeic acid: a greenish-blue fluorescent zone	
	A bluish fluorescent zone
	A greenish fluorescent zone
	A yellowish-green fluorescent zone
	A bluish fluorescent zone
Hyperoside: a yellowish-brown fluorescent zone	
	A greenish fluorescent zone
Rutin: a yellowish-brown fluorescent zone	
Reference solution	**Test solution**

D. Boil 1.0 g of the powdered drug (355) (*2.9.12*) with 15 mL of *water R* for 1 min. Filter. Add 1 mL of *hydrochloric acid R* and boil for 1 min. A greenish-blue colour develops and, after a few minutes, cloudiness appears and then a blackish precipitate (iridoids).

TESTS

Foreign matter (*2.8.2*)

Maximum 5 per cent of brown petals and maximum 2 per cent of fragments of the calyx and other foreign matter, determined on 20 g.

Swelling index (*2.8.4*)

Minimum 9, determined on the powdered drug (710) (*2.9.12*), moistened with 2 mL of *ethanol (96 per cent) R*.

Loss on drying (*2.2.32*)

Maximum 12.0 per cent, determined on 1.000 g of the powdered drug (710) (*2.9.12*) by drying in an oven at 105 °C for 2 h.

Total ash (*2.4.16*)

Maximum 6.0 per cent.

Ash insoluble in hydrochloric acid (*2.8.1*)

Maximum 2.0 per cent.

STORAGE

In an airtight container.

———————————————————————— *Ph Eur*

Myrrh

(*Ph Eur monograph 1349*)

Preparation
Myrrh Tincture

Ph Eur —————————————————————————————

DEFINITION

Gum-resin, hardened in air, obtained by incision or produced by spontaneous exudation from the stem and branches of *Commiphora molmol* Engler and/or other species of *Commiphora*.

CHARACTERS

Bitter taste.

IDENTIFICATION

A. The light or dark orange-brown, irregular or roundish grains or pieces of different size show components of various colours. Their surface is mostly covered with grey or yellowish-brown dust.

B. Reduce to a powder (355) (*2.9.12*). The powder is brownish-yellow or reddish-brown. Examine under a microscope, using *chloral hydrate solution R*. The powder shows the following diagnostic characters: a few tissue fragments from the original plants including: reddish-brown cork fragments; single or grouped polyhedral or elongated stone cells with partly strongly thickened, pitted and lignified walls with a brownish content; fragments of thin-walled parenchyma and sclerenchymatous fibres; irregular prismatic or polyhedral crystals of calcium oxalate, about 10-25 µm in size.

C. Examine the chromatograms obtained in the test for *Commiphora mukul*.

Detection Spray with *anisaldehyde solution R*, and examine in daylight while heating at 100-105 °C for 10 min.

Results The chromatogram obtained with the reference solution shows in the lower third an orange-red zone (thymol) and in the middle third a violet zone (anethole). The chromatogram obtained with the test solution shows an intense violet zone (furanoeudesma-1,3-diene), exceeding the other zones in size and intensity, above the zone of anethole in the chromatogram obtained with the reference solution; a violet zone similar in position to the zone of anethole in the chromatogram obtained with the reference solution; 2 intense violet zones similar in position to the zone of thymol in the chromatogram obtained with the reference solution, the upper one due to curzerenone and the lower one to

2-methoxyfuranodiene. Further mostly violet zones are present in the chromatogram obtained with the test solution.

TESTS

Commiphora mukul

Thin-layer chromatography (2.2.27).

Test solution   To 0.5 g of the powdered drug (355) (2.9.12) add 5.0 mL of *ethanol (96 per cent) R* and warm the mixture on a water-bath for 2-3 min. Cool and filter.

Reference solution   Dissolve 10 mg of *thymol R* and 40 µL of *anethole R* in 10 mL of *ethanol (96 per cent) R*.

Plate   *TLC silica gel plate R*.

Mobile phase   ethyl acetate R, toluene R (2:98 V/V).

Application   10 µL, as bands.

Development   Over a path of 15 cm.

Drying   In air.

Detection   Examine in ultraviolet light at 365 nm.

Results   The chromatogram obtained with the test solution shows no blue or violet fluorescent zones in the lower third of the chromatogram.

Matter insoluble in ethanol

Maximum 70 per cent.

Place 1.00 g of the powdered drug (250) (2.9.12) in a flask. Add 30 mL of *ethanol (96 per cent) R* and shake vigorously for 10 min. Filter the supernatant through a tared sintered-glass filter (16) (2.1.2) avoiding the transfer of sediment from the flask. Repeat the extraction with 2 quantities, each of 20 mL, of *ethanol (96 per cent) R*. Quantitatively transfer the sediment to the filter by rinsing the flask with *ethanol (96 per cent) R*. Dry the filter and the residue in an oven at 100-105 °C and weigh.

Loss on drying (2.2.32)

Maximum 15.0 per cent, determined on 1.000 g of powdered drug (355) (2.9.12) by drying in an oven at 105 °C for 2 h.

Total ash (2.4.16)

Maximum 7.0 per cent.

_____ *Ph Eur*

Myrrh Tincture

(*Ph Eur monograph 1877*)

Ph Eur _____

DEFINITION

Tincture produced from *Myrrh (1349)*.

PRODUCTION

The tincture is produced from 1 part of the drug and 5 parts of ethanol (90 per cent V/V) by a suitable procedure.

CHARACTERS

Clear yellowish-brown or orange-brown liquid.

IDENTIFICATION

Thin-layer chromatography (2.2.27).

Test solution   Dilute 5 mL of the tincture to be examined to 10 mL with *alcohol R*.

Reference solution   Dissolve 10 mg of *thymol R* and 40 µL of *anethole R* in 10 mL of *ether R*.

Plate   *TLC silica gel plate R*.

Mobile phase   ethyl acetate R, toluene R (2:98 V/V).

Application   10 µL, as bands.

Development   Over a path of 15 cm.

Drying   In air.

Detection   Spray with *anisaldehyde solution R* and examine in daylight whilst heating at 100-105 °C for 10 min.

Results   See below the sequence of the zones present in the chromatograms obtained with the reference solution and the test solution. Furthermore, other zones mostly violet, are present in the chromatogram obtained with the test solution.

Top of the plate	
	An intense violet zone exceeding the others in size and intensity (furanoeudesma-1,3-diene)
Anethole: a violet zone	A violet zone
Thymol: an orange-red zone	Two intense violet zones (curzerenone and below 2-methoxyfuranodiene)
Reference solution	**Test solution**

TESTS

Ethanol content (2.9.10)

82 per cent V/V to 88 per cent V/V.

Methanol and 2-propanol (2.9.11)

Maximum 0.05 per cent V/V of methanol and maximum 0.05 per cent V/V of 2-propanol.

Dry residue (2.8.16)

Minimum 4.0 per cent m/m.

STORAGE

Plastic containers are not recommended.

_____ *Ph Eur*

Cineole Type Niaouli Oil

(*Ph Eur monograph 2468*)

Ph Eur _____

DEFINITION

Essential oil obtained by steam distillation from young leafy branches of *Melaleuca quinquenervia* (Cav.) S.T.Blake.

CHARACTERS

Appearance

Colourless or pale yellow liquid.

Aromatic odour of cineole.

IDENTIFICATION

First identification   B.

Second identification   A.

A. Thin-layer chromatography (2.2.27).

Test solution   Dissolve 100 µL of the oil to be examined in *toluene R* and dilute to 10.0 mL with the same solvent.

Reference solution   Dissolve 25 µL of *trans-nerolidol R* and 50 µL of *cineole R* in *toluene R* and dilute to 5.0 mL with the same solvent.

Plate   *TLC silica gel plate R* (5-40 µm) [or *TLC silica gel plate R* (2-10 µm)].

Mobile phase   ethyl acetate R, toluene R (5:95 V/V).

Application   10 µL [or 2 µL] as bands of 10 mm [or 8 mm].

Development   Over a path of 15 cm [or 6 cm].

Drying   In air.

Detection   Treat with *anisaldehyde solution R* and heat at 100-105 °C for 3 min; examine in daylight.

Results   See below the sequence of zones present in the chromatograms obtained with the reference solution and the test solution. Furthermore, other faint zones may be present in the chromatogram obtained with the test solution.

Top of the plate	
——— ———	———
	A faint grey zone
	A purple zone
1,8-Cineole: a violet-brown zone	An intense violet-brown zone (1,8-cineole)
trans-Nerolidol: a dark violet zone	
——— ———	———
	An intense violet-brown zone
	A violet-brown zone
Reference solution	**Test solution**

TESTS

Relative density (*2.2.5*)
0.904 to 0.925.

Refractive index (*2.2.6*)
1.463 to 1.472.

Optical rotation (*2.2.7*)
−4° to + 1°.

Methyleugenol and isomethyleugenol
Gas chromatography (*2.2.28*) as described in the test for chromatographic profile with the following modifications.

Reference solution   Dissolve 5 µL of *methyleugenol R* and 5 µL of *isomethyleugenol R* in *heptane R* and dilute to 50.0 mL with the same solvent. Dilute 0.5 mL of the solution to 5.0 mL with *heptane R*.

Elution order   Order indicated in the composition of the reference solution; record the retention times of methyleugenol and isomethyleugenol.

Identification of peaks   Using the retention times determined from the chromatogram obtained with the reference solution, locate the components of the reference solution in the chromatogram obtained with the test solution.

Limits:
— *methyleugenol*: maximum 0.05 per cent;
— *isomethyleugenol*: maximum 0.05 per cent.

Chromatographic profile
Gas chromatography (*2.2.28*): use the normalisation procedure.

Test solution   Dilute 0.2 mL of the oil to be examined to 10.0 mL with *heptane R*.

Reference solution (a)   Dilute 10 µL of *α-pinene R*, 5 µL of *β-pinene R*, 10 µL of *limonene R*, 50 µL of *cineole R*, 5 µL of *ρ-cymene R*, 5 µL of *benzaldehyde R*, 5 mg of *α-terpineol R* and 5 µL of *trans-nerolidol R* in *heptane R* and dilute to 10 mL with the same solvent.

Reference solution (b)   Dissolve 5 µL of *limonene R* in *heptane R* and dilute to 50.0 mL with the same solvent. Dilute 0.5 mL of the solution to 5.0 mL with *heptane R*.

Column:
— *material*: fused silica;
— *size*: *l* = 60 m, Ø = 0.25 mm;
— *stationary phase*: *macrogol 20 000 R* (film thickness 0.25 µm).

Carrier gas   helium for chromatography R.

Flow rate   1.3 mL/min.

Split ratio   1:50.

Temperature:

	Time (min)	Temperature (°C)
Column	0 - 5	65
	5 - 65	65 → 185
	65 - 80	185 → 230
Injection port		230
Detector		250

Detection   Flame ionisation.

Injection   1 µL.

Elution order   Order indicated in the composition of reference solution (a); record the retention times of these substances.

Identification of peaks   Using the retention times determined from the chromatogram obtained with reference solution (a), locate the components of reference solution (a) in the chromatogram obtained with the test solution; the peak due to viridiflorol elutes with a relative retention of about 1.02 with reference to *trans*-nerolidol.

System suitability   Reference solution (a):
— *resolution*: minimum 1.5 between the peaks due to limonene and 1,8-cineole.

Determine the percentage content of each of the following components. The limits are within the following ranges:
— *α-pinene*: 5.0 per cent to 15.0 per cent;
— *β-pinene*: 1.0 per cent to 4.0 per cent;
— *limonene*: 5.0 per cent to 10.0 per cent;
— *1,8-cineole*: 45.0 per cent to 65.0 per cent;
— *p-cymene*: 0.05 per cent to 4.0 per cent;
— *benzaldehyde*: 0.05 per cent to 0.5 per cent;
— *α-terpineol*: 3.0 per cent to 8.0 per cent;
— *trans-nerolidol*: 0.05 per cent to 1.5 per cent;
— *viridiflorol*: 2.5 per cent to 9.0 per cent;
— *disregard limit*: the area of the principal peak in the chromatogram obtained with reference solution (b) (0.05 per cent).

STORAGE

At a temperature not exceeding 25 °C.

Neroli Oil

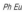

(*Ph Eur monograph 1175*)

Ph Eur _____

DEFINITION

Neroli oil is obtained by steam distillation from the fresh flowers of *Citrus aurantium* L. subsp. *aurantium* L. (*C. aurantium* L. subsp. *amara* Engl.).

CHARACTERS

Appearance

Clear, pale-yellow or dark-yellow liquid.

Characteristic odour.

IDENTIFICATION

First identification   B.

Second identification   A.

A. Examine the chromatograms obtained in the test for bergapten.

Results A   See below the sequence of zones present in the chromatograms obtained with the reference solution and the test solution. Furthermore other zones may be present in the chromatograms obtained with the test solution.

Top of the plate	
Methyl anthranilate: a blue fluorescent zone	A faint blue fluorescent zone (methyl anthranilate)
Bergapten: a greenish-yellow fluorescent zone	
Reference solution	**Test solution**

Detection B   Spray with *anisaldehyde solution R*; heat at 100-105 °C for 10 min; examine the chromatograms in ultraviolet light at 365 nm.

Results B   See below the sequence of zones present in the chromatograms obtained with the reference solution and the test solution. In the chromatogram obtained with the test solution the zone due to linalol is more intense than the zone due to linalyl acetate.

Top of the plate	
	A brown fluorescent zone
Linalyl acetate: a brownish-red fluorescent zone	An intense brownish-red fluorescent zone (linalyl acetate)
Methyl anthranilate: a blue fluorescent zone	A faint blue fluorescent zone (methyl anthranilate)
	A faint brownish-red fluorescent zone
Linalol: a brownish-red fluorescent zone	A brownish-red fluorescent zone (linalol)
Bergapten: a greenish-yellow fluorescent zone	
	Several blue and brownish-red fluorescent zones
Reference solution	**Test solution**

B. Examine the chromatograms obtained in the test for chromatographic profile.

Results   The principal peaks in the chromatogram obtained with the test solution are similar in retention time to the principal peaks in the chromatogram obtained with the reference solution.

TESTS

Relative density (*2.2.5*)

0.863 to 0.880.

Refractive index (*2.2.6*)

1.464 to 1.474.

Optical rotation (*2.2.7*)

+ 1.5° to + 11.5°.

Acid value (*2.5.1*)

Maximum 2.0.

Bergapten

Thin-layer chromatography (*2.2.27*).

Test solution   Dissolve 0.1 g of the substance to be examined in *ethanol (96 per cent) R* and dilute to 5.0 mL with the same solvent.

Reference solution   Dissolve 2 µL of *methyl anthranilate R*, 10 µL of *linalyl acetate R*, 20 µL of *linalol R* and 5 mg of *bergapten R* in *ethanol (96 per cent) R* and dilute to 10.0 mL with the same solvent.

Plate   *TLC silica gel plate R* (5-40 µm) [or *TLC silica gel plate R* (2-10 µm)].

Mobile phase   *ethyl acetate R*, *toluene R* (15:85 *V/V*).

Application   10 µL [or 2 µL] as bands.

Development   Over a path of 15 cm [or 8 cm].

Drying   In air.

Detection   Examine in ultraviolet light at 365 nm.

Results   The chromatogram obtained with the test solution does not show a zone corresponding to the zone due to bergapten in the chromatogram obtained with the reference solution.

Chromatographic profile

Gas chromatography (*2.2.28*): use the normalisation procedure.

Test solution   The substance to be examined.

Reference solution (a)   Dissolve 20 µL of *β-pinene R*, 5 mg of *sabinene R*, 40 µL of *limonene R*, 40 µL of *linalol R*, 20 µL of *linalyl acetate R*, 5 mg of α-terpineol R, 5 µL of *neryl acetate R*, 5 µL of *geranyl acetate R*, 5 µL of *trans-nerolidol R*, 5 µL of *methyl anthranilate R* and 5 µL *(E,E)-farnesol R* in 2 mL of *heptane R*.

Reference solution (b)   Dissolve 5 µL of *methyl anthranilate R* in *heptane R* and dilute to 10 mL with the same solvent.

Column:

— *material*: fused silica,

— *size*: *l* = 60 m, Ø = 0.25 mm,

— *stationary phase*: *macrogol 20 000 R* (film thickness 0.25 µm).

Carrier gas   *helium for chromatography R*.

Flow rate   1.5 mL/min.

Split ratio   1:100.

Temperature:

	Time (min)	Temperature (°C)
Column	0 - 4	75
	4 - 42.8	75 → 230
	42.8 - 63	230
Injection port		270
Detector		270

Detection   Flame ionisation.

Injection   0.2 µL.

Elution order   Order indicated in the composition of reference solution (a). Record the retention times of these substances.

System suitability   Reference solution (a):
— *resolution*: minimum 1.5 between the peaks due to β-pinene and sabinene.

Using the retention times determined from the chromatogram obtained with reference solution (a), locate the components of reference solution (a) in the chromatogram obtained with the test solution.

Limits:
— *β-pinene*: 7.0 per cent to 17.0 per cent,
— *limonene*: 9.0 per cent to 18.0 per cent,
— *linalol*: 28.0 per cent to 44.0 per cent,
— *linalyl acetate*: 2.0 per cent to 15.0 per cent,
— *α-terpineol*: 2.0 per cent to 5.5 per cent,
— *neryl acetate*: maximum 2.5 per cent,
— *geranyl acetate*: 1.0 per cent to 5.0 per cent,
— *trans-nerolidol*: 1.0 per cent to 5.0 per cent,
— *methyl anthranilate*: 0.1 per cent to 1.0 per cent,
— *(E,E)-farnesol*: 0.8 per cent to 4.0 per cent,
— *disregard limit*: area of the peak in the chromatogram obtained with reference solution (b).

Chiral purity

Gas chromatography (*2.2.28*).

Test solution   Dissolve 20 mg of the substance to be examined in *pentane R* and dilute to 10.0 mL with the same solvent.

Reference solution   To 10 µL of *linalol R* add 10 µL of *linalyl acetate R*. Dilute to 10.0 mL with *pentane R*.

Column:
— *material*: fused silica,
— *size*: $l = 25$ m, $\varnothing = 0.25$ mm,
— *stationary phase*: modified β-cyclodextrin for chiral chromatography R (film thickness 0.25 µm).

Carrier gas   helium for chromatography R.

Flow rate   1.3 mL/min.

Split ratio   1:30.

Temperature:

	Time (min)	Temperature (°C)
Column	0 - 65	50 → 180
Injection port		230
Detector		230

Detection   Flame ionisation.

Injection   1 µL.

System suitability   Reference solution:
— *resolution*: minimum 5.5 between the peaks due to (R)(−)-linalol (1st peak) and (S)(+)-linalol (2nd peak); minimum 2.7 between the peaks due to (R)(−)-linalyl acetate (3rd peak) and (S)(+)-linalyl acetate 4th peak).

Calculate the percentage content of the specified (S)-enantiomers from the following expression:

$$\frac{A_1}{A_1 + A_2} \times 100$$

A_1 = area of the corresponding (S)-enantiomer,
A_2 = area of the corresponding (R)-enantiomer.

Limits:
— (S)(+)-linalol: maximum 30 per cent,
— (S)(+)-linalyl acetate: maximum 5 per cent.

STORAGE

At a temperature not exceeding 25 °C.

Ph Eur

Nettle Leaf

(Ph Eur monograph 1897)

Ph Eur

DEFINITION

Whole or cut dried leaves of *Urtica dioica* L., *Urtica urens* L., or a mixture of the 2 species.

Content

Minimum 0.3 per cent for the sum of caffeoylmalic acid and chlorogenic acid, expressed as chlorogenic acid ($C_{16}H_{18}O_9$; M_r 354.3) (dried drug).

IDENTIFICATION

A. The leaves are dark green, dark greyish-green or brownish-green on the upper surface, paler on the lower surface; scattered stinging hairs occur on both surfaces, also small covering trichomes that are more numerous along the margins and on the veins on the lower surface. The lamina is strongly shrunken, ovate or oblong, up to 100 mm long and 50 mm wide, with a coarsely serrate margin and a cordate or rounded base. The venation is reticulate and distinctly prominent on the lower surface. The petiole is green or brownish-green, rounded or flattened, about 1 mm wide, longitudinally furrowed and twisted; it bears stinging hairs and covering trichomes.

B. Reduce to a powder (355) (*2.9.12*). The powder is green or greyish-green. Examine under a microscope using *chloral hydrate solution R*. The powder shows the following diagnostic characters (Figure 1897.-1): fragments of unicellular stinging hairs [A, B, C], up to 2 mm long, composed of an elongated tapering cell with a slightly swollen stinging tip that readily breaks off, arising from a raised, multicellular base [Ca]; small glandular trichomes [F] (35-65 µm), with a uni- or bicellular stalk and a bi- or quadricellular head, isolated [Fa], or on fragments of the epidermis [Fb]; fragments of the upper epidermis of the leaves in surface view [G] or in transverse section [D] showing slightly sinuous cells [Da, Gc], unicellular, straight or slightly curved covering trichomes, enlarged at the base, up to 700 µm long [Dc, Ga] and abundant large cystoliths [Db, Ea, Gb], empty or containing dense, granular masses of calcium carbonate; palisade parenchyma in surface view [E], with rounded cells [Eb] surrounding cystoliths (Ea), or in transverse section [Dd]; fragments of lower epidermis of leaves showing sinuous or wavy-walled cells [H], anomocytic [Ha] or anisocytic stomata [Hb] (*2.8.3*) accompanied by spongy mesophyll in surface view [Hc] and in transverse section [De] containing small cluster crystals of calcium oxalate in surface view [Hd] and in transverse section [Df]; occasional small groups of vessels, accompanied by parenchyma containing cluster crystals of calcium oxalate [J].

Top of the plate	
	2 red zones
Scopoletin: an intense blue fluorescent zone	A blue fluorescent zone (scopoletin)
	A blue fluorescent zone
_____	_____
_____	_____
Chlorogenic acid: a blue fluorescent zone	A blue fluorescent zone (chlorogenic acid)
	A brownish-yellow zone
Reference solution	**Test solution**

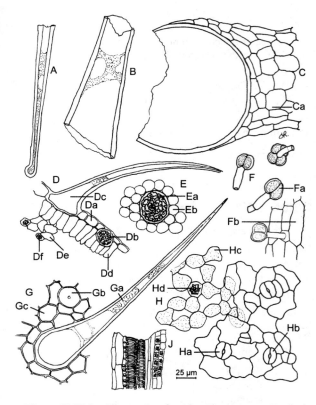

Figure 1897.-1.– *Illustration for identification test B of powdered herbal drug of nettle leaf*

C. Thin-layer chromatography (*2.2.27*).

Test solution To 1 g of the powdered drug (355) (*2.9.12*) add 10 mL of *methanol R*. Boil under a reflux condenser for 15 min. Cool and filter. Evaporate to dryness *in vacuo* at 40 °C. Dissolve the residue in 2 mL of *methanol R*.

Reference solution Dissolve 1 mg of *scopoletin R* and 2 mg of *chlorogenic acid R* in 20 mL of *methanol R*.

Plate TLC silica gel plate R (5-40 μm) [or TLC silica gel plate R (2-10 μm)].

Mobile phase anhydrous formic acid R, methanol R, water R, ethyl acetate R (2.5:4:4:50 V/V/V/V).

Application 10 μL [or 4 μL] as bands of 10 mm [or 8 mm].

Development Over a path of 8 cm [or 6 cm].

Drying In air.

Detection Heat at 100 °C for 5 min; spray the still-warm plate with a 10 g/L solution of *diphenylboric acid aminoethyl ester R* in *methanol R*; examine in ultraviolet light at 365 nm.

Results See below the sequence of zones present in the chromatograms obtained with the reference solution and the test solution. Furthermore, other faint blue or yellow fluorescent zones may be present in the lower half of the chromatogram obtained with the test solution.

TESTS

Foreign matter (*2.8.2*)
Maximum 5 per cent of stems and maximum 5 per cent of other foreign matter (including inflorescences).

Loss on drying (*2.2.32*)
Maximum 12.0 per cent, determined on 1.000 g of the powdered drug (355) (*2.9.12*) by drying in an oven at 105 °C for 2 h.

Total ash (*2.4.16*)
Maximum 20.0 per cent.

Ash insoluble in hydrochloric acid (*2.8.1*)
Maximum 4.0 per cent.

ASSAY

Liquid chromatography (*2.2.29*).

Test solution To 0.200 g of the powdered drug (355) (*2.9.12*) add 25.0 mL of a 40 per cent *V/V* solution of *methanol R*. Extract for 30 min in an ultrasonic bath at 40 °C and filter.

Reference solution Dissolve 10.0 mg of *chlorogenic acid CRS* in 100.0 mL of a 40 per cent *V/V* solution of *methanol R*. Dilute 5.0 mL of this solution to 25.0 mL with a 40 per cent *V/V* solution of *methanol R*.

Precolumn:
— size: l = 4 mm, Ø = 4 mm;
— stationary phase: end-capped octadecylsilyl silica gel for chromatography R (5 μm).

Column:
— size: l = 0.125 m, Ø = 4 mm;
— stationary phase: end-capped octadecylsilyl silica gel for chromatography R (5 μm);
— temperature: 25 °C.

Mobile phase:
— mobile phase A: mix 15 volumes of *methanol R* and 85 volumes of *water R* and adjust to pH 2.0 with *dilute phosphoric acid R*;
— mobile phase B: *methanol R*;

Time (min)	Mobile phase A (per cent V/V)	Mobile phase B (per cent V/V)
0 - 1	100	0
1 - 25	100 → 85	0 → 15
25 - 35	85	15
35 - 36	85 → 0	15 → 100

Flow rate 1 mL/min.

Detection Spectrophotometer at 330 nm.

Injection   20 µL.

Relative retention   With reference to chlorogenic acid (retention time = about 13 min):
caffeoylmalic acid = about 2.2.

Calculate the percentage content of caffeoylmalic acid and chlorogenic acid, expressed as chlorogenic acid, using the following expression:

$$\frac{A_1 \times m_2 \times p}{A_2 \times m_1 \times 20}$$

A_1 = sum of the areas of the peaks due to caffeoylmalic acid and chlorogenic acid in the chromatogram obtained with the test solution;

A_2 = area of the peak due to chlorogenic acid in the chromatogram obtained with the reference solution;

m_1 = mass of the drug to be examined used to prepare the test solution, in grams;

m_2 = mass of *chlorogenic acid CRS* used to prepare the reference solution, in grams;

p = percentage content of chlorogenic acid in *chlorogenic acid CRS*.

Ph Eur

Notoginseng Root

(Ph Eur monograph 2383)

Ph Eur

DEFINITION

Whole or fragmented taproot, without secondary roots, of *Panax pseudoginseng* Wall. var. *notoginseng* (Burk.) Hoo et Tseng [*Panax notoginseng* (Burk.) F.H. Chen ex C.Y. Wu et K.M. Feng] treated with steam and dried.

Content

Minimum 3.8 per cent for the sum of ginsenosides Rg1 ($C_{42}H_{72}O_{14},2H_2O$; M_r 837) and Rb1 ($C_{54}H_{92}O_{23},3H_2O$; M_r 1163) (dried drug).

IDENTIFICATION

A. The primary root is conical, subconical or cylindrical, up to 6 cm long and 4 cm in diameter. The outer surface, showing shallow transverse striations and secondary root scars, is brownish-grey or yellowish-grey. The aerial stem scar is surrounded by warty protuberances at the crown. The texture of the root is compact. The fracture is smooth, shiny, brownish-grey and shows a yellowish-grey ring (cambial zone) and many radial striations.

B. Reduce to a powder (355) (*2.9.12*). The powder is light yellowish-grey. Examine under a microscope using *chloral hydrate solution R*. The powder shows the following diagnostic characters: abundant fragments of thin-walled parenchymatous cells; fragments of secretory canals containing yellowish-brown resin; rare lignified vessels about 30 µm in diameter, reticulate or pitted; rare cork fragments. Examine under a microscope using a 50 per cent *V/V* solution of *glycerol R*. The starch granules, often deformed, are very abundant, single or in groups of 2-3, and 1-10 µm in diameter.

C. Examine the chromatogram obtained in the test for *Panax ginseng* or *Panax quinquefolium*.

Results   See below the sequence of zones present in the chromatograms obtained with the reference solution and the

test solution. Furthermore, other faint zones may be present in the chromatogram obtained with the test solution.

Top of the plate	
	A violet zone (at the solvent front)
	A violet zone
Arbutin: a brown zone	
————	————
	A violet zone (ginsenosides Rg1 + Rg2)
	2 violet zones
	2 faint violet zones
————	————
Aescin: a grey zone	A violet zone
	Several violet and greenish zones
Reference solution	**Test solution**

TESTS

Panax ginseng or *Panax quinquefolium*

Thin-layer chromatography (*2.2.27*).

Test solution   To 1.0 g of the powdered drug (355) (*2.9.12*) add 10 mL of a 70 per cent *V/V* solution of *methanol R* and boil under a reflux condenser for 15 min. Filter after cooling and dilute to 10.0 mL with *methanol R*.

Reference solution   Dissolve 5.0 mg of *aescin R* and 5.0 mg of *arbutin R* in 1 mL of *methanol R*.

Plate   *TLC silica gel plate R* (5-40 µm) [or *TLC silica gel plate R* (2-10 µm)].

Mobile phase   ethyl acetate R, water R, butanol R (25:50:100 *V/V/V*); allow to stand for 10 min and use the upper layer.

Application   20 µL, as bands of 15 mm [or 4 µL of the test solution and 2 µL of the reference solution, as bands of 8 mm].

Development   In an unsaturated tank, over a path of 10 cm [or 5 cm].

Drying   In air for 30 min.

Detection   Spray with *anisaldehyde solution R* and heat at 105-110 °C for 5-10 min; examine in daylight.

Results   In the chromatogram obtained with the test solution, the absence of a violet zone immediately above the zone due to arbutin in the chromatogram obtained with the reference solution suggests the presence of *Panax ginseng*; in the chromatogram obtained with the test solution, the presence of a brown zone immediately below the violet zone due to the ginsenosides Rg1 + Rg2 suggests the presence of *Panax quinquefolium*.

Loss on drying (*2.2.32*)

Maximum 12.0 per cent, determined on 1.000 g of the powdered drug (355) (*2.9.12*) by drying in an oven at 105 °C for 2 h.

Total ash (*2.4.16*)

Maximum 6.0 per cent.

Ash insoluble in hydrochloric acid (*2.8.1*)

Maximum 1.0 per cent.

ASSAY

Liquid chromatography (*2.2.29*).

Test solution   Reduce about 50 g to a powder (355) (*2.9.12*). Place 0.250 g of the powdered drug and 70 mL of a 50 per cent *V/V* solution of *methanol R* in a 250 mL round-bottomed flask. After adding a few grains of pumice, boil on a water-bath under a reflux condenser for 1 h. After cooling, centrifuge and collect the supernatant liquid. Treat the residue as described above. Mix the collected liquids and evaporate to dryness under reduced pressure at a temperature not exceeding 60 °C. Take up the residue with 10.0 mL of a buffer solution, adjusted to pH 4.5, containing 3.5 g of *sodium dihydrogen phosphate R* and 7.2 g of *potassium dihydrogen phosphate R* in 1000 mL of *water R* (solution A). Wash a cartridge containing about 0.36 g of *octadecylsilyl silica gel for chromatography R* with 5 mL of *methanol R* followed by 20 mL of *water for chromatography R*. Apply 5.0 mL of solution A to the cartridge. Elute with 20 mL of *water for chromatography R*, followed by 15 mL of a 30 per cent *V/V* solution of *methanol R*. Discard the eluates after confirming that no ginsenosides are present, otherwise repeat the assay with another type of cartridge. Elute the cartridge with 20 mL of *methanol R* and evaporate the eluate to dryness. Take up the residue with 5.0 mL of *methanol R*.

Reference solution   Dissolve 3.0 mg of *ginsenoside Rb1 R*, 3.0 mg of *ginsenoside Rg1 R* and 3.0 mg of *ginsenoside Rf R* in *methanol R* and dilute to 5.0 mL with the same solvent.

Column:
— *size: l* = 0.10 m, Ø = 4.6 mm;
— *stationary phase: aminopropylsilyl silica gel for chromatography R* (3 μm).

Mobile phase:
— *mobile phase A*: acetonitrile *R*;
— *mobile phase B*: water for chromatography *R*;

Time (min)	Mobile phase A (per cent *V/V*)	Mobile phase B (per cent *V/V*)
0 - 14	90	10
14 - 18	90 → 80	10 → 20
18 - 55	80	20

Flow rate   2 mL/min.

Detection   Spectrophotometer at 203 nm.

Injection   20 μL.

System suitability   Reference solution:
— *resolution*: minimum 3.0 between the peaks due to ginsenosides Rf and Rg1.

Calculate the sum of the percentage contents of ginsenosides Rb1 and Rg1 using the following expression:

$$\frac{A_1 \times m_2 \times 2 \times p_1}{m_1 \times A_3} + \frac{A_2 \times m_3 \times 2 \times p_2}{m_1 \times A_4}$$

A_1 = area of the peak due to ginsenoside Rb1 in the chromatogram obtained with the test solution;
A_2 = area of the peak due to ginsenoside Rg1 in the chromatogram obtained with the test solution;
A_3 = area of the peak due to ginsenoside Rb1 in the chromatogram obtained with the reference solution;
A_4 = area of the peak due to ginsenoside Rg1 in the chromatogram obtained with the reference solution;
m_1 = mass of the dried drug to be examined, in grams;
m_2 = mass of *ginsenoside Rb1 R* in the reference solution, in grams;
m_3 = mass of *ginsenoside Rg1 R* in the reference solution, in grams;

p_1 = percentage content of ginsenoside Rb1 in *ginsenoside Rb1 R*;
p_2 = percentage content of ginsenoside Rg1 in *ginsenoside Rg1 R*

_____ *Ph Eur*

Nutmeg Oil

(*Ph Eur monograph 1552*)

Ph Eur _____

DEFINITION

Essential oil obtained by steam distillation of the dried and crushed kernels of *Myristica fragrans* Houtt.

CHARACTERS

Appearance

Colourless or pale yellow liquid.

Spicy odour.

IDENTIFICATION

First identification   B.

Second identification   A.

A. Thin-layer chromatography (*2.2.27*).

Test solution   Dissolve 1 mL of the substance to be examined in *toluene R* and dilute to 10 mL with the same solvent.

Reference solution   Dissolve 20 μL of *myristicine R* in 10 mL of *toluene R*.

Plate   TLC silica gel plate R.

Mobile phase   ethyl acetate *R*, toluene *R* (5:95 *V/V*).

Application   10 μL as bands.

Development   Over a path of 15 cm.

Drying   In air.

Detection   Spray with *vanillin reagent R*, heat at 100-105 °C for 10 min and examine in daylight.

Results   The chromatogram obtained with the reference solution shows in the upper third a pink or reddish-brown zone (myristicine); the chromatogram obtained with the test solution shows a series of zones of which 1 is similar in position and colour to the zone in the chromatogram obtained with the reference solution; above this zone a brownish zone (safrole) and a violet zone (hydrocarbons) are present; below the myristicine zone, 5 blue zones of variable intensity are present.

B. Examine the chromatograms obtained in the test for chromatographic profile.

Results   The principal peaks in the chromatogram obtained with the test solution are similar in retention time to those in the chromatogram obtained with the reference solution.

TESTS

Relative density (*2.2.5*)
0.885 to 0.905.

Refractive index (*2.2.6*)
1.475 to 1.485.

Optical rotation (*2.2.7*)
+ 8° to + 18°.

Chromatographic profile
Gas chromatography (*2.2.28*): use the normalisation procedure.

Test solution   The substance to be examined.

Reference solution   Dissolve 15 μL of *α-pinene R*, 15 μL of *β-pinene R*, 15 μL of *sabinene R*, 5 μL of *car-3-ene R*, 5 μL of *limonene R*, 5 μL of *γ-terpinene R*, 5 μL of *terpinen-4-ol R*, 5 μL of *safrole R* and 10 μL of *myristicine R* in 1 mL of *hexane R*.

Column:
— *material*: fused silica;
— *size*: l = 25-60 m, Ø = about 0.3 mm;
— *stationary phase*: bonded *macrogol 20 000 R*.

Carrier gas   helium for chromatography R.

Flow rate   1.5 mL/min.

Split ratio   1:100.

Temperature:

	Time (min)	Temperature (°C)
Column	0 - 10	50
	10 - 75	50 → 180
	75 - 130	180
Injection port		200 - 220
Detector		240 - 250

Detection   Flame ionisation.

Injection   0.2 μL.

Elution order   Order indicated in the composition of the reference solution; record the retention times of these substances.

System suitability   Reference solution:
— *resolution*: minimum 1.5 between the peaks due to β-pinene and sabinene.

Identification of components   Using the retention times determined from the chromatogram obtained with the reference solution, locate the components of the reference solution in the chromatogram obtained with the test solution. Determine the percentage content of each of these components. The percentages are within the following ranges:
— *α-pinene*: 15 per cent to 28 per cent;
— *β-pinene*: 13 per cent to 18 per cent;
— *sabinene*: 14 per cent to 29 per cent;
— *car-3-ene*: 0.5 per cent to 2.0 per cent;
— *limonene*: 2.0 per cent to 7.0 per cent;
— *γ-terpinene*: 2.0 per cent to 6.0 per cent;
— *terpinen-4-ol*: 2.0 per cent to 6.0 per cent;
— *safrole*: maximum 2.5 per cent;
— *myristicine*: 5.0 per cent to 12.0 per cent.

STORAGE

Protected from heat.

———————————————————————— *Ph Eur*

Oak Bark

(*Ph Eur monograph 1887*)

Ph Eur ————————————————————————

DEFINITION

Cut and dried bark from the fresh young branches of *Quercus robur* L., *Q. petraea* (Matt.) Liebl. and *Q. pubescens* Willd.

Content

Minimum 3.0 per cent of tannins, expressed as pyrogallol ($C_6H_6O_3$; M_r 126.1) (dried drug).

IDENTIFICATION

A. The bark occurs in channelled or quilled pieces, not more than 3 mm thick. The outer surface is light grey or greenish-grey, rather smooth, with occasional lenticels. The inner surface is dull brown or reddish-brown and has slightly raised longitudinal striations about 0.5-1 mm wide. The fracture is splintery and fibrous.

B. Reduce to a powder (355) (*2.9.12*). The powder is light brown or reddish-brown and fibrous. Examine under a microscope using *chloral hydrate solution R*. The powder shows the following diagnostic characters: groups of thick-walled fibres surrounded by a moderately thickened parenchymatous sheath containing prism crystals of calcium oxalate; fragments of cork composed of thin-walled tabular cells filled with brownish or reddish contents; abundant sclereids, isolated and in groups, some large with thick, stratified walls and branching pits, others smaller and thinner-walled with simple pits, often with dense brown contents; fragments of parenchyma containing cluster crystals of calcium oxalate; occasional fragments of sieve tissue, thin-walled, some showing sieve areas on the oblique end-walls.

C. To 1 g of the powdered drug (710) (*2.9.12*) add 10 mL of *ethanol (30 per cent V/V) R* and heat the mixture under a reflux condenser on a water-bath for 30 min. Cool and filter. To 1 mL of this solution add 2 mL of a 10 g/L solution of *vanillin R* in *hydrochloric acid R*. A red colour develops.

TESTS

Loss on drying (*2.2.32*)

Maximum 10.0 per cent, determined on 1.000 g of the powdered drug (710) (*2.9.12*) by drying in an oven at 105 °C for 2 h.

Total ash (*2.4.16*)

Maximum 8.0 per cent.

ASSAY

Carry out the determination of tannins in herbal drugs (*2.8.14*). Use 0.700 g of the powdered drug (710) (*2.9.12*).

———————————————————————— *Ph Eur*

Olive Leaf

(*Ph Eur monograph 1878*)

Preparation

Olive Leaf Dry Extract

Ph Eur ————————————————————————

DEFINITION

Dried leaf of *Olea europaea* L.

Content

Minimum 5.0 per cent of oleuropein ($C_{25}H_{32}O_{13}$; M_r 540.5) (dried drug).

IDENTIFICATION

A. The leaf is simple, thick and coriaceous, lanceolate to obovate, 30-50 mm long and 10-15 mm wide, with a mucronate apex and tapering at the base to a short petiole; the margins are entire and reflexed abaxially. The upper surface is greyish-green, smooth and shiny, the lower surface paler and pubescent, particularly along the midrib and main lateral veins.

B. Reduce to a powder (355) (*2.9.12*). The powder is yellowish-green. Examine under a microscope using *chloral hydrate solution R*. The powder shows the following diagnostic characters: fragments of the epidermis in surface view with small, thick-walled polygonal cells and, in the lower epidermis only, small anomocytic stomata (*2.8.3*); fragments of the lamina in sectional view showing a thick cuticle, a palisade composed of 3 layers of cells and a small-celled spongy parenchyma; numerous sclereids, very thick-walled and mostly fibre-like with blunt or, occasionally, forked ends, isolated or associated with the parenchyma of the mesophyll; abundant, very large peltate trichomes, with a central unicellular stalk from which radiate some 10-30 thin-walled cells that become free from the adjoining cells at the margin of the shield, giving an uneven, jagged appearance.

C. Thin-layer chromatography (*2.2.27*).

Test solution   To 1.0 g of the powdered drug (355) (*2.9.12*) add 10 mL of *methanol R*. Boil under a reflux condenser for 15 min. Cool and filter.

Reference solution   Dissolve 10 mg of *oleuropein R* and 1 mg of *rutin R* in 1 mL of *methanol R*.

Plate   TLC silica gel plate R.

Mobile phase   *water R*, *methanol R*, *methylene chloride R* (1.5:15:85 *V/V/V*).

Application   10 µL, as bands.

Development   Over a path of 10 cm.

Drying   In air.

Detection   Spray with *vanillin reagent R* and heat at 100-105 °C for 5 min; examine in daylight.

Results   See below the sequence of zones present in the chromatograms obtained with the reference solution and the test solution. Furthermore, other faint zones may be present in the chromatogram obtained with the test solution.

Top of the plate	
	A dark violet-blue zone (solvent front)
	A dark violet-blue zone
_____	_____
Oleuropein: a brownish-green zone	A brownish-green zone (oleuropein)
_____	_____
Rutin: a brownish-yellow zone	
Reference solution	**Test solution**

TESTS

Loss on drying (*2.2.32*)
Maximum 10.0 per cent, determined on 1.000 g of the powdered drug (355) (*2.9.12*) by drying in an oven at 105 °C for 2 h.

Total ash (*2.4.16*)
Maximum 9.0 per cent.

ASSAY

Liquid chromatography (*2.2.29*).

Test solution   In a flask, place 1.000 g of the powdered drug (355) (*2.9.12*) and add 50 mL of *methanol R*. Heat in a water-bath at 60 °C for 30 min with shaking. Allow to cool and filter into a 100 mL volumetric flask. Rinse the flask and the filter with *methanol R* and dilute to 100.0 mL with the same solvent. Dilute 2.5 mL of this solution to 25.0 mL with *water R*.

Reference solution   Dissolve 5.0 mg of *oleuropein CRS* in 5.0 mL of *methanol R*. Dilute 1.0 mL of this solution to 25.0 mL with *water R*.

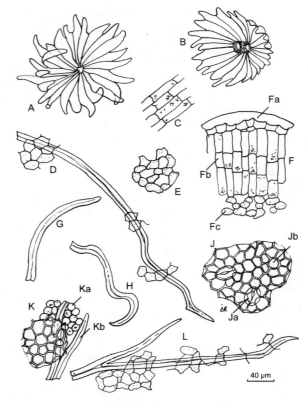

A. Peltate trichome, seen from above
B. Peltate trichome, seen from below
C. Palisade parenchyma
D, G, H and L. Fibre-like sclereids, some accompanied by parenchymatous fragments of the spongy mesophyll
E. Spongy parenchyma

F. Fragment of the lamina, in transverse section, showing a thick cuticle (Fa), palisade parenchyma composed of 3 layers of cells (Fb), and spongy parenchyma (Fc)

J. Fragment of lower epidermis with anomocytic stomata (Ja) and cicatrix of peltate trichome (Jb)

K. Fragment of upper epidermis, in surface view, with underlying palisade parenchyma (Ka) and sclereids of the spongy mesophyll (Kb)

Figure 1878.-1. – *Illustration of powdered herbal drug of olive leaf (see Identification B)*

Column:
— *size*: l = 0.15 m, Ø = 3.9 mm;
— *stationary phase*: octadecylsilyl silica gel for chromatography R (5 µm);
— *temperature*: 25 °C.

Mobile phase:
— *mobile phase A*: dilute 1.0 mL of *glacial acetic acid R* to 100 mL with *water R*;
— *mobile phase B*: methanol R;

Time (min)	Mobile phase A (per cent *V/V*)	Mobile phase B (per cent *V/V*)
0 - 5	85 → 40	15 → 60
5 - 12	40 → 20	60 → 80
12 - 15	20 → 85	80 → 15

Flow rate   1 mL/min.

Detection   Spectrophotometer at 254 nm.

Injection   20 µL.

Retention time   Oleuropein = about 9 min.

Calculate the percentage content of oleuropein using the following expression:

$$\frac{A_1 \times m_2 \times p \times 8}{A_2 \times m_1}$$

A_1 = area of the peak due to oleuropein in the chromatogram obtained with the test solution;

A_2 = area of the peak due to oleuropein in the chromatogram obtained with the reference solution;

m_1 = mass of the drug to be examined in the test solution, in grams;

m_2 = mass of *oleuropein CRS* in the reference solution, in grams;

p = percentage content of oleuropein in *oleuropein CRS*.

_____ *Ph Eur*

Olive Leaf Dry Extract

(*Ph Eur monograph 2313*)

Ph Eur _____

DEFINITION

Dry extract produced from *Olive leaf (1878)*.

Content

Minimum 16.0 per cent of oleuropein ($C_{25}H_{32}O_{13}$; M_r 540.5) (dried extract).

PRODUCTION

The extract is produced from the herbal drug by a suitable procedure using ethanol (65-96 per cent *V/V*).

CHARACTERS

Appearance

Greenish-brown or brown, amorphous powder.

IDENTIFICATION

Thin-layer chromatography (*2.2.27*).

Test solution   To 0.25 g of the extract to be examined add 10 mL of *methanol R*. Sonicate for 15 min and filter.

Reference solution   Dissolve 5 mg of *oleuropein R* and 1 mg of *rutin R* in 1 mL of *methanol R*.

Plate   *TLC silica gel plate R* (5-40 μm) [or *TLC silica gel plate R* (2-10 μm)].

Mobile phase   *water R, anhydrous formic acid R, ethyl acetate R* (7:13:80 *V/V/V*).

Application   10 μL [or 2 μL] as bands of 10 mm [or 8 mm].

Development   Over a path of 10 cm [or 6 cm].

Drying   In air.

Detection   Spray with *anisaldehyde solution R* and heat at 100-105 °C for 5 min; examine in daylight.

Results   See below the sequence of zones present in the chromatograms obtained with the reference solution and the test solution. Furthermore, other faint zones may be present in the chromatogram obtained with the test solution.

Top of the plate	
	A dark violet-blue zone
—————	—————
Oleuropein: a brownish-green zone	A brownish-green zone (oleuropein)
—————	—————
Rutin: a yellow zone	
Reference solution	**Test solution**

TESTS

Loss on drying (*2.8.17*)
Maximum 8.0 per cent.

ASSAY

Liquid chromatography (*2.2.29*). *Prepare the solutions immediately before use.*

Test solution   To 0.250 g of the extract to be examined add 50 mL of *methanol R*. Sonicate for 15 min and filter into a 100 mL volumetric flask. Rinse the flask and the filter with 2 mL of *methanol R* and dilute to 100.0 mL with *water R*.

Reference solution (a)   Dissolve 10.0 mg of *oleuropein CRS* in 10.0 mL of *methanol R* and dilute to 25.0 mL with *water R*.

Reference solution (b)   Dissolve 4 mg of *rutin R* in 10 mL of reference solution (a).

Column:
— *size*: l = 0.15 m, Ø = 4.6 mm;
— *stationary phase*: *end-capped octadecylsilyl silica gel for chromatography R* (5 μm);
— *temperature*: 25 °C.

Mobile phase   *trifluoroacetic acid R, methanol R, water R* (1:400:600 *V/V/V*).

Flow rate   1 mL/min.

Detection   Spectrophotometer at 233 nm.

Injection   20 μL.

Run time   Twice the retention time of oleuropein.

Relative retention   With reference to oleuropein (retention time = about 11 min): rutin = about 0.7.

System suitability   Reference solution (b):
— *resolution*: minimum 3.0 between the peaks due to rutin and oleuropein.

Calculate the percentage content of oleuropein using the following expression:

$$\frac{A_1 \times m_2 \times p \times 4}{A_2 \times m_1}$$

A_1 = area of the peak due to oleuropein in the chromatogram obtained with the test solution;

A_2 = area of the peak due to oleuropein in the chromatogram obtained with reference solution (a);

m_1 = mass of the extract to be examined used to prepare the test solution, in grams;

m_2 = mass of *oleuropein CRS* used to prepare reference solution (a), in grams;

p = percentage content of oleuropein in *oleuropein CRS*.

_____ *Ph Eur*

Opium

(*Raw Opium, Ph Eur monograph 0777*)

Preparations

Opium Tincture

Prepared Opium

Standardised Opium

Standardised Opium Tincture

Ph Eur _____

DEFINITION

Raw opium is intended only as starting material for the manufacture of galenical preparations. It is not dispensed as such.

Air-dried latex obtained by incision from the unripe capsules of *Papaver somniferum* L.

Content:
— *morphine* ($C_{17}H_{19}NO_3$; M_r 285.3): minimum 10.0 per cent (dried drug);
— *codeine* ($C_{18}H_{21}NO_3$; M_r 299.4): minimum 2.0 per cent (dried drug).

CHARACTERS
Characteristic odour.

Appearance
Blackish-brown masses of various sizes, which tend to be soft and shiny and, after drying, become hard and brittle.

IDENTIFICATION
Strip off any covering, cut the substance to be examined into thin slices, dry at about 60 °C for 48 h, if necessary, and reduce to a powder (500) (2.9.12).

A. Examined under a microscope, a suspension of raw opium in a 20 g/L solution of *potassium hydroxide R* shows the following diagnostic characters: granules of latex agglomerated in irregular masses, and light-brown elongated filaments. Some fragments of vessels and rather elongated, refringent crystals are also visible, as well as a smaller number of round pollen grains and fragments of elongated fibres. Hairs of various lengths with sharp points and a few grains of starch introduced during the handling of the latex may be present. Fragments of epicarp consisting of polygonal cells with thick walls defining a stellate lumen may also be present.

B. Thin-layer chromatography (*2.2.27*).

Test solution Triturate 0.10 g of the powdered drug with 5 mL of *ethanol (70 per cent V/V) R*, add 3 mL of *ethanol (70 per cent V/V) R*, transfer to a 25 mL conical flask and heat in a water-bath at 50-60 °C with stirring for 30 min. Cool, filter, wash the filter with *ethanol (70 per cent V/V) R* and dilute the filtrate to 10 mL with the same solvent.

Reference solution Dissolve 2.0 mg of *papaverine hydrochloride R*, 12.0 mg of *codeine phosphate R*, 12.0 mg of *noscapine hydrochloride R* and 25.0 mg of *morphine hydrochloride R* in *ethanol (70 per cent V/V) R* and dilute to 25.0 mL with the same solvent.

Plate TLC *silica gel G plate R*.

Mobile phase *concentrated ammonia R*, *ethanol (96 per cent) R*, *acetone R*, *toluene R* (2:6:40:40 *V/V/V/V*); use a freshly prepared mixture.

Application 20 μL, as bands of 20 mm by 3 mm.

Development Over a path of 15 cm.

Drying At 100-105 °C for 15 min, then allow to cool.

Detection Spray with *potassium iodobismuthate solution R2* and then with a 4 g/L solution of *sulfuric acid R*.

Results The chromatogram obtained with the reference solution shows in the lower part an orange-red or red zone (morphine) with a similarly coloured zone (codeine) above it, and in the upper part an orange-red or red zone (papaverine) with a similarly coloured zone (noscapine) above that; the chromatogram obtained with the test solution shows orange-red or red zones corresponding to those in the chromatogram obtained with the reference solution, and may also show a dark red zone (thebaine) situated between those due to codeine and papaverine.

C. To 1.0 g of the powdered drug add 5 mL of *water R*, shake for 5 min and filter. To the filtrate add 0.25 mL of *ferric chloride solution R2*. A red colour develops that does not disappear upon the addition of 0.5 mL of *dilute hydrochloric acid R*.

TESTS
Thebaine
Liquid chromatography (*2.2.29*).

Test solution Suspend 1.00 g of the substance to be examined, cut into thin slices, in 50 mL of *ethanol (50 per cent V/V) R*, mix with the aid of ultrasound for 1 h, allow to cool and dilute to 100.0 mL with the same solvent. Allow to stand. To 10.0 mL of the supernatant liquid add 5 mL of *ammonium chloride buffer solution pH 9.5 R*, dilute to 25.0 mL with *water R* and mix. Transfer 20.0 mL of this solution to a chromatography column about 0.15 m long and about 30 mm in internal diameter containing 15 g of *kieselguhr for chromatography R*. Allow to stand for 15 min. Elute with 2 quantities, each of 40 mL, of a mixture of 15 volumes of *2-propanol R* and 85 volumes of *methylene chloride R*. Evaporate the eluate to dryness *in vacuo* at 40 °C. Transfer the residue to a volumetric flask with the aid of the mobile phase and dilute to 25.0 mL with the mobile phase.

Reference solution Dissolve 25.0 mg of *thebaine R* in the mobile phase and dilute to 25.0 mL with the mobile phase. Dilute 10.0 mL of this solution to 100.0 mL with the mobile phase.

Precolumn:
— *size*: l = 4 mm, Ø = 4.0 mm;
— *stationary phase*: *octylsilyl silica gel for chromatography R* (5 μm).

Column:
— *size*: l = 0.25 m, Ø = 4.0 mm;
— *stationary phase*: *octylsilyl silica gel for chromatography R* (5 μm).

Mobile phase Dissolve 1.0 g of *sodium heptanesulfonate monohydrate R* in 420 mL of *water R*, adjust to pH 3.2 with phosphoric acid (4.9 g/L H_3PO_4) (about 5 mL) and add 180 mL of *acetonitrile R*.

Flow rate 1.5 mL/min.

Detection Spectrophotometer at 280 nm.

Injection A suitable volume with a loop injector.

System suitability Reference solution:
— *number of theoretical plates*: minimum 3000;
— *mass distribution ratio*: minimum 3.0 for the peak due to thebaine.

Calculate the percentage content of the alkaloid using the following expression:

$$\frac{m_1 \times A_2 \times 625}{m_2 \times A_1 \times 5} \times \frac{100}{100 - h}$$

m_1 = mass of the alkaloid used to prepare the reference solution, in grams;

m_2 = mass of the substance to be examined used to prepare the test solution, in grams;

A_1 = area of the peak due to the alkaloid in the chromatogram obtained with the reference solution;

A_2 = area of the peak due to the alkaloid in the chromatogram obtained with the test solution;

h = percentage loss on drying.

Limit:
— *thebaine*: maximum 3.0 per cent (dried drug).

Loss on drying *(2.2.32)*
Maximum 15.0 per cent, determined on 1.000 g of the substance to be examined cut into thin slices, by drying in an oven at 105 °C for 4 h.

Total ash *(2.4.16)*
Maximum 6.0 per cent.

ASSAY
Liquid chromatography *(2.2.29)* as described in the test for thebaine with the following modifications.

Reference solution Dissolve 0.100 g of *morphine hydrochloride R* and 25.0 mg of *codeine R* in the mobile phase and dilute to 25.0 mL with the mobile phase. Dilute 10.0 mL of this solution to 100.0 mL with the mobile phase.

System suitability Reference solution:
— *resolution*: minimum 2.5 between the peaks due to morphine and codeine; if necessary, adjust the volume of acetonitrile in the mobile phase;
— *repeatability*: maximum relative standard deviation of 1.0 per cent for the area of the peak due to morphine after 6 injections.

Calculate the percentage content of morphine and codeine from the expression given in the test for thebaine.

For the calculation, 1 mg of *morphine hydrochloride R* is equivalent to 0.759 mg of morphine, and 1 mg of *codeine R* is equivalent to 0.943 mg of codeine.

Ph Eur

Prepared Opium

(Ph Eur monograph 1840)

Ph Eur

DEFINITION
Raw opium powdered (180) *(2.9.12)*, and dried at a temperature not exceeding 70 °C.

Content:
— *morphine* ($C_{17}H_{19}NO_3$; M_r 285.3): 9.8 per cent to 10.2 per cent (drug dried at 100-105 °C for 4 h),
— *codeine* ($C_{18}H_{21}NO_3$; M_r 299.4): minimum 1.0 per cent (drug dried at 100-105 °C for 4 h).

Content adjusted if necessary by adding a suitable excipient or raw opium powder.

CHARACTERS
Appearance
Yellowish-brown or dark brown powder.

IDENTIFICATION
A. Examine under a microscope using a 20 g/L solution of *potassium hydroxide R*. It is seen to consist of granules of latex agglomerated in irregular masses, and of light brown elongated filaments. Some fragments of vessels and rather elongated, refringent crystals are also visible, as well as a smaller number of round pollen grains and fragments of elongated fibres. Hairs of various lengths with sharp points and fragments of epicarp consisting of polygonal cells with thick walls defining a stellate lumen may be present. Examine under a microscope using *glycerol (85 per cent) R*. Particles of excipient and a few grains of starch introduced during the handling of the latex may be seen.

B. Thin-layer chromatography *(2.2.27)*.

Test solution Triturate 0.10 g of the drug to be examined with 5 mL of *ethanol (70 per cent V/V) R*, rinse with 3 mL of *ethanol (70 per cent V/V) R*, transfer to a 25 mL conical flask. Heat in a water-bath at 50-60 °C with stirring for 30 min. Cool, filter, wash the filter with *ethanol (70 per cent V/V) R* and dilute the filtrate to 10 mL with the same solvent.

Reference solution Dissolve 2.0 mg of *papaverine hydrochloride R*, 12.0 mg of *codeine phosphate R*, 12.0 mg of *noscapine hydrochloride R* and 25.0 mg of *morphine hydrochloride R* in *ethanol (70 per cent V/V) R* and dilute to 25.0 mL with the same solvent.

Plate TLC silica gel G plate R.

Mobile phase concentrated ammonia R, ethanol (96 per cent) R, acetone R, toluene R (2:6:40:40 V/V/V/V). Use a freshly prepared mixture.

Application 20 μL, as bands of 20 mm by 3 mm.

Development Over a path of 15 cm.

Drying At 100-105 °C for 15 min.

Detection Allow to cool and spray with *potassium iodobismuthate solution R2* and then with a 4 g/L solution of *sulfuric acid R*, examine in daylight.

Results See below the sequence of the zones present in the chromatograms obtained with the reference solution and the test solution. Furthermore, a dark red zone (thebaine) situated between the codeine zone and the papaverine zone may be present in the chromatogram obtained with the test solution.

Top of the plate	
Noscapine: an orange-red or red zone	An orange-red or red zone (noscapine)
Papaverine: an orange-red or red zone	An orange-red or red zone (papaverine)
Codeine: an orange-red or red zone	An orange-red or red zone (codeine)
Morphine: an orange-red or red zone	An orange-red or red zone (morphine)
Reference solution	**Test solution**

C. To 1.0 g of the drug to be examined add 5 mL of *water R*, shake for 5 min and filter. To the filtrate add 0.25 mL of *ferric chloride solution R2*. A red colour develops which does not disappear on the addition of 0.5 mL of *dilute hydrochloric acid R*.

TESTS
Thebaine
Liquid chromatography *(2.2.29)*.

Test solution Suspend 1.00 g of the drug to be examined in 50 mL of *ethanol (50 per cent V/V) R*, mix using sonication for 1 h, allow to cool and dilute to 100.0 mL with the same solvent. Allow to stand. To 10.0 mL of the supernatant liquid, add 5 mL of *ammonium chloride buffer solution pH 9.5 R*, dilute to 25.0 mL with *water R* and mix. Transfer 20.0 mL of the solution to a chromatography column about 0.15 m long and about 30 mm in internal diameter containing 15 g of *kieselguhr for chromatography R*. Allow to stand for 15 min. Elute with 2 quantities, each of 40 mL, of a mixture of 15 volumes of *2-propanol R* and 85 volumes of *methylene chloride R*. Evaporate the eluate to dryness *in vacuo* at 40 °C. Transfer the residue to a volumetric flask with the aid of the mobile phase and dilute to 25.0 mL with the mobile phase.

Reference solution   Dissolve 25.0 mg of *thebaine R* in the mobile phase and dilute to 25.0 mL with the mobile phase. Dilute 10.0 mL of the solution to 100.0 mL with the mobile phase.

Precolumn:
— *size*: l = 4 mm, Ø = 4.0 mm,
— *stationary phase*: octylsilyl silica gel for chromatography *R* (5 µm).

Column:
— *size*: l = 0.25 m, Ø = 4.0 mm,
— *stationary phase*: octylsilyl silica gel for chromatography *R* (5 µm).

Mobile phase   Dissolve 1.0 g of *sodium heptanesulfonate monohydrate R* in 420 mL of *water R*, adjust to pH 3.2 with phosphoric acid (4.9 g/L H_3PO_4) (about 5 mL) and add 180 mL of *acetonitrile R*.

Flow rate   1.5 mL/min.

Detection   Spectrophotometer at 280 nm.

Injection   A suitable volume with a loop injector.

System suitability   Reference solution:
— *mass distribution ratio*: minimum 3.0 for the peak due to thebaine.

Calculate the percentage content of alkaloid from the expression:

$$\frac{m_1 \times A_2 \times 125}{m_2 \times A_1} \times \frac{100}{100 - h}$$

m_1 = mass of the alkaloid in the reference solution, in grams,
m_2 = mass of the substance to be examined in the test solution, in grams,
A_1 = area of the peak due to the alkaloid in the chromatogram obtained with the reference solution,
A_2 = area of the peak due to the alkaloid in the chromatogram obtained with the test solution,
h = percentage loss on drying.

Limit:
— *thebaine*: maximum 3.0 per cent (dried drug).

Loss on drying (*2.2.32*)
Maximum 8.0 per cent, determined on 1.000 g by drying in an oven at 105 °C for 4 h.

Total ash (*2.4.16*)
Maximum 6.0 per cent.

ASSAY
Liquid chromatography (*2.2.29*) as described in the test for thebaine with the following modifications.

Reference solution   Dissolve 0.100 g of *morphine hydrochloride R* and 25.0 mg of *codeine R* in the mobile phase and dilute to 25.0 mL with the mobile phase. Dilute 10.0 mL of the solution to 100.0 mL with the mobile phase.

System suitability   Reference solution:
— *resolution*: minimum 2.5 between the peaks due to morphine and codeine; if necessary, adjust the volume of acetonitrile in the mobile phase,
— *repeatability*: maximum relative standard deviation of 1.0 per cent for the peak area due to morphine, determined on 6 replicate injections.

Calculate the percentage content of morphine and codeine from the expression given in the test for thebaine. For the calculation, 1 mg of *morphine hydrochloride R* is taken to be

equivalent to 0.759 mg of morphine and 1 mg of *codeine R* is taken to be equivalent to 0.943 mg of codeine.

Ph Eur

Standardised Opium Dry Extract

(*Ph Eur monograph 1839*)

Ph Eur

DEFINITION
Standardised dry extract produced from *Raw opium (0777)*.

Content:
— *morphine* ($C_{17}H_{19}NO_3$; M_r 285.3): 19.6 per cent to 20.4 per cent (dried extract);
— *codeine* ($C_{18}H_{21}NO_3$; M_r 299.4): minimum 2.0 per cent (dried extract).

Content adjusted if necessary by adding a suitable excipient (e.g. lactose, dextrin).

PRODUCTION
It is produced from the drug and water by a suitable procedure.

CHARACTERS
Appearance: brown, amorphous powder.

IDENTIFICATION
A. Thin-layer chromatography (*2.2.27*).

Test solution   Triturate 0.05 g of the extract to be examined with 5 mL of *ethanol (70 per cent V/V) R*. Transfer to a 25 mL conical flask. Rinse with 3 mL of *ethanol (70 per cent V/V) R* and transfer to the same 25 mL conical flask. Heat in a water-bath at 50-60 °C, with stirring, for 30 min. Cool, filter, wash the filter with *ethanol (70 per cent V/V) R* and dilute the combined filtrate and washings to 10 mL with the same solvent.

Reference solution   Dissolve 5 mg of *morphine hydrochloride R* in the solution prepared as follows and dilute to 5 mL with the same solution: dissolve 2 mg of *papaverine hydrochloride R*, 12 mg of *codeine phosphate R* and 12 mg of *noscapine hydrochloride R* in *ethanol (70 per cent V/V) R* and dilute to 25 mL with the same solvent.

Plate   TLC silica gel plate *R* (5-40 µm) [or TLC silica gel plate *R* (2-10 µm)].

Mobile phase   concentrated ammonia *R*, ethanol (96 per cent) *R*, acetone *R*, toluene *R* (2:6:40:40 *V/V/V/V*). Use a freshly prepared mixture.

Application   20 µL [or 6 µL] as bands.

Development   Over a path of 15 cm [or 8 cm].

Drying   At 100-105 °C for 15 min.

Detection   Allow to cool and spray with *potassium iodobismuthate solution R2* and then with a 4 g/L solution of *sulfuric acid R*; examine in daylight.

Results   See below the sequences of zones present in the chromatograms obtained with the reference solution and the test solution. A dark red zone (thebaine) situated between the zone due to codeine and the zone due to papaverine may be present in the chromatogram obtained with the test solution. Furthermore, other faint zones may be present in the chromatogram obtained with the test solution.

Top of the plate	
Noscapine: an orange-red or red zone	An orange-red or red zone (noscapine)
———	———
Papaverine: an orange-red or red zone	An orange-red or red zone (papaverine)
———	———
Codeine: an orange-red or red zone	An orange-red or red zone (codeine)
Morphine: an orange-red or red zone	An orange-red or red zone (morphine)
Reference solution	**Test solution**

B. To 0.5 g of the extract to be examined add 5 mL of *water R*, shake for 5 min and filter. To the filtrate add 0.25 mL of *ferric chloride solution R2*. A red colour develops, which does not disappear on the addition of 0.5 mL of *dilute hydrochloric acid R*.

TESTS
Thebaine
Liquid chromatography (*2.2.29*).

Test solution Suspend 0.500 g of the extract to be examined in 50 mL of *ethanol (50 per cent V/V) R*, mix with the aid of ultrasound for 1 h, allow to cool and dilute to 100.0 mL with the same solvent. Allow to stand. To 10.0 mL of the supernatant liquid, add 5 mL of *ammonium chloride buffer solution pH 9.5 R*, dilute to 25.0 mL with *water R* and mix. Transfer 20.0 mL of this solution to a chromatography column about 0.15 m long and about 30 mm in internal diameter containing 15 g of *kieselguhr for chromatography R*. Allow to stand for 15 min. Elute with 2 quantities, each of 40 mL, of a mixture of 15 volumes of *2-propanol R* and 85 volumes of *methylene chloride R*. Evaporate the eluate to dryness *in vacuo* at 40 °C. Transfer the residue to a volumetric flask with the aid of the mobile phase and dilute to 25.0 mL with the mobile phase.

Reference solution (a) Dissolve 5.0 mg of *thebaine CRS* in the mobile phase and dilute to 50.0 mL with the mobile phase.

Reference solution (b) Dissolve 12.0 mg of *morphine hydrochloride CRS* in the mobile phase and dilute to 15.0 mL with the mobile phase (solution A). Dissolve 10.0 mg of *codeine CRS* in the mobile phase and dilute to 50.0 mL with the mobile phase. To 10.0 mL of this solution add 10.0 mL of solution A and mix.

Precolumn:
— *size*: $l = 4$ mm, Ø = 4.0 mm;
— *stationary phase*: *octylsilyl silica gel for chromatography R* (5 μm).

Column:
— *size*: $l = 0.25$ m, Ø = 4.0 mm;
— *stationary phase*: *octylsilyl silica gel for chromatography R* (5 μm).

Mobile phase Dissolve 1.0 g of *sodium heptanesulfonate monohydrate R* in 420 mL of *water R*, adjust to pH 3.2 with a 4.9 g/L solution of *phosphoric acid R* and add 180 mL of *acetonitrile R*.

Flow rate 1.5 mL/min.

Detection Sectrophotometer at 280 nm.

Injection 20 μL.

System suitability:
— *resolution*: minimum 2.5 between the peaks due to morphine and codeine in the chromatogram obtained with reference solution (b);

— *mass distribution ratio*: minimum 3.0 for the peak due to thebaine in the chromatogram obtained with reference solution (a).

Calculate the percentage content of thebaine using the following expression:

$$\frac{A_1 \times m_2 \times F \times p}{A_2 \times m_1}$$

A_1 = area of the peak due to the relevant alkaloid in the chromatogram obtained with the test solution;
A_2 = area of the peak due to the relevant alkaloid in the chromatogram obtained with the reference solution;
m_1 = mass of the extract to be examined in the test solution, in grams;
m_2 = mass of the relevant alkaloid in the reference solution, in grams;
p = percentage content of the alkaloid in the relevant alkaloid CRS;
F = 6.250 for the determination of thebaine.

Limit:
— *thebaine*: maximum 6.0 per cent (dried extract).

Loss on drying (*2.2.32*)
Maximum 5.0 per cent, determined on 1.000 g by drying in an oven at 105 °C for 4 h.

ASSAY
Liquid chromatography (*2.2.29*) as described in the test for thebaine with the following modifications.

Injection Test solution and reference solution (b).

System suitability:
— *repeatability*: maximum relative standard deviation of 1.0 per cent for the area of the peak due to morphine after 6 injections of reference solution (b).

Calculate the percentage content of morphine and codeine from the expression given in the test for thebaine, assigning F as 10.417 for morphine and as 3.125 for codeine.

_____ *Ph Eur*

Standardised Opium Tincture

(*Ph Eur monograph 1841*)

Ph Eur _____

DEFINITION
Standardised tincture produced from *Raw opium (0777)*.

Content:
— *morphine* ($C_{17}H_{19}NO_3$; M_r 285.3): 0.95 per cent to 1.05 per cent;
— *codeine* ($C_{18}H_{21}NO_3$; M_r 299.4): minimum 0.1 per cent.

PRODUCTION
It is produced from the drug and equal volumes of ethanol (70 per cent *V/V*) and water by an appropriate procedure.

CHARACTERS
Appearance
Reddish-brown liquid.

IDENTIFICATION
Thin-layer chromatography (*2.2.27*).

Test solution Dilute 1.0 mL of the tincture to be examined to 10 mL with *ethanol (70 per cent V/V) R*.

Reference solution Dissolve 5 mg of *morphine hydrochloride R* in the solution prepared as follows and dilute to 5 mL with the same solution: dissolve 2 mg of *papaverine hydrochloride R*, 12 mg of *codeine phosphate R* and 12 mg of *noscapine hydrochloride R* in *ethanol (70 per cent V/V) R* and dilute to 25 mL with the same solvent.

Plate TLC silica gel plate R (5-40 μm) [or *TLC silica gel plate R* (2-10 μm)].

Mobile phase *concentrated ammonia R*, *ethanol (96 per cent) R*, *acetone R*, *toluene R* (2:6:40:40 *V/V/V/V*). Use a freshly prepared mixture.

Application 20 μL [or 6 μL] as bands.

Development Over a path of 15 cm [or 8 cm].

Drying At 100-105 °C for 15 min.

Detection Allow to cool and spray the plate with *potassium iodobismuthate solution R2* and then with a 4 g/L solution of *sulfuric acid R*; examine in daylight.

Results See below the sequence of zones present in the chromatograms obtained with the reference solution and the test solution. A dark red zone (thebaine) situated between the zone due to codeine and the zone due to papaverine may be present in the chromatogram obtained with the test solution. Furthermore, other faint zones may be present in the chromatogram obtained with the test solution.

Top of the plate	
Noscapine: an orange-red or red zone	An orange-red or red zone (noscapine)
———	———
Papaverine: an orange-red or red zone	An orange-red or red zone (papaverine)
———	———
Codeine: an orange-red or red zone	An orange-red or red zone (codeine)
Morphine: an orange-red or red zone	An orange-red or red zone (morphine)
Reference solution	**Test solution**

TESTS

Ethanol *(2.9.10)*

31 per cent *V/V* to 34 per cent *V/V*.

Thebaine

Liquid chromatography *(2.2.29)*.

Test solution Dilute 2.000 g of the tincture to be examined to 25.0 mL with *ethanol (50 per cent V/V) R*. To 10.0 mL of the solution add 5 mL of *ammonium chloride buffer solution pH 9.5 R*, dilute to 25.0 mL with *water R* and mix. Transfer 20.0 mL of this solution to a chromatography column about 0.15 m long and about 30 mm in internal diameter containing 15 g of *kieselguhr for chromatography R*. Allow to stand for 15 min. Elute with 2 quantities, each of 40 mL, of a mixture of 15 volumes of *2-propanol R* and 85 volumes of *methylene chloride R*. Evaporate the eluate to dryness *in vacuo* at 40 °C. Transfer the residue to a volumetric flask with the aid of the mobile phase and dilute to 25.0 mL with the mobile phase.

Reference solution (a) Dissolve 5.0 mg of *thebaine CRS* in the mobile phase and dilute to 50.0 mL with the mobile phase.

Reference solution (b) Dissolve 12.0 mg of *morphine hydrochloride CRS* in the mobile phase and dilute to 15.0 mL with the mobile phase (solution A). Dissolve 10.0 mg of *codeine CRS* in the mobile phase and dilute to 50.0 mL with the mobile phase. To 10.0 mL of this solution add 10.0 mL of solution A and mix.

Precolumn:
— *size*: $l = 4$ mm, $\emptyset = 4.0$ mm;
— *stationary phase*: octylsilyl silica gel for chromatography R (5 μm).

Column:
— *size*: $l = 0.25$ m, $\emptyset = 4.0$ mm;
— *stationary phase*: octylsilyl silica gel for chromatography R (5 μm).

Mobile phase Dissolve 1.0 g of *sodium heptanesulfonate monohydrate R* in 420 mL of *water R*, adjust to pH 3.2 with a 4.9 g/L solution of *phosphoric acid R* and add 180 mL of *acetonitrile R*.

Flow rate 1.5 mL/min.

Detection Spectrophotometer at 280 nm.

Injection 20 μL.

System suitability Reference solution (b):
— *resolution*: minimum 2.5 between the peaks due to morphine and codeine.

Calculate the percentage content of thebaine using the following expression:

$$\frac{A_1 \times m_2 \times F \times p}{A_2 \times m_1}$$

A_1 = area of the peak due to the relevant alkaloid in the chromatogram obtained with the test solution;

A_2 = area of the peak due to the relevant alkaloid in the chromatogram obtained with the reference solution;

m_1 = mass of the tincture to be examined in the test solution, in grams;

m_2 = mass of the relevant alkaloid in the reference solution, in grams;

p = percentage content of the alkaloid in the relevant alkaloid CRS;

F = 1.563 for the determination of thebaine.

Limit:
— *thebaine*: maximum 0.3 per cent.

Dry residue *(2.8.16)*

Minimum 4.0 per cent *m/m*, determined on 3.00 g.

ASSAY

Liquid chromatography *(2.2.29)* as described in the test for thebaine with the following modifications.

Injection Test solution and reference solution (b).

System suitability:
— *repeatability*: maximum relative standard deviation of 1.0 per cent for the area of the peak due to morphine after 6 injections of reference solution (b).

Calculate the percentage content of morphine and codeine from the expression given in the test for thebaine, assigning F as 2.604 for morphine and 0.781 for codeine.

Ph Eur

Opium Tincture

DEFINITION

Opium, sliced	200 g
Ethanol (90 per cent)	A sufficient quantity
Purified Water	A sufficient quantity

Extemporaneous preparation

The following directions apply.

Pour 500 mL of boiling Purified Water on to the Opium and allow to stand for 6 hours; add 500 mL of Ethanol (90 per cent), mix thoroughly and allow to stand in a covered vessel for 24 hours; strain, press the marc, mix the liquids and allow to stand for not less than 24 hours; filter.

Determine the concentration of morphine, calculated as anhydrous morphine, in the tincture so prepared by the Assay. To the remainder of the liquid add sufficient of a mixture of equal volumes of Ethanol (90 per cent) and Purified Water to produce an Opium Tincture containing 1% w/v of anhydrous morphine.

The tincture complies with the requirements for Tinctures stated under Extracts and with the following requirements.

Content of anhydrous morphine, $C_{17}H_{19}NO_3$

0.925 to 1.075% w/v.

TESTS

Ethanol content

41 to 46% v/v, Appendix VIII F, Method III.

Relative density

0.898 to 0.969, Appendix V G.

ASSAY

Dilute 5 mL to 100 mL with *ethanol (45%)*. To 10 mL of the resulting solution add 5 mL of *water* and 1 mL of 5M *ammonia* and extract with 30 mL of a mixture of equal volumes of *ethanol (96%)* and *chloroform* and then with two 22.5 mL quantities of a mixture of 2 volumes of *chloroform* and 1 volume of *ethanol (96%)*, washing each extract with the same 20 mL of a mixture of equal volumes of *ethanol (96%)* and *water*. Evaporate the combined extracts just to dryness, extract the residue with two 5 mL quantities of *calcium hydroxide solution*, filter and wash the filter with 10 mL of *calcium hydroxide solution*. To the combined filtrate and washings add 0.1 g of *ammonium sulfate*, extract with two 10 mL quantities of *ethanol-free chloroform*, wash the combined extracts with 10 mL of *water* and discard the chloroform solution. To the combined alkaline liquid and aqueous washings add 10 mL of 1M *hydrochloric acid*, heat on a water bath to remove any chloroform, cool and dilute to 100 mL with *water*. To 10 mL of this solution add 10 mL of 0.1M *hydrochloric acid* and 8 mL of a freshly prepared 1.0% w/v solution of *sodium nitrite*, allow to stand for 15 minutes, add 12 mL of 5M *ammonia*, dilute to 50 mL with *water* and measure the *absorbance* of a 4-cm layer of the resulting solution at the maximum at 442 nm, Appendix II B, using in the reference cell a solution prepared at the same time and in the same manner but using 8 mL of *water* in place of the solution of sodium nitrite. Calculate the content of $C_{17}H_{19}NO_3$ taking 124 as the value of A(1%, 1 cm) at the maximum at 442 nm.

Concentrated Camphorated Opium Tincture

DEFINITION

Opium Tincture	400 mL
Benzoic Acid	40 g
Racemic Camphor	24 g
Anise Oil or Star Anise Oil	24 mL
Ethanol (96 per cent)	400 mL
Water	Sufficient to produce 1000 mL

Extemporaneous preparation

The following directions apply.

Dissolve the Benzoic Acid, the Racemic Camphor and the Anise Oil or Star Anise Oil in the Ethanol (96 per cent), add the Opium Tincture and sufficient Water to produce 1000 mL, mix and filter if necessary.

The tincture complies with the requirements for Tinctures stated under Extracts and with the following requirements.

Content of anhydrous morphine, $C_{17}H_{19}NO_3$

0.36 to 0.44% w/v.

TESTS

Ethanol content

54 to 59% v/v, Appendix VIII F, Method III.

Relative density

0.912 to 0.930, Appendix V G.

ASSAY

Dilute 10 mL to 100 mL with *ethanol (50%)* and carry out the Assay described under Camphorated Opium Tincture using 10 mL of the diluted solution.

Camphorated Opium Tincture

DEFINITION

Opium Tincture	50 mL
Benzoic Acid	5 g
Racemic Camphor	3 g
Anise Oil or Star Anise Oil	3 mL
Ethanol (60 per cent)	Sufficient to produce 1000 mL

Extemporaneous preparation

The following directions apply.

Dissolve the Benzoic Acid, the Racemic Camphor and the Anise Oil or Star Anise Oil in 900 mL of Ethanol (60 per cent), add the Opium Tincture and sufficient Ethanol (60 per cent) to produce 1000 mL and mix. Filter, if necessary.

The tincture complies with the requirements for Tinctures stated under Extracts and with the following requirements.

Content of anhydrous morphine, $C_{17}H_{19}NO_3$

0.045 to 0.055% w/v.

TESTS

Ethanol content

56 to 60% v/v, Appendix VIII F, Method III.

Relative density

0.90 to 0.92, Appendix V G.

ASSAY

To 10 mL add 5 mL of *water* and 1 mL of 5M *ammonia* and extract with 30 mL of a mixture of equal volumes of *ethanol (96%)* and *chloroform* and then with two 22.5-mL quantities of a mixture of 2 volumes of *chloroform* and 1 volume of *ethanol (96%)*, washing each extract with the same 20 mL of

Herbal Drugs

a mixture of equal volumes of *ethanol* (*96%*) and *water*. Evaporate the combined extracts almost to dryness, extract the residue with 10 mL of *calcium hydroxide solution*, filter and wash the filter with 10 mL of *calcium hydroxide solution*. To the combined filtrate and washings add 0.1 g of *ammonium sulfate*, extract with two 10 mL quantities of *ethanol-free chloroform*, wash the combined extracts with 10 mL of *water* and discard the chloroform solution. To the combined alkaline liquid and aqueous washings add 10 mL of 1M *hydrochloric acid*, heat on a water bath to remove any chloroform, cool and dilute to 100 mL with *water*. To 10 mL of this solution add 10 mL of 0.1M *hydrochloric acid* and 8 mL of a freshly prepared 1.0% w/v solution of *sodium nitrite*, allow to stand for 15 minutes, add 12 mL of 5M *ammonia*, dilute to 50 mL with *water* and measure the *absorbance* of a 4-cm layer of the resulting solution at the maximum at 442 nm, Appendix II B, using in the reference cell a solution prepared at the same time and in the same manner but using 8 mL of *water* in place of the solution of sodium nitrite. Calculate the content of $C_{17}H_{19}NO_3$ taking 124 as the value of A(1%, 1 cm) at the maximum at 442 nm.

Bitter-Orange Flower

(*Ph Eur monograph 1810*)

Ph Eur ————————————————

DEFINITION

Whole, dried, unopened flower of *Citrus aurantium* L. ssp. *aurantium* (*C. aurantium* L. ssp. *amara* Engl.).

Content

Minimum 8.0 per cent of total flavonoids, expressed as naringin ($C_{27}H_{32}O_{14}$; M_r 580.5) (dried drug).

IDENTIFICATION

A. The flower buds are white or yellowish-white and may reach up to 25 mm in length. The dialypetalous corolla is composed of 5 thick, oblong and concave petals dotted with oil glands visible under a hand lens; the short, yellowish-green persistent gamosepalous calyx has 5 spreading sepals, connate at the base and forming a star-shaped structure attached to the yellowish-green peduncle, which is about 5-10 mm long. The flower buds contain at least 20 stamens with yellow anthers and with filaments fused at the base into groups of 4 or 5; the ovary is superior, brownish-black and spherical, consists of 8-10 multi-ovular loculi and is surrounded at the base by an annular granular hypogynous disc; the thick, cylindrical style ends in a capitate stigma.

B. Microscopic examination (*2.8.23*). The powder is brownish-yellow. Examine under a microscope using *chloral hydrate solution R*. The powder shows the following diagnostic characters (Figure 1810.-1): very numerous spherical pollen grains, with a finely pitted exine and 3-5 germinal pores [H, K]; fragments of the epidermis of the sepals in surface view [D] and in transverse section [A, C], accompanied by underlying mesophyll [B], some cells of which contain prisms of calcium oxalate [Aa, Ba, Db], unicellular covering trichomes [Ca] and numerous anomocytic stomata (*2.8.3*) [Da]; fragments of the epidermis of the petals in surface view [F, G, J], with a distinctly striated cuticle; fragments of large schizolysigenous oil glands in transverse section [E], which measure up to 100 µm in diameter. Examine under a microscope using a 20 g/L solution of *potassium hydroxide R*.

The mounting medium becomes yellow because of the presence of hesperidin in the drug.

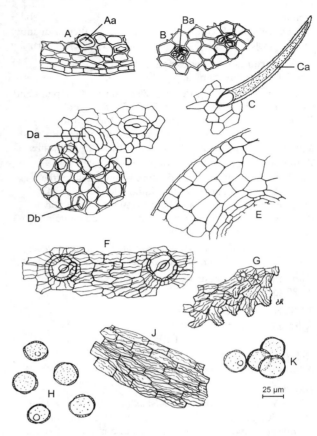

Figure 1810.-1. – *Illustration for identification test B of powdered herbal drug of bitter-orange flower*

C. Examine the chromatograms obtained in the test for sweet-orange flower.

Results See below the sequence of zones present in the chromatograms obtained with the reference solution and the test solution.

Top of the plate	
	A weak yellow fluorescent zone
	A weak yellow fluorescent zone
Hesperidin: a greenish-yellow fluorescent zone	A greenish-yellow fluorescent zone (hesperidin)
Naringin: a yellow fluorescent zone	A yellow fluorescent zone (naringin)
	A red fluorescent zone (neoeriocitrin)
	A yellow fluorescent zone (diosmin and neodiosmin)
Reference solution	**Test solution**

TESTS

Sweet-orange flower

Thin-layer chromatography (*2.2.27*).

Test solution To 0.5 g of the powdered herbal drug (355) (*2.9.12*) add 5 mL of *methanol R*. Heat with stirring at 40 °C for 10 min. Filter.

Reference solution Dissolve 3.0 mg of *naringin R* and 3.0 mg of *hesperidin R* in 10 mL of *methanol R*.

Plate   TLC silica gel plate R.

Mobile phase   water R, anhydrous formic acid R, ethyl acetate R (10:15:75 V/V/V).

Application   10 µL as bands.

Development   Over a path of 10 cm.

Drying   In air; heat in an oven at 110-120 °C for 5 min.

Detection   Spray the hot plate with a 10 g/L solution of *diphenylboric acid aminoethyl ester R* in *methanol R* and then with a 50 g/L solution of *macrogol 400 R* in *methanol R*; after at least 1 h, examine in ultraviolet light at 365 nm.

Results   The chromatogram obtained with the test solution shows a yellow zone similar in position to the zone of naringin in the chromatogram obtained with the reference solution, and immediately below it a red zone (neoeriocitrin).

Loss on drying (*2.2.32*)
Maximum 11.0 per cent, determined on 1.000 g of the powdered herbal drug (355) (*2.9.12*) by drying in an oven at 105 °C.

Total ash (*2.4.16*)
Maximum 10.0 per cent.

ASSAY

Stock solution   To 0.175 g of the powdered herbal drug (355) (*2.9.12*) add 95 mL of *ethanol (50 per cent V/V) R*. Heat on a water-bath under a reflux condenser for 30 min. Allow to cool and filter through a sintered-glass filter (*2.1.2*). Rinse the filter with 5 mL of *ethanol (50 per cent V/V) R*. Combine the filtrate and the rinsings in a volumetric flask and dilute to 100.0 mL with *ethanol (50 per cent V/V) R*.

Test solution   Into a test tube (10 mm × 180 mm) introduce 0.150 g of powdered *magnesium R (250)* (*2.9.12*), a magnetic stirring bar 25 mm long and 2.00 mL of the stock solution. Maintain the test tube upright, centrifuge at 125 *g* and carefully add dropwise, especially at the beginning, 2.0 mL of *hydrochloric acid R*, and then 6.0 mL of *ethanol (50 per cent V/V) R*. Stopper the tube and mix by inverting.

Compensation solution   Into a 2nd test tube, introduce 2.00 mL of the stock solution and carefully add dropwise, especially at the beginning, 2.0 mL of *hydrochloric acid R* and then 6.0 mL of *ethanol (50 per cent V/V) R*.

After 10 min, measure the absorbance (*2.2.25*) of the test solution at 530 nm.

Calculate the percentage content of total flavonoids, expressed as naringin, using the following expression:

$$\frac{A \times 9.62}{m}$$

i.e. taking the specific absorbance of the reaction product of naringin to be 52.

A =   absorbance at 530 nm;
m =   mass of the substance to be examined, in grams.

———————————————————— *Ph Eur*

Orange Oil

DEFINITION
Orange Oil is obtained by mechanical means from the fresh peel of the sweet orange, *Citrus sinensis* (L.) Osbeck.

CHARACTERISTICS
A yellow to yellowish brown liquid, visibly free from water; odour, that of orange.

TESTS
Optical rotation
+94° to +99°, Appendix V F. On distillation, the first 10% of the distillate has an optical rotation the same as, or only slightly lower than, the original oil.

Refractive index
1.472 to 1.476, Appendix V E.

Residue on evaporation
1.0 to 5.0% when determined by the method for *residue on evaporation of volatile oils*, Appendix X M. Use 2 g and heat for 4 hours.

Solubility in ethanol
Soluble at 20°, in 7 parts of *ethanol (90%)*, Appendix X M. A bright solution is rarely obtained due to the presence of waxy non-volatile substances.

Weight per mL
0.842 to 0.848 g, Appendix V G.

Content of aldehydes
Not less than 1.0% w/w, calculated as decanal, $C_{10}H_{20}O$. Carry out the method for the *determination of aldehydes*, Appendix X K, using 10 g, omitting the *toluene* and using a volume, not less than 7 mL, of *alcoholic hydroxylamine solution* that exceeds by 1 to 2 mL the volume of 0.5M *potassium hydroxide in ethanol (60%) VS* required. Each mL of 0.5M *potassium hydroxide in ethanol (60%) VS* is equivalent to 78.76 mg of $C_{10}H_{20}O$.

STORAGE
Orange Oil should be kept in a well-filled container and protected from light.

Sweet Orange Oil

(*Ph Eur monograph 1811*)

Ph Eur ——————————————————————

DEFINITION
Essential oil obtained without heating, by suitable mechanical treatment from the fresh peel of the fruit of *Citrus sinensis* (L.) Osbeck (*Citrus aurantium* L. var. *dulcis* L.). A suitable antioxidant may be added.

CHARACTERS
Appearance
Clear, pale yellow or orange, mobile liquid, which may become cloudy when chilled.

Characteristic odour of fresh orange peel.

IDENTIFICATION
First identification   B.
Second identification   A.

A. Thin-layer chromatography (*2.2.27*).

Examine the chromatograms obtained in the test for bergapten.

Results A   See below the sequence of the zones present in the chromatograms obtained with the reference solution and the test solution.

Top of the plate	
	———
Bergaptene: a greenish-yellow fluorescent zone	
———	
	Many blue fluorescent zones
Reference solution	Test solution

Results B   See below the sequence of the zones present in the chromatograms obtained with the reference solution and the test solution.

Top of the plate	
	A brown fluorescent zone
Linalyl acetate: a brownish-orange fluorescent zone	A faint brownish-orange fluorescent zone (linalyl acetate)
———	———
	Many orange fluorescent zones
Linalol: a brownish-orange fluorescent zone	A brownish-orange fluorescent zone (linalol)
Bergaptene: a faint greenish-yellow fluorescent zone	
	Many brownish-orange fluorescent zones
———	———
	Many blue fluorescent zones
Reference solution	Test solution

B. Examine the chromatograms obtained in the test for chromatographic profile.

Results   The characteristic peaks in the chromatogram obtained with the test solution are similar in retention time to those in the chromatogram obtained with the reference solution.

TESTS

Relative density (2.2.5)
0.842 to 0.850.

Refractive index (2.2.6)
1.470 to 1.476.

Optical rotation (2.2.7)
+ 94° to + 99°.

Peroxide value (2.5.5, Method B)
Maximum 20.

Fatty oils and resinified essential oils (2.8.7)
It complies with the test for fatty oils and resinified essential oils.

Bergaptene

Thin-layer chromatography (2.2.27).

Test solution   Dilute 0.2 mL of the substance to be examined in 1 mL of alcohol R.

Reference solution   Dissolve 2 mg of bergaptene R, 10 µL of linalol R and 20 µL of linalyl acetate R in 10 mL of alcohol R.

Plate   TLC silica gel plate R.

Mobile phase   ethyl acetate R, toluene R (15:85 V/V).

Application   10 µL, as bands.

Development   Over a path of 15 cm.

Drying   In air.

Detection A   Examine in ultraviolet light at 365 nm.

Results A   The chromatogram obtained with the test solution shows no greenish-yellow fluorescent zone present in the chromatogram obtained with the reference solution.

Detection B   Spray with anisaldehyde solution R and heat at 100-105 °C for 10 min; examine the plate in ultraviolet light at 365 nm.

Chromatographic profile
Gas chromatography (2.2.28): use the normalisation procedure.

Test solution   Dilute 300 µL of the substance to be examined to 1 mL with acetone R.

Reference solution (a)   Dilute 10 µL of α-pinene R, 10 µL of β-pinene R, 10 µL of sabinene R, 20 µL of β-myrcene R, 800 µL of limonene R, 10 µL of octanal, 10 µL of decanal R, 10 µL of linalol R, 10 µL of citral R (composed of neral and geranial) and 10 µL of valencene R in 1 mL of acetone R.

Reference solution (b)   Dissolve 5 µL of β-pinene R in 10 mL of acetone R. Dilute 0.5 mL to 10 mL with acetone R.

Column:
— material: fused silica,
— size: l = 30 m, Ø = 0.53 mm,
— stationary phase: macrogol 20 000 R (film thickness 1 µm).

Carrier gas   helium for chromatography R.

Flow rate   1 mL/min.

Split ratio   1:100.

Temperature:

	Time (min)	Temperature (°C)
Column	0 - 6	50
	6 - 31	50 → 150
	31 - 41	150 → 180
	41 - 55	180
Injection port		250
Detector		250

Detection   Flame ionisation.

Injection   0.5 µL.

Elution order   Order indicated in the composition of reference solution (a). Record the retention times of these substances.

System suitability   Reference solution (a)
— resolution: minimum 3.9 between the peaks due to β-pinene and sabinene and minimum 1.5 between the peaks due to valencene and geranial.

Using the retention times determined from the chromatogram obtained with reference solution (a), locate the components of reference solution (a) in the chromatogram obtained with the test solution.

Determine the percentage content of these components. The limits are within the following ranges:
— α-pinene: 0.4 per cent to 0.6 per cent,
— β-pinene: 0.02 per cent to 0.3 per cent,
— sabinene: 0.2 per cent to 1.1 per cent,
— β-myrcene: 1.7 per cent to 2.5 per cent,
— limonene: 92.0 per cent to 97.0 per cent,
— octanal: 0.1 per cent to 0.4 per cent,
— decanal: 0.1 per cent to 0.4 per cent,
— linalol: 0.2 per cent to 0.7 per cent,
— neral: 0.02 per cent to 0.10 per cent,
— valencene: 0.02 per cent to 0.5 per cent,

— geranial: 0.03 per cent to 0.20 per cent.
— *disregard limit*: area of the peak in the chromatogram obtained with reference solution (b) (0.01 per cent).

Residue on evaporation

1.0 per cent to 5.0 per cent.

Evaporate 5.0 g to dryness on a water-bath and dry at 100-105 °C for 4 h.

STORAGE

At a temperature not exceeding 25 °C.

Ph Eur

Terpeneless Orange Oil

Preparation

Compound Orange Spirit

DEFINITION

Terpeneless Orange Oil may be prepared by concentrating orange oil under reduced pressure until most of the terpenes have been removed or by solvent partition.

CHARACTERISTICS

A clear, yellow or orange-yellow liquid, visibly free from water.

TESTS

Optical rotation

Not more than +60°, Appendix V F.

Refractive index

1.461 to 1.473, Appendix V E.

Solubility in ethanol

Soluble, at 20°, in 1 part of *ethanol (90%)*, Appendix X M.

Weight per mL

0.855 to 0.880 g, Appendix V G.

Content of aldehydes

Not less than 18% w/w, calculated as decanal, $C_{10}H_{20}O$. Carry out the method for the *determination of aldehydes*, Appendix X K, using 1.5 g, omitting the *toluene* and using a volume, not less than 7 mL, of *alcoholic hydroxylamine solution* that exceeds by 1 to 2 mL the volume of 0.5M *potassium hydroxide in ethanol (60%) VS* required. Each mL of 0.5M *potassium hydroxide in ethanol (60%) VS* is equivalent to 78.76 mg of $C_{10}H_{20}O$.

STORAGE

Terpeneless Orange Oil should be kept in a well-filled container and protected from light.

Compound Orange Spirit

DEFINITION

Terpeneless Orange Oil	2.5 mL
Terpeneless Lemon Oil	1.3 mL
Anise Oil or Star Anise Oil	4.25 mL
Coriander Oil	6.25 mL
Ethanol (90 per cent)	Sufficient to produce 1000 mL

The spirit complies with the requirements stated under Spirits and with the following requirements.

TESTS

Ethanol content

86 to 90% v/v, Appendix VIII F.

Weight per mL

0.828 to 0.841 g, Appendix V G.

Dried Bitter-Orange Peel

(Bitter-Orange Epicarp and Mesocarp, Ph Eur monograph 1603)

Preparations

Orange Peel Infusion

Orange Tincture

Ph Eur

DEFINITION

Dried epicarp and mesocarp of the ripe fruit of *Citrus aurantium* L. ssp. *aurantium* (*C. aurantium* L. ssp. *amara* Engl.) partly freed from the white spongy tissue of the mesocarp and endocarp.

Content

Minimum 20 mL/kg of essential oil (anhydrous drug).

CHARACTERS

Aromatic odour and spicy bitter taste.

IDENTIFICATION

A. The drug consists of elliptical or irregular pieces 5-8 cm long, 3-5 cm broad and about 3 mm thick. The outer surface is yellowish or reddish-brown and distinctly punctate, the inner surface is yellowish or brownish-white.

B. Reduce to a powder (355) (*2.9.12*). The powder is light brown. Examine under a microscope using *chloral hydrate solution R*. The powder shows the following diagnostic characters: small polygonal cells with slightly thickened anticlinal walls, filled with orange-red chromatophores, and very occasional anomocytic stomata (*2.8.3*); fragments of the hypodermis showing collenchymatous thickening; groups of parenchyma with each cell containing a prism crystal of calcium oxalate; fragments of lysigenous oil glands; parenchyma containing crystals of hesperidin which dissolve in a 20 g/L *potassium hydroxide R* solution giving a yellow colour.

C. Thin-layer chromatography (*2.2.27*).

Test solution   To 1.0 g of the powdered drug (710) (*2.9.12*) add 10 mL of *methanol R* and heat in a water-bath at 65 °C for 5 min shaking frequently. Allow to cool and filter.

Reference solution   Dissolve 1.0 mg of *naringin R* and 1.0 mg of *caffeic acid R* in 1 mL of *methanol R*.

Plate   TLC silica gel plate R.

Mobile phase   water R, anhydrous formic acid R, ethyl acetate R (10:15:75 *V/V/V*).

Application   20 µL as bands.

Development   Over a path of 10 cm.

Drying   In air, and heat in an oven at 110-120 °C for 5 min.

Detection   Spray the warm plate with a 10 g/L solution of *diphenylboric acid aminoethyl ester R* in *methanol R* and then with a 50 g/L solution of *macrogol 400 R* in *methanol R*. After at least 1 h, examine in ultraviolet light at 365 nm.

Results   See below the sequence of zones present in the chromatograms obtained with the reference and test solutions. Furthermore, other fluorescent zones are present in the chromatogram obtained with the test solution.

Top of the plate		
	A light blue fluorescent zone	
	A light blue fluorescent zone	
Caffeic acid: a light blue fluorescent zone		
	A light blue fluorescent zone	
	A light blue fluorescent zone	
Naringin: a dark green fluorescent zone	A dark green fluorescent zone (naringin)	
	A red fluorescent zone (neoeriocitrin)	
	An orange fluorescent zone	
Reference solution	Test solution	

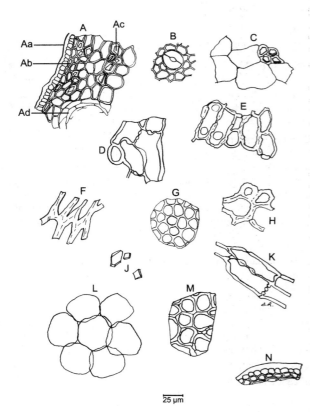

A. Fragment in transverse section showing epicarp with thick cuticle (Aa), collenchymatous hypodermis (Ab) and part of the mesocarp parenchyma containing prism crystals (Ac) of calcium oxalate and fragment of an oil gland (Ad)

B. Fragment of epicarp with anomocytic stoma, in surface view

C. Group of cells of the mesocarp, some containing calcium oxalate crystals

D, E, F, H, K and M. Fragments of mesocarp

G. Sub-epicarpal collenchymatous cells

J. Prism crystals of calcium oxalate

L. Group of parenchymatous cells

N. Fragment of epicarp with thick cuticle and hypodermis showing collenchymatous thickening, in transverse section

Figure 1603.-1. – *Illustration of powdered herbal drug of bitter-orange epicarp and mesocarp (see Identification B)*

TESTS

Water (*2.2.13*)
Maximum 10.0 per cent, determined by distillation on 20.0 g of powdered drug (355) (*2.9.12*).

Total ash (*2.4.16*)
Maximum 7.0 per cent.

Extractable matter
Minimum 6.0 per cent.

To 2.000 g of the powdered drug (250) (*2.9.12*) add a mixture of 3 mL of *water R* and 7 mL of *ethanol (96 per cent) R* and extract for 2 h, shaking frequently. Filter, evaporate 2.000 g of the filtrate to dryness on a water-bath and dry in an oven at 100-105 °C for 3 h. Allow to cool in a desiccator over *diphosphorus pentoxide R* and weigh. The residue weighs a minimum of 120 mg.

ASSAY
Carry out the determination of essential oil in herbal drugs (*2.8.12*). Use a 500 mL round-bottomed flask, 200 mL of *water R* as the distillation liquid and 0.5 mL of *xylene R* in the graduated tube. Reduce the drug to a powder (710) (*2.9.12*) and immediately use 15.0 g for the determination. Distil at a rate of 2-3 mL/min for 90 min.

———————————— Ph Eur

Orange Peel Infusion

DEFINITION

Concentrated Orange Peel Infusion	100 mL
Water	Sufficient to produce 1000 mL

The infusion complies with the requirements stated under Infusions.

CONCENTRATED ORANGE PEEL INFUSION

DEFINITION

Dried Bitter-Orange Peel, cut small	500 g
Ethanol (25 per cent)	1350 mL

Extemporaneous preparation
The following directions apply.

Macerate the Dried Bitter-Orange Peel in a covered vessel for 48 hours with 1000 mL of the Ethanol (25 per cent) and press out the liquid. To the pressed marc add 350 mL of the Ethanol (25 per cent), macerate for 24 hours, press and add the liquid to the product of the first pressing. Allow to stand for not less than 14 days and filter.

TESTS
Ethanol content
18 to 23% v/v, Appendix VIII F.

Total solids
10 to 15% w/v, Appendix XI A. Use 1 mL.

Weight per mL
1.01 to 1.04 g, Appendix V G.

Orange Tincture

*(Bitter-Orange Epicarp and Mesocarp Tincture,
Ph Eur monograph 1604)*

Ph Eur _____

DEFINITION
Tincture produced from *Bitter-orange epicarp* and
mesocarp (1603).

PRODUCTION
The tincture is produced from 1 part of the freshly powdered
drug (2000) *(2.9.12)* and 5 parts of alcohol
(70 per cent V/V/V) by an appropriate procedure.

CHARACTERS
Liquid with a bitter taste.

IDENTIFICATION
Examine by thin-layer chromatography *(2.2.27)*.

Test solution   The tincture to be examined.

Reference solution   Dissolve 1.0 mg of *naringin R* and 1.0 mg
of *caffeic acid R* in 1 mL of *methanol R*.

Plate   TLC silica gel plate R.

Mobile phase   water R, anhydrous formic acid R, ethyl acetate R
(10:15:75 V/V/V).

Application   20 µL, as bands.

Development   Over a path of 10 cm.

Drying   In air, and heat in an oven at 110-120 °C for 5 min.

Detection   Spray the warm plate with a 10 g/L solution of
diphenylboric acid aminoethyl ester R in *methanol R* and then
with a 50 g/L solution of *macrogol 400 R* in *methanol R*. After
1 h, examine in ultraviolet light at 365 nm.

Results   See below the sequence of the zones present in the
chromatograms obtained with the reference and test
solutions. Furthermore, other zones are present in the
chromatogram obtained with the test solution.

Top of the plate	
	A light blue fluorescent zone
	A light blue fluorescent zone
Caffeic acid: a light blue fluorescent zone	
	A light blue fluorescent zone
	A light blue fluorescent zone
Naringin: a dark green fluorescent zone	A dark green fluorescent zone (naringin)
	A red fluorescent zone (neoeriocitrin)
	An orange fluorescent zone
Reference solution	**Test solution**

TESTS
Ethanol content *(2.9.10)*
63 per cent to 67 per cent *V/V*.

Methanol and 2-propanol *(2.9.11)*
Maximum 0.05 per cent *V/V* of methanol and maximum
0.05 per cent *V/V* of 2-propanol.

Dry residue
Minimum 6.0 per cent *m/m*, determined on 2.00 g of
tincture to be examined.

_____ *Ph Eur*

Orange Syrup

DEFINITION
Orange Tincture	60 mL
Syrup	Sufficient to produce 1000 mL

*The syrup complies with the requirements stated under Oral
Liquids and with the following requirement.*

TESTS
Weight per mL
1.29 to 1.31 g, Appendix V G.

Oregano

(Ph Eur monograph 1880)

Ph Eur _____

DEFINITION
Dried leaves and flowers separated from the stems of
Origanum onites L. or *Origanum vulgare* L. subsp. *hirtum*
(Link) Ietsw., or a mixture of both species.

Content:
— *essential oil*: minimum 25 mL/kg (anhydrous drug);
— *sum of the contents of carvacrol and thymol* (both $C_{10}H_{14}O$;
  M_r 150.2): minimum 60 per cent in the essential oil.

IDENTIFICATION
A. *O. onites*. The leaf is yellowish-green, usually 4-22 mm
long and 3-14 mm wide. It has a long or short petiole or is
sessile. The lamina is ovate, elliptic or ovate-lanceolate.
Margins are entire or serrate, the apex is acute or obtuse.
The veins are yellowish and conspicuous on the adaxial
surface. Flowers are solitary or seen as broken parts of the
corymb. The calyx is bract-like and inconspicuous.
The corolla is white, on top of inflorescences or single
flowers, or inconspicuous. The bracts are imbricate and
green like the leaves. The drug contains yellowish or
yellowish-brown stem parts.

O. vulgare (subsp. *hirtum*). The leaf is green and usually
3-28 mm long and 2.5-19 mm wide. It is petiolate or sessile.
The lamina is ovate or ovate-eliptic. The margins are entire
or serrate, the apex is acute or obtuse. Flowers are rare,
found as broken parts of the corymbs. Bracts are greenish-
yellow and imbricate. The calyx is corolla-like and
inconspicuous. The corolla is white, on top of inflorescences,
slightly conspicuous or inconspicuous.

B. Reduce to a powder (710) *(2.9.12)*. The powder is green
(*O. vulgare*) or yellowish-green (*O. onites*). Examine under a
microscope using *chloral hydrate solution R* (Figure 1880.-1).

O. onites powder shows fragments of leaf epidermis [A, D, G]
composed of cells with sinuous walls, diacytic stomata *(2.8.3)*
[Ga], covering trichomes and glandular trichomes; there are
2 types of glandular trichomes: some of lamiaceous type with
8-16 cells, in surface view [Da], and a very common type
with a unicellular head and uni- [Gc], bi- [H] or tricellular
stalk; the covering trichomes have smooth, thick walls; some
are multicellular [B, Gb], often broken [Aa], and contain
prisms of calcium oxalate, while others, which are rare, are
unicellular and conical [C]; scars from covering and
glandular trichomes are visible on the epidermises [Gd, Ge];
pollen grains, with smooth exine, are frequent [E, F].

O. vulgare subsp. *hirtum* powder shows fragments of the
upper epidermis with cells with sinuous, beaded walls,
accompanied by palisade parenchyma [J]; fragments of the
lower epidermis [N] composed of cells with finely and

HERBAL DRUGS

irregularly thickened walls, diacytic stomata (2.8.3) [Na], covering trichomes and glandular trichomes; there are 2 types of glandular trichomes: some of lamiaceous type with 12 cells, in surface view [Nb], and a rare type with a unicellular head [Nc] and bi- or tricellular stalk; the covering trichomes have thick, warty walls and contain fine needles of calcium oxalate; some are conical, multicellular and serrate [L, M], while others, which are rare, are unicellular [K]; there are occasional pollen grains, with smooth exine [E, F].

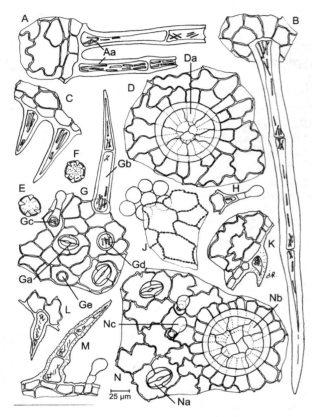

Figure 1880.-1.– Illustration for identification test B of powdered herbal drug of oregano

C. Thin-layer chromatography (2.2.27).

Test solution   To 1.0 g of the powdered drug (355) (2.9.12) add 5 mL of *methylene chloride R* and shake for 3 min, then filter through about 2 g of *anhydrous sodium sulfate R*.

Reference solution   Dissolve 1 mg of *thymol R* and 10 µL of *carvacrol R* in 10 mL of *methylene chloride R*.

Plate   TLC silica gel plate R.

Mobile phase   methylene chloride R.

Application   20 µL as bands.

Development   Over a path of 15 cm.

Drying   In air.

Detection   Spray with *anisaldehyde solution R* using 10 mL for a plate 200 mm square and heat at 100-105 °C for 10 min.

Results   See below the sequence of zones present in the chromatograms obtained with the reference solution and the test solution. Furthermore, other zones are present in the lower third and upper part of the chromatogram obtained with the test solution.

Top of the plate	
	A bluish-purple zone
———	———
	A pale green zone
Thymol: a pink zone	A pink zone (thymol)
Carvacrol: a pale violet zone	A pale violet zone (carvacrol)
	———
	A pale purple zone
	A grey zone
	A pale green zone
	A bluish-purple zone
	An intense brown zone
Reference solution	**Test solution**

TESTS

Water (2.2.13)
Maximum 120 mL/kg, determined on 20.0 g of the powdered drug (355) (2.9.12).

Total ash (2.4.16)
Maximum 15.0 per cent.

Ash insoluble in hydrochloric acid (2.8.1)
Maximum 4.0 per cent.

ASSAY

Essential oil (2.8.12)
Use 30.0 g of the drug to be examined, a 1000 mL round-bottomed flask and 400 mL of *water R* as the distillation liquid. Distil at a rate of 2-3 mL/min for 2 h without *xylene R* in the graduated tube.

Carvacrol and thymol
Gas chromatography (2.2.28): use the normalisation procedure.

Test solution   Filter the essential oil obtained in the assay of essential oil over a small amount of *anhydrous sodium sulfate R* and dilute to 5.0 mL with *heptane R* by rinsing the apparatus and the anhydrous sodium sulfate.

Reference solution   Dissolve 0.20 g of *thymol R* and 50 mg of *carvacrol R* in *heptane R* and dilute to 5.0 mL with the same solvent.

Column:
— *material*: fused silica;
— *size*: l = 60 m, Ø = 0.25 mm;
— *stationary phase*: macrogol 20 000 R (film thickness 0.25 µm).

Carrier gas   nitrogen for chromatography R or *helium for chromatography R*.

Flow rate   1.5 mL/min.

Split ratio   1:100.

Temperature:

	Time (min)	Temperature (°C)
Column	0 - 45	40 → 250
Injection port		190
Detector		210

Detection   Flame ionisation.

Injection   0.2 µL.

Elution order   Order indicated in the composition of the reference solution; record the retention times of these substances.

System suitability   Reference solution:
— *resolution*: minimum 1.5 between the peaks due to thymol and carvacrol.

Using the retention times determined from the chromatogram obtained with the reference solution, locate the components of the reference solution in the chromatogram obtained with the test solution.

Determine the percentage content of the sum of carvacrol and thymol.

_____ *Ph Eur*

Orientvine Stem

(*Ph Eur monograph 2450*)

Ph Eur _____

DEFINITION
Dried, whole or fragmented stem of *Sinomenium acutum* (Thunb.) Rehder et E.H.Wilson, collected in late autumn and early winter.

Content
Minimum 0.5 per cent of sinomenine ($C_{19}H_{23}NO_4$; M_r 329.4) (dried drug).

IDENTIFICATION
A. *Whole drug*. Long cylindrical stem, somewhat curved, 60 cm long or more, 0.5-2 cm in diameter. The outer bark is greenish-brown or brown, sometimes greyish-brown, with relatively wide longitudinal striations and prominent verrucose lenticels; the nodes are slightly swollen and branched. The texture is light, hard and difficult to break; the fracture is uneven, greyish-yellow or pale greyish-brown; the bark is thin (about 1/10 of the diameter); the medullary rays are very conspicuous; the pith is yellowish-white or pale yellowish-brown.

Fragmented drug. Fragments of stems, in discs, about 1.5 cm in diameter and 0.3 cm thick, with greenish-brown, brown or greyish-brown outer surface; a transverse section shows a narrow, pale yellow cortical zone, it is mainly occupied by the vascular system (about 3/4 of the section) consisting of very numerous vascular bundles (about 15-20) in a circle around the yellowish-white or pale yellowish-brown, small, circular pith; each bundle is delimited on the outside by a narrow and continuous, wavy, light brown zone and is separated from the next bundle by a narrow, light brown medullary ray; the xylem vessels with a relatively wide interior lumen are clearly visible.

B. Microscopic examination (*2.8.23*). The powder is yellowish-brown or greyish-brown. Examine under a microscope using chloral hydrate solution R. The powder shows the following diagnostic characters: rare fragments of epidermis with polyhedral cells, in surface view, covered with a thick, pale yellow cuticle about 50 µm in diameter; sclereids isolated or in groups, of various sizes and shapes (subsquare, fusiform, elliptical or irregular), with thickened, pitted walls with conspicuous pit canals, free or included in fragments of parenchyma; pale yellow or yellow fibres, 30-70 µm in diameter with thick, distinctly channelled walls and a very narrow lumen; fragments of parenchyma with thin-walled cells containing fine, needle-shaped crystals of calcium oxalate; fragments of xylem consisting of reticulate or pitted vessels, up to 200 µm in diameter, accompanied by ligneous parenchyma with slightly and regularly thickened and pitted cells. Examine under a microscope using a 50 per cent *V/V* solution of *glycerol R*. The powder shows simple, spherical starch granules about 10 µm in diameter, free or contained in parenchymatous cells.

C. Thin-layer chromatography (*2.2.27*).

Test solution   To 2 g of the powdered herbal drug (355) (*2.9.12*) add 25 mL of *ethanol (96 per cent) R* and heat under reflux for 1 h. Filter and evaporate the filtrate to dryness. Dissolve the residue in 2 mL of *ethanol (96 per cent) R*.

Reference solution   Dissolve 5 mg of *sinomenine R* and 5 mg of *papaverine hydrochloride R* in 5 mL of *ethanol (96 per cent) R*.

Plate   TLC silica gel F_{254} plate R (2-10 µm).

Mobile phase   concentrated ammonia R, water R, toluene R, methanol R, ethyl acetate R (2:10:20:30:40 *V/V/V/V/V*).

Application   8 µL as bands of 8 mm.

Development   Over a path of 6 cm.

Drying   In air.

Detection A   Examine in ultraviolet light at 254 nm.

Results A   See below the sequence of zones present in the chromatograms obtained with the reference solution and the test solution. Furthermore, other faint fluorescent zones may be present in the chromatogram obtained with the test solution.

Top of the plate	
Papaverine: a quenching zone	A quenching zone
___	___
Sinomenine: a quenching zone	A quenching zone (sinomenine)
	___
	A dark blue fluorescent zone
Reference solution	**Test solution**

Detection B   Treat with a 10 g/L solution of *sodium nitrite R* in *potassium iodobismuthate solution R5* and allow to dry in air. Examine in daylight.

Results B   See below the sequence of zones present in the chromatograms obtained with the reference solution and the test solution. Furthermore, other faint zones may be present in the chromatogram obtained with the test solution.

Top of the plate	
Papaverine: an orange zone	An orange zone
___	___
	3 light orange zones
Sinomenine: an orange zone	An orange zone (sinomenine)
___	___
	2 orange zones
	A light orange zone
Reference solution	**Test solution**

TESTS

Loss on drying *(2.2.32)*

Maximum 10.0 per cent, determined on 1.000 g of the powdered herbal drug (355) *(2.9.12)* by drying in an oven at 105 °C for 3 h.

Total ash *(2.4.16)*

Maximum 6.0 per cent.

Aristolochic acids *(2.8.21, Method A)*

It complies with the test.

ASSAY

Liquid chromatography *(2.2.29)*.

Test solution Disperse 0.500 g of the powdered herbal drug (355) *(2.9.12)* in 20.0 mL of *ethanol (70 per cent V/V) R* in a conical flask and weigh. Sonicate for 20 min. Cool and weigh again. Compensate the loss of solvent with *ethanol (70 per cent V/V) R* and stopper the flask. Shake thoroughly and filter through a membrane filter (nominal pore size 0.45 μm).

Reference solution (a) Dissolve 3.0 mg of *sinomenine CRS* in *methanol R* and dilute to 10.0 mL with the same solvent.

Reference solution (b) Disperse 0.250 g of *orientvine stem HRS* in 10.0 mL of *ethanol (70 per cent V/V) R* in a conical flask and weigh. Sonicate for 20 min. Cool and weigh again. Compensate the loss of solvent with *ethanol (70 per cent V/V) R* and stopper the flask. Shake thoroughly and filter through a membrane filter (nominal pore size 0.45 μm).

Column:
— *size: l* = 0.15 m, Ø = 4.6 mm;
— *stationary phase: end-capped octadecylsilyl silica gel for chromatography R* (5 μm).

Mobile phase Adjust a 1.8 g/L solution of *disodium hydrogen phosphate R* to pH 8.0 with a 0.8 g/L solution of *sodium dihydrogen phosphate R*, then adjust to pH 9.0 with a 10 g/L solution of *triethylamine R*. Mix 60 volumes of this solution with 40 volumes of *acetonitrile R*.

Flow rate 1.0 mL/min.

Detection Spectrophotometer at 262 nm.

Injection 20 μL.

Retention time Sinomenine = about 3 min.

System suitability Reference solution (b):
— *resolution*: minimum 1.5 between peak 1 and the peak due to sinomenine; identify peak 1 using the chromatogram supplied with *orientvine stem HRS*.

Calculate the percentage content of sinomenine using the following expression:

$$\frac{A_1 \times m_2 \times 2 \times p}{A_2 \times m_1}$$

A_1 = area of the peak due to sinomenine in the chromatogram obtained with the test solution;

A_2 = area of the peak due to sinomenine in the chromatogram obtained with reference solution (a);

m_1 = mass of the herbal drug to be examined used to prepare the test solution, in grams;

m_2 = mass of *sinomenine CRS* used to prepare reference solution (a), in grams;

p = assigned percentage content of sinomenine in *sinomenine CRS*.

Ph Eur

Wild Pansy

*(Wild Pansy (Flowering Aerial Parts),
Ph Eur monograph 1855)*

Ph Eur

DEFINITION

Dried flowering aerial parts of *Viola arvensis* Murray and/or *Viola tricolor* L.

Content

Minimum 1.5 per cent of flavonoids, expressed as violanthin ($C_{27}H_{30}O_{14}$; M_r 578.5) (dried drug).

IDENTIFICATION

A. The stem is angular and hollow. The leaves are oval, petiolate, with a cordate base or elongated and obtuse, with lyrate stipules, divided in the middle. The flowers, with a long peduncle, are zygomorphic, with 5 oval, lanceolate sepals, an appendage pointed outwards and 5 petals of which the lower one bears a spur; in *Viola arvensis*, the petals are shorter than the calyx, the lower petal is cream coloured, with black lines, the 4 upper petals may be cream coloured or violet blue; in *Viola tricolor*, the petals are longer than the calyx and violet coloured, more or less tinged with yellow. The androecium consisting of 5 stamens bears at the apex a membranous connective appendage with 2 spurs. The trilocular ovary shows a short style and globular stigmata. The fruit are navicular capsules, three-lobed, yellowish brown, 5 mm to 10 mm long. The pale yellow, pyriform seeds are about 1 mm long, bearing a caruncle.

B. Reduce to a powder (355) *(2.9.12)*. The powder is greenish. Examine under a microscope using *chloral hydrate solution R*. The powder shows the following diagnostic characters: fragments of the epidermis of the leaves in surface view with wavy-walled cells and anomocytic stomata *(2.8.3)*; conical unicellular covering trichomes, widened at the base and sharply pointed at the apex, with a striated cuticle; glandular trichomes with a multicellular head, and a short, multicellular stalk in the indentations of the leaf margins; cluster crystals of calcium oxalate, sometimes included in parenchyma; fragments of the corolla with wavy-walled epidermal cells, those from the mid-region papillose and with some extended to form flask or bottle-shaped projections, those from the base of the petals with covering trichomes up to about 300 μm long with characteristic hump-like swellings along their length; spherical or polyhedral pollen grains, 60 μm to 80 μm in diameter, with finely pitted exines and 5 pores (*Viola arvensis*) or 4 pores (*Viola tricolor*); occasional fragments of spiral and reticulate vessels and groups of fibres from the stem.

C. Thin-layer chromatography *(2.2.27)*.

Test solution Heat in a water-bath at 65 °C for 5 min, with frequent stirring, 2.0 g of the powdered drug (355) *(2.9.12)* in 10 mL of *alcohol (70 per cent V/V) R*. Cool and filter.

Reference solution Dissolve 2.5 mg of *rutin R*, 2.5 mg of *hyperoside R* and 1.0 mg of *caffeic acid R* in *methanol R* and dilute to 10 mL with the same solvent.

Plate *TLC silica gel plate R*.

Mobile phase *anhydrous formic acid R*, *acetic acid R*, *water R*, *ethyl acetate R* (11:11:27:100 *V/V/V/V*).

Application 10 μL, as bands.

Development Over a path of 12 cm.

Drying At 100-105 °C.

Detection Spray with a solution containing 10 g/L of *diphenylboric acid aminoethyl ester R* and 50 g/L of *macrogol*

400 R in *methanol R*. Allow the plate to dry in air for 30 min. Examine in ultraviolet light at 365 nm.

Results   See below the sequence of the zones present in the chromatograms obtained with the reference solution and the test solution. Furthermore, other zones may be present in the chromatogram obtained with the test solution.

Top of the plate	
Caffeic acid: a greenish-blue to light blue fluorescent zone	A blue fluorescent zone
———	———
Hyperoside: a yellowish-brown fluorescent zone	A yellowish-green fluorescent zone
———	———
Rutin: a yellowish-brown fluorescent zone	An intense yellowish-brown fluorescent zone (rutin)
	A yellowish-green fluorescent zone
	A yellowish-green fluorescent zone
	A yellowish-green fluorescent zone
Reference solution	**Test solution**

TESTS

Foreign matter (*2.8.2*)
Maximum 3 per cent.

Swelling index (*2.8.4*)
Minimum 9, determined on the powdered drug (355) (*2.9.12*).

Loss on drying (*2.2.32*)
Maximum 12.0 per cent, determined on 1.000 g of the powdered drug (355) (*2.9.12*) by drying in an oven at 105 °C for 2 h.

Total ash (*2.4.16*)
Maximum 15.0 per cent.

ASSAY

Stock solution   In a 200 mL flask, introduce 0.300 g of the powdered drug (250) (*2.9.12*) and 40 mL of *alcohol (60 per cent V/V)* R. Heat in a water-bath at 60 °C for 10 min, shaking frequently. Allow to cool and filter through a plug of absorbent cotton into a 100 mL volumetric flask. Transfer the absorbent cotton with the drug residue back into the 200 mL flask, add 40 mL of *alcohol (60 per cent V/V) R* and heat again in a water-bath at 60 °C for 10 min, shaking frequently. Allow to cool and filter into the same 100 mL volumetric flask as used previously. Rinse the 200 mL flask with a further quantity of *alcohol (60 per cent V/V) R*, filter and transfer to the same 100 mL volumetric flask. Dilute to volume with *alcohol (60 per cent V/V) R* and filter.

Test solution   Introduce 5.0 mL of the stock solution into a round-bottomed flask and evaporate to dryness under reduced pressure. Take up the residue with 8 mL of a mixture of 10 volumes of *methanol R* and 100 volumes of *glacial acetic acid R* and transfer into a 25 mL volumetric flask. Rinse the round-bottomed flask with 3 mL of a mixture of 10 volumes of *methanol R* and 100 volumes of *glacial acetic acid R* and transfer into the same 25 mL volumetric flask as used previously. Add 10.0 mL of a solution containing 25.0 g/L of *boric acid R* and 20.0 g/L of *oxalic acid R* in *anhydrous formic acid R* and dilute to 25.0 mL with *anhydrous acetic acid R*.

Compensation liquid   Introduce 5.0 mL of the stock solution into a round-bottomed flask and evaporate to dryness under reduced pressure. Take up the residue with 8 mL of a mixture of 10 volumes of *methanol R* and 100 volumes of *glacial acetic acid R* and transfer into a 25 mL volumetric flask. Rinse the round-bottomed flask with 3 mL of a mixture of 10 volumes of *methanol R* and 100 volumes of *glacial acetic acid R* and transfer into the same 25 mL volumetric flask as used previously. Add 10.0 mL of *anhydrous formic acid R* and dilute to 25.0 mL with *anhydrous acetic acid R*.

Measure the absorbance (*2.2.25*) of the test solution at 405 nm after 30 min.

Calculate the percentage content of total flavonoids, expressed as violanthin from the expression:

$$\frac{A \times 1.25}{m}$$

taking the specific absorbance of violanthin to be 400.
A = measured absorbance at 405 nm
m = mass of the drug to be examined, in grams

——————————————————— *Ph Eur*

Passion Flower

Passiflora

(*Ph Eur monograph 1459*)

Preparation
Passion Flower Dry Extract

Ph Eur ——————————————————————————

DEFINITION

Fragmented or cut, dried aerial parts of *Passiflora incarnata L.* It may also contain flowers and/or fruits.

Content
Minimum 1.5 per cent of total flavonoids, expressed as vitexin ($C_{21}H_{20}O_{10}$; M_r 432.4) (dried drug).

IDENTIFICATION

A. The green or greenish-grey or brownish stem is ligneous, hollow, longitudinally striated, glabrous or very slightly pubescent, with a diameter that is generally less than 8 mm. The green or greenish-brown leaves are alternate, finely dentate and pubescent, deeply divided into 3 acute lobes of which the central lobe is the largest. The midrib is much more prominent on the lower surface. The petiole is pubescent and bears 2 dark nectaries near the lamina. The tendrils are very numerous and grow from the axils of the leaves; they are fine, smooth, round and terminated in cylindrical spirals. The radiate flowers, if present, have 3 small bracts and a corolla consisting of 5 white, elongated petals with several rows of filiform, petaloid appendices. If present, the greenish or brownish fruit is flattened and oval; it contains several flattened, brownish-yellow, pitted seeds.

B. Reduce to a powder (355) (2.9.12). The powder is light green. Examine under a microscope using *chloral hydrate solution R*. The powder shows the following diagnostic characters: fragments of the leaf epidermis with sinuous walls and anomocytic stomata (2.8.3); numerous cluster crystals of calcium oxalate isolated or aligned along the veins; many isolated or grouped fibres from the stems associated with pitted vessels and tracheids; uniseriate trichomes with 1-3 thin-walled cells, straight or slightly curved, ending in a point or sometimes a hook. In addition, the powder shows, if flowers are present, papillose epidermises of the petals and appendages and pollen grains with a reticulate exine; and if mature fruits are present, scattered brown tannin cells and brownish-yellow, pitted fragments of the testa.

C. Examine the chromatograms obtained in the test for other species of *Passiflora*.

Results The chromatogram obtained with the test solution shows below the zone due to rutin in the chromatogram obtained with the reference solution a zone of intense yellow fluorescence, above it a zone of green fluorescence (diglycosylflavone), below the zone due to hyperoside in the chromatogram obtained with the reference solution a zone of yellow fluorescence (iso-orientin) and above a zone of green fluorescence (isovitexin), above the zone due to hyperoside in the chromatogram obtained with the reference solution a zone of brownish-yellow fluorescence (orientin) and above it a zone of green fluorescence (vitexin). These latter 2 zones may be absent. Further zones may be present.

TESTS

Other species of *Passiflora*
Thin-layer chromatography (2.2.27).

Test solution To 1.0 g of the powdered drug (355) (2.9.12) add 5 mL of *methanol R*. Heat to boiling under a reflux condenser for 10 min. Cool and filter.

Reference solution Dissolve with heating 2.0 mg of *rutin R* and 2.0 mg of *hyperoside R* in 10 mL of *methanol R*.

Plate TLC silica gel plate R.

Mobile phase anhydrous formic acid R, water R, methyl ethyl ketone R, ethyl acetate R (10:10:30:50 V/V/V/V).

Application 10 µL, as bands.

Development Over a path of 15 cm.

Drying In air.

Detection Spray with a 10 g/L solution of *diphenylboric acid aminoethyl ester R* in *methanol R* and then with a 50 g/L solution of *macrogol 400 R* in *methanol R*. Allow to dry in air for 30 min. Examine in ultraviolet light at 365 nm.

Results The chromatogram obtained with the reference solution shows in the lower third a zone of yellowish-brown fluorescence due to rutin and in the middle third a zone of yellowish-brown fluorescence due to hyperoside. The chromatogram obtained with the test solution shows no intense zones of greenish-yellow or orange-yellow fluorescence between the zone due to diglycosylflavones and that due to iso-orientin (*P. coerulea* and *P. edulis*).

Total ash (2.4.16)
Maximum 13.0 per cent.

Loss on drying (2.2.32)
Maximum 10.0 per cent, determined on 1.000 g of the powdered drug (355) (2.9.12) by drying in an oven at 105 °C for 2 h.

ASSAY

Stock solution In a 100 mL round-bottomed flask, introduce 0.200 g of the powdered drug (250) (2.9.12) and add 40 mL of *ethanol (60 per cent V/V) R*. Heat in a water-bath at 60 °C under a reflux condenser for 30 min while shaking frequently. Allow to cool and filter the mixture through a plug of absorbent cotton in a 100 mL flask. Transfer the absorbent cotton with the drug residue into the round-bottomed flask. Add 40 mL of *ethanol (60 per cent V/V) R* and heat again in a water-bath at 60 °C under reflux for 10 min. Allow to cool and filter the mixture and the first filtrate from the 100 mL flask through a filter paper into the 100 mL volumetric flask. Dilute to 100 mL with the same solvent, while rinsing the flask, round-bottomed flask and filter.

Test solution Introduce 5.0 mL of stock solution into a flask. Evaporate to dryness under reduced pressure and take up the residue with 10 mL of a mixture of 10 volumes of *methanol R* and 100 volumes of *glacial acetic acid R*. Add 10 mL of a solution consisting of 25 g/L of *boric acid R* and 20 g/L of oxalic acid in *anhydrous formic acid R* and dilute to 25.0 mL with *anhydrous acetic acid R*.

Compensation liquid Introduce 5.0 mL of the stock solution into a second flask. Evaporate to dryness under reduced pressure and take up the residue with 10 mL of a mixture of 10 volumes of *methanol R* and 100 volumes of *glacial acetic acid R*. Add 10 mL of *anhydrous formic acid R* and dilute to 25.0 mL with *anhydrous acetic acid R*.

After 30 min, measure the absorbance (2.2.25) of the test solution at 401 nm, by comparison with the compensation liquid.

Calculate the percentage content of total flavonoids, expressed as vitexin, using the following expression:

$$\frac{A \times 0.8}{m}$$

i.e. taking the specific absorbance of vitexin to be 628.
A = absorbance at 401 nm,
m = mass of the drug to be examined, in grams.

_____ *Ph Eur*

Passion Flower Dry Extract

(*Ph Eur monograph 1882*)

Ph Eur _____

DEFINITION
Dry extract produced from *Passion flower (1459)*.

Content
Minimum 2.0 per cent of flavonoids, expressed as vitexin ($C_{21}H_{20}O_{10}$; M_r 432.4) (dried extract).

PRODUCTION
The extract is produced from the herbal drug and ethanol (40 per cent V/V to 90 per cent V/V), methanol (60 per cent V/V) or acetone (40 per cent V/V) by an appropriate procedure.

CHARACTERS
Appearance
Greenish-brown amorphous powder.

IDENTIFICATION
Thin-layer chromatography (2.2.27).

Test solution To 0.25 g of the extract to be examined add *methanol R*. Shake, filter and dilute to 5 mL with *methanol R*.

Reference solution   Dissolve 2.0 mg of *hyperoside R* and 2.0 mg of *rutin R* in *methanol R* and dilute to 10 mL with the same solvent.

Plate   TLC silica gel plate *R* (5-40 µm) [or *TLC silica gel plate R* (2-10 µm)].

Mobile phase   anhydrous formic acid *R*, water *R*, methyl ethyl ketone *R*, ethyl acetate *R* (10:10:30:50 *V/V/V/V*).

Application   10 µL [or 5 µL] as bands.

Development   Over a path of 15 cm [or 5 cm].

Drying   At 100-105 °C.

Detection   Spray with a 10 g/L solution of *diphenylboric acid aminoethyl ester R* in *methanol R*. Subsequently spray with a 50 g/L solution of *macrogol 400 R* in *methanol R*. Allow the plate to dry in air for about 30 min. Examine in ultraviolet light at 365 nm.

Results   See below the sequence of zones present in the chromatograms obtained with the reference solution and the test solution. Other fluorescent zones may be present in the chromatogram obtained with the test solution.

Top of the plate	
____	____
Hyperoside: a yellowish-orange fluorescent zone	
	A green fluorescent zone
	A yellow fluorescent zone
Rutin: a yellowish-orange fluorescent zone	
____	____
	A green fluorescent zone
Reference solution	**Test solution**

TESTS

Loss on drying (*2.8.17*)
Maximum 5.0 per cent, determined on 0.500 g.

ASSAY

Stock solution   To 50 mg of the extract to be examined add *ethanol (60 per cent V/V) R*. Shake, filter and dilute to 100.0 mL with *ethanol (60 per cent V/V) R*.

Test solution   Introduce 5.0 mL of the stock solution into a round-bottomed flask and evaporate to dryness under reduced pressure. Take up the residue with 8 mL of a mixture of 10 volumes of *methanol R* and 100 volumes of *glacial acetic acid R* and transfer into a 25 mL volumetric flask. Rinse the round-bottomed flask with 3 mL of a mixture of 10 volumes of *methanol R* and 100 volumes of *glacial acetic acid R* and transfer into the 25 mL volumetric flask. Add 10.0 mL of a solution containing 25.0 g/L of *boric acid R* and 20.0 g/L of *oxalic acid R* in *anhydrous formic acid R* and dilute to 25.0 mL with *anhydrous acetic acid R*.

Compensation liquid   Introduce 5.0 mL of the stock solution into a round-bottomed flask and evaporate to dryness under reduced pressure. Take up the residue with 8 mL of a mixture of 10 volumes of *methanol R* and 100 volumes of *glacial acetic acid R* and transfer into a 25 mL volumetric flask. Rinse the round-bottomed flask with 3 mL of a mixture of 10 volumes of *methanol R* and 100 volumes of

glacial acetic acid R and transfer into the 25 mL volumetric flask. Add 10.0 mL of *anhydrous formic acid R* and dilute to 25.0 mL with *anhydrous acetic acid R*.

After 30 min, measure the absorbance (*2.2.25*) of the test solution at 401 nm.

Calculate the percentage content of total flavonoids, expressed as vitexin, from the following expression:

$$\frac{A \times 0.8}{m}$$

i.e. taking the specific absorbance of vitexin to be 628.
A =   absorbance at 401 nm,
m =   mass of the extract to be examined, in grams.

Ph Eur

Pelargonium Root

(*Ph Eur monograph 2264*)

Ph Eur

DEFINITION

Dried, usually fragmented, underground organs of *Pelargonium sidoides* DC and/or *Pelargonium reniforme* Curt.

Content
Minimum 2.0 per cent of tannins, expressed as pyrogallol ($C_6H_6O_3$; M_r 126.1) (dried drug).

IDENTIFICATION

A. The root is covered with dark, partly reddish-brown, longitudinally fissured bark. The transverse section shows, underneath the cork layer, yellow or white wood, which clearly shows partly brownish medullary rays.

B. Reduce to a powder (355 (*2.9.12*)). The powder is brownish-red. Examine under a microscope using *chloral hydrate solution R*. The powder shows the following diagnostic characters: multilayer cork cells consisting of almost uniform, rectangular cells; fragments of parenchyma underneath the cork containing sclereids with a wide lumen; numerous calcium oxalate cluster crystals. Examine under a microscope using a 50 per cent *V/V* solution of *glycerol R*. The powder shows simple starch granules without striations or cracks.

C. Thin-layer chromatography (*2.2.27*).

Test solution   To 0.5 g of the powdered drug (355) (*2.9.12*) add 10 mL of *methanol R*, shake for 15 min and filter.

Reference solution   Dissolve 1 mg of *scopoletin R* and 2 mg of *esculin R* in 20 mL of *methanol R*.

Plate   TLC silica gel F_{254} plate *R* (5-40 µm) [or *TLC silica gel F_{254} plate R* (2-10 µm)].

Mobile phase   water *R*, methanol *R*, ethyl acetate *R* (10:14:76 *V/V/V*).

Application   10 µL [or 5 µL] as bands.

Development   Over a path of 10 cm [or 6 cm].

Drying   In air.

Detection   Spray with *alcoholic potassium hydroxide solution R*. Examine in ultraviolet light at 365 nm.

Results   See below the sequence of zones present in the chromatograms obtained with the reference solution and the test solution. Furthermore, other blue fluorescent zones may be present in the chromatogram obtained with the test solution.

Top of the plate		
	A blue fluorescent zone	
Scopoletin: a very bright blue fluorescent zone	A weak blue fluorescent zone (scopoletin)	
———	———	
	One or two bright blue fluorescent zones	
Esculin: a very bright blue fluorescent zone		
	A blue fluorescent zone	
	A weak blue fluorescent zone	
———	———	
	A blue fluorescent zone	
Reference solution	Test solution	

TESTS

Loss on drying (*2.2.32*)

Maximum 12.0 per cent, determined on 1.000 g of the powdered drug (355) (*2.9.12*) by drying in an oven at 105 °C.

Total ash (*2.4.16*)

Maximum 12.0 per cent.

Ash insoluble in hydrochloric acid (*2.8.1*)

Maximum 3.0 per cent.

ASSAY

Carry out the determination of tannins in herbal drugs (*2.8.14*). Use 0.750 g of the powdered drug (180) (*2.9.12*).

——————————————————————— *Ph Eur*

White Peony Root

DEFINITION

White Peony Root is the dried whole root of *Paeonia lactiflora* Pallas (*Paeonia albiflora* Pallas; *Paeonia edulis* Salisb.; *Paeonia officinalis* Thunb.). It contains not less than 1.6% of paeoniflorin ($C_{23}H_{28}O_{11}$), calculated with reference to the dried material.

It is collected in summer and autumn, washed clean, with the two ends and rootlet removed and dried.

IDENTIFICATION

A. Cylindrical, straight or slightly curved, two ends truncate, 5 to 20 cm long, 1 to 2.5 cm in diameter. Externally light brown to reddish brown, with longitudinal wrinkles, rootlet scars and with laterally elongated lenticels. Texture compact, easily broken, fracture relatively even, internally whitish or pale brownish-red. Cambium ring distinct and rays radial.

B. Reduce to a powder. The powder is pale yellow. Examine under a microscope using *chloral hydrate solution*. The powder shows abundant rounded, rectangular or elongated parenchymatous cells which occur singly or in groups, some with pitted or slightly beaded walls; single cluster crystals of calcium oxalate, 11 to 35 μm in diameter, isolated or packed in rows in parenchymatous cells, sometimes with several crystals in each cell; fragments of lignified vessels, 20 to 65 μm in diameter, usually reticulately thickened but occasionally bordered-pitted; fibres occur rarely, usually accompanying the vessel fragments, they are 15 to 40 μm in diameter, with thickened, slightly lignified and frequently pitted walls. Examine under a microscope using a 50% v/v

solution of *glycerol* in *water*. Many of the parenchymatous cells contain masses of starch grains which may also be found scattered throughout the powder.

C. In the Assay, the chromatogram obtained with solution (1) shows a peak with the same retention time as the principal peak in the chromatogram obtained with solution (2).

D. Carry out the method for *thin-layer chromatography*, Appendix III A, using the following solutions.

(1) Shake 0.5 g of the powdered root with 10 mL of *ethanol* for 5 minutes, filter and evaporate the filtrate to dryness and dissolve the residue in 1 mL of *absolute ethanol*.

(2) 0.1% w/v each of *paeoniflorin BPCRS* and *4'-hydroxyacetophenone BPCRS* in *ethanol*.

CHROMATOGRAPHIC CONDITIONS

(a) Use as the coating *silica gel* (Merck silica gel 60 precoated plates are suitable).

(b) Use the mobile phase described below.

(c) Apply 10 μL for each solution, as a band.

(d) Develop the plate to 15 cm.

(e) Dry the plate in air. Spray with a 5% w/v solution of *vanillin* in *sulfuric acid*, heat at 105° for 5 minutes and examine immediately.

MOBILE PHASE

0.2 volumes of *formic acid*, 5 volumes of *ethyl acetate*, 10 volumes of *methanol* and 40 volumes of *dichloromethane*.

SYSTEM SUITABILITY

The test is not valid unless, in the chromatogram obtained with solution (2), two clearly separated bands are observed.

CONFIRMATION

The bluish-purple band with an Rf value of approximately 0.4 in the chromatogram obtained with solution (1) corresponds in colour and position to that in the chromatogram obtained with solution (2). Other bands are present in the chromatogram obtained with solution (1) as shown below.

Top of the plate	
A dark pink band	
Several bluish bands	4'-hydroxyacetophenone: an orange band
A bluish-purple band	Paeoniflorin: a bluish-purple band
Solution (1)	**Solution (2)**

TESTS

Tree Peony

In the Assay, the chromatogram obtained with solution (1) shows no peak with a relative retention of approximately 1.2 with reference to paeoniflorin.

Loss on drying

When dried for 3 hours at 100° to 105°, loses not more than 12.0% of its weight. Use 1 g.

Acid-insoluble ash

Not more than 0.5%, Appendix XI K.

Ash

Not more than 6.5%, Appendix XI J.

Cadmium

Maximum 3 ppm, Appendix VII.

Lead

Maximum 5 ppm, Appendix VII.

ASSAY

Carry out the method for *liquid chromatography*, Appendix III D, using the following solutions prepared in 0.05M *potassium dihydrogen orthophosphate* (solution A).

(1) Finely powder not less than 5 g of the herbal drug being examined. Mix 0.15 g of the powdered drug with 3 mL of *methanol* and place in an ultrasonic bath for 30 minutes. Dilute to 10 mL with solution A, mix, filter through a 0.45-µm filter and use the filtrate.

(2) Dissolve a quantity of *paeoniflorin BPCRS* in *methanol* and dilute with solution A to produce a solution containing 0.05% w/v in 3 volumes of *methanol* and 7 volumes of solution A and mix.

(3) Dissolve a quantity of *4′-hydroxyacetophenone BPCRS* in solution (2) to produce a solution containing 0.05% w/v of 4′-hydroxyacetophenone.

CHROMATOGRAPHIC CONDITIONS

(a) Use a stainless steel column (15 cm × 4.6 mm) packed with *octadecylsilyl silica gel for chromatography* (5 µm) (Luna C18 is suitable).

(b) Use isocratic elution and the mobile phase described below.

(c) Use a flow rate of 1 mL per minute.

(d) Use a column temperature of 30°.

(e) Use a detection wavelength of 230 nm.

(f) Inject 10 µL of each solution.

MOBILE PHASE

30 volumes of *methanol* and 70 volumes of solution A.

SYSTEM SUITABILITY

The test is not valid unless, in the chromatogram obtained with solution (3), the number of *theoretical plates* for the peak due to paeoniflorin is at least 3000, the *symmetry factor* for the peak due to paeoniflorin is not more than 1.3 and the *resolution factor* between the two peaks is not less than 1.7.

DETERMINATION OF CONTENT

Using the retention time and the peak area from the chromatograms obtained with solution (2), locate and integrate the peak due to paeoniflorin in the chromatogram obtained with solution (1).

Calculate the content of $C_{23}H_{28}O_{11}$ in the sample, using the declared content of paeoniflorin ($C_{23}H_{28}O_{11}$) in *paeoniflorin BPCRS* and the following expression:

$$\frac{A_1}{A_2} \times \frac{m_2}{V_2} \times \frac{V_1}{m_1} \times p \times \frac{100}{100 - d}$$

A_1 = Area of the peak due to paeoniflorin in the chromatogram obtained with solution (1).

A_2 = Area of the peak due to paeoniflorin in the chromatogram obtained with solution (2).

m_1 = Weight of the drug being examined in mg.

m_2 = Weight of *paeoniflorin BPCRS* in mg.

V_1 = Dilution volume of solution (1) in mL.

V_2 = Dilution volume of solution (2) in mL.

p = Percentage content of $C_{23}H_{28}O_{11}$ in *paeoniflorin BPCRS*.

d = Percentage loss on drying of the herbal drug being examined.

STORAGE

White Peony Root should be protected from moisture.

Processed White Peony Root

DEFINITION

Processed White Peony Root is White Peony Root that has been the boiled, peeled and dried. It contains not less than 1.6% of paeoniflorin ($C_{23}H_{28}O_{11}$), calculated with reference to the dried material.

PRODUCTION

It is collected in summer and autumn, washed clean, with the two ends and rootlets removed, either peeled after boiling in water or boiled in water after peeling and dried in the sun. The dried root is washed and soaked thoroughly prior to being sliced transversely or longitudinally and dried.

IDENTIFICATION

A. The root slices are greyish-white to pale brown, darker at the edges, and up to about 2 mm thick. They are smooth and compact with a short and even fracture. Those that have been cut transversely occur in oval pieces up to about 4.5 cm in diameter and the cut surface shows a distinctly radiate xylem with narrow lines of vascular tissue separated by wide medullary rays. The longitudinally cut slices are up to 10 cm long and 1.5 cm wide and the cut surface shows raised strands of vascular tissue running longitudinally.

B. Reduce to a powder. The powder is pale yellow. Examine under a microscope using *chloral hydrate solution*. The powder shows abundant rounded, rectangular or elongated parenchymatous cells which occur singly or in groups, some with pitted or slightly beaded walls; many of the cells contain pale yellow or pinkish masses of gelatinised starch which are also found scattered throughout the powder; single cluster crystals of calcium oxalate, 11 to 35 µm in diameter, isolated or packed in rows in parenchymatous cells, sometimes with several crystals in each cell; fragments of lignified vessels, 20 to 65 µm in diameter, usually reticulately thickened but occasionally bordered-pitted; fibres occur rarely, usually accompanying the vessel fragments, they are 15 to 40 µm in diameter, with thickened, slightly lignified and frequently pitted walls.

C. In the Assay, the chromatogram obtained with solution (1) shows a peak with the same retention time as the principal peak in the chromatogram obtained with solution (2).

D. Carry out the method for *thin-layer chromatography*, Appendix III A, using the following solutions.

(1) Shake 0.5 g of the powdered root with 10 mL of *ethanol* for 5 minutes, filter, evaporate the filtrate to dryness and dissolve the residue in 1 mL of ethanol.

(2) 0.1% w/v each of *paeoniflorin BPCRS* and *4′-hydroxyacetophenone BPCRS* in *ethanol*.

CHROMATOGRAPHIC CONDITIONS

(a) Use as the coating *silica gel* (Merck silica gel 60 precoated plates are suitable).

(b) Use the mobile phase described below.

(c) Apply 10 µL of each solution, as a band.

(d) Develop the plate to 15 cm.

(e) Dry the plate in air. Spray with a 5% w/v solution of *vanillin* in *sulfuric acid*, heat at 105° for 5 minutes and examine immediately.

MOBILE PHASE

A mixture of 0.2 volumes of *formic acid*, 5 volumes of *ethyl acetate*, 10 volumes of *methanol* and 40 volumes of *dichloromethane*.

SYSTEM SUITABILITY

The test is not valid unless, in the chromatogram obtained with solution (2), two clearly separated spots are observed.

CONFIRMATION

The bluish-purple spot with an Rf value of approximately 0.4 in the chromatogram obtained with solution (1) corresponds in colour and position to that in the chromatogram obtained with solution (2). Other spots are present in the chromatogram obtained with solution (1) as shown below.

Top of the plate	
A dark pink band	
Several bluish bands	4'-hydroxyacetophenone: an orange band
A bluish-purple band	Paeoniflorin: a bluish-purple band
Solution (1)	**Solution (2)**

TESTS

Tree Peony

In the Assay, the chromatogram obtained with solution (1) shows no peak with a relative retention of approximately 1.2 with reference to paeoniflorin.

Loss on drying

When dried for 3 hours at 100° to 105°, loses not more than 12.0% of its weight. Use 1 g.

Acid-insoluble ash

Not more than 0.5%, Appendix XI K.

Ash

Not more than 6.5%, Appendix XI J.

Cadmium

Maximum 3 ppm, Appendix VII.

Lead

Maximum 5 ppm, Appendix VII.

ASSAY

Carry out the method for *liquid chromatography*, Appendix III D, using the following solutions prepared in 0.05M *potassium dihydrogen orthophosphate* (solution A).

(1) Finely powder not less than 5 g of the herbal drug being examined. Mix 0.15 g of the powdered drug with 3 mL of *methanol* and place in an ultrasonic bath for 30 minutes. Dilute to 10 mL with solution A, mix, filter through a 0.45-µm filter and use the filtrate.

(2) Dissolve a quantity of *paeoniflorin BPCRS* in *methanol* and dilute with solution A to produce a solution containing 0.05% w/v in 3 volumes of methanol and 7 volumes of solution A and mix.

(3) Dissolve a quantity of *4'-hydroxyacetophenone BPCRS* in solution (2) to produce a solution containing 0.05% w/v of *4'-hydroxyacetophenone*.

CHROMATOGRAPHIC CONDITIONS

(a) Use a stainless steel column (15 cm × 4.6 mm) packed with *octadecylsilyl silica gel for chromatography* (5 µm) (Luna C18 is suitable).

(b) Use isocratic elution and the mobile phase described below.

(c) Use a flow rate of 1 mL per minute.

(d) Use a column temperature of 30°.

(e) Use a detection wavelength of 230 nm.

(f) Inject 10 µL of each solution.

MOBILE PHASE

A mixture of 30 volumes of *methanol* and 70 volumes of solution A.

SYSTEM SUITABILITY

The test is not valid unless, in the chromatogram obtained with solution (3), the number of *theoretical plates* for each peak due to paeoniflorin is at least 3000, the *symmetry factor* for the peak due to paeoniflorin is not more than 1.3 and the *resolution factor* between the two peaks is not less than 1.7.

DETERMINATION OF CONTENT

Using the retention time and the peak area from the chromatograms obtained with solution (2), locate and integrate the peak due to paeoniflorin in the chromatogram obtained with solution (1).

Calculate the content of $C_{23}H_{28}O_{11}$ in the sample, using the declared content of paeoniflorin ($C_{23}H_{28}O_{11}$) in *paeoniflorin BPCRS* and the following expression:

$$\frac{A_1}{A_2} \times \frac{m_2}{V_2} \times \frac{V_1}{m_1} \times p \times \frac{100}{100-d}$$

A_1 = Area of the peak due to paeoniflorin in the chromatogram obtained with solution (1).

A_2 = Area of the peak due to paeoniflorin in the chromatogram obtained with solution (2).

m_1 = Weight of the drug being examined in mg.

m_2 = Weight of *paeoniflorin BPCRS* in mg.

V_1 = Dilution volume of solution (1) in mL.

V_2 = Dilution volume of solution (2) in mL.

p = Percentage content of $C_{23}H_{28}O_{11}$ in *paeoniflorin BPCRS*.

d = Percentage loss on drying of the herbal drug being examined.

STORAGE

Processed White Peony Root should be protected from moisture.

Pepper

(*Ph Eur monograph 2477*)

Ph Eur ____

DEFINITION

Dried, ripe or nearly ripe fruit of *Piper nigrum* L. with an unbroken pericarp (black pepper) or with the outer layers of the pericarp removed (white pepper).

Content:
— *essential oil*: minimum 25 mL/kg (anhydrous drug);
— *piperine* ($C_{17}H_{19}NO_3$; M_r 285.3): minimum 3.0 per cent (anhydrous drug).

IDENTIFICATION

A. *White pepper*. Spheroid berries, 3-5 mm in diameter, slightly flattened at one pole and with a small protuberance at the other, with smooth, externally matt, brownish-grey, greyish-white or pale yellowish-white surface, with numerous pale, linear striations between apex and base.

Black pepper. Spheroid berries, 3-6 mm in diameter, externally blackish-brown, with raised reticular wrinkles, bearing fine remains of the style at the apex and a scar of the peduncle at the base. The texture is hard, the epicarp can be stripped, the endocarp is greyish-white or pale yellow. The fracture is greyish-white, starchy, possessing a small space at the centre.

B. Microscopic examination (*2.8.23*).

White pepper. The powder is light grey. Examine under a microscope using *chloral hydrate solution R*. The powder shows the following diagnostic characters (Figure 2477.-1): fragments of the endocarp in surface view, consisting of more or less polygonal sclereids about 20-30 µm in diameter, which have irregularly thickened walls [Ac, C, Fa] and which may or may not be associated with the testa [A, F], consisting of a layer of indistinct, reddish-brown pigmented cells constituting the 'pigmented layer' [Ab, Fb] and a layer of very thin-walled polygonal cells constituting the 'hyaline layer' [Aa]; fragments of the endocarp, in transverse section [G], showing sclereids with thickened inner walls on the 3 lower sides [Ga], usually associated with the testa (pigmented layer [Gb] and hyaline layer [Gc]); fragments of the parenchyma of the mesocarp [D] containing large oil cells 50-75 µm in diameter [Da]; numerous thin-walled, ovoid or polygonal cells of the parenchyma of the seed [E]; rare, elongated sclereids, with thickened walls, from the fruit peduncle [B]; a few fragments of vascular tissue with narrow spiral vessels [J]. Examine under a microscope using a 50 per cent *V/V* solution of *glycerol R*. Rounded, compound starch granules [H], about 30 µm in diameter, made up of tiny individual granules, ovoid or polyhedral by compression, free [Hb] or included in the parenchymatous cells of the seed [Ha].

Black pepper. The powder is grey. Examine under a microscope using *chloral hydrate solution R*. In addition to the diagnostic characters described for white pepper, the powdered black pepper shows the following diagnostic characters (Figure 2477.-1): fragments of the epicarp [K] with extremely thin-walled, brownish-red pigmented, polygonal or ovoid cells, which contain small prisms of calcium oxalate [Ka], and which are associated with the outer layers of the mesocarp consisting of groups of sclereids with strongly thickened walls [Kb].

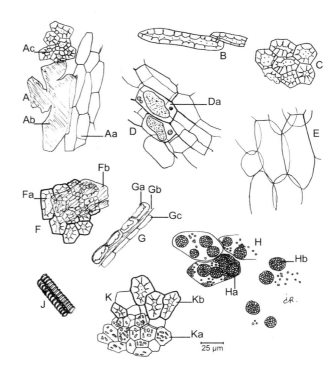

Figure 2477.-1. − *Illustration for identification test B of powdered herbal drug of pepper*

C. Thin-layer chromatography (*2.2.27*).

Test solution   To 0.5 g of the powdered herbal drug (355) (*2.9.12*) add 5 mL of *methanol R*. Sonicate for 10 min, centrifuge and use the supernatant.

Reference solution   Dissolve 10 mg of *borneol R* and 15 mg of *piperine R* in 10 mL of *methanol R*.

Plate   TLC silica gel F_{254} plate R (5-40 µm) [or TLC silica gel F_{254} plate R (2-10 µm)].

Mobile phase   ethyl acetate R, cyclohexane R (30:50 *V/V*).

Application   10 µL [or 5 µL] as bands of 10 mm [or 8 mm].

Development   Over a path of 15 cm [or 6 cm].

Drying   In air.

Detection A   Examine in ultraviolet light at 254 nm.

Results A   See below the sequence of zones present in the chromatograms obtained with the reference solution and the test solution. Furthermore, other faint quenching zones may be present in the chromatogram obtained with the test solution.

Top of the plate	
─────── ───────	3 quenching zones
───────	───────
	A quenching zone
Piperine: a quenching zone	A strong quenching zone (piperine)
Reference solution	**Test solution**

Detection B   Treat with *anisaldehyde solution R* and heat at 100 °C for 5 min; examine in daylight.

Results B See below the sequence of zones present in the chromatograms obtained with the reference solution and the test solution. Furthermore, other zones may be present in the chromatogram obtained with the test solution.

Top of the plate		
	A strong purple zone	
	A purple zone	
————		————
Borneol: a yellowish-brown zone		
	A purple-grey zone	
————		————
	A violet-grey zone	
	A grey zone	
Piperine: a green or brownish zone	A green or brownish zone (piperine)	
	A grey zone	
Reference solution	**Test solution**	

TESTS

Foreign matter (*2.8.2*)
Maximum 3 per cent.

Water (*2.2.13*)
Maximum 120 mL/kg, determined on 20.0 g of the freshly, coarsely powdered herbal drug (1400) (*2.9.12*) reduced using a knife mill.

Total ash (*2.4.16*)
Maximum 6.0 per cent.

ASSAY

Essential oil (*2.8.12*)
Use 10.0 g of the freshly, coarsely powdered herbal drug (1400) (*2.9.12*), a 1000 mL round-bottomed flask, 400 mL of *water R* as the distillation liquid and 0.5 mL of *xylene R* in the graduated tube. Distil at a rate of 2-3 mL/min for 3 h.

Piperine
Liquid chromatography (*2.2.29*). *Carry out the assay protected from light.*

Test solution Disperse 0.250 g of the powdered herbal drug (355) (*2.9.12*) in 40 mL of *ethanol (96 per cent) R*. Sonicate for 20 min and filter. Rinse the flask and the filter with 5 mL of *ethanol (96 per cent) R*, combine the filtrate and washings and dilute to 50.0 mL with the same solvent. Filter through a membrane filter (nominal pore size 0.45 μm).

Reference solution (a) Dissolve 15.0 mg of *piperine CRS* in *ethanol (96 per cent) R* and dilute to 100.0 mL with the same solvent.

Reference solution (b) Disperse 0.250 g of *long pepper for system suitability HRS* (355) (*2.9.12*) in 40 mL of *ethanol (96 per cent) R*. Sonicate for 20 min and filter. Rinse the flask and the filter with 5 mL of *ethanol (96 per cent) R*, combine the filtrate and washings and dilute to 50.0 mL with the same solvent. Filter through a membrane filter (nominal pore size 0.45 μm).

Column:
— *size: l* = 0.15 m, Ø = 4.6 mm;
— *stationary phase: end-capped octadecylsilyl silica gel for chromatography R* (5 μm).

Mobile phase:
— *mobile phase A: water R;*
— *mobile phase B: acetonitrile R;*

Time (min)	Mobile phase A (per cent *V/V*)	Mobile phase B (per cent *V/V*)
0 - 5	50	50
5 - 20	50 → 5	50 → 95
20 - 22	5 → 0	95 → 100

Flow rate 1.0 mL/min.

Detection Spectrophotometer at 343 nm.

Injection 10 μL.

Retention time Piperine = about 10 min.

Identification of peaks Use the chromatogram supplied with *long pepper for system suitability HRS* and the chromatogram obtained with reference solution (b) to identify the peak due to piperine and peak 2.

System suitability Reference solution (b):
— *peak-to-valley ratio:* minimum 4, where H_p = height above the baseline of peak 2 and H_v = height above the baseline of the lowest point of the curve separating the peak due to piperine from peak 2.

Calculate the percentage content of piperine using the following expression:

$$\frac{A_1 \times m_2 \times p}{A_2 \times m_1 \times 2}$$

A_1 = area of the peak due to piperine in the chromatogram obtained with the test solution;

A_2 = area of the peak due to piperine in the chromatogram obtained with reference solution (a);

m_1 = mass of the herbal drug to be examined used to prepare the test solution, in grams;

m_2 = mass of *piperine CRS* used to prepare reference solution (a), in grams;

p = percentage content of piperine in *piperine CRS*.

———————— Ph Eur

Peppermint Leaf

(*Ph Eur monograph 0406*)

Preparation
Peppermint Leaf Dry Extract

Ph Eur ————————

DEFINITION

Whole or cut dried leaves of *Mentha × piperita* L.

Content
Minimum 12 mL/kg of essential oil for the whole drug and minimum 9 mL/kg of essential oil for the cut drug.

CHARACTERS

Characteristic and penetrating odour.

Characteristic aromatic taste.

Peppermint leaf is green or brownish-green, with brownish-violet veins in some varieties. The petioles are green or brownish-violet.

IDENTIFICATION

A. The leaf is entire, broken or cut, thin, fragile and often crumpled; the entire leaf is 3-9 cm long and 1-3 cm wide. The lamina is oval or lanceolate, the apex acuminate, the margin sharply dentate and the base asymmetrical. Venation is pinnate, prominent on the lower surface, with lateral veins leaving the midrib at about 45°. The lower surface is slightly pubescent and secretory trichomes are visible under a lens (6×) as bright yellowish points. The petiole is grooved, usually up to 1 mm in diameter and 0.5-1 cm long.

B. Reduce to a powder (355) (*2.9.12*). The powder is brownish-green. Examine under a microscope using *chloral hydrate solution R*. The powder shows the following diagnostic characters (Figure 0406.-1): fragments of epidermises bearing covering and glandular trichomes; adaxial epidermis, in surface view [B, H], having cells with sinuous-wavy walls [Ha] and cuticle striated over the veins (B) associated with palisade parenchyma [Hb]; abaxial epidermis [C] with diacytic stomata (*2.8.3*) [Ca]; covering trichomes are usually fragmented, elongated, uniseriate with 3-8 cells with striated cuticle [A, E]; glandular trichomes of 2 types: a) unicellular stalk with small, rounded unicellular head 15-25 μm in diameter, in surface view [Ba, Cb] or in transverse section [D], b) unicellular stalk with enlarged oval head 55-70 μm in diameter composed of 8 radiating cells, in surface view [Bb] or in transverse section [Ga]; fragments from near the leaf margin [F] with isodiametric cells whose anticlinal walls are more-or-less straight and beaded [Fa] and short, conical, unicellular or bicellular covering trichomes [Fb]; dorsiventral mesophyll fragments, in transverse section [G], with a single palisade layer [Gc] and 4-6 layers of spongy parenchyma [Gb]. Yellowish crystals of menthol under the cuticle of secretory cells may be present.

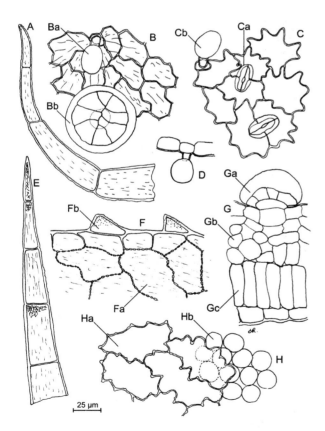

Figure 0406.-1.– *Illustration for identification test B of powdered herbal drug of peppermint leaf*

C. Thin-layer chromatography (*2.2.27*).

Test solution To 0.2 g of the recently powdered drug add 2 mL of *methylene chloride R*, shake for a few minutes and filter. Evaporate the filtrate to dryness at about 40 °C and dissolve the residue in 0.1 mL of *toluene R*.

Reference solution Dissolve 50 mg of *menthol R*, 20 μL of *cineole R*, 10 mg of *thymol R* and 10 μL of *menthyl acetate R* in *toluene R* and dilute to 10 mL with the same solvent.

Plate TLC silica gel GF$_{254}$ plate R.

Mobile phase *ethyl acetate R*, *toluene R* (5:95 *V/V*).

Application 10 μL of the reference solution and 20 μL of the test solution, as bands.

Development Over a path of 15 cm.

Drying In air until the solvent has evaporated.

Detection A Examine in ultraviolet light at 254 nm.

Results A See below the sequence of zones present in the chromatograms obtained with the reference solution and the test solution. Furthermore, other weak quenching zones may be present in the chromatogram obtained with the test solution.

Top of the plate	
	———
Thymol: a quenching zone	
	Quenching zones may be present (carvone, pulegone)
———	———
Reference solution	**Test solution**

Detection B Spray with *anisaldehyde solution R* and examine in daylight while heating for 5-10 min at 100-105 °C.

Results B See below the sequence of zones present in the chromatograms obtained with the reference solution and the test solution. Furthermore, other faint zones may be present in the chromatogram obtained with the test solution.

Top of the plate	
	An intense violet-red zone (near the solvent front) (hydrocarbons)
Menthyl acetate: a violet-blue zone	A violet-blue zone (menthyl acetate)
	A greenish-blue zone (menthone)
Thymol: a pink zone	
	Light pink or greyish-blue or greyish-green zones may be present (carvone, pulegone, isomenthone)
Cineole: a violet-blue or brown zone	A faint violet-blue or brown zone (cineole)
	———
Menthol: an intense blue or violet zone	An intense blue or violet zone (menthol)
Reference solution	**Test solution**

TESTS

Foreign matter (*2.8.2*)

Maximum 5 per cent stems, whose diameter is not greater than 1.5 mm; maximum 2 per cent foreign elements; not more than 8 per cent of the leaves show brown stains due to *Puccinia menthae*.

Carry out the determination using 10 g of the drug.

Water (*2.2.13*)
Maximum 110 mL/kg, determined on 20.0 g.

Total ash (*2.4.16*)
Maximum 15.0 per cent.

Ash insoluble in hydrochloric acid (*2.8.1*)
Maximum 1.5 per cent.

ASSAY
Carry out the determination of essential oils in herbal drugs
(*2.8.12*). Use 20.0 g of crushed drug, a 500 mL flask,
200 mL of *water R* as the distillation liquid and 0.50 mL of
xylene R in the graduated tube. Distil at a rate of 3-4 mL/min
for 2 h.

———————————————————————— *Ph Eur*

Peppermint Oil

(*Ph Eur monograph 0405*)

Preparations
Gastro-resistant Peppermint Oil Capsules
Concentrated Peppermint Emulsion
Peppermint Spirit

Ph Eur ————————————————————————

DEFINITION
Essential oil obtained by steam distillation from the fresh
aerial parts of the flowering plant of *Mentha × piperita* L.

CHARACTERS
Appearance
Colourless, pale yellow or pale greenish-yellow liquid.
Characteristic odour and taste followed by a sensation of
cold.

Solubility
Miscible with ethanol (96 per cent) and with methylene
chloride.

IDENTIFICATION
First identification B.

Second identification A.

A. Examine the chromatograms obtained in test A for mint
oil.

Results A See below the sequence of zones present in the
chromatograms obtained with the reference solution and the
test solution.

Top of the plate	
———	———
Thymol: a quenching zone	
	Quenching zones may be present (carvone, pulegone)
———	———
Reference solution	**Test solution**

Results B See below the sequence of zones present in the
chromatograms obtained with the reference solution and the
test solution. Furthermore, other less intensely coloured
zones may be present in the chromatogram obtained with the
test solution.

Top of the plate	
	An intense violet-red zone (near the solvent front) (hydrocarbons)
	A brownish-yellow zone (menthofuran)
Menthyl acetate: a violet-blue zone	A violet-blue zone (menthyl acetate)
	A greenish-blue zone (menthone)
Thymol: a pink zone	
	Light pink or greyish-blue or greyish-green zones may be present (carvone, pulegone, isomenthone)
1,8-Cineole: a violet-blue or brown zone	A faint violet-blue or brown zone (1,8-cineole)
———	———
Menthol: an intense blue or violet zone	An intense blue or violet zone (menthol)
Reference solution	**Test solution**

B. Examine the chromatograms obtained in the test for
chromatographic profile.

Results The characteristic peaks due to limonene,
1,8-cineole, menthone, menthofuran, isomenthone, menthyl
acetate and menthol in the chromatogram obtained with the
test solution are similar in retention time to those in the
chromatogram obtained with reference solution (a).
Isopulegol, pulegone and carvone may be present in the
chromatogram obtained with the test solution.

TESTS
Relative density (*2.2.5*)
0.900 to 0.916.

Refractive index (*2.2.6*)
1.457 to 1.467.

Optical rotation (*2.2.7*)
−30° to −10°.

Acid value (*2.5.1*)
Maximum 1.4, determined on 5.0 g diluted in 50 mL of the
prescribed mixture of solvents.

Fatty oils and resinified essential oils (*2.8.7*)
It complies with the test for fatty oils and resinified essential
oils.

Mint oil
A. Thin-layer chromatography (*2.2.27*).

Test solution Mix 0.1 g of the substance to be examined
with *toluene R* and dilute to 10 mL with the same solvent.

Reference solution Dissolve 50 mg of *menthol R*, 20 μL of
cineole R, 10 mg of *thymol R* and 10 μL of *menthyl acetate R*
in *toluene R* and dilute to 10 mL with the same solvent.

Plate TLC silica gel F_{254} plate R (5-40 μm) [or *TLC silica gel
F_{254} plate R* (2-10 μm)].

Mobile phase ethyl acetate R, toluene R (5:95 *V/V*).

Application 10 μL [or 1 μL] of the reference solution and
20 μL [or 2 μL] of the test solution, as bands of 10 mm [or
8 mm].

Development Over a path of 15 cm [or 6 cm].

Drying In air.

Detection A Examine in ultraviolet light at 254 nm.

Detection B Treat with *anisaldehyde solution R* and heat at
100-105 °C for 5-10 min; examine immediately in daylight.

Results B   The chromatogram obtained with the test solution shows no blue zone between the zones due to 1,8-cineole and menthol.

B. Examine the chromatograms obtained in the test for chromatographic profile.

Results   The chromatogram obtained with the test solution does not show a peak with the retention time of isopulegol that has an area of more than 0.2 per cent of the total area.

Chromatographic profile   Gas chromatography (*2.2.28*): use the normalisation procedure.

Test solution   Mix 0.20 mL of the substance to be examined with *heptane R* and dilute to 10.0 mL with the same solvent.

Reference solution (a)   Dissolve 10 μL of *limonene R*, 20 μL of *cineole R*, 40 μL of *menthone R*, 10 μL of *menthofuran R*, 10 μL of *isomenthone R*, 40 μL of *menthyl acetate R*, 20 μL of *isopulegol R*, 60 mg of *menthol R*, 20 μL of *pulegone R*, 10 μL of *piperitone R* and 10 μL of *carvone R* in *heptane R* and dilute to 10.0 mL with the same solvent.

Reference solution (b)   Dissolve 5 μL of *isopulegol R* in *heptane R* and dilute to 10.0 mL with the same solvent. Dilute 0.1 mL of the solution to 5.0 mL with *heptane R*.

Column:
— *material*: fused silica;
— *size: l* = 60 m, Ø = 0.25 mm;
— *stationary phase: macrogol 20 000 R* (film thickness 0.25 μm).

Carrier gas   *helium for chromatography R.*

Flow rate   1.5 mL/min.

Split ratio   1:50.

Temperature:

	Time (min)	Temperature (°C)
Column	0 - 10	60
	10 - 70	60 → 180
	70 - 75	180
Injection port		200
Detector		220

Detection   Flame ionisation.

Injection   1 μL.

Elution order   Order indicated in the composition of reference solution (a); record the retention times of these substances.

Identification of peaks   Using the retention times determined from the chromatogram obtained with reference solution (a), locate the components of reference solution (a) in the chromatogram obtained with the test solution.

System suitability   Reference solution (a):
— *resolution*: minimum 1.5 between the peaks due to limonene and 1,8-cineole; minimum 1.5 between the peaks due to piperitone and carvone.

Determine the percentage content of each of the following components. The limits are within the following ranges:
— *limonene*: 1.0 per cent to 3.5 per cent;
— *1,8-cineole*: 3.5 per cent to 8.0 per cent;
— *menthone*: 14.0 per cent to 32.0 per cent;
— *menthofuran*: 1.0 per cent to 8.0 per cent;
— *isomenthone*: 1.5 per cent to 10.0 per cent;
— *menthyl acetate*: 2.8 per cent to 10.0 per cent;
— *isopulegol*: maximum 0.2 per cent;
— *menthol*: 30.0 per cent to 55.0 per cent;
— *pulegone*: maximum 3.0 per cent,

— *carvone*: maximum 1.0 per cent;
— *disregard limit*: the area of the principal peak in the chromatogram obtained with reference solution (b) (0.05 per cent).

The ratio of 1,8-cineole content to limonene content is minimum 2.

STORAGE

At a temperature not exceeding 25 °C.

———————————————————————— *Ph Eur*

Concentrated Peppermint Emulsion

DEFINITION

Concentrated Peppermint Emulsion is a 2% v/v dispersion of Peppermint Oil in a suitable vehicle containing a non-ionic surface-active agent.

Extemporaneous preparation

The following formula and directions apply.

Peppermint Oil	20 mL
Polysorbate 20	1 mL
Double-strength Chloroform Water	500 mL
Purified Water, freshly boiled and cooled	Sufficient to produce 1000 mL

Shake the Peppermint Oil with the Polysorbate 20 and add gradually, shaking well after each addition, the Double-strength Chloroform Water and sufficient Purified Water to produce 1000 mL.

Peppermint Spirit

Peppermint Essence

DEFINITION

Peppermint Oil	100 mL
Ethanol (90 per cent)	Sufficient to produce 1000 mL

Extemporaneous preparation

The following directions apply.

Dissolve the Peppermint Oil in Ethanol (90 per cent) and add sufficient Ethanol (90 per cent) to produce 1000 mL. If the solution is not clear, shake with previously sterilised Purified Talc and filter.

The spirit complies with the requirements stated under Spirits and with the following requirements.

TESTS

Ethanol content

78 to 82% v/v, Appendix VIII F.

Weight per mL

0.830 to 0.840 g, Appendix V G.

Content of oil

9.0 to 11.0% v/v when determined by the following method. Add 25 mL of the spirit and 5 mL of *xylene* to 90 mL of a 10% w/v solution of *sodium chloride* containing 1.0% v/v of *hydrochloric acid* in a flask of about 150 mL capacity with a long neck graduated in 0.1 mL increments and of such a diameter that a 15-cm length has a capacity of 10 mL. Shake the mixture for about 30 minutes, allow to separate and raise the undissolved oily layer into the graduated part of the neck of the flask by the gradual addition of more of the acidified sodium chloride solution, allow to stand for 2 hours or until

Herbal Drugs

there is no further change in volume of the oily layer and measure the volume of the oily layer. The volume of the oily layer, after the subtraction of 5 mL, is taken to be the volume of oil.

Gastro-resistant Peppermint Oil Capsules

DEFINITION

Gastro-resistant Peppermint Oil Capsules contain Peppermint Oil. They are enteric capsules.

The capsules comply with the requirements stated under Capsules and with the following requirements.

IDENTIFICATION

A. Carry out the method for *thin-layer chromatography*, Appendix III A, using a *TLC silica gel GF$_{254}$* plate and a mixture of 5 volumes of *ethyl acetate* and 95 volumes of *toluene* as the mobile phase. Apply separately to the plate as bands 20 µL of solution (1) and 10 µL of solution (2). For solution (1) dissolve a quantity of the contents of the capsules containing 0.1 g of Peppermint Oil in sufficient *toluene* to produce 10 mL. For solution (2) dissolve 10 mg of *thymol*, 10 µL of *menthyl acetate*, 20 µL of *cineole* and 50 mg of *menthol* in *toluene* and dilute to 10 mL with the same solvent. Allow the plate to dry in air until the solvent has evaporated and examine under *ultraviolet light (254 nm)*. The chromatogram obtained with solution (1) may show quenching zones (carvone, pulegone) situated just below the level of the zone (thymol) in the chromatogram obtained with solution (2). Spray with *anisaldehyde solution* and examine in daylight for 5 to 10 minutes while heating at 100° to 105°. The chromatogram obtained with solution (2) shows, in order of increasing Rf value, an intense blue to violet zone (menthol) in the lower third; a violet-blue to brown zone (cineole); a pink zone (thymol); and a violet-blue zone (menthyl acetate). In the chromatogram obtained with solution (1) there is a zone due to menthol (the most intense) and a faint zone due to cineole; at Rf values between those of the cineole and thymol zones in the chromatogram obtained with solution (2), there may be light pink or greyish-blue or greenish-grey zones (carvone, pulegone, isomenthone); in the middle of the chromatogram, there is a violet-blue zone (menthyl acetate) and just below it a greenish-blue zone (menthone); an intense violet-red zone (hydrocarbons) appears near the solvent front and below it there may be a brownish-yellow zone (menthofuran); other less intensely coloured zones may also appear.

B. Examine the chromatograms obtained in the test for Chromatographic profile. The retention time of the principal peaks in the chromatogram obtained with solution (1) is similar to that of the principal peaks in the chromatogram obtained with solution (2). Carvone and pulegone may be absent from the chromatogram obtained with solution (1).

TESTS

Disintegration test

Complies with the requirements stated under Gastro-resistant Capsules.

Refractive index

1.457 to 1.467, determined on the contents of the capsules, Appendix V G.

Relative density

0.900 to 0.916, determined on the contents of the capsules, Appendix V E.

Composition of peppermint oil

Carry out the method for *gas chromatography*, Appendix III B, using the following solutions. For solution (1) use the contents of the capsules. For solution (2) dissolve 0.1 g of *limonene*, 0.2 g of *cineole*, 0.4 g of *menthone*, 0.1 g of *menthofuran*, 0.1 g of *isomenthone*, 0.4 g of *menthyl acetate*, 0.6 g of *menthol*, 0.2 g of *pulegone* and 0.1 g of *carvone* in 1 mL of *hexane*. Prepare immediately before use.

The chromatographic procedure may be carried out using (a) a fused-silica capillary column (60 m × 0.25 mm) coated with *macrogol 20,000* as the bonded phase, maintaining the temperature of the column at 60° for 10 minutes, then raising the temperature at a rate of 2° per minute to 180° and maintaining at 180° for 5 minutes, a split injection system with a split ratio of 100 to 1 and maintaining the temperature of the injection port and of the detector at 220° and (b) *helium* as the carrier gas at a flow rate of 1.5 mL per minute.

Inject about 0.2 µL of solution (2). When the chromatograms are recorded in the prescribed conditions, the components elute in the order indicated in the composition of solution (2); a type chromatogram is reproduced in the monograph for Peppermint Oil. Record the retention times of these substances.

The test is not valid unless the number of *theoretical plates* calculated from the limonene peak at 110° is at least 30,000 and the *resolution factor* between the peaks corresponding to limonene and cineole is at least 1.5.

Inject about 0.2 µL of solution (1). Using the retention times determined from the chromatogram obtained with solution (2), locate the components of solution (2) on the chromatogram obtained with solution (1) (disregard the peak due to hexane).

Determine the percentage content of the components by the normalisation procedure.

The percentages are within the following ranges:

Limonene	1.0 to 5.0%,
Cineole	3.5 to 14.0%,
Menthone	14.0 to 32.0%,
Menthofuran	1.0 to 9.0%,
Isomenthone	1.5 to 10.0%,
Menthyl acetate	2.8 to 10.0%,
Menthol	30.0 to 55.0%,
Pulegon	Not more than 4.0%,
Carvone	Not more than 1.0%.

The ratio of cineole content to limonene content is greater than 2.

STORAGE

Gastro-resistant Peppermint Oil Capsules should be protected from light.

Peppermint Leaf Dry Extract

(*Ph Eur monograph 2382*)

Ph Eur ───────

DEFINITION
Dry extract produced from *Peppermint leaf (0406)*.

Content
Minimum 0.5 per cent of rosmarinic acid ($C_{18}H_{16}O_8$; M_r 360.33) (dried extract).

PRODUCTION
The extract is produced from the herbal drug by a suitable procedure using ethanol (30-50 per cent *V/V*) or water of minimum 60 °C.

CHARACTERS
Appearance
Brown, amorphous powder.

IDENTIFICATION
Thin-layer chromatography (*2.2.27*).

Test solution   To 0.2 g of the extract to be examined add 5 mL of *methanol R*. Sonicate for 5 min and filter.

Reference solution   Dissolve 5 mg of *rosmarinic acid R*, 1 mg of *hyperoside R* and 1 mg of *rutin R* in 10 mL of *methanol R*.

Plate   TLC silica gel plate R (5-40 µm) [or *TLC silica gel plate R* (2-10 µm)].

Mobile phase   anhydrous formic acid R, water R, ethyl acetate R (6:6:90 *V/V/V*).

Application   10 µL [or 4 µL] as bands of 15 mm [or 8 mm].

Development   Over a path of 8 cm [or 6 cm].

Drying   In air.

Detection   Heat at 100 °C for 5 min and spray the hot plate with a 5 g/L solution of *diphenylboric acid aminoethyl ester R* in *ethyl acetate R*; examine in ultraviolet light at 365 nm.

Results   See below the sequence of zones present in the chromatograms obtained with the reference solution and the test solution. Furthermore, other faint zones may be present in the chromatogram obtained with the test solution.

Top of the plate	
Rosmarinic acid: a light blue fluorescent zone	A light blue fluorescent zone (rosmarinic acid)
───────	───────
Hyperoside: an orange fluorescent zone	
	A yellow fluorescent zone
	A brown fluorescent zone
Rutin: an orange fluorescent zone	A yellow fluorescent zone
Reference solution	**Test solution**

ASSAY
Liquid chromatography (*2.2.29*).

Test solution   Use brown glass flasks. To 0.400 g of the extract to be examined add 15 mL of *ethanol (50 per cent V/V) R*, sonicate for 10 min and filter into a 20 mL volumetric flask. Rinse the flask and the filter with *ethanol (50 per cent V/V) R* and dilute to 20.0 mL with the same solvent.

Reference solution (a)   Dissolve 10.0 mg of *rosmarinic acid CRS* in ethanol (50 per cent V/V) R and dilute to 100.0 mL with the same solvent.

Reference solution (b)   Dissolve 5 mg of *ferulic acid R* in reference solution (a) and dilute to 50 mL with the same solution.

Column:
— *size*: l = 0.25 m, Ø = 4.6 mm;
— *stationary phase*: octadecylsilyl silica gel for chromatography R (5 µm).

Mobile phase:
— *mobile phase A*: phosphoric acid R, acetonitrile R, water R (1:19:80 *V/V/V*);
— *mobile phase B*: phosphoric acid R, methanol R, acetonitrile R (1:40:59 *V/V/V*);

Time (min)	Mobile phase A (per cent *V/V*)	Mobile phase B (per cent *V/V*)
0 - 20	100 → 55	0 → 45
20 - 25	55 → 0	45 → 100
25 - 30	0 → 100	100 → 0

Flow rate   1.2 mL/min.

Detection   Spectrophotometer at 330 nm.

Injection   20 µL.

Relative retention   With reference to rosmarinic acid (retention time = about 11 min): ferulic acid = about 0.8.

System suitability   Reference solution (b):
— *resolution*: minimum 4.0 between the peaks due to ferulic acid and rosmarinic acid.

Calculate the percentage content of rosmarinic acid using the following expression:

$$\frac{A_1 \times m_2 \times p \times 0.2}{A_2 \times m_1}$$

A_1 =   area of the peak due to rosmarinic acid in the chromatogram obtained with the test solution;

A_2 =   area of the peak due to rosmarinic acid in the chromatogram obtained with reference solution (a);

m_1 =   mass of the extract to be examined used to prepare the test solution, in grams;

m_2 =   mass of *rosmarinic acid CRS* used to prepare reference solution (a), in grams;

p =   percentage content of rosmarinic acid in *rosmarinic acid CRS*.

─────── *Ph Eur*

Peru Balsam

(*Ph Eur monograph 0754*)

Ph Eur ───────

DEFINITION
Balsam obtained from the scorched and wounded trunk of *Myroxylon balsamum* (L.) Harms var. *pereirae* (Royle) Harms.

Content
45.0 per cent *m/m* to 70.0 per cent *m/m* of esters, mainly benzyl benzoate and benzyl cinnamate.

CHARACTERS
Appearance
Dark brown, viscous liquid which is transparent and yellowish-brown when viewed in a thin layer; it is not sticky, non-drying and does not form threads.

Solubility

Practically insoluble in water, freely soluble in anhydrous ethanol, not miscible with fatty oils, except for castor oil.

IDENTIFICATION

A. Dissolve 0.20 g in 10 mL of *ethanol (96 per cent) R*. Add 0.2 mL of *ferric chloride solution R1*. A green or yellowish-green colour develops.

B. Thin-layer chromatography (*2.2.27*).

Test solution Dissolve 0.5 g of the substance to be examined in 10 mL of *ethyl acetate R*.

Reference solution Dissolve 4 mg of *thymol R*, 30 mg of *benzyl cinnamate R* and 80 μL of *benzyl benzoate R* in 5 mL of *ethyl acetate R*.

Plate TLC silica gel GF$_{254}$ plate R.

Mobile phase glacial acetic acid R, ethyl acetate R, hexane R (0.5:10:90 V/V/V).

Application 10 μL, as bands of 20 mm by 3 mm.

Development Twice over a path of 10 cm.

Drying In air.

Detection A Examine in ultraviolet light at 254 nm and mark the quenching zones.

Results A The chromatogram obtained with the reference solution shows in the upper third 2 quenching zones, the higher one due to benzyl benzoate and the lower one due to benzyl cinnamate. The chromatogram obtained with the test solution shows 2 quenching zones at the same levels and of approximately the same size.

Detection B Spray with a freshly prepared 200 g/L solution of *phosphomolybdic acid R* in *ethanol (96 per cent) R*, using 10 mL for a plate 200 mm square and examine in daylight while heating at 100-105 °C for 5-10 min.

Results B The zones due to benzyl benzoate and benzyl cinnamate are blue against a yellow background. The chromatogram obtained with the reference solution shows at about the middle a violet-grey zone (thymol). In the chromatogram obtained with the test solution, a blue zone (nerolidol) is seen just below the level of the zone due to thymol in the chromatogram obtained with the reference solution. Just below the zone due to nerolidol, no blue zone is seen corresponding to a quenching zone seen when examined in ultraviolet light at 254 nm (colophony). In the upper and lower part of the chromatogram obtained with the test solution, other faint blue zones may be seen.

TESTS

Relative density (*2.2.5*)
1.14 to 1.17.

Saponification value (*2.5.6*)
230 to 255, determined on the residue obtained in the assay.

Artificial balsams
Shake 0.20 g with 6 mL of *light petroleum R1*. The light petroleum solution is clear and colourless and the whole of the insoluble parts of the balsam stick to the wall of the test-tube.

Fatty oils
Shake 1 g with 3 mL of a 1000 g/L solution of *chloral hydrate R*. The resulting solution is as clear as the 1000 g/L solution of *chloral hydrate R*.

Turpentine
Evaporate to dryness 4 mL of the solution obtained in the test for artificial balsams. The residue has no odour of turpentine.

ASSAY

To 2.50 g in a separating funnel add 7.5 mL of *dilute sodium hydroxide solution R* and 40 mL of *peroxide-free ether R* and shake vigorously for 10 min. Separate the lower layer and shake it with 3 quantities, each of 15 mL, of *peroxide-free ether R*. Combine the ether layers, dry over 10 g of *anhydrous sodium sulfate R* and filter. Wash the sodium sulfate with 2 quantities, each of 10 mL, of *peroxide-free ether R*. Combine the ether layers and evaporate to dryness. Dry the residue (esters) at 100-105 °C for 30 min and weigh.

STORAGE

Protected from light.

Ph Eur

Phyllanthus Emblica Pericarp

DEFINITION

Phyllanthus Emblica Pericarp is the pericarp of dried mature fruits of *Phyllanthus emblica* L. (syn. *Emblica officinalis* Gaertn.)

It contains not less than 6.0% tannins, expressed as pyrogallol (C$_6$H$_6$O$_3$. M_r 126.1), calculated with reference to the dried drug.

IDENTIFICATION

A. Irregular pieces of the pericarp showing a dark brownish to black outer surface, much wrinkled and grooved with occasional greyish-white patches; the underlying brown mesocarp is about 2 to 3 mm wide surrounding a thin, paler brown endocarp. Infrequently whole seeds, or portions of the creamish white testa may be present, attached to the endocarp; whole seeds are subspherical, about 1 cm in diameter and the testa is marked with 6 equidistant longitudinal ridges. Occasional whole fruits may also be present; they are spherical to ovoid or irregular, about 2 cm in diameter and show a depression at one end.

B. The powder is yellow-green or pale brown. It shows small polygonal cells from the exocarp covered with a thick cuticle, numerous mesocarp, some filled with amorphous grey birefractive masses, some with mucilage, and some with calcium oxalate crystals in the form of needles, large prism or microsphenoids; thick-walled, pitted sclereids from the mesocarp found singly and usually surrounded by parenchyma, and fragments of the endocarp consisting of a thick layer of pitted fibres and sclereids.

C. Carry out the method for *thin-layer chromatography*, Appendix III A, using the following solutions.

(1) Add 25 mL of *ethanol* to 1.0 g of the powdered herbal drug, sonicate for 30 minutes and filter.

(2) 0.1% w/v of *ellagic acid* and 0.1% w/v of *gallic acid* in *methanol*.

CHROMATOGRAPHIC CONDITIONS

(a) Use as the coating *silica gel 60 F$_{254}$* or high-performance *silica gel 60 F$_{254}$* (Merck silica gel 60 F$_{254}$ HPTLC plates are suitable).

(b) Use the mobile phase as described below.

(c) Apply 10 μL [or 2 μL] of each solution, as bands.

(d) Develop the plate to 15 cm [or 7 cm].

(e) After removal of the plate, dry in air, spray with a 5% w/v solution of *iron(III) chloride* in *ethanol* and examine in daylight.

MOBILE PHASE

1.5 volumes of *toluene*, 3 volumes of *acetic acid*, 4 volumes of *formic acid* and 30 volumes of *ethyl acetate*.

SYSTEM SUITABILITY

The test is not valid unless the chromatogram obtained with solution (2) shows two clearly separated bands.

CONFIRMATION

The chromatogram obtained with solution (1) shows a dark blue band with an Rf value of 0.6 corresponding in colour and position to the band obtained with ellagic acid in solution (2) and a dark blue band with an Rf value of approximately 0.9 corresponding in position to the dark blue band obtained with gallic acid in solution (2). Two or three separated blue or faint blue bands with Rf values of between 0.2 and 0.3 are also present. Other bands may be present in solution (1).

Top of the plate	
Dark blue band	Gallic acid: a dark blue band
Dark blue band	Ellagic acid: a dark blue band
Blue/faint blue band Blue/faint blue band	
Solution (1)	**Solution (2)**

TESTS

Ethanol-soluble extractive

Not less than 15.0%, Appendix XI B1

Foreign matter

Not more than 5% of foreign matter including seed material, Appendix XI D.

Water-soluble extractive

Not less than 50%, Appendix XI B2.

Ash

Not more than 7.0%, Appendix XI J, method II.

Loss on drying

Not more than 10.0%, Appendix IX D. Use 1 g.

ASSAY

Carry out the determination of *tannins in herbal drugs*, Appendix XI M. Use 1.0 g of powdered drug.

Dwarf Pine Oil

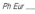

(*Ph Eur monograph 2377*)

Ph Eur

DEFINITION

Essential oil obtained by steam distillation of the fresh leaves and twigs of *Pinus mugo* Turra. A suitable antioxidant may be added.

CHARACTERS

Appearance

Clear, colourless or pale yellow liquid.

IDENTIFICATION

First identification   B.

Second identification   A.

A. Thin-layer chromatography (*2.2.27*).

Test solution   Dilute 1 mL of the substance to be examined to 10 mL with *toluene R*.

Reference solution   Dissolve 10 mg of *borneol R* and 10 µL of *bornyl acetate R* in *toluene R* and dilute to 10 mL with the same solvent.

Plate   TLC silica gel plate R (5-40 µm) [or *TLC silica gel plate R* (2-10 µm)].

Mobile phase   ethyl acetate R, toluene R (5:95 *V/V*).

Application   10 µL [or 2 µL], as bands.

Development   Over a path of 15 cm [or 6 cm].

Drying   In air.

Detection   Spray with *anisaldehyde solution R* and heat at 100-105 °C for 5-10 min; examine in daylight.

Results   See below the sequence of zones present in the chromatograms obtained with the reference solution and the test solution. Furthermore, other zones may be present in the chromatogram obtained with the test solution.

Top of the plate	
	A pink zone
———	———
Bornyl acetate: a brown or greyish-brown zone	A brown or greyish-brown zone (bornyl acetate) A pink zone
———	———
Borneol: a brown or greyish-brown zone	A cluster of violet zones
Reference solution	**Test solution**

B. Examine the chromatograms obtained in the test for chromatographic profile.

Results   The characteristic peaks in the chromatogram obtained with the test solution are similar in retention time to those in the chromatogram obtained with reference solution (a).

TESTS

Relative density (*2.2.5*)
0.857 to 0.868.

Refractive index (*2.2.6*)
1.474 to 1.480.

Optical rotation (*2.2.7*)
− 7° to − 15°.

Acid value (*2.5.1*)
Maximum 1.0.

Peroxide value (*2.5.5*)
Maximum 20.

Fatty oils and resinified oils (*2.8.7*)
It complies with the test.

Chromatographic profile
Gas chromatography (*2.2.28*): use the normalisation procedure.

Test solution   Dilute 200 µL of the substance to be examined to 10.0 mL with *heptane R*.

Reference solution (a)   Dilute 30 µL of *α-pinene R*, 5 mg of *camphene R*, 10 µL of *β-pinene R*, 20 µL of *car-3-ene R*, 5 µL of *β-myrcene R*, 10 µL of *limonene R*, 5 µL of *p-cymene R*, 10 µL of *terpinolene R*, 5 µL of *bornyl acetate R* and 5 µL of *β-caryophyllene R* in *heptane R* and dilute to 5 mL with the same solvent.

Reference solution (b)   Dissolve 5 mg of *camphene R* in *heptane R* and dilute to 50.0 mL with the same solvent. Dilute 1.0 mL of this solution to 10.0 mL with *heptane R*.

Column:
— *material*: fused silica;
— *size*: *l* = 60 m, Ø = 0.25 mm;
— *stationary phase*: *macrogol 20 000 R* (film thickness 0.25 µm).

Carrier gas   *helium for chromatography R.*

Flow rate   1.5 mL/min.

Split ratio   1:50.

Temperature:

	Time (min)	Temperature (°C)
Column	0 - 10	65
	10 - 41	65 → 220
	41 - 50	220
Injection port		220
Detector		250

Detection   Flame ionisation.

Injection   1 µL.

Elution order   Order indicated in the composition of reference solution (a); record the retention times of these substances.

System suitability   Reference solution (a):
— *resolution*: minimum 1.5 between the peaks due to car-3-ene and β-myrcene.

Identification of components   Using the retention times determined from the chromatogram obtained with reference solution (a), locate the components of reference solution (a) in the chromatogram obtained with the test solution; the peak due to β-phellandrene is eluted after the peak due to limonene with a relative retention of about 1.03 with reference to limonene.

Determine the percentage content of each of these components. The limits are within the following ranges:
— *α-pinene*: 10.0 per cent to 30.0 per cent;
— *camphene*: maximum 2.0 per cent;
— *β-pinene*: 3.0 per cent to 14.0 per cent;
— *car-3-ene*: 10.0 per cent to 20.0 per cent;
— *β-myrcene*: 3.0 per cent to 12.0 per cent;
— *limonene*: 8.0 per cent to 14.0 per cent;
— *β-phellandrene*: 10.0 per cent to 19.0 per cent;
— *p-cymene*: maximum 2.5 per cent;
— *terpinolene*: maximum 8.0 per cent;
— *bornyl acetate*: 0.5 per cent to 5.0 per cent;
— *β-caryophyllene*: 0.5 per cent to 5.0 per cent;
— *disregard limit*: the area of the principal peak in the chromatogram obtained with reference solution (b) (0.05 per cent).

STORAGE

In an inert container and at a temperature not exceeding 25 °C.

_____ *Ph Eur*

Pine Silvestris Oil

(Ph Eur monograph 1842)

Ph Eur _____

DEFINITION

Essential oil obtained by steam distillation of the fresh leaves and branches of *Pinus sylvestris* L. A suitable antioxidant may be added.

CHARACTERS

Appearance

Clear, colourless or pale yellow liquid.

Characteristic odour.

IDENTIFICATION

First identification   B.

Second identification   A.

A. Thin-layer chromatography (*2.2.27*).

Test solution   Dilute 1 mL of the substance to be examined to 10 mL with *toluene R*.

Reference solution   Dissolve 10 mg of *borneol R* and 10 µL of *bornyl acetate R* in *toluene R* and dilute to 10 mL with the same solvent.

Plate   *TLC silica gel plate R* (5-40 µm) [or *TLC silica gel plate R* (2-10 µm)].

Mobile phase   *ethyl acetate R*, *toluene R* (5:95 *V/V*).

Application   10 µL [or 2 µL] as bands.

Development   Over a path of 15 cm [or 6 cm].

Drying   In air.

Detection   Treat with *anisaldehyde solution R*, heat at 100-105 °C for 5-10 min and examine in daylight.

Results   See below the sequence of the zones present in the chromatograms obtained with the reference solution and the test solution. Furthermore other faint zones may be present in the chromatogram obtained with the test solution.

Top of the plate	
	A pink zone (hydrocarbons)
	_____
Bornyl acetate: a brown or grey-brown zone	A brown or grey-brown zone (bornyl acetate)
	A pink zone
	_____
Borneol: a brown or grey-brown zone	A cluster of violet zones
Reference solution	**Test solution**

B. Examine the chromatograms obtained in the test for chromatographic profile.

Results   The characteristic peaks in the chromatogram obtained with the test solution are similar in retention time to those in the chromatogram obtained with reference solution (a).

TESTS

Relative density (*2.2.5*)

0.855 to 0.875.

Refractive index (*2.2.6*)

1.465 to 1.480.

Optical rotation (2.2.7)
− 9° to − 30°.

Acid value (2.5.1)
Maximum 1.0.

Peroxide value (2.5.5)
Maximum 20.

Fatty oils and resinified oils (2.8.7)
It complies with the test.

Chromatographic profile
Gas chromatography (2.2.28): use the normalisation procedure.

Test solution   The substance to be examined.

Reference solution (a)   Dissolve 30 μL of α-*pinene R*, 10 mg of *camphene R*, 20 μL of β-*pinene R*, 10 μL of *car-3-ene R*, 10 μL of β-*myrcene R*, 20 μL of *limonene R*, 10 μL of *p-cymene R*, 10 μL of *terpinolene R*, 10 μL of *bornyl acetate R* and 10 μL of β-*caryophyllene R* in 1 mL of *heptane R*.

Reference solution (b)   Dissolve 10 mg of *camphene R* in *heptane R* and dilute to 2 mL with the same solvent. Dilute 0.1 mL of the solution to 1 mL with *heptane R*.

Column:
— *material*: fused silica,
— *size*: $l = 60$ m, $\varnothing = 0.22$ mm,
— *stationary phase*: macrogol 20 000 R (0.2 μm).

Carrier gas   helium for chromatography R.

Flow rate   1.5 mL/min.

Split ratio   1:100.

Temperature:

	Time (min)	Temperature (°C)
Column	0 - 10	65
	10 - 41	65 → 220
	41 - 50	220
Injection port		220
Detector		250

Detection   Flame ionisation.

Injection   0.2 μL.

Elution order   Order indicated in the preparation of reference solution (a). Record the retention times of these substances.

System suitability   Reference solution (a):
— *resolution*: minimum 1.5 between the peaks due to car-3-ene and β-myrcene.

Identification of components   Using the retention times determined from the chromatogram obtained with reference solution (a), locate the components of reference solution (a) in the chromatogram obtained with the test solution. The peak due to β-phellandrene is eluted after the peak due to limonene with a relative retention of about 1.03 with reference to limonene.

Determine the percentage content of these components. The limits are within the following ranges:
— α-*pinene*: 32.0 per cent to 60.0 per cent,
— *camphene*: 0.5 per cent to 2.0 per cent,
— β-*pinene*: 5.0 per cent to 22.0 per cent,
— *car-3-ene*: 6.0 per cent to 18.0 per cent,
— β-*myrcene*: 1.5 per cent to 10.0 per cent,
— *limonene*: 7.0 per cent to 12.0 per cent,
— β-*phellandrene*: maximum 2.5 per cent,
— *p-cymene*: maximum 2.0 per cent,
— *terpinolene*: maximum 4.0 per cent,
— *bornyl acetate*: 1.0 per cent to 4.0 per cent,

— β-*caryophyllene*: 1.0 per cent to 6.0 per cent,
— *disregard limit*: the area of the principal peak in the chromatogram obtained with reference solution (b).

STORAGE
At a temperature not exceeding 25 °C.

_____ Ph Eur

Plantain

(Ribwort Plantain, Ph Eur monograph 1884)

Ph Eur _____

DEFINITION
Whole or fragmented, dried leaf and scape of *Plantago lanceolata* L. s.l.

Content
Minimum 1.5 per cent of total *ortho*-dihydroxycinnamic acid derivatives expressed as acteoside ($C_{29}H_{36}O_{15}$; M_r 624.6) (dried drug).

IDENTIFICATION
A. The leaf is up to 30 cm long and 4 cm wide, yellowish-green to brownish-green, with a prominent, whitish-green, almost parallel venation on the abaxial surface. It consists of a lanceolate lamina narrowing at the base into a channelled petiole. The margin is indistinctly dentate and often undulate. It has 3, 5 or 7 primary veins, nearly equal in length and running almost parallel. Hairs may be almost absent, sparsely scattered or sometimes abundant, especially on the lower surface and over the veins. The scape is brownish-green, longer than the leaves, 3-4 mm in diameter and is deeply grooved longitudinally, with 5-7 conspicuous ribs. The surface is usually covered with fine hairs.

B. Microscopic examination (2.8.23). The powder is yellowish-green. Examine under a microscope using *chloral hydrate solution R*. The powder shows the following diagnostic characters (Figure 1884.-1): fragments of epidermis, composed of cells with irregularly sinuous anticlinal walls, the fragments of the upper epidermis of the lamina in surface view [H] and in transverse section [D] are accompanied by palisade parenchyma [Da, Ha], and those of the lower epidermis in surface view [G] show stomata (2.8.3) mostly of the diacytic type [Ga] and sometimes of the anomocytic type [Gb]; the multicellular, uniseriate, conical covering trichomes are highly characteristic, whole [C] or mostly fragmented [A], with a basal cell larger than the other epidermal cells followed by a short cell supporting 2 or more elongated cells with the lumen narrow and variable, occluded at intervals corresponding to slight swellings in the trichome and giving a jointed appearance, the terminal cell has an acute apex and a filiform lumen; the glandular trichomes have a unicellular, cylindrical stalk and a multicellular, elongated, conical head consisting of several rows of small cells and a single terminal cell [B, Gc]; dense groups of lignified fibro-vascular tissue with narrow, spirally and annularly thickened vessels and slender, moderately thickened fibres [F]; fragments of the scape [E] with cells with thickened walls and a coarsely ridged cuticle, stomata [Ec], multicellular, uniseriate covering trichomes [Eb] and glandular trichomes [Ea] of the type previously described.

C. Examine the chromatograms obtained in the test for *Digitalis lanata* leaves.

Results A   See below the sequence of zones present in the chromatogram obtained with the reference solution and the

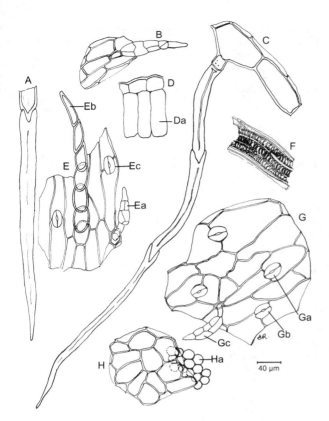

Figure 1884.-1. – *Illustration for identification test B of powdered herbal drug of ribwort plantain*

test solution. Furthermore, other zones may be present in the chromatogram obtained with the test solution.

Top of the plate	
Acteoside: a yellow zone	A yellow zone (acteoside)
Aucubin: a blue zone	A blue zone (aucubin)
Reference solution	**Test solution**

TESTS

Digitalis lanata leaves

Thin-layer chromatography (*2.2.27*).

Solvent mixture water R, methanol R (30:70 *V/V*).

Test solution Use a freshly prepared solution. To 1 g of the powdered herbal drug (355) (*2.9.12*) in a 25 mL flask, add 10 mL of the solvent mixture and shake for 30 min. Filter, rinse the flask and the filter with 2 quantities, each of 5 mL, of the solvent mixture. Dilute to 25 mL with the solvent mixture.

Reference solution Dissolve 1 mg of *acteoside R* and 1 mg of *aucubin R* in 1 mL of the solvent mixture.

Plate TLC silica gel F_{254} plate R.

Mobile phase anhydrous formic acid R, glacial acetic acid R, water R, ethyl acetate R (11:11:27:100 *V/V/V/V*).

Application 10 µL as bands.

Development Over a path of 8 cm; heat immediately after development at about 120 °C for 5-10 min.

Detection A Examine in daylight.

Detection B Examine in ultraviolet light at 365 nm.

Results B The chromatogram obtained with the test solution shows no bright blue fluorescent zone just below the reddish-brown fluorescent zone corresponding to aucubin in the chromatogram obtained with the reference solution.

Foreign matter (*2.8.2*)
Maximum 5 per cent of leaves of different colour and maximum 2 per cent of other foreign matter.

Loss on drying (*2.2.32*)
Maximum 10.0 per cent, determined on 1.000 g of the powdered herbal drug (355) (*2.9.12*) by drying in an oven at 105 °C for 2 h.

Total ash (*2.4.16*)
Maximum 14.0 per cent.

ASSAY

Stock solution In a flask, place 1.000 g of the powdered herbal drug (355) (*2.9.12*) and add 90 mL of *ethanol (50 per cent V/V) R*. Boil in a water-bath under a reflux condenser for 30 min. Allow to cool and filter into a 100 mL volumetric flask. Rinse the flask and the filter with 10 mL of *ethanol (50 per cent V/V) R*. Combine the filtrate and the rinsings and dilute to 100.0 mL with *ethanol (50 per cent V/V) R*.

Test solution To a 10 mL volumetric flask add, mixing after each addition, 1.0 mL of the stock solution, 2 mL of *0.5 M hydrochloric acid*, 2 mL of a solution prepared by dissolving 10 g of *sodium nitrite R* and 10 g of *sodium molybdate R* in 100 mL of *water R*, and 2 mL of *dilute sodium hydroxide solution R*. Dilute to 10.0 mL with *water R*.

Immediately measure the absorbance (*2.2.25*) of the test solution at 525 nm using as compensation liquid a solution prepared as follows: to a 10 mL volumetric flask add 1.0 mL of the stock solution, 2 mL of *0.5 M hydrochloric acid* and 2 mL of *dilute sodium hydroxide solution R*, and dilute to 10.0 mL with *water R*.

Calculate the percentage content of total *ortho*-dihydroxycinnamic acid derivatives, expressed as acteoside, using the following expression:

$$\frac{A \times 1000}{185 \times m}$$

i.e. taking the specific absorbance to be 185 for acteoside at 525 nm.

A = absorbance of the test solution at 525 nm;

m = mass of the substance to be examined, in grams.

_____ *Ph Eur*

Podophyllum Resin

Podophyllin

Action and use

Used in treatment of warts.

Preparation

Compound Podophyllin Paint

DEFINITION

Podophyllum Resin is the resin obtained from rhizomes and roots of *Podophyllum hexandrum* Royle (*P. emodi* Wall.). It contains not less than 50.0% of total aryltetralin lignans, calculated as podophyllotoxin.

CHARACTERISTICS

An amorphous powder varying in colour from light brown to greenish yellow, or brownish grey masses; odour, characteristic; caustic.

Partly soluble in hot *water*, from which it is precipitated on cooling, in *chloroform*, in *ether* and in 5M *ammonia*.

IDENTIFICATION

Carry out the method for *thin-layer chromatography*, Appendix III A, using the following solutions in *methanol*.

(1) 1% w/v of the substance being examined.

(2) 0.5% w/v of *podophyllotoxin*.

(3) 0.1% w/v of *phenazone*.

CHROMATOGRAPHIC CONDITIONS

(a) Use as the coating *silica gel GF$_{254}$*.

(b) Use the mobile phase as described below.

(c) Apply as bands 10 µL of each solution.

(d) Develop the plate to 10 cm.

(e) After removal of the plate, allow it to dry in air and examine under *ultraviolet light (254 nm)*. Spray the plate with *methanolic sulfuric acid (50%)* and heat at 130° for 10 minutes.

MOBILE PHASE

1 volume of *methanol* and 25 volumes of *chloroform*.

CONFIRMATION

When viewed under *ultraviolet light (254 nm)*, the chromatogram obtained with solution (1) exhibits quenching zones corresponding in position to the principal quenching zones in the chromatograms obtained with solutions (2) and (3). Other quenching zones may be present.

When viewed after spraying, the chromatogram obtained with solution (1) exhibits a purplish zone (podophyllotoxin) corresponding in position and colour to the principal zone in solution (2) and a purplish zone (4′-demethylpodophyllotoxin) corresponding in position to the quenching zone found in solution (3). Other coloured zones may be present.

TESTS

Matter insoluble in ethanol (96%)

Shake 1 g, finely powdered, with 20 mL of *ethanol (96%)* for 5 minutes, filter through a sintered-glass crucible (ISO 4793, porosity grade 2, is suitable), wash the filter with *ethanol (96%)* and dry at 105°. The residue weighs not more than 25 mg.

Matter insoluble in 5m ammonia

Shake 0.5 g, finely powdered, with 30 mL of 5M *ammonia* for 30 minutes at about 20°; filter through a sintered-glass crucible (ISO 4793, porosity grade 2, is suitable) and wash the flask and filter with 30 mL of *water*, the time taken for filtering and washing being not more than 10 minutes. Dry the filter and residue to constant weight at 105°. The residue weighs not less than 0.18 g and not more than 0.30 g.

Loss on drying

When dried to constant weight at 105°, loses not more than 5.0% of its weight. Use 1 g.

Sulfated ash

Not more than 1.0%, Appendix IX A.

ASSAY

Dissolve 0.5 g in sufficient *ethanol (96%)* to produce 100 mL. To 10 mL of this solution in a separating funnel add 190 mL of *water* and extract with six 30-mL quantities of *dichloromethane*. Combine the dichloromethane layers, extract with 10 mL of 0.2M *sodium hydroxide* followed by five 10-mL quantities of *water* and wash each of the six aqueous layers separately with the same 20-mL quantity of *dichloromethane*. Combine the dichloromethane solutions, filter through absorbent cotton and evaporate the filtrate to dryness. Dissolve the residue in sufficient *ethanol (96%)* to produce 100 mL, dilute 10 mL of this solution to 50 mL with *ethanol (96%)* and measure the *absorbance* of the resulting solution at the maximum at 292 nm, Appendix II B. Calculate the content of total aryltetralin lignans expressed as podophyllotoxin, taking 105.4 as the value of A(1%, 1 cm) at the maximum at 292 nm.

STORAGE

Podophyllum Resin should be protected from light. On exposure to light, or to temperatures above 25°, it becomes darker in colour.

LABELLING

The label states the botanical source.

Compound Podophyllin Paint

Compound Podophyllin Cutaneous Solution

DEFINITION

Compound Podophyllin Paint is a *cutaneous solution*.

Podophyllum Resin	150 g
Compound Benzoin Tincture	Sufficient to produce 1000 mL

In making the Compound Benzoin Tincture used to prepare Compound Podophyllin Paint, the Ethanol (90 per cent) may be replaced by Industrial Methylated Spirit[1] diluted so as to be of equivalent ethanolic strength.

The paint complies with the requirements stated under Liquids for Cutaneous Application and with the following requirements.

IDENTIFICATION

Carry out the method for *thin-layer chromatography*, Appendix III A, using the following solutions in *methanol*.

(1) 7% v/v of the paint.

(2) 0.5% w/v of *podophyllotoxin*.

(3) 0.1% w/v of *phenazone*.

CHROMATOGRAPHIC CONDITIONS

(a) Use as the coating *silica gel GF$_{254}$*.

(b) Use the mobile phase as described below.

(c) Apply 10 µL of each solution.

(d) Develop the plate to 10 cm.

(e) After removal of the plate, dry in air and examine under *ultraviolet light (254 nm)* to locate the quenching zone due to phenazone in solution (3). Spray the plate with *methanolic sulfuric acid (50%)* and heat at 130° for 10 minutes.

MOBILE PHASE

1 volume of *methanol* and 25 volumes of *chloroform*.

CONFIRMATION

The chromatogram obtained with solution (1) exhibits a purplish zone (podophyllotoxin) corresponding in position and colour to the principal zone in solution (2) and a purplish zone (4'-demethylpodophyllotoxin) corresponding in position to the quenching zone found in solution (3). Other coloured zones are present in the chromatogram obtained with solution (1).

TESTS

Weight per mL

0.925 to 0.975 g, Appendix V G.

Total solids

27.0 to 33.0% w/v when determined by evaporating 1 mL to dryness on a water bath and drying the residue at 105° for 4 hours.

---

[1]The *law and the statutory regulations governing the use of Industrial Methylated Spirit must be observed.*

Red Poppy Petals

(*Ph Eur monograph 1881*)

Ph Eur

DEFINITION

Dried, whole or fragmented petals of *Papaver rhoeas* L.

IDENTIFICATION

A. The petal is dark red or dark violet-brown, very thin, floppy, wrinkled, often crumpled into a ball and velvety to the touch. It is broadly ovate with an entire margin, about 6 cm long and 4-6 cm wide, narrowing at the base where there is a black spot. The vascular bundles radiate from the base and they anastomose in a continuous arc, all at the same short distance from the margin.

B. Reduce to a powder (355) (*2.9.12*). Examine under a microscope using *chloral hydrate solution R*. The powder has an intense reddish-pink colour and shows the following diagnostic characters (Figure 1881.-1): fragments of epidermis composed of elongated, sinuous-walled cells [B, D, G] with small, rounded, anomocytic stomata (*2.8.3*) [Ba]; numerous vascular bundles with spiral vessels [E] embedded in the parenchyma; occasional fragments of the fibrous layer of the anthers [F]; rounded pollen grains, about 30 μm in diameter, with 3 pores and a finely verrucose exine [A, C, H].

C. Thin-layer chromatography (*2.2.27*).

Test solution To 1.0 g of the powdered drug (355) (*2.9.12*) add 10 mL of *ethanol (60 per cent V/V) R*. Stir for 15 min. Filter through a filter paper.

Reference solution Dissolve 1 mg of *quinaldine red R* and 1 mg of *sulfan blue R* in 2 mL of *methanol R*.

Plate TLC silica gel plate R.

Mobile phase anhydrous formic acid R, water R, butanol R (10:12:40 *V/V/V*).

Application 10 μL as bands.

Development Over a path of 10 cm.

Drying In air.

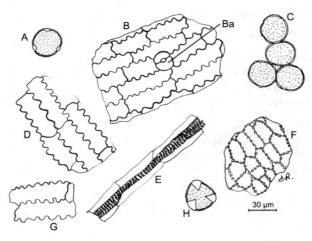

Figure 1881.-1.– *Illustration for identification test B of powdered herbal drug of red poppy petals*

Detection Examine in daylight.

Results See below the sequence of zones present in the chromatograms obtained with the reference solution and the test solution. Furthermore, other zones may be present in the chromatogram obtained with the test solution.

Top of the plate	
	2 yellow zones
Quinaldine red: an orange-red zone	
	A violet principal zone A violet zone A yellow zone
Sulfan blue: a blue zone	
	A compact group of violet zones
Reference solution	**Test solution**

TESTS

Foreign matter (*2.8.2*)

Maximum 2.0 per cent of capsules and maximum 1.0 per cent of other foreign matter.

Loss on drying (*2.2.32*)

Maximum 12.0 per cent, determined on 1.000 g of the powdered drug (355) (*2.9.12*) by drying in an oven at 105 °C for 2 h.

Total ash (*2.4.16*)

Maximum 11.0 per cent.

Colouring intensity

Place 1.0 g of the powdered drug (355) (*2.9.12*) in a 250 mL flask and add 100 mL of *ethanol (30 per cent V/V) R*. Allow to macerate for 4 h with frequent stirring. Filter and discard the first 10 mL. To 10.0 mL of the filtrate add 2 mL of *hydrochloric acid R* and dilute to 100.0 mL with *ethanol (30 per cent V/V) R*. Allow to stand for 10 min. The absorbance (*2.2.25*) measured at 523 nm using *ethanol (30 per cent V/V) R* as the compensation liquid is not less than 0.6.

Ph Eur

Poria

(Ph Eur monograph 2475)

Ph Eur _____

DEFINITION

Dried sclerotium without skin of *Wolfiporia extensa* (Peck)
Ginns (syn. *Poria cocos* (Schw.) Wolf; *Wolfiporia cocos* (F.A.
Wolf) Ryvarden & Gilb.).

IDENTIFICATION

A. Square, rectangular or polyhedral pieces, or slices, varying
in length and thickness; whitish with a pale brown hue, flat
and smooth, square, rectangular or polyhedral pieces, with
no brown skin, difficult to break; slices easily broken, rough
fracture with granular or farinaceous texture.

B. Microscopic examination (*2.8.23*). The powder is whitish
with a pale brown hue. Examine under a microscope using
chloral hydrate solution R. The powder shows the following
diagnostic characters: irregularly shaped and occasionally
branched colourless particles, which dissolve gradually in
chloral hydrate solution R. Examine under a microscope using
a 50 g/L solution of *potassium hydroxide R*. The powder
shows the following diagnostic characters: fragments of
hyphae, colourless, slender, slightly curved, sometimes with
septa, branched, 3-16 μm in diameter.

C. Thin-layer chromatography (*2.2.27*).

Test solution   To 1 g of the powdered herbal drug (250)
(*2.9.12*) add a mixture of 2 mL of *ethyl acetate R* and 3 mL
of *methanol R*. Sonicate for 10 min, centrifuge and use the
supernatant.

Reference solution   Dissolve 10 mg of *4-aminobenzoic acid R*,
10 mg of *coumarin R* and 10 mg of *thymol R* in 10 mL of
methanol R.

Plate   TLC silica gel F$_{254}$ plate R (2-10 μm).

Mobile phase   glacial acetic acid R, 2-propanol R, cyclohexane R
(10:10:80 *V/V/V*).

Application   5 μL as bands of 8 mm.

Development   Over a path of 6 cm.

Drying   In air.

Detection   Examine in ultraviolet light at 254 nm.

Results   See below the sequence of zones present in the
chromatograms obtained with the reference solution and the
test solution. Furthermore, other faint quenching zones may
be present in the chromatogram obtained with the test
solution between the zones due to 4-aminobenzoic acid and
coumarin in the chromatogram obtained with the reference
solution.

Top of the plate	
Thymol: a quenching zone	
	2 quenching zones
Coumarin: a quenching zone	
4-Aminobenzoic acid: a quenching zone	
Reference solution	**Test solution**

D. The herbal drug sticks to the pestle when moistened with
water R and pressed into a mortar.

E. To a small piece of the herbal drug add 1 drop of
iodinated potassium iodide solution R1. A deep red colour is
produced.

TESTS

Foreign matter (*2.8.2*)
Maximum 0.1 per cent of brown skins and roots of conifer
and maximum 2 per cent of other foreign matter.

Loss on drying (*2.2.32*)
Maximum 13.0 per cent, determined on 1.000 g of the
powdered herbal drug (355) (*2.9.12*) by drying in an oven at
105 °C for 2 h.

Total ash (*2.4.16*)
Maximum 1.0 per cent.

Water-soluble extractive
Minimum 1.5 per cent.

To 5.00 g of the powdered herbal drug (355) (*2.9.12*) add
100 mL of boiling *water R*. Allow to stand for 10 min,
shaking occasionally. Allow to cool, dilute to 100.0 mL with
water R and filter. Evaporate 25.0 mL of the filtrate to
dryness on a water-bath. Dry the residue in an oven at
100-105 °C. The residue weighs a minimum of 18.75 mg.

_____ *Ph Eur*

Primula Root

(Ph Eur monograph 1364)

Ph Eur _____

DEFINITION

Whole or cut, dried rhizome and root of *Primula veris* L.
or *Primula elatior* Hill.

IDENTIFICATION

A. The coarsely torose, greyish-brown rhizome is straight or
slightly curved, about 1-5 cm long and about 2-4 mm thick.
The rhizome crown often bears the remains of stems and
leaves. Attached to the rhizome are numerous brittle roots,
about 1 mm thick and usually 6-8 cm long. The root of *P.
elatior* is light brown or reddish-brown, that of *P. veris* light
yellow or yellowish-white. The fracture is smooth.

B. Microscopic examination (*2.8.23*). The powder is greyish-
brown. Examine under a microscope using *chloral hydrate
solution R*. The powder shows the following diagnostic
characters (Figure 1364.-1): fragments of parenchyma from
the bark of the root or the rhizome and from the medulla of
the rhizome [G, H], consisting of rounded or ovoid cells with
irregularly thickened and pitted walls; brownish fragments
from the dermal tissue of the root showing absorbent hairs
[C]; yellow or brownish fragments of the epidermis of the
rhizome covered by a striated cuticle, in surface view [A], or
in transverse section [F] accompanied by parenchyma from
the bark [Fa]; reticulate vessels [B] sometimes accompanied
by spiral vessels [J]; groups of large, strongly pitted,
yellowish-green sclereids from the medullary parenchyma of
the rhizome [E], which are characteristic of *P. elatior*.
Examine under a microscope using a 50 per cent *V/V*
solution of *glycerol R*. The powder shows simple or
compound starch granules of various shapes and sizes [D].

HERBAL DRUGS

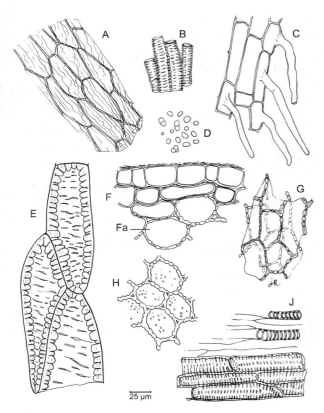

Figure 1364.-1. – *Illustration for identification test B of powdered herbal drug of primula root*

C. Thin-layer chromatography (*2.2.27*) as described in the test for *Vincetoxicum hirundinaria* Medik. root with the following modifications.

Detection Treat with *anisaldehyde solution R*, heat at 100-105 °C for 5-10 min and examine in daylight.

Results The main zone (aescin) in the chromatogram obtained with the reference solution is bluish-violet and is situated near the boundary between the lower and middle thirds. The chromatogram obtained with the test solution shows 1-2 strong dark violet zones a little below the zone due to aescin in the chromatogram obtained with the reference solution; further pale violet, yellowish or brownish-green zones may be visible.

TESTS

Vincetoxicum hirundinaria Medik. root

Thin-layer chromatography (*2.2.27*).

Test solution To 1.0 g of the powdered herbal drug (500) (*2.9.12*) add 10 mL of *ethanol (70 per cent V/V) R* and heat under a reflux condenser for 15 min. Cool and filter.

Reference solution Dissolve 10 mg of *aescin R* in 1.0 mL of *ethanol (70 per cent V/V) R*.

Plate TLC silica gel F_{254} plate R.

Mobile phase glacial acetic acid R, water R, butanol R (10:40:50 *V/V/V*); use the upper layer.

Application 20 μL as bands.

Development Over a path of 12 cm.

Drying In an oven at 100-105 °C.

Detection A Examine in ultraviolet light at 254 nm.

Results A The chromatograms obtained with the reference solution and the test solution show a quenching zone (aescin)

near the boundary between the lower and the middle thirds. Mark this zone.

Detection B Examine in ultraviolet light at 365 nm.

Results B In the chromatogram obtained with the test solution no zones of light-blue or greenish fluorescence occur below the main zone due to aescin in the chromatogram obtained with the reference solution.

Loss on drying (*2.2.32*)

Maximum 10.0 per cent, determined on 1.000 g of the powdered herbal drug (355) (*2.9.12*) by drying in an oven at 105 °C for 2 h.

Total ash (*2.4.16*)

Maximum 9.0 per cent.

Ash insoluble in hydrochloric acid (*2.8.1*)

Maximum 3.0 per cent.

———————————————————— *Ph Eur*

Psyllium Seed

(*Ph Eur monograph 0858*)

Ph Eur ————————————————————

DEFINITION

Ripe, whole, dry seeds of *Plantago afra* L. (*Plantago psyllium* L.) or *Plantago indica* L. (*Plantago arenaria* Waldstein and Kitaibel).

CHARACTERS

Sweet taste.

IDENTIFICATION

P. afra seeds are light brown to very dark brown but never black, smooth and shiny having an elliptical oblong shape. They are 2-3 mm long and 0.8-1.0 mm wide, one end being wider than the other. Towards the middle of the dorsal surface there is a fairly marked transverse constriction of light colour. On the ventral surface, there is a linear lighter-coloured groove in the middle of which is a clear spot corresponding to the hilum and bounded by swollen edges.

P. indica seeds are almost identical to the seeds of *P. afra*, but a little less shiny; they are 2-3 mm long and have a maximum diameter of 1.5 mm.

TESTS

Swelling index (*2.8.4*)

Minimum 10.

Foreign matter (*2.8.2*)

Maximum 1.0 per cent, determined on 10.0 g of the drug, including greenish unripe seeds. Psyllium seed does not contain seeds having a dark central spot on the groove (*Plantago lanceolata* L. and *P. major* L.) or seeds with brownish-grey or pinkish outer coats (*P. ovata* Forssk. and *P. sempervirens* Crantz).

Loss on drying (*2.2.32*)

Maximum 14.0 per cent, determined on 1.000 g of drug by drying in an oven at 105 °C for 2 h.

Total ash (*2.4.16*)

Maximum 4.0 per cent.

STORAGE

Store protected from moisture.

———————————————————— *Ph Eur*

Pygeum Bark

(*Pygeum Africanum Bark*, *Ph Eur monograph 1886*)

Ph Eur _____

DEFINITION

Whole or cut, dried bark of the stems and branches of *Prunus africana* (Hook f.) Kalkm. (syn. *Pygeum africanum* Hook f.).

IDENTIFICATION

A. The dark brown to reddish-brown bark occurs in curved, hard, irregular pieces. The outer surface has a wrinkled dark reddish-brown cork with areas of adhering lichen.
The reddish-brown to dark brown inner surface bears longitudinal striations. It may also occur in rolled fragments with a fibrous fracture.

B. Reduce to a powder (355) (*2.9.12*). The powder is reddish-brown. Examine under a microscope using *chloral hydrate solution R*. The powdered drug shows thick-walled sclereids, solitary or in groups; calcium oxalate cluster crystals of different size; numerous lignified fibres, thick-walled and with narrow lumen, some of them solitary and most in groups with forked ends; fragments of pigmented polygonal cells of reddish-brown colour; fragments of cork. Examine under a microscope using a 50 per cent *V/V* solution of *glycerol R*, the powder shows some isolated small starch grains that stain bluish-black against *iodine solution R1*.

C. Thin-layer chromatography (*2.2.27*).

Test solution   Extract 15.0 g of powdered drug (250) (*2.9.12*) with *methylene chloride R* for 30 min in a continuous extraction apparatus (Soxhlet type). Filter. Evaporate the solvent to dryness under reduced pressure. Dissolve the residue in 1 mL of *methylene chloride R*.

Reference solution   Dissolve 20 mg of *β-sitosterol R* and 20 mg of *ursolic acid R* in 10 mL of a mixture of equal volumes of *methanol R* and *methylene chloride R*.

Plate   *TLC silica gel plate R*.

Mobile phase   *methanol R*, *methylene chloride R* (10:90 *V/V*).

Application   10 µL, as 1 cm bands.

Development   Over a path of 15 cm.

Drying   In air.

Detection   Spray with *vanillin reagent R*. Heat the plate at 100-105 °C for 10 min and allow to cool; examine in daylight.

Results   See below the sequence of the zones present in the chromatograms obtained with the reference solution and the test solution. Furthermore, other zones may be present in the chromatogram obtained with the test solution.

Top of the plate		
	A violet zone	
	Several weak violet, blue or grey zones	
		_____
β-Sitosterol: a violet zone	A violet zone (β-sitosterol)	
Ursolic acid: a blue zone	A blue zone (ursolic acid)	
	Several weak violet, blue or grey zones	
		_____
	A violet zone (β-sitosterol glucoside)	
Reference solution	**Test solution**	

TESTS

Foreign matter (*2.8.2*)
Maximum 3.0 per cent.

Loss on drying (*2.2.32*)
Maximum 12.0 per cent, determined on 1.000 g of powdered drug (355) (*2.9.12*) by drying in an oven at 105 °C for 2 h.

Total ash (*2.4.16*)
Maximum 10.0 per cent.

Extractable matter
Minimum 0.5 per cent.

Extract 20.0 g of the powdered drug (250) (*2.9.12*) with *methylene chloride R* for 4 h in a continuous extraction apparatus (Soxhlet type). Evaporate the solution to dryness on a water-bath *in vacuo* and then dry the residue at 80 °C for 2 h. The residue weighs a minimum of 0.10 g.

_____ *Ph Eur*

Quillaia

Quillaia Bark

Preparation
Quillaia Liquid Extract

When Powdered Quillaia is prescribed or demanded, material complying with the appropriate requirements below shall be dispensed or supplied.

DEFINITION

Quillaia is the dried inner part of the bark of *Quillaja saponaria* Molina and of other species of *Quillaja*.

IDENTIFICATION

A. Pieces flat, up to about 1 metre long, 10 to 20 cm broad and 3 to 10 mm, usually 6 mm, thick. Outer surface brownish white or pale reddish brown, longitudinally striated or coarsely reticulated, with occasional blackish brown patches of adherent outer bark; inner surface yellowish white, smooth and very hard; fracture splintery and laminated, the broken surface showing numerous large prisms of calcium oxalate as glistening points. Smoothed transversely cut surface appearing chequered, with delicate radial lines representing medullary rays and tangential lines formed by alternating tangential bands of fibrous and non-fibrous phloem.

B. Outer bark, when present, consisting of reddish brown cork cells alternating with bands of brown parenchyma containing numerous groups of phloem fibres and large prisms of calcium oxalate. Inner bark consisting of alternating bands of tortuous fibres, irregularly enlarged at intervals, about 500 to 1000 µm long and 20 to 50 µm wide and of sieve tissue mixed with parenchyma. Medullary rays mostly three to four, but sometimes up to six cells wide, with occasional pitted, subrectangular sclereids adjacent to the bundles of phloem fibres. Starch granules 5 to 20 µm, usually about 10 µm, in diameter and prisms of calcium oxalate usually 50 to 170 µm long and up to 30 µm wide present in the parenchymatous cells.

TESTS

Extractive soluble in ethanol (45%)
Not less than 22.0%, Appendix XI B1.

Acid-insoluble ash
Not more than 1.0%, Appendix XI K.

Foreign matter
Complies with the test for *foreign matter*, Appendix XI D.

Quillaia Bark

(*Ph Eur monograph 1843*)

Ph Eur _____

DEFINITION

Whole or fragmented, dried bark, with the cork and underlying parenchyma removed, of *Quillaja saponaria* Molina *s.l.*

Content

Minimum 6.5 per cent of triterpene glycosides, expressed as quillaia saponin III ($C_{104}H_{168}O_{55}$; M_r 2298) (dried drug).

IDENTIFICATION

A. Large, flat pieces of variable length and width, 3-10 mm thick, or smaller, splintered pieces. The outer surface is brownish-white or pale reddish-brown, longitudinally striated or coarsely reticulated, with occasional blackish-brown patches of incompletely removed outer bark. The inner surface is yellowish-white and smooth. The fracture is splintery and laminated, the surface often glistening due to the presence of numerous large prisms of calcium oxalate.

B. Microscopic examination (*2.8.23*). The powder is pale pinkish-yellow. Examine under a microscope using *chloral hydrate solution R*. The powder shows the following diagnostic characters (Figure 1843.-1): abundant phloem fibres [E, F], up to 1 mm long, isolated or, more usually, in groups, each fibre irregular in outline with lignified walls of varying thickness and an uneven lumen; numerous, multiseriate medullary rays, spindle-shaped in tangential section [Ca, Fb], accompanied by either phloem fibres [Fa] or phloem parenchyma [Cb]; very numerous prisms of calcium oxalate, up to 200 µm long, free, whole or, more usually, fragmented [A] or included in phloem parenchyma cells [Cc, Cd]; occasional sclereids of 2 types: the 1st type is sub-rectangular with pitted, slightly thickened walls, isolated [G] or included in phloem parenchyma cells [H], while the 2nd type has an irregularly shaped outline and very thick walls [J], sometimes adjacent to the bundles of phloem fibres; occasional dark brown or reddish-brown fragments of cork [D]. Examine under a microscope using a 50 per cent *V/V* solution of *glycerol R*. The powder shows numerous, small (5-20 µm), mainly simple, spherical starch granules, either scattered or as compacted masses in parenchyma cells [B].

C. Thin-layer chromatography (*2.2.27*).

Test solution   To 1.0 g of the powdered herbal drug (355) (*2.9.12*) add 5 mL of *methanol R* and 5 mL of *water R*. Sonicate for 10 min and filter.

Reference solution   Dissolve 10 mg of *purified quillaia saponins R* and 2 mg of *sucrose R* in 1 mL of *water R* and mix with 1 mL of *methanol R*.

Plate   *TLC silica gel plate R* (2-10 µm).

Mobile phase   anhydrous acetic acid R, ethyl acetate R, water R, propanol R (1.5:30:30:40 *V/V/V/V*).

Application   5 µL as bands of 6 mm.

Development   Over a path of 6 cm.

Drying   In hot air.

Detection   Treat with a 10 per cent *V/V* solution of *sulfuric acid R* in *methanol R*; heat at 120 °C for 5 min and examine in daylight.

Results   See below the sequence of zones present in the chromatograms obtained with the reference solution and the test solution. Furthermore, other faint zones may be present in the chromatogram obtained with the test solution.

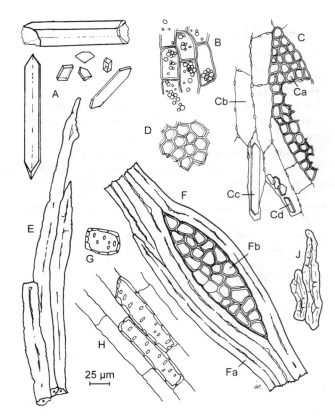

Figure 1843.-1. – *Illustration for identification test B of powdered herbal drug of quillaia bark*

Top of the plate	
	——— ———
Quillaia saponins: 3 or more green or brown zones	3 or more green or brown zones (quillaia saponins)
	A blue zone
Sucrose: a brown or blue zone	A brown or blue zone (sucrose)
	——— ———
Reference solution	**Test solution**

TESTS

Loss on drying (*2.2.32*)

Maximum 10.0 per cent, determined on 1.000 g of the powdered herbal drug (355) (*2.9.12*) by drying in an oven at 105 °C for 2 h.

Total ash (*2.4.16*)

Maximum 10.0 per cent.

Ash insoluble in hydrochloric acid (*2.8.1*)

Maximum 1.0 per cent.

ASSAY

Liquid chromatography (*2.2.29*).

Test solution   Introduce 0.500 g of the powdered herbal drug (355) (*2.9.12*) into a round-bottomed flask, add 20 mL of a 20 g/L solution of *potassium hydroxide R* and heat under a reflux condenser in a water-bath for 2 h. After cooling, add 2 mL of *phosphoric acid R* and filter through a plug of absorbent cotton. Add the absorbent cotton to the residue, add 25 mL of *ethanol (96 per cent) R* and shake thoroughly.

Filter. Combine the filtrates and dilute to 50.0 mL with *water R*. Filter through a membrane filter (nominal pore size 0.45 μm).

Reference solution (a)   Dissolve 12.0 mg of *quillaia saponin for assay CRS* (containing monoammonium glycyrrhizate) in a mixture of equal volumes of *ethanol (96 per cent) R* and a 10 g/L solution of *phosphoric acid R*, and dilute to 50.0 mL with the same mixture of solvents.

Reference solution (b)   Introduce 12 mg of *purified quillaia saponins HRS* into a 50 mL round-bottomed flask, add 20 mL of a 20 g/L solution of *potassium hydroxide R* and heat under a reflux condenser in a water-bath for 2 h. After cooling, add 2 mL of *phosphoric acid R*. Add 25 mL of *ethanol (96 per cent) R* and shake thoroughly. Dilute to 50.0 mL with *water R*. Filter through a membrane filter (nominal pore size 0.45 μm).

Column:
— *size: l* = 0.25 m, Ø = 4.6 mm;
— *stationary phase: octadecylsilyl silica gel for chromatography R* (5 μm);
— *temperature*: 30 ± 2 °C.

Mobile phase   acetonitrile R1, 1 g/L solution of *phosphoric acid R* (35:65 *V/V*).

Flow rate   1.0 mL/min.

Detection   Spectrophotometer at 210 nm.

Injection   50 μL.

Run time   1.2 times the retention time of glycyrrhizic acid.

Identification of peaks   Use the chromatogram supplied with *purified quillaia saponins HRS* and the chromatogram obtained with reference solution (b) to identify the peaks due to monodesmosidic quillaia saponins 1 and 3; a minor peak due to monodesmosidic quillaia saponin 2 may be present between the peaks due to monodesmosidic quillaia saponins 1 and 3.

Retention time   Monodesmosidic quillaia saponin 1 = about 9 min; monodesmosidic quillaia saponin 3 = about 10 min; glycyrrhizic acid = about 13 min.

Calculate the percentage content of triterpene glycosides, expressed as quillaia saponin III, using the following expression:

$$\frac{A_1 \times m_2 \times p \times 2298 \times 0.6}{A_2 \times m_1 \times 957}$$

A_1 = sum of the areas of the peaks due to monodesmosidic quillaia saponins (1, 2 and 3) in the chromatogram obtained with the test solution;

A_2 = area of the peak due to glycyrrhizic acid derived from monoammonium glycyrrhizate in the chromatogram obtained with reference solution (a);

m_1 = mass of the herbal drug to be examined used to prepare the test solution, in grams;

m_2 = mass of *quillaia saponin for assay CRS* used to prepare reference solution (a), in grams;

p = percentage content of monoammonium glycyrrhizate in *quillaia saponin for assay CRS*;

0.6 = response factor between monoammonium glycyrrhizate and monodesmosidic quillaia saponin 3;

2298 = molecular mass of quillaia saponin III;

957 = molecular mass of monodesmosidic quillaia saponin 3.

Quillaia Liquid Extract

DEFINITION
Quillaia Liquid Extract is prepared by extracting Quillaia with Ethanol (45 per cent).

Extemporaneous preparation
The following formula and directions apply.

Quillaia, in *moderately fine powder*	1000 g
Ethanol (45 per cent)	A sufficient quantity

Exhaust the Quillaia in *moderately fine powder* with Ethanol (45 per cent) by *percolation*, Appendix XI F, and reserve the first 850 mL of percolate. Evaporate the subsequent percolate to the consistence of a soft extract, dissolve it in the reserved portion and add sufficient Ethanol (45 per cent) to produce 1000 mL. Allow to stand for not less than 24 hours; filter.

The extract complies with the requirements stated under Extracts and with the following requirements.

TESTS
Ethanol content
28 to 34% v/v, Appendix VIII F, Method III.

Dry residue
20 to 30% w/v.

Relative density
1.02 to 1.06, Appendix V G.

Quillaia Tincture

DEFINITION

Quillaia Liquid Extract	50 mL
Ethanol (45 per cent)	Sufficient to produce 1000 mL

Extemporaneous preparation
The following directions apply.

Mix, allow to stand for not less than 12 hours and filter.

The tincture complies with the requirements for Tinctures stated under Extracts and with the following requirements.

TESTS
Ethanol content
43 to 45% v/v, Appendix VIII F, Method III.

Dry residue
1.0 to 1.5% w/v. Use 10 mL.

Relative density
0.940 to 0.955, Appendix V G.

Restharrow Root

(Ph Eur monograph 1879)

Ph Eur _____

DEFINITION
Whole or cut, dried root of *Ononis spinosa* L.

IDENTIFICATION
A. The root is more or less flattened, twisted and branched, deeply wrinkled, brown and grooved longitudinally.
The transversely cut surface shows a thin bark and a xylem cylinder with a conspicuously radiate structure. The fracture of the root is short and fibrous.

B. Reduce to a powder (355) (*2.9.12*). The powder is light brown or brown. Examine under a microscope using *chloral hydrate solution R.* The powder shows the following diagnostic characters: brown fragments of cork composed of thin-walled polygonal cells; groups of thick-walled narrow fibres, often accompanied by a parenchymatous crystal sheath containing prisms of calcium oxalate; fragments of vessels with numerous small bordered pits; parenchymatous cells with single prisms of calcium oxalate. Examine under a microscope using a mixture of equal volumes of *glycerol R* and *water R.* The powder shows numerous simple, round starch granules, 5-10 µm in diameter.

C. Thin-layer chromatography (*2.2.27*).

Test solution   To 1.0 g of the powdered drug (180) (*2.9.12*) add 15.0 mL of *methanol R* and boil under a reflux condenser for 30 min. Cool and filter.

Reference solution   Dissolve 10 mg of *resorcinol R* and 50 mg of *vanillin R* in 10 mL of *methanol R.*

Plate   TLC silica gel F$_{254}$ plate R.

Mobile phase   ethanol (96 per cent) R, methylene chloride R, toluene R (10:45:45 *V/V/V*).

Application   20 µL, as bands.

Development   Over a path of 15 cm.

Drying   In air.

Detection A   Examine in ultraviolet light at 254 nm and 365 nm.

Results A   See below the sequence of the zones present in the chromatograms obtained with the reference solution and the test solution. Furthermore, other fluorescent zones are present in the middle third of the chromatogram obtained with the test solution.

Top of the plate	
Vanillin: a zone visible at 254 nm	
Resorcinol: a zone visible at 254 nm	An intense blue fluorescent zone visible at 365 nm
Reference solution	**Test solution**

Detection B   Spray with *anisaldehyde solution R.* Heat at 100-105 °C for 5-10 min. Examine in daylight.

Results B   See below the sequence of the zones present in the chromatograms obtained with the reference solution and the test solution.

Top of the plate	
Vanillin: a greyish-violet zone	
	A violet zone (onocol)
Resorcinol: a red zone	
Reference solution	**Test solution**

TESTS

Loss on drying (*2.2.32*)
Maximum 10.0 per cent, determined on 1.000 g of the powdered drug (355) (*2.9.12*) by drying in an oven at 105 °C for 2 h.

Total ash (*2.4.16*)
Maximum 8.0 per cent.

Extractable matter
Minimum 15.0 per cent.

To 2.00 g of the powdered drug (250) (*2.9.12*) add a mixture of 8 g of *water R* and 12 g of *ethanol (96 per cent) R* and allow to macerate for 2 h, shaking frequently. Filter, evaporate 5 g of the filtrate to dryness on a water-bath and dry in an oven at 100-105 °C for 2 h. The residue weighs a minimum of 75 mg.

———— Ph Eur

Rhatany Root

Krameria

(*Ph Eur monograph 0289*)

Preparation
Rhatany Tincture

When Powdered Rhatany Root is prescribed or demanded, material complying with the requirements below with the exception of Identification test A and the test for Foreign matter shall be dispensed or supplied.

Ph Eur ————————————————

DEFINITION

Dried, usually fragmented, underground organs of *Krameria triandra* Ruiz and Pavon, known as Peruvian rhatany.

Content
Minimum 5.0 per cent of tannins, expressed as pyrogallol (C$_6$H$_6$O$_3$; M_r 126.1) (dried drug).

IDENTIFICATION

A. The taproot is dark reddish-brown and has a thick, knotty crown. The secondary roots are the same colour and nearly straight or somewhat tortuous. The bark is rugged or scaly in the older pieces and smooth with sharp, transverse fissures in the younger pieces; it separates readily from the wood. The fracture is fibrous in the bark and splintery in the wood. The smooth, transversely cut surface shows a dark brownish-red bark about one third of the radius in thickness; a dense, pale reddish-brown and finely porous wood is present with numerous fine medullary rays; the central heartwood is often darker.

B. Reduce to a powder (355) (*2.9.12*). The powder is brownish-red. Examine under a microscope using *chloral hydrate solution R.* The powder shows the following diagnostic characters: cork cells containing dark brown phlobaphenes; fragments of unlignified phloem fibres, usually 12-30 µm in diameter with moderately thick walls; phloem parenchyma cells in files containing prisms and microcrystals of calcium oxalate; fragments of vessels usually 20-60 µm in diameter with bordered pits; fragments of tracheids up to 20 µm wide with slit-shaped pits. Examine under a microscope using a 50 per cent *V/V* solution of *glycerol R.* The powder shows rounded starch granules, simple or 2- to 4-compound, an individual granule measuring up to 30 µm in diameter and some granules being found in the cells of the medullary rays and in the parenchyma.

C. Thin-layer chromatography (*2.2.27*).

Test solution   To 1.0 g of the powdered drug (355) (*2.9.12*) add 10 mL of a mixture of 3 volumes of *water R* and 7 volumes of *ethanol (96 per cent) R*, shake for 10 min and filter. To the filtrate add 10 mL of *light petroleum R* and shake. Separate the light petroleum layer, add 2 g of *anhydrous sodium sulfate R*, shake and filter. Evaporate the filtrate to dryness. Dissolve the residue in 0.5 mL of *methanol R*.

Reference solution   Dissolve 5.0 mg of *Sudan red G R* in 10 mL of *methanol R*.

Plate   *TLC silica gel plate R*.

Mobile phase   ethyl acetate R, toluene R (2:98 *V/V*).

Application   10 µL, as bands.

Development   Over a path of 15 cm.

Drying   In air.

Detection   Spray with a 5 g/L solution of *fast blue B salt R*. Allow to dry in air and spray with *0.1 M ethanolic sodium hydroxide*; examine in daylight.

Results   The chromatogram obtained with the reference solution shows in the lower third a red zone due to Sudan red G. The chromatogram obtained with the test solution shows a violet zone due to rhatany phenol I similar in position to the zone of Sudan red G in the chromatogram obtained with the reference solution, below it the brownish zone due to rhatany phenol II and below this the bluish-grey zone due to rhatany phenol III. Further zones may be present.

TESTS

Foreign matter (*2.8.2*)
Maximum 2 per cent of foreign matter and maximum 5 per cent of fragments of crown or root exceeding 25 mm in diameter. Root without bark may be present in very small quantities.

Loss on drying (*2.2.32*)
Maximum 12.0 per cent, determined on 1.000 g of the powdered drug (355) (*2.9.12*) by drying in an oven at 105 °C.

Total ash (*2.4.16*)
Maximum 5.5 per cent.

ASSAY
Carry out the determination of tannins in herbal drugs (*2.8.14*). Use 0.750 g of powdered drug (180) (*2.9.12*).

———————————————————— Ph Eur

Rhatany Tincture

(*Ph Eur monograph 1888*)

Ph Eur ———————————————————————

DEFINITION
Tincture produced from *Rhatany root (0289)*.

Content
Minimum 1.0 per cent *m/m* of tannins, expressed as pyrogallol ($C_6H_6O_3$; M_r 126.1).

PRODUCTION
The tincture is produced from 1 part of the drug and 5 parts of ethanol (70 per cent *V/V*) by a suitable procedure.

CHARACTERS
Appearance
Reddish-brown liquid.

IDENTIFICATION
Thin-layer chromatography (*2.2.27*).

Test solution   To 5 mL of the tincture to be examined, add 10 mL of *light petroleum R* and shake. Separate the light petroleum layer, add 2 g of *anhydrous sodium sulfate R*, shake

and filter. Evaporate the filtrate to dryness. Dissolve the residue in 0.5 mL of *methylene chloride R*.

Reference solution   Dissolve 5 mg of *thymol R* and 10 mg of *dichlorophenolindophenol, sodium salt R* in 10 mL of *alcohol (60 per cent V/V) R*.

Plate   *TLC silica gel plate R*.

Mobile phase   methylene chloride R.

Application   10 µL, as bands.

Development   Over a path of 10 cm.

Drying   In air.

Detection   Spray with a 5 g/L solution of *fast blue B salt R*; allow the plate to dry in air and spray with *0.1 M ethanolic sodium hydroxide*; examine in daylight.

Results   See below the sequence of the zones present in the chromatograms obtained with the reference solution and the test solution. Furthermore, other zones may be present in the chromatogram obtained with the test solution.

Top of the plate	
	A violet zone
Thymol: an orange brownish-yellow zone	
	A greenish-grey zone
	A bluish-grey zone
	A yellowish-brown zone
Dichlorophenolindophenol: a greyish-blue zone	A violet zone
Reference solution	**Test solution**

TESTS
Ethanol (*2.9.10*)
63 per cent *V/V* to 67 per cent *V/V*.

Methanol and 2-propanol (*2.9.11*)
Maximum 0.05 per cent *V/V* of methanol and maximum 0.05 per cent *V/V* of 2-propanol.

ASSAY
Carry out the determination of tannins in herbal drugs (*2.8.14*) using 2.500 g of the tincture to be examined.

———————————————————— Ph Eur

Rhubarb

(*Ph Eur monograph 0291*)

Preparation
Compound Rhubarb Tincture

When Powdered Rhubarb is prescribed or demanded, material complying with the requirements below with the exception of Identification test A and the test for Foreign matter shall be dispensed or supplied.

Ph Eur ———————————————————————

DEFINITION
Rhubarb consists of the whole or cut, dried underground parts of *Rheum palmatum* L. or of *Rheum officinale* Baillon or of hybrids of these two species or of a mixture.
The underground parts are often divided; the stem and most of the bark with the rootlets are removed. It contains not less than 2.2 per cent of hydroxyanthracene derivatives, expressed

as rhein ($C_{15}H_8O_6$, M_r 284.2), calculated with reference to the dried drug.

CHARACTERS
Characteristic, aromatic odour.

IDENTIFICATION
A. The appearance is variable: disc-shaped pieces up to 10 cm in diameter and 1 cm to 5 cm in thickness; cylindrical pieces; oval or planoconvex pieces. The surface has a pinkish tinge and is usually covered with a layer of brownish-yellow powder. It shows, especially after moistening, a reticulum of darker lines. This structure causes the marbled appearance of the drug. The fracture is granular. The transverse section of the rhizome shows a narrow outer zone of radiating brownish-red lines. These medullary rays are crossed perpendicularly by a dark cambial ring. Inside this zone is a ring of small star-spot formations of anomalous vascular bundles. The root shows a more radiate structure.

B. Reduce to a powder (355) (*2.9.12*). The powder is orange to brownish-yellow. Examine under a microscope using *chloral hydrate solution R*. The powder shows the following diagnostic characters: large calcium oxalate cluster crystals, which may measure more than 100 µm, and their fragments; reticulately thickened non-lignified vessels measuring up to 175 µm. Numerous groups of rounded or polygonal, thin-walled parenchyma cells. Sclereids and fibres are absent. Examine under a microscope using a 50 per cent *V/V* solution of *glycerol R*. The powder shows simple, rounded or compound (2 to 4) starch granules with a star-shaped hilum.

C. Examine by thin-layer chromatography (*2.2.27*), using a suitable silica gel as the coating substance.

Test solution   Heat 50 mg of the powdered drug (180) (*2.9.12*) in a water-bath for 15 min with a mixture of 1 mL of *hydrochloric acid R* and 30 mL of *water R*. Allow to cool and shake the liquid with 25 mL of *ether R*. Dry the ether layer over *anhydrous sodium sulfate R* and filter. Evaporate the ether layer to dryness and dissolve the residue in 0.5 mL of *ether R*.

Reference solution   Dissolve 5 mg of *emodin R* in 5 mL of *ether R*.

Apply separately to the plate as bands 20 µL of each solution. Develop over a path of 10 cm using a mixture of 1 volume of *anhydrous formic acid R*, 25 volumes of *ethyl acetate R* and 75 volumes of *light petroleum R*. Allow the plate to dry in air and examine in ultraviolet light at 365 nm. The chromatogram obtained with the reference solution shows in its central part a zone of orange fluorescence (emodin). The chromatogram obtained with the test solution shows: a zone due to emodin; above the emodin zone, two zones of similar fluorescence (physcione and chrysophanol, in order of increasing R_F value); below the emodin zone, also two zones of similar fluorescence (rhein and aloe-emodin, in order of decreasing R_F value). Spray with a 100 g/L solution of *potassium hydroxide R* in *methanol R*. All the zones become red to violet.

D. To about 50 mg of the powdered drug (180) (*2.9.12*) add 25 mL of *dilute hydrochloric acid R* and heat the mixture on a water-bath for 15 min. Allow to cool, shake with 20 mL of *ether R* and discard the aqueous layer. Shake the ether layer with 10 mL of *dilute ammonia R1*. The aqueous layer becomes red to violet.

TESTS

Rheum rhaponticum
Examine by thin-layer chromatography (*2.2.27*), using *silica gel G R* as the coating substance.

Test solution   To 0.2 g of the powdered drug (180) (*2.9.12*) add 2 mL of *methanol R* and boil for 5 min under a reflux condenser. Allow to cool and filter. Use the filtrate as the test solution.

Reference solution   Dissolve 10 mg of *rhaponticin R* in 10 mL of *methanol R*.

Apply separately to the plate, as bands not more than 20 mm by 3 mm, 20 µL of each solution. Develop over a path of 12 cm using a mixture of 20 volumes of *methanol R* and 80 volumes of *methylene chloride R*. Allow the plate to dry in air and spray with *phosphomolybdic acid solution R*. The chromatogram obtained with the test solution does not show a blue zone near the line of application (rhaponticin) corresponding to the zone in the chromatogram obtained with the reference solution.

Loss on drying (*2.2.32*)
Not more than 12.0 per cent, determined on 1.000 g of the powdered drug (180) (*2.9.12*) by drying in an oven at 105 °C.

Total ash (*2.4.16*)
Not more than 12.0 per cent.

Ash insoluble in hydrochloric acid (*2.8.1*)
Not more than 2.0 per cent.

ASSAY
Carry out the assay protected from bright light.

Introduce 0.100 g of the powdered drug (180) (*2.9.12*) into a 100 mL flask. Add 30.0 mL of *water R*, mix and weigh. Heat in a water-bath under a reflux condenser for 15 min. Allow to cool, add 50 mg of *sodium hydrogen carbonate R*, weigh and adjust to the original mass with *water R*. Centrifuge and transfer 10.0 mL of the liquid to a 100 mL round-bottomed flask with a ground-glass neck. Add 20 mL of *ferric chloride solution R1* and mix. Heat under a reflux condenser on a water-bath for 20 min, add 1 mL of *hydrochloric acid R* and heat for a further 20 min, shaking frequently. Cool, transfer to a separating funnel and shake with three quantities, each of 25 mL, of *ether R* previously used to rinse the flask. Combine the ether extracts and wash with two quantities, each of 15 mL, of *water R*. Filter the ether extracts through a plug of absorbent cotton into a volumetric flask and dilute to 100.0 mL with *ether R*. Evaporate 10.0 mL carefully to dryness on a water-bath and dissolve the residue in 10.0 mL of a 5 g/L solution of *magnesium acetate R* in *methanol R*. Measure the absorbance (*2.2.25*) at 515 nm, using *methanol R* as the compensation liquid.

Calculate the percentage content of rhein from the expression:

$$\frac{A \times 0.64}{m}$$

i.e. taking the specific absorbance of rhein to be 468, calculated on the basis of the specific absorbance of barbaloin.

A = absorbance at 515 nm;
m = mass of the drug used, in grams.

Compound Rhubarb Tincture

DEFINITION

Rhubarb, in *moderately coarse powder*	100 g
Cardamom Oil	0.40 mL
Coriander Oil	0.03 mL
Glycerol	100 mL
Ethanol (60 per cent)	Sufficient to produce 1000 mL

Extemporaneous preparation

The following directions apply.

Moisten the Rhubarb with a sufficient quantity of Ethanol (60 per cent) and prepare 850 mL of tincture by *percolation*, Appendix XI F. Add the Cardamom Oil, the Coriander Oil and the Glycerol and sufficient Ethanol (60 per cent) to produce 1000 mL. Mix and filter, if necessary.

The tincture complies with the requirements for Tinctures stated under Extracts and with the following requirements.

TESTS

Ethanol content

48 to 53% v/v, Appendix VIII F, Method III.

Glycerol

9.0 to 11.0% v/v when determined by the following method. Dilute 20 mL to 100 mL with *water*; to 10 mL of this solution add 100 mL of *water* and 1 g of *activated charcoal* and boil under a reflux condenser for 15 minutes. Filter, wash the filter and charcoal with sufficient *water* to produce 150 mL, add 0.25 mL of *bromocresol purple solution* and neutralise with 0.1M *sodium hydroxide* or 0.05M *sulfuric acid* to the blue colour of the indicator. Add 1.4 g of *sodium periodate*, allow to stand for 15 minutes, add 3 mL of *propane-1,2-diol*, shake and allow to stand for 5 minutes. Add 0.25 mL of *bromocresol purple solution* and titrate with 0.1M *sodium hydroxide VS* to the same blue colour. Each mL of 0.1M *sodium hydroxide VS* is equivalent to 9.210 mg of glycerol. Calculate the percentage v/v of glycerol, taking 1.260 g as its weight per mL.

Relative density

0.958 to 0.977, Appendix V G.

Roselle

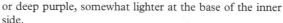

(Ph Eur monograph 1623)

Ph Eur _____

DEFINITION

Whole or cut dried calyces and epicalyces of *Hibiscus sabdariffa* L. collected during fruiting.

Content

Minimum 13.5 per cent of acids, expressed as citric acid ($C_6H_8O_7$; M_r 192.1) (dried drug).

CHARACTERS

Acidic taste.

IDENTIFICATION

A. The calyx is joined in the lower half to form an urceolate structure, the upper half dividing to form 5 long acuminate recurved tips. The tips have a prominent, slightly protruding midrib and a large, thick nectary gland about 1 mm in diameter. The epicalyx consists of 8-12 small, obovate leaflets, which are adnate to the base of the calyx. The calyx and epicalyx are fleshy, dry, easily fragmented and bright red or deep purple, somewhat lighter at the base of the inner side.

B. Microscopic examination (*2.8.23*). The powder is red or violet-red. Examine under a microscope using *chloral hydrate solution R*. The powder shows the following diagnostic characters (Figure 1623.-1): predominantly red fragments [A, F] consisting of polygonal epidermal cells with very irregularly thickened walls, in surface view [Ac, Fa], some containing cluster crystals of calcium oxalate [Fb], with underlying parenchyma consisting of ovoid cells with slightly thickened walls [Aa], some containing cluster crystals of calcium oxalate [Ab] whilst others are filled with mucilage, unicellular, long, flexuous, twisted covering trichomes [Ad], rigid, straight, unicellular covering trichomes, simple or in groups of 2-4 [Fd], glandular trichomes with a unicellular stalk and a globular or oval, multicellular and biseriate head [Fe] and stomata usually of the anisocytic type (*2.8.3*) [Fc]; numerous fragments of vascular bundles [D] with spiral or reticulate vessels [Da], sometimes accompanied by sclerenchymatous fibres with a wide lumen [Db], and parenchyma [Dc], of which some cells contain cluster crystals of calcium oxalate [Dd], whilst others are mucilage-filled [De]; rare, rectangular, parenchymatous sclereids [H]; numerous fragments of rigid [C, G] or flexuous [J] covering trichomes; free cluster crystals of calcium oxalate [B] and glandular trichomes [E]; exceptionally, spherical pollen grains, about 200 μm in diameter, with a spiny exine.

C. Thin-layer chromatography (*2.2.27*).

Test solution To 1 g of the powdered herbal drug (355) (*2.9.12*) add 10 mL of *ethanol (60 per cent V/V) R*. Shake for 15 min and filter.

Reference solution Dissolve 2.5 mg of *quinaldine red R* and 2.5 mg of *sulfan blue R* in 10 mL of *methanol R*.

Plate TLC silica gel plate R (5-40 μm) [or TLC silica gel plate R (2-10 μm)].

Mobile phase anhydrous formic acid R, water R, butanol R (10:12:40 V/V/V).

Application 5 μL [or 2 μL] as bands of 10 mm [or 8 mm].

Development Over a path of 10 cm [or 6 cm].

Drying In air.

Examine immediately in daylight.

Results See below the sequence of zones present in the chromatograms obtained with the reference solution and the test solution. Furthermore, other faint zones may be present in the chromatogram obtained with the test solution.

Top of the plate	
	An intense violet zone
Quinaldine red: an orange-red zone	
Sulfan blue: a blue zone	
	An intense violet-blue zone
Reference solution	**Test solution**

TESTS

Foreign matter (*2.8.2*)

Maximum 2 per cent of fragments of fruits (red funicles and parts of the 5-caverned capsule with yellowish-grey pericarp, whose thin walls consist of several layers of differently

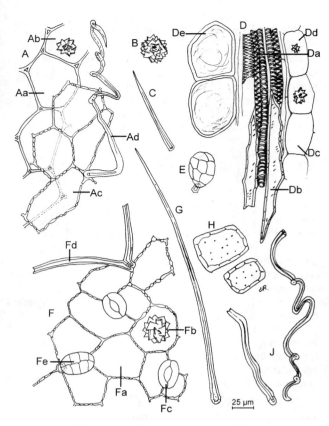

Figure 1623.-1. – *Illustration for identification test B of powdered herbal drug of roselle*

directed fibres; flattened, reniform seeds with a dotted surface) and maximum 2 per cent of other foreign matter.

Loss on drying (*2.2.32*)
Maximum 11.0 per cent, determined on 1.000 g of the powdered herbal drug (355) (*2.9.12*) by drying in an oven at 105 °C for 2 h.

Total ash (*2.4.16*)
Maximum 10.0 per cent.

Colouring intensity
Reduce 100 g to a coarse powder (1400) (*2.9.12*) and homogenise. Reduce about 10 g of this mixture to a very fine powder (355) (*2.9.12*). To 1.0 g of this powder in a 100 mL flask add 25 mL of boiling *water R* and heat for 15 min on a water-bath with frequent shaking. Filter the hot mixture into a 50 mL graduated flask; rinse successively the 100 mL flask and the filter with 3 quantities, each of 5 mL, of warm *water R*. After cooling, dilute to 50 mL with *water R*. Dilute 5 mL of this solution to 50 mL with *water R*. Measure the absorbance (*2.2.25*) at 520 nm using *water R* as the compensation liquid. The absorbance is not less than 0.350 for the whole drug and not less than 0.250 for the cut drug.

ASSAY
Shake 1.00 g of the powdered herbal drug (355) (*2.9.12*) with 100.0 mL of *carbon dioxide-free water R* for 15 min. Filter. To 50.0 mL of the filtrate add 100 mL of *carbon dioxide-free water R*. Titrate with *0.1 M sodium hydroxide* to pH 7.0, determining the end-point potentiometrically (*2.2.20*).

1 mL of *0.1 M sodium hydroxide* is equivalent to 6.4 mg of citric acid.

Rosemary Leaf

(*Ph Eur monograph 1560*)

Ph Eur

DEFINITION
Whole, dried leaf of *Rosmarinus officinalis* L.

Content:
— minimum 12 mL/kg of essential oil (anhydrous drug);
— minimum 3 per cent of total hydroxycinnamic derivatives, expressed as rosmarinic acid ($C_{18}H_{16}O_8$; M_r 360.3) (anhydrous drug).

CHARACTERS
Strongly aromatic odour.

IDENTIFICATION
A. The leaves are sessile, tough, linear or linear-lanceolate, 1-4 cm long and 2-4 mm wide, with recurved edges. The upper surface is dark green, glabrous and grainy, the lower surface is greyish-green and densely tomentose with a prominent midrib.

B. Microscopic examination (*2.8.23*). The powder is greyish-green or yellowish-green. Examine under a microscope using *chloral hydrate solution R*. The powder shows the following diagnostic characters (Figure 1560.-1): fragments of the lower epidermis in surface view [B, J] with straight or sinuous-walled cells [Ba] and numerous diacytic stomata (*2.8.3*) [Bb] and glandular trichomes [Ja] or covering trichomes or their scars [Bc, Bd]; numerous multicellular, mostly branched, covering trichomes of the lower epidermis, usually fragmented [A, C, D]; fragments of the upper epidermis in surface view [F] with cells with straight, thickened and pitted walls [Fa], and an underlying hypodermis composed of large, irregular cells with thickened and beaded anticlinal walls [Fb]; fragments of the lamina in transverse section [G], showing the epidermis covered by a very thick cuticle [Ga], hypodermal cells extending across the mesophyll [Gb] at intervals, separating 1 or 2 layers of palisade parenchyma into large, crescent-shaped areas [Gc]; glandular trichomes of 2 types, the majority with a short, unicellular stalk and a radiate head composed of 8 cells, in surface view [E] and in side view [H], others, less abundant, with a uni- or bicellular stalk and a spherical, unicellular head [Ja, K].

C. Thin-layer chromatography (*2.2.27*).

Test solution Dissolve 20 µL of the oil obtained in the assay in 1 mL of *hexane R*.

Reference solution Dissolve 5 mg of *borneol R*, 5 mg of *bornyl acetate R* and 10 µL of *cineole R* in 1 mL of *hexane R*.

Plate TLC silica gel plate R.

Mobile phase ethyl acetate R, toluene R (5:95 *V/V*).

Application 10 µL as bands.

Development Over a path of 15 cm.

Drying In air.

Detection Treat with *anisaldehyde solution R*, heat at 100-105 °C for 10 min and examine in daylight.

Results See below the sequence of zones present in the chromatograms obtained with the reference solution and the test solution.

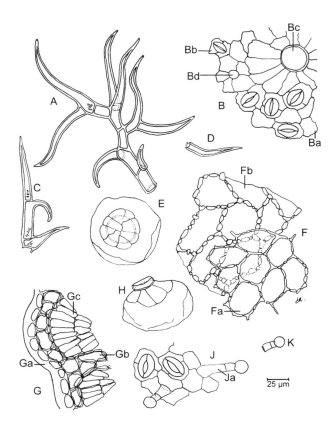

Figure 1560.-1. – *Illustration for identification test B of powdered herbal drug of rosemary leaf*

Top of the plate	
	A red zone
Bornyl acetate: a yellowish-brown zone	A yellowish-brown zone of low intensity
	A coloured zone of low intensity
Cineole: a violet zone	A violet zone
	Coloured zones of low intensity
Borneol: a violet-brown zone	A violet-brown zone
	A coloured zone of low intensity
Reference solution	**Test solution**

D. Thin-layer chromatography (*2.2.27*).

Test solution   Grind 1.0 g of the herbal drug in 10 mL of *methanol R* and filter.

Reference solution   Dissolve 1.0 mg of *caffeic acid R* and 5.0 mg of *rosmarinic acid R* in 10 mL of *methanol R*.

Plate   *TLC silica gel plate R.*

Mobile phase   *anhydrous formic acid R, acetone R, methylene chloride R* (8.5:25:85 *V/V/V*).

Application   10 µL of the test solution and 20 µL of the reference solution, as bands.

Development   Over a path of 8 cm.

Drying   In air.

Detection   Examine in ultraviolet light at 365 nm.

Results   See below the sequence of zones present in the chromatograms obtained with the reference solution and the test solution.

Top of the plate	
	A pink fluorescent zone
Caffeic acid: a light blue fluorescent zone	A blue fluorescent zone of low intensity
Rosmarinic acid: a light blue fluorescent zone	An intense light blue fluorescent zone
Reference solution	**Test solution**

TESTS

Foreign matter (*2.8.2*)
Maximum 5 per cent of stems and maximum 2 per cent of other foreign matter.

Water (*2.2.13*)
Maximum 100 mL/kg, determined on 20.0 g of the powdered herbal drug (355) (*2.9.12*).

Total ash (*2.4.16*)
Maximum 9.0 per cent.

ASSAY

Total hydroxycinnamic derivatives

Stock solution   To 0.200 g of the powdered herbal drug (355) (*2.9.12*) add 80 mL of *ethanol (50 per cent V/V) R*. Boil in a water-bath under a reflux condenser for 30 min. Allow to cool and filter. Rinse the filter with 10 mL of *ethanol (50 per cent V/V) R*. Combine the filtrate and the rinsings in a volumetric flask and dilute to 100.0 mL with *ethanol (50 per cent V/V) R*.

Test solution   To 1.0 mL of the stock solution add 2 mL of *0.5 M hydrochloric acid*, 2 mL of a solution prepared by dissolving 10 g of *sodium nitrite R* and 10 g of *sodium molybdate R* in 100 mL of *water R*, and then add 2 mL of *dilute sodium hydroxide solution R* and dilute to 10.0 mL with *water R*; mix.

Compensation solution   Dilute 1.0 mL of the stock solution to 10.0 mL with *water R*.

Measure immediately the absorbance (*2.2.25*) of the test solution at 505 nm.

Calculate the percentage content of total hydroxycinnamic derivatives, expressed as rosmarinic acid, using the following expression:

$$\frac{A \times 2.5}{m}$$

i.e. taking the specific absorbance of rosmarinic acid to be 400.

A = absorbance of the test solution at 505 nm;
m = mass of the substance to be examined, in grams.

Essential oil (*2.8.12*)
Use 25.0 g of the crushed herbal drug, a 1000 mL flask and 300 mL of *water R* as the distillation liquid. Distil at a rate of 2-3 mL/min for 3 h.

_____ *Ph Eur*

HERBAL DRUGS

Rosemary Oil

(Ph Eur monograph 1846)

Ph Eur

DEFINITION
Essential oil obtained by steam distillation from the flowering aerial parts of *Rosmarinus officinalis* L.

CHARACTERS
Appearance
Clear, mobile, colourless or pale yellow liquid.
Characteristic odour.

IDENTIFICATION
First identification B.
Second identification A.

A. Thin-layer chromatography (*2.2.27*).

Test solution Dissolve 0.5 mL of the substance to be examined in *toluene R* and dilute to 10 mL with the same solvent.

Reference solution Dissolve 50 mg of *borneol R*, 50 mg of *bornyl acetate R* and 100 µL of *cineole R* in *toluene R* and dilute to 10 mL with the same solvent.

Plate TLC silica gel plate R.

Mobile phase ethyl acetate R, toluene R (5:95 V/V).

Application 10 µL, as bands.

Development Over a path of 15 cm.

Drying In air.

Detection Spray the plate with *vanillin reagent R* and heat the plate at 100-105 °C for 10 min. Examine immediately in daylight.

Results See below the sequence of the zones present in the chromatograms obtained with the reference solution and the test solution. Furthermore, several violet-blue to violet-grey zones of medium intensity (terpene alcohols) are present in the lower third of the chromatogram obtained with the test solution.

Top of the plate	
	An intense violet zone
	A violet-grey zone
Bornyl acetate: a bluish-grey zone of low intensity	A bluish-grey zone of low intensity (bornyl acetate)
	A violet-pink zone
Cineole: an intense blue zone	An intense blue zone (cineole)
Borneol: a violet-blue zone of medium intensity	A violet-blue zone of medium intensity (borneol)
Reference solution	**Test solution**

B. Examine the chromatograms obtained in the test for chromatographic profile.

Results The characteristic peaks in the chromatogram obtained with the test solution are similar in retention time to those in the chromatogram obtained with the reference solution.

TESTS
Relative density (*2.2.5*)
0.895 to 0.920.

Refractive index (*2.2.6*)
1.464 to 1.473.

Optical rotation (*2.2.7*)
− 5° to + 8°.

Acid value (*2.5.1*)
Maximum 1.0.

Chromatographic profile
Gas chromatography (*2.2.28*): use the normalisation procedure.

Test solution Dissolve 0.20 mL of the substance to be examined in *hexane R* and dilute to 10.0 mL with the same solvent.

Reference solution Dissolve 20 µL of α-*pinene R*, 10 mg of camphene R, 20 µL of β-*pinene R*, 10 µL of β-*myrcene R*, 20 µL of limonene R, 50 µL of cineole R, 10 µL of p-cymene R, 50 mg of camphor R, 30 mg of bornyl acetate R, 10 mg of α-*terpineol R*, 10 mg of borneol R and 10 µL of verbenone R in *hexane R* and dilute to 10.0 mL with the same solvent.

Column:
— *material*: fused silica,
— *size*: l = 30 m (a film thickness of 1 µm may be used) to 60 m (a film thickness of 0.2 µm may be used), Ø = 0.25-0.53 mm,
— *stationary phase*: macrogol 20 000 R.

Carrier gas helium for chromatography R.

Flow rate 1 mL/min.

Split ratio 1:50.

Temperature:

	Time (min)	Temperature (°C)
Column	0 - 10	50
	10 - 85	50 → 200
	85 - 110	200
Injection port		200
Detector		250

Detection Flame ionisation.

Injection 1 µL.

Elution order Order indicated in the composition of the reference solution. Record the retention times of these substances.

System suitability Reference solution:
— *resolution*: minimum 1.5 between the peaks due to limonene and cineole and minimum 1.5 between the peaks due to α-terpineol and borneol.

Using the retention times determined from the chromatogram obtained with the reference solution, locate the components of the reference solution in the chromatogram obtained with the test solution.

Determine the percentage content of these components.

For rosemary oil, Spanish type, the percentages are within the following ranges:
— α-*pinene*: 18 per cent to 26 per cent,
— *camphene*: 8.0 per cent to 12.0 per cent,
— β-*pinene*: 2.0 per cent to 6.0 per cent,
— β-*myrcene*: 1.5 per cent to 5.0 per cent,
— *limonene*: 2.5 per cent to 5.0 per cent,
— *cineole*: 16.0 per cent to 25.0 per cent,
— *p-cymene*: 1.0 per cent to 2.2 per cent,
— *camphor*: 13.0 per cent to 21.0 per cent,
— *bornyl acetate*: 0.5 per cent to 2.5 per cent,
— α-*terpineol*: 1.0 per cent to 3.5 per cent,

— *borneol*: 2.0 per cent to 4.5 per cent,
— *verbenone*: 0.7 per cent to 2.5 per cent.

For rosemary oil, Moroccan and Tunisian type, the percentages are within the following ranges:
— *α-pinene*: 9.0 per cent to 14.0 per cent,
— *camphene*: 2.5 per cent to 6.0 per cent,
— *β-pinene*: 4.0 per cent to 9.0 per cent,
— *β-myrcene*: 1.0 per cent to 2.0 per cent,
— *limonene*: 1.5 per cent to 4.0 per cent,
— *cineole*: 38.0 per cent to 55.0 per cent,
— *p-cymene*: 0.8 per cent to 2.5 per cent,
— *camphor*: 5.0 per cent to 15.0 per cent,
— *bornyl acetate*: 0.1 per cent to 1.5 per cent,
— *α-terpineol*: 1.0 per cent to 2.6 per cent,
— *borneol*: 1.5 per cent to 5.0 per cent,
— *verbenone*: maximum 0.4 per cent.

STORAGE

At a temperature not exceeding 25 °C.

LABELLING

The label states that the content is Spanish type or Moroccan and Tunisian type.

Ph Eur

Safflower Flower

(*Ph Eur monograph 2386*)

Ph Eur

DEFINITION

Dried flower of *Carthamus tinctorius* L.

Content

Minimum 1.0 per cent of total flavonoids, expressed as hyperoside ($C_{21}H_{20}O_{12}$; M_r 464.4) (dried drug).

IDENTIFICATION

A. The orange-yellow or reddish-orange, tubular, gametalous, actinomorphic florets are separate from the capitulum. Each consists of a long, filiform tube, about 1 cm long divided into 5 equal, narrow, lanceolate lobes, about 0.5 cm long. From the opening of the tube emerges the hollow cylinder formed by the fused yellow anthers, in which the filiform style persists, thickened near the apex.

B. Reduce to a powder (355) (*2.9.12*). The powder is orange-yellow. Examine under a microscope using *chloral hydrate solution R*. The powder shows fragments of the corolla tube with epidermis consisting of elongated, thin-walled polygonal cells; fragments of the lobes of the corolla showing at their apices a large number of small, rounded, very prominent papillae; fragments of parenchyma containing vascular bundles surrounded by secretory canals with reddish-brown contents; fragments of anthers consisting of irregularly shaped cells whose walls show thickenings in characteristic bands; fragments of the style, whose lower part consists of elongated cells and which ends in a stigma, bristling with rather long, conical, confluent papillae; rounded or elliptical triporate pollen grains up to 60 μm in diameter with an echinulate exine; calcium oxalate prisms, either isolated or present in parenchyma cells.

C. Thin-layer chromatography (*2.2.27*).

Test solution To 1.0 g of the powdered drug (355) (*2.9.12*) add 10 mL of *methanol R*. Sonicate for 10 min and centrifuge.

Reference solution Dissolve 1 mg of *rutin R* and 5 mg of *quercetin dihydrate R* in 50 mL of *methanol R*.

Plate TLC silica gel plate R (5-40 μm) [or *TLC silica gel plate R* (2-10 μm)].

Mobile phase acetic acid R, anhydrous formic acid R, water R, ethyl acetate R (11:11:27:100 V/V/V/V).

Application 25 μL as bands of 15 mm [or 10 μL as bands of 8 mm].

Development Over a path of 12 cm [or 7 cm].

Drying In air.

Detection A Examine in daylight.

Results A See below the sequence of the zones present in the chromatograms obtained with the reference solution and the test solution. Furthermore, other faint zones may be present in the chromatogram obtained with the test solution.

Top of the plate	
Quercetin: a light yellow zone	
———	———
———	———
Rutin: a light yellow zone	
	A red zone
	A yellow zone
	A yellow zone
Reference solution	**Test solution**

Detection B Heat at 100 °C for 3 min; spray the plate whilst still hot with a 10 g/L solution of *diphenylboric acid aminoethyl ester R* in *methanol R* and then with a 50 g/L solution of *macrogol 400 R* in *methanol R*; allow to dry in air for about 30 min; examine in ultraviolet light at 365 nm.

Results B See below the sequence of zones present in the chromatograms obtained with the reference solution and the test solution. Furthermore, other faint zones may be present in the chromatogram obtained with the test solution.

Top of the plate	
Quercetin: an orange fluorescent zone	
	A blue fluorescent zone
———	———
	A green fluorescent zone
	A brown fluorescent zone
	A green fluorescent zone
———	———
Rutin: a yellow fluorescent zone	
	A yellow fluorescent zone
	A green fluorescent zone
	A brown fluorescent zone
Reference solution	**Test solution**

TESTS

Absorbance (2.2.25)

A. *Yellow pigment*: macerate 0.1 g of the powdered drug (355) (2.9.12) in 150 mL of *water R*, stir for 1 h, filter through a sintered-glass filter (40) (2.1.2) and dilute to 500.0 mL, washing the residue, with *water R*. The absorbance is not less than 0.40 at 401 nm.

B. *Red pigment*: to 0.25 g of the powdered drug (355) (2.9.12) add 50 mL of a mixture of 20 volumes of *water R* and 80 volumes of *acetone R*. Heat on a water-bath at 50 °C for 90 min. Allow to cool, filter through a sintered-glass filter (40) (2.1.2) and dilute to 100.0 mL, washing the residue with a mixture of 20 volumes of *water R* and 80 volumes of *acetone R*. The absorbance is not less than 0.40 at 518 nm.

Loss on drying (2.2.32)

Maximum 11.0 per cent, determined on 1.000 g of the powdered drug (355) (2.9.12) by drying in an oven at 105 °C for 2 h.

Total ash (2.4.16)

Maximum 10.0 per cent.

Ash insoluble in hydrochloric acid (2.8.1)

Maximum 3.0 per cent.

ASSAY

Solution A   Place 0.250 g of the powdered drug (180) (2.9.12) in a 250 mL flask and add 95 mL of *methanol R*. Heat under a reflux condenser on a water-bath for 30 min. Allow to cool and filter. Rinse the filter with 5 mL of *methanol R*. Combine the filtrate and the rinsing solution in a volumetric flask and dilute to 100.0 mL with *methanol R*.

Test solution   Place 5.0 mL of solution A in a volumetric flask and dilute to 20.0 mL with a 20 g/L solution of *aluminium chloride R* in *methanol R*.

Compensation solution   Place 5.0 mL of solution A in a volumetric flask and dilute to 20.0 mL with *methanol R*.

After exactly 15 min, measure the absorbance (2.2.25) of the test solution at 420 nm by comparison with the compensation solution. Calculate the percentage content of total flavonoids, expressed as hyperoside, using the following expression:

$$\frac{A}{m}$$

taking the specific absorbance of hyperoside at 420 nm to be 400.

A = absorbance of the test solution, at 420 nm;
m = mass of the substance to be examined, in grams.

_____ *Ph Eur*

Sage Leaf

(*Sage Leaf (Salvia officinalis)*, Ph Eur monograph 1370)

Preparation
Sage Tincture

Ph Eur _____

DEFINITION

Whole or cut dried leaves of *Salvia officinalis* L.

Content

Minimum 15 mL/kg of essential oil for the whole drug and minimum 10 mL/kg of essential oil for the cut drug (anhydrous drug).

CHARACTERS

Sage leaf (*Salvia officinalis*) oil is rich in thujone.

IDENTIFICATION

A. The lamina of whole sage leaf (*Salvia officinalis*) is about 2 cm to 10 cm long and 1 cm to 2 cm wide, oblong-ovate, elliptical. The margin is finely crenate to smooth. The apex is rounded or subacute and the base is shrunken at the petiole and rounded or cordate. The upper surface is greenish-grey and finely granular; the lower surface is white and pubescent and shows a dense network of raised veinlets.

B. Reduce to a powder (355) (2.9.12). The powder is light grey to brownish-green. Examine under a microscope using *chloral hydrate solution R*. The powder shows the following diagnostic characters: very numerous articulated and bent trichomes with narrow elongated cells and a very thick cell at the base as well as fragments of these trichomes; fragments of the upper epidermis with pitted, somewhat polygonal cells; fragments of the lower epidermis with sinuous cells and numerous diacytic stomata (2.8.3); rare single glandular trichomes with a uni- or bicellular head and a stalk consisting of 1 to 4 cells; abundant glandular trichomes with a unicellular stalk and a head composed of 8 radiating cells with a raised common cuticle.

C. Thin-layer chromatography (2.2.27).

Test solution   Shake 0.5 g of the freshly powdered drug (355) (2.9.12) with 5 mL of *ethanol R* for 5 min.

Reference solution   Dissolve 20 μL of *thujone R* and 25 μL of *cineole R* in 20 mL of *ethanol R*.

Plate   TLC silica gel plate R.

Mobile phase   ethyl acetate R, toluene R (5:95 *V/V*).

Application   20 μL, as bands.

Development   Over a path of 15 cm.

Drying   In air.

Detection   Spray the plate with a 200 g/L solution of *phosphomolybdic acid R* in *ethanol R* and heat at 100-105 °C for 10 min. Examine in daylight.

Results   See below the sequence of the zones present in the chromatograms obtained with the reference solution and the test solution. Furthermore, other zones are present in the chromatogram obtained with the test solution.

Top of the plate	
	A blue zone (near the solvent front)
	_____
α-Thujone and β-thujone: 2 pinkish-violet zones	2 pinkish-violet zones (α-thujone and β-thujone)
Cineole: a blue zone	A blue zone (cineole)
	_____
	Blue zones
Reference solution	**Test solution**

TESTS

Foreign matter (2.8.2)

Maximum 3 per cent of stems and maximum 2 per cent of other foreign matter.

Water (2.2.13)

Maximum 100 mL/kg, determined on 20.0 g.

Total ash (2.4.16)

Maximum 10.0 per cent.

ASSAY

Carry out the determination of essential oils in herbal drugs (*2.8.12*). Use 20.0 g of the substance to be examined, cut, if necessary, immediately before the assay, a 500 mL flask, 250 mL of *water R* as the distillation liquid and 0.5 mL of *xylene R* in the graduated tube. Distil at a rate of 2-3 mL/min for 2 h.

———————————————— Ph Eur

Sage Tincture

(*Ph Eur monograph 1889*)

Ph Eur _____

DEFINITION

Tincture produced from *Sage leaf (Salvia officinalis) (1370)*.

Content

Minimum 0.1 per cent *m/m* of essential oil.

PRODUCTION

The tincture is produced from 1 part of comminuted drug and 10 parts of ethanol (70 per cent *V/V*) by a suitable procedure.

CHARACTERS

Appearance

Brownish liquid with a characteristic odour.

IDENTIFICATION

Thin-layer chromatography (*2.2.27*).

Test solution   The tincture to be examined.

Reference solution   Dissolve 20 μL of *thujone R* and 25 μL of *cineole R* in 20 mL of *ethanol R*.

Plate   TLC silica gel plate R.

Mobile phase   ethyl acetate R, toluene R (5:95 *V/V*).

Application   20 μL, as bands.

Development   Over a path of 15 cm.

Drying   In air.

Detection   Spray with a 200 g/L solution of *phosphomolybdic acid R* in *ethanol R* and heat at 100-105 °C for 10 min. Examine in daylight.

Results   See below the sequence of the zones present in the chromatograms obtained with the reference solution and the test solution. Furthermore, other zones are present in the chromatogram obtained with the test solution.

Top of the plate	
	A blue zone (near the solvent front)
α-Thujone and β-thujone: 2 pinkish-violet zones Cineole: a blue zone	2 pinkish-violet zones (α-thujone and β-thujone) A blue zone (cineole)
	Blue zones
Reference solution	**Test solution**

TESTS

Ethanol content (*2.9.10*)
64 per cent *V/V* to 69 per cent *V/V*.

Methanol and 2-propanol (*2.9.11*)
Maximum 0.05 per cent *V/V* of methanol and maximum 0.05 per cent of 2-propanol.

Dry residue (*2.8.16*)
Minimum 2.0 per cent *m/m*, determined on 3.00 g.

ASSAY

In a 500 mL round-bottomed flask, place 30.0 g of the tincture and add 100 mL of *water R*. Distil, using a descending condenser, into a separating funnel which has been marked beforehand at 50 mL. Stop the distillation process as soon as the distillate reaches the 50 mL mark. Rinse the condenser with 10 mL of *pentane R*. Dissolve in the distillate sufficient *sodium chloride R* to produce a saturated solution. Shake with 3 quantities, each of 20 mL, of *pentane R*. Dry the combined pentane layers, including the pentane from rinsing the condenser, over *anhydrous sodium sulfate R* and filter through a plug of absorbent cotton into a weighed 100 mL round-bottomed flask. Wash the sodium sulfate several times with small quantities of *pentane R*. Remove the pentane carefully at a temperature not exceeding 40 °C. Dry the residue in a desiccator over *diphosphorus pentoxide R* and hard paraffin at atmospheric pressure and at room temperature for 2 h. Weigh the residue (essential oil).

———————————————— Ph Eur

Three-lobed Sage Leaf

(*Ph Eur monograph 1561*)

Ph Eur _____

DEFINITION

Whole or cut, dried leaves of *Salvia fructicosa* Mill. (*S. triloba* L. fil).

Content

Minimum 18 mL/kg of essential oil in the whole drug (anhydrous drug) and minimum 12 mL/kg of essential oil in the cut drug (anhydrous drug).

CHARACTERS

Spicy odour when ground, similar to eucalyptus oil.

IDENTIFICATION

A. The lamina of the whole three-lobed sage leaf is about 8-50 mm long and about 4-20 mm wide, and oblong-ovate or lanceolate. The margin is finely crenate and undulate but indistinct owing to the dense hairy covering on both surfaces. The base is obtuse and sometimes bears 1 or 2 more or less developed lobes. The upper surface is grey-tomentose pubescent, the lower surface is densely white-tomentose pubescent; the venation is indistinct. The densely white-tomentose pubescent petiole is about 1 mm in diameter.

B. Reduce to a powder (355) (*2.9.12*). The powder is greyish-green and tomentose. Examine under a microscope using *chloral hydrate solution R*. The powder shows the following diagnostic characters: very numerous, whole or fragmented, covering and glandular trichomes, scattered and attached to fragments of the epidermises; covering trichomes articulated, uniseriate, thick-walled and bluntly tapering, those on the upper epidermis straight, those on the lower epidermis longer, tortuous and more densely packed; glandular trichomes, some with a unicellular or bicellular head and a stalk consisting of from 1-4 cells, the majority having a short, unicellular stalk and a head composed of 8 radiating cells with a raised common cuticle; the upper epidermis with pitted and beaded cells, somewhat polygonal, with a few diacytic stomata (*2.8.3*); the lower epidermis with sinuous or wavy-walled cells and numerous diacytic stomata.

C. Examine the chromatogram obtained in the test for thujone.

Results The chromatogram obtained with the test solution shows a blue zone due to cineole, equal or greater in size and intensity to the zone in the chromatogram obtained with the reference solution. Further zones are present.

TESTS
Thujone
Thin-layer chromatography (*2.2.27*).

Test solution Shake 0.3 g of the freshly powdered drug (355) (*2.9.12*) with 5.0 mL of *anhydrous ethanol R* for 5 min.

Reference solution Dissolve 20 µL of *thujone R* and 25 µL of *cineole R* in 20 mL of *anhydrous ethanol R*.

Plate TLC silica gel plate R.

Mobile phase ethyl acetate R, toluene R (5:95 *V/V*).

Application 20 µL, as bands.

Development Over a path of 15 cm.

Drying In air.

Detection Spray with a 200 g/L solution of *phosphomolybdic acid R* in *anhydrous ethanol R* and heat at 100-105 °C for 10 min. Examine in daylight.

Results The chromatogram obtained with the reference solution shows in the middle part a blue zone (cineole) and in the upper part a pink-blue zone (thujone).
The chromatogram obtained with the test solution shows no zone or a very faint pink-blue zone due to thujone.

Foreign matter (*2.8.2*)
Maximum 8 per cent of stems and maximum 2 per cent of other foreign matter.

Water (*2.2.13*)
Maximum 100 mL/kg, determined on 20.0 g.

Total ash (*2.4.16*)
Maximum 10.0 per cent.

ASSAY
Carry out the determination of essential oils in herbal drugs (*2.8.12*). Use 20.0 g of drug, if necessary cut immediately before the assay, a 500 mL flask, 250 mL of *water R* as the distillation liquid. Add 0.50 mL of *xylene R* in the graduated tube. Distil at a rate of 2-3 mL/min for 2 h.

_____ Ph Eur

Sage Oil

(*Clary Sage Oil, Ph Eur monograph 1850*)

Ph Eur _____

DEFINITION
Essential oil obtained by steam distillation from the fresh or dried flowering stems of *Salvia sclarea* L.

CHARACTERS
Appearance
Colourless or brownish-yellow liquid, usually pale yellow.
Characteristic odour.

IDENTIFICATION
First identification B.
Second identification A.

A. Thin-layer chromatography (*2.2.27*).

Test solution Dissolve 1 mL of the substance to be examined in *toluene R* and dilute to 10 mL with the same solvent.

Reference solution Dissolve 60 µL of *linalol R*, 200 µL of *linalyl acetate R* and 60 µL of *α-terpineol R* in *toluene R* and dilute to 10 mL with the same solvent.

Plate TLC silica gel plate R.

Mobile phase ethyl acetate R, toluene R (5:95 *V/V*).

Application 5 µL of the test solution and 10 µL of the reference solution, as bands.

Development Over a path of 15 cm.

Drying In air.

Detection Spray with *vanillin reagent R* and heat at 100-105 °C for 5-10 min; examine in daylight within 5 min.

Results See below the sequence of the zones present in the chromatograms obtained with the reference solution and the test solution. Furthermore, other faint zones are present in the chromatogram obtained with the test solution.

Top of the plate	
α-Terpineol: a dark violet zone	A dark violet zone
_____	
Linalyl acetate: a dark violet zone	A dark violet zone
_____	_____
Linalol: a dark violet zone	A dark violet zone
Reference solution	**Test solution**

B. Examine the chromatograms obtained in the test for chromatographic profile.

Results The chromatogram obtained with the test solution shows 5 peaks similar in position to the 5 peaks in the chromatogram obtained with the reference solution. The 2 peaks corresponding to α- and β-thujone may be absent.

TESTS
Relative density (*2.2.5*)
0.890 to 0.908.

Refractive index (*2.2.6*)
1.456 to 1.466.

Optical rotation (*2.2.7*)
− 26° to − 10°.

Acid value (*2.5.1*)
Maximum 1.0.

Chromatographic profile
Gas chromatography (*2.2.28*): use the normalisation procedure.

Test solution The substance to be examined.

Reference solution To 1 g of *hexane R*, add 5 µL of *thujone R*, 5 µL of *linalol R*, 100 µL of *linalyl acetate R*, 10 µL of *α-terpineol R* and 25 mg (± 20 per cent) of *sclareol R*. Mix thoroughly by stirring.

Column:
— *material*: fused silica,
— *size*: *l* = 30 m (a film thickness of 1 µm may be used) to 60 m (a film thickness of 0.2 µm may be used), Ø = 0.25-0.53 mm,
— *stationary phase: macrogol 20 000 R*.

Carrier gas helium for chromatography R.

Split ratio 1:100.

Temperature:

	Time (min)	Temperature (°C)
Column	0 - 10	60
	10 - 75	60 → 190
	75 - 120	190
Injection port		220
Detector		240

Detection   Flame ionisation.

Injection   0.2 µL.

Elution order   Order indicated in the composition of the reference solution. Record the retention times of these substances.

System suitability   Reference solution:
— *resolution*: minimum 1.5 between the peaks due to linalol and linalyl acetate,

Using the retention times determined from the chromatogram obtained with the reference solution, locate the components of the reference solution in the chromatogram obtained with the test solution (disregard any peak due to hexane). *Thujone R* is a mixture of α- and β-thujone. α-Thujone elutes before β-thujone under the described conditions.

Determine the percentage content of each of these components.

Also determine the percentage content of germacrene-D. The germacrene-D peak can be identified in the chromatogram obtained with the test solution by its relative retention of 1.23 with reference to linalol under the described operating conditions.

The percentages are within the following ranges:
— *α- and β-thujone*: maximum 0.2 per cent,
— *linalol*: 6.5 per cent to 24 per cent,
— *linalyl acetate*: 56 per cent to 78 per cent,
— *α-terpineol*: maximum 5.0 per cent,
— *germacrene-D*: 1.0 per cent to 12 per cent,
— *sclareol*: 0.4 per cent to 2.6 per cent.

STORAGE

At a temperature not exceeding 25 °C.

_____ *Ph Eur*

Spanish Sage Oil

(Ph Eur monograph 1849)

Ph Eur _____

DEFINITION

Essential oil obtained by steam distillation from the aerial parts of *Salvia lavandulifolia* Vahl, collected at the flowering stage.

CHARACTERS

Appearance

Clear, colourless or pale yellow, mobile liquid.

Camphor-like odour.

IDENTIFICATION

First identification   B.

Second identification   A.

A. Thin-layer chromatography (*2.2.27*).

Test solution   Dissolve 0.1 mL of the oil to be examined in 10 mL of *toluene R*.

Reference solution   Dissolve 20 µL of *thujone R* and 30 µL of *cineole R* in 10 mL of *toluene R*.

Plate   TLC silica gel plate R (5-40 µm) [or *TLC silica gel plate R* (2-10 µm)].

Mobile phase   ethyl acetate R, toluene R (5:95 *V/V*).

Application   10 µL [or 3 µL] as bands of 10 mm [or 6 mm].

Development   Over a path of 15 cm [or 6 cm].

Drying   In air.

Detection   Spray with a freshly prepared 200 g/L solution of *phosphomolybdic acid R* in *ethanol (96 per cent) R* and heat at 105 °C for 10 min; examine in daylight.

Results   See below the sequence of zones present in the chromatograms obtained with the reference solution and the test solution. Furthermore, other faint zones may be present in the chromatogram obtained with the test solution.

Top of the plate	
	A blue zone
	———
Thujone: 2 pinkish-violet zones	
Cineole: a blue zone	A blue zone (cineole)
	———
	3 blue zones
Reference solution	**Test solution**

B. Examine the chromatograms obtained in the test for chromatographic profile.

Results   The characteristic peaks in the chromatogram obtained with the test solution are similar in retention time to those in the chromatogram obtained with reference solution (a).

TESTS

Relative density (*2.2.5*)

0.907 to 0.932.

Refractive index (*2.2.6*)

1.465 to 1.473.

Optical rotation (*2.2.7*)

+ 7° to + 17°.

Acid value (*2.5.1*)

Maximum 2.0, determined on 5.00 g.

Solubility in alcohol (*2.8.10*)

1 volume is soluble in 2 volumes and more of *ethanol (80 per cent V/V) R*.

Chromatographic profile

Gas chromatography (*2.2.28*): use the normalisation procedure.

Test solution   Dissolve 0.200 g of the oil to be examined in *heptane R* and dilute to 10.0 mL with the same solvent.

Reference solution (a)   Dissolve 0.200 g of *Spanish sage oil for peak identification CRS* in *heptane R* and dilute to 10.0 mL with the same solvent.

Reference solution (b)   Dissolve 5 µL of *limonene R* in *heptane R* and dilute to 50.0 mL with the same solvent. Dilute 0.5 mL of this solution to 5.0 mL with *heptane R*.

Column:
— *material*: fused silica;
— *size*: l = 60 m, Ø = 0.25 mm;

— stationary phase: macrogol 20 000 R (film thickness 0.25 µm).

Carrier gas   *helium for chromatography R.*

Flow rate   1.5 mL/min.

Split ratio   1:50.

Temperature:

	Time (min)	Temperature (°C)
Column	0 - 43	60 → 232
Injection port		250
Detector		250

Detection   Flame ionisation.

Injection   1 µL.

System suitability   Reference solution (a):
— the chromatogram obtained is similar to the chromatogram supplied with *Spanish sage oil for peak identification CRS*;
— *resolution*: minimum 1.5 between the peaks due to limonene and 1,8-cineole and minimum 1.5 between the peaks due to α-terpinyl acetate and borneol.

Use the chromatogram supplied with *Spanish sage oil for peak identification CRS* and the chromatogram obtained with reference solution (a) to locate the peaks due to α-pinene, sabinene, limonene, 1,8-cineole, thujone, camphor, linalol, linalyl acetate, terpinen-4-ol, sabinyl acetate, α-terpinyl acetate and borneol.

Determine the percentage content of each of these components. The percentages are within the following ranges:
— *α-pinene*: 4.0 per cent to 11.0 per cent;
— *sabinene*: 0.1 per cent to 3.5 per cent;
— *limonene*: 2.0 per cent to 6.5 per cent;
— *1,8-cineole*: 10.0 per cent to 30.5 per cent;
— *thujone*: maximum 0.5 per cent;
— *camphor*: 11.0 per cent to 36.0 per cent;
— *linalol*: 0.3 per cent to 4.0 per cent;
— *linalyl acetate*: maximum 5.0 per cent;
— *terpinen-4-ol*: maximum 2.0 per cent;
— *sabinyl acetate*: 0.5 per cent to 9.0 per cent;
— *α-terpinyl acetate*: 0.5 per cent to 9.0 per cent;
— *borneol*: 1.0 per cent to 7.0 per cent;
— *disregard limit*: the area of the principal peak in the chromatogram obtained with reference solution (b) (0.05 per cent).

STORAGE

At a temperature not exceeding 25 °C.

Ph Eur

Salvia Miltiorrhiza Root and Rhizome

(Ph Eur monograph 2663)

Ph Eur

DEFINITION

Dried, whole or fragmented rhizome and root of *Salvia miltiorrhiza* Bunge, collected in spring or autumn.

Content:
— *salvianolic acid B* ($C_{36}H_{30}O_{16}$; M_r 719): minimum 3.0 per cent (dried drug);
— *tanshinone IIA* ($C_{19}H_{18}O_3$; M_r 294.3): minimum 0.12 per cent (dried drug).

IDENTIFICATION

A. The rhizome is short and thick, sometimes with stem remnants at the apex. The roots are numerous, about 10-20 cm long and 0.3-1 cm in diameter, cylindrical and slightly curved; some are branched, with secondary roots and rootlets. The outer surface is reddish-brown or dark reddish-brown, marked with longitudinal striations. The bark of old roots comes off usually as purplish-brown scales. The texture is hard and fragile. The fracture is soft, fissured or slightly even and dense, with a reddish-brown outer part and a greyish-yellow or purplish-brown wood, showing bundles of yellowish-white vessels, arranged radially.

Cultivars are relatively stout, about 0.5-1.5 cm in diameter. The outer surface is brownish-red, longitudinally wrinkled. The bark adheres closely to the wood and is difficult to remove. The texture is compact; the fracture is relatively even.

B. Microscopic examination (*2.8.23*). The powder is brownish-red. Examine under a microscope using *chloral hydrate solution R*. The powder shows the following diagnostic characters: fragments of cork in surface view, consisting of subrectangular or polygonal cells, up to 150 µm in diameter, containing yellowish-brown pigment; fragments of parenchyma consisting of polygonal or elongated, thin-walled cells that may contain yellowish-brown pigment; xylem fibres usually in bundles, long and fusiform, with pitted walls showing oblique or criss-cross striations; very numerous reticulate or pitted vessels, 3-120 µm in diameter, free, in bundles or sometimes accompanying the fibres.

C. Thin-layer chromatography (*2.2.27*).

Test solution   To 1 g of the powdered herbal drug (355) (*2.9.12*) add 40 mL of *methanol R*. Sonicate for 15 min. Filter. Evaporate the filtrate to 1 mL.

Reference solution   Dissolve 2 mg of *salvianolic acid B R* and 2 mg of *tanshinone IIₐ R* in 1 mL of *methanol R*.

Plate   TLC silica gel F_{254} plate R (5-40 µm) [or TLC silica gel F_{254} plate R (2-10 µm)].

Mobile phase   methanol R, anhydrous formic acid R, toluene R, methylene chloride R, ethyl acetate R (5:20:20:30:40 *V/V/V/V/V*).

Application   5 µL [or 5 µL] as bands of 8 mm [or 8 mm].

Development   Over a path of 8 cm [or 6 cm].

Drying   In air.

Detection A   Examine in daylight.

Results A   See below the sequence of zones present in the chromatograms obtained with the reference solution and the test solution. Furthermore, other faint zones may be present in the upper third and middle part of the chromatogram obtained with the test solution.

Top of the plate	
Tanshinone IIₐ: a prominent red zone	A prominent red zone (tanshinone IIₐ)
	An orange zone
	A faint brownish-green zone
Salvianolic acid B: a faint grey zone	A faint grey zone (salvianolic acid B)
Reference solution	**Test solution**

Detection B Examine in ultraviolet light at 254 nm.

Results See below the sequence of zones present in the chromatograms obtained with the reference solution and the test solution. Furthermore, other faint zones may be present in the upper third and middle part of the chromatogram obtained with the test solution.

Top of the plate	
Tanshinone II$_A$: a prominent quenching zone	A prominent quenching zone (tanshinone II$_A$)
	A quenching zone
_ _ _	_ _ _
	A quenching zone
Salvianolic acid B: a prominent quenching zone	A prominent quenching zone (salvianolic acid B)
	_ _ _
Reference solution	**Test solution**

TESTS

Loss on drying *(2.2.32)*
Maximum 10.0 per cent, determined on 1.000 g of the powdered herbal drug (355) *(2.9.12)* by drying in an oven at 105 °C for 2 h.

Total ash *(2.4.16)*
Maximum 10.0 per cent.

Ash insoluble in hydrochloric acid *(2.8.1)*
Maximum 3.0 per cent.

ASSAY

Liquid chromatography *(2.2.29)*. *Protect the solutions from light.*

Test solution Disperse 0.30 g of the powdered herbal drug (355) *(2.9.12)* in 50.0 mL of a 70 per cent *V/V* solution of *methanol R*. Sonicate for 1 h. Filter through a membrane filter (nominal pore size 0.45 μm).

Reference solution (a) Dissolve 5.0 mg of *tanshinone IIA CRS* in *methanol R* and dilute to 50.0 mL with the same solvent. Dilute 2.0 mL of the solution to 10.0 mL with *methanol R*.

Reference solution (b) Dissolve 5.0 mg of *salvianolic acid B CRS* in *methanol R* and dilute to 25.0 mL with the same solvent.

Reference solution (c) Dissolve 1 mg of *rosmarinic acid R* in *methanol R*, add 5 mL of reference solution (b) and dilute to 10.0 mL with *methanol R*.

Column:
— *size: l = 0.25 m, Ø = 4.6 mm;*
— *stationary phase: end-capped octadecylsilyl silica gel for chromatography R (5 μm).*

Mobile phase:
— *mobile phase A: 0.1 per cent V/V solution of anhydrous formic acid R;*
— *mobile phase B: acetonitrile for chromatography R;*

Time (min)	Mobile phase A (per cent *V/V*)	Mobile phase B (per cent *V/V*)
0 - 10	79 → 71	21 → 29
10 - 15	71 → 65	29 → 35
15 - 25	65 → 28	35 → 72
25 - 37	28 → 0	72 → 100

Flow rate 1.0 mL/min.

Detection Spectrophotometer at 280 nm.

Injection 10 μL.

Relative retention With reference to tanshinone IIA (retention time = about 33 min):
rosmarinic acid = about 0.3; salvianolic acid B = about 0.4.

System suitability Reference solution (c):
— *resolution*: minimum 5.0 between the peaks due to rosmarinic acid and salvianolic acid B.

Calculate the percentage content of tanshinone II$_A$ using the following expression:

$$\frac{A_1 \times m_2 \times p_1}{A_2 \times m_1 \times 5}$$

A_1 = area of the peak due to tanshinone II$_A$ in the chromatogram obtained with the test solution;

A_2 = area of the peak due to tanshinone II$_A$ in the chromatogram obtained with reference solution (a);

m_1 = mass of the herbal drug to be examined used to prepare the test solution, in grams;

m_2 = mass of *tanshinone II$_A$ CRS* used to prepare reference solution (a), in grams;

p_1 = percentage content of tanshinone II$_A$ in *tanshinone II$_A$ CRS*.

Calculate the percentage content of salvianolic acid B using the following expression:

$$\frac{A_3 \times m_3 \times p_2 \times 2}{A_4 \times m_1}$$

A_3 = area of the peak due to salvianolic acid B in the chromatogram obtained with the test solution;

A_4 = area of the peak due to salvianolic acid B in the chromatogram obtained with reference solution (b);

m_1 = mass of the herbal drug to be examined used to prepare the test solution, in grams;

m_3 = mass of *salvianolic acid B CRS* used to prepare reference solution (b), in grams;

p_2 = percentage content of salvianolic acid B in *salvianolic acid B CRS*.

_____ *Ph Eur*

Processed Salvia Miltiorrhiza Rhizome and Root

DEFINITION

Processed Salvia Miltiorrhiza Rhizome and Root is Salvia Miltiorrhiza Rhizome and Root that has been processed. It contains not less than 0.04% of tanshinone II$_A$ ($C_{19}H_{18}O_3$), not less than 0.17% of rosmarinic acid ($C_{18}H_{16}O_8$) and not less than 3.0% of salvianolic acid B ($C_{36}H_{36}O_{16}$), calculated with reference to the dried material.

PRODUCTION

It is collected in spring or autumn, separated from soil, washed clean, softened thoroughly, sliced longitudinally or transversely and dried. It may be stir baked with wine.

IDENTIFICATION

A. The longitudinally-sliced pieces are up to about 5 cm long, 1.5 cm wide and 1 to 2 mm thick; those cut from the thinner roots show the dark brown striated cork covering one longitudinal surface and the yellowish to cream inner tissues on the other; slices cut from the thicker rhizomes are usually cut obliquely so that parts of the outer and inner tissues are included on both longitudinal surfaces. The transversely-cut slices are irregularly elliptical to nearly circular, 4 to 12 mm wide and 2 to 3 mm thick; the outer surface is dark brown and uneven; the smoothed transverse surface shows the outer layers about 1 to 2 mm wide separated by a darker line from the yellowish white, radiate vascular tissue; some pieces show a small, light brown central pith.

B. Reduce to a powder (355). The powder is reddish-brown. Examine under a microscope using chloral hydrate solution. The powder shows a surface view of cork cells almost rectangular or polygonal, containing yellowish-brown pigment, 12 to 151 μm in diameter. Parenchymatous cells in cortex squarish or polygonal, containing reddish-brown pigmental sediments. Xylem fibres usually in bundles, long fusiform, with oblique or criss-cross striations, 11 to 60 μm in diameter, vivid yellow when examined under a polarizing microscope. Numerous mainly bordered or reticulated vessels, 3 to 120 μm in diameter.

C. Carry out the method for thin-layer chromatography, Appendix III A, using the following solutions.

(1) Place 2 g of the powdered drug (355) in a cellulose fingerstall in a continuous extraction apparatus (Soxhlet type). Add 75 mL of *methanol* and heat for 1 hour. Evaporate the extract to 20 mL, cool and filter if necessary.

(2) 0.1% w/v each of *tanshinone II*$_A$ *CRS*, *rosmarinic acid CRS* and *salvianolic acid B CRS* in *methanol*.

CHROMATOGRAPHIC CONDITIONS

(a) Use as the coating *silica gel F*$_{254}$.

(b) Use the mobile phase described below.

(c) Apply as bands 8 μL of solution (1) and 5 μL of solution (2).

(d) Develop the plate to 15 cm.

(e) After removal of the plate, dry in air and examine under *ultraviolet light (366 nm)*.

MOBILE PHASE

10 volumes of *water*, 13.5 volumes of *methanol* and 100 volumes of *ethyl acetate*.

SYSTEM SUITABILITY

The chromatogram obtained with solution (2) shows three clearly separated bands.

CONFIRMATION

The blue fluorescent bands with Rf values of approximately 0.7 (tanshinone II$_A$), 0.2 (rosmarinic acid) and 0.06 (salvianolic acid B) in the chromatogram obtained with solution (1) correspond in colour and position to those in the chromatogram obtained with solution (2). Other bands may be present in the chromatogram obtained with solution (1) as shown below.

Top of the plate	
A fluorescent band	Tanshinone II$_A$: a fluorescent band
Several fluorescent bands	
A fluorescent band	Rosmarinic acid: a fluorescent band
A fluorescent band	Salvianolic acid B: a fluorescent band
Solution (1)	**Solution (2)**

TESTS

Total ash

Not more than 10%, Appendix XI J.

Acid-insoluble ash

Not more than 2.0%, Appendix XI K.

Loss on drying

When dried for 2 hours at 105°, loses not more than 12.0% of its weight. Use 1 g.

ASSAY

For tanshinone II$_A$

Carry out the method for *liquid chromatography*, Appendix III D, using the following solutions.

(1) Finely powder about 5.0 g of the herbal drug being examined. Transfer 0.5 g of the powder into a 25 mL volumetric flask and add 20 mL of the mobile phase given below. Shake and mix with the aid of ultrasound for 30 minutes, shaking intermittently. Add the mobile phase to give a total volume of 25 mL. Filter through a 0.45-μm filter.

(2) 0.002% w/v of *tanshinone II*$_A$ *CRS* in the mobile phase.

CHROMATOGRAPHIC CONDITIONS

(a) Use a stainless steel column (25 cm × 4.6 mm) packed with *octadecylsilyl silica gel for chromatography* (5 μm) (Nucleosil ODS is suitable).

(b) Use isocratic elution and the mobile phase described below.

(c) Use a flow rate of 1 mL per minute.

(d) Use an ambient column temperature.

(e) Use a detection wavelength of 270 nm.

(f) Inject 20 μL of each solution.

MOBILE PHASE

0.01M *sodium octyl sulfonate* in a mixture of 25 volumes of *water* and 75 volumes of *methanol* adjusted to pH 5.0 with *acetic acid*.

SYSTEM SUITABILITY

The test is not valid, unless in the chromatogram obtained with solution (2):

— the *symmetry factor* of the peak due to tanshinone II$_A$ is less than 1.2;

— the number of *theoretical plates* is not less than 4500.

DETERMINATION OF CONTENT

Using the retention time and peak area from the chromatograms obtained with solution (2), locate and integrate the peak due to tanshinone II$_A$ in the chromatogram obtained with solution (1).

Calculate the content of tanshinone II$_A$ in the sample using the declared content of tanshinone II$_A$ ($C_{19}H_{18}O_3$) in *tanshinone II*$_A$ *CRS* and the following expression:

$$\frac{A_1}{A_2} \times \frac{m_2}{V_2} \times \frac{V_1}{m_1} \times p \times \frac{100}{100-d}$$

A_1 = Area of the peak due to tanshinone II$_A$ in the chromatogram obtained with solution (1).

A_2 = Area of the peak due to tanshinone II$_A$ in the chromatogram obtained with solution (2).

m_1 = Weight of the drug in mg.

m_2 = Weight of *tanshinone II*$_A$ *CRS* in mg.

V_1 = Dilution volume of solution (1) in mL.

V_2 = Dilution volume of solution (2) in mL.

p = Percentage content of tanshinone II$_A$ in *tanshinone II*$_A$ *CRS*.

d   =   Percentage loss on drying of the herbal drug being examined.

For rosmarinic acid and salvianolic acid B
Carry out the method for *liquid chromatography*, Appendix III D, using the following solutions prepared immediately before use.

(1) Finely powder about 5.0 g of the herbal drug being examined. Transfer 0.5 g of the powder into a 25-mL volumetric flask and add 20 mL of the mobile phase given below. Shake and mix with ultrasound for 30 minutes, shaking intermittently. Add the mobile phase to give a total volume of 25 mL. Filter through a 0.45-µm filter.

(2) 0.003% w/v each of *rosmarinic acid CRS* and *ferulic acid* in *water*.

(3) 0.06% w/v of *salvianolic acid B CRS* in the mobile phase.

CHROMATOGRAPHIC CONDITIONS

(a) Use a stainless steel column (25 cm × 4.6 mm) packed with *octadecylsilyl silica gel for chromatography* (5 µm) (Nucleosil ODS is suitable).

(b) Use isocratic elution and the mobile phase described below.

(c) Use a flow rate of 1 mL per minute.

(d) Use an ambient column temperature.

(e) Use a detection wavelength of 330 nm.

(f) Inject 20 µL of each solution.

MOBILE PHASE

22 volumes of *acetonitrile* and 78 volumes of 0.4% v/v of *formic acid*.

SYSTEM SUITABILITY

The test is not valid unless, in the chromatogram obtained with solution (2), the *resolution factor* between the two main peaks, rosmarinic acid and ferulic acid, is at least 5.0.

DETERMINATION OF CONTENT

Rosmarinic acid Using the retention time and peak area from the chromatogram obtained with solution (2), locate and integrate the peak due to rosmarinic acid in the chromatogram obtained with solution (1).

Calculate the content of rosmarinic acid in the sample using the declared content of rosmarinic acid ($C_{18}H_{16}O_8$) in *rosmarinic acid CRS* and the following expression:

$$\frac{A_1}{A_2} \times \frac{m_2}{V_2} \times \frac{V_1}{m_1} \times p \times \frac{100}{100-d}$$

A_1 =   Area of the peak due to rosmarinic acid in the chromatogram obtained with solution (1).

A_2 =   Area of the peak due to rosmarinic acid in the chromatogram obtained with solution (2).

m_1 =   Weight of the drug in mg.

m_2 =   Weight of *rosmarinic acid CRS* in mg.

V_1 =   Dilution volume of solution (1) in mL.

V_2 =   Dilution volume of solution (2) in mL.

p =   Percentage content of rosmarinic acid in *rosmarinic acid CRS*.

d =   Percentage loss on drying of the herbal drug being examined.

Salvianolic acid B Using the retention time and peak area from the chromatogram obtained with solution (3), locate and integrate the peak due to salvianolic acid B in the chromatogram obtained with solution (1).

Calculate the content of salvianolic acid B in the sample using the declared content of salvianolic acid B ($C_{36}H_{36}O_{16}$) in *salvianolic acid B CRS* and the following expression:

$$\frac{A_1}{A_2} \times \frac{m_2}{V_2} \times \frac{V_1}{m_1} \times p \times \frac{100}{100-d}$$

A_1 =   Area of the peak due to salvianolic acid in the chromatogram obtained with solution (1).

A_2 =   Area of the peak due to salvianolic acid in the chromatogram obtained with solution (3).

m_1 =   Weight of the drug in mg.

m_2 =   Weight of *salvianolic acid B CRS* in mg.

V_1 =   Dilution volume of solution (1) in mL.

V_2 =   Dilution volume of solution (2) in mL.

p =   Percentage content of salvianolic acid B in *salvianolic acid B CRS*.

d =   Percentage loss on drying of the herbal drug being examined.

STORAGE
Processed Salvia Miltiorrhiza Rhizome and Root should be protected from moisture.

Saw Palmetto Fruit

(Ph Eur monograph 1848)

Ph Eur _____

DEFINITION
Dried ripe fruit of *Serenoa repens* (W. Bartram) Small (Syn. *Sabal serrulata* (Michaux) T. Nuttal ex Schultes & Schultes).

Content
Minimum 11.0 per cent of total fatty acids (dried drug).

CHARACTERS
Odour
Strong but not rancid.

IDENTIFICATION
First identification   A, B, D.
Second identification   A, B, C.

A. The fruit is an ovoid or subspherical drupe, with a dark brown or blackish, roughly wrinkled surface and more or less coppery sheen, up to 2.5 cm long and 1.5 cm in diameter. The apex sometimes bears the remains of the style and tubular calyx, with 3 teeth, and the base bears a small depression with the scar of the stalk. The epicarp and underlying mesocarp form a thin fragile layer, which partially peels off, revealing the thin, hard, pale brown endocarp, which is fibrous and easily separable. The seed is irregularly spherical or ovoid, up to 12 mm long and 8 mm in diameter, with a hard, smooth or finely pitted surface which is reddish-brown with a paler, raised and membranous area over the raphe and micropyle; cut transversely, the seed has a thin testa, narrow perisperm and a large area of dense, horny, greyish-white endosperm, with the embryo positioned to one side.

B. Microscopic examination (*2.8.23*). Reduce to a powder (710) (*2.9.12*). The powder is reddish or blackish-brown and oily. Examine under a microscope using *chloral hydrate solution R*. The powder shows the following diagnostic characters: fragments of epicarp composed of several layers of thin-walled, reddish-brown, pigmented, polyhedral cells

(10-40 µm) which are strongly cuticularised; those of the outer layers are much smaller than those of the inner layers. Parenchyma cells of the mesocarp may be large and filled with oil droplets, or smaller and containing nodules of silica. Groups of xylem tissue of the mesocarp show small lignified, annular or spirally thickened vessels. Stone cells of the mesocarp (20-200 µm) may be found scattered, usually singly but sometimes in small groups, the walls are moderately thickened, distinctly striated and finely pitted. Fragments of endocarp contain groups of elongated sclereids about 300 µm long, with strongly thickened walls and numerous pits. The seed testa consists of small, thin-walled cells with brownish contents and underlying sclereids; albumen cells are thick-walled with large conspicuous pits and contain aleurone grains and fixed oil.

C. Thin-layer chromatography (*2.2.27*).

Test solution   To 1.5 g of the powdered herbal drug (710) (*2.9.12*), add 20 mL of *ethanol (96 per cent) R* and stir for 15 min. Filter.

Reference solution   Dissolve 4 mg of *β-amyrin R* and 10 mg of *β-sitosterol R* in 10 mL of *ethanol (96 per cent) R*.

Plate   *TLC silica gel plate R* (5-40 µm) [or *TLC silica gel plate R* (2-10 µm)].

Mobile phase   acetic acid R, ethyl acetate R, toluene R (1:30:70 *V/V/V*).

Application   10 µL [or 2 µL] as bands of 10 mm [or 8 mm].

Development   Over a path of 10 cm [or 6 cm].

Drying   In air.

Detection   Treat with *anisaldehyde solution R*; heat at 100-105 °C for 5-10 min; examine in daylight.

Results   See below the sequence of zones present in the chromatograms obtained with the reference solution and the test solution. Furthermore, other faint zones may be present, especially in the lower third, in the chromatogram obtained with the test solution.

Top of the plate	
	A strong blue zone
————	————
	2 faint blue zones
β-Amyrin: a blue zone	
	A strong bluish-violet zone
β-Sitosterol: a blue zone	A faint blue zone
————	————
	A faint blue zone
Reference solution	**Test solution**

D. Examine the chromatograms obtained in the assay of total fatty acids.

Results   The peaks due to caproic, caprylic, capric, lauric, myristic, palmitoleic, palmitic, linoleic, linolenic, oleic and stearic acids in the chromatogram obtained with the test solution are similar in retention time to the corresponding peaks in the chromatogram obtained with reference solution (b); the principal peaks are due to lauric acid and oleic acid.

TESTS

Loss on drying (*2.2.32*)
Maximum 12.0 per cent, determined on 1.000 g of the powdered herbal drug (710) (*2.9.12*) by drying in an oven at 105 °C for 2 h.

Total ash (*2.4.16*)
Maximum 5.0 per cent.

ASSAY

Total fatty acids
Gas chromatography (*2.2.28*).

Internal standard solution   Dissolve 0.47 g of *methyl margarate R* in 20.0 mL of *dimethylformamide R* and dilute to 100.0 mL with the same solvent.

Test solution   Reduce 50 g of the herbal drug to a powder (200) (*2.9.12*). Disperse 4.00 g of the powdered herbal drug in 60 mL of *dimethylformamide R*. Sonicate for 15 min and then shake for 30 min. Dilute to 100.0 mL with *dimethylformamide R*. Allow to stand for a few minutes and filter. To 20.0 mL of this solution add 4.0 mL of the internal standard solution and dilute to 25.0 mL with *dimethylformamide R*. Mix 0.4 mL of this solution and 0.6 mL of an 18.84 g/L solution of *trimethylsulfonium hydroxide R* in *methanol R*.

Reference solution (a)   Dissolve 0.699 g of *lauric acid CRS* and 0.870 g of *oleic acid CRS* in *dimethylformamide R* and dilute to 10.0 mL with the same solvent. To 1.0 mL of the solution add 4.0 mL of the internal standard solution and dilute to 25.0 mL with *dimethylformamide R*. Mix 0.4 mL of this solution and 0.6 mL of an 18.84 g/L solution of *trimethylsulfonium hydroxide R* in *methanol R*.

Reference solution (b)   Disperse 0.25 g of *saw palmetto extract HRS* in 10 mL of *dimethylformamide R*. Add 4.0 mL of the internal standard solution and dilute to 25.0 mL with *dimethylformamide R*. Mix 0.4 mL of this solution and 0.6 mL of an 18.84 g/L solution of *trimethylsulfonium hydroxide R* in *methanol R*.

Column:
— *material*: fused silica;
— *size*: $l = 25$ m, $\varnothing = 0.20$ mm;
— *stationary phase*: *poly(dimethyl)siloxane R* (film thickness 0.33 µm).

Carrier gas   helium for chromatography R.

Flow rate   0.5 mL/min.

Split ratio   1:40.

Temperature:

	Time (min)	Temperature (°C)
Column	0 - 2	150
	2 - 7	150 → 190
	7 - 12	190
	12 - 22	190 → 220
	22 - 32	220
Injection port		300
Detector		300

Detection   Flame ionisation.

Injection   1 µL.

Identification of peaks   Use the chromatogram supplied with *saw palmetto extract HRS* and the chromatogram obtained with reference solution (b) to identify the peaks due to caproic, caprylic, capric, lauric, myristic, palmitoleic, palmitic, linoleic, linolenic, oleic and stearic acids and methyl margarate.

System suitability   Reference solution (b):
— *peak-to-valley ratio*: minimum 1.2, where H_p = height above the baseline of the peak due to linolenic acid and H_v = height above the baseline of the lowest point of the curve separating this peak from the peak due to linoleic acid.

Calculate the percentage content of total fatty acids, where caproic, caprylic, capric, lauric, myristic, palmitoleic, palmitic and stearic acids are expressed as lauric acid ($C_{12}H_{24}O_2$; M_r 200.3) and linoleic, linolenic and oleic acids are expressed as oleic acid ($C_{18}H_{34}O_2$; M_r 282.5), using the following expression:

$$\frac{A_1 \times A_4 \times m_2 \times p_1 \times 0.5}{A_2 \times A_3 \times m_1} + \frac{A_5 \times A_4 \times m_3 \times p_2 \times 0.5}{A_6 \times A_3 \times m_1}$$

A_1 = sum of the areas of the peaks due to caproic, caprylic, capric, lauric, myristic, palmitoleic, palmitic and stearic acids in the chromatogram obtained with the test solution;

A_2 = area of the peak due to lauric acid in the chromatogram obtained with reference solution (a);

A_3 = area of the peak due to methyl margarate in the chromatogram obtained with the test solution;

A_4 = area of the peak due to methyl margarate in the chromatogram obtained with reference solution (a);

A_5 = sum of the areas of the peaks due to linoleic, linolenic and oleic acids in the chromatogram obtained with the test solution;

A_6 = area of the peak due to oleic acid in the chromatogram obtained with reference solution (a);

m_1 = mass of the herbal drug to be examined used to prepare the test solution, in grams;

m_2 = mass of *lauric acid CRS* used to prepare reference solution (a), in grams;

m_3 = mass of *oleic acid CRS* used to prepare reference solution (a), in grams;

p_1 = percentage content of lauric acid in *lauric acid CRS*;

p_2 = percentage content of oleic acid in *oleic acid CRS*.

Ph Eur

Schisandra Fruit

(*Ph Eur monograph 2428*)

Ph Eur

DEFINITION
Whole, dried or steamed and dried, ripe fruit of *Schisandra chinensis* (Turcz.) Baill.

Content
Minimum 0.40 per cent of schisandrin ($C_{24}H_{32}O_7$; M_r 432.5) (dried drug).

IDENTIFICATION
A. The berry is more or less spherical, up to 8 mm in diameter; red, reddish-brown or blackish outer surface, sometimes covered in a whitish frost; strongly shrivelled pericarp; presence of 1-2 reniform, yellowish-brown, lustrous seeds, with thin seed-coat.

B. Reduce to a powder (355) (*2.9.12*). The powder is reddish-brown. Examine under a microscope using *chloral hydrate solution R*. The powder shows the following diagnostic characters: reddish-brown fragments of pericarp, consisting of 1 layer of thin-walled epicarp cells, accompanied by sparse oil cells and several layers of ovoid, more-or-less flattened mesocarp cells; fragments of the outer testa of the seed consisting of thick-walled, finely channelled sclereids, polygonal in surface view (15-50 μm in diameter) and in palisade arrangement in side view; fragments of the inner testa with sclereids, isolated or in small groups, about 80 μm in diameter, with slightly thickened and markedly channelled walls; fragments of endosperm consisting of polyhedral cells containing oil droplets and aleurone grains. Examine under a microscope using a 50 per cent *V/V* solution of *glycerol R*: the powder shows parenchymatous cells of the mesocarp containing numerous small, round starch granules.

C. Examine the chromatograms obtained in the test for *Schisandra sphenanthera*.

Results A   See below the sequence of quenching zones present in the chromatograms obtained with the reference solution and the test solution. Furthermore, other weak quenching zones may be present in the chromatogram obtained with the test solution.

Top of the plate	
γ-Schisandrin: a quenching zone	A quenching zone (γ-schisandrin)
———	———
	A weak quenching zone
———	———
Schisandrin: a quenching zone	A quenching zone (schisandrin)
Reference solution	**Test solution**

Results B   See below the sequence of zones present in the chromatograms obtained with the reference solution and the test solution. Furthermore, other faint zones may be present in the chromatogram obtained with the test solution.

Top of the plate	
γ-Schisandrin: a brown zone	A brown zone (γ-schisandrin)
———	———
———	———
Schisandrin: an intense, brownish-green zone	An intense, brownish-green zone (schisandrin)
Reference solution	**Test solution**

TESTS
Schisandra sphenanthera
Thin-layer chromatography (*2.2.27*).

Test solution   To 2.5 g of the powdered drug (355) (*2.9.12*) add 10 mL of *methanol R*. Extract at 25 °C in an ultrasonic bath for 5 min and centrifuge.

Reference solution   Dissolve 5 mg of *schisandrin R* and 5 mg of *γ-schisandrin R* in 5 mL of *methanol R*.

Plate   *TLC silica gel F_{254} plate R* (5-40 μm) [or *TLC silica gel F_{254} plate R* (2-10 μm)].

Mobile phase   acetic acid R, ethyl acetate R, toluene R (2:22:46 *V/V/V*).

Application   5 μL [or 2 μL] as bands of 10 mm [or 6 mm].

Development   Over a path of 10 cm [or 7 cm].

Drying In air.

Detection A Examine in ultraviolet light at 254 nm.

Detection B Spray with a 100 g/L solution of *sulfuric acid R* in *methanol R* and heat in an oven at 120 °C for 7 min; examine in daylight.

Results B The chromatogram obtained with the test solution shows a zone due to schisandrin and a zone due to γ-schisandrin; the chromatogram shows no intense violet-pink zone in the middle third.

Loss on drying *(2.2.32)*
Maximum 10.0 per cent, determined on 1.000 g of the powdered drug (355) *(2.9.12)* by drying in an oven at 105 °C for 2 h.

Total ash *(2.4.16)*
Maximum 6.0 per cent.

ASSAY
Liquid chromatography *(2.2.29)*.

Test solution Weigh 1.250 g of the powdered drug (355) *(2.9.12)* into a 250 mL conical flask, add 90 mL of *methanol R* and sonicate for 30 min. Filter the solution into a volumetric flask, add 10 mL of *methanol R* whilst rinsing the filter and dilute to 100.0 mL with the same solvent.

Reference solution Dissolve 5.0 mg of *schisandrin R* in *methanol R* and dilute to 100.0 mL with the same solvent.

Column:
— *size: l = 0.25 m, Ø = 4.6 mm;*
— *stationary phase: end-capped octadecylsilyl silica gel for chromatography R;*
— *temperature: 25 °C.*

Mobile phase:
— *mobile phase A: water R, methanol R (35:65 V/V);*
— *mobile phase B: methanol R;*

Time (min)	Mobile phase A (per cent *V/V*)	Mobile phase B (per cent *V/V*)
0 - 10	100	0
10 - 16	100 → 58	0 → 42
16 - 26	58	42

Flow rate 1 mL/min.

Detection Spectrophotometer at 250 nm.

Injection 10 μL.

Retention time Schisandrin = about 8 min.

System suitability:
— *number of theoretical plates*: minimum 5000, calculated for the peak due to schisandrin in the chromatogram obtained with the reference solution.

Calculate the percentage content of schisandrin using the following expression:

$$\frac{A_1 \times m_2 \times p}{A_2 \times m_1}$$

A_1 = area of the peak due to schisandrin in the chromatogram obtained with the test solution;
A_2 = area of the peak due to schisandrin in the chromatogram obtained with the reference solution;
m_1 = mass of the drug to be examined used to prepare the test solution, in grams;
m_2 = mass of *schisandrin R* used to prepare the reference solution, in grams;
p = percentage content of schisandrin in *schisandrin R*.

Scutellariae Baicalensis Root

(Baical Skullcap Root, Ph Eur monograph 2438)

Ph Eur

DEFINITION
Dried, peeled, usually fragmented root of *Scutellaria baicalensis* Georgi without rootlets. It is collected in spring or autumn.

Content
Not less than 9.0 per cent of baicalin ($C_{21}H_{18}O_{11}$; M_r 446.4) (dried drug).

IDENTIFICATION
A. The root is conical, twisted and, if not reduced in size, 8-25 cm long and 1-3 cm in diameter. The outer surface is brownish-yellow or dark yellow, bearing sparse, warty traces of rootlets, the upper part rough, with twisted longitudinal wrinkles or irregular reticula, the lower part with longitudinal striations and fine wrinkles. Texture hard and fragile, easily broken, fracture yellow, reddish-brown in the centre; the central part of an old root dark brown or brownish-black, withered or hollowed.

B. Microscopic examination *(2.8.23)*. The powder is yellow or light brown. Examine under a microscope using *chloral hydrate solution R*. The powder shows the following diagnostic characters: phloem fibres, single or in bundles, fusiform, 60-250 μm long, 9-33 μm in diameter, with thick, channelled walls; stone cells sub-spherical, square or rectangular with rounded edges, with thickened walls, sometimes heavily; cork cells polygonal and brownish-yellow; numerous reticulated vessels, 24-72 μm in diameter; lignified fibres frequently broken, about 12 μm in diameter, with sparse, oblique pits. Examine under a microscope using a 50 per cent *V/V* solution of *glycerol R*. The powder shows abundant starch granules, simple, spheroidal, 2-10 μm in diameter, with a distinct hilum, or compound with 2-3 components.

C. Thin-layer chromatography *(2.2.27)*.

Test solution To 1 g of the powdered herbal drug (355) *(2.9.12)* add 10 mL of *methanol R* and sonicate for 10 min. Centrifuge and use the supernatant.

Reference solution Dissolve 1 mg of *baicalin R* and 1 mg of *acteoside R* in 10 mL of *methanol R*.

Plate TLC silica gel F_{254} plate R (2-10 μm).

Mobile phase acetic acid R, formic acid R, water R, ethyl acetate R (1:1:2:15 *V/V/V/V*).

Application 10 μL as bands.

Development Over a path of 6 cm.

Drying In air.

Detection Heat at 100-105 °C for 3 min, treat with a 10 g/L solution of *diphenylboric acid aminoethyl ester R* in *methanol R*, then treat with a 50 g/L solution of *macrogol 400 R* in *methanol R*, allow to dry in air for 30 min and examine in ultraviolet light at 365 nm.

Results See below the sequence of zones present in the chromatograms obtained with the reference solution and the test solution. Furthermore, other faint blue fluorescent zones may be present in the chromatogram obtained with the test solution.

Top of the plate	
	3-4 fluorescent zones
	2 fluorescent zones
Verbascoside: a blue fluorescent zone	A strong blue fluorescent zone
	A blue fluorescent zone
Baicalin: a black zone	A black zone
	A weak yellow fluorescent zone
Reference solution	**Test solution**

TESTS

Loss on drying (*2.2.32*)
Maximum 12.0 per cent, determined on 1.000 g of the powdered herbal drug (355) (*2.9.12*) by drying in an oven at 105 °C for 2 h.

Total ash (*2.4.16*)
Maximum 6.0 per cent.

Ash insoluble in hydrochloric acid (*2.8.1*)
Maximum 2.0 per cent.

ASSAY

Liquid chromatography (*2.2.29*).

Test solution   To 0.300 g of the powdered herbal drug (355) (*2.9.12*) add 40 mL of *ethanol (70 per cent V/V) R*, heat under a reflux condenser on a water bath for 3 h, cool and filter. Transfer the filtrate to a 100 mL volumetric flask. Wash both the container and the residue several times with a small volume of *ethanol (70 per cent V/V) R* and filter the washings into the same flask. Dilute to 100.0 mL with *ethanol (70 per cent V/V) R*. Mix well. Dilute 1.0 mL of the solution to 10.0 mL with *methanol R*. Mix well.

Reference solution (a)   Dissolve 5.0 mg of *baicalin CRS* in *methanol R* and dilute to 100.0 mL with the same solvent.

Reference solution (b)   Dissolve 2 mg of *methyl parahydroxybenzoate R* in *methanol R*, add 20 mL of reference solution (a) and dilute to 100 mL with *methanol R*.

Column:
— *size*: l = 0.125 m, Ø = 4 mm;
— *stationary phase*: *octadecylsilyl silica gel for chromatography R* (5 μm).

Mobile phase:
— *mobile phase A*: 0.1 per cent *V/V* solution of *phosphoric acid R*;
— *mobile phase B*: *acetonitrile R*;

Time (min)	Mobile phase A (per cent *V/V*)	Mobile phase B (per cent *V/V*)
0 - 30	90 → 60	10 → 40

Flow rate   1.0 mL/min.

Detection   Spectrophotometer at 280 nm.

Injection   10 μL.

Retention time   Methyl parahydroxybenzoate = about 15 min; baicalin = about 16 min.

System suitability   Reference solution (b):
— *resolution*: minimum 3 between the peaks due to methyl parahydroxybenzoate and baicalin.

Calculate the percentage content of baicalin using the following expression:

$$\frac{m_2 \times S_1 \times 10 \times p}{S_2 \times m_1}$$

m_1 = mass of the herbal drug, in grams;
m_2 = mass of baicalin used to prepare reference solution (a), in grams;
S_1 = area of the peak due to baicalin in the chromatogram obtained with the test solution;
S_2 = area of the peak due to baicalin in the chromatogram obtained with reference solution (a);
p = percentage content of baicalin in *baicalin CRS*.

STORAGE
Protected from moisture.

Ph Eur

Selfheal Fruit-Spike

(*Common Selfheal Fruit-Spike,*
Ph Eur monograph 2439)

Ph Eur

DEFINITION
Dried fruit-spike of *Prunella vulgaris* L.

Content
Minimum 0.12 per cent of the sum of oleanolic acid ($C_{30}H_{48}O_3$; M_r 456.7) and ursolic acid ($C_{30}H_{48}O_3$; M_r 456.7), expressed as ursolic acid, of which not less than 70.0 per cent consists of ursolic acid (dried drug).

IDENTIFICATION
A. Cylindrical, somewhat flattened, 1.5-8 cm long, 0.8-1.5 cm in diameter, accompanied by remains of the stem up to 15 cm long, pale brown or brownish-red. The whole spike is composed of up to 10 or more whorls of persistent calyx and bracts, each whorl with 2 opposite bracts, fan-shaped, apex acuminate, striations of vein distinct, the outer surface with white hairs. Each bract is accompanied by 3 flowers, with a persistent bilabiate calyx, and whose corolla is often missing, and by 4 small brown ovoid nutlets, white and convex at the acute end. Calyx closed in the fruit stage.

B. Microscopic examination (*2.8.23*). The powder is reddish-brown or brown. Examine under a microscope using *chloral hydrate solution R*. The powder shows the following diagnostic characters: very numerous covering trichomes, multicellular, scattered, usually broken, sometimes exceeding 1 mm long and 125 μm wide at the base, with spiny walls, upper cell usually short and acuminate, fine needle-shaped crystals may be visible in the cells; fragments of the bracts, in surface view, with lobed epidermal cells, trichomes mostly unicellular and occasionally bi- or tricellular, conical, acute, short, serrate; diacytic stomata (*2.8.3*) usually accompanied by 2 subsidiary cells very unequal in size and rare glandular trichomes with a unicellular stalk and a bicellular head; fragments of the bracts and/or calyx margins with numerous serrate trichomes pointing towards the same direction; fragments of the calyx, in surface view, composed of lobed cells strongly thickened and deeply grooved; fragments of reticulate or bordered pitted vessels from the stems; rare fragments of the nucules having a pericarp composed of palisade-like mucilaginous cells accompanied by polygonal cells with thickened walls and granular coloured contents;

fragments of endosperm with oily contents; very numerous oil droplets; glandular trichomes of laminaceous type with 4 secretory cells may be present.

C. Thin-layer chromatography (2.2.27).

Test solution   To 0.5 g of the powdered herbal drug (355) (2.9.12) add 5 mL of *methanol R*, sonicate for 10 min and centrifuge; use the supernatant.

Reference solution   Dissolve 1 mg of *β-sitosterol R* and 1 mg of *ursolic acid R* in 2 mL of *methanol R*.

Plate   *TLC silica gel F₂₅₄ plate R* (5-40 µm) [or *TLC silica gel F₂₅₄ plate R* (2-10 µm)].

Mobile phase   glacial acetic acid R, ethyl acetate R, cyclohexane R (0.5:8:20 V/V/V).

Application   10 µL [or 4 µL] as bands of 10 mm [or 8 mm].

Development   Over a path of 12 cm [or 6 cm].

Drying   In air.

Detection   Treat with a 10 per cent *V/V* solution of *sulfuric acid R* in *anhydrous ethanol R* and heat at 100 °C for 3 min; examine in ultraviolet light at 365 nm.

Results   See below the sequence of zones present in the chromatograms obtained with the reference solution and the test solution. Furthermore, other faint zones may be present in the chromatogram obtained with the test solution.

Top of the plate	
	A pale violet fluorescent zone
———	———
	2 faint yellow fluorescent zones
β-sitosterol: a violet fluorescent zone	
Ursolic acid: a yellowish-orange fluorescent zone	A yellowish-orange fluorescent zone (ursolic acid)
———	———
	2 faint green fluorescent zones
Reference solution	Test solution

if

TESTS

Foreign matter (2.8.2)
Maximum 5 per cent of stems longer than 15 cm and maximum 2 per cent of other foreign matter.

Loss on drying (2.2.32)
Maximum 12.0 per cent, determined on 1.000 g of the powdered herbal drug (355) (2.9.12) by drying in an oven at 105 °C.

Total ash (2.4.16)
Maximum 12.0 per cent.

Ash insoluble in hydrochloric acid (2.8.1)
Maximum 4.0 per cent.

ASSAY

Liquid chromatography (2.2.29).

Solvent mixture   methanol R, 1,1-dimethylethyl methyl ether R (20:80 V/V).

Test solution   Disperse 2.000 g of the powdered herbal drug (355) (2.9.12) in 20 mL of the solvent mixture, heat under reflux at 80 °C for 30 min and filter. Repeat the extraction twice. Combine the filtrates and dilute to 100.0 mL with the solvent mixture. Evaporate 50.0 mL of this solution to dryness at 40 °C. Dissolve the residue in 1.0 mL of

1,1-dimethylethyl methyl ether R. Rinse the flask 4 times with 1.0 mL of *1,1-dimethylethyl methyl ether R*. Pre-condition a 3 mL solid phase extraction column, containing 500 mg of *aminopropylsilyl silica gel for chromatography R1*, using 2 mL of *methanol R* followed by 2 mL of *1,1-dimethylethyl methyl ether R*. Subsequently apply the solution and the washings to the pre-conditioned column. Wash the column with 1.0 mL of *1,1-dimethylethyl methyl ether R* followed by 5 quantities, each of 1.0 mL, of *methanol R*. Apply 1.0 mL of a 2 per cent *V/V* solution of *anhydrous formic acid R* in *methanol R* and elute after 5 min. Repeat the elution 3 times and dilute the eluates to 5.0 mL with a 2 per cent *V/V* solution of *anhydrous formic acid R* in *methanol R*.

Solution A   Dissolve 10.0 mg of *ursolic acid CRS* in *methanol R* and dilute to 10.0 mL with the same solvent.

Reference solution (a)   Dilute 1.0 mL of solution A to 10.0 mL with a 2 per cent *V/V* solution of *anhydrous formic acid R* in *methanol R*.

Reference solution (b)   Dissolve 10.0 mg of *oleanolic acid R* in *methanol R* and dilute to 10.0 mL with the same solvent. Mix 1.0 mL of the solution and 1.0 mL of solution A and dilute to 10.0 mL with a 2 per cent *V/V* solution of *anhydrous formic acid R* in *methanol R*.

Column:
— *size: l = 0.15 m, Ø = 4.6 mm;*
— *stationary phase: octadecylsilyl silica gel for chromatography R* (5 µm).

Mobile phase   Mix 25 volumes of a 4.6 g/L solution of *ammonium dihydrogen phosphate R* adjusted to pH 6.0 with *strong sodium hydroxide solution R*, 35 volumes of *methanol R1* and 40 volumes of *acetonitrile R1*.

Flow rate   1.0 mL/min.

Detection   Spectrophotometer at 205 nm.

Injection   20 µL.

Run time   1.1 times the retention time of ursolic acid.

Elution order   Oleanolic acid, ursolic acid.

Relative retention   With reference to ursolic acid (retention time = about 28 min): oleanolic acid = about 0.9.

System suitability   Reference solution (b):
— *resolution*: minimum 1.5 between the peaks due to oleanolic acid and ursolic acid.

Calculate the percentage contents of ursolic acid and oleanolic acid, expressed as ursolic acid, using the following equations:

$$n_1 = \frac{A_1 \times m_2 \times p \times 0.1}{A_2 \times m_1}$$

$$n_2 = \frac{A_3 \times m_2 \times p \times 0.1}{A_2 \times m_1}$$

n_1 = percentage content of ursolic acid;
n_2 = percentage content of oleanolic acid;
A_1 = area of the peak due to ursolic acid in the chromatogram obtained with the test solution;
A_2 = area of the peak due to ursolic acid in the chromatogram obtained with reference solution (a);
A_3 = area of the peak due to oleanolic acid in the chromatogram obtained with the test solution;
m_1 = mass of the herbal drug to be examined used to prepare the test solution, in grams;
m_2 = mass of *ursolic acid CRS* used to prepare solution A, in grams;

p = assigned percentage content of ursolic acid in *ursolic acid CRS*.

Calculate the sum of the percentage contents of ursolic acid and oleanolic acid ($n_1 + n_2$) and the relative content of ursolic acid using the following expression:

$$\frac{n_1 \times 100}{(n_1 + n_2)}$$

——————————————————————— Ph Eur

Senega Root

Senega

(*Ph Eur monograph 0202*)

When Powdered Senega Root is prescribed or demanded, material complying with the requirements below with the exception of Identification test A and the test for Foreign matter shall be dispensed or supplied.

Ph Eur ————————————————————————

DEFINITION

Dried and usually fragmented root and root crown of *Polygala senega* L. or of certain other closely related species or of a mixture of these *Polygala* species.

CHARACTERS

Faint, sweet odour, slightly rancid or reminiscent of methyl salicylate.

Reduced to a powder, it is irritant and sternutatory. Shaken with water, the powder produces a copious froth.

IDENTIFICATION

A. The root crown is greyish-brown and wider than the root; it forms an irregular head consisting of numerous remains of stems and tightly packed purplish-brown buds. The taproot is brown or yellow, occasionally branched, sometimes flexuous, usually tortuous and without secondary roots, except in the Japanese varieties and species, which contain numerous fibrous rootlets. The diameter is usually 1-8 mm at the crown, gradually tapering to the tip; the surface is transversely and longitudinally striated and often shows a more or less distinct decurrent, elongated spiral keel. The fracture is short and shows a yellowish cortex of varying thickness surrounding a paler central woody area somewhat circular or irregular in shape depending on the species.

B. Examine under a microscope using *chloral hydrate solution R*. The transverse section of the root shows the following diagnostic characters: cork formed from several layers of thin-walled cells, phelloderm of slightly collenchymatous cells containing droplets of oil; the phloem and xylem arrangement is usually normal, especially near the crown but where a keel is present this is formed by increased development of phloem; other anomalous secondary development sometimes occurs, resulting in the formation of 1 or 2 large wedge-shaped rays in the phloem and xylem, the parenchymatous cells of which contain droplets of oil. The xylem is usually central and consists of vessels up to 60 µm in diameter associated with numerous thin-walled tracheids and a few small lignified parenchymatous cells.

C. Reduce to a powder (355) (*2.9.12*). The powder is light brown. Examine under a microscope using *chloral hydrate solution R*. The powder shows the following diagnostic characters: longitudinal fragments of lignified tissue made up of pitted tracheids and somewhat larger vessels with numerous bordered pits or with reticulate thickening;

yellowish parenchyma and collenchymatous cells containing droplets of oil; occasional fragments of cork, and of epidermal tissue with stomata and unicellular trichomes from the bud scales. Crystals and stone cells are absent.

D. Thin-layer chromatography (*2.2.27*).

Test solution To 1.0 g of the powdered drug (355) (*2.9.12*) add 10 mL of *ethanol (70 per cent V/V) R*, boil under a reflux condenser for 15 min, filter and allow to cool.

Reference solution Dissolve 10 mg of *aescin R* in *ethanol (70 per cent V/V) R* and dilute to 10 mL with the same solvent.

Plate TLC *silica gel G plate R*.

Mobile phase The upper layer of a mixture of 10 volumes of *glacial acetic acid R*, 40 volumes of *water R* and 50 volumes of *butanol R*.

Application 10 µL of the test solution and 10 µL and 40 µL of the reference solution, as bands of 20 mm by 3 mm.

Development Over a path of 12 cm.

Drying At 100-105 °C.

Detection A Spray with about 10 mL of *anisaldehyde solution R* for a plate 200 mm square and heat again at 100-105 °C until red zones due to saponosides appear in the chromatogram obtained with the test solution.

Results A In the chromatogram obtained with the test solution, 3-5 red zones appear in the lower and middle parts, similar in position to the grey-violet zones due to aescin in the chromatogram obtained with the reference solution.

Detection B Spray with about 10 mL of a 200 g/L solution of *phosphomolybdic acid R* in *anhydrous ethanol R* and heat at 100-105 °C until the zones due to saponosides become blue.

Results B The intensity and size of the zones in the chromatogram obtained with the test solution are between those of the 2 bands due to aescin in the chromatograms obtained with 10 µL and 40 µL of the reference solution.

TESTS

Total ash (*2.4.16*)

Maximum 6.0 per cent.

Ash insoluble in hydrochloric acid (*2.8.1*)

Maximum 3.0 per cent.

STORAGE

Store protected from humidity.

——————————————————————— Ph Eur

Alexandrian Senna Fruit

(*Alexandrian Senna Pods, Ph Eur monograph 0207*)

Preparations

Senna Liquid Extract

Standardised Senna Granules

Senna Tablets

When Powdered Alexandrian Senna Fruit is prescribed or demanded, material complying with the requirements below, with the exception of Identification test A and the test for Foreign matter, shall be dispensed or supplied.

Ph Eur ————————————————————————

DEFINITION

Dried fruit of *Cassia senna* L. (*C. acutifolia* Delile).

Content

Minimum 3.4 per cent of hydroxyanthracene glycosides, expressed as sennoside B ($C_{42}H_{38}O_{20}$; M_r 863) (dried drug).

CHARACTERS
Slight odour.

IDENTIFICATION
A. Flattened reniform pods, green or greenish-brown with brown patches at the positions corresponding to the seeds, usually 40-50 mm long and at least 20 mm wide. At one end is a stylar point and at the other a short stalk. The pods contain 6-7 flattened and obovate seeds, green or pale brown, with a continuous network of prominent ridges on the testa.

B. Reduce to a powder (355) (*2.9.12*). The powder is brown. Examine under a microscope using *chloral hydrate solution R*. The powder shows the following diagnostic characters: epicarp with polygonal cells and a small number of conical warty trichomes and occasional anomocytic or paracytic stomata (*2.8.3*); fibres in 2 crossed layers accompanied by a crystal sheath of calcium oxalate prisms; characteristic palisade cells in the seed and stratified cells in the endosperm; clusters and prisms of calcium oxalate.

C. Thin-layer chromatography (*2.2.27*).

Test solution   To 0.5 g of the powdered drug (180) (*2.9.12*) add 5 mL of a mixture of equal volumes of *ethanol (96 per cent) R* and *water R* and heat to boiling. Centrifuge and use the supernatant liquid.

Reference solution   Dissolve 10 mg of *senna extract CRS* in 1 mL of a mixture of equal volumes of *ethanol (96 per cent) R* and *water R* (a slight residue remains).

Plate   TLC *silica gel G plate R*.

Mobile phase   *glacial acetic acid R*, *water R*, *ethyl acetate R*, *propanol R* (1:30:40:40 *V/V/V/V*).

Application   10 µL, as bands of 20 mm by 2 mm.

Development   Over a path of 10 cm.

Drying   In air.

Detection   Spray with a 20 per cent *V/V* solution of *nitric acid R* and heat at 120 °C for 10 min; allow to cool and spray with a 50 g/L solution of *potassium hydroxide R* in *ethanol (50 per cent V/V) R* until the zones appear.

Results   The principal zones in the chromatogram obtained with the test solution are similar in position (sennosides B, A, D and C in order of increasing R_F value), colour and size to the principal zones in the chromatogram obtained with the reference solution; between the zones due to sennosides D and C, a red zone due to rhein-8-glucoside may be visible; the zones due to sennosides D and C are faint in the chromatogram obtained with the test solution.

D. Place about 25 mg of the powdered drug (180) (*2.9.12*) in a conical flask and add 50 mL of *water R* and 2 mL of *hydrochloric acid R*. Heat in a water-bath for 15 min, cool and shake with 40 mL of *ether R*. Separate the ether layer, dry over *anhydrous sodium sulfate R*, evaporate 5 mL to dryness and to the cooled residue add 5 mL of *dilute ammonia R1*. A yellow or orange colour develops. Heat on a water-bath for 2 min. A reddish-violet colour develops.

TESTS
Foreign matter (*2.8.2*)
Maximum 1 per cent.

Loss on drying (*2.2.32*)
Maximum 12.0 per cent, determined on 1.000 g of the powdered drug (355) (*2.9.12*) by drying in an oven at 105 °C for 2 h.

Total ash (*2.4.16*)
Maximum 9.0 per cent.

Ash insoluble in hydrochloric acid (*2.8.1*)
Maximum 2.0 per cent.

ASSAY
Carry out the assay protected from bright light.

Place 0.150 g of the powdered drug (180) (*2.9.12*) in a 100 mL flask. Add 30.0 mL of *water R*, mix, weigh and place in a water-bath. Heat under a reflux condenser for 15 min. Allow to cool, weigh and adjust to the original mass with *water R*. Centrifuge and transfer 20.0 mL of the supernatant liquid to a 150 mL separating funnel. Add 0.1 mL of *dilute hydrochloric acid R* and shake with 3 quantities, each of 15 mL, of *chloroform R*. Allow to separate and discard the chloroform layer. Add 0.10 g of *sodium hydrogen carbonate R* and shake for 3 min. Centrifuge and transfer 10.0 mL of the supernatant liquid to a 100 mL round-bottomed flask with a ground-glass neck. Add 20 mL of *ferric chloride solution R1* and mix. Place the flask in a water-bath so that the water level is above that of the liquid in the flask, and heat under a reflux condenser for 20 min. Add 1 mL of *hydrochloric acid R* and heat for a further 20 min, with frequent shaking, to dissolve the precipitate. Cool, transfer the mixture to a separating funnel and shake with 3 quantities, each of 25 mL, of *ether R* previously used to rinse the flask. Combine the 3 ether layers and wash with 2 quantities, each of 15 mL, of *water R*. Transfer the ether layers to a volumetric flask and dilute to 100.0 mL with *ether R*. Evaporate 10.0 mL carefully to dryness and dissolve the residue in 10.0 mL of a 5 g/L solution of *magnesium acetate R* in *methanol R*. Measure the absorbance (*2.2.25*) at 515 nm using *methanol R* as the compensation liquid.

Calculate the percentage content of hydroxyanthracene glycosides, expressed as sennoside B, using the following expression:

$$\frac{A \times 1.25}{m}$$

i.e. taking the specific absorbance of sennoside B to be 240.
A = absorbance at 515 nm;
m = mass of the substance to be examined, in grams.

STORAGE
Protected from moisture.

_____ *Ph Eur*

Tinnevelly Senna Fruit

(*Tinnevelly Senna Pods, Ph Eur monograph 0208*)

Preparations
Senna Liquid Extract

Senna Tablets

When Powdered Tinnevelly Senna Fruit is prescribed or demanded, material complying with the requirements below with the exception of Identification test A and the test for Foreign matter shall be dispensed or supplied.

Ph Eur _____

DEFINITION
Dried fruit of *Cassia angustifolia* Vahl.

Content
Minimum 2.2 per cent of hydroxyanthracene glycosides, expressed as sennoside B ($C_{42}H_{38}O_{20}$; M_r 863) (dried drug).

CHARACTERS
Slight odour.

IDENTIFICATION
A. Flattened, slightly reniform pods, yellowish-brown or brown with dark brown patches at the positions corresponding to the seeds, usually 35-60 mm long and 14-18 mm wide. At one end is a stylar point and at the other a short stalk. The pods contain 5-8 flattened and obovate seeds, green or pale brown, with incomplete, wavy, transverse ridges on the testa.

B. Reduce to a powder (355) (*2.9.12*). The powder is brown. Examine under a microscope using *chloral hydrate solution R*. The powder shows the following diagnostic characters: epicarp with polygonal cells and a small number of conical warty trichomes and occasional anomocytic or paracytic stomata (*2.8.3*); fibres in 2 crossed layers accompanied by a crystal sheath of calcium oxalate prisms; characteristic palisade cells in the seed and stratified cells in the endosperm; clusters and prisms of calcium oxalate.

C. Thin-layer chromatography (*2.2.27*).

Test solution To 0.5 g of the powdered drug (180) (*2.9.12*) add 5 mL of a mixture of equal volumes of *ethanol (96 per cent) R* and *water R* and heat to boiling. Centrifuge and use the supernatant liquid.

Reference solution Dissolve 10 mg of *senna extract CRS* in 1 mL of a mixture of equal volumes of *ethanol (96 per cent) R* and *water R* (a slight residue remains).

Plate *TLC silica gel G plate R*.

Mobile phase glacial acetic acid R, water R, ethyl acetate R, propanol R (1:30:40:40 *V/V/V/V*).

Application 10 μL, as bands of 20 mm by 2 mm.

Development Over a path of 10 cm.

Drying In air.

Detection Spray with a 20 per cent *V/V* solution of *nitric acid R* and heat at 120 °C for 10 min; allow to cool and spray with a 50 g/L solution of *potassium hydroxide R* in *ethanol (50 per cent V/V) R* until the zones appear.

Results The principal zones in the chromatogram obtained with the test solution are similar in position (sennosides B, A, D and C in the order of increasing R_F value), colour and size to the principal zones in the chromatogram obtained with the reference solution. Between the zones due to sennosides D and C a red zone due to rhein-8-glucoside may be visible. The zones due to sennosides D and C are faint in the chromatogram obtained with the test solution.

D. Place about 25 mg of the powdered drug (180) (*2.9.12*) in a conical flask and add 50 mL of *water R* and 2 mL of *hydrochloric acid R*. Heat in a water-bath for 15 min, cool and shake with 40 mL of *ether R*. Separate the ether layer, dry over *anhydrous sodium sulfate R*, evaporate 5 mL to dryness and to the cooled residue add 5 mL of *dilute ammonia R1*. A yellow or orange colour develops. Heat on a water-bath for 2 min. A reddish-violet colour develops.

TESTS
Foreign matter (*2.8.2*)
Maximum 1 per cent.

Loss on drying (*2.2.32*)
Maximum 12.0 per cent, determined on 1.000 g of the powdered drug (355) (*2.9.12*) by drying in an oven at 105 °C for 2 h.

Total ash (*2.4.16*)
Maximum 9.0 per cent.

Ash insoluble in hydrochloric acid (*2.8.1*)
Maximum 2.0 per cent.

ASSAY
Carry out the assay protected from bright light.

Place 0.150 g of the powdered drug (180) (*2.9.12*) in a 100 mL flask. Add 30.0 mL of *water R*, mix, weigh and place in a water-bath. Heat under a reflux condenser for 15 min. Allow to cool, weigh and adjust to the original mass with *water R*. Centrifuge and transfer 20.0 mL of the supernatant liquid to a 150 mL separating funnel. Add 0.1 mL of *dilute hydrochloric acid R* and shake with 3 quantities, each of 15 mL, of *chloroform R*. Allow to separate and discard the chloroform layer. Add 0.10 g of *sodium hydrogen carbonate R* and shake for 3 min. Centrifuge and transfer 10.0 mL of the supernatant liquid to a 100 mL round-bottomed flask with a ground-glass neck. Add 20 mL of *ferric chloride solution R1* and mix. Heat for 20 min in a water-bath under a reflux condenser, with the water level above that of the liquid in the flask; add 1 mL of *hydrochloric acid R* and heat for a further 20 min, with frequent shaking, to dissolve the precipitate. Cool, transfer the mixture to a separating funnel and shake with 3 quantities, each of 25 mL, of *ether R* previously used to rinse the flask. Combine the 3 ether layers and wash with 2 quantities, each of 15 mL, of *water R*. Transfer the ether layer to a volumetric flask and dilute to 100.0 mL with *ether R*. Carefully evaporate 10.0 mL to dryness and dissolve the residue in 10.0 mL of a 5 g/L solution of *magnesium acetate R* in *methanol R*. Measure the absorbance (*2.2.25*) at 515 nm using *methanol R* as the compensation liquid.

Calculate the percentage content of hydroxyanthracene glycosides, expressed as sennoside B, using the following expression:

$$\frac{A \times 1.25}{m}$$

taking the specific absorbance of sennoside B to be 240.
A = absorbance at 515 nm;
m = mass of the substance to be examined, in grams.

STORAGE
Protected from moisture.

_____ *Ph Eur*

Senna Liquid Extract

DEFINITION

Senna Fruit, Alexandrian or Tinnevelly, crushed	1000 g
Coriander Oil	6 mL
Ethanol (90 per cent)	250 mL
Purified Water, freshly boiled and cooled	A sufficient quantity

Extemporaneous preparation
The following directions apply.

Macerate the crushed Senna Fruit in 5 litres of Purified Water for 8 hours, decant the clear liquid and strain; repeat the process twice using 2 litres of Purified Water for each maceration. Lightly press the marc, strain the expressed liquid, mix the strained liquid with the previously decanted liquid and heat the combined liquids at 80° for 3 minutes in a covered vessel. Allow to stand for not less than 24 hours; filter.

Evaporate the filtrate to 750 mL under reduced pressure at a temperature not exceeding 60°. Separately, dissolve the Coriander Oil in the Ethanol (90 per cent), add the solution to the evaporated filtrate and add sufficient Purified Water to produce 1000 mL. Allow to stand for not less than 24 hours; filter.

The extract complies with the requirements stated under Extracts and with the following requirements.

TESTS

Ethanol content
21 to 24% v/v, Appendix VIII F, Method III.

Dry residue
17 to 25% w/v.

Relative density
1.02 to 1.09, Appendix V G.

Standardised Senna Granules

DEFINITION

Standardised Senna Granules contain Alexandrian Senna Fruit in powder form with suitable excipients. The granules contain 0.55% w/w of sennosides, calculated as sennoside B.

The granules comply with the requirements stated under Granules and with the following requirements.

Content of sennosides calculated as sennoside B
0.467 to 0.633% w/w.

IDENTIFICATION

A. To 25 mg, in *No. 180 powder*, add 50 mL of *water* and 2 mL of *hydrochloric acid*, heat in a water bath for 15 minutes, allow to cool and shake with 40 mL of *ether*. Dry the ether layer over *anhydrous sodium sulfate*, filter, evaporate 5 mL of the filtrate to dryness, cool and add 5 mL of 6M *ammonia* to the residue; a yellow or orange colour is produced. Heat on a water bath for 2 minutes; a reddish violet colour is produced.

B. In the Assay, the chromatogram obtained with solution (1) exhibits two peaks corresponding to the peaks due to sennoside A and sennoside B in the chromatogram obtained with solution (2).

Loss on drying
When dried at 105° for 5 hours, lose not more than 2.0% of their weight. Use 5 g.

ASSAY

Carry out the method for *liquid chromatography*, Appendix III D, using the following solutions.

(1) Shake 2 g of the granules with 50 mL of a 0.3% v/v solution of *acetic acid* adjusted to pH 5.9 with 1M *sodium hydroxide* for 30 minutes, centrifuge, filter through a glass fibre paper (Whatman GF/C is suitable) and use the filtrate.

(2) Prepare solution (2) in the same manner as solution (1) but using a quantity of *Alexandrian senna fruit powder BPCRS* 1 mg of sennoside B.

CHROMATOGRAPHIC CONDITIONS

(a) Use a stainless steel column (15 cm × 4.6 mm) packed with *end-capped octadecylsilyl silica gel for chromatography* (5 µm) (Spherisorb ODS 2 is suitable).

(b) Use isocratic elution and the mobile phase described below.

(c) Use a flow rate of 2 mL per minute.

(d) Use an ambient column temperature.

(e) Use a detection wavelength of 350 nm.

(f) Inject 20 µL of each solution.

MOBILE PHASE

17 volumes of *acetonitrile* and 83 volumes of a 1% v/v solution of *glacial acetic acid*.

DETERMINATION OF CONTENT

Calculate the total content of sennosides A and B as sennoside B in the granules using the declared content of sennosides in *Alexandrian senna fruit powder BPCRS*.

STORAGE

Standardised Senna Granules should be kept in an airtight container.

LABELLING

The quantity of active ingredient is stated in terms of the equivalent amount of sennoside B.

Senna Tablets

DEFINITION

Senna Tablets contain the powdered pericarp of Senna Fruit, Alexandrian or Tinnevelly.

The tablets comply with the requirements stated under Tablets and with the following requirements.

Content of total sennosides, calculated as sennoside B
85.0 to 115.0% of the stated amount.

IDENTIFICATION

The powdered tablets exhibit diagnostic structures of senna pericarp. External epidermis of isodiametric cells with very thick outer walls. Occasional stomata. Trichomes few, unicellular, conical and warty. Parenchymatous cells from inner part of a two-to five-layered zone subjacent to the epidermis, each containing a single prism of calcium oxalate. Thick-walled fibres in two to four layers, the fibres of the outer and inner zones respectively with their long axes at right angles to each other. Sutural vascular strands sheathed by cells containing prisms of calcium oxalate; elements of seed tissue may also be present.

TESTS

Disintegration
Maximum time, 60 minutes, Appendix XII A.

ASSAY

Weigh and powder 20 tablets. Carry out the following procedure protected from light. To a quantity of the powder containing the equivalent of 7.5 mg of total sennosides add 30 mL of *water*, weigh, heat under a reflux condenser on a water bath for 15 minutes, allow to cool, weigh and restore the original weight with *water*. Centrifuge, transfer 20 mL of the supernatant liquid to a separating funnel, add 0.1 mL of 2M *hydrochloric acid*, shake with two 15 mL quantities of *chloroform*, allow to separate and discard the chloroform layers. Add 0.10 g of *sodium hydrogen carbonate* and shake for 3 minutes; centrifuge and transfer 10 mL of the liquid to a round-bottomed flask fitted with a ground-glass neck. Add a mixture of 8 mL of *iron(III) chloride solution* and 12 mL of *water* and mix. Heat under a reflux condenser on a water bath for 20 minutes, add 1 mL of *hydrochloric acid* and continue heating for a further 20 minutes, shaking frequently, until the precipitate is dissolved. Allow to cool, transfer the mixture to a separating funnel and extract with three 25-mL quantities of *ether* previously used to rinse the flask. Wash the combined ether extracts with two 15-mL quantities of *water* and add sufficient *ether* to produce 100 mL. Evaporate 10 mL just to dryness on a water-bath and dissolve the residue in 10 mL of 1M *potassium hydroxide*, filtering if necessary through a sintered-glass filter (ISO 4793, porosity grade 3, is suitable). Measure the *absorbance* of the resulting solution without delay at the maximum at 500 nm, Appendix II B. Calculate the content of total sennosides, as sennoside B, taking 200 as the value of A(1%, 1 cm) at the maximum at 500 nm.

LABELLING
The quantity of active ingredient is stated in terms of total sennosides expressed as the equivalent content of sennoside B.

Senna Leaf

(Ph Eur monograph 0206)

Preparation
Standardised Senna Leaf Dry Extract

When Powdered Senna Leaf is prescribed or demanded, material complying with the requirements below with the exception of Identification test A and the test for Foreign matter shall be dispensed or supplied.

Ph Eur _____

DEFINITION
Dried leaflets of *Cassia senna* L. (*C. acutifolia* Delile), known as Alexandrian or Khartoum senna, or *Cassia angustifolia* Vahl, known as Tinnevelly senna, or a mixture of the 2 species.

Content
Minimum 2.5 per cent of hydroxyanthracene glycosides, expressed as sennoside B ($C_{42}H_{38}O_{20}$; M_r 863) (dried drug).

CHARACTERS
Slight characteristic odour.

IDENTIFICATION
A. *C. senna* occurs as greyish-green or brownish-green, thin, fragile leaflets, lanceolate, mucronate, asymmetrical at the base, usually 15-40 mm long and 5-15 mm wide, the maximum width being at a point slightly below the centre; the lamina is slightly undulant with both surfaces covered with fine, short trichomes. Pinnate venation is visible mainly on the lower surface, with lateral veins leaving the midrib at an angle of about 60° and anastomosing to form a ridge near the margin.

Stomatal index (2.8.3) 10-12.5-15.

C. angustifolia occurs as yellowish-green or brownish-green leaflets, elongated and lanceolate, slightly asymmetrical at the base, usually 20-50 mm long and 7-20 mm wide at the centre. Both surfaces are smooth with a very small number of short trichomes and are frequently marked with transverse or oblique lines.

Stomatal index (2.8.3) 14-17.5-20

B. Reduce to a powder (355) *(2.9.12)*. The powder is light green or greenish-yellow. Examine under a microscope using *chloral hydrate solution R*. The powder shows the following diagnostic characters: polygonal epidermal cells showing paracytic stomata *(2.8.3)*; unicellular trichomes, conical in shape, with warted walls, isolated or attached to fragments of epidermis; fibres with a crystal sheath of prismatic crystals of calcium oxalate; cluster crystals isolated or in fragments of parenchyma.

C. Thin-layer chromatography *(2.2.27)*.

Test solution To 0.5 g of the powdered drug (180) *(2.9.12)* add 5 mL of a mixture of equal volumes of *ethanol (96 per cent) R* and *water R* and heat to boiling. Centrifuge and use the supernatant liquid.

Reference solution Dissolve 10 mg of *senna extract CRS* in 1 mL of a mixture of equal volumes of *ethanol (96 per cent) R* and *water R* (a slight residue remains).

Plate TLC silica gel G plate R.

Mobile phase glacial acetic acid R, water R, ethyl acetate R, propanol R (1:30:40:40 *V/V/V/V*).

Application 10 µL, as bands of 20 mm by 2 mm.

Development Over a path of 10 cm.

Drying In air.

Detection Spray with a 20 per cent *V/V* solution of *nitric acid R* and heat at 120 °C for 10 min. Allow to cool and spray with a 50 g/L solution of *potassium hydroxide R* in *alcohol (50 per cent V/V) R* until the zones appear.

Results The principal zones in the chromatogram obtained with the test solution are similar in position (sennosides B, A, D and C in the order of increasing R_F value), colour and size to the principal zones in the chromatogram obtained with the reference solution. Between the zones due to sennosides D and C a red zone due to rhein-8-glucoside may be visible.

D. Place about 25 mg of the powdered drug (180) *(2.9.12)* in a conical flask and add 50 mL of *water R* and 2 mL of *hydrochloric acid R*. Heat in a water-bath for 15 min, cool and shake with 40 mL of *ether R*. Separate the ether layer, dry over *anhydrous sodium sulfate R*, evaporate 5 mL to dryness and to the cooled residue add 5 mL of *dilute ammonia R1*. A yellow or orange colour develops. Heat on a water-bath for 2 min. A reddish-violet colour develops.

TESTS
Foreign matter *(2.8.2)*
Maximum 3 per cent of foreign organs and maximum 1 per cent of foreign elements.

Loss on drying *(2.2.32)*
Maximum 12.0 per cent, determined on 1.000 g of the powdered drug (355) *(2.9.12)* by drying in an oven at 105 °C for 2 h.

Total ash *(2.4.16)*
Maximum 12.0 per cent.

Ash insoluble in hydrochloric acid *(2.8.1)*
Maximum 2.5 per cent.

ASSAY
Carry out the assay protected from bright light.

Place 0.150 g of the powdered drug (180) *(2.9.12)* in a 100 mL flask. Add 30.0 mL of *water R*, mix, weigh and place in a water-bath. Heat under a reflux condenser for 15 min. Allow to cool, weigh and adjust to the original mass with *water R*. Centrifuge and transfer 20.0 mL of the supernatant liquid to a 150 mL separating funnel. Add 0.1 mL of *dilute hydrochloric acid R* and shake with 3 quantities, each of 15 mL, of *chloroform R*. Allow to separate and discard the chloroform layer. Add 0.10 g of *sodium hydrogen carbonate R* and shake for 3 min. Centrifuge and transfer 10.0 mL of the supernatant liquid to a 100 mL round-bottomed flask with a ground-glass neck. Add 20 mL of *ferric chloride solution R1* and mix. Heat for 20 min in a water-bath under a reflux condenser with the water level above that of the liquid in the flask; add 1 mL of *hydrochloric acid R* and heat for a further 20 min, with frequent shaking, to dissolve the precipitate.

Cool, transfer the mixture to a separating funnel and shake with 3 quantities, each of 25 mL, of *ether R* previously used to rinse the flask. Combine the 3 ether layers and wash with 2 quantities, each of 15 mL, of *water R*. Transfer the ether layer to a volumetric flask and dilute to 100.0 mL with *ether R*. Evaporate 10.0 mL carefully to dryness and dissolve the residue in 10.0 mL of a 5 g/L solution of *magnesium acetate R* in *methanol R*. Measure the absorbance (*2.2.25*) at 515 nm, using *methanol R* as the compensation liquid.

Calculate the percentage content of hydroxyanthracene glycosides, expressed as sennoside B, using the following expression:

$$\frac{A \times 1.25}{m}$$

i. e. taking the specific absorbance of sennoside B to be 240.
A = absorbance at 515 nm,
m = mass of the substance to be examined, in grams.

STORAGE

Protected from moisture.

──────────────── Ph Eur

Standardised Senna Leaf Dry Extract

(*Ph Eur monograph 1261*)

Ph Eur _____

DEFINITION

Standardised dry extract produced from *Senna leaf (0206)*.

Content

5.5 per cent to 8.0 per cent of hydroxyanthracene glycosides, expressed as sennoside B ($C_{42}H_{38}O_{20}$; M_r 863) (dried extract). The measured content does not deviate from the value stated on the label by more than ± 10 per cent.

PRODUCTION

The extract is produced from the herbal drug by a suitable procedure using ethanol (50-80 per cent *V/V*).

CHARACTERS

Appearance

Brownish or brown powder.

IDENTIFICATION

A. Thin-layer chromatography (*2.2.27*).

Solvent mixture ethanol (96 per cent) *R*, water *R* (50:50 *V/V*).

Test solution To 0.1 g of the extract to be examined add 5 mL of the solvent mixture and heat to boiling. Cool and centrifuge. Use the supernatant liquid.

Reference solution Dissolve 10 mg of *senna extract CRS* in 1 mL of the solvent mixture (a slight residue remains).

Plate TLC silica gel plate *R*.

Mobile phase glacial acetic acid *R*, water *R*, ethyl acetate *R*, 1-propanol *R* (1:30:40:40 *V/V/V/V*).

Application 10 μL as bands.

Development Over a path of 10 cm.

Drying In air.

Detection Spray with a 20 per cent *V/V* solution of *nitric acid R* and heat at 120 °C for 10 min; allow to cool and spray with a 50 g/L solution of *potassium hydroxide R* in *ethanol (50 per cent V/V) R* until the zones appear.

Results The principal zones in the chromatogram obtained with the test solution are similar in position, colour and size to the principal zones in the chromatogram obtained with the reference solution. The chromatograms show in the lower third a prominent brown zone due to sennoside B and above it a yellow zone followed by another prominent brown zone due to sennoside A. In the upper half of the chromatograms are visible, in order of increasing R_F value, a prominent reddish-brown zone and an orange-brown zone followed by a faint pink zone and 2 yellow zones. Close to the solvent front a dark pink zone appears, which may be followed by several faint zones.

B. Place about 25 mg of the extract to be examined in a conical flask and add 50 mL of *water R* and 2 mL of *hydrochloric acid R*. Heat in a water-bath for 15 min, cool and shake with 40 mL of *ether R*. Separate the ether layer, dry over *anhydrous sodium sulfate R*, evaporate 5 mL to dryness and to the cooled residue add 5 mL of *dilute ammonia R1*. A yellow or orange colour develops. Heat on a water-bath for 2 min. A reddish-violet colour develops.

TESTS

Loss on drying (*2.8.17*)

Maximum 5.0 per cent.

Microbial contamination

TAMC: acceptance criterion 10^4 CFU/g (*2.6.12*).
TYMC: acceptance criterion 10^2 CFU/g (*2.6.12*).
Absence of *Escherichia coli* (*2.6.13*).
Absence of *Salmonella* (*2.6.13*).

ASSAY

Carry out the assay protected from bright light.

Place 0.150 g of the extract to be examined in a 100 mL flask, dissolve in *water R* and dilute to 100.0 mL with the same solvent. Filter the solution, discard the first 10 mL of the filtrate. Transfer 20.0 mL of the filtrate to a 150 mL separating funnel. Add 0.1 mL of *dilute hydrochloric acid R* and shake with 3 quantities, each of 15 mL, of *ether R*. Allow the layers to separate and discard the ether layer. Add 0.10 g of *sodium hydrogen carbonate R* to the aqueous layer and shake for 3 min. Centrifuge and transfer 10.0 mL of the supernatant liquid to a 100 mL round-bottomed flask with a ground-glass neck. Add 20 mL of *ferric chloride solution R1* and mix. Heat for 20 min under a reflux condenser in a water-bath with the water level above that of the liquid in the flask; add 3 mL of *hydrochloric acid R* and heat for a further 30 min with frequent shaking to dissolve the precipitate. Cool, transfer the mixture to a separating funnel and shake with 3 quantities, each of 25 mL, of *ether R* previously used to rinse the flask. Combine the ether layers and wash with 2 quantities, each of 15 mL, of *water R*. Transfer the ether layers to a volumetric flask and dilute to 100.0 mL with *ether R*. Evaporate 10.0 mL carefully to dryness and dissolve the residue in 10.0 mL of a 5.0 g/L solution of *magnesium acetate R* in *methanol R*. Measure the absorbance (*2.2.25*) at 515 nm using *methanol R* as the compensation liquid.

Calculate the percentage content of hydroxyanthracene glycosides expressed as sennoside B using the following expression:

$$\frac{A \times 4.167}{m}$$

i.e. taking the specific absorbance of sennoside B to be 240.
A = absorbance at 515 nm;
m = mass of the herbal drug to be examined, in grams.

LABELLING

The label states the content of hydroxyanthracene glycosides.

_____ *Ph Eur*

Sophora Flower

(*Ph Eur monograph 2639*)

Ph Eur _____

DEFINITION

Dried, opened flower of *Styphnolobium japonicum* (L.) Schott (syn. *Sophora japonica* L.).

Content:

— minimum 8.0 per cent of total flavonoids, expressed as rutin ($C_{27}H_{30}O_{16}$; M_r 611) (dried drug);
— minimum 6.0 per cent of rutin ($C_{27}H_{30}O_{16}$; M_r 611) (dried drug).

IDENTIFICATION

A. The opened flower is crumpled, rolled, and has a very thin and short pedicel. The dark green or brown, campanulate calyx is about 3-4 mm long and consists of 5 fused sepals with longitudinal striations at the base, divided at the apex into 5 slightly bilabiate lobes. The pale yellow or light yellowish-brown, papilionaceous type corolla is often broken and measures about 10-15 mm; the upper petal is the largest, subrounded, with a reflexed apex and a bright yellow unguis at its internal base. The other 4 petals are oblong. There are 10 free stamens surrounding a cylindrical and curved central style.

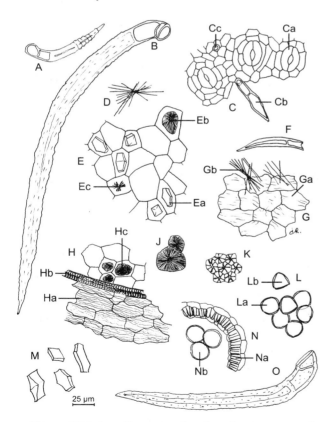

Figure 2639.-1. – *Illustration for identification test B of powdered herbal drug of sophora flower*

B. Microscopic examination (*2.8.23*). The powder is yellowish-green. Examine under a microscope using *chloral hydrate solution R*. The powder shows the following diagnostic characters (Figure 2639.-1): roundish [La] or triangular [Lb] pollen grains [L] with 3 pores and a smooth exine, about 18 μm in diameter; isolated covering trichomes [A, B, F, O] of varying lengths (60-660 μm), slightly flexed, usually consisting of 1 or 2 basal cells and a long pointed distal cell, with smooth or slightly warty walls; fragments of sepals [C] composed of anomocytic stomata (*2.8.3*) with 4-8 subsidiary cells [Ca], covering trichomes [Cb] or their scars [Cc]; fragments of petals [G, H] with cells covered by a finely striated cuticle [Ga, Ha], sometimes accompanied by fine annular or spiral vessels [Hb] and parenchyma with some cells containing crystalline masses of rutin [Hc]; fragments of parenchyma [E] from the sepals containing prisms of calcium oxalate [Ea] and crystalline masses of rutin [Eb]; fragments of anthers [N] showing the characteristic fibrous layer, in transverse section [Na] or in surface view [K], and immature pollen grains [Nb]; free prisms of calcium oxalate [M]. Examine under a microscope using *chloral hydrate solution R*, without heating the preparation: brownish-yellow rutin crystals are visible, free or included in cells, as crystalline masses [Eb, Hc, J] or in fan-shaped aggregates of very fine needles [D, Ec, Gb].

C. Thin-layer chromatography (*2.2.27*).

Test solution To 1 g of the powdered herbal drug (355) (*2.9.12*) add 5.0 mL of *methanol R*, sonicate for 10 min and filter.

Reference solution Dissolve 10 mg of *hyperoside R* and 10 mg of *rutin R* in 10 mL of *methanol R*.

Plate TLC silica gel plate R (5-40 μm) [or TLC silica gel plate R (2-10 μm)].

Mobile phase anhydrous formic acid R, water R, ethyl acetate R (10:10:80 *V/V/V*).

Application 10 μL [or 5 μL] as bands of 10 mm [or 8 mm].

Development Over a path of 10 cm [or 6 cm].

Drying In air.

Detection Treat with a 10 g/L solution of *diphenylboric acid aminoethyl ester R* in *methanol R* and then with a 50 g/L solution of *macrogol 400 R* in *methanol R*, allow to dry in air for about 30 min, and examine in ultraviolet light at 365 nm.

Results See below the sequence of fluorescent zones present in the chromatograms obtained with the reference solution and the test solution. Furthermore, other faint fluorescent zones may be present in the chromatogram obtained with the test solution.

Top of the plate	
	An orange-yellow zone
_____	_____
	A brown zone
Hyperoside: a yellowish-orange zone	
_____	_____
	2 green zones
Rutin: an orange-yellow zone	A very intense orange-yellow zone (rutin)
Reference solution	**Test solution**

TESTS

Foreign matter (2.8.2)
Maximum 5 per cent of flower buds and maximum
2 per cent of other foreign matter.

Loss on drying (2.2.32)
Maximum 11.0 per cent, determined on 1.000 g of the
powdered herbal drug (355) (2.9.12) by drying in an oven at
105 °C for 2 h.

Total ash (2.4.16)
Maximum 9.0 per cent.

ASSAY

Total flavonoids

Stock solution   Place 2.000 g of the powdered herbal drug
(355) (2.9.12) in the cartridge of a continuous-extraction
apparatus (Soxhlet type). Add 100 mL of *heptane R* and heat
under a reflux condenser until the extraction liquid is
colourless. Allow to cool and discard the heptane.
Add 90 mL of *methanol R* and continue the extraction with
heating under a reflux condenser until the extraction liquid is
colourless. Allow to cool. Transfer the methanolic solution to
a 100 mL volumetric flask. Rinse the extraction flask with a
few millilitres of *methanol R*. Combine the methanolic
solutions and dilute to 100.0 mL with *methanol R*. Dilute
10.0 mL of this solution to 100.0 mL with *water R* and shake
vigorously.

Test solution   Dilute 10.0 mL of the stock solution to
100.0 mL with a 20 g/L solution of *aluminium chloride R* in
methanol R.

Compensation solution   Dilute 10.0 mL of the stock solution
to 100.0 mL with *methanol R*.

Measure the absorbance (2.2.25) of the test solution after
15 min by comparison with the compensation solution at
425 nm.

Calculate the percentage content of total flavonoids,
expressed as rutin, using the following expression:

$$\frac{A \times 1000}{m \times 37}$$

i.e. taking the specific absorbance of rutin to be 370.

A = absorbance of the test solution at 425 nm;
m = mass of the herbal drug to be examined, in grams.

Rutin

Liquid chromatography (2.2.29).

Test solution   Place 0.500 g of the powdered herbal drug
(355) (2.9.12) in a conical flask and add 50.0 mL of
methanol R. Weigh, sonicate for 30 min and allow to cool.
Weigh and compensate for the loss of solvent with
methanol R. Shake vigorously, filter, and dilute 2.0 mL of the
filtrate to 10.0 mL with *methanol R*.

Reference solution (a)   Dissolve 10.0 mg of *rutoside
trihydrate CRS* in 2 mL of *methanol R* and dilute to 10.0 mL
with a 50 per cent *V/V* solution of *methanol R*. Dilute 2.0 mL
of this solution to 10.0 mL with a 50 per cent *V/V* solution
of *methanol R*.

Reference solution (b)   Dissolve 10.0 mg of *apigenin
7-glucoside R* and 10.0 mg of *rutin R* in 2 mL of *methanol R*
and dilute to 10.0 mL with a 50 per cent *V/V* solution of
methanol R. Dilute 2.0 mL of this solution to 10.0 mL with a
50 per cent *V/V* solution of *methanol R*.

Column:
— *size: l* = 0.25 m, Ø = 4.6 mm;

— *stationary phase: octadecylsilyl silica gel for chromatography R*
(5 µm).

Mobile phase:
— *mobile phase A*: 1 per cent *V/V* solution of *glacial acetic
acid R*;
— *mobile phase B: methanol R*;

Time (min)	Mobile phase A (per cent V/V)	Mobile phase B (per cent V/V)
0 - 5	68	32
5 - 20	68 → 50	32 → 50
20 - 30	50 → 0	50 → 100
30 - 35	0	100

Flow rate   1.3 mL/min.

Detection   Spectrophotometer at 350 nm.

Injection   20 µL.

Relative retention   With reference to rutin (retention
time = about 17 min): apigenin 7-glucoside = about 1.1.

System suitability   Reference solution (b):
— *resolution*: minimum 1.5 between the peaks due to rutin
and apigenin 7-glucoside.

Calculate the percentage content of rutin using the following
expression:

$$\frac{A_1 \times m_2 \times p \times 5}{A_2 \times m_1}$$

A_1 = area of the peak due to rutin in the chromatogram
obtained with the test solution;
A_2 = area of the peak due to rutin in the chromatogram
obtained with reference solution (a);
m_1 = mass of the herbal drug to be examined used to
prepare the test solution, in grams;
m_2 = mass of *rutoside trihydrate CRS* used to prepare
reference solution (a), in grams;
p = assigned percentage content of rutin in *rutoside
trihydrate CRS*.

_____ Ph Eur

Sophora Flower-Bud

(Ph Eur monograph 2427)

Ph Eur _____

DEFINITION

Whole, dried flower bud of *Styphnolobium japonicum* (L.)
Schott (syn. *Sophora japonica* L.).

Content:
— minimum 20.0 per cent of total flavonoids, expressed as
rutin ($C_{27}H_{30}O_{16}$; Mr 611) (dried drug);
— minimum 15.0 per cent of rutin ($C_{27}H_{30}O_{16}$; Mr 611)
(dried drug).

IDENTIFICATION

A. The flat flower bud, ovoid or ellipsoid, has a very thin and
short pedicel and is about 7-10 mm long and 3-4 mm thick.
The dark green or brown calyx, forming the lower part of the
bud, is about 3-4 mm long and consists of 5 fused sepals
with longitudinal striations at the base. The pale yellow or
brownish-yellow corolla, unopened, delicate, extends beyond
the calyx and contains 10 free stamens surrounding a central
style.

B. Microscopic examination (*2.8.23*). The powder is pale yellow. Examine under a microscope using *chloral hydrate solution R*. The powder shows the following diagnostic characters (Figure 2427.-1): roundish [La] or triangular [Lb] pollen grains [L] with 3 pores and a smooth exine, about 18 μm in diameter; isolated covering trichomes [A, B, F, O] of varying lengths (60-660 μm), slightly flexed, usually consisting of 1 or 2 basal cells and a long pointed distal cell, with smooth or slightly warty walls; fragments of sepals [C] composed of anomocytic stomata (*2.8.3*) with 4-8 subsidiary cells [Ca], covering trichomes [Cb] or their scars [Cc]; fragments of petals [G, H] with cells covered by a finely striated cuticle [Ga, Ha], sometimes accompanied by fine annular or spiral vessels [Hb] and parenchyma with some cells containing crystalline masses of rutin [Hc]; fragments of parenchyma [E] from the sepals containing prisms of calcium oxalate [Ea] and crystalline masses of rutin [Eb]; fragments of anthers [N] showing the characteristic fibrous layer, in transverse section [Na] or in surface view [K], and immature pollen grains [Nb]; free prisms of calcium oxalate [M]. Examine under a microscope using *chloral hydrate solution R*, without heating the preparation: brownish-yellow rutin crystals are visible, free or included in cells, as crystalline masses [Eb, Hc, J] or in fan-shaped aggregates of very fine needles [D, Ec, Gb].

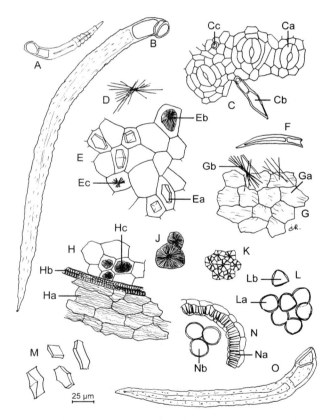

Figure 2427.-1. – *Illustration for identification test B of powdered herbal drug of sophora flower-bud*

C. Thin-layer chromatography (*2.2.27*).

Test solution   To 0.2 g of the powdered herbal drug (355) (*2.9.12*) add 5.0 mL of *methanol R*, sonicate for 10 min and filter.

Reference solution   Dissolve 10 mg of *hyperoside R* and 10 mg of *rutin R* in 10 mL of *methanol R*.

Plate   *TLC silica gel plate R* (5-40 μm) [or *TLC silica gel plate R* (2-10 μm)].

Mobile phase   anhydrous *formic acid R*, *water R*, *ethyl acetate R* (10:10:80 *V/V/V*).

Application   10 μL [or 5 μL] as bands of 10 mm [or 8 mm].

Development   Over a path of 10 cm [or 6 cm].

Drying   In air.

Detection   Treat with a 10 g/L solution of *diphenylboric acid aminoethyl ester R* in *methanol R* and then with a 50 g/L solution of *macrogol 400 R* in *methanol R*, allow to dry in air for about 30 min, and examine in ultraviolet light at 365 nm.

Results   See below the sequence of fluorescent zones present in the chromatograms obtained with the reference solution and the test solution. Furthermore, other faint fluorescent zones may be present in the chromatogram obtained with the test solution.

Top of the plate	
	An orange-yellow zone
———	———
	A brown zone
Hyperoside: a yellowish-orange zone	
———	———
	2 green zones
Rutin: an orange-yellow zone	A very intense orange-yellow zone (rutin)
Reference solution	**Test solution**

TESTS

Foreign matter (*2.8.2*)
Maximum 5 per cent of opened flowers and maximum 2 per cent of other foreign matter.

Loss on drying (*2.2.32*)
Maximum 11.0 per cent, determined on 1.000 g of the powdered herbal drug (355) (*2.9.12*) by drying in an oven at 105 °C for 2 h.

Total ash (*2.4.16*)
Maximum 9.0 per cent.

ASSAY

Total flavonoids

Stock solution   Place 1.00 g of the powdered herbal drug (355) (*2.9.12*) in the cartridge of a continuous-extraction apparatus (Soxhlet type). Add 100 mL of *heptane R* and heat under a reflux condenser until the extraction liquid is colourless. Allow to cool and discard the heptane. Add 90 mL of *methanol R* and continue the extraction with heating under a reflux condenser until the extraction liquid is colourless. Allow to cool. Transfer the methanolic solution to a 100 mL volumetric flask. Rinse the extraction flask with a few millilitres of *methanol R*. Combine the methanolic solutions and dilute to 100.0 mL with *methanol R*. Dilute 10.0 mL of this solution to 100.0 mL with *water R* and shake vigorously.

Test solution   Dilute 10.0 mL of the stock solution to 100.0 mL with a 20 g/L solution of *aluminium chloride R* in *methanol R*.

Compensation solution   Dilute 10.0 mL of the stock solution to 100.0 mL with methanol R.

Measure the absorbance (*2.2.25*) of the test solution after 15 min by comparison with the compensation solution at 425 nm.

Calculate the percentage content of total flavonoids, expressed as rutin, using the following expression:

$$\frac{A \times 1000}{m \times 37}$$

i.e. taking the specific absorbance of rutin to be 370.

A = absorbance of the test solution at 425 nm;

m = mass of the herbal drug to be examined, in grams.

Rutin

Liquid chromatography (*2.2.29*).

Test solution Place 0.200 g of the powdered herbal drug (355) (*2.9.12*) in a conical flask and add 50.0 mL of *methanol R*. Weigh, sonicate for 30 min and allow to cool. Weigh and compensate for the loss of solvent with *methanol R*. Shake vigorously, filter, and dilute 2.0 mL of the filtrate to 10.0 mL with *methanol R*.

Reference solution (a) Dissolve 10.0 mg of *rutoside trihydrate CRS* in 2 mL of *methanol R* and dilute to 10.0 mL with a 50 per cent *V/V* solution of *methanol R*. Dilute 2.0 mL of this solution to 10.0 mL with a 50 per cent *V/V* solution of *methanol R*.

Reference solution (b) Dissolve 10.0 mg of *apigenin 7-glucoside R* and 10.0 mg of *rutin R* in 2 mL of *methanol R* and dilute to 10.0 mL with a 50 per cent *V/V* solution of *methanol R*. Dilute 2.0 mL of this solution to 10.0 mL with a 50 per cent *V/V* solution of *methanol R*.

Column:
— *size: l* = 0.25 m, Ø = 4.6 mm;
— *stationary phase: octadecylsilyl silica gel for chromatography R* (5 µm).

Mobile phase:
— *mobile phase A*: 1 per cent *V/V* solution of *glacial acetic acid R*;
— *mobile phase B: methanol R*;

Time (min)	Mobile phase A (per cent *V/V*)	Mobile phase B (per cent *V/V*)
0 - 5	68	32
5 - 20	68 → 50	32 → 50
20 - 30	50 → 0	50 → 100
30 - 35	0	100

Flow rate 1.3 mL/min.

Detection Spectrophotometer at 350 nm.

Injection 20 µL.

Relative retention With reference to rutin (retention time = about 17 min): apigenin 7-glucoside = about 1.1.

System suitability Reference solution (b):
— *resolution*: minimum 1.5 between the peaks due to rutin and apigenin 7-glucoside.

Calculate the percentage content of rutin using the following expression:

$$\frac{A_1 \times m_2 \times p \times 5}{A_2 \times m_1}$$

A_1 = area of the peak due to rutin in the chromatogram obtained with the test solution;

A_2 = area of the peak due to rutin in the chromatogram obtained with reference solution (a);

m_1 = mass of the herbal drug to be examined used to prepare the test solution, in grams;

m_2 = mass of *rutoside trihydrate CRS* used to prepare reference solution (a), in grams;

p = assigned percentage content of rutin in *rutoside trihydrate CRS*.

Ph Eur

Spearmint Oil

DEFINITION

Spearmint Oil is obtained by distillation from fresh flowering plants of *Mentha spicata* L. and *Mentha × cardiaca* (Gray) Bak.

CHARACTERISTICS

A clear, colourless, pale yellow or greenish yellow liquid when recently distilled, but becoming darker and viscous on keeping; visibly free from water; odour, that of spearmint.

IDENTIFICATION

Examine the chromatograms obtained in the test for Chromatographic profile. The retention times of the principal peaks in the chromatogram obtained with solution (1) are similar to those of the principal peaks in the chromatogram obtained with solution (2).

TESTS

Optical rotation
American-type oil, −45° to −60°; Chinese-type oil, −50° to −62°; Appendix V F.

Refractive index
1.484 to 1.491, Appendix V E.

Solubility in ethanol
Soluble, at 20°, in 1 part of *ethanol (80%)*, Appendix X M. The solution may become cloudy when diluted.

Weight per mL
American-type oil, 0.917 to 0.934 g; Chinese-type oil, 0.935 to 0.952 g, Appendix V G.

Chromatographic profile
Carry out the method for *gas chromatography*, Appendix III B, using the following solutions. Solution (1) is the substance being examined. For solution (2) mix carefully 0.1 g of *limonene*, 0.2 g of *cineole*, 0.4 g of *menthone*, 0.1 g of (+)-*isomenthone*, 0.4 g of *menthyl acetate*, 0.2 g of *pulegone*, 0.6 g of *menthol* and 0.1 g of *carvone* with 1 g of *hexane*.

The chromatographic procedure may be carried out using (a) a glass capillary column (25 m to 60 m × about 0.25 mm) coated with *polyethylene glycol 20,000* as bonded phase (Carbowax 20M is suitable) and (b) *helium* as the carrier gas at a flow rate of 1.5 mL per minute. Maintain the temperature of the column at 55° for 6 minutes then increase it at the rate of 4° per minute to 180°; keep the injection port temperature at 220° and the detector at 230°.

Inject 0.1 µL of solution (2). When the chromatograms are recorded in the prescribed conditions, the components elute in the order indicated in the composition of the reference solution. Record the retention times of these substances. The test is not valid unless the number of *theoretical plates* calculated from the limonene peak is at least 30,000 and the *resolution factor* between the peaks corresponding to limonene and cineole is at least 1.5.

Inject 0.1 µL of solution (1). Using the retention times determined from the chromatogram obtained with solution (2) locate the components of the reference solution on the chromatogram obtained with solution (1) (disregard the peak due to hexane). Determine the percentage content of the components by *normalisation*. The percentages are within the following ranges:

Limonene 2.0 to 25.0%.

Cineole less than 2.5%.

Menthone less than 2.5%.

Isomenthone less than 1.0%.

Menthyl acetate less than 1.0%.

Pulegone less than 0.5%.

Menthol less than 2.0%.

Carvone Not less than 55.0%.

STORAGE
Spearmint Oil should be kept in a well-filled container and protected from light.

LABELLING
The label states whether the oil is American-type oil or Chinese-type oil.

Squill

Preparations
Squill Liquid Extract

Squill Oxymel

When Powdered Squill is prescribed or demanded, material complying with the appropriate requirements below shall be dispensed or supplied.

DEFINITION
Squill consists of the bulb of *Drimia maritima* (L.) Stearn, collected soon after the plant has flowered, divested of its dry, outer, membranous coats, cut into transverse slices and dried. It is known in commerce as white squill.

IDENTIFICATION
A. Transverse slices, about 5 to 8 mm thick, occurring as straight or curved triangular pieces about 5 to 50 mm long and 3 to 8 mm wide at mid-point, tapering towards each end, yellowish white, texture horny, somewhat translucent, breaking with an almost glassy fracture when quite dry, but readily absorbing moisture when exposed to the air and becoming tough and flexible; transversely cut surface showing a single row of prominent, vascular bundles near the concave edge and numerous smaller bundles scattered throughout the mesophyll.

B. Epidermis: cells polygonal and axially elongated, 1 to 2 times longer than wide, cuticle thick, stratified; stomata very rare, *anomocytic*, Appendix XI H, and nearly circular in outline, about 50 to 60 μm in diameter; mesophyll of colourless, thin-walled parenchyma containing very occasional starch granules, many cells containing bundles of acicular crystals of calcium oxalate embedded in mucilage, crystals up to about 1 mm long and about 1 to 15 μm wide; other cells containing sinistrin; vascular bundles collateral, scattered throughout the mesophyll; xylem vessels with spiral and annular wall thickening; trichomes absent.

C. The mucilage contained in the cells of the mesophyll is stained red with alkaline *corallin* solution but produces no red colour with *ruthenium red* solution and no purple colour with 0.01M *iodine*.

TESTS
Acid-insoluble ash
Not more than 1.5%, Appendix XI K, Method I.

Extractive soluble in ethanol (60%)
Not less than 68.0%, Appendix XI B1. Use material that has been dried for 1 hour at 105° and powdered.

STORAGE
Squill should be stored in a dry place.

Indian Squill

Preparation
Squill Oxymel

When Powdered Indian Squill is prescribed or demanded, material complying with the appropriate requirements below shall be dispensed or supplied.

DEFINITION
Indian Squill consists of the bulb of *Drimia indica* (Roxb.) J P Jessop, collected soon after the plant has flowered, divested of dry, outer membranous coats and usually cut longitudinally into slices and dried.

CHARACTERISTICS
Odourless or almost odourless.

Macroscopical
Curved or irregularly shaped strips, about 10 to 50 mm long, 3 to 10 mm wide and 1 to 3 mm thick, frequently tapering towards the ends, occasionally grouped three or four together and attached to a portion of the axis; ridged in the direction of their length and varying in colour from pale yellowish brown to buff; brittle when dry, but tough and flexible when exposed to air.

Microscopical
Epidermis: cells tetrahedral to hexahedral, thin-walled, three to five times longer than wide, having a thick, striated cuticle; stomata rare, *anomocytic*, Appendix XI H, circular in outline, 40 to 42 μm in diameter; mesophyll of thin-walled polygonal cells containing mucilage, some cells also containing bundles of acicular crystals of calcium oxalate, 20 to 900 μm in length; vascular bundles collateral, scattered throughout the mesophyll; xylem vessels with spiral and annular wall thickening; trichomes and starch absent.

IDENTIFICATION
The mucilage contained in the cells of the mesophyll is stained red with *alkaline corallin solution* and reddish purple with 0.01M *iodine*.

TESTS
Ash
Not more than 6.0%, Appendix XI J.

STORAGE
Indian Squill should be stored in a dry place.

Squill Liquid Extract

DEFINITION
Squill Liquid Extract is prepared by extracting Squill with Ethanol (70 per cent).

Extemporaneous preparation
The following formula and directions apply.

Squill, in *coarse powder*	1000 g
Ethanol (70 per cent)	A sufficient quantity

Exhaust the Squill, in *coarse powder*, with Ethanol (70 per cent) by *percolation*, Appendix XI F. Reserve the first 850 mL of the percolate; evaporate the subsequent percolate to the consistence of a soft extract and dissolve it in the reserved portion. Add sufficient Ethanol (70 per cent) to produce 1000 mL and filter.

The extract complies with the requirements stated under Extracts and with the following requirements.

TESTS

Ethanol content
34 to 50% v/v, Appendix VIII F, Method III.

Dry residue
40 to 55% w/v.

Relative density
1.00 to 1.14, Appendix V G.

Squill Oxymel

DEFINITION

Squill, bruised or Indian Squill, bruised	50 g
Acetic Acid (33 per cent)	90 mL or a sufficient quantity
Purified Water, freshly boiled and cooled	250 mL
Purified Honey	A sufficient quantity

Extemporaneous preparation
The following directions apply.

Macerate the Squill or the Indian Squill with the Acetic Acid (33 per cent) and the Purified Water for 7 days with occasional agitation, strain, press out the liquid, heat the mixed liquids to boiling, filter whilst hot, cool, determine the content of acetic acid, add sufficient Acetic Acid (33 per cent) to the remainder of the filtrate to produce a solution containing about 8.5% w/v of acetic acid and mix. To every three volumes of the resulting solution add seven volumes of Purified Honey and mix thoroughly.

Content of acetic acid, $C_2H_4O_2$
2.2 to 2.7% w/v.

TESTS

Optical rotation
+0.6° to -3.0°, Appendix V F, when measured in a 25% w/v solution in *water* decolourised, if necessary, with *activated charcoal*.

Weight per mL
1.260 to 1.270 g, Appendix V G.

ASSAY

Dilute 20 mL with 20 mL of *carbon dioxide-free water* and titrate with 1M *sodium hydroxide VS* using *phenolphthalein solution R1* as indicator. Each mL of 1M *sodium hydroxide VS* is equivalent to 60.05 mg of $C_2H_4O_2$.

Opiate Squill Linctus

Compound Squill Linctus; Gee's Linctus; Opiate Squill Oral Solution

DEFINITION

Opiate Squill Linctus is an opalescent *oral solution* containing 33% v/v each of Squill Oxymel and Camphorated Opium Tincture in a suitable vehicle with a tolu flavour.

Extemporaneous preparation
The following formula applies.

Squill Oxymel	300 mL
Camphorated Opium Tincture	300 mL
Tolu Syrup	300 mL

The linctus complies with the requirements stated under Oral Liquids and with the following requirements.

Content of anhydrous morphine, $C_{17}H_{19}NO_3$
0.013 to 0.020% w/v.

TESTS

Ethanol content
18.0 to 22.0% v/v, Appendix VIII F.

ASSAY

To 12 g add 5 mL of *water* and 1 mL of 5M *ammonia* and extract with 30 mL of a mixture of equal volumes of *ethanol* (*96%*) and *chloroform* and then with two 22.5-mL quantities of a mixture of 2 volumes of *chloroform* and 1 volume of *ethanol* (*96%*), washing each extract with the same 20 mL of a mixture of equal volumes of *ethanol* (*96%*) and *water*. Evaporate the combined extracts, extract the residue with 10 mL of *calcium hydroxide solution*, filter and wash the filter with 10 mL of *calcium hydroxide solution*. To the combined filtrate and washings add 0.1 g of *ammonium sulfate*, extract with two 10 mL quantities of *ethanol-free chloroform*, wash the combined extracts with 10 mL of *water* and discard the chloroform solution. To the combined alkaline liquid and aqueous washings add 10 mL of 1M *hydrochloric acid*, heat on a water bath to remove any chloroform, cool and dilute to 100 mL with *water*. To 20 mL of this solution add 8 mL of a freshly prepared 1.0% w/v solution of *sodium nitrite*, allow to stand for 15 minutes, add 12 mL of 5M *ammonia*, dilute to 50 mL with *water* and measure the *absorbance* of a 4-cm layer of the resulting solution at the maximum at 442 nm, Appendix II B, using in the reference cell a solution prepared in the same manner and at the same time but using 8 mL of *water* in place of the solution of sodium nitrite. Calculate the content of $C_{17}H_{19}NO_3$ from a calibration curve prepared using quantities of 2, 4, 6 and 8 mL of a 0.008% w/v solution of *anhydrous morphine* in 0.1M *hydrochloric acid*, each diluted to 20 mL with 0.1M *hydrochloric acid* and using the method described above beginning at the words 'add 8 mL ...'. Determine the *weight per mL* of the linctus, Appendix V G, and calculate the content of $C_{17}H_{19}NO_3$, weight in volume.

Paediatric Opiate Squill Linctus

Opiate Linctus for Infants; Paediatric Opiate Squill Oral Solution

DEFINITION

Paediatric Opiate Squill Linctus is an *oral solution* containing 6% v/v each of Squill Oxymel and Camphorated Opium Tincture in a suitable vehicle with a tolu flavour.

Extemporaneous preparation
The following formula applies.

Squill Oxymel	60 mL
Camphorated Opium Tincture	60 mL
Tolu Syrup	60 mL
Glycerol	200 mL
Syrup	Sufficient to produce 1000 mL

The linctus complies with the requirements stated under Oral Liquids and with the following requirements.

Content of anhydrous morphine, $C_{17}H_{19}NO_3$
0.0024 to 0.0036% w/v.

ASSAY

To 32 g add 5 mL of *water* and 1 mL of 5M *ammonia* and extract with 30 mL of a mixture of equal volumes of *ethanol (96%)* and *chloroform* and then with two 22.5-mL quantities of a mixture of 2 volumes of *chloroform* and 1 volume of *ethanol (96%)*, washing each extract with the same 20 mL of a mixture of equal volumes of *ethanol (96%)* and *water*. Evaporate the combined extracts, extract the residue with 10 mL of *calcium hydroxide solution*, filter and wash the filter with 10 mL of *calcium hydroxide solution*. To the combined filtrate and washings add 0.1 g of *ammonium sulfate*, extract with two 10 mL quantities of *ethanol-free chloroform*, wash the combined extracts with 10 mL of *water* and discard the chloroform solution. To the combined alkaline liquid and aqueous washings add 5 mL of 1M *hydrochloric acid*, heat on a water bath to remove any chloroform, cool and dilute to 50 mL with *water*. To 20 mL of this solution add 8 mL of a freshly prepared 1.0% w/v solution of *sodium nitrite*, allow to stand for 15 minutes, add 12 mL of 5M *ammonia*, dilute to 50 mL with *water* and measure the *absorbance* of a 4-cm layer of the resulting solution at the maximum at 442 nm, Appendix II B, using in the reference cell a solution prepared in the same manner and at the same time but using 8 mL of *water* in place of the solution of sodium nitrite. Calculate the content of $C_{17}H_{19}NO_3$ from a calibration curve prepared using quantities of 2, 4, 6 and 8 mL of a 0.008% w/v solution of *anhydrous morphine* in 0.1M *hydrochloric acid*, each diluted to 20 mL with 0.1M *hydrochloric acid* and using the method described above beginning at the words 'add 8 mL ...'. Determine the *weight per mL* of the linctus, Appendix V G, and calculate the content of $C_{17}H_{19}NO_3$, weight in volume.

St. John's Wort

Hypericum

(Ph Eur monograph 1438)

Preparation

St. John's Wort Dry Extract, Quantified

Ph Eur _____

DEFINITION

Whole or fragmented, dried flowering tops of *Hypericum perforatum* L., harvested during flowering time.

Content

Minimum 0.08 per cent of total hypericins, expressed as hypericin ($C_{30}H_{16}O_8$; M_r 504.4) (dried drug).

IDENTIFICATION

A. The branched and bare stem shows 2 more or less prominent longitudinal ridges. The leaves are opposite, sessile, exstipulate, oblong-oval and 15-30 mm long; present on the leaf margins are glands which appear as black dots and over all the surface of the leaves many small, strongly translucent excretory glands which are visible in transmitted light. The flowers are regular and form corymbose clusters at the apex of the stem. They have 5 green, acute sepals, with black secretory glands on the margins; 5 orange-yellow petals, also with black secretory glands on the margins; 3 staminal blades, each divided into many orange-yellow stamens and 3 carpels surmounted by red styles.

The drug may also show the following: immature and ripe fruits and seeds. Immature fruits are green or yellowish, seeds are whitish. Occasional ripe fruits may be present; these are dry trilocular capsules containing numerous seeds, brown, broad or small-ovate, 5-10 mm long, with broad linear or punctiform glands, irregularly striated ducts, conducting secretions. Ripe seeds are 1-1.3 mm long, cylindrical or trigonous, shortly pointed at both ends, brown or almost black, minutely pitted longitudinally.

B. Microscopic examination *(2.8.23)*. The powder is greenish-yellow. Examine under a microscope using *chloral hydrate solution R*. The powder shows the following diagnostic characters (Figure 1438.-1): fragments of the leaf epidermis [A, B] or stems [H] with paracytic [Ab, Ha], anisocytic [Ac, Bb, Hb] or anomocytic [Ae] stomata (*2.8.3*); fragments of the leaf epidermis often accompanied by palisade parenchyma [Ad, Bc]; polygonal cells of the upper epidermis with thickened and beaded walls [Ba]; more or less sinuous, thin-walled cells of the lower epidermis [Aa]; fragments of the leaf and sepal [E] with large, red-pigmented oil glands [Ea] associated with palisade parenchyma [Eb] and small vessels [Ec]; elongated cells of fragments of the petal epidermis with straight or wavy anticlinal walls [J]; vessels [D] with reticulate or pitted walls [Da] and groups of thick-walled fibres [Db]; fragments of the central parenchyma of the stems [K] with lignified and pitted rectangular cells [Ka] sometimes associated with vessels [Kb]; fragments of the anthers [F] showing the central part consisting of small cells containing cluster crystals of calcium oxalate [Fb] and cells from the fibrous layer [Fa]; fragments of the staminal filament with elongated, thin-walled cells with a striated cuticle [C]; numerous pollen grains with 3 germinal pores and a smooth exine, occurring singly [G] or in dense groups.

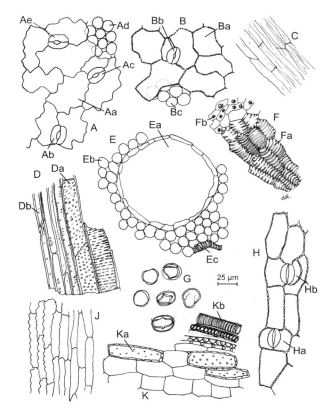

Figure 1438.-1. – *Illustration for identification test B of powdered herbal drug of St. John's wort*

C. Thin-layer chromatography (*2.2.27*).

Test solution Stir 0.5 g of the powdered herbal drug (500) (*2.9.12*) in 10 mL of *methanol R* in a water-bath at 60 °C for 10 min and filter.

Reference solution Dissolve 5 mg of *hyperoside R* and 5 mg of *rutin R* in *methanol R*, then dilute to 5 mL with the same solvent.

Plate *TLC silica gel plate R*.

Mobile phase anhydrous formic acid R, water R, ethyl acetate R (6:9:90 *V/V/V*).

Application 10 µL of the test solution and 5 µL of the reference solution, as bands of 10 mm.

Development Over a path of 10 cm.

Drying At 100-105 °C for 10 min.

Detection Treat with a 10 g/L solution of *diphenylboric acid aminoethyl ester R* in *methanol R* and then with a 50 g/L solution of *macrogol 400 R* in *methanol R*. After about 30 min, examine in ultraviolet light at 365 nm.

Results The chromatogram obtained with the reference solution shows in the lower third a zone due to rutin and above it a zone due to hyperoside, both with yellow-orange fluorescence. The chromatogram obtained with the test solution shows in the lower third 2 reddish-orange fluorescent zones due to rutin and hyperoside, and in the lower part of the upper third a zone due to pseudohypericin and above it a zone due to hypericin, both with red fluorescence. Other yellow or blue fluorescent zones are visible.

TESTS

Foreign matter (*2.8.2*)
Maximum 3 per cent of stems with a diameter greater than 5 mm and maximum 2 per cent of other foreign matter.

Loss on drying (*2.2.32*)
Maximum 10.0 per cent, determined on 1.000 g of the powdered herbal drug (500) (*2.9.12*) by drying in an oven at 105 °C for 2 h.

Total ash (*2.4.16*)
Maximum 7.0 per cent.

ASSAY

Test solution In a 100 mL round-bottomed flask, introduce 0.800 g of the powdered herbal drug (500) (*2.9.12*), 60 mL of a mixture of 20 volumes of *water R* and 80 volumes of *tetrahydrofuran R* and a magnetic stirrer. Boil the mixture in a water-bath at 70 °C under a reflux condenser for 30 min. Centrifuge (2 min at 700 g) and decant the supernatant into a 250 mL flask. Take up the residue with 60 mL of a mixture of 20 volumes of *water R* and 80 volumes of *tetrahydrofuran R*. Heat again under a reflux condenser for 30 min. Centrifuge (2 min at 700 g) and decant the supernatant. Combine the extracts and evaporate to dryness. Take up the residue with 15 mL of *methanol R* with the help of ultrasound and transfer to a 25 mL measuring flask. Rinse the 250 mL flask with *methanol R* and dilute to 25.0 mL with the same solvent. Centrifuge again, filter 10 mL through a syringe filter (0.2 µm). Discard the first 2 millilitres of the filtrate. Introduce 5.0 mL of the filtrate into a measuring flask and dilute to 25.0 mL with *methanol R*.

Compensation liquid *methanol R*.

Measure the absorbance (*2.2.25*) at 590 nm of the test solution, by comparison with the compensation liquid.

Calculate the percentage content of total hypericins, expressed as hypericin, using the following expression:

$$\frac{A \times 125}{m \times 870}$$

i.e. taking the specific absorbance of hypericin to be 870.
A = absorbance at 590 nm;
m = mass of the herbal drug to be examined, in grams.

———————————— *Ph Eur*

Quantified St. John's Wort Dry Extract

(*Ph Eur monograph 1874*)

Ph Eur ————————————————————————

DEFINITION
Quantified dry extract obtained from *St. John's wort (1438)*.

Content:
— *total hypericins, expressed as hypericin* ($C_{30}H_{16}O_8$; M_r 504.5): 0.10 per cent to 0.30 per cent (anhydrous extract);
— *flavonoids, expressed as rutin* ($C_{27}H_{30}O_{16}$; M_r 610.5): minimum 6.0 per cent (anhydrous extract);
— *hyperforin* ($C_{35}H_{52}O_4$; M_r 536.8): maximum 6.0 per cent (anhydrous extract) and not more than the content stated on the label.

PRODUCTION
The extract is produced from the herbal drug by a suitable procedure using ethanol (50-80 per cent *V/V*) or methanol (50-80 per cent *V/V*).

CHARACTERS
Appearance: brownish-grey powder.

IDENTIFICATION
Thin-layer chromatography (*2.2.27*).

Test solution Disperse 0.25 g of the extract to be examined in 5 mL of *methanol R*.

Reference solution Dissolve 5 mg of *rutin R* and 5 mg of *hyperoside R* in *methanol R* and dilute to 10 mL with the same solvent.

Plate *TLC silica gel plate R* (5-40 µm) [or *TLC silica gel plate R* (2-10 µm)].

Mobile phase anhydrous formic acid R, water R, ethyl acetate R (6:9:90 *V/V/V*).

Application 10 µL [or 5 µL] as bands of 10 mm [or 8 mm].

Development Over a path of 10 cm [or 7.5 cm].

Drying At 100-105 °C for 10 min.

Detection Treat with a 10 g/L solution of *diphenylboric acid aminoethyl ester R* in *methanol R* and then with a 50 g/L solution of *macrogol 400 R* in *methanol R*. Examine after about 30 min in ultraviolet light at 365 nm.

Results See below the sequence of zones present in the chromatograms obtained with the reference solution and the test solution. Furthermore, other fluorescent zones may be present in the chromatogram obtained with the test solution.

Top of the plate	
	A yellowish-orange fluorescent zone
	2 red fluorescent zones (hypericin and pseudohypericin)
_____	_____
	3 yellowish-orange fluorescent zones
_____	_____
Hyperoside: a yellowish-orange fluorescent zone	A yellowish-orange fluorescent zone (hyperoside)
	Yellow and blue possibly superimposed fluorescent zones
Rutin: a yellowish-orange fluorescent zone	A yellowish-orange fluorescent zone (rutin)
Reference solution	**Test solution**

TESTS

Water (*2.5.12*)
Maximum 4.0 per cent, determined on 0.5 g.

ASSAY

Total hypericins
Liquid chromatography (*2.2.29*).

Test solution   Dissolve 70.0 mg of the extract to be examined in 25.0 mL of *methanol R*. Sonicate and centrifuge the solution. Expose the solution to a xenon lamp at about 765 W/m² for 8 min.

Reference solution   Dissolve a quantity of *St. John's wort dry extract HRS* corresponding to 0.15 mg of hypericin in 25.0 mL of *methanol R*. Sonicate and centrifuge. Expose the solution to a xenon lamp at about 765 W/m² for 8 min.

Column:
— *size*: l = 0.15 m, Ø = 4.6 mm;
— *stationary phase*: *octadecylsilyl silica gel for chromatography R* (5 μm);
— *temperature*: 40 °C.

Mobile phase   Mix 39 volumes of *ethyl acetate R*, 41 volumes of a 15.6 g/L solution of *sodium dihydrogen phosphate R* adjusted to pH 2 with *phosphoric acid R* and 160 volumes of *methanol R*.

Flow rate   1.0 mL/min.

Detection   Spectrophotometer at 590 nm.

Injection   20 μL.

Run time   15 min.

Identification of peaks   Use the chromatogram supplied with *St. John's wort dry extract HRS* and the chromatogram obtained with the reference solution to identify the peaks due to pseudohypericin and hypericin.

System suitability   Reference solution:
— the chromatogram obtained is similar to the chromatogram supplied with *St. John's wort dry extract HRS*;
— *resolution*: minimum 2 between the peaks due to pseudohypericin and hypericin.

Calculate the percentage content of total hypericins, expressed as hypericin, using the following expression:

$$\frac{(A_1 + A_2) \times m_2 \times p}{A_3 \times m_1}$$

A_1 =   area of the peak due to pseudohypericin in the chromatogram obtained with the test solution;

A_2 =   area of the peak due to hypericin in the chromatogram obtained with the test solution;

A_3 =   area of the peak due to hypericin in the chromatogram obtained with the reference solution;

m_1 =   mass of the extract to be examined used to prepare the test solution, in grams;

m_2 =   mass of *St. John's wort dry extract HRS* used to prepare the reference solution, in grams;

p =   percentage content of hypericin in *St. John's wort dry extract HRS*.

Hyperforin and flavonoids
Liquid chromatography (*2.2.29*). *Carry out the assay protected from light.*

Solvent mixture   water R, methanol R (20:80 *V/V*).

Test solution   Dissolve 75.0 mg of the extract to be examined in 20.0 mL of the solvent mixture. Sonicate and centrifuge.

Reference solution (a)   Dissolve 20.0 mg of *rutoside trihydrate CRS* in 200.0 mL of the solvent mixture.

Reference solution (b)   Dissolve 75.0 mg of *St. John's wort dry extract HRS* in 20.0 mL of the solvent mixture. Sonicate and centrifuge.

Column:
— *size*: l = 0.15 m, Ø = 4.6 mm;
— *stationary phase*: *octadecylsilyl silica gel for chromatography R* (3 μm).

Mobile phase:
— *mobile phase A*: *phosphoric acid R, water R* (3:1000 *V/V*);
— *mobile phase B*: *phosphoric acid R, acetonitrile R* (3:1000 *V/V*);

Time (min)	Mobile phase A (per cent *V/V*)	Mobile phase B (per cent *V/V*)	Flow rate (mL/min)
0 - 8	82	18	0.8
8 - 18	82 → 47	18 → 53	0.8
18 - 18.1	47 → 3	53 → 97	0.8
18.1 - 19	3	97	0.8 → 1.2
19 - 31	3	97	1.2

Detection   Spectrophotometer at 360 nm, then at 275 nm after the elution of biapigenin (about 22 min).

Injection   10 μL.

Identification of peaks   Use the chromatogram supplied with *St. John's wort dry extract HRS* and the chromatogram obtained with reference solution (b) to identify the peaks due to rutin, hyperoside, isoquercitroside, quercitroside, quercetin, biapigenin, hyperforin and adhyperforin.

System suitability   Reference solution (b):
— the chromatogram obtained is similar to the chromatogram supplied with *St. John's wort dry extract HRS*;
— *resolution*: minimum 2.0 between the peaks due to rutin and hyperoside, and minimum 2.0 between the peaks due to hyperforin and adhyperforin.

Calculate the percentage content of hyperforin using the following expression:

$$\frac{A_4 \times m_4 \times p \times 2.3}{A_5 \times m_3 \times 10}$$

A_4 =   area of the peak due to hyperforin in the chromatogram obtained with the test solution;

A_5 = area of the peak due to rutin in the chromatogram obtained with reference solution (a);

m_3 = mass of the extract to be examined used to prepare the test solution, in grams;

m_4 = mass of *rutoside trihydrate CRS* used to prepare reference solution (a), in grams;

2.3 = correction factor for hyperforin with respect to rutin;

p = percentage content of rutin in *rutoside trihydrate CRS*.

Calculate the percentage content of flavonoids, expressed as rutin, using the following expression:

$$\frac{m_4 \times p \times (A_6 + A_7 + A_8 + A_9 + A_{10} + A_{11})}{m_3 \times A_5 \times 10}$$

A_5 = area of the peak due to rutin in the chromatogram obtained with reference solution (a);

A_6 = area of the peak due to rutin in the chromatogram obtained with the test solution;

A_7 = area of the peak due to hyperoside in the chromatogram obtained with the test solution;

A_8 = area of the peak due to isoquercitroside in the chromatogram obtained with the test solution;

A_9 = area of the peak due to quercitroside in the chromatogram obtained with the test solution;

A_{10} = area of the peak due to quercetin in the chromatogram obtained with the test solution;

A_{11} = area of the peak due to biapigenin in the chromatogram obtained with the test solution;

m_3 = mass of the extract to be examined used to prepare the test solution, in grams;

m_4 = mass of *rutoside trihydrate CRS* used to prepare reference solution (a), in grams;

p = percentage content of rutin in *rutoside trihydrate CRS*.

LABELLING
The label states the content of hyperforin.

———————————————————— Ph Eur

Stephania Tetrandra Root

(*Fourstamen Stephania Root,*
Ph Eur monograph 2478)

Ph Eur ——————

DEFINITION
Scraped, cut and dried root of *Stephania tetrandra* S.Moore.

Content
Minimum 1.6 per cent of the sum of tetrandrine and fangchinoline, expressed as tetrandrine ($C_{38}H_{42}N_2O_6$; M_r 623) (dried drug).

IDENTIFICATION
A. The root is found as slices or irregularly cylindrical or semi-cylindrical pieces, mostly tortuous, about 0.5-1 cm thick and 1-5 cm in diameter. The greyish-yellow outer surface usually shows deep and sinuous transversal striations; the curved parts are knotty and bumpy. The texture is dense and compact. The cut surface is greyish-white and shows radial striations.

B. Reduce to a powder (355) (*2.9.12*). The powder is whitish-grey. Examine under a microscope using *chloral hydrate solution R*. The powder shows the following diagnostic characters: numerous fragments of parenchyma with cells having slightly thickened and moniliform walls; reticulate or pitted xylem vessels accompanied by fibres; fragments of phelloderm containing sclereids; rare cork fragments; rare, fine, rod-shaped calcium oxalate crystals. Examine under a microscope using a 50 per cent *V/V* solution of *glycerol R*. The powder shows very many round or truncated, simple or 2- or 3-compound starch granules, 10-20 μm in diameter, with a punctiform hilum.

C. Thin-layer chromatography (*2.2.27*).

Test solution To 0.4 g of the powdered herbal drug (355) (*2.9.12*) add 10 mL of a mixture of 1 volume of *anhydrous formic acid R*, 9 volumes of *water R* and 40 volumes of *methanol R*. Sonicate at 25 °C for 10 min and filter.

Reference solution Dissolve 10 mg of *protopine hydrochloride R* and 10 mg of *tetrandrine R* in *methanol R* and dilute to 10 mL with the same solvent.

Plate *TLC silica gel plate R* (5-40 μm) [or *TLC silica gel plate R* (2-10 μm)].

Mobile phase concentrated ammonia R, methanol R, ethyl acetate R, toluene R (0.3:5:10:10 *V/V/V/V*).

Application 10 μL [or 5 μL] as bands of 10 mm [or 8 mm].

Development Over a path of 10 cm [or 6 cm].

Drying In a current of warm air for 5 min.

Detection Treat with a 5 g/L solution of *iodine R* in *ethanol (96 per cent) R* until the background becomes yellow; examine in daylight after the yellow colour has disappeared.

Results See below the sequence of zones present in the chromatograms obtained with the reference solution and the test solution. Furthermore, other faint zones may be present in the chromatogram obtained with the test solution.

Top of the plate	
Protopine: an orange zone	
———	
Tetrandrine: an orange zone	An orange zone (tetrandrine)
	An orange zone
Reference solution	**Test solution**

TESTS
Aristolochia fangchi
Test for aristolochic acids in herbal drugs (*2.8.21*). The drug to be examined complies with method A.

Loss on drying (*2.2.32*)
Maximum 10.0 per cent, determined on 1.000 g of the powdered herbal drug (355) (*2.9.12*) by drying in an oven at 105 °C for 2 h.

Total ash (*2.4.16*)
Maximum 4.0 per cent.

Ash insoluble in hydrochloric acid (*2.8.1*)
Maximum 1.0 per cent.

ASSAY
Tetrandrine and fangchinoline
Liquid chromatography (*2.2.29*).

Test solution In a 50 mL round-bottomed flask, weigh 0.500 g of the powdered herbal drug (355) (*2.9.12*). Add 25 mL of a 2 per cent *V/V* solution of *hydrochloric acid R* in *methanol R*. Weigh. Heat under a reflux condenser on a water-bath at 60 °C for 30 min. Cool and weigh. Adjust to the initial weight using a 2 per cent V/V solution of *hydrochloric acid R* in *methanol R*. Filter. Dilute 5.0 mL of the filtrate to 10.0 mL with the mobile phase.

Reference solution   Dissolve 10.0 mg of *tetrandrine CRS* in 5 mL of *methanol R* and dilute to 10.0 mL with the mobile phase.

Column:
— *size: l* = 0.25 m, Ø = 4.6 mm;
— *stationary phase: octadecylsilyl silica gel for chromatography R* (5 µm).

Mobile phase   4.1 g/L solution of *sodium laurylsulfonate for chromatography R* in a mixture of 1 volume of *glacial acetic acid R*, 30 volumes of *methanol R*, 30 volumes of *water R* and 40 volumes of *acetonitrile R*.

Flow rate   2.0 mL/min.

Detection   Spectrophotometer at 280 nm.

Injection   20 µL.

Run time   30 min.

Relative retention   With reference to tetrandrine (retention time = about 18 min): fangchinoline = about 0.7.

System suitability   Test solution:
— *resolution*: minimum 3.0 between the peaks due to fangchinoline and tetrandrine.

Calculate the percentage content of tetrandrine and fangchinoline, expressed as tetrandrine, using the following expression:

$$\frac{(A_1 + A_3) \times m_2 \times p \times 5}{A_2 \times m_1}$$

A_1 = area of the peak due to tetrandrine in the chromatogram obtained with the test solution;

A_2 = area of the peak due to tetrandrine in the chromatogram obtained with the reference solution;

A_3 = area of the peak due to fangchinoline in the chromatogram obtained with the test solution;

m_1 = mass of the herbal drug to be examined used to prepare the test solution, in grams;

m_2 = mass of *tetrandrine CRS* used to prepare the reference solution, in grams;

p = assigned percentage content of tetrandrine in *tetrandrine CRS*.

_____ *Ph Eur*

Sterculia

Sterculia Gum; Karaya Gum

Preparation
Sterculia Granules

When Powdered Sterculia is prescribed or demanded, material complying with the appropriate requirements below and containing not less than 10.0% of volatile acid shall be dispensed or supplied.

DEFINITION
Sterculia is the gum obtained from *Sterculia urens* Roxb. and other species of *Sterculia*.

CHARACTERISTICS
It has the macroscopical and microscopical characters described under Identification tests A and B.

Sparingly soluble in *water*, but swells into a homogeneous, adhesive, gelatinous mass. Practically insoluble in *ethanol (96%)*.

IDENTIFICATION
A. Irregular or vermiform pieces, about 5 to 20 mm thick; greyish white with a brown or pink tinge; surface striated.

B. When powdered and mounted in *ethanol (96%)* it appears as small, transparent, angular particles of various sizes and shapes; the particles lose their sharp edges when *water* is added and each gradually swells until a large, indefinite, almost structureless mass results; when mounted in *ruthenium red solution* the particles are stained red; no blue coloured particles (starch) are visible when mounted in *iodine solution R1*.

C. Add 1 g to 80 mL of *water* and allow to stand for 24 hours, shaking occasionally. A tacky and viscous granular mucilage is produced. Retain the mucilage for use in test D.

D. Boil 4 mL of the mucilage obtained in test C with 0.5 mL of *hydrochloric acid*, add 1 mL of 5M *sodium hydroxide*, filter, add 3 mL of *cupri-tartaric solution R1* to the filtrate and heat. A red precipitate is produced.

E. Warm 0.5 g with 2 mL of 5M *sodium hydroxide*. A brown colour is produced.

TESTS
Acid-insoluble ash
Not more than 1.0%, Appendix XI K.

Foreign matter
Complies with the *test for foreign matter*, Appendix XI D.

Ash
Not more than 7.0%, Appendix XI J.

Volatile acid
Not less than 14.0%, calculated as acetic acid, $C_2H_4O_2$, when determined by the following method. To 1 g contained in a 700 mL Kjeldahl flask add 100 mL of *water* and 5 mL of *orthophosphoric acid*, allow to stand for several hours, or until the gum is completely swollen, and boil gently under a reflux condenser for 2 hours. Steam distil until 800 mL of distillate is obtained and the acid residue measures about 20 mL and titrate the distillate with 0.1M *sodium hydroxide VS* using *phenolphthalein solution R1* as indicator. Repeat the operation without the substance being examined.
The difference between the titrations represents the amount of alkali required to neutralise the volatile acid. Each mL of 0.1M *sodium hydroxide VS* is equivalent to 6.005 mg of volatile acid, calculated as $C_2H_4O_2$.

Microbial contamination
1.0 g is free from *Escherichia coli*, Appendix XVI B1.

STORAGE
Sterculia should be stored in a dry place.

Sterculia Granules

DEFINITION
Sterculia Granules are Sterculia in granule form.

The granules comply with the requirements stated under Granules and with the following requirements.

CHARACTERISTICS
White or buff with a distinct odour of acetic acid; transparent, irregular shaped granules of about 1 to 4 mm which swell when treated with water.

IDENTIFICATION

A. Irregular or vermiform pieces, about 5 to 20 mm thick; greyish white with a brown or pink tinge; surface striated.

B. When powdered and mounted in *ethanol (96%)* it appears as small, transparent, angular particles of various sizes and shapes; the particles lose their sharp edges when *water* is added and each gradually swells until a large, indefinite, almost structureless mass results; when mounted in *ruthenium red solution* the particles are stained red; no blue coloured particles (starch) are visible when mounted in *iodine solution R1*.

C. Add 1 g to 80 mL of *water* and allow to stand for 24 hours, shaking occasionally. A tacky and viscous granular mucilage is produced. Retain the mucilage for use in test D.

D. Boil 4 mL of the mucilage obtained in test C with 0.5 mL of *hydrochloric acid*, add 1 mL of 5M *sodium hydroxide*, filter, add 3 mL of *cupri-tartaric solution R1* to the filtrate and heat. A red precipitate is produced.

TESTS

Acid-insoluble ash

Not more than 1.0%, Appendix XI K.

Ash

Not more than 7.0%, Appendix XI J.

Volatile acid

Not less than 13.0%, calculated as acetic acid, $C_2H_4O_2$, when determined by the following method. To 1 g contained in a 700 mL Kjeldahl flask add 100 mL of *water* and 5 mL of *orthophosphoric acid*, allow to stand for several hours, or until the granules are completely swollen, and boil gently under a reflux condenser for 2 hours. Steam distil until 800 mL of the distillate is obtained and the acid residue measures about 20 mL and titrate the distillate with 0.1M *sodium hydroxide VS* using *phenolphthalein solution R1* as indicator. Repeat the operation without the substance being examined. The difference between the titrations represents the amount of alkali required to neutralise the volatile acid. Each mL of 0.1M *sodium hydroxide VS* is equivalent to 6.005 mg of volatile acid, calculated as $C_2H_4O_2$.

Loss on drying

The powdered granules, when dried to constant weight at 105°, lose not more than 20.0% of their weight. Use 1 g.

Microbial contamination

1.0 g is free from *Escherichia coli*, Appendix XVI B1.

STORAGE

Sterculia Granules should be stored in a dry place.

Stramonium Leaf

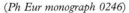

(*Ph Eur monograph 0246*)

Preparation

Prepared Stramonium

When Stramonium Leaf or Powdered Stramonium Leaf is prescribed, Prepared Stramonium shall be dispensed.

Ph Eur

DEFINITION

Dried leaf or dried leaf and flowering, and occasionally fruit-bearing, tops of *Datura stramonium* L. and its varieties.

Content

Minimum 0.25 per cent of total alkaloids, expressed as hyoscyamine ($C_{17}H_{23}NO_3$; M_r 289.4) (dried drug).

The alkaloids consist mainly of hyoscyamine with varying proportions of hyoscine (scopolamine).

CHARACTERS

Unpleasant odour.

IDENTIFICATION

A. The leaves are dark brownish-green or dark greyish-green with a short petiole, often much twisted and shrunken during drying, thin and brittle, ovate or triangular-ovate, dentately lobed with an acuminate apex and often unequal at the base. Young leaves are pubescent on the veins, older leaves are nearly glabrous. Stems are green or purplish-green, slender, curved and twisted, wrinkled longitudinally and sometimes wrinkled transversely, branched dichasially, with a single flower or an immature fruit in the fork. Flowers, on short pedicels, have a gamosepalous calyx with 5 lobes and trumpet-shaped brownish-white or purplish corolla. The fruit is a capsule, usually covered with numerous short, stiff emergences; seeds are brown or black with a minutely pitted testa.

B. Microscopic examination (*2.8.23*). The powder is greyish-green. Examine under a microscope using *chloral hydrate solution R*. The powder shows the following diagnostic characters (Figure 0246.-1): fragments of upper [A] and lower [C] epidermises of the lamina, in surface view, showing cells with slightly wavy anticlinal walls and a smooth cuticle accompanied by palisade [Aa] and spongy [Ca] parenchyma; anisocytic [Ac, Cb] and anomocytic [Ab] stomata (*2.8.3*), more frequent on the lower epidermis; fragments of covering trichomes, conical [E], uniseriate with 3-5 cells with warty walls, some of them collapsed [Ea]; glandular trichomes, short and clavate, in side view [B] with heads formed by 2-7 cells; dorsiventral mesophyll in transverse section [F], with a single layer of palisade cells [Fa] and a spongy parenchyma [Fb] containing cluster crystals of calcium oxalate [Fc]; fragments of spongy parenchyma [D] with some cells containing small cluster crystals of calcium oxalate [Db], associated with annularly and spirally thickened vessels [Da], in surface view. The powdered drug may also show: fibres and reticulately thickened vessels from the stems; subspherical pollen grains about 60-80 μm in diameter with 3 germinal pores and a nearly smooth exine [G]; fragments of the corolla [H] with wavy-walled cells [Ha] and underlying mesophyll [Hb] with some cells containing prisms [Hc] or cluster crystals [Hd] of calcium oxalate; seed fragments containing yellowish-brown, sinuous, thick-walled sclereids of the testa [J], and occasional prisms and microsphenoidal crystals of calcium oxalate.

C. Examine the chromatograms obtained in the chromatography test.

Results   The principal zones in the chromatograms obtained with the test solution are similar in position, colour and size to the principal zones in the chromatogram obtained with the same volume of the reference solution.

D. Shake 1 g of the powdered herbal drug (180) (*2.9.12*) with 10 mL of *0.05 M sulfuric acid* for 2 min. Filter and add to the filtrate 1 mL of *concentrated ammonia R* and 5 mL of *water R*. Shake cautiously with 15 mL of *peroxide-free ether R*, avoiding the formation of an emulsion. Separate the ether layer and dry over *anhydrous sodium sulfate R*. Filter and evaporate the ether in a porcelain dish. Add 0.5 mL of *nitric acid R* and evaporate to dryness on a water-bath. Add 10 mL of *acetone R* and, dropwise, a 30 g/L solution of *potassium hydroxide R* in *ethanol (96 per cent) R*. A deep violet colour develops.

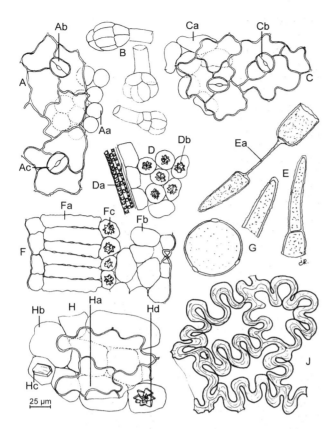

Figure 0246.-1. – *Illustration for identification test B of powdered herbal drug of stramonium leaf*

TESTS
Chromatography
Thin-layer chromatography (*2.2.27*).

Test solution   To 1.0 g of the powdered herbal drug (180) (*2.9.12*) add 10 mL of *0.05 M sulfuric acid*, shake for 15 min and filter. Wash the filter with *0.05 M sulfuric acid* until 25 mL of filtrate is obtained. To the filtrate add 1 mL of *concentrated ammonia R* and shake with 2 quantities, each of 10 mL, of *peroxide-free ether R*. If necessary, separate by centrifugation. Dry the combined ether layers over *anhydrous sodium sulfate R*, filter and evaporate to dryness on a water-bath. Dissolve the residue in 0.5 mL of *methanol R*.

Reference solution   Dissolve 50 mg of *hyoscyamine sulfate R* in 9 mL of *methanol R*. Dissolve 15 mg of *hyoscine hydrobromide R* in 10 mL of *methanol R*. Mix 3.8 mL of the hyoscyamine sulfate solution and 4.2 mL of the hyoscine hydrobromide solution and dilute to 10 mL with *methanol R*.

Plate   *TLC silica gel G plate R*.

Mobile phase   concentrated ammonia R, water R, acetone R (3:7:90 *V/V/V*).

Application   10 µL and 20 µL, as bands of 20 mm by 3 mm, leaving 1 cm between the bands.

Development   Over a path of 10 cm.

Drying   At 100-105 °C for 15 min; allow to cool.

Detection A   Spray with *potassium iodobismuthate solution R2*, using about 10 mL for a plate 200 mm square, until the orange or brown zones become visible against a yellow background.

Results A   The zones in the chromatograms obtained with the test solution are similar in position (hyoscyamine in the lower third, hyoscine in the upper third of the chromatograms) and colour to those in the chromatograms obtained with the reference solution. The zones in the chromatograms obtained with the test solution are at least equal in size to the corresponding zones in the chromatogram obtained with the same volume of the reference solution. Faint secondary zones may appear, particularly in the middle of the chromatogram obtained with 20 µL of the test solution or near the point of application in the chromatogram obtained with 10 µL of the test solution.

Detection B   Spray with *sodium nitrite solution R* until the coating is transparent; examine after 15 min.

Results B   The zones due to hyoscyamine in the chromatograms obtained with the reference solution and the test solution change from brown to reddish-brown but not to greyish-blue (atropine) and any secondary zones disappear.

Foreign matter (*2.8.2*)
Maximum 3 per cent of stems with a diameter greater than 5 mm.

Total ash (*2.4.16*)
Maximum 20.0 per cent.

Ash insoluble in hydrochloric acid (*2.8.1*)
Maximum 4.0 per cent.

ASSAY
a) Determine the loss on drying (*2.2.32*) on 2.000 g of the powdered herbal drug (180) (*2.9.12*) by drying in an oven at 105 °C.

b) Moisten 10.0 g of the powdered herbal drug (180) (*2.9.12*) with a mixture of 5 mL of *ammonia R*, 10 mL of *ethanol (96 per cent) R* and 30 mL of *peroxide-free ether R* and mix thoroughly. Transfer the mixture to a suitable percolator, if necessary with the aid of the extracting mixture. Allow to macerate for 4 h and percolate with a mixture of 1 volume of *chloroform R* and 3 volumes of *peroxide-free ether R* until the alkaloids are completely extracted. Evaporate to dryness a few millilitres of the liquid flowing from the percolator, dissolve the residue in *0.25 M sulfuric acid* and verify the absence of alkaloids using *potassium tetraiodomercurate solution R*. Concentrate the percolate to about 50 mL by distilling on a water-bath and transfer it to a separating funnel, rinsing with *peroxide-free ether R*. Add a quantity of *peroxide-free ether R* equal to at least 2.1 times the volume of the percolate to produce a liquid of a density well below that of water. Shake the solution with no fewer than 3 quantities, each of 20 mL, of *0.25 M sulfuric acid*, separate the 2 layers by centrifugation if necessary and transfer the acid layers to a 2nd separating funnel. Make the acid layer alkaline with *ammonia R* and shake with 3 quantities, each of 30 mL, of *chloroform R*. Combine the chloroform layers, add 4 g of *anhydrous sodium sulfate R* and allow to stand for 30 min with occasional shaking. Decant the chloroform and wash the anhydrous sodium sulfate with 3 quantities, each of 10 mL, of *chloroform R*. Add the washings to the chloroform extract, evaporate to dryness on a water-bath and heat in an oven at 100-105 °C for 15 min. Dissolve the residue in a few millilitres of *chloroform R*, add 20.0 mL of *0.01 M sulfuric acid* and remove the chloroform by evaporation on a water-bath. Titrate the excess of acid with *0.02 M sodium hydroxide* using *methyl red mixed solution R* as indicator.

Calculate the percentage content of total alkaloids, expressed as hyoscyamine, using the following expression:

$$\frac{57.88 \times (20 - n)}{(100 - d) \times m}$$

d = loss on drying, as a percentage;
n = volume of *0.02 M sodium hydroxide*, in millilitres;
m = mass of the powdered herbal drug, in grams.

STORAGE

Protected from moisture.

————————————————————————— *Ph Eur*

Prepared Stramonium

(*Ph Eur monograph 0247*)

Ph Eur _____

DEFINITION

Stramonium leaf powder (180) (*2.9.12*) adjusted, if necessary, by the addition of powdered lactose or stramonium leaf of lower content of total alkaloids.

Content

0.23 per cent to 0.27 per cent of total alkaloids, expressed as hyoscyamine ($C_{17}H_{23}NO_3$; M_r 289.4) (dried drug).

CHARACTERS

Appearance

Greyish-green powder.

Unpleasant odour.

IDENTIFICATION

A. Examine under a microscope using *chloral hydrate solution R*. The powder shows the following diagnostic characters: fragments of leaf lamina showing epidermal cells with slightly wavy anticlinal walls and smooth cuticle; stomata are more frequent on the lower epidermis (anisocytic and anomocytic) (*2.8.3*); covering trichomes are conical, uniseriate with 3-5 cells and warty walls; glandular trichomes are short and clavate with heads formed by 2-7 cells; dorsiventral mesophyll, with a single layer of palisade cells and a spongy parenchyma containing cluster crystals of calcium oxalate; annularly and spirally thickened vessels. The powdered drug may also show the following diagnostic characters: fibres and reticulately thickened vessels from the stems; subspherical pollen grains usually about 60-80 µm in diameter with 3 germinal pores and nearly smooth exine; fragments of the corolla with papillose epidermis; seed fragments containing yellowish-brown, sinuous, thick-walled sclereids of testa; occasional prisms and microsphenoidal crystals of calcium oxalate. Examined in *glycerol (85 per cent) R*, it may be seen to contain lactose crystals.

B. Examine the chromatograms obtained in the Chromatography test.

Results The principal zones in the chromatogram obtained with the test solution are similar in position, colour and size to the principal zones in the chromatogram obtained with the same volume of the reference solution.

C. Shake 1 g with 10 mL of *0.05 M sulfuric acid* for 2 min. Filter and add to the filtrate 1 mL of *concentrated ammonia R* and 5 mL of *water R*. Shake cautiously with 15 mL of *peroxide-free ether R*, avoiding the formation of an emulsion. Separate the ether layer and dry over *anhydrous sodium sulfate R*. Filter and evaporate the ether in a porcelain dish. Add 0.5 mL of *nitric acid R* and evaporate to dryness on a water-bath. Add 10 mL of *acetone R* and, dropwise, a 30 g/L solution of *potassium hydroxide R* in *ethanol (96 per cent) R*. A deep violet colour develops.

TESTS

Chromatography

Thin-layer chromatography (*2.2.27*).

Test solution To 1.0 g of the drug to be examined add 10 mL of *0.05 M sulfuric acid*, shake for 15 min and filter. Wash the filter with *0.05 M sulfuric acid* until 25 mL of filtrate is obtained. To the filtrate add 1 mL of *concentrated ammonia R* and shake with 2 quantities, each of 10 mL, of *peroxide-free ether R*. If necessary, separate by centrifugation. Dry the combined ether layers over *anhydrous sodium sulfate R*, filter and evaporate to dryness on a water-bath. Dissolve the residue in 0.5 mL of *methanol R*.

Reference solution Dissolve 50 mg of *hyoscyamine sulfate R* in 9 mL of *methanol R*. Dissolve 15 mg of *hyoscine hydrobromide R* in 10 mL of *methanol R*. Mix 3.8 mL of the hyoscyamine sulfate solution and 4.2 mL of the hyoscine hydrobromide solution and dilute to 10 mL with *methanol R*.

Plate TLC silica gel G plate R.

Mobile phase concentrated ammonia R, water R, acetone R (3:7:90 *V/V/V*).

Application 10 µL and 20 µL of each solution as bands of 20 mm by 3 mm, leaving 1 cm between the bands.

Development Over a path of 10 cm.

Drying At 100-105 °C for 15 min and allow to cool.

Detection A Spray with *potassium iodobismuthate solution R2*, using about 10 mL for a plate 200 mm square, until the orange or brown zones become visible against a yellow background.

Results A The zones in the chromatograms obtained with the test solution are similar in position (hyoscyamine in the lower third, hyoscine in the upper third of the chromatogram) and colour to those in the chromatograms obtained with the reference solution. The zones in the chromatograms obtained with the test solution are at least equal in size to the corresponding zones in the chromatogram obtained with the same volume of the reference solution. Faint secondary zones may appear, particularly in the middle of the chromatogram obtained with 20 µL of the test solution or near the point of application in the chromatogram obtained with 10 µL of the test solution.

Detection B Spray with *sodium nitrite solution R* until the coating is transparent; examine after 15 min.

Results B The zones due to hyoscyamine in the chromatograms obtained with the test solution and the reference solution change from brown to reddish-brown but not to greyish-blue (atropine) and any secondary zones disappear.

Loss on drying (*2.2.32*)

Maximum 5.0 per cent, determined on 1.000 g by drying in an oven at 105 °C.

Total ash (*2.4.16*)

Maximum 20.0 per cent.

Ash insoluble in hydrochloric acid (*2.8.1*)

Maximum 4.0 per cent.

ASSAY

a) Determine the loss on drying (*2.2.32*) on 2.000 g by drying in an oven at 105 °C.

b) Moisten 10.0 g with a mixture of 5 mL of *ammonia R*, 10 mL of *ethanol (96 per cent) R* and 30 mL of *peroxide-free ether R* and mix thoroughly. Transfer the mixture to a suitable percolator, if necessary with the aid of the extracting mixture. Allow to macerate for 4 h and percolate with a mixture of 1 volume of *chloroform R* and 3 volumes of *peroxide-free ether R* until the alkaloids are completely extracted. Evaporate to dryness a few millilitres of the liquid flowing from the percolator, dissolve the residue in *0.25 M sulfuric acid* and verify the absence of alkaloids using *potassium tetraiodomercurate solution R*. Concentrate the percolate to about 50 mL by distilling on a water-bath and transfer it to a separating funnel, rinsing with *peroxide-free ether R*. Add a quantity of *peroxide-free ether R* equal to at least 2.1 times the volume of the percolate to produce a liquid of a density well below that of water. Shake the solution with no fewer than 3 quantities, each of 20 mL, of *0.25 M sulfuric acid*, separate the 2 layers by centrifugation if necessary and transfer the acid layers to a 2nd separating funnel. Make the acid layer alkaline with *ammonia R* and shake with 3 quantities, each of 30 mL, of *chloroform R*. Combine the chloroform layers, add 4 g of *anhydrous sodium sulfate R* and allow to stand for 30 min with occasional shaking. Decant the chloroform and wash the sodium sulfate with 3 quantities, each of 10 mL, of *chloroform R*. Add the washings to the chloroform extract, evaporate to dryness on a water-bath and heat in an oven at 100-105 °C for 15 min. Dissolve the residue in a few millilitres of *chloroform R*, add 20.0 mL of *0.01 M sulfuric acid* and remove the chloroform by evaporation on a water-bath. Titrate the excess of acid with *0.02 M sodium hydroxide* using *methyl red mixed solution R* as indicator.

Calculate the percentage content of total alkaloids, expressed as hyoscyamine, using the following expression:

$$\frac{57.88\,(20 - n)}{(100 - d)\,m}$$

d = loss on drying, as a percentage;
n = volume of *0.02 M sodium hydroxide*, in millilitres;
m = mass of drug, in grams.

STORAGE
In an airtight container.

———————————————————————————— *Ph Eur*

Tea Tree Oil

Melaleuca Oil

(Ph Eur monograph 1837)

Ph Eur ————————————————————————————

DEFINITION
Essential oil obtained by steam distillation from the foliage and terminal branchlets of *Melaleuca alternifolia* (Maiden and Betch) Cheel, *M. linariifolia* Smith, *M. dissitiflora* F. Mueller and/or other species of *Melaleuca*.

CHARACTERS
Appearance
Clear, mobile, colourless or pale yellow liquid.
Characteristic odour.

IDENTIFICATION
First identification B.
Second identification A.
A. Thin-layer chromatography (*2.2.27*).

Test solution Dissolve 0.1 mL of the substance to be examined in 5 mL of *heptane R*.

Reference solution Dissolve 30 µL of *cineole R*, 60 µL of *terpinen-4-ol R* and 10 mg of *α-terpineol R* in 10 mL of *heptane R*.

Plate TLC silica gel plate R.

Mobile phase ethyl acetate R, heptane R (20:80 *V/V*).

Application 10 µL, as bands.

Development Over a path of 10 cm.

Drying In air.

Detection Spray with *anisaldehyde solution R*. Heat at 100-105 °C for 5-10 min while observing. Examine in daylight.

Results See below the sequence of the zones present in the chromatograms obtained with the reference solution and the test solution. Furthermore, other zones are present in the chromatogram obtained with the test solution.

Top of the plate	
Cineole: a violet-brown zone	A violet-brown zone, less intense (cineole)
Terpinen-4-ol: a brownish-violet zone	A brownish-violet zone terpinen-4-ol)
α-terpineol: a violet or brownish-violet zone	A violet or brownish-violet zone (α-terpineol)
Reference solution	**Test solution**

B. Examine the chromatograms obtained in the test for chromatographic profile.

Results The characteristic peaks in the chromatogram obtained with the test solution are similar in retention time to those in the chromatogram obtained with the reference solution.

TESTS
Relative density (*2.2.5*)
0.885 to 0.906.

Refractive index (*2.2.6*)
1.475 to 1.482.

Optical rotation (*2.2.7*)
+ 5° to + 15°.

Chromatographic profile
Gas chromatography (*2.2.28*): use the normalisation procedure.

Test solution Dissolve 0.15 mL of the substance to be examined in 10 mL of *hexane R*.

Reference solution Dissolve 5 µL of *α-pinene R*, 5 µL of *sabinene R*, 15 µL of *α-terpinene R*, 5 µL of *limonene R*, 5 µL of *cineole R*, 30 µL of *γ-terpinene R*, 5 µL of *p-cymene R*, 5 µL of *terpinolene R*, 60 µL of *terpinen-4-ol R*, 5 µL of *aromadendrene R* and 5 mg of *α-terpineol R* in 10 mL of *hexane R*.

Column:
— *material*: fused silica,
— *size*: $l = 30$ m (a film thickness of 1 µm may be used) to 60 m (a film thickness of 0.2 µm may be used), Ø = 0.25-0.53 mm,
— *stationary phase*: macrogol 20 000 R.

Carrier gas helium for chromatography R.

Flow rate 1.3 mL/min.

Split ratio 1:50.

Temperature:

	Time (min)	Temperature (°C)
Column	0 - 1	50
	1 - 37	50 → 230
	37 - 45	230
Injection port		240
Detector		240

Detection   Flame ionisation.

Injection   1 µL.

Elution order   Order indicated in the composition of the reference solution. Record the retention times of these substances.

System suitability   Reference solution:
— *resolution*: minimum 2.7 between the peaks due to terpinen-4-ol and aromadendrene.

Using the retention times determined from the chromatogram obtained with the reference solution, locate the components of the reference solution in the chromatogram obtained with the test solution. Disregard the peak due to hexane.

Determine the percentage content of these components. The percentages are within the following ranges:
— *α-pinene*: 1.0 per cent to 6.0 per cent,
— *sabinene*: maximum 3.5 per cent,
— *α-terpinene*: 5.0 per cent to 13.0 per cent,
— *limonene*: 0.5 per cent to 4.0 per cent,
— *cineole*: maximum 15.0 per cent,
— *γ-terpinene*: 10.0 per cent to 28.0 per cent,
— *p-cymene*: 0.5 per cent to 12.0 per cent,
— *terpinolene*: 1.5 per cent to 5.0 per cent,
— *terpinen-4-ol*: minimum 30.0 per cent,
— *aromadendrene*: maximum 7.0 per cent,
— *α-terpineol*: 1.5 per cent to 8.0 per cent.

STORAGE

At a temperature not exceeding 25 °C.

_____ *Ph Eur*

Terminalia Arjuna Stem Bark

DEFINITION

Terminalia Arjuna Stem Bark consists of cut dried bark of the stems of *Terminalia arjuna* W. and A. It contains not less than 6% of tannins, expressed as pyrogallol, calculated with reference to the dried drug.

IDENTIFICATION

A. Irregularly flattened or slightly curved or recurved pieces, up to about 8 cm long, 4 cm wide and 1 cm thick; outer surface uneven, dark brown or sometimes mottled greyish-brown, smooth or, more frequently, irregularly striated longitudinally with occasional transverse ridges; inner surface pink to reddish brown with longitudinal striations and occasional paler brown patches. Fracture short and starchy in the inner part, the outer part frequently laminated.

B. Reduce to a powder (355). The powder is reddish-brown. Examine under a microscope using *chloral hydrate solution*. The powder shows a variety of parenchymatous cells, some thin-walled, square or round and others yellowish, polygonal and thick-walled. Rectangular or polygonal, pitted, thin-walled, light brown, lightly lignified cells from the cork layer or outer areas of the cortex are present.

Fibres occur singly and in small or large groups, individual cells narrowing to highly pointed ends, and possibly showing wavy invaginations of the walls where surrounding cells have become detached; degree of lignification varies; walls are yellowish brown, some pitted, others not. Single fibres may be complete, but those in groups are usually fragmented, individual cells being straight or noticeably curved in places. Rounded cells of the medullary rays, which are one cell wide, intersperse the fibres.

Small, calcium oxalate cluster crystals occur scattered throughout as well as being found within parenchymatous cells, some forming a crystal sheath alongside the fibres. Other crystals are very large and less well defined, and usually free.

Examine under a microscope using 50% v/v of *glycerol*. Starch granules are frequent, but not abundant, mainly free, but some in parenchymatous cells. They are small, simple, round, oval or irregular in shape, and occasionally in 2 to 3 compound granules, without visible hila. More or less frequent scattered lumps of brown pigment may be found sometimes in parenchymatous cells.

C. Carry out the method for *thin-layer chromatography*, Appendix III A, using the following solutions.

(1) Shake 1.0 g of the powdered drug with 10 mL of *absolute ethanol*, centrifuge at 3000 rpm for 5 minutes and filter (Whatman GF/C is suitable).

(2) 0.01% w/v each of *arjunolic acid* and *gallic acid* in *absolute ethanol*.

CHROMATOGRAPHIC CONDITIONS

(a) Use as the coating high performance silica gel (Merck silica gel 60 HPTLC plates are suitable).

(b) Use the mobile phase described below.

(c) Apply as bands 8 µL of each solution.

(d) Develop the plate to 8 cm.

(e) Remove the plate and allow it to dry in air for 5 minutes. Spray the plate with *anisaldehyde solution*, heat at 100° to 105° for 5 minutes and examine in daylight.

MOBILE PHASE

15 volumes of *ethyl acetate*, 15 volumes of *formic acid* and 70 volumes of *toluene*.

SYSTEM SUITABILITY

The test is not valid unless the chromatogram obtained with solution (2) shows two clearly separated bands.

CONFIRMATION

The chromatogram obtained with solution (1) shows a band with an Rf value of approximately 0.30 corresponding in colour and position to the band obtained for arjunolic acid in solution (2); two clearly separated dark bands with an Rf value of approximately 0.2; a band with an Rf value of 0.63 is present. Other bands may be present.

TESTS

Ash

Not more than 25%, Appendix XI J.

Loss on drying

When dried for 2 hours at 100° to 105°, loses not more than 10% of its weight. Use 1 g.

Water soluble extractive

Not less than 20%, Appendix XI B2.

Top of the plate	
Dark band	
Dark band	Dark band: arjunolic acid
Two separated dark bands	Yellow band: gallic acid
Solution (1)	**Solution (2)**

ASSAY

Carry out the determination of *tannins in herbal drugs*, Appendix XI M. Use 1.0 g of powdered drug.

Terminalia Belerica Fruit

DEFINITION

Terminalia Belerica Fruit consists of pericarp of dried ripe fruits of *Terminalia belerica* Roxb. It contains not less than 10% of tannins, expressed as pyrogallol, calculated with reference to the dried drug.

IDENTIFICATION

A. The dried fruits are spherical to subspherical, about 3 to 5 cm in diameter, slightly depressed at the upper end and more or less tapering to the scar of the pedicel at the lower end. The surface is brown to yellowish brown with a grey velvety sheen, irregularly wrinkled and sometimes with faint, incomplete, longitudinal ridges. Cut transversely, the fruit shows the pericarp about 4 to 5 mm thick enclosing a very hard, yellowish-white seed.

B. Reduce to a powder (355). The powder is light-brown. Examine under a microscope using *chloral hydrate solution*. The powder shows many free, unicellular, straight or slightly bent trichomes from the epicarp. A variety of thick–walled, heavily pitted, lignified fibro-sclereids of elongated and spherical shapes occur in large and small groups; occasional medium sized reticulate vessels; heavily pitted, lignified parenchymatous cells and others with reticulate thickenings; many lignified, pitted, thin walled sclereids and groups of fragmented, thick-walled, pitted, fibres are present. Rarely oil globules, starch granules, and calcium oxalate crystals may be found in the parenchymatous cells from the embryo. Examine under a microscope using 50% v/v of *glycerol*. The powder shows minute, either single or 2 to 4 compound starch granules, some scattered, but mainly filling parenchymatous cells. Some have slit or stellate hila; simple granules are often not perfectly spherical. Larger calcium oxalate crystals, with fewer small ones, are scattered or in parenchymatous cells.

C. Carry out the method for *thin-layer chromatography*, Appendix III A, using the following solutions.

(1) Add 10 mL of *absolute ethanol* to 1.0 g of the powdered drug, centrifuge at 3000 rpm for 5 minutes and filter (Whatman GF/C is suitable).

(2) 0.01% w/v each of *arjunolic acid*, *gallic acid* and *ellagic acid* in *absolute ethanol*.

CHROMATOGRAPHIC CONDITIONS

(a) Use as the coating high performance silica gel F_{254} (Merck silica gel 60 F_{254} HPTLC plates are suitable).

(b) Use the mobile phase described below.

(c) Apply as bands 8 µL of each solution.

(d) Develop the plate to 8 cm.

(e) Remove the plate and allow it to dry in air for 5 minutes. Examine under *ultraviolet light (254 nm)*. Spray the plate with *anisaldehyde solution*, heat at 100° to 105° for 5 minutes and examine in daylight.

MOBILE PHASE

15 volumes of *ethyl acetate*, 15 volumes of *formic acid* and 70 volumes of *toluene*.

SYSTEM SUITABILITY

The test is not valid unless the chromatogram obtained with solution (2) shows two clearly separated bands under both *ultraviolet light (254 nm)* and daylight.

CONFIRMATION

Under *ultraviolet light (254 nm)* the chromatogram obtained with solution (1) shows bands with Rf values of approximately 0.11 and 0.15 corresponding in colour and position to the bands obtained with ellagic acid and gallic acid in solution (2) and light blue bands with Rf values of approximately 0.04 and 0.36. Other bands may be present.

Top of the plate	
Light blue band	
Blue band	Blue band: gallic acid
Dark band	Dark band: ellagic acid
Light blue band	
Solution (1)	**Solution (2)**

Under daylight after spraying with *anisaldehyde solution* the chromatogram obtained with solution (1) shows a band with an Rf value of approximately 0.15 corresponding in colour and position to the band obtained gallic acid in solution (2); a dark band with an Rf value of 0.36; several dark bands in the upper part of the plate.

Top of the plate	
Several dark bands	
Dark band	
	Dark band: arjunolic acid
Light brown band	Light brown band: gallic acid
Solution (1)	**Solution (2)**

TESTS

Ash

Not more than 7%, Appendix XI J.

Loss on drying

When dried for 2 hours at 100° to 105°, loses not more than 5.0% of its weight. Use 1 g.

Water soluble extractive

Not less than 45%, Appendix XI B2.

ASSAY

Carry out the determination of *tannins in herbal drugs*, Appendix XI M. Use 1.0 g of powdered drug.

Terminalia Chebula Fruit

DEFINITION

Terminalia Chebula Fruit consists of pericarp of mature fruits of *Terminalia chebula* Retz. It contains not less than 20% of tannins, expressed as pyrogallol, calculated with reference to the dried drug.

IDENTIFICATION

A. The dried fruits are sub-globular to ovoid, 3 to 4 cm long and 1.5 to 2 cm wide, bluntly pointed at the tip and tapering towards the base. The surface is yellowish to greenish, sometimes brown, shiny and more or less wrinkled and has distinct longitudinal ridges. Cut transversely, the fruit shows the pericarp about 3 to 4 mm thick, non-adherent to the very hard, creamy-white seed.

B. Reduce to a powder (355). The powder is yellowish brown. Examine under a microscope using *chloral hydrate solution*. The powder shows round, oval or elongated, thin-walled parenchymatous cells in groups. Occasional narrow-walled, unpitted, lightly lignified fibres occur in small or larger groups, some forming wave-like arrangements. Large groups of fragmented, heavily lignified and pitted fibres also occur. A variety of thick–walled, heavily pitted, lignified fibro-sclereids of elongated, rectangular, and irregular shapes occur in large and small groups. Fewer pitted, lignified parenchyma, or thinner-walled, less lignified and pitted sclereids, with broad lumens, are also found. There are very occasional small, spiral, lignified vessel fragments. Small, greenish, thick-walled polygonal epicarp cells are seen in surface view. Parenchymatous cells with reticulate thickenings across the surface are rare, as are others without such thickenings, but containing oil globules. Examine under a microscope using 50% v/v of *glycerol*. The powder shows minute, either single or 2 to 4 compound granules, some scattered, but mainly filling parenchymatous cells. Some have slit or stellate hila; simple granules are often not perfectly spherical. Larger calcium oxalate crystals, with fewer small ones, are scattered or in parenchymatous cells.

C. Carry out the method for *thin-layer chromatography*, Appendix III A, using the following solutions.

(1) To 1.0 g of the powdered drug, add 10 mL of *absolute ethanol*, centrifuge at 3000 rpm for 5 minutes and filter (Whatman GF/C is suitable).

(2) 0.01% w/v each of *arjunolic acid, gallic acid* and *ellagic acid* in *absolute ethanol*.

CHROMATOGRAPHIC CONDITIONS

(a) Use as the coating high performance silica gel F_{254} (Merck silica gel 60 F_{254} HPTLC plates are suitable).

(b) Use the mobile phase described below.

(c) Apply as bands 8 µL of each solution.

(d) Develop the plate to 8 cm.

(e) Remove the plate and allow it to dry in air for 5 minutes. Examine under *ultraviolet light (254 nm)*. Spray the plate with *anisaldehyde solution*, heat at 100° to 105° for 5 minutes and examine in daylight.

MOBILE PHASE

A mixture of 15 volumes of *ethyl acetate*, 15 volumes of *formic acid* and 70 volumes of *toluene*.

SYSTEM SUITABILITY

The test is not valid unless the chromatogram obtained with solution (2) shows two clearly separated bands under both *ultraviolet light (254 nm)* and daylight.

VALIDITY

When examined under *ultraviolet light (254 nm)* the chromatogram obtained with solution (1) shows bands with Rf values of approximately 0.11 and 0.15 corresponding in colour and position to the bands obtained with gallic acid and ellagic acid in solution (2).

Top of the plate	
Blue band	Blue band: gallic acid
Dark band	Dark band: ellagic acid
Solution (1)	Solution (2)

When examined under daylight after spraying with *anisaldehyde solution* the chromatogram obtained with solution (1) shows a band with an Rf value of approximately 0.15 corresponding in colour and position to the band obtained for gallic acid in solution (2) and a dark band with an Rf value of approximately 0.30. There may be some faint brown bands with Rf values of approximately 0.40 and 0.70.

Top of the plate	
Dark band	Dark band: arjunolic acid
Light brown band	Light brown band: gallic acid
Solution (1)	Solution (2)

TESTS

Ash
Not more than 5%, Appendix XI J.

Loss on drying
When dried for 2 hours at 100° to 105°, loses not more than 10% of its weight. Use 1 g.

Water soluble extractive
Not less than 50%, Appendix XI B2.

ASSAY
Carry out the determination of *tannins in herbal drugs*, Appendix XI M. Use 1.0 g of powdered drug.

Thyme

(Ph Eur monograph 0865)

Ph Eur _____

DEFINITION
Whole leaves and flowers separated from the previously dried stems of *Thymus vulgaris* L. or *Thymus zygis* L. or a mixture of both species.

Content:
— *essential oil*: minimum 12 mL/kg (anhydrous drug);
— *sum of the contents of thymol and carvacrol* (both $C_{10}H_{14}O$; M_r 150.2): minimum 40 per cent in the essential oil.

CHARACTERS
Strong aromatic odour reminiscent of thymol.

IDENTIFICATION
A. The leaf of *Thymus vulgaris* is usually 4-12 mm long and up to 3 mm wide, sessile or with a very short petiole. The lamina is tough, entire, lanceolate or ovate, covered on both surfaces by a grey or greenish-grey indumentum; the edges are markedly rolled up towards the abaxial surface. The midrib is depressed on the adaxial surface and is very prominent on the abaxial surface. The calyx is green, often with violet spots and is tubular; at the end are 2 lips of which the upper one is bent back and at the end has 3 lobes, the lower is longer and has 2 hairy teeth. After flowering, the calyx tube is closed by a crown of long, stiff hairs. The corolla, about twice as long as the calyx, is usually brownish in the dry state and is slightly bilabiate.

The leaf of *Thymus zygis* is usually 1.7-6.5 mm long and 0.4-1.2 mm wide; it is acicular or linear-lanceolate and the edges are markedly rolled towards the abaxial surface. Both surfaces of the lamina are green or greenish-grey and the midrib is sometimes violet; the edges, in particular at the base, have long, white hairs. The dried flowers are very similar to those of *Thymus vulgaris*.

B. Reduce to a powder (355) (*2.9.12*). The powder of both species is greyish-green or greenish-brown. Examine under a microscope using *chloral hydrate solution R*. The epidermises of the leaves have cells with anticlinal walls which are sinuous and beaded and the stomata are diacytic (*2.8.3*); numerous secretory trichomes made up of 12 secretory cells, the cuticle of which is generally raised by the secretion to form a globular or ovoid bladder-like covering; the glandular trichomes have a unicellular stalk and a globular or ovoid head; the covering trichomes of the adaxial surface are common to both species; they have warty walls and are shaped as pointed teeth; the warty covering trichomes of the abaxial surface are of many types: unicellular, straight or slightly curved, and bicellular or tricellular, articulated and often elbow-shaped (*Thymus vulgaris*); bicellular or tricellular, more or less straight (*Thymus zygis*). Fragments of calyx are covered by numerous, uniseriate, articulated trichomes with 5-6 cells and with a weakly striated cuticle. Fragments of the corolla have numerous uniseriate covering trichomes, often collapsed, and secretory trichomes generally with 12 cells. Pollen grains are relatively rare, spherical and smooth with 6 germinal slit-like pores, measuring about 35 μm in diameter. The powder of *Thymus zygis* also contains numerous thick bundles of fibres from the main veins and from fragments of stems.

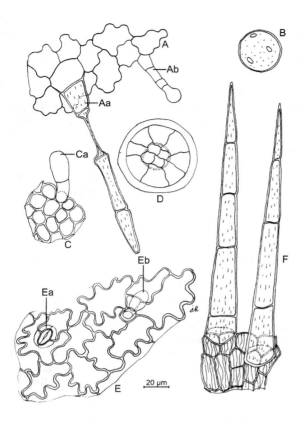

A. Epidermis of the outer surface of the corolla, in surface view, showing a covering trichome with one cell collapsed (Aa), and a unicellular-headed glandular trichomes (Ab)

B. Pollen grain with 6 germinal pores (of which only 3 are visible in the illustration)

C. Epidermis of the lower corolla with glandular trichome (Ca)

D. Secretory trichome with 12 cells

E. Outer epidermis of the upper corolla, in surface view, with diacytic stomata (Ea) and glandular trichome (Eb)

F. Epidermis of the calyx, in surface view, with covering trichomes

Figure 0865.-1. – *Illustration of powdered herbal drug of Thymus vulgaris L. (see Identification B)*

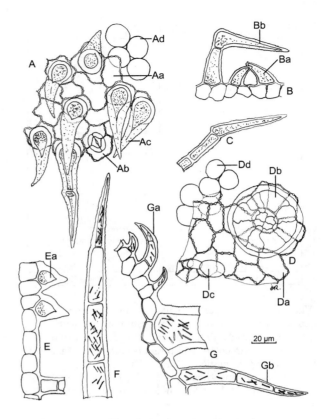

A. Upper epidermis, in surface view, with beaded cells (Aa), diacytic stomata (Ab) and covering trichomes with warty walls (Ac) and underlying palisade parenchyma (Ad)

B and E. Epidermis, in transverse section, with unicellular covering trichomes (Ba, Ea) and articulated bicellular covering trichome (Bb)

C. Articulated tricellular covering trichome

D. Upper epidermis, in surface view, with beaded cells (Da), secretory trichome made up of 12 secretory cells (Db), and glandular trichome with a unicellular head (Dc) and underlying palisade parenchyma (Dd)

F. Multicellular covering trichome from the base of the lamina (T. zygis)

G. Epidermis, in transverse section, with bicellular (Ga) and tricellular (Gb) covering trichomes (T. zygis)

Figure 0865.-2. – *Illustration of powdered herbal drug of Thymus zygis L. (see Identification B)*

C. Thin-layer chromatography (*2.2.27*).

Test solution To 1.0 of the powdered drug (355) (*2.9.12*) add 5 mL of *methylene chloride R* and shake for 3 min, filter through about 2 g of *anhydrous sodium sulfate R*.

Reference solution Dissolve 5 mg of *thymol R* and 10 μL of *carvacrol R* in 10 mL of *methylene chloride R*.

Plate TLC silica gel F_{254} plate R.

Mobile phase methylene chloride R.

Application 20 μL as bands.

Development Over a path of 15 cm.

Drying In air.

Detection A Examine in ultraviolet light at 254 nm.

Results A See below the sequence of the zones present in the chromatograms obtained with the reference solution and the test solution.

Top of the plate	
—	—
	A prominent quenching zone
	A quenching zone (thymol)
Thymol: a quenching zone	
—	—
	Quenching zones
Reference solution	**Test solution**

Detection B Spray with *anisaldehyde solution R* using 10 mL for a plate 200 mm square and heat at 100-105 °C for 10 min.

Results B See below the sequence of the zones present in the chromatograms obtained with the reference solution and the test solution. Furthermore, other zones are present in the lower third of the chromatogram obtained with the test solution. The intensity of the zones due to thymol and carvacrol depends upon the species examined.

Top of the plate	
———	———
Thymol: a brownish-pink zone	A brownish-pink zone (thymol)
Carvacrol: a pale violet zone	A pale violet zone (carvacrol)
———	———
	A greyish-pink zone
	A violet zone (cineole and linalol)
	A greyish-brown zone (borneol)
	A violet-blue zone
	An intense violet zone
Reference solution	Test solution

D. Examine the chromatograms obtained in the assay for thymol and carvacrol.

Results   The characteristic peaks in the chromatogram obtained with the test solution are similar in retention time to those in the chromatogram obtained with the reference solution.

TESTS

Foreign matter (*2.8.2*)

Maximum 10 per cent of stems and maximum 2 per cent of other foreign matter. Stems must not be more than 1 mm in diameter and 15 mm in length. Leaves with long trichomes at their base and with weakly pubescent other parts (*Thymus serpyllum L.*) are absent.

Water (*2.2.13*)

Maximum 100 mL/kg, determined on 20.0 g of the powdered drug (355) (*2.9.12*).

Total ash (*2.4.16*)

Maximum 15.0 per cent.

Ash insoluble in hydrochloric acid (*2.8.1*)

Maximum 3.0 per cent.

ASSAY

Essential oil (*2.8.12*)

Use 30.0 g of the drug, a 1000 mL round-bottomed flask and 400 mL of *water R* as the distillation liquid. Distil at a rate of 2-3 mL/min for 2 h without *xylene R* in the graduated tube.

Thymol and carvacrol

Gas chromatography (*2.2.28*): use the normalisation procedure.

Test solution   Filter the essential oil obtained in the determination of essential oil over a small amount of *anhydrous sodium sulfate R* and dilute to 5.0 mL with *hexane R* by rinsing the apparatus and the anhydrous sodium sulfate.

Reference solution   Dissolve 0.20 g of *thymol R* and 50 mg of *carvacrol R* in *hexane R* and dilute to 5.0 mL with the same solvent.

Column:
— *material*: fused silica;
— *size*: l = 30-60 m, Ø = 0.25 mm;
— *stationary phase*: *macrogol 20 000 R* (film thickness 0.25 μm).

Carrier gas   *nitrogen for chromatography R* or *helium for chromatography R*.

Flow rate   1-2 mL/min.

Split ratio   1:100.

Temperature:

	Time (min)	Temperature (°C)
Column	0 - 45	40 → 220
Injection port		190
Detector		210

Detection   Flame ionisation.

Injection   0.2 μL.

Elution order   Order indicated in the composition of the reference solution. Record the retention times of these substances.

System suitability   Reference solution:
— *resolution*: minimum 1.5 between the peaks due to thymol and carvacrol.

Using the retention times determined from the chromatogram obtained with the reference solution, locate the components of the reference solution in the chromatogram obtained with the test solution.

Determine the percentage content of thymol and carvacrol.

_____ *Ph Eur*

Thyme Oil, Thymol Type

(*Ph Eur monograph 1374*)

Ph Eur _____

DEFINITION

Essential oil obtained by steam distillation from the fresh flowering aerial parts of *Thymus vulgaris* L., *T. zygis* L. or a mixture of both species.

CHARACTERS

Appearance

Clear, yellow or very dark reddish-brown, mobile liquid.

Odour reminiscent of thymol.

Solubility

Miscible with anhydrous ethanol and with light petroleum.

IDENTIFICATION

First identification   B.

Second identification   A.

A. Thin-layer chromatography (*2.2.27*).

Test solution   Dissolve 0.2 mL of the substance to be examined in *methylene chloride R* and dilute to 10 mL with the same solvent.

Reference solution   Dissolve 5 mg of *thymol R* and 10 μL of *carvacrol R* in *methylene chloride R* and dilute to 10 mL with the same solvent.

Plate   *TLC silica gel plate R* (5-40 μm) [or *TLC silica gel plate R* (2-10 μm)].

Mobile phase   methylene chloride R.

Application   10 μL [or 4 μL] as bands of 10 mm [or 8 mm].

Development   Over a path of 12 cm [or 6 cm].

Drying   In air.

Detection   Treat with *anisaldehyde solution R* and heat at 100-105 °C for 5-10 min; examine in daylight.

Results   See below the sequence of zones present in the chromatograms obtained with the reference solution and the test solution. Furthermore, other faint zones may be present in the chromatogram obtained with the test solution.

Top of the plate	
	A pink zone
———	———
Thymol: an orange-brown zone	An intense orange-brown zone (thymol)
Carvacrol: an orange-grey zone	A faint orange-grey zone (carvacrol) may be present
———	
	A pink zone
	A violet zone
	A brownish-grey zone
Reference solution	Test solution

B. Examine the chromatograms obtained in the test for chromatographic profile.

Results The characteristic peaks in the chromatogram obtained with the test solution are similar in retention time to those in the chromatogram obtained with reference solution (a).

TESTS

Relative density (*2.2.5*)
0.915 to 0.935.

Refractive index (*2.2.6*)
1.490 to 1.505.

Chromatographic profile
Gas chromatography (*2.2.28*): use the normalisation procedure.

Test solution Dissolve 200 µL of the substance to be examined in *heptane R* and dilute to 10.0 mL with the same solvent.

Reference solution (a) Dissolve 5 µL of *β-myrcene R*, 5 µL of α-terpinene R, 20 µL of *p-cymene R*, 10 µL of *γ-terpinene R*, 5 µL of *linalol R*, 5 µL of *terpinen-4-ol R*, 40 mg of *thymol R* and 5 µL of *carvacrol R* in 5 mL of *heptane R*.

Reference solution (b) Dissolve 10 µL of *carvacrol R* in *heptane R* and dilute to 10.0 mL with the same solvent. Dilute 100 µL of the solution to 10.0 mL with *heptane R*.

Column:
— *material*: fused silica;
— *size*: $l = 60$ m, Ø = 0.25 mm;
— *stationary phase*: *poly(dimethyl)(diphenyl)siloxane R* (film thickness 0.25 µm).

Carrier gas *helium for chromatography R*.

Flow rate 1.5 mL/min.

Split ratio 1:50.

Temperature:

	Time (min)	Temperature (°C)
Column	0 - 75	65 → 215
Injection port		230
Detector		250

Detection Flame ionisation.

Injection 1 µL.

Elution order Order indicated in the composition of reference solution (a); record the retention times of these substances.

System suitability Reference solution (a):

— *resolution*: minimum 1.5 between the peaks due to thymol and carvacrol.

Identification of peaks

Using the retention times determined from the chromatogram obtained with reference solution (a), locate the components of reference solution (a) in the chromatogram obtained with the test solution. The peak due to α-thujene elutes with a relative retention of about 0.8 with reference to β-myrcene. The peak due to carvacrol methyl ether elutes with a relative retention of about 0.9 with reference to thymol.

Determine the percentage content of these components. The limits are within the following ranges:
— *α-thujene*: 0.2 per cent to 1.5 per cent;
— *β-myrcene*: 1.0 per cent to 3.0 per cent;
— *α-terpinene*: 0.9 per cent to 2.6 per cent;
— *p-cymene*: 14.0 per cent to 28.0 per cent;
— *γ-terpinene*: 4.0 per cent to 12.0 per cent;
— *linalol*: 1.5 per cent to 6.5 per cent;
— *terpinen-4-ol*: 0.1 per cent to 2.5 per cent;
— *carvacrol methyl ether*: 0.05 per cent to 1.5 per cent;
— *thymol*: 37.0 per cent to 55.0 per cent;
— *carvacrol*: 0.5 per cent to 5.5 per cent;
— *disregard limit*: the area of the principal peak in the chromatogram obtained with reference solution (b) (0.05 per cent).

STORAGE
At a temperature not exceeding 25 °C.

_____ *Ph Eur*

Wild Thyme

(*Ph Eur. monograph 1891*)

Ph Eur _____

DEFINITION
Whole or cut, dried, flowering aerial parts of *Thymus serpyllum* L.s.l.

Content
Minimum 3.0 mL/kg of essential oil (dried drug).

IDENTIFICATION
A. The stem is much branched, up to about 1.5 mm in diameter, cylindrical or indistinctly quadrangular, green, reddish or purplish, the older stems brown and woody, the younger stems pubescent. The leaves are opposite, 3 mm to 12 mm long and up to 4 mm wide, elliptical to ovate-lanceolate with an obtuse apex, cuneate and shortly petiolate at the base; the margin is entire and markedly ciliate, especially near the base; both surfaces are more or less glabrous but distinctly punctate. The inflorescence is composed of about 6 to 12 flowers in rounded to ovoid, terminal heads. The calyx is tubular, two-lipped with the upper lip dividing to form 3 teeth, the lower lip with 2 teeth, edged with long hairs; inner surfaces strongly pubescent, the hairs forming a closed tube after flowering. The corolla is purplish-violet to red, two-lipped, the lower lip with 3 lobes, upper lip notched, inner surface strongly pubescent; stamens 4, epipetalous, projecting from the corolla tube.

B. Reduce to a powder (355) (*2.9.12*). The powder is greyish-green to brownish-green. Examine under a microscope using *chloral hydrate solution R*. The powder shows the following diagnostic characters: fragments of the leaf epidermises with sinuous, slightly thickened anticlinical walls and stomata of the diacytic type (*2.8.3*); numerous covering trichomes on both epidermises and along the leaf margins, the majority short, conical, unicellular, with thickened and warty walls, fewer long, uniseriate, composed of up to 8 cells, slightly swollen at the joints, with moderately thickened walls; abundant glandular trichomes, mostly multicellular with a small, rounded, unicellular stalk and a large globular head composed of a number of indistinct, radiating cells containing brown secretion, others smaller, capitate, with unicellular stalk and a unicellular, globoid or ovoid head; purplish-violet fragments of the corolla, the outer epidermis with numerous covering and glandular trichomes, inner epidermis papillose; pollen grains spherical to elliptical, 30 µm to 40 µm in diameter, with a finely grained exine and 6 germinal pores.

C. Thin-layer chromatography (*2.2.27*).

Test solution   To 1.0 g of the powdered drug (355) (*2.9.12*) add 5 mL of *methylene chloride R* and shake for 3 min. Filter through about 2 g of *anhydrous sodium sulfate R*.

Reference solution   Dissolve 5 mg of *thymol R* and 10 µL of *carvacrol R* in 10 mL of *methylene chloride R*.

Plate   *TLC silica gel F$_{254}$ plate R*.

Mobile phase   *methylene chloride R*.

Application   20 µL, as bands.

Development   Over a path of 15 cm.

Drying   In air.

Detection A   Examine in ultraviolet light at 254 nm.

Results A   See below the sequence of the zones present in the chromatograms obtained with the reference solution and the test solution.

Top of the plate	
	A prominent quenching zone
Thymol: a quenching zone	A quenching zone (thymol)
	Quenching zones
Reference solution	**Test solution**

Detection B   Spray with *anisaldehyde solution R* using 10 mL for a plate 200 mm square and heat at 100-105 °C for 10 min.

Results B   See below the sequence of the zones present in the chromatograms obtained with the reference solution and the test solution. Furthermore, other zones are present in the lower third of the chromatogram obtained with the test solution. The intensity of the zones due to thymol and carvacrol depends upon the sample examined (chemotypes).

Top of the plate	
Thymol: a brownish-pink zone	A brownish-pink zone (thymol)
Carvacrol: a pale violet zone	A pale violet zone (carvacrol)
Reference solution	**Test solution**

TESTS

Foreign matter (*2.8.2*)
Maximum 3 per cent, determined on 30 g.

Foreign matter may also consist of acicular to linear-lanceolate leaves with a strongly bent margin, the adaxial surface showing covering trichomes shaped as pointed teeth with warty walls, the abaxial surface showing many types of warty covering trichomes: unicellular, straight or slightly curved, bicellular or tricellular, often elbow-shaped, and bicellular or tricellular, more or less straight (*Thymus vulgaris, Thymus zygis*).

Loss on drying (*2.2.32*)
Maximum 10.0 per cent, determined on 1.000 g of the powdered drug (355) (*2.9.12*) by drying in an oven at 105 °C for 2 h.

Total ash (*2.4.16*)
Maximum 10.0 per cent.

Ash insoluble in hydrochloric acid (*2.8.1*)
Maximum 3.0 per cent.

ASSAY
Carry out the determination of essential oils in herbal drugs (*2.8.12*). Use 50.0 g of the cut drug, a 1000 mL round-bottomed flask and 500 mL of *water R* as the distillation liquid. Distil at a rate of 2-3 mL/min for 2 h without *xylene R* in the graduated tube.

_____*Ph Eur*

Tolu Balsam

(*Ph Eur monograph 1596*)

Ph Eur _____

DEFINITION
Oleo-resin obtained from the trunk of *Myroxylon balsamum* (L.) Harms var. *balsamum*.

Content
25.0 per cent to 50.0 per cent of free or combined acids, expressed as cinnamic acid ($C_9H_8O_2$; M_r 148.2) (dried drug).

CHARACTERS

Appearance
Hard, friable, brownish to reddish-brown mass; thin fragments are brownish-yellow when examined against the light.

Reminiscent odour of vanillin.

Solubility
Practically insoluble in water, very soluble to freely soluble in alcohol, practically insoluble in light petroleum.

IDENTIFICATION
Thin-layer chromatography (*2.2.27*).

Test solution   Stir 0.40 g of the fragmented drug with 10 mL of *methylene chloride R* for 5 min and filter.

Reference solution   Dissolve 50 mg of *benzyl cinnamate R* in *methylene chloride R*, add 50 µL of *benzyl benzoate R* and dilute to 10 mL with *methylene chloride R*.

Plate   *TLC silica gel G plate R*.

Mobile phase   *light petroleum R, toluene R* (5:95 *V/V*).

Application   20 µL, as bands.

Development   Over a path of 15 cm.

Drying   In air.

Detection Spray with *vanillin reagent R* and heat at 100-105 °C for 5 min. Examine in daylight.

Results See below the sequence of the zones present in the chromatograms obtained with the test and reference solutions. Furthermore, other coloured zones are present in the chromatogram obtained with the test solution.

Top of the plate	
Benzyl benzoate: a greyish-blue zone	a greyish-blue zone
Benzyl cinnamate: a greyish-green zone	a greyish-green zone
Reference solution	Test solution

TESTS

Acid value

100 to 160.

Dissolve 0.5 g of the fragmented drug in 50 mL of *alcohol R*. Add 0.5 mL of *acid blue 93 solution R* and 5.0 mL of *0.5 M alcoholic potassium hydroxide*. Stir vigorously and titrate with *0.5 M hydrochloric acid* until the colour changes from brownish-red to blackish-green ($n1$ mL of *0.5 M hydrochloric acid*). Carry out a blank test in the same manner ($n2$ mL of *0.5 M hydrochloric acid*). Calculate the acid value in the same manner as the saponification value (*2.5.6*).

Matter insoluble in alcohol

Maximum 5 per cent.

Boil 2.0 g of the fragmented drug with 25 mL of *alcohol (90 per cent V/V) R* and filter. Wash the residue with *alcohol (90 per cent V/V) R*, boiling until completely extracted, then dry the residue at 100-105 °C. Weigh the residue.

Loss on drying (*2.2.32*)

Maximum 5.0 per cent, determined on 2.000 g of the fragmented drug by spreading on a flat evaporating dish 9 cm in diameter and allowing to dry *in vacuo* for 4 h.

Total ash (*2.4.16*)

Maximum 0.3 per cent.

ASSAY

Boil 1.500 g under a reflux condenser with 25 mL of *0.5 M alcoholic potassium hydroxide* for 1 h. Evaporate the ethanol and heat the residue with 50 mL of *water R* until the substance is homogeneously distributed. After cooling, add 80 mL of *water R* and a solution of 1.5 g of *magnesium sulfate R* in 50 mL of *water R*. Mix, and allow to stand for 10 min. Filter through a pleated filter paper and wash the residue with 20 mL of *water R*. Combine the filtrate and the washings, acidify with *hydrochloric acid R* and extract with 4 quantities, each of 40 mL, of *ether R*. Discard the aqueous layer. Combine the organic extracts and wash with 2 quantities, each of 20 mL, and with 3 quantities, each of 10 mL, of a 50 g/L solution of *sodium bicarbonate R*. Discard the ether layer. Combine the aqueous extracts, acidify with *hydrochloric acid R* and stir once with 30 mL, twice with 20 mL and once with 10 mL of *methylene chloride R*. Dry the combined methylene chloride extracts over *anhydrous sodium sulfate R*. Filter through a pleated filter and wash the residue with 10 mL of *methylene chloride R*. Reduce the combined methylene chloride extracts to 10 mL by distillation and eliminate the remaining methylene chloride in a current of air. Dissolve the residue with heating in 10 mL of *alcohol R* previously neutralised to *phenol red solution R*. After cooling, titrate with *0.1 M sodium hydroxide*, using the same indicator.

1 mL of *0.1 M sodium hydroxide* is equivalent to 14.82 mg of total acids, expressed as cinnamic acid.

STORAGE

Do not store in powdered form.

_____ *Ph Eur*

Tolu-flavour Solution

DEFINITION

Cinnamic Acid	5.0 g
Benzoic Acid	2.5 g
Ethyl Cinnamate	0.3 g
Vanillin	0.1 g
Cinnamon Oil	0.02 mL
Sucrose	500 g
Ethanol (96 per cent)	350 mL
Water	Sufficient to produce 1000 mL

Extemporaneous preparation

The following directions apply.

Dissolve the Sucrose in 320 mL of Water. Add 250 mL of the Ethanol (96 per cent), with mixing. Dissolve the Cinnamic Acid, Benzoic Acid, Ethyl Cinnamate, Vanillin and Cinnamon Oil in the remaining 100 mL of Ethanol (96 per cent), add this solution to the sucrose solution with mixing, dilute to 1000 mL with Water and mix. Allow to stand for a few hours before use.

IDENTIFICATION

Carry out the method for *thin-layer chromatography*, Appendix III A, using the following solutions.

(1) The solution being examined.

(2) 0.5% w/v of *cinnamic acid*, 0.25% w/v of *benzoic acid* and 0.03% v/v of *ethyl cinnamate* in *ethanol (90%)*.

CHROMATOGRAPHIC CONDITIONS

(a) Use as the coating *silica gel GF$_{254}$*.

(b) Use the mobile phase as described below.

(c) Apply 5 μL of each solution.

(d) Develop the plate to 15 cm.

(e) After removal of the plate, dry in air for 15 minutes and repeat the development using the same mobile phase. Remove the plate, allow the solvent to evaporate and examine under *ultraviolet light (254 nm)*.

MOBILE PHASE

15 volumes of *glacial acetic acid*, 25 volumes of *hexane* and 75 volumes of n-*pentane*.

CONFIRMATION

The spots in the chromatogram obtained with solution (1) are similar in size and correspond in position to those in the chromatogram obtained with solution (2).

TESTS

Ethanol content

31 to 36% v/v, Appendix VIII F.

Weight per mL

1.125 to 1.155 g, Appendix V G.

Tolu Syrup

DEFINITION

| Tolu-flavour Solution | 100 mL |
| Syrup | Sufficient to produce 1000 mL |

The syrup complies with the requirements stated under Oral Liquids and with the following requirement.

Weight per mL
1.29 to 1.32 g, Appendix V G.

Paediatric Compound Tolu Linctus

Paediatric Compound Tolu Oral Solution

DEFINITION

Paediatric Compound Tolu Linctus is an *oral solution* containing 0.6% w/v of Citric Acid Monohydrate in a suitable vehicle with a tolu flavour.

The linctus complies with the requirements stated under Oral Liquids and with the following requirements.

Content of total acid, calculated as citric acid monohydrate, $C_6H_8O_7,H_2O$
0.60 to 0.66% w/v.

ASSAY

To 15 g add 100 mL of *water* and titrate with 0.1M *sodium hydroxide VS* using *phenolphthalein solution R1* as indicator. Each mL of 0.1M *sodium hydroxide VS* is equivalent to 7.005 mg of $C_6H_8O_7,H_2O$. Determine the *weight per mL* of the linctus, Appendix V G, and calculate the content of $C_6H_8O_7,H_2O$, weight in volume.

Tormentil

(Ph Eur monograph 1478)

Preparation
Tormentil Tincture

Ph Eur _____

DEFINITION

Whole or cut, dried rhizome, freed from the roots, of *Potentilla erecta* (L.) Raeusch. (*P. tormentilla* Stokes).

Content

Minimum 7 per cent of tannins, expressed as pyrogallol ($C_6H_6O_3$; M_r 126.1) (dried drug).

IDENTIFICATION

A. The rhizome is cylindrically spindle-shaped, with a very irregular appearance, often forming, twisted, knotty tubers, up to 10 cm long and 1-2 cm thick, very hard and scarcely branched. The surface is brown to reddish-brown, rugose and has remains of roots and transversely elongated depressed whitish scars from the stems. At the top of the rhizome the remains of numerous aerial stems may be present. The fracture is short and granular, dark red to brownish-yellow.

B. Reduce to a powder (355) (*2.9.12*). The powder is reddish-brown. Examine under a microscope using *chloral hydrate solution R*. The powder shows the following diagnostic characters: coarsely serrate cluster crystals of calcium oxalate, up to 60 μm in diameter; fragments of thin-walled parenchyma containing reddish-brown tannin; groups of narrow, bordered-pitted vessels with lateral pores; thick-walled and pitted, polygonal parenchyma; groups and fragments of sclerenchymatous thick-walled fibres; occasional fragments of cork with thin-walled, brown, tabular cells. Examine under a microscope using a 50 per cent *V/V* solution of *glycerol R*. The powder shows spherical or elliptical starch granules, up to about 20 μm in length.

C. Thin-layer chromatography (*2.2.27*).

Test solution   To 0.5 g of the powdered drug (355) (*2.9.12*) add 10 mL of *water R*, shake for 10 min and filter. Shake the filtrate with 2 quantities, each of 10 mL, of *ethyl acetate R* and filter the combined upper phases over 6 g of *anhydrous sodium sulfate R*. Evaporate the filtrate to dryness under reduced pressure and dissolve the residue in 1.0 mL of *ethyl acetate R*.

Reference solution   Dissolve 1.0 mg of *catechin R* in 1.0 mL of *methanol R*.

Plate   TLC silica gel plate R.

Mobile phase   glacial acetic acid R, ether R, hexane R, ethyl acetate R (20:20:20:40 *V/V/V/V*).

Application   10 μL as bands.

Development   Over a path of 10 cm.

Drying   In air for 10-15 min.

Detection   Spray with a freshly prepared 5 g/L solution of *fast blue B salt R*. Reddish zones appear. Expose the plate to ammonia vapour, the zones become more intense turning reddish-brown. Examine in daylight.

Results   See below the sequence of the zones present in the chromatograms obtained with the reference solution and the test solution. Furthermore, other fainter zones are present in the chromatogram obtained with the test solution.

Top of the plate	
	A more intense reddish-brown zone (catechin)
Catechin: an intense reddish-brown zone	A fainter zone
	An intense zone
	Fainter zones
Reference solution	**Test solution**

TESTS

Foreign matter (*2.8.2*)
Maximum 3 per cent of root and stems as well as rhizomes with black fracture and maximum 2 per cent of other foreign matter.

Cadmium (*2.4.27*)
Maximum 2.0 ppm.

Loss on drying (*2.2.32*)
Maximum 12.0 per cent, determined on 1.000 g of the powdered drug (355) (*2.9.12*) by drying in an oven at 105 °C for 2 h.

Total ash (*2.4.16*)
Maximum 5.0 per cent.

ASSAY

Carry out the determination of tannins in herbal drugs (*2.8.14*). Use 0.500 g of the powdered drug (180) (*2.9.12*).

Ph Eur _____

Tormentil Tincture

(Ph Eur monograph 1895)

Ph Eur

DEFINITION
Tincture produced from *Tormentil (1478)*.

Content
Minimum 1.5 per cent *m/m* of tannins, expressed as pyrogallol ($C_6H_6O_3$; M_r 126.1).

PRODUCTION
The tincture is produced from 1 part of comminuted drug and 5 parts of ethanol (70 per cent *V/V*) by a suitable procedure.

CHARACTERS
Red or reddish-brown liquid.

IDENTIFICATION
Thin-layer chromatography (*2.2.27*).

Test solution   Mix 1.0 mL of the tincture to be examined with 1.0 mL of *alcohol (70 per cent V/V) R*.

Reference solution   Dissolve 1.0 mg of *catechin R* in 1.0 mL of *methanol R*.

Plate   *TLC silica gel plate R*.

Mobile phase   *ether R, glacial acetic acid R, hexane R, ethyl acetate R* (20:20:20:40 *V/V/V/V*).

Application   10 µL as bands.

Development   Over a path of 10 cm.

Drying   In air for 10-15 min.

Detection   Spray with a freshly prepared 5 g/L solution of *fast blue B salt R*. Reddish zones appear. Expose the plate to ammonia vapour, the zones become more intense, turning reddish-brown. Examine in daylight.

Results   See below the sequence of the zones present in the chromatograms obtained with the reference solution and the test solution.

Top of the plate	
	___
Catechin: an intense zone	An intense zone (catechin)
___	
	A fainter zone
	An intense zone
	Fainter zones
Reference solution	**Test solution**

TESTS
Ethanol content (*2.9.10*)
64 per cent *V/V* to 69 per cent *V/V*.

Methanol and 2-propanol (*2.9.11*)
Maximum 0.05 per cent *V/V* of methanol and maximum 0.05 per cent *V/V* of 2-propanol.

ASSAY
Carry out the determination of tannins in herbal drugs (*2.8.14*). Use 2.50 g of the tincture to be examined.

_____ *Ph Eur*

Trachyspermum Ammi

DEFINITION
Trachyspermum Ammi is the dried ripe fruit of *Trachyspermum ammi* (L.) Sprague (syn. *C.* [*Carum*] *copticum* (L) Benth. & Hook.f. ex C.B. Clarke).

Content
It contains not less than 2.5% v/w of essential oil calculated with reference to the anhydrous drug.

IDENTIFICATION
A. The dried fruits occur mainly as entire cremocarps with carpophore present, yellowish green, ovoid, laterally compressed, 1 to 3 mm in length and 1 to 2.8 mm in diameter, usually with pedicel attached; styles remaining as a curved, bifid stylopod at the apex. Each fruit composed of two mericarps, dorsal surface convex with five distinct ridges, surface warty; commissural surface flat; vittae visible as two darker longitudinal bands.

B. Reduce to a powder (355). The powder is greenish brown. Examine under a microscope using *chloral hydrate solution*. The powder contains numerous fragments of the papillose epicarp, also showing cuticular striations, with attached or detached whole or fragmented unicellular, warty-walled trichomes; parquetry layer of endocarp in surface view; endosperm of thick-walled cells containing oil globules and aleurone grains with embedded microrosette crystals of calcium oxalate; fragments of yellowish-brown septate vittae; bicollateral vascular bundles with associated lignified, reticulate or pitted parenchyma.

C. Examine the chromatograms obtained in the test for Chromatographic profile. The retention times of the principal peaks in the chromatogram obtained with solution (1) are similar to those in the chromatogram obtained with solution (3).

TESTS
Water
Not more than 10% w/w, Appendix IX C. Use 10.0 g.

Total Ash
Not more than 10%, Appendix XI J, Method II.

Chromatographic profile
Carry out the method for *gas chromatography*, Appendix III B, using the following solutions.

(1) Use the essential oil-toluene mixture obtained in the determination of essential oil.

(2) 0.4% v/v each of γ-*terpinene* and p-*cymene* in *toluene*.

(3) 0.1% v/v each of p-*cymene* and γ-*terpinene* and 0.1% w/v of *thymol* in *toluene*.

(4) 0.01% v/v of γ-*terpinene* in *toluene*.

CHROMATOGRAPHIC CONDITIONS

(a) Use a fused silica column (30 m × 0.53 mm) bonded with a 1 µm film thickness and coated with *polyethylene glycol 20,000* as the bonded phase (DB-Wax is suitable).

(b) Use *helium* as the carrier gas at 1.5 mL per minute.

(c) Use the temperature gradient described below.

(d) Inject 1.0 µL of each solution.

(e) Use a split ratio of 1:50.

(f) Record the chromatogram for a sufficient length of time to elute all the peaks in the chromatogram obtained with solution (1).

	Time (Minutes)	Temperature (°)
column	0→5	60
	5→68	60→250
	68→75	250
Inject port		250
Detector		260

SYSTEM SUITABILITY

The test is not valid unless in the chromatogram obtained with solution (2), the *resolution factor* between the peaks due to γ-terpinene and p-cymene is at least 2.5.

In the chromatogram obtained with solution (3), the peaks elute in the following order:
γ-terpinene, p-cymene and thymol.

DETERMINATION OF CONTENT

Using the retention times determined from the chromatogram obtained with solution (3), locate the components of solution (3) in the chromatogram obtained with solution (1) and calculate the content of p-cymene, γ-terpinene and thymol by normalisation.

Limits:
— p-*cymene* 10 to 25%,
— γ-*terpinene* 10 to 30%,
— *thymol* 45 to 70%.

Disregard any peak with an area less than the peak in the chromatogram obtained with solution (4).

ASSAY

Essential oil

Carry out the method for *Essential Oils in Herbal Drugs*, Appendix XI E, using 15 g of the powdered drug with 1000 mL of *water* as distillation liquid. Distil at a rate of 2 to 3 mL per minute for 2 hours using 0.5 mL of *toluene* in the graduated tube. Measure the quantity of essential oil distilled and use for the test for Chromatographic profile.

Tragacanth

(*Ph Eur monograph 0532*)

9000-65-1

When Powdered Tragacanth is prescribed or demanded, material complying with the requirements below with the exception of Identification test A shall be dispensed or supplied.

Ph Eur _____

DEFINITION

Air-hardened, gummy exudate, flowing naturally or obtained by incision from the trunk and branches of *Astragalus gummifer* Labill. and certain other species of *Astragalus* from western Asia.

IDENTIFICATION

A. Tragacanth occurs in thin, flattened, ribbon-like, white or pale yellow, translucent strips, about 30 mm long and 10 mm wide and up to 1 mm thick, more or less curved, horny, with a short fracture; the surface is marked by fine longitudinal striae and concentric transverse ridges. It may also contain pieces similar in shape but somewhat thicker, more opaque and more difficult to fracture.

B. Reduce to a powder (355) (*2.9.12*). The powder is white or almost white and forms a mucilaginous gel with about 10 times its mass of *water R*. Examine under a microscope using a 50 per cent *V/V* solution of *glycerol R*. The powder shows in the gummy mass numerous stratified cellular membranes that turn slowly violet when treated with *iodinated zinc chloride solution R*. The gummy mass includes starch grains, isolated or in small groups, usually rounded in shape and sometimes deformed, with diameters varying between 4 μm and 10 μm, occasionally up to 20 μm, and a central hilum visible between crossed nicol prisms.

C. Examine the chromatograms obtained in the test for acacia.

Results The chromatogram obtained with the test solution shows 3 zones due to galactose, arabinose and xylose. A faint yellowish zone at the solvent front and a greyish-green zone between the zones due to galactose and arabinose may be present.

D. Moisten 0.5 g of the powdered drug (355) (*2.9.12*) with 1 mL of *ethanol (96 per cent) R* and add gradually, while shaking, 50 mL of *water R* until a homogeneous mucilage is obtained. To 5 mL of the mucilage add 5 mL of *water R* and 2 mL of *barium hydroxide solution R*. A slight flocculent precipitate is formed. Heat on a water-bath for 10 min. An intense yellow colour develops.

TESTS

Acacia

Thin-layer chromatography (*2.2.27*).

Test solution To 100 mg of the powdered drug (355) (*2.9.12*) in a thick-walled centrifuge test-tube, add 2 mL of a 100 g/L solution of *trifluoroacetic acid R*, shake vigorously to dissolve the forming gel, stopper the test-tube and heat the mixture at 120 °C for 1 h. Centrifuge the resulting hydrolysate, transfer the clear supernatant carefully into a 50 mL flask, add 10 mL of *water R* and evaporate the solution to dryness under reduced pressure. To the resulting clear film add 0.1 mL of *water R* and 0.9 mL of *methanol R*. Centrifuge to separate the amorphous precipitate, collect the supernatant and, if necessary, dilute to 1 mL with *methanol R*.

Reference solution Dissolve 10 mg of *arabinose R*, 10 mg of *galactose R*, 10 mg of *rhamnose R* and 10 mg of *xylose R* in 1 mL of *water R* and dilute to 10 mL with *methanol R*.

Plate TLC silica gel plate R.

Mobile phase 16 g/L solution of *sodium dihydrogen phosphate R*, butanol R, acetone R (10:40:50 V/V/V).

Application 10 μL as bands.

Development A Over a path of 10 cm.

Drying A In a current of warm air for a few minutes.

Development B Over a path of 15 cm using the same mobile phase.

Drying B At 110 °C for 10 min.

Detection Spray with *anisaldehyde solution R* and dry at 110 °C for 10 min.

Results The chromatogram obtained with the reference solution shows 4 clearly separated coloured zones due to galactose (greyish-green or green), arabinose (yellowish-green), xylose (greenish-grey or yellowish-grey) and rhamnose (yellowish-green), in order of increasing RF value; the chromatogram obtained with the test solution does not show a yellowish-green zone corresponding to the zone of rhamnose in the chromatogram obtained with the reference solution.

Methylcellulose

Examine the chromatograms obtained in the test for acacia.

Results   The chromatogram obtained with the test solution does not show a red zone near the solvent front.

Sterculia gum

A. Place 0.2 g of the powdered drug (355) (*2.9.12*) in a 10 mL ground-glass-stoppered cylinder graduated in 0.1 mL. Add 10 mL of *ethanol (60 per cent V/V) R* and shake. Any gel formed occupies not more than 1.5 mL.

B. To 1.0 g of the powdered drug (355) (*2.9.12*) add 100 mL of *water R* and shake. Add 0.1 mL of *methyl red solution R*. Not more than 5.0 mL of *0.01 M sodium hydroxide* is required to change the colour of the indicator.

Foreign matter

Maximum 1.0 per cent.

Place 2.0 g of the powdered drug (355) (*2.9.12*) in a 250 mL round-bottomed flask and add 95 mL of *methanol R*. Swirl to moisten the powder and add 60 mL of *hydrochloric acid R1*. Add a few glass beads about 4 mm in diameter and heat on a water-bath under a reflux condenser for 3 h, shaking occasionally. Remove the glass beads and filter the hot suspension *in vacuo* through a sintered-glass filter (160) (*2.1.2*). Rinse the flask with a small quantity of *water R* and pass the rinsings through the filter. Wash the residue on the filter with about 40 mL of *methanol R* and dry to constant mass at 110 °C (about 1 h). Allow to cool in a desiccator and weigh. The residue weighs a maximum of 20 mg.

Flow time

Minimum 10 s, or minimum 50 s if the substance to be examined is to be used for the preparation of emulsions.

Place 1.0 g of the powdered drug (125-250) (*2.9.12*) in a 1000 mL round-bottomed flask with a ground-glass stopper, add 8.0 mL of *ethanol (96 per cent) R* and close the flask. Disperse the suspension over the inner surface of the flask by shaking, taking care not to wet the stopper. Open the flask and add as a single portion 72.0 mL of *water R*. Stopper the flask and shake vigorously for 3 min. Allow to stand for 24 h and shake vigorously again for 3 min. Eliminate air bubbles by applying vacuum above the mucilage for 5 min. Transfer the mucilage to a 50 mL cylinder. Dip in the mucilage a piece of glass tubing 200 mm long and 6.0 mm in internal diameter and graduated at 20 mm and 120 mm from the lower end; the tubing must not be rinsed with surface-active substances. When the mucilage has reached the upper mark, close the tube with a finger. Withdraw the closed tube, remove the finger and measure with a stop-watch the time needed for the meniscus to reach the lower graduation. Carry out this operation 4 times and determine the average value of the last 3 determinations.

Total ash (*2.4.16*)

Maximum 4.0 per cent.

Microbial contamination

TAMC: acceptance criterion 10^4 CFU/g (*2.6.12*).

TYMC: acceptance criterion 10^2 CFU/g (*2.6.12*).

Absence of *Escherichia coli* (*2.6.13*).

Absence of *Salmonella* (*2.6.13*).

LABELLING

The label states whether or not the contents are suitable for preparing emulsions.

_____ *Ph Eur*

Javanese Turmeric

(*Ph Eur monograph 1441*)

Ph Eur _____

DEFINITION

Dried rhizome, cut in slices, of *Curcuma xanthorrhiza* Roxb. (*C. xanthorrhiza* D. Dietrich).

Content:
— *essential oil*: minimum 50 mL/kg (anhydrous drug);
— *dicinnamoyl methane derivatives, expressed as curcumin* ($C_{21}H_{20}O_6$; M_r 368.4): minimum 1.0 per cent (anhydrous drug).

CHARACTERS

Aromatic odour.

IDENTIFICATION

A. Orange-yellow or yellowish-brown or greyish-brown slices, mostly peeled 1.5-6 mm thick and 15-50 mm, more rarely up to 70 mm, in diameter. Fragments of the brownish-grey cork are sporadically present. The transverse surface is yellow with dark spots in the paler centre. The fracture is short and finely grained.

B. Reduce to a powder (355) (*2.9.12*). The powder is reddish-brown. Examine under a microscope, using *chloral hydrate solution R*. The powder shows the following diagnostic characters: fragments of colourless parenchyma with orange-yellow or yellowish-brown secretory cells; fragments of reticulate and other vessels; rare fragments of cork and epidermis and fragments of thick-walled unicellular acute trichomes. Examine under a microscope using a 50 per cent *V/V* solution of *glycerol R*. The powder shows numerous stratified, ovoid or irregular starch granules, about 30-50 μm long and about 10-30 μm wide, with an eccentric hilum and marked, concentric striations.

C. Thin-layer chromatography (*2.2.27*) as described in the test for *Curcuma domestica* with the following modifications.

Detection   Spray with a freshly prepared 0.4 g/L solution of *dichloroquinonechlorimide R* in *2-propanol R*. Expose to ammonia vapour until the zone due to thymol becomes bluish-violet.

Results   The chromatogram obtained with the reference solution shows almost in the middle a bluish-violet zone (thymol) and in the lower part a yellow zone (fluorescein). The chromatogram obtained with the test solution shows a blue zone (xanthorrhizol) slightly above the zone due to thymol in the chromatogram obtained with the reference solution and 2 yellowish-brown or brown zones (curcumin and demethoxycurcumin) between the zones due to thymol and fluorescein in the chromatogram obtained with the reference solution.

TESTS

Curcuma domestica

Thin-layer chromatography (*2.2.27*).

Test solution   Shake 0.5 g of the freshly powdered drug (500) (*2.9.12*) with 5 mL of *methanol R* for 30 min and filter.

Reference solution   Dissolve 5 mg of *fluorescein R* and 10 mg of *thymol R* in 10 mL of *methanol R*.

Plate   TLC silica gel plate R.

Mobile phase   glacial acetic acid R, toluene R (20:80 *V/V*).

Application   10 μL, as bands.

Development   Over a path of 10 cm.

Drying   In air.

Detection   Spray with a mixture of 1 volume of *sulfuric acid R* and 9 volumes of *acetic anhydride R*. Examine in ultraviolet light at 365 nm.

Results   In the chromatogram obtained with the test solution, no yellowish-red fluorescent zone (bisdemethoxycurcumin) appears slightly above the greenish-blue fluorescent zone due to fluorescein in the chromatogram obtained with the reference solution.

Water (*2.2.13*)
Maximum 120 mL/kg, determined on 20.0 g of the powdered drug (500) (*2.9.12*).

Total ash (*2.4.16*)
Maximum 8.0 per cent.

ASSAY
Essential oil
Carry out the determination of essential oils in herbal drugs (*2.8.12*). Use a 500 mL round-bottomed flask, 200 mL of *water R* as the distillation liquid and 0.5 mL of *xylene R* in the graduated tube. Reduce the drug to a powder (500) (*2.9.12*) and immediately use 5.0 g for the determination. Distil at a rate of 3-4 mL/min for 3 h.

Dicinnamoyl methane derivatives
To 0.100 g of the powdered drug (180) (*2.9.12*) add 60 mL of *glacial acetic acid R* and heat in a water-bath at 90 °C for 60 min. Add 2.0 g of *boric acid R* and 2.0 g of *oxalic acid R* and heat in a water-bath at 90 °C for 10 min. Allow to cool, dilute to 100.0 mL with *glacial acetic acid R* and shake. Dilute 5.0 mL of the clear supernatant to 50.0 mL with *glacial acetic acid R*. Measure the absorbance (*2.2.25*) at 530 nm, using *glacial acetic acid R* as the compensation liquid.

Calculate the percentage content of dicinnamoyl methane derivatives, expressed as curcumin, using the following expression:

$$\frac{A \times 0.426}{m}$$

i.e. taking the specific absorbance of curcumin to be 2350.
A = absorbance at 530 nm
m = mass of the drug to be examined, in grams

_____ *Ph Eur*

Turmeric Rhizome

(*Ph Eur monograph 2543*)

Ph Eur _____

DEFINITION
Whole, cured (by boiling or steaming), dried rhizome of *Curcuma longa* L. (syn. *C. domestica* Valeton) with roots and outer surface removed.

Content:
— *essential oil*: minimum 25 mL/kg (anhydrous drug);
— *dicinnamoyl methane derivatives, expressed as curcumin* ($C_{21}H_{20}O_6$; M_r 368.4): minimum 2.0 per cent (anhydrous drug).

CHARACTERS
Spicy odour.

IDENTIFICATION
A. The rhizome is ovate, oblong-ovoid, pyriform or cylindrical, often shortly branched, up to 6 cm long and 15 mm thick. The primary rhizome shows scars from the lateral branches. The surface is slightly dusty, spotted and brownish-yellow, yellow or brownish-grey, finely striated. The fracture is granular, smooth, non-fibrous, slightly glossy, uniformly orange-yellow; it shows a narrow cortex that is darker on the outside.

B. Microscopic examination (*2.8.23*). The powder is orange-yellow. Examine under a microscope using *chloral hydrate solution R*. The powder shows the following diagnostic characters: fragments of parenchyma sometimes coloured yellow by curcumin; reticulate or pitted vessels; rare fragments of brown cork; rare oil droplets. Examine under a microscope using a 50 per cent *V/V* solution of *glycerol R*. The powder shows starch granules, free or included in parenchymatous cells, usually gelatinised and agglomerated; rare ovoid starch granules, with a punctiform hilum in the narrow part, are also present.

C. Thin-layer chromatography (*2.2.27*).

Test solution   To 1 g of the freshly powdered herbal drug (355) (*2.9.12*) add 10 mL of *ethanol (96 per cent) R*, shake, allow to stand for 30 min with occasional shaking and filter; use the filtrate.

Reference solution   Dissolve 20 mg of *curcuminoids R* and 10 mg of *thymol R* in 10 mL of *ethanol (96 per cent) R*.

Plate   TLC silica gel plate R (5-40 μm) [or *TLC silica gel plate R* (2-10 μm)].

Mobile phase   glacial acetic acid R, toluene R (20:80 *V/V*).

Application   10 μL [or 3 μL] as bands of 10 mm [or 8 mm].

Development   Over a path of 10 cm [or 6 cm].

Drying   In air.

Detection A   Examine in ultraviolet light at 365 nm.

Results A   See below the sequence of zones present in the chromatograms obtained with the reference solution and the test solution. Furthermore, other faint zones may be present in the chromatogram obtained with the test solution.

Top of the plate	
___	___
Curcuminoids: a greenish fluorescent zone	A greenish fluorescent zone (curcuminoids)
___	___
Curcuminoids: 2 greenish fluorescent zones	2 greenish fluorescent zones (curcuminoids)
Reference solution	**Test solution**

Detection B   Treat with *anisaldehyde solution R* and heat at 100-105 °C for 10 min; examine in ultraviolet light at 365 nm.

Results B   See below the sequence of zones present in the chromatograms obtained with the reference solution and the test solution. Furthermore, other faint zones may be present in the chromatogram obtained with the test solution.

Top of the plate	
	A faint pink zone
	An intense reddish zone
———	———
Thymol: a dark zone	
	A pinkish-red zone
Curcuminoids: a brown zone	A brown zone (curcuminoids)
———	———
Curcuminoids: 2 yellow zones	2 yellow zones (curcuminoids)
Reference solution	Test solution

TESTS

Curcuma zanthorrhiza Roxb
Examine the chromatogram obtained in Identification C, detection B.

Results B   The chromatogram obtained with the test solution shows no dark zone just above the zone due to thymol in the chromatogram obtained with the reference solution.

Water (*2.2.13*)
Maximum 120 mL/kg, determined on 15.0 g of the powdered herbal drug (500) (*2.9.12*).

Total ash (*2.4.16*)
Maximum 7.0 per cent.

ASSAY

Essential oil
Carry out the determination of essential oils in herbal drugs (*2.8.12*). Use 2.5 g of the freshly powdered herbal drug (500) (*2.9.12*), a 2 L round-bottomed flask, 400 mL of *water R* as the distillation liquid and 0.5 mL of *xylene R* in the graduated tube. Distil at a rate of 2 mL/min for 3 h.

Dicinnamoyl methane derivatives
Disperse 0.500 g of the powdered herbal drug (500) (*2.9.12*) in 30 mL of *ethanol (96 per cent) R* in a 100 mL round-bottomed flask. Heat under a reflux condenser for 2.5 h. Cool and filter into a volumetric flask, rinse the round-bottomed flask and the filter with *ethanol (96 per cent) R* and dilute to 100.0 mL with the same solvent. Dilute 1.0 mL of the solution to 50.0 mL with *ethanol (96 per cent) R*. Measure the absorbance (*2.2.25*) at 425 nm using *ethanol (96 per cent) R* as the compensation liquid.

Calculate the percentage content of dicinnamoyl methane derivatives, expressed as curcumin, using the following expression:

$$\frac{A \times 5000}{1607 \times m}$$

i.e. taking the specific absorbance of curcumin to be 1607.
A = absorbance at 425 nm;
m = mass of the herbal drug to be examined, in grams.

——————————————— *Ph Eur*

Turpentine Oil

Preparation
White Liniment

DEFINITION
Turpentine Oil is obtained by distillation from the oleoresin obtained from various species of *Pinus* and rectified.

CHARACTERISTICS
A clear, bright, colourless liquid, visibly free from water; odour, characteristic.

TESTS
Refractive index
1.467 to 1.477, Appendix V E.

Solubility in ethanol
Soluble, at 20°, in 7 volumes of *ethanol (90%)* and in 3 volumes of *ethanol (96%)*, Appendix X M.

Weight per mL
0.855 to 0.868 g, Appendix V G.

Residue on evaporation
Not more than 1.0% when determined by the method for *residue on evaporation of volatile oils*, Appendix X M. Use 2 g and heat for 4 hours.

STORAGE
Turpentine Oil should be kept in a well-filled container and protected from light.

Pinus Pinaster Type Turpentine Oil

(*Turpentine Oil, Pinus Pinaster Type, Ph Eur monograph 1627*)

Ph Eur ———————————————————————

DEFINITION
Essential oil obtained by steam distillation, followed by rectification at a temperature below 180 °C, from the oleoresin obtained by tapping *Pinus pinaster* Aiton. A suitable antioxidant may be added.

CHARACTERS
Appearance
Clear, colourless or pale yellow liquid.
Characteristic odour.

IDENTIFICATION
First identification   B.
Second identification   A.

A. Thin-layer chromatography (*2.2.27*).

Test solution   Mix 1 mL of the substance to be examined with *toluene R* and dilute to 10 mL with the same solvent.

Reference solution   Mix 10 µL of *β-pinene R* and 10 µL of *linalol R* with *toluene R* and dilute to 10 mL with the same solvent.

Plate   TLC silica gel plate R.

Mobile phase   ethyl acetate R, toluene R (5:95 V/V).

Application   10 µL, as bands.

Development   Over a path of 15 cm.

Drying   In air.

Detection   Spray with anisaldehyde solution R and heat at 100-105 °C for 5-10 min. Examine in daylight.

Results See below the sequence of the zones present in the chromatograms obtained with the reference solution and the test solution.

Top of the plate	
β-Pinene: a pink zone	A pink zone (β-pinene)
	A pink zone
Linalol: a pinkish-grey zone	
	3 faint violet zones
	A faint yellow zone
Reference solution	**Test solution**

B. Examine the chromatograms obtained in the test for chromatographic profile.

Results The peaks in the chromatogram obtained with the test solution are similar in retention time to those in the chromatogram obtained with the reference solution.

TESTS
Relative density (*2.2.5*)
0.856 to 0.872.

Refractive index (*2.2.6*)
1.465 to 1.475.

Optical rotation (*2.2.7*)
– 40° to – 28°.

Acid value (*2.5.1*)
Maximum 1.0.

Peroxide value (*2.5.5, Method B*)
Maximum 20.

Fatty oils and resinified essential oils (*2.8.7*)
It complies with the test for fatty oils and resinified essential oils.

Chromatographic profile
Gas chromatography (*2.2.28*): use the normalisation procedure.

Test solution The substance to be examined.

Reference solution (a) Dissolve 30 μL of *α-pinene R*, 10 mg of *camphene R*, 20 μL of *β-pinene R*, 10 μL of *car-3-ene R*, 10 μL of *β-myrcene R*, 20 μL of *limonene R*, 10 μL of *longifolene R*, 10 μL of *β-caryophyllene R* and 10 mg of *caryophyllene oxide R* in 1 mL of *hexane R*.

Reference solution (b) Dissolve 5 μL of *β-caryophyllene R* in *hexane R* and dilute to 1 mL with the same solvent. Dilute 0.1 mL to 1 mL with *hexane R*.

Column:
— *material*: fused silica;
— *size*: *l* = 60 m, Ø = 0.25 mm;
— *stationary phase*: *macrogol 20 000 R* (film thickness 0.25 μm).

Carrier gas *helium for chromatography R.*

Flow rate 1.0 mL/min.

Split ratio 1:63.

Temperature:

		Time (min)	Temperature (°C)
Column		0 - 10	60
		10 - 80	60 → 200
		80 - 120	200
Injection port			200
Detector			250

Detection Flame ionisation.

Injection 0.5 μL.

Elution order Order indicated in the composition of the reference solution (a); record the retention times of these substances.

System suitability:
— *resolution*: minimum 1.5 between the peaks due to car-3-ene and β-myrcene in the chromatogram obtained with reference solution (a).

Using the retention times determined from the chromatogram obtained with reference solution (a), locate the components of reference solution (a) in the chromatogram obtained with the test solution.

Determine the percentage content of these components. The limits are within the following ranges:
— *α-pinene*: 70.0 per cent to 85.0 per cent;
— *camphene*: 0.5 per cent to 1.5 per cent;
— *β-pinene*: 11.0 per cent to 20.0 per cent;
— *car-3-ene*: maximum 1.0 per cent;
— *β-myrcene*: 0.4 per cent to 1.5 per cent;
— *limonene*: 1.0 per cent to 7.0 per cent;
— *longifolene*: 0.2 per cent to 2.5 per cent;
— *β-caryophyllene*: 0.1 per cent to 3.0 per cent;
— *caryophyllene oxide*: maximum 1.0 per cent;
— *disregard limit*: area of the peak in the chromatogram obtained with reference solution (b) (0.05 per cent).

Residue on evaporation (*2.8.9*)
Maximum 2.5 per cent, determined after heating on a water-bath for 3 h.

STORAGE
At a temperature not exceeding 25 °C.
_____ *Ph Eur*

Valerian

(*Valerian Root, Ph Eur monograph 0453*)

Preparations
Valerian Dry Extract
Valerian Dry Hydroalcoholic Extract
Valerian Tincture

When Powdered Valerian is prescribed or demanded, material complying with the appropriate requirements below shall be dispensed or supplied.

Ph Eur _____

DEFINITION
Dried, whole or fragmented underground parts of *Valeriana officinalis* L. *s.l.*, including the rhizome surrounded by the roots and stolons.

Content:
— *essential oil*: minimum 4 mL/kg (dried drug);

— *sesquiterpenic acids*: minimum 0.17 per cent *m/m*, expressed as valerenic acid ($C_{15}H_{22}O_2$; M_r 234.3) (dried drug);

IDENTIFICATION

A. The rhizome is yellowish-grey or pale brownish-grey, obconical or cylindrical, up to about 50 mm long and 30 mm in diameter; the base is elongated or compressed, usually entirely covered by numerous roots. The apex usually exhibits a cup-shaped scar from the aerial parts; stem bases are rarely present. When cut longitudinally, the pith exhibits a central cavity transversed by septa. The roots are numerous, almost cylindrical, of the same colour as the rhizome, 1-3 mm in diameter and sometimes more than 100 mm long. A few filiform fragile secondary roots are present. The fracture is short. The stolons show prominent nodes separated by longitudinally striated internodes, each 20-50 mm long, with a fibrous fracture.

B. Reduce to a powder (355) (*2.9.12*). The powder is pale yellowish-grey or pale greyish-brown. Examine under a microscope using *chloral hydrate solution R*. The powder shows the following diagnostic characters: cells containing a pale brown resin or droplets of essential oil; groups of small, rectangular sclereids with thick walls and a narrow, channelled branched lumen; occasional groups of larger, thinner-walled sclereids from the stem bases; lignified, reticulately-thickened vessels, singly or in small groups; thin-walled, elongated cells of the piliferous layer, some with root hairs; occasional fragments of cork. Examine under a microscope using a 50 per cent *V/V* solution of *glycerol R*. The powder shows abundant starch granules, mainly compound with up to 4-6 components but frequently separated to form single granules, rounded or irregular and up to about 15 µm in diameter; most of the granules show a rather indistinct cleft or radiate hilum.

C. Thin-layer chromatography (*2.2.27*).

Test solution Suspend 1 g of the powdered drug (355) (*2.9.12*) in 10 mL of *methanol R* and sonicate for 10 min. Filter the supernatant through a membrane filter (nominal pore size 0.45 µm). Use the filtrate as the test solution.

Reference solution Dissolve 5 mg of *acetoxyvalerenic acid R* and 5 mg of *valerenic acid R* in 20 mL of *methanol R*.

Plate *TLC silica gel plate R* (5-40 µm) [or *TLC silica gel plate R* (2-10 µm)].

Mobile phase glacial acetic acid R, ethyl acetate R, cyclohexane R (2:38:60 *V/V/V*).

Application 20 µL [or 5 µL] as bands of 10 mm [or 8 mm].

Development Over a path of 10 cm [or 6 cm].

Drying In air.

Detection Spray with *anisaldehyde solution R* and heat at 100-105 °C for 5-10 min; examine in daylight.

Results See below the sequence of zones present in the chromatograms obtained with the reference solution and the test solution. Furthermore, other violet zones may be present in the chromatogram obtained with the test solution.

Top of the plate	
___	___
Valerenic acid: a violet zone	A violet zone (valerenic acid)
Acetoxyvalerenic acid: a violet zone	A violet zone (acetoxyvalerenic acid)
	___
	2 faint or very faint violet zones
Reference solution	**Test solution**

TESTS

Foreign matter (*2.8.2*)
Maximum 5 per cent of stem bases and maximum 2 per cent of other foreign matter.

Loss on drying (*2.2.32*)
Maximum 12.0 per cent, determined on 1.000 g of well homogenised powdered drug (355) (*2.9.12*) by drying in an oven at 105 °C for 2 h.

Total ash (*2.4.16*)
Maximum 12.0 per cent.

Ash insoluble in hydrochloric acid (*2.8.1*)
Maximum 5.0 per cent.

ASSAY

Essential oil (*2.8.12*)
Use 40.0 g of freshly powdered drug (500) (*2.9.12*), a 2000 mL flask, 500 mL of *water R* as the distillation liquid and 0.50 mL of *xylene R* in the graduated tube. Distil at a rate of 3-4 mL/min for 4 h.

Sesquiterpenic acids
Liquid chromatography (*2.2.29*).

Test solution Place 1.50 g of the powdered drug (710) (*2.9.12*) in a 100 mL round-bottomed flask with a ground-glass neck. Add 20 mL of *methanol R1*. Mix and heat on a water-bath under a reflux condenser for 30 min. Allow to cool and filter. Place the filter with the residue in the 100 mL round-bottomed flask. Add 20 mL of *methanol R1* and heat on a water-bath under the reflux condenser for 15 min. Allow to cool and filter. Combine the filtrates and dilute to 50.0 mL with *methanol R1*, rinsing the round-bottomed flask and the filter.

Reference solution Dissolve an amount of *valerian dry extract HRS* corresponding to 1.0 mg of valerenic acid in *methanol R1* and dilute to 10.0 mL with the same solvent. Sonicate for 10 min and filter through a membrane filter (nominal pore size 0.45 µm).

Column:
— *size*: l = 0.25 m, Ø = 4.6 mm;
— *stationary phase*: octadecylsilyl silica gel for chromatography R (5 µm).

Mobile phase:
— *mobile phase A*: acetonitrile R1, 5 g/L solution of *phosphoric acid R* (20:80 *V/V*);
— *mobile phase B*: 5 g/L solution of *phosphoric acid R*, acetonitrile R1 (20:80 *V/V*);

Time (min)	Mobile phase A (per cent *V/V*)	Mobile phase B (per cent *V/V*)
0 - 5	55	45
5 - 18	55 → 20	45 → 80
18 - 22	20	80

Flow rate 1.5 mL/min.

Detection Spectrophotometer at 220 nm.

Injection 20 µL.

Peak identification Use the chromatogram supplied with *valerian dry extract HRS* and the chromatogram obtained with the reference solution to identify the peaks due to acetoxyvalerenic acid and valerenic acid.

System suitability Reference solution:
— *relative retention* with reference to valerenic acid (retention time = about 19 min):
acetoxyvalerenic acid = about 0.5.

Calculate the percentage content of sesquiterpenic acids, expressed as valerenic acid, using the following expression:

$$\frac{(A_1 + A_2) \times m_2 \times p \times 5}{A_3 \times m_1}$$

A_1 = area of the peak due to acetoxyvalerenic acid in the chromatogram obtained with the test solution;

A_2 = area of the peak due to valerenic acid in the chromatogram obtained with the test solution;

A_3 = area of the peak due to valerenic acid in the chromatogram obtained with the reference solution;

m_1 = mass of the drug to be examined used to prepare the test solution, in grams;

m_2 = mass of *valerian dry extract HRS*, used to prepare the reference solution, in grams;

p = percentage content of valerenic acid in *valerian dry extract HRS*.

_____ *Ph Eur*

Cut Valerian

(*Valerian Root, Cut Ph Eur monograph 2526*)

Ph Eur _____

DEFINITION
Dried, cut underground parts of *Valeriana officinalis* L. *s.l.*, including the rhizome, roots and stolons.

It is produced from *Valerian root (0453)* for the purpose of being used in herbal teas.

Content:
— *essential oil*: minimum 3 mL/kg (dried drug);
— *sesquiterpenic acids*: minimum 0.10 per cent *m/m* expressed as valerenic acid ($C_{15}H_{22}O_2$; M_r 234.3) (dried drug).

IDENTIFICATION
A. Reduce to a powder (355) (*2.9.12*). The powder is pale yellowish-grey or pale greyish-brown. Examine under a microscope using *chloral hydrate solution R*. The powder shows the following diagnostic characters: cells containing a pale brown resin or droplets of essential oil; groups of small, rectangular sclereids with thick walls and a narrow, channelled branched lumen; occasional groups of larger, thin-walled sclereids from the stem bases; lignified, reticulately-thickened vessels, singly or in small groups; thin-walled, elongated cells of the piliferous layer, some with root hairs; occasional fragments of cork. Examine under a microscope using a 50 per cent *V/V* solution of *glycerol R*. The powder shows abundant starch granules, mainly compound with up to 4-6 components but frequently separated to form single granules, rounded or irregular and up to about 15 µm in diameter; most of the granules show a rather indistinct cleft or radiate hilum.

B. Thin-layer chromatography (*2.2.27*).

Test solution Suspend 1 g of the powdered drug (355) (*2.9.12*) in 10 mL of *methanol R* and sonicate for 10 min. Filter the supernatant through a membrane filter (nominal pore size 0.45 µm). Use the filtrate as the test solution.

Reference solution Dissolve 5 mg of *acetoxyvalerenic acid R* and 5 mg of *valerenic acid R* in 20 mL of *methanol R*.

Plate *TLC silica gel plate R* (5-40 µm) [or *TLC silica gel plate R* (2-10 µm)].

Mobile phase glacial acetic acid R, ethyl acetate R, cyclohexane R (2:38:60 *V/V/V*).

Application 20 µL [or 5 µL] as bands of 10 mm [or 8 mm].

Development Over a path of 10 cm [or 6 cm].

Drying In air.

Detection Spray with *anisaldehyde solution R* and heat at 100-105 °C for 5-10 min; examine in daylight.

Results See below the sequence of zones present in the chromatograms obtained with the reference solution and the test solution. Furthermore, other violet zones may be present in the chromatogram obtained with the test solution.

Top of the plate	
Valerenic acid: a violet zone	A violet zone (valerenic acid)
Acetoxyvalerenic acid: a violet zone	A violet zone (acetoxyvalerenic acid)
	2 faint or very faint violet zones
Reference solution	**Test solution**

TESTS
Foreign matter (*2.8.2*)
Maximum 5 per cent of stem bases and maximum 2 per cent of other foreign matter, determined on the herbal drug prior to cutting.

Loss on drying (*2.2.32*)
Maximum 12.0 per cent, determined on 1.000 g of well homogenised powdered drug (355) (*2.9.12*) by drying in an oven at 105 °C for 2 h.

Total ash (*2.4.16*)
Maximum 12.0 per cent.

Ash insoluble in hydrochloric acid (*2.8.1*)
Maximum 5.0 per cent.

ASSAY
Essential oil (*2.8.12*)
Use 40.0 g of freshly powdered drug (500) (*2.9.12*), a 2000 mL flask, 500 mL of *water R* as the distillation liquid and 0.50 mL of *xylene R* in the graduated tube. Distil at a rate of 3-4 mL/min for 4 h.

Sesquiterpenic acids
Liquid chromatography (*2.2.29*).

Test solution Place 1.50 g of the powdered drug (710) (*2.9.12*) in a 100 mL round-bottomed flask with a ground-glass neck. Add 20 mL of *methanol R1*. Mix and heat on a water-bath under a reflux condenser for 30 min. Allow to cool and filter. Place the filter with the residue in the 100 mL round-bottomed flask. Add 20 mL of *methanol R1* and heat on a water-bath under the reflux condenser for 15 min. Allow to cool and filter. Combine the filtrates and dilute to

50.0 mL with *methanol R1*, rinsing the round-bottomed flask and the filter.

Reference solution   Dissolve an amount of *valerian dry extract HRS* corresponding to 1.0 mg of valerenic acid in *methanol R1* and dilute to 10.0 mL with the same solvent. Sonicate for 10 min and filter through a membrane filter (nominal pore size 0.45 μm).

Column:
— *size*: l = 0.25 m, Ø = 4.6 mm;
— *stationary phase*: *octadecylsilyl silica gel for chromatography R* (5 μm).

Mobile phase:
— *mobile phase A*: *acetonitrile R1*, 5 g/L solution of *phosphoric acid R* (20:80 *V/V*);
— *mobile phase B*: 5 g/L solution of *phosphoric acid R*, *acetonitrile R1* (20:80 *V/V*);

Time (min)	Mobile phase A (per cent *V/V*)	Mobile phase B (per cent *V/V*)
0 - 5	55	45
5 - 18	55 → 20	45 → 80
18 - 22	20	80

Flow rate   1.5 mL/min.

Detection   Spectrophotometer at 220 nm.

Injection   20 μL.

Peak identification   Use the chromatogram supplied with *valerian dry extract HRS* and the chromatogram obtained with the reference solution to identify the peaks due to acetoxyvalerenic acid and valerenic acid.

System suitability   Reference solution:
— *relative retention* with reference to valerenic acid (retention time = about 19 min):
  acetoxyvalerenic acid = about 0.5.

Calculate the percentage content of sesquiterpenic acids, expressed as valerenic acid, using the following expression:

$$\frac{(A_1 + A_2) \times m_2 \times p \times 5}{A_3 \times m_1}$$

A_1 = area of the peak due to acetoxyvalerenic acid in the chromatogram obtained with the test solution;

A_2 = area of the peak due to valerenic acid in the chromatogram obtained with the test solution;

A_3 = area of the peak due to valerenic acid in the chromatogram obtained with the reference solution;

m_1 = mass of the drug to be examined used to prepare the test solution, in grams;

m_2 = mass of *valerian dry extract HRS*, used to prepare the reference solution, in grams;

p = percentage content of valerenic acid in *valerian dry extract HRS*.

Ph Eur

Valerian Dry Aqueous Extract

(Ph Eur monograph 2400)

Ph Eur

DEFINITION

Extract produced from *Valerian root (0453)*.

Content

Minimum 0.02 per cent of sesquiterpenic acids, expressed as valerenic acid ($C_{15}H_{22}O_2$; M_r 234.3) (dried extract).

PRODUCTION

The extract is produced from the herbal drug by a suitable procedure using water at not less than 60 °C.

CHARACTERS

Appearance

Brown or brownish, hygroscopic powder.

IDENTIFICATION

Thin-layer chromatography (*2.2.27*).

Test solution   Suspend 1.0 g of the extract to be examined in 10 mL of *methanol R* and sonicate for 10 min. Filter the supernatant through a membrane filter (nominal pore size 0.45 μm). Use the filtrate as the test solution.

Reference solution   Dissolve 5 mg of *acetoxyvalerenic acid R* and 5 mg of *valerenic acid R* in 20 mL of *methanol R*.

Plate   *TLC silica gel plate R* (5-40 μm) [or *TLC silica gel plate R* (2-10 μm)].

Mobile phase   glacial acetic acid R, ethyl acetate R, cyclohexane R (2:38:60 *V/V/V*).

Application   20 μL [or 5 μL] as bands of 10 mm [or 8 mm].

Development   Over a path of 10 cm [or 6 cm].

Drying   In air.

Detection   Spray with *anisaldehyde solution R* and heat at 100-105 °C for 5-10 min; examine in daylight.

Results   See below the sequence of zones present in the chromatograms obtained with the reference solution and the test solution. A faint violet zone due to valerenic acid may be present in the chromatogram obtained with the test solution. Furthermore, other zones may be present in the chromatogram obtained with the test solution.

Top of the plate		
———		———
Valerenic acid: a violet zone		
Acetoxyvalerenic acid: a violet zone	A violet zone (acetoxyvalerenic acid)	
	A violet zone (hydroxyvalerenic acid)	———
———		
Reference solution	**Test solution**	

TESTS

Loss on drying (*2.8.17*)
Maximum 6.0 per cent.

ASSAY

Liquid chromatography (*2.2.29*).

Solvent mixture   methanol R, water R (50:50 *V/V*).

Test solution   In a 300 mL conical flask suspend 1.00 g of the extract to be examined in 40 mL of *water R* whilst swirling. Add 40 mL of *methanol R* and swirl for 1 h at 200 r/min. Filter the suspension into a volumetric flask and rinse the conical flask with 3 quantities, each of 5 mL, of the solvent mixture. Dilute to 100.0 mL with the solvent mixture.

Reference solution (a)   Dissolve a quantity of *valerian dry extract HRS* corresponding to 1.0 mg of valerenic acid in *methanol R* and dilute to 10.0 mL with the same solvent. Sonicate for 10 min and filter through a membrane filter (nominal pore size 0.45 μm).

Reference solution (b)   Dilute 1.0 mL of reference solution (a) to 50.0 mL with *methanol R*.

Column:
— *size: l* = 0.25 m, Ø = 4 mm;
— *stationary phase: octadecylsilyl silica gel for chromatography R* (5 μm).

Mobile phase:
— *mobile phase A: acetonitrile R1*, 5 g/L solution of *phosphoric acid R* (20:80 *V/V*);
— *mobile phase B*: 5 g/L solution of *phosphoric acid R*, *acetonitrile R1* (20:80 *V/V*);

Time (min)	Mobile phase A (per cent *V/V*)	Mobile phase B (per cent *V/V*)
0 - 5	55	45
5 - 18	55 → 20	45 → 80
18 - 22	20	80

Flow rate   1.5 mL/min.

Detection   Spectrophotometer at 220 nm.

Injection   20 μL.

Identification of peaks   Use the chromatogram supplied with *valerian dry extract HRS* and the chromatogram obtained with reference solution (a) to identify the peaks due to acetoxyvalerenic acid and hydroxyvalerenic acid.

Relative retention   With reference to valerenic acid (retention time = about 19 min): hydroxyvalerenic acid = about 0.2; acetoxyvalerenic acid = about 0.5.

Calculate the percentage content of sesquiterpenic acids, expressed as valerenic acid, using the following expression:

$$\frac{(A_1 + A_2) \times m_2 \times p \times 0.2}{A_3 \times m_1}$$

A_1 = area of the peak due to hydroxyvalerenic acid in the chromatogram obtained with the test solution;

A_2 = area of the peak due to acetoxyvalerenic acid in the chromatogram obtained with the test solution;

A_3 = area of the peak due to valerenic acid in the chromatogram obtained with reference solution (b);

m_1 = mass of the extract to be examined used to prepare the test solution, in grams;

m_2 = mass of *valerian dry extract HRS* used to prepare reference solution (a), in grams;

p = percentage content of valerenic acid in *valerian dry extract HRS*.

_____ *Ph Eur*

Valerian Dry Hydroalcoholic Extract

(Ph Eur monograph 1898)

Ph Eur ___

DEFINITION
Extract produced from *Valerian root (0453)*.

Content
Minimum 0.25 per cent *m/m* of sesquiterpenic acids, expressed as valerenic acid ($C_{15}H_{22}O_2$; M_r 234.3) (dried extract).

PRODUCTION
The extract is produced from the herbal drug by a suitable procedure using ethanol (30-90 per cent *V/V*) or methanol (40-55 per cent *V/V*).

CHARACTERS
Appearance
Brown, hygroscopic powder.

IDENTIFICATION
Thin-layer chromatography (*2.2.27*).

Test solution   Suspend 1 g of the extract to be examined in 10 mL of *methanol R* and sonicate for 10 min. Filter the supernatant through a membrane filter (nominal pore size 0.45 μm). Use the filtrate as the test solution.

Reference solution   Dissolve 5 mg of *acetoxyvalerenic acid R* and 5 mg of *valerenic acid R* in 20 mL of *methanol R*.

Plate   *TLC silica gel plate R* (5-40 μm) [or *TLC silica gel plate R* (2-10 μm)].

Mobile phase   glacial acetic acid R, ethyl acetate R, cyclohexane R (2:38:60 *V/V/V*).

Application   20 μL [or 5 μL] as bands of 10 mm [or 8 mm].

Development   Over a path of 10 cm [or 6 cm].

Drying   In air.

Detection   Spray with *anisaldehyde solution R* and heat at 100-105 °C for 5-10 min; examine in daylight.

Results   See below the sequence of zones present in the chromatograms obtained with the reference solution and the test solution. Furthermore, other violet zones may be present in the chromatogram obtained with the test solution.

Top of the plate	
Valerenic acid: a violet zone	A violet zone (valerenic acid)
Acetoxyvalerenic acid: a violet zone	A violet zone (acetoxyvalerenic acid)
	2 faint or very faint violet zones
Reference solution	**Test solution**

TESTS
Loss on drying (*2.8.17*)
Maximum 6.0 per cent.

ASSAY
Liquid chromatography (*2.2.29*).

Test solution   Suspend 1.00 g of the extract to be examined in 50.0 mL of *methanol R1*, sonicate for 10 min and filter through a membrane filter (nominal pore size 0.45 μm).

Reference solution   Dissolve an amount of *valerian dry extract HRS* corresponding to 0.5 mg of valerenic acid in *methanol R1* and dilute to 10.0 mL with the same solvent. Sonicate for 10 min and filter through a membrane filter (nominal pore size 0.45 μm).

Column:
— *size: l* = 0.25 m, Ø = 4.6 mm;
— *stationary phase: octadecylsilyl silica gel for chromatography R* (5 μm).

Mobile phase:
— *mobile phase A: acetonitrile R1*, 5 g/L solution of *phosphoric acid R* (20:80 *V/V*);
— *mobile phase B*: 5 g/L solution of *phosphoric acid R*, *acetonitrile R1* (20:80 *V/V*);

Time (min)	Mobile phase A (per cent *V/V*)	Mobile phase B (per cent *V/V*)
0 - 5	55	45
5 - 18	55 → 20	45 → 80
18 - 22	20	80

Flow rate 1.5 mL/min.

Detection Spectrophotometer at 220 nm.

Injection 20 μL.

Identification of peaks Use the chromatogram supplied with *valerian dry extract HRS* and the chromatogram obtained with the reference solution to identify the peaks due to hydroxyvalerenic acid, acetoxyvalerenic acid and valerenic acid.

System suitability Reference solution:
— relative retention with reference to valerenic acid (retention time = about 19 min): hydroxyvalerenic acid = about 0.2; acetoxyvalerenic acid = about 0.5.

Calculate the percentage content of sesquiterpenic acids, expressed as valerenic acid, using the following expression:

$$\frac{(A_1 + A_2 + A_3) \times m_2 \times p \times 5}{A_4 \times m_1}$$

A_1 = area of the peak due to hydroxyvalerenic acid in the chromatogram obtained with the test solution;

A_2 = area of the peak due to acetoxyvalerenic acid in the chromatogram obtained with the test solution;

A_3 = area of the peak due to valerenic acid in the chromatogram obtained with the test solution;

A_4 = area of the peak due to valerenic acid in the chromatogram obtained with the reference solution;

m_1 = mass of the extract to be examined used to prepare the test solution, in grams;

m_2 = mass of *valerian dry extract HRS* used to prepare the reference solution, in grams;

p = percentage content of valerenic acid in *valerian dry extract HRS*.

Ph Eur

Valerian Tincture

(Ph Eur monograph 1899)

Ph Eur

DEFINITION
Tincture produced from *Valerian root (0453)*.

Content
Minimum 0.015 per cent *m/m* of sesquiterpenic acids, expressed as valerenic acid ($C_{15}H_{22}O_2$; M_r 234.3).

PRODUCTION
The tincture is produced from 1 part of the drug and 5 parts of ethanol (60 to 80 per cent *V/V*) by an appropriate procedure.

CHARACTERS
Appearance
Brown liquid.

IDENTIFICATION
Thin-layer chromatography (2.2.27).

Test solution Dilute 5 mL of the tincture to be examined with 5 mL of *ethanol (70 per cent V/V) R*.

Reference solution Dissolve 5 mg of *acetoxyvalerenic acid R* and 5 mg of *valerenic acid R* in 20 mL of *methanol R*.

Plate TLC silica gel plate R (5-40 μm) [or *TLC silica gel plate R* (2-10 μm)].

Mobile phase glacial acetic acid R, ethyl acetate R, cyclohexane R (2:38:60 *V/V/V*).

Application 20 μL [or 5 μL] as bands of 10 mm [or 8 mm].

Development Over a path of 10 cm [or 6 cm].

Drying In air.

Detection Spray with *anisaldehyde solution R* and heat at 100-105 °C for 5-10 min; examine in daylight.

Results See below the sequence of zones present in the chromatograms obtained with the reference solution and the test solution. Furthermore, other violet zones may be present in the chromatogram obtained with the test solution.

Top of the plate	
Valerenic acid: a violet zone	A violet zone (valerenic acid)
Acetoxyvalerenic acid: a violet zone	A violet zone (acetoxyvalerenic acid)
	2 faint or very faint violet zones
Reference solution	**Test solution**

TESTS
Ethanol (2.9.10)
95 per cent to 105 per cent of the quantity stated on the label.

ASSAY
Liquid chromatography (2.2.29).

Test solution Dilute 10.0 g of the tincture to be examined to 50.0 mL with *methanol R1*.

Reference solution Dissolve an amount of *valerian dry extract HRS* corresponding to 1.0 mg of valerenic acid in *methanol R1* and dilute to 10.0 mL with the same solvent. Sonicate for 10 min and filter through a membrane filter (nominal pore size 0.45 μm).

Column:
— *size: l* = 0.25 m, Ø = 4.6 mm;
— *stationary phase: octadecylsilyl silica gel for chromatography R* (5 μm).

Mobile phase:
— *mobile phase A: acetonitrile R1*, 5 g/L solution of *phosphoric acid R* (20:80 *V/V*);
— *mobile phase B*: 5 g/L solution of *phosphoric acid R*, *acetonitrile R1* (20:80 *V/V*);

Time (min)	Mobile phase A (per cent V/V)	Mobile phase B (per cent V/V)
0 - 5	55	45
5 - 18	55 → 20	45 → 80
18 - 22	20	80

Flow rate   1.5 mL/min.

Detection   Spectrophotometer at 220 nm.

Injection   20 µL.

Peak identification   Use the chromatogram supplied with *valerian dry extract HRS* and the chromatogram obtained with the reference solution to identify the peaks due to acetoxyvalerenic acid and valerenic acid.

System suitability   Reference solution:
— *relative retention* with reference to valerenic acid (retention time = about 19 min):
acetoxyvalerenic acid = about 0.5.

Calculate the percentage content of sesquiterpenic acids, expressed as valerenic acid, using the following expression:

$$\frac{(A_1 + A_2) \times m_2 \times p \times 5}{A_3 \times m_1}$$

A_1 = area of the peak due to acetoxyvalerenic acid in the chromatogram obtained with the test solution;

A_2 = area of the peak due to valerenic acid in the chromatogram obtained with the test solution;

A_3 = area of the peak due to valerenic acid in the chromatogram obtained with the reference solution;

m_1 = mass of the tincture to be examined used to prepare the test solution, in grams;

m_2 = mass of *valerian dry extract HRS* used to prepare the reference solution, in grams;

p = percentage content of valerenic acid in *valerian dry extract HRS*.

———————————————— Ph Eur

Verbena Herb

(Ph Eur monograph 1854)

Ph Eur —————————————————————

DEFINITION
Whole or fragmented, dried aerial parts of *Verbena officinalis* L. collected during flowering.

Content
Minimum 1.5 per cent of verbenalin ($C_{17}H_{24}O_{10}$; M_r 388.4) (dried drug).

IDENTIFICATION
A. The stem is greenish-brown, quadrangular, longitudinally grooved and roughly hairy, especially on the angles.
The larger leaves are petiolate and deeply pinnately lobed, with bluntly dentate margins, the smaller leaves are sessile, not lobed, with crenate or dentate margins; the surfaces are rough and covered with bristly hairs, particularly over the veins, which are prominent on the lower surface. The flowers are numerous, arranged in a slender spike in the axils of leaf-like bracts; the tubular calyx has 5 acutely pointed lobes with the pale pink or lilac corolla forming a tube about twice as long as the calyx.

B. Microscopic examination (*2.8.23*). The powder is greenish-brown. Examine under a microscope using *chloral*

hydrate solution R. The powder shows the following diagnostic characters (Figure 1854.-1): fragments of the leaves, which in surface view [C] show sinuous-walled epidermal cells [Ca] with anisocytic [Cb] or anomocytic [Cc] stomata (*2.8.3*), more numerous on the lower epidermis; fragments of stem epidermis [A] consisting of long, polygonal or rectangular epidermal cells [Aa] with thickened walls and stomata [Ab]; covering trichomes, unicellular, thick-walled, up to 500 µm long, wide at the base and arising from the centre of a single ring of domed, spherical epidermal cells, in surface view [B] or in side view [D]; occasional glandular trichomes of 2 types: (a) long stalk with a flattened head about 35 µm in diameter and consisting of 4-8 radiating cells in side view [E] or in surface view of the head [G], and (b) short unicellular stalk and an enlarged ovate head composed of 4 radiating cells in surface view [Cd] or in transverse section [K]; triangular-ovoid or rounded pollen grains about 30 µm in diameter, with 3 pores and a smooth exine [J]; many fragments of stems [F] consisting of groups of fibres [Fb], vessels [Fa] and fragments of parenchyma [Fc]; isolated fragments of fibres [H].

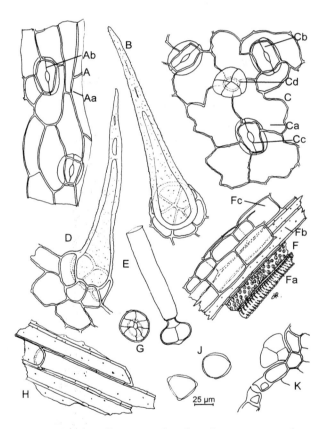

Figure 1854.-1. – *Illustration for identification test B of powdered herbal drug of verbena herb*

C. Examine the chromatograms obtained in test B for *Aloysia citrodora*.

Results   See below the sequence of zones present in the chromatograms obtained with the reference solution and the test solution. Furthermore, other zones may be present in the chromatogram obtained with the test solution.

Top of the plate	
────	────
	A brown or green zone
Arbutin: a blue or brown zone	
	An intense brownish-grey zone
Rutin: a dark brownish-yellow zone	
────	────
Reference solution	**Test solution**

TESTS

Aloysia citrodora

A. A lemon-like odour indicates the presence of *Aloysia citrodora*.

B. Thin-layer chromatography (*2.2.27*).

Test solution To 0.5 g of the powdered herbal drug (710) (*2.9.12*) add 5 mL of *methanol R*. Heat in a water-bath at 60 °C for 10 min. Cool and filter.

Reference solution Dissolve 10 mg of *arbutin R* and 10 mg of *rutin R* in *methanol R* and dilute to 10 mL with the same solvent.

Plate *TLC silica gel plate R* (5-40 μm) [or *TLC silica gel plate R* (2-10 μm)].

Mobile phase anhydrous formic acid R, glacial acetic acid R, water R, ethyl acetate R (11:11:27:100 *V/V/V/V*).

Application 20 μL [or 5 μL] as bands of 10 mm [or 8 mm].

Development Over a path of 12 cm [or 6 cm].

Drying In air.

Detection Spray with *anisaldehyde solution R* and heat at 100-105 °C for about 10 min; examine in daylight.

Results The chromatogram obtained with the test solution shows no intense blue or violet zone approximately at the position of rutin in the chromatogram obtained with the reference solution.

Loss on drying (*2.2.32*)
Maximum 10.0 per cent, determined on 1.000 g of the powdered herbal drug (710) (*2.9.12*) by drying in an oven at 105 °C for 2 h.

Total ash (*2.4.16*)
Maximum 10.0 per cent.

Ash insoluble in hydrochloric acid (*2.8.1*)
Maximum 2.0 per cent.

ASSAY

Liquid chromatography (*2.2.29*).

Internal standard solution Dissolve 10.0 mg of *ferulic acid R* in *ethanol (60 per cent V/V) R* and dilute to 100.0 mL with the same solvent.

Test solution To 1.00 g of the powdered herbal drug (710) (*2.9.12*) add 50.0 mL of the internal standard solution and stir with a magnetic stirrer for 2 h. Centrifuge for 15 min and filter the supernatant using a membrane filter (nominal pore size 0.45 μm).

Reference solution Dissolve the contents of a vial of *verbenalin CRS* in the internal standard solution and dilute to 5.0 mL with the same solution.

Precolumn:
— *size: l* = 0.01 m, Ø = 4.0 mm;
— *stationary phase*: octadecylsilyl silica gel for chromatography R (5 μm).

Column:
— *size: l* = 0.25 m, Ø = 4.0 mm;
— *stationary phase*: octadecylsilyl silica gel for chromatography R (5 μm);
— *temperature*: 20 °C.

Mobile phase:
— *mobile phase A*: 0.3 per cent *V/V* solution of *phosphoric acid R*;
— *mobile phase B*: *acetonitrile R*;

Time (min)	Mobile phase A (per cent *V/V*)	Mobile phase B (per cent *V/V*)
0 - 20	93 → 83	7 → 17
20 - 30	83	17
30 - 35	83 → 75	17 → 25

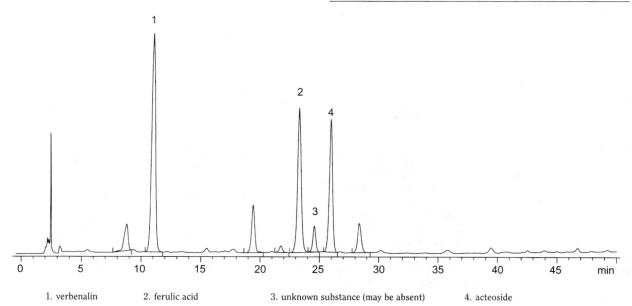

1. verbenalin   2. ferulic acid   3. unknown substance (may be absent)   4. acteoside

Figure 1854.-2. – *Chromatogram for the assay of verbena herb: test solution*

Flow rate 1.0 mL/min.

Detection Spectrophotometer at 240 nm.

Injection 20 μL.

System suitability Test solution:
— the chromatogram obtained is similar to the chromatogram shown in Figure 1854.-2;
— *resolution*: minimum 3.5 between the peaks due to ferulic acid and acteoside.

Calculate the percentage content of verbenalin using the following expression:

$$\frac{A_1 \times A_4 \times m_2 \times 1000}{A_2 \times A_3 \times m_1}$$

A_1 = area of the peak due to verbenalin in the chromatogram obtained with the test solution;

A_2 = area of the peak due to verbenalin in the chromatogram obtained with the reference solution;

A_3 = area of the peak due to ferulic acid in the chromatogram obtained with the test solution;

A_4 = area of the peak due to ferulic acid in the chromatogram obtained with the reference solution;

m_1 = mass of the herbal drug used to prepare the test solution, in grams;

m_2 = mass of verbenalin in the reference solution, in grams.

_____ *Ph Eur*

Willow Bark

(*Ph Eur monograph 1583*)

Preparation
Willow Bark Dry Extract

Ph Eur _____

DEFINITION

Whole or fragmented dried bark of young branches or whole dried pieces of current-year twigs of various species of genus *Salix* including *S. purpurea* L., *S. daphnoides* Vill. and *S. fragilis* L.

Content

Minimum 1.5 per cent of total salicylic derivatives, expressed as salicin ($C_{13}H_{18}O_7$; M_r 286.3) (dried drug).

IDENTIFICATION

A. The bark is 1-2 mm thick and occurs in flexible, elongated, quilled or curved pieces. The outer surface is smooth or slightly wrinkled longitudinally and greenish-yellow or brownish-grey. The inner surface is smooth or finely striated longitudinally and white, pale yellow or reddish-brown, depending on the species. The fracture is short in the outer part and coarsely fibrous in the inner region. The diameter of current-year twigs is not greater than 10 mm. The wood is white or pale yellow.

B. Microscopic examination (*2.8.23*). The powder is pale yellow, greenish-yellow or light brown. Examine under a microscope using *chloral hydrate solution R*. The powder shows the following diagnostic characters (Figure 1583.-1): bundles [B, C] of narrow fibres [Ba, Ca], up to about 600 μm long, with very thick walls and surrounded by a crystal sheath containing prisms of calcium oxalate [Bb, Cb]; parenchymatous cells of the cortex [D, J], with thick, pitted and deeply beaded walls [Da], and containing large cluster crystals of calcium oxalate [Ga, Ja]; some parenchyma cells are collenchymatous [G]; uniseriate medullary rays, in tangential section [Db]; thickened cork cells, in surface view [F]; numerous scattered prism crystals [E] and cluster crystals [A] of calcium oxalate; fragments of brownish collenchyma from the buds may also be present. Twigs show, additionally, wood fragments [H] composed of lignified fibres [Ha] and vessels [Hb], sometimes accompanied by medullary rays [Hc].

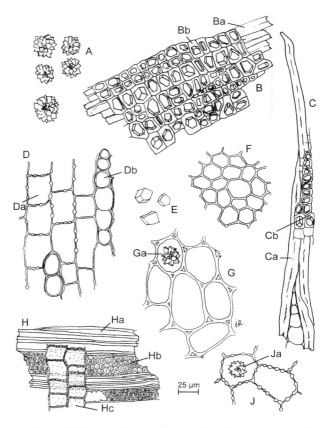

Figure 1583.-1. – *Illustration for identification test B of powdered herbal drug of willow bark*

C. Thin-layer chromatography (*2.2.27*).

Test solution (a) To 1.0 g of the powdered herbal drug (355) (*2.9.12*) add 10 mL of *methanol R*. Heat on a water-bath at about 50 °C, with frequent shaking, for 10 min. Cool and filter.

Test solution (b) To 5.0 mL of test solution (a) add 1.0 mL of a 50 g/L solution of *anhydrous sodium carbonate R* and heat in a water-bath at about 60 °C for 10 min. Cool and filter if necessary.

Reference solution Dissolve 2 mg of *salicin R* and 2 mg of *chlorogenic acid R* in 1.0 mL of *methanol R*.

Plate TLC silica gel plate R (5-40 μm) [or *TLC silica gel plate R* (2-10 μm)].

Mobile phase water R, methanol R, ethyl acetate R (8:15:77 *V/V/V*).

Application 10 μL [or 2 μL] as bands.

Development Over a path of 15 cm [or 6 cm].

Drying In a current of warm air.

Detection Treat with a mixture of 5 volumes of *sulfuric acid R* and 95 volumes of *methanol R*. Heat at 100-105 °C for 5 min and examine in daylight.

Results See below the sequence of zones present in the chromatograms obtained with the reference solution and test solutions (a) and (b). Furthermore, other zones may be present in the chromatograms obtained with test solutions (a) and (b).

Top of the plate		
	Several reddish-violet zones may be present	
Salicin: a reddish-violet zone	A weak reddish-violet zone (salicin)	A reddish-violet zone (salicin)
Chlorogenic acid: a brown zone		
Reference solution	Test solution (a)	Test solution (b)

TESTS

Foreign matter (*2.8.2*)
Maximum 3 per cent of twigs with a diameter greater than 10 mm and maximum 2 per cent of other foreign matter.

Cadmium (*2.4.27*)
Maximum 2.0 ppm.

Loss on drying (*2.2.32*)
Maximum 11 per cent, determined on 1.000 g of the powdered herbal drug (355) (*2.9.12*) by drying in an oven at 105 °C for 2 h.

Total ash (*2.4.16*)
Maximum 10 per cent.

ASSAY

Liquid chromatography (*2.2.29*).

Test solution To 1.000 g of the powdered herbal drug (355) (*2.9.12*) add 40 mL of *methanol R* and 40.0 mL of a 4.2 g/L solution of *sodium hydroxide R*. Heat in a water-bath at about 60 °C under a reflux condenser, with frequent shaking, for about 1 h. After cooling, add 4.0 mL of a 103.0 g/L solution of *hydrochloric acid R*. Filter the suspension into a 100 mL volumetric flask, wash and dilute to 100.0 mL with a mixture of equal volumes of *methanol R* and *water R*. Filter through a membrane filter (nominal pore size 0.45 µm).

Reference solution Dissolve 5.0 mg of *picein R* in 25.0 mL of a mixture of 20 volumes of *water R* and 80 volumes of *methanol R* (solution A). Dissolve 15.0 mg of *salicin CRS* in 25 mL of a mixture of 20 volumes of *water R* and 80 volumes of *methanol R*; add 5.0 mL of solution A and dilute to 50.0 mL with *water R*.

Column:
— *size: l* = 0.10 m, Ø = 4.6 mm;
— *stationary phase: octadecylsilyl silica gel for chromatography R* (3 µm).

Mobile phase:
— *mobile phase A: tetrahydrofuran R*, 0.5 per cent *V/V* solution of *phosphoric acid R* (1.8:98.2 *V/V*);
— *mobile phase B: tetrahydrofuran R*;

Time (min)	Mobile phase A (per cent *V/V*)	Mobile phase B (per cent *V/V*)
0 - 15	100	0
15 - 17	100 → 90	0 → 10
17 - 23	90	10

Flow rate 1.0 mL/min.

Detection Spectrophotometer at 270 nm.

Injection 10 µL.

Retention time Salicin = about 6.4 min; picein = about 7.7 min.

System suitability Reference solution:
— *resolution*: minimum 1.5 between the peaks due to salicin and picein.

Calculate the percentage content of total salicylic derivatives, expressed as salicin, using the following expression:

$$\frac{A_1 \times m_2 \times p \times 2}{A_2 \times m_1}$$

A_1 = area of the peak due to salicin in the chromatogram obtained with the test solution;

A_2 = area of the peak due to salicin in the chromatogram obtained with the reference solution;

m_1 = mass of the herbal drug to be examined used to prepare the test solution, in grams;

m_2 = mass of *salicin CRS* used to prepare the reference solution, in grams;

p = percentage content of salicin in *salicin CRS*.

_____ Ph Eur

Willow Bark Dry Extract

(*Ph Eur monograph 2312*)

Ph Eur _____

DEFINITION

Dry extract produced from *Willow bark (1583)*.

Content

Minimum 5.0 per cent of total salicylic derivatives, expressed as salicin ($C_{13}H_{18}O_7$; M_r 286.3) (dried extract).

PRODUCTION

The extract is produced from the herbal drug by a suitable procedure using either water or a hydroalcoholic solvent equivalent in strength to a maximum of 80 per cent *V/V* ethanol.

CHARACTERS

Appearance

Yellowish-brown amorphous powder.

IDENTIFICATION

Thin-layer chromatography (*2.2.27*).

Test solution (a) To 0.200 g of the extract to be examined add 5 mL of *methanol R*. Sonicate for 5 min, filter and dilute to 10 mL with *methanol R*.

Test solution (b) To 5.0 mL of test solution (a) add 1.0 mL of a 50 g/L solution of *anhydrous sodium carbonate R* and heat in a water-bath at about 60 °C for 10 min. Cool and filter if necessary.

Reference solution Dissolve 2.0 mg of *salicin R* and 2.0 mg of *chlorogenic acid R* in 1.0 mL of *methanol R*.

Plate *TLC silica gel plate R* (5-40 μm) [or *TLC silica gel plate R* (2-10 μm)].

Mobile phase *water R*, *methanol R*, *ethyl acetate R* (8:15:77 V/V/V).

Application 10 μL [or 2 μL] as bands.

Development Over a path of 15 cm [or 6 cm].

Drying In a current of warm air.

Detection Spray with a mixture of 5 volumes of *sulfuric acid R* and 95 volumes of *methanol R*. Heat at 100-105 °C for 5 min and examine in daylight.

Results See below the sequence of the zones present in the chromatograms obtained with the reference solution and test solutions (a) and (b). Furthermore, other zones may be present in the chromatogram obtained with test solutions (a) and (b).

Top of the plate		
	Several reddish-violet zones may be present	A reddish-violet zone (salicin)
Salicin: a reddish-violet zone	A weak reddish-violet zone (salicin)	
Chlorogenic acid: a brown zone		
Reference solution	**Test solution (a)**	**Test solution (b)**

ASSAY

Liquid chromatography (*2.2.29*).

Test solution To 0.300 g of the extract to be examined add 40 mL of *methanol R* and 40.0 mL of *0.1 M sodium hydroxide*. Heat in a water-bath at about 60 °C under a reflux condenser, with frequent shaking, for about 1 h. After cooling, add 4.0 mL of *1 M hydrochloric acid*. Filter the suspension into a 100 mL volumetric flask, then wash and dilute to 100.0 mL with a mixture of equal volumes of *water R* and *methanol R*. Filter through a membrane filter (nominal pore size 0.45 μm).

Reference solution Dissolve 5.0 mg of *picein R* in 25.0 mL of a mixture of 20 volumes of *water R* and 80 volumes of *methanol R* (solution A). Dissolve 15.0 mg of *salicin CRS* in 25 mL of a mixture of 20 volumes of *water R* and 80 volumes of *methanol R*. Add 5.0 mL of solution A and dilute to 50.0 mL with *water R*.

Column:
— *size*: l = 0.10 m, Ø = 4.6 mm;
— *stationary phase*: *octadecylsilyl silica gel for chromatography R* (3 μm).

Mobile phase:
— *mobile phase A*: *tetrahydrofuran R*, 0.5 per cent V/V solution of *phosphoric acid R* (1.8:98.2 V/V);
— *mobile phase B*: *tetrahydrofuran R*;

Time (min)	Mobile phase A (per cent V/V)	Mobile phase B (per cent V/V)
0 - 15	100	0
15 - 17	100 → 90	0 → 10
17 - 23	90	10
23 - 25	90 → 100	10 → 0
25 - 40	100	0

Flow rate 1.0 mL/min.

Detection Spectrophotometer at 270 nm.

Injection 10 μL.

Retention time Salicin = about 6.4 min; picein = about 7.7 min.

System suitability Reference solution:
— *resolution*: minimum 1.5 between the peaks due to salicin and picein.

Calculate the percentage content of total salicylic derivatives, expressed as salicin, from the following expression:

$$\frac{A_1 \times m_2 \times p \times 2}{A_2 \times m_1}$$

A_1 = area of the peak due to salicin in the chromatogram obtained with the test solution

A_2 = area of the peak due to salicin in the chromatogram obtained with the reference solution;

m_1 = mass of the extract to be examined used to prepare the test solution, in grams

m_2 = mass of *salicin CRS* used to prepare the reference solution, in grams

p = percentage content of salicin in *salicin CRS*.

Ph Eur

Withania Somnifera Root

DEFINITION

Withania Somnifera Root consists of the dried mature roots of *Withania somnifera* (L.) Dunal.

It contains not less than 0.01% withaferin A ($C_{28}H_{38}O_6$) and not less than 0.01% withanolide A ($C_{29}H_{42}O_7$).

PRODUCTION

It is collected in winter, washed, dried and cut into short pieces.

IDENTIFICATION

A. Pieces of root, cut into lengths of up to 8 cm, varying in diameter from 2 mm to 1 cm, with some narrower pieces of rhizome, often cut at the transition zone. Outer surface pale greyish-brown, somewhat darker brown in larger specimens. Fracture short, showing a whitish interior. The cut surface of the root may show a distinction between the xylem and other tissues marked by a faint yellow-green cambial ring.

B. Reduce to a powder (355). Examine under a microscope using *chloral hydrate solution*. Cork cells in surface view polygonal, in sectional view rectangular, thin-walled, yellowish brown, often broken. Parenchymatous cells in groups, elongated, rectangular, or oval to round, filled with starch; some pitted, lightly lignified, found alongside vascular fragments; parenchyma of the medullary rays, one or two cells wide shown crossing xylem elements at right angles; Occasional fragments of spiral, scalariform or pitted vessels with broad lumen; tracheids and vessels usually heavily lignified, reticulate or bordered pitted, single or in small groups. Fibres often accompanying vessels, thick walled, heavily pitted, and lignified; others less pitted and lignified, thin walled, either found singly or in groups of two or three. Microcrystals of calcium oxalate scattered or occasionally in idioblasts. Examine under a microscope using a 50% v/v solution of *glycerol*. Starch granules abundant, simple or 2 to 4 compound, round to oval, with a point, stellate or cleft hilum.

C. Carry out the method for *thin-layer chromatography*, Appendix III A, using the following solutions.

(1) Shake 0.5 g of freshly powdered (355) drug with 1 mL of *dilute ammonia R4*, add 10 mL of *methanol*, sonicate for 10 seconds, heat on a water-bath for 3 minutes, cool, filter, evaporate the filtrate to dryness at 60° and dissolve the dried residue in 1 mL of *methanol*. Filter through a 0.45 µm filter.

(2) 0.1% w/v each of *withaferin A CRS, withanolide B CRS* and *β-sitosterol* in *methanol*.

CHROMATOGRAPHIC CONDITIONS

(a) Use a *silica gel F$_{254}$* precoated high performance plate (Merck silica gel F$_{254}$ HPTLC plates are suitable).

(b) Use the mobile phase described below.

(c) Apply 2 µL of each of solution, as 6 mm bands.

(d) Develop the plate to 8 cm.

(e) After removal of the plate, dry in air and examine under *ultraviolet light (254 nm)*. Immerse the plate in 5% v/v of *methanolic sulfuric acid* for 1 second, allow to dry in air, heat at 110° for 2 minutes and examine immediately in daylight. Examine the derivatised plate under *ultraviolet light (366 nm)*.

MOBILE PHASE

5 volumes of *anhydrous formic acid*, 15 volumes of *ethyl acetate* and 50 volumes of *toluene*.

SYSTEM SUITABILITY

The test is not valid unless the chromatogram obtained with solution (2) shows three clearly separated bands.

CONFIRMATION

The bands with Rf values of approximately 0.1 (withaferin A), 0.26 (withanolide B) and 0.57 (β-sitosterol) in the chromatogram obtained with solution (1) correspond in colour and position to those in the chromatogram obtained with solution (2).

TESTS

Absence of *Withania coagulans*

In Identification test C, the derivatised plate under *ultraviolet light (366 nm)* shows no orange band with an Rf of approximately 0.2 in the chromatogram obtained with solution (1).

Ash

Not more than 7.0%, Appendix XI J.

Acid-insoluble ash

Not more than 1.0%, Appendix XI K.

Loss on drying

When dried for 2 hours at 105°, loses not more than 12.0% of its weight. Use 1 g.

ASSAY

Carry out the method for *liquid chromatography*, Appendix III D, using the following solutions.

(1) Extract 1 g of the powdered drug with 3.0 mL of *methanol* with the aid of ultrasound for 10 minutes, centrifuge at 3000 rpm for 5 minutes and retain the supernatant extract. The extraction is repeated twice as described. Combine the three supernatant extracts, adjust the total volume of the combined extracts to 20.0 ml with *methanol* and filter through a 0.45-µm filter.

(2) 0.02% w/v each of *withaferin A CRS* and *withanolide A CRS* and 0.01% w/v of *withanolide B CRS* in *methanol*.

CHROMATOGRAPHIC CONDITIONS

(a) Use a stainless steel column (15 cm × 4.6 mm) packed with *dodecylsilyl silica gel for chromatography* (4 µm) (Phenomenex Synergi Max-RP 80Å is suitable).

(b) Use gradient elution and the mobile phases described below. Equilibrate the column with a mixture of 65% mobile phase A and 35% mobile phase B for at least 15 minutes.

(c) Use a flow rate of 1 mL per minute.

(d) Use a column temperature of 50°.

(e) Use a detection wavelength of 230 nm.

(f) Inject 20 µL of each solution.

MOBILE PHASE

Mobile phase A   *water.*

Mobile phase B   Equal volumes of *ethanol (96%)* and *methanol.*

Time (Minutes)	Mobile phase A % v/v	Mobile phase B % v/v	Comments
0-5	65	35	isocratic
5-30	65→55	35→45	linear gradient
30-31	55→0	45→100	linear gradient
31-36	0	100	isocratic
36-37	0→65	100→35	linear gradient
37-45	65	35	re-equilibration

SYSTEM SUITABILITY

The test is not valid unless, in the chromatogram obtained with solution (2), the *resolution factor* between the first two main peaks, of withaferin A and withanolide A is at least 5.0 and the *symmetry factor* for both peaks is less than 1.3.

DETERMINATION OF CONTENT

Withaferin A Using the retention time and peak area of the peak due to withaferin A in the chromatogram obtained with solution (2), locate and integrate the peak due to withaferin A in the chromatogram obtained with solution (1).

Calculate the content of withaferin A in the sample using the declared content withaferin A ($C_{28}H_{38}O_6$) in *withaferin A CRS* and the following expression:

$$\frac{A_1}{A_2} \times \frac{m_2}{V_2} \times \frac{V_1}{m_1} \times p \times \frac{100}{100-d}$$

A_1 = Area of the peak due to withaferin A in the chromatogram obtained with solution (1).

A_2 = Area of the peak due to withaferin A in the chromatogram obtained with solution (2).

m_1 = Weight of the drug being examined in mg.

m_2 = Weight of *withaferin A CRS* in mg.

V_1 = Dilution volume of solution (1) in mL.

V_2 = Dilution volume of solution (2) in mL.

p = Percentage content of withaferin A in *withaferin A CRS*.

d = Percentage loss on drying of the herbal drug being examined.

Withanolide A Using the retention time and peak area of the peak due to withanolide A in the chromatogram obtained with solution (2), locate and integrate the peak due to withanolide A in the chromatogram obtained with solution (1).

Calculate the content of withanolide A in the sample using the declared content of withanolide A ($C_{29}H_{42}O_7$) in *withanolide A CRS* and the following expression:

$$\frac{A_1}{A_2} \times \frac{m_2}{V_2} \times \frac{V_1}{m_1} \times p \times \frac{100}{100 - d}$$

A_1 = Area of the peak due to withanolide A in the chromatogram obtained with solution (1).

A_2 = Area of the peak due to withanolide A in the chromatogram obtained with solution (2).

m_1 = Weight of the drug in mg.

m_2 = Weight of *withanolide A CRS* in mg.

V_1 = Dilution volume of solution (1) in mL.

V_2 = Dilution volume of solution (2) in mL.

p = Percentage content withanolide A in *withanolide A CRS*.

d = Percentage loss on drying of the herbal drug being examined.

STORAGE

Withania Somnifera Root should be protected from moisture.

Wormwood

(Ph Eur monograph 1380)

Ph Eur ⎯⎯⎯⎯⎯⎯⎯⎯⎯⎯⎯⎯⎯⎯⎯⎯⎯

DEFINITION

Basal leaves or slightly leafy, flowering tops, or mixture of these dried, whole or cut organs of *Artemisia absinthium* L.

Content

Minimum 2 mL/kg of essential oil (dried drug).

IDENTIFICATION

A. The leaves are greyish or greenish, densely tomentose on both surfaces. The basal leaves, with long petioles, have triangular or oval bipinnatisect or tripinnatisect lamina, with rounded or lanceolate segments. The cauline leaves are less segmented and the apical leaves are lanceolate. The stem of the flower-bearing region is greenish-grey, tomentose, up to 2.5 mm in diameter and usually with 5 flattened longitudinal grooves. The capitula are arranged as loose, axillary panicles, inserted at the level of the lanceolate or slightly pinnatisect leaves; they are spherical or flattened hemispherical, 2-4 mm in diameter and consist of a grey, tomentose involucre, the outer bracts linear, inner layer ovate, blunt at the apices with scarious margins, a receptacle with very long paleae up to 1 mm or more long, numerous yellow, tubular, hermaphroditic florets about 2 mm long and few yellow, ray florets.

B. Microscopic examination (*2.8.23*). The powder is greenish-grey. Examine under a microscope using *chloral hydrate solution R*. The powder shows the following diagnostic characters (Figure 1380.-1.): many T-shaped trichomes [A] with a short uniseriate stalk consisting of 1-5 small cells, perpendicularly capped by a very long, undulating terminal cell tapering at the ends; fragments of epidermises in surface view [D] with sinuous or wavy walls, anomocytic stomata (*2.8.3*) [Da], covering trichomes [Db] and glandular trichomes containing oil [Dc] or not containing oil [Dd], each with a short, biseriate, 2-celled stalk and a biseriate

head with 2-4 cells; free glandular trichomes in side view [C]; fragments of the corollas of the tubular and ray florets, some containing small cluster crystals of calcium oxalate [H]; numerous paleae each composed of a small cell forming a stalk and a very long, cylindrical and thin-walled terminal cell about 1-1.5 mm long, either whole [E] or limited to the distal part [B]; spheroidal pollen grains, about 30 μm in diameter, with 3 pores and a finely warty exine [G]; fragments of vascular tissue from the leaves [F] or the stems [J] consisting of vessels with spiral or annular thickenings [Fa], or with bordered pits [Ja], fibres [Fb, Jb] and parenchymatous cells with pitted, moderately thickened walls [Fc, Jc].

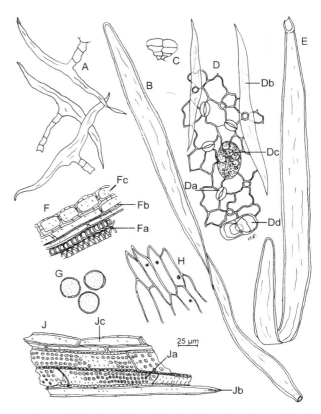

Figure 1380.-1. − *Illustration for identification test B of powdered herbal drug of wormwood*

C. Thin-layer chromatography (*2.2.27*).

Test solution Place 2 g of the powdered drug (355) (*2.9.12*) in 50 mL of boiling *water R* and allow to stand for 5 min, shaking the flask several times. After cooling, add 5 mL of a 100 g/L solution of *lead acetate R*. Mix and filter. Rinse the flask and the residue on the filter with 20 mL of *water R*. Shake the filter with 50 mL of *methylene chloride R*. Separate the organic layer, dry over *anhydrous sodium sulfate R*, filter and evaporate the filtrate to dryness on a water-bath. Dissolve the residue in 0.5 mL of *ethanol (96 per cent) R*.

Reference solution Dissolve 2 mg of *methyl red R* and 2 mg of *resorcinol R* in 10.0 mL of *methanol R*.

Plate TLC silica gel plate R.

Mobile phase acetone R, glacial acetic acid R, toluene R, methylene chloride R (10:10:30:50 *V/V/V/V*).

Application 10 μL as bands.

Development Over a path of 15 cm.

Drying In air.

Detection A Spray with *acetic anhydride - sulfuric acid solution R* and examine in daylight.

Results A The chromatogram obtained with the test solution shows a blue zone due to artabsin shortly above a red zone due to methyl red in the chromatogram obtained with the reference solution.

Detection B Examine in daylight while heating at 100-105 °C for 5 min.

Results B The chromatogram obtained with the reference solution shows in the middle third a red zone due to methyl red and below it a light pink zone due to resorcinol. The chromatogram obtained with the test solution shows an intense red or brownish-red zone due to absinthin with a similar R_F value to that of the zone due to resorcinol in the chromatogram obtained with the reference solution. Other zones are visible, but less intense than that due to absinthin.

TESTS

Foreign matter (*2.8.2*)
Maximum 5 per cent of stems with a diameter greater than 4 mm and maximum 2 per cent of other foreign matter.

Bitterness value (*2.8.15*)
Minimum 10 000.

Loss on drying (*2.2.32*)
Maximum 10.0 per cent, determined on 1.000 g of the powdered herbal drug (355) (*2.9.12*) by drying in an oven at 105 °C for 2 h.

Total ash (*2.4.16*)
Maximum 12.0 per cent.

Ash insoluble in hydrochloric acid (*2.8.1*)
Maximum 1.0 per cent.

ASSAY

Carry out the determination of essential oil in herbal drugs (*2.8.12*). Use 50.0 g of the cut drug, a 1000 mL round-bottomed flask and 500 mL of *water R* as the distillation liquid. Add 0.5 mL of *xylene R* in the graduated tube. Distil at a rate of 2-3 mL/min for not less than 3 h.

—————————————————— Ph Eur

Yarrow

(*Ph Eur monograph 1382*)

Ph Eur _____

DEFINITION

Whole or cut, dried flowering tops of *Achillea millefolium* L.

Content:

— *essential oil*: minimum 2 mL/kg (dried drug);
— *proazulenes, expressed as chamazulene* ($C_{14}H_{16}$; M_r 184.3): minimum 0.02 per cent (dried drug).

IDENTIFICATION

A. The leaves are green or greyish-green, faintly pubescent on the upper surface and more pubescent on the lower surface, 2-3 pinnately divided with linear lobes and a finely pointed whitish tip. The capitula are arranged in a corymb at the end of the stem. Each capitulum, 3-5 mm in diameter, consists of the receptacle, usually 4-5 ligulate ray-florets and 3-20 tubular disk-florets. The involucre consists of 3 rows of imbricate lanceolate, pubescent green bracts arranged with a brownish or whitish, membranous margin. The receptacle is slightly convex and, in the axillae of paleae, bears ligulate ray-florets with a three-lobed, whitish or reddish ligule and

tubular disk-florets with a radial, five-lobed, yellowish or light brownish corolla. The pubescent green, partly brown or violet stems are longitudinally furrowed, up to 3 mm thick with a light-coloured medulla.

B. Microscopic examination (*2.8.23*). The powder is green or greyish-green. Examine under a microscope using *chloral hydrate solution R*. The powder shows the following diagnostic characters (Figure 1382.-1): fragments of the stem epidermis, in surface view [K], with cells having a smooth cuticle and anomocytic stomata (*2.8.3*); fragments of leaf and bract epidermises, in surface view [B], with cells having wavy and irregularly thickened walls, a finely striated cuticle and anomocytic stomata (*2.8.3*); very rare glandular trichomes with a short stalk and a head formed of 2 rows of 3-5 cells enclosed in a bladder-like membrane [H]; uniseriate, whole or fragmented covering trichomes [A] consisting of 4-6 small, more or less isodiametric cells at the base and a thick-walled, often somewhat tortuous terminal cell, about 400 µm to greater than 1000 µm long; fragments of the ligulate corolla with papillary epidermal cells [D]; fragments of the corolla tubes, in surface view, with sinuous epidermal cells, covered by a thin striated cuticle [F]; small-celled parenchyma from the corolla tubes containing cluster crystals of calcium oxalate [E]; groups of lignified and pitted cells from the bracts [G]; spherical pollen grains, about 30 µm in diameter, with 3 germinal pores and a spiny exine [C]; groups of sclerenchymatous fibres and small vessels with spiral or annular thickening, from the stem [J].

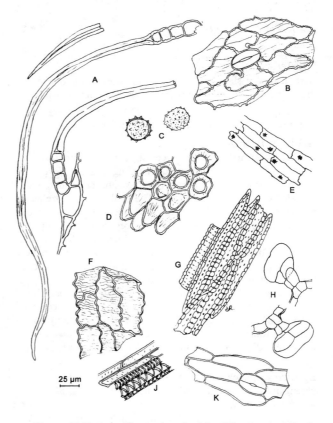

25 µm

Figure 1382.-1. – *Illustration for identification test B of powdered herbal drug of yarrow*

C. To 2.0 g of the powdered herbal drug (710) (*2.9.12*) add 25 mL of *ethyl acetate R*, shake for 5 min and filter. Evaporate to dryness on a water-bath and dissolve the residue in 0.5 mL of *toluene R* (solution A). To 0.1 mL of this solution add 2.5 mL of *dimethylaminobenzaldehyde solution R8* and heat on a water-bath for 2 min. Allow to cool. Add 5 mL of *light petroleum R* and shake the mixture vigorously. The aqueous layer shows a blue or greenish-blue colour.

D. Thin-layer chromatography (*2.2.27*).

Test solution   Use solution A prepared in identification test C.

Reference solution   Dissolve 10 mg of *cineole R* and 10 mg of *guaiazulene R* in 20 mL of *toluene R*.

Plate   *TLC silica gel plate R.*

Mobile phase   *ethyl acetate R, toluene R* (5:95 *V/V*).

Application   20 µL as bands.

Development   Over a path of 10 cm.

Drying   In air.

Detection   Spray with *anisaldehyde solution R*, heat at 100-105 °C for 5-10 min and examine in daylight.

Results   The chromatogram obtained with the reference solution shows in the upper part a red zone (guaiazulene) and in the middle part a blue or greyish-blue zone (cineole). The chromatogram obtained with the test solution shows a violet zone a little above the zone due to guaiazulene in the chromatogram obtained with the reference solution; below this zone a reddish-violet zone; below which, 1-2 not clearly separated greyish-violet or greyish zones (which changes to greenish-grey after a few hours) and a reddish-violet zone a little above the zone due to cineole in the chromatogram obtained with the reference solution. Further faint zones may be present.

TESTS

Foreign matter (*2.8.2*)
Maximum 5 per cent of stems with a diameter greater than 3 mm and maximum 2 per cent of other foreign matter.

Loss on drying (*2.2.32*)
Maximum 12.0 per cent, determined on 0.500 g of powdered herbal drug (355) (*2.9.12*) by drying in an oven at 105 °C for 2 h.

Total ash (*2.4.16*)
Maximum 10.0 per cent.

Ash insoluble in hydrochloric acid (*2.8.1*)
Maximum 2.5 per cent.

ASSAY

Essential oil
Carry out the determination of essential oils in herbal drugs (*2.8.12*). Use 20.0 g of cut drug, a 1000 mL round-bottomed flask and 500 mL of a mixture of 1 volume of *water R* and 9 volumes of *ethylene glycol R* as the distillation liquid. Add 0.2 mL of *xylene R* in the graduated tube. Distil at a rate of 2-3 mL/min for 2 h.

Stop cooling at the end of distillation and continue distilling until the blue, steam-volatile components have reached the lower end of the cooler. Immediately start cooling again, taking care to avoid warming the separation space. Stop the distillation after 5 min. Replace the 1000 mL round-bottomed flask by a 250 mL round-bottomed flask containing a mixture of 0.4 mL of *xylene R* and 50 mL of *water R*. Distil for 15 min. After 10 min read the total volume. To determine the blank value, use 0.2 mL of *xylene R* in the graduated tube and distil a mixture of 0.4 mL of *xylene R* and 50 mL of *water R* for 15 min.

Proazulenes
To ensure that as little water as possible is transferred, transfer the blue essential oil-xylene mixture obtained in the assay of essential oil into a 50 mL volumetric flask with the aid of small portions of *xylene R*, rinsing the graduated tube of the apparatus with *xylene R* and dilute to 50.0 mL with the same solvent. Measure the absorbance (*2.2.25*) at 608 nm using *xylene R* as the compensation liquid.

Calculate the percentage content of proazulenes, expressed as chamazulene, using the following expression:

$$\frac{A \times 2.1}{m}$$

i.e. taking the specific absorbance of chamazulene to be 23.8.
A =   absorbance at 608 nm;
m =   mass of the herbal drug to be examined, in grams.

Ph Eur

Monographs

Materials for use in the Manufacture of Homoeopathic Preparations

Homoeopathic Preparations

(*Ph Eur monograph 1038*)

Ph Eur ___

DEFINITION

Homoeopathic preparations are prepared from substances, products or preparations called stocks, in accordance with a homoeopathic manufacturing procedure. A homoeopathic preparation is usually designated by the Latin name of the stock, followed by an indication of the degree of dilution.

Raw materials

Raw materials for the production of homoeopathic preparations may be of natural or synthetic origin.

For raw materials of zoological or human origin, adequate measures are taken to minimise the risk of agents of infection, including viruses (*5.1.7*), in the homoeopathic preparations. For this purpose, it is demonstrated that:

— the method of production includes a step or steps that have been shown to remove or inactivate agents of infection;
— where applicable, raw materials of zoological origin comply with the monograph *Products with risk of transmitting agents of animal spongiform encephalopathies (1483)*;
— where applicable, the animals and the tissues used to obtain the raw materials comply with the health requirements of the competent authorities for animals for human consumption;
— for materials of human origin, the donor follows the recommendations applicable to human blood donors and to donated blood (see *Human plasma for fractionation (0853)*), unless otherwise justified and authorised.

A raw material of botanical, zoological or human origin may be used either in the fresh state or in the dried state. Where appropriate, fresh material may be kept deep-frozen. Raw materials of botanical origin comply with the requirements of the monograph *Herbal drugs for homoeopathic preparations (2045)*.

Where justified and authorised for transportation or storage purposes, fresh plant material may be kept in ethanol (96 per cent) or in alcohol of a suitable concentration, provided the whole material including the storage medium is used for processing.

Raw materials comply with any requirements of the relevant monographs of the European Pharmacopoeia.

Vehicles

Vehicles are excipients used for the preparation of certain stocks or for the potentisation process. They may include, for example: purified water, alcohol of a suitable concentration, glycerol and lactose.

Vehicles comply with any requirements of the relevant monographs of the European Pharmacopoeia.

Stocks

Stocks are substances, products or preparations used as starting materials for the production of homoeopathic preparations. A stock is usually one of the following: a mother tincture or a glycerol macerate, for raw materials of botanical, zoological or human origin, or the substance itself, for raw materials of chemical or mineral origin.

Mother tinctures comply with the requirements of the monograph *Mother tinctures for homoeopathic preparations (2029)*.

Glycerol macerates are liquid preparations obtained from raw materials of botanical, zoological or human origin by using glycerol or a mixture of glycerol and either alcohol of a suitable concentration or a solution of sodium chloride of a suitable concentration.

Potentisation

Dilutions and triturations are obtained from stocks by a process of potentisation in accordance with a homoeopathic manufacturing procedure: this means successive dilutions and succussions, or successive appropriate triturations, or a combination of the 2 processes.

The potentisation steps are usually one of the following:

— 1 part of the stock plus 9 parts of the vehicle; they may be designated as 'D', 'DH' or 'X' (decimal);
— 1 part of the stock plus 99 parts of the vehicle; they may be designated as 'C' or 'CH' (centesimal).

The number of potentisation steps defines the degree of dilution; for example, 'D3', '3 DH' or '3X' means 3 decimal potentisation steps, and 'C3', '3 CH' or '3C' means 3 centesimal potentisation steps.

'LM-' (or 'Q-') potencies are manufactured according to a specific procedure.

Dosage forms

A dosage form of a homoeopathic preparation complies with any relevant dosage form monograph in the European Pharmacopoeia, and with the following:

— for the purpose of dosage forms for homoeopathic use, 'active substances' are considered to be 'dilutions or triturations of homoeopathic stocks';
— these dosage forms are prepared using appropriate excipients;
— the test for uniformity of content (*2.9.6*) or uniformity of dosage units (*2.9.40*) is normally not appropriate; however, in certain circumstances, it is required by the competent authority.

Homoeopathic dosage form 'pillule'

Pillules for homoeopathic use are solid preparations obtained from sucrose, lactose or other suitable excipients. They may be prepared by impregnation of preformed pillules with a dilution or dilutions of homoeopathic stocks or by progressive addition of these excipients and the addition of a dilution or dilutions of homoeopathic stocks. They are intended for oral or sublingual use.

Homoeopathic dosage form 'tablet'

Tablets for homoeopathic use are solid preparations obtained from sucrose, lactose or other suitable excipients according to the monograph *Tablets (0478)*. They may either be prepared by compressing one or more solid active substances with the excipients or by impregnating preformed tablets with a dilution or dilutions of homoeopathic stocks. The preformed tablets for impregnation are obtained from sucrose, lactose or other suitable excipients according to the monograph *Tablets (0478)*. They are intended for oral or sublingual use.

Manufacturing methods

Homoeopathic preparations are manufactured using a range of methods of preparation and are presented in various dosage forms (covered by general dosage form monographs). The methods of preparation are described in the monograph *Methods of preparation of homoeopathic stocks and potentisation (2371)*. The use of certain preparations obtained using the methods listed below is restricted to certain dosage forms as indicated in Table 1038.-1.

Table 1038.-1.

Manufacturing methods	Dosage forms
2.1.2	Eye drops Solutions for injection Nasal preparations
2.2.1, 2.2.2, 2.2.3	Eye drops Pillules (globuli velati) Solutions for injection Nasal preparations Ointments, creams and gels Oral powders (triturations) Suppositories
2.2.4	Solutions for injection
3.1.2, 3.2.2	Eye drops Pillules (globuli velati) Solutions for injection Nasal preparations Ointments, creams and gels Suppositories

The competent authority has the right to accept or reject particular combinations of manufacturing method and substance.

—————————————————————— *Ph Eur*

Herbal Drugs for Homoeopathic Preparations

Herbal Drugs for Homoeopathic Use

(*Ph Eur monograph 2045*)

Ph Eur —————————————————————————

DEFINITION

Herbal drugs for homoeopathic preparations are mainly whole plants or parts of plants, fragmented or broken, and include algae, fungi or lichens, in an unprocessed state, usually in fresh form. The state, fresh or dried, in which the drug is used, is defined in the individual monograph of the European Pharmacopoeia or, in its absence, in the individual monograph of an official national pharmacopoeia of a member state. In the absence of such a monograph, the state in which the herbal drug is used has to be defined. Certain exudates that have not been subjected to a specific treatment are also considered to be herbal drugs for homoeopathic preparations. Herbal drugs for homoeopathic preparations are precisely defined by the botanical scientific name of the source species according to the binomial system (genus, species, variety and author).

Whole describes a herbal drug for homoeopathic preparations that has not been reduced in size and is presented, dried or undried, as harvested.

Fragmented describes a herbal drug for homoeopathic preparations that has been reduced in size after harvesting to permit ease of handling, drying and/or packaging.

Broken describes a herbal drug for homoeopathic preparations in which the more fragile parts of the plant have broken during drying, packaging or transportation.

For dried herbal drugs for homoeopathic preparations, *cut* describes size reduction, other than powdering, that reduces the particle size below that which is described in the macroscopic identity of the herbal drug for homoeopathic preparations.

PRODUCTION

Herbal drugs for homoeopathic preparations are obtained from cultivated or wild plants. Suitable collection, cultivation, harvesting, sorting, drying, fragmentation and storage conditions are essential to guarantee the quality of herbal drugs for homoeopathic preparations.

Herbal drugs for homoeopathic preparations are, as far as possible, free from impurities such as soil, dust, dirt and other contaminants such as fungal, insect and other animal contaminants. They do not present signs of decay.

If a decontaminating treatment has been used, it is necessary to demonstrate that the constituents of the plant are not affected and that no harmful residues remain. The use of ethylene oxide is prohibited for the decontamination of herbal drugs for homoeopathic preparations.

Fresh herbal drugs are processed as rapidly as possible after harvesting. Where justified and authorised for transportation or storage purposes, fresh plant material may be deep-frozen; it may also be kept in ethanol (96 per cent) or in ethanol of a suitable concentration, provided the whole material including the storage medium is used for processing.

Adequate measures have to be taken in order to ensure that the microbiological quality of homoeopathic preparations containing 1 or more herbal drugs comply with the recommendations given in general chapter *5.1.4. Microbiological quality of non-sterile pharmaceutical preparations and substances for pharmaceutical use.*

IDENTIFICATION

Herbal drugs for homoeopathic preparations are identified using their macroscopic and, where necessary, microscopic descriptions and any further tests that may be required (for example, thin-layer chromatography).

TESTS

The tests for foreign matter and loss on drying should be performed before any further processing of the fresh plant.

Foreign matter (*2.8.2*)

Where a fresh plant is used as a starting material for the manufacture of homoeopathic preparations, the content of foreign matter is as low as possible; if necessary, the maximum content of foreign matter is indicated in the individual monograph.

Where a dried plant is used as a starting material for the manufacture of homoeopathic preparations, carry out a test for foreign matter, unless otherwise prescribed in the individual monograph. The content of foreign matter is not more than 2 per cent *m/m*, unless otherwise prescribed or justified and authorised.

Adulteration

A specific appropriate test may apply to herbal drugs for homoeopathic preparations liable to be falsified.

Loss on drying (*2.2.32*)

Carry out a test for loss on drying on dried herbal drugs for homoeopathic preparations.

If a fresh plant is processed more than 24 h after harvesting, a test for loss on drying should be carried out. The minimum limit is indicated in the individual monograph.

Water (*2.2.13*)

A determination of water is carried out on herbal drugs for homoeopathic preparations with a high essential oil content.

Pesticides (*2.8.13*)

Herbal drugs for homoeopathic preparations comply with the requirements for pesticide residues. The requirements take into account the origin and the nature of the plant, where necessary the preparation in which the plant might be used and, where available, knowledge of the complete record of treatment of the batch of the plant. Where justified, the test for pesticides may be performed on the mother tincture according to the requirements of the general monograph *Mother tinctures for homoeopathic preparations (2029)*.

If appropriate, herbal drugs for homoeopathic preparations comply with other tests, such as the following, for example.

Total ash *(2.4.16)*.

Bitterness value *(2.8.15)*.

Heavy metals *(2.4.27)*
Unless otherwise stated in an individual monograph or unless otherwise justified and authorised:
— *cadmium*: maximum 1.0 ppm;
— *lead*: maximum 5.0 ppm;
— *mercury*: maximum 0.1 ppm.

If justified by the nature or origin of the herbal drug or if required by the competent authority, suitable limits for the content of other heavy metals such as arsenic or nickel are defined.

Where justified, the test for heavy metals may be performed on the mother tincture according to the requirements of the general monograph *Mother tinctures for homoeopathic preparations (2029)*.

Aflatoxin B₁ *(2.8.18)*
Where appropriate, limits for aflatoxins may be required.

Ochratoxin A *(2.8.22)*
Where appropriate, a limit for ochratoxin A may be required.

Radioactive contamination
In some specific circumstances, the risk of radioactive contamination is to be considered.

ASSAY
Where applicable, herbal drugs for homoeopathic preparations are assayed by an appropriate method.

STORAGE
Store dried herbal drugs protected from light.

_____ *Ph Eur*

Methods of Preparation of Homoeopathic Stocks and Potentisation

(Ph Eur monograph 2371)

Ph Eur _____

Homoeopathic stocks are prepared, using suitable methods, from raw materials that comply with the requirements of the monograph *Homoeopathic preparations (1038)*. The methods described below, combined with established methods for potentisation, are examples of methods, but other methods described in an official national pharmacopoeia of a Member State may equally be used.

Where material of animal origin is to be used, particular reference is made to the requirements concerning the use of raw material of zoological or human origin in the monograph *Homoeopathic preparations (1038)*.

In the preparation of liquid dilutions, the ethanol of the concentration prescribed in the method may, if necessary, be replaced by ethanol (36 per cent *V/V*) [ethanol (30 per cent

m/m)] or ethanol (18 per cent *V/V*) [ethanol (15 per cent *m/m*)].

When the individual monograph allows that the mother tincture be prepared from more than one plant species, the mother tincture can be prepared from the specified parts of an individual plant species or from any mixture thereof.

Unless otherwise stated, mother tinctures are prepared by maceration. Maceration lasts not less than 10 days and not more than 30 days.

Maceration may be replaced by long maceration (maximum 60 days) or very long maceration (maximum 180 days), provided it is demonstrated that the quality of the resulting mother tincture is the same as that of the mother tincture prepared by maceration.

Unless otherwise stated in the individual monograph, the term 'part(s)' denotes 'mass part(s)'. Unless otherwise stated in the method, the maximum temperature for the preparation is 25 °C.

1. MOTHER TINCTURES
METHOD 1.1

Method 1.1.1 (EQUIVALENT TO HOMÖOPATHISCHES ARZNEIBUCH (HAB) 1a: MOTHER TINCTURES AND LIQUID DILUTIONS)
Method 1.1.1 is used for fresh herbal drugs containing generally more than 70 per cent of expressed juice and no essential oil or resin or mucilage. Mother tinctures prepared according to Method 1.1.1 are mixtures of equal parts of expressed juices and ethanol (90 per cent *V/V*) [ethanol (86 per cent *m/m*)].

Express the comminuted herbal drug. Immediately mix the expressed juice with an equal mass of ethanol (90 per cent *V/V*) [ethanol (86 per cent *m/m*)]. Allow to stand in a closed container at a temperature not exceeding 20 °C for not less than 5 days, then filter.

Adjustment to any value specified in the individual monograph
Determine the percentage dry residue *(2.8.16)* or, where prescribed, the percentage assay content of the above-mentioned filtrate. Calculate the amount (A_1), in kilograms, of ethanol (50 per cent *V/V*) [ethanol (43 per cent *m/m*)] required, using the following expression:

$$\frac{m \times (N_x - N_0)}{N_0}$$

m = mass of filtrate, in kilograms;
N_0 = percentage dry residue or percentage assay content as required in the individual monograph;
N_x = percentage dry residue or percentage assay content of the filtrate.

Mix the filtrate with the calculated amount of ethanol (50 per cent *V/V*) [ethanol (43 per cent *m/m*)]. Allow to stand at a temperature not exceeding 20 °C for not less than 5 days, then filter if necessary.

Potentisation
The 1ˢᵗ 'decimal' dilution (D1) is made from:
— 2 parts of the mother tincture;
— 8 parts of ethanol (50 per cent *V/V*) [ethanol (43 per cent *m/m*)].
The 2ⁿᵈ decimal dilution (D2) is made from:
— 1 part of the 1ˢᵗ 'decimal' dilution;
— 9 parts of ethanol (50 per cent *V/V*) [ethanol (43 per cent *m/m*)].
Subsequent decimal dilutions are produced as stated for D2.

The 1st 'centesimal' dilution (C1) is made from:
— 2 parts of the mother tincture;
— 98 parts of ethanol (50 per cent V/V) [ethanol (43 per cent m/m)].

The 2nd centesimal dilution (C2) is made from:
— 1 part of the 1st 'centesimal' dilution;
— 99 parts of ethanol (50 per cent V/V) [ethanol 43 per cent m/m)].

Subsequent centesimal dilutions are produced as stated for C2.

Method 1.1.2 (EQUIVALENT TO HAB 1b: MOTHER TINCTURES AND LIQUID DILUTIONS)

Method 1.1.2 is used where the latex of a herbal drug is to be processed.

Mother tinctures prepared according to Method 1.1.2 are mixtures of fresh plant latex with ethanol (36 per cent V/V) [ethanol (30 per cent m/m)]. Mix the fresh latex with 2 parts by mass of ethanol (36 per cent V/V) [ethanol (30 per cent m/m)] and filter.

Adjustment to any value specified in the individual monograph

Determine the percentage dry residue (*2.8.16*) or, where prescribed, the percentage assay content of the above-mentioned filtrate. Calculate the amount (A_1), in kilograms, of ethanol (36 per cent V/V) [ethanol (30 per cent m/m)] required, using the following expression:

$$\frac{m \times (N_x - N_0)}{N_0}$$

m = mass of filtrate, in kilograms;
N_0 = percentage dry residue or percentage assay content as required in the individual monograph;
N_x = percentage dry residue or percentage assay content of the filtrate.

Mix the filtrate with the calculated amount of ethanol (36 per cent V/V) [ethanol (30 per cent m/m)]. Allow to stand at a temperature not exceeding 20 °C for not less than 5 days, then filter if necessary.

Potentisation

The 1st 'decimal' dilution (D1) is made from:
— 3 parts of the mother tincture;
— 7 parts of ethanol (36 per cent V/V) [ethanol (30 per cent m/m)].

The 2nd decimal dilution (D2) is made from:
— 1 part of the 1st 'decimal' dilution;
— 9 parts of ethanol (18 per cent V/V) [ethanol (15 per cent m/m)].

Subsequent decimal dilutions are produced as stated for D2.

Method 1.1.3 (EQUIVALENT TO HAB 2a: MOTHER TINCTURES AND LIQUID DILUTIONS)

Method 1.1.3 is used for fresh herbal drugs containing generally less than 70 per cent of expressed juice and more than 60 per cent moisture (loss on drying) and no essential oil or resin.

Mother tinctures prepared according to Method 1.1.3 (ethanol content approximately 50 per cent V/V or 43 per cent m/m) are prepared by maceration as described below.

Comminute the herbal drug. Take a sample and determine the loss on drying (*2.2.32*). Unless otherwise prescribed, determine the loss on drying on 2.00-5.00 g of comminuted raw material in a flat-bottomed tared vessel, 45-55 mm in diameter, that has been previously dried as indicated for the raw material. Dry the raw material at 105 °C for 2 h then allow to cool in a desiccator.

To the comminuted herbal drug immediately add not less than half the mass of ethanol (90 per cent V/V) [ethanol (86 per cent m/m)] and store in well-closed containers at a temperature not exceeding 20 °C.

Use the following expression to calculate the amount (A_2), in kilograms, of ethanol (90 per cent V/V) [ethanol (86 per cent m/m)] required for the mass (m) of raw material, then subtract the amount of ethanol (90 per cent V/V) [ethanol (86 per cent m/m)] already added and add the difference to the mixture.

$$\frac{m \times T}{100}$$

m = mass of raw material, in kilograms;
T = percentage loss on drying of the sample.

Allow to stand at a temperature not exceeding 20 °C for not less than 10 days, swirling from time to time, then express the mixture and filter the resulting liquid.

Adjustment to any value specified in the individual monograph

Determine the percentage dry residue (*2.8.16*) or, where prescribed, the percentage assay content of the above-mentioned filtrate. Calculate the amount (A_1), in kilograms, of ethanol (50 per cent V/V) [ethanol (43 per cent m/m)] required, using the following expression:

$$\frac{m \times (N_x - N_0)}{N_0}$$

m = mass of filtrate, in kilograms;
N_0 = percentage dry residue or percentage assay content as required in the individual monograph;
N_x = percentage dry residue or percentage assay content of the filtrate.

Mix the filtrate with the calculated amount of ethanol (50 per cent V/V) [ethanol (43 per cent m/m)]. Allow to stand at a temperature not exceeding 20 °C for not less than 5 days, then filter if necessary.

Potentisation

The 1st 'decimal' dilution (D1) is made from:
— 2 parts of the mother tincture;
— 8 parts of ethanol (50 per cent V/V) [ethanol (43 per cent m/m)].

The 2nd decimal dilution (D2) is made from:
— 1 part of the 1st 'decimal' dilution;
— 9 parts of ethanol (50 per cent V/V) [ethanol (43 per cent m/m)].

Subsequent decimal dilutions are produced as stated for D2.

The 1st 'centesimal' dilution (C1) is made from:
— 2 parts of the mother tincture;
— 98 parts of ethanol (50 per cent V/V) [ethanol (43 per cent m/m)].

The 2nd centesimal dilution (C2) is made from:
— 1 part of the 1st 'centesimal' dilution;
— 99 parts of ethanol (50 per cent V/V) [ethanol (43 per cent m/m)].

Subsequent centesimal dilutions are produced as stated for C2.

Method 1.1.4 (EQUIVALENT TO HAB 2b: MOTHER TINCTURES AND LIQUID DILUTIONS)

Method 1.1.4 is used for fresh herbal drugs containing generally less than 70 per cent of expressed juice and more than 60 per cent moisture (loss on drying) and no essential oil or resin.

Mother tinctures prepared according to Method 1.1.4 (ethanol content approximately 36 per cent V/V or 30 per cent m/m) are prepared by maceration as described below.

Comminute the herbal drug. Take a sample and determine the loss on drying (2.2.32). Unless otherwise prescribed, determine the loss on drying on 2.00-5.00 g of comminuted raw material in a flat-bottomed tared vessel, 45-55 mm in diameter, that has been previously dried as indicated for the raw material. Dry the raw material at 105 °C for 2 h then allow to cool in a desiccator.

To the comminuted herbal drug immediately add not less than half the mass of ethanol (70 per cent V/V) [ethanol (62 per cent m/m)] and store in well-closed containers at a temperature not exceeding 20 °C.

Use the following expression to calculate the amount (A_2), in kilograms, of ethanol (70 per cent V/V) [ethanol (62 per cent m/m)] required for the mass (m) of raw material, then subtract the amount of ethanol (70 per cent V/V) [ethanol (62 per cent m/m)] already added and add the difference to the mixture.

$$\frac{m \times T}{100}$$

m = mass of raw material, in kilograms;
T = percentage loss on drying of the sample.

Allow to stand at a temperature not exceeding 20 °C for not less than 10 days, swirling from time to time, then express the mixture and filter the resulting liquid.

Adjustment to any value specified in the individual monograph

Determine the percentage dry residue (2.8.16) or, where prescribed, the percentage assay content of the above-mentioned filtrate. Calculate the amount (A_1), in kilograms, of ethanol (36 per cent V/V) [ethanol (30 per cent m/m)] required, using the following expression:

$$\frac{m \times (N_x - N_0)}{N_0}$$

m = mass of filtrate, in kilograms;
N_0 = percentage dry residue or percentage assay content as required in the individual monograph;
N_x = percentage dry residue or percentage assay content of the filtrate.

Mix the filtrate with the calculated amount of ethanol (36 per cent V/V) [ethanol (30 per cent m/m)]. Allow to stand at a temperature not exceeding 20 °C for not less than 5 days, then filter if necessary.

Potentisation

The 1st 'decimal' dilution (D1) is made from:
— 2 parts of the mother tincture;
— 8 parts of ethanol (36 per cent V/V) [ethanol (30 per cent m/m)].

The 2nd decimal dilution (D2) is made from:
— 1 part of the 1st 'decimal' dilution;
— 9 parts of ethanol (18 per cent V/V) [ethanol (15 per cent m/m)].

Subsequent decimal dilutions are produced as stated for D2.

Method 1.1.5 (EQUIVALENT TO HAB 3a: MOTHER TINCTURES AND LIQUID DILUTIONS)

Method 1.1.5 is used for fresh herbal drugs containing essential oil or resin, or generally less than 60 per cent moisture (loss on drying).

Mother tinctures prepared according to Method 1.1.5 (ethanol content approximately 68 per cent V/V or 60 per cent m/m) are prepared by maceration as described below.

Comminute the herbal drug. Take a sample and determine the loss on drying (2.2.32). Unless otherwise prescribed, determine the loss on drying on 2.00-5.00 g of comminuted raw material in a flat-bottomed tared vessel, 45-55 mm in diameter, that has been previously dried as indicated for the raw material. Dry the raw material at 105 °C for 2 h then allow to cool in a desiccator.

To the comminuted herbal drug immediately add not less than half the mass of ethanol (90 per cent V/V) [ethanol (86 per cent m/m)] and store in well-closed containers at a temperature not exceeding 20 °C.

Use the following expression to calculate the amount (A_3), in kilograms, of ethanol (90 per cent V/V) [ethanol (86 per cent m/m)] required for the mass (m) of raw material, then subtract the amount of ethanol (90 per cent V/V) [ethanol (86 per cent m/m)] already added and add the difference to the mixture.

$$\frac{2 \times m \times T}{100}$$

m = mass of raw material, in kilograms;
T = percentage loss on drying of the sample.

Allow to stand at a temperature not exceeding 20 °C for not less than 10 days, swirling from time to time, then express the mixture and filter the resulting liquid.

Adjustment to any value specified in the individual monograph

Determine the percentage dry residue (2.8.16) or, where prescribed, the percentage assay content of the above-mentioned filtrate. Calculate the amount (A_1), in kilograms, of ethanol (70 per cent V/V) [ethanol (62 per cent m/m)] required, using the following expression:

$$\frac{m \times (N_x - N_0)}{N_0}$$

m = mass of filtrate, in kilograms;
N_0 = percentage dry residue or percentage assay content as required in the individual monograph;
N_x = percentage dry residue or percentage assay content of the filtrate.

Mix the filtrate with the calculated amount of ethanol (70 per cent V/V) [ethanol (62 per cent m/m)]. Allow to stand at a temperature not exceeding 20 °C for not less than 5 days, then filter if necessary.

Potentisation

The 1st 'decimal' dilution (D1) is made from:
— 3 parts of the mother tincture;
— 7 parts of ethanol (70 per cent V/V) [ethanol (62 per cent m/m)].

The 2nd decimal dilution (D2) is made from:
— 1 part of the 1st 'decimal' dilution;

— 9 parts of ethanol (70 per cent V/V) [ethanol (62 per cent m/m)].

Subsequent decimal dilutions are produced as stated for D2. Use ethanol (50 per cent V/V) [ethanol (43 per cent m/m)] for dilutions from D4 onwards.

The 1st 'centesimal' dilution (C1) is made from:
— 3 parts of the mother tincture;
— 97 parts of ethanol (70 per cent V/V) [ethanol (62 per cent m/m)].

The 2nd centesimal dilution (C2) is made from:
— 1 part of the 1st 'centesimal' dilution;
— 99 parts of ethanol (50 per cent V/V) [ethanol (43 per cent m/m)].

Subsequent centesimal dilutions are produced as stated for C2.

Method 1.1.6 (EQUIVALENT TO HAB 3b: MOTHER TINCTURES AND LIQUID DILUTIONS)

Method 1.1.6 is used for fresh herbal drugs containing essential oils or resins or generally less than 60 per cent moisture (loss on drying).

Mother tinctures prepared according to Method 1.1.6 (ethanol content approximately 50 per cent V/V or 43 per cent m/m) are prepared by maceration as described below.

Comminute the herbal drug. Take a sample and determine the loss on drying (2.2.32). Unless otherwise prescribed, determine the loss on drying on 2.00-5.00 g of comminuted raw material in a flat-bottomed tared vessel, 45-55 mm in diameter, that has been previously dried as indicated for the raw material. Dry the raw material at 105 °C for 2 h then allow to cool in a desiccator.

To the comminuted herbal drug immediately add not less than half the mass of ethanol (80 per cent V/V) [ethanol (73 per cent m/m)] and store in well-closed containers at a temperature not exceeding 20 °C.

Use the following expression to calculate the amount (A_3), in kilograms, of ethanol (80 per cent V/V) [ethanol (73 per cent m/m)] required for the mass (m) of raw material, then subtract the amount of ethanol (80 per cent V/V) [ethanol (73 per cent m/m)] already added and add the difference to the mixture.

$$\frac{2 \times m \times T}{100}$$

m = mass of raw material, in kilograms;
T = percentage loss on drying of the sample.

Allow to stand at a temperature not exceeding 20 °C for not less than 10 days, swirling from time to time, then express the mixture and filter the resulting liquid.

Adjustment to any value specified in the individual monograph

Determine the percentage dry residue (2.8.16) or, where prescribed, the percentage assay content of the above-mentioned filtrate. Calculate the amount (A_1), in kilograms, of ethanol (50 per cent V/V) [ethanol (43 per cent m/m)] required, using the following expression:

$$\frac{m \times (N_x - N_0)}{N_0}$$

m = mass of filtrate, in kilograms;
N_0 = percentage dry residue or percentage assay content as required in the individual monograph;

N_x = percentage dry residue or percentage assay content of the filtrate.

Mix the filtrate with the calculated amount of ethanol (50 per cent V/V) [ethanol (43 per cent m/m)]. Allow to stand at a temperature not exceeding 20 °C for not less than 5 days, then filter if necessary.

Potentisation

The 1st 'decimal' dilution (D1) is made from:
— 3 parts of the mother tincture;
— 7 parts of ethanol (50 per cent V/V) [ethanol (43 per cent m/m)].

The 2nd decimal dilution (D2) is made from:
— 1 part of the 1st 'decimal' dilution;
— 9 parts of ethanol (36 per cent V/V) [ethanol (30 per cent m/m)].

The 3rd decimal dilution (D3) is made from:
— 1 part of the 2nd decimal dilution;
— 9 parts of ethanol (18 per cent V/V) [ethanol (15 per cent m/m)].

Subsequent decimal dilutions are produced as stated for D3.

Method 1.1.7 (EQUIVALENT TO HAB 3c: MOTHER TINCTURES AND LIQUID DILUTIONS)

Method 1.1.7 is used for fresh herbal drugs containing generally less than 60 per cent moisture (loss on drying).

Mother tinctures prepared according to Method 1.1.7 (ethanol content approximately 36 per cent V/V or 30 per cent m/m) are prepared by maceration as described below.

Comminute the herbal drug. Take a sample and determine the loss on drying (2.2.32). Unless otherwise prescribed, determine the loss on drying on 2.00-5.00 g of comminuted raw material in a flat-bottomed tared vessel, 45-55 mm in diameter, that has been previously dried as indicated for the raw material. Dry the raw material at 105 °C for 2 h then allow to cool in a desiccator.

To the comminuted herbal drug immediately add not less than half the mass of ethanol (50 per cent V/V) [ethanol (43 per cent m/m)] and store in well-closed containers at a temperature not exceeding 20 °C.

Use the following expression to calculate the amount (A_3), in kilograms, of ethanol (50 per cent V/V) [ethanol (43 per cent m/m)] required for the mass (m) of raw material, then subtract the amount of ethanol (50 per cent V/V) [ethanol (43 per cent m/m)] already added and add the difference to the mixture.

$$\frac{2 \times m \times T}{100}$$

m = mass of raw material, in kilograms;
T = percentage loss on drying of the sample.

Allow to stand at a temperature not exceeding 20 °C for not less than 10 days, swirling from time to time, then express the mixture and filter the resulting liquid.

Adjustment to any value specified in the individual monograph

Determine the percentage dry residue (2.8.16) or, where prescribed, the percentage assay content of the above-mentioned filtrate. Calculate the amount (A_1), in kilograms, of ethanol (36 per cent V/V) [ethanol (30 per cent m/m)] required, using the following expression:

$$\frac{m \times (N_x - N_0)}{N_0}$$

m = mass of filtrate, in kilograms;
N_0 = percentage dry residue or percentage assay content as required in the individual monograph;
N_x = percentage dry residue or percentage assay content of the filtrate.

Mix the filtrate with the calculated amount of ethanol (36 per cent V/V) [ethanol (30 per cent m/m)]. Allow to stand at a temperature not exceeding 20 °C for not less than 5 days, then filter if necessary.

Potentisation
The 1st 'decimal' dilution (D1) is made from:
— 3 parts of the mother tincture;
— 7 parts of ethanol (36 per cent V/V) [ethanol (30 per cent m/m)].

The 2nd decimal dilution (D2) is made from:
— 1 part of the 1st 'decimal' dilution;
— 9 parts of ethanol (18 per cent V/V) [ethanol (15 per cent m/m)].

Subsequent decimal dilutions are produced as stated for D2.

METHOD 1.1.8 (EQUIVALENT TO HAB 4a: MOTHER TINCTURES AND LIQUID DILUTIONS)
Method 1.1.8 is generally used for dried herbal drugs.

Mother tinctures prepared according to Method 1.1.8 are prepared by maceration or percolation as described below, using 1 part of dried herbal drug and 10 parts of ethanol of the appropriate concentration (anhydrous, 96 per cent V/V - 94 per cent m/m, 90 per cent V/V - 86 per cent m/m, 80 per cent V/V - 73 per cent m/m, 70 per cent V/V - 62 per cent m/m, 50 per cent V/V - 43 per cent m/m, 36 per cent V/V - 30 per cent m/m, 18 per cent V/V - 15 per cent m/m), unless otherwise prescribed in the individual monograph.

Production by maceration   Unless otherwise prescribed, comminute the herbal drug, mix thoroughly with ethanol of the appropriate concentration and allow to stand in a closed container for an appropriate time. Separate the residue from the ethanol and, if necessary, press out. In the latter case, combine the 2 liquids obtained.

Production by percolation   If necessary, comminute the herbal drug. Mix thoroughly with a portion of ethanol of the appropriate concentration and allow to stand for an appropriate time. Transfer to a percolator and allow the percolate to flow slowly, at room temperature, making sure that the herbal drug to be extracted is always covered with the remaining ethanol. The residue may be pressed out and the expressed liquid combined with the percolate.

If adjustment to a given concentration is necessary, calculate the amount (A_1), in kilograms, of ethanol of the appropriate concentration required to obtain the concentration specified or used for production, using the following expression:

$$\frac{m \times (N_x - N_0)}{N_0}$$

m = mass of percolate or macerate, in kilograms;
N_0 = percentage dry residue or percentage assay content as required in the individual monograph;
N_x = percentage dry residue or percentage assay content of the percolate or macerate.

Mix the macerate or percolate with the calculated amount of ethanol of the appropriate concentration. Allow to stand at a temperature not exceeding 20 °C for not less than 5 days, then filter if necessary.

Potentisation
The mother tincture corresponds to the 1st decimal dilution (Ø = D1).
The 2nd decimal dilution (D2) is made from:
— 1 part of the mother tincture (D1);
— 9 parts of ethanol of the same concentration.
The 3rd decimal dilution (D3) is made from:
— 1 part of the 2nd decimal dilution;
— 9 parts of ethanol of the same concentration.

Unless a different ethanol concentration is specified, use ethanol (50 per cent V/V) [ethanol (43 per cent m/m)] for subsequent decimal dilutions from D4 onwards and proceed as stated for D3.

The 1st 'centesimal' dilution (C1) is made from:
— 10 parts of the mother tincture (D1);
— 90 parts of ethanol of the same concentration.
The 2nd centesimal dilution (C2) is made from:
— 1 part of the 1st 'centesimal' dilution;
— 99 parts of ethanol (50 per cent V/V) [ethanol (43 per cent m/m)], unless a different ethanol concentration is specified.

Subsequent centesimal dilutions are produced as stated for C2.

METHOD 1.1.9 (EQUIVALENT TO HAB 4b: MOTHER TINCTURES AND LIQUID DILUTIONS)
Method 1.1.9 is generally used for animal matter.

Mother tinctures prepared according to Method 1.1.9 are prepared by maceration or percolation as described below, using 1 part of animal matter and 10 parts of ethanol of the appropriate concentration (anhydrous, 96 per cent V/V - 94 per cent m/m, 90 per cent V/V - 86 per cent m/m, 80 per cent V/V - 73 per cent m/m, 70 per cent V/V - 62 per cent m/m, 50 per cent V/V - 43 per cent m/m, 36 per cent V/V - 30 per cent m/m, 18 per cent V/V - 15 per cent m/m), unless otherwise prescribed in the individual monograph.

Production by maceration. Unless otherwise prescribed, comminute the animal matter, mix thoroughly with ethanol of the appropriate concentration and allow to stand in a closed container for an appropriate time. Separate the residue from the ethanol and, if necessary, press out. In the latter case, combine the 2 liquids obtained.

Production by percolation. If necessary, comminute the animal matter. Mix thoroughly with a portion of ethanol of the appropriate concentration and allow to stand for an appropriate time. Transfer to a percolator and allow the percolate to flow slowly at room temperature, making sure that the animal matter to be extracted is always covered with the remaining ethanol. The residue may be pressed out and the expressed liquid combined with the percolate.

If adjustment to a given concentration is necessary, calculate the amount (A_1), in kilograms, of ethanol of the appropriate concentration required to obtain the concentration specified or used for production, using the following expression:

$$\frac{m \times (N_x - N_0)}{N_0}$$

m = mass of percolate or macerate, in kilograms;
N_0 = percentage dry residue or percentage assay content as required in the individual monograph;
N_x = percentage dry residue or percentage assay content of the percolate or macerate.

Mix the macerate or percolate with the calculated amount of ethanol of the appropriate concentration. Allow to stand at a temperature not exceeding 20 °C for not less than 5 days, then filter if necessary.

Potentisation

The mother tincture corresponds to the 1st decimal dilution (Ø = D1).

The 2nd decimal dilution (D2) is made from:
— 1 part of the mother tincture (D1);
— 9 parts of ethanol of the same concentration.

The 3rd decimal dilution (D3) is made from:
— 1 part of the 2nd decimal dilution;
— 9 parts of ethanol of the same concentration.

Unless a different ethanol concentration is specified, use ethanol (50 per cent *V/V*) [ethanol (43 per cent *m/m*)] for subsequent decimal dilutions from D4 onwards and proceed as stated for D3.

The 1st 'centesimal' dilution (C1) is made from:
— 10 parts of the mother tincture (D1);
— 90 parts of ethanol of the same concentration.

The 2nd centesimal dilution (C2) is made from:
— 1 part of the 1st 'centesimal' dilution;
— 99 parts of ethanol (50 per cent *V/V*) [ethanol (43 per cent *m/m*)], unless a different ethanol concentration is specified.

Subsequent centesimal dilutions are produced as stated for C2.

METHOD 1.1.10 (FRENCH PHARMACOPOEIA)

Method 1.1.10 is generally used for herbal drugs. The state of the herbal drug, fresh or dried, is specified in the individual monograph.

Mother tinctures prepared according to Method 1.1.10 are prepared by maceration.

Comminute appropriately the herbal drug. Take a sample and determine the loss on drying at 105 °C for 2 h (*2.2.32*) or the water content (*2.2.13*). Taking this value into account, calculate and add to the herbal drug the quantities of ethanol of the appropriate concentration required to produce, unless otherwise prescribed, a 1 in 10 mother tincture (1:10 mother tincture) with a suitable ethanol content. Allow to macerate for at least 10 days, with sufficient shaking.

Separate the residue from the ethanol and strain under pressure if necessary. Allow the combined liquids to stand for 48 h and filter. For mother tinctures with a required assay content, adjustment may be carried out, if necessary, by adding ethanol of the same concentration as used for the preparation of the tincture.

Potentisation

The 1st decimal dilution (D1) is made from:
— 1 part of the mother tincture;
— 9 parts of ethanol of the appropriate concentration.

The 2nd decimal dilution (D2) is made from:
— 1 part of the 1st decimal dilution;
— 9 parts of ethanol of the appropriate concentration.

Subsequent decimal dilutions are produced as stated for D2, using ethanol of the appropriate concentration.

The 1st centesimal dilution (C1) is made from:
— 1 part of the mother tincture;
— 99 parts of ethanol of the appropriate concentration.

The 2nd centesimal dilution (C2) is made from:
— 1 part of the 1st centesimal dilution;
— 99 parts of ethanol of the appropriate concentration.

Subsequent centesimal dilutions are produced as stated for C2, using ethanol of the appropriate concentration.

METHOD 1.1.11 (FRENCH PHARMACOPOEIA)

Method 1.1.11 is generally used for animal matter.

Mother tinctures prepared according to Method 1.1.11 are prepared by maceration.

The mass ratio of raw material to mother tincture is usually 1 to 20. To the raw material, appropriately comminuted, add the quantity of ethanol of the appropriate concentration required to produce a 1 in 20 mother tincture. Allow to macerate for at least 10 days, with sufficient shaking. Decant and filter. Allow to stand for 48 h and filter again.

For mother tinctures with a required assay content, adjustment may be carried out, if necessary, by adding ethanol of the same concentration as used for the preparation of the tincture.

Potentisation

The 1st decimal dilution (D1) is made from:
— 1 part of the mother tincture;
— 9 parts of ethanol of the appropriate concentration.

The 2nd decimal dilution (D2) is made from:
— 1 part of the 1st decimal dilution;
— 9 parts of ethanol of the appropriate concentration.

Subsequent decimal dilutions are produced as stated for D2, using ethanol of the appropriate concentration.

The 1st centesimal dilution (C1) is made from:
— 1 part of the mother tincture;
— 99 parts of ethanol of the appropriate concentration.

The 2nd centesimal dilution (C2) is made from:
— 1 part of the 1st centesimal dilution;
— 99 parts of ethanol of the appropriate concentration.

Subsequent centesimal dilutions are produced as stated for C2, using ethanol of the appropriate concentration.

2. GLYCEROL MACERATES

METHOD 2.1

Method 2.1 is used for maceration of raw materials of animal or herbal origin in glycerol (85 per cent) or glycerol/ethanol mixtures of appropriate concentration. Pathological material is excluded.

The raw materials are finely minced before use, where appropriate.

METHODS 2.1.1, 2.1.2 (EQUIVALENT TO HAB 42a AND 42b: MOTHER TINCTURES AND LIQUID DILUTIONS THEREOF)

Raw materials of animal origin - freshly killed animals or parts thereof - are used. Animals are processed immediately after being killed.

Maceration

Disperse 1 part of finely minced animal material in:
— 9 parts (decimal dilutions) or 99 parts (centesimal dilutions) of glycerol (85 per cent) for Method 2.1.1,
— or 2.1 parts of glycerol (85 per cent) for Method 2.1.2.

Allow to macerate for at least 2 h, then succuss. Filter when necessary.

Where justified, 1 part of glycerol (85 per cent) may be added to 1 part of animal material before mincing. Where very small amounts of animal material are used, the dilution may be prepared by dispersing 1 part of finely minced animal material in 99 parts of glycerol (85 per cent) (C1 or 'D2' if to be used for further decimal dilutions).

Potentisation

Method 2.1.1

The 2nd decimal dilution (D2) is made from:
— 1 part of the glycerol macerate D1;
— 9 parts of glycerol (85 per cent) or ethanol (18 per cent V/V) [ethanol (15 per cent m/m)].

Subsequent decimal dilutions are produced as stated for D2 but with ethanol (18 per cent V/V) [ethanol (15 per cent m/m)] as the vehicle.

The 2nd centesimal dilution (C2) is made from:
— 1 part of the glycerol macerate C1;
— 99 parts of ethanol (18 per cent V/V) [ethanol 15 per cent m/m)].

Subsequent centesimal dilutions are produced as stated for C2.

Method 2.1.2

The 1st 'decimal' dilution (D1) is made from:
— 3 parts of the glycerol macerate;
— 7 parts of water for injections.

The 2nd decimal dilution (D2) is made from:
— 1 part of D1;
— 9 parts of water for injections.

Subsequent decimal dilutions are produced as stated for D2.

METHOD 2.1.3 (FRENCH PHARMACOPOEIA)

Raw materials of herbal or animal origin are used.

Maceration

Comminute the raw material appropriately. Take a sample and determine the loss on drying at 105 °C for 2 h (*2.2.32*) or the water content (*2.2.13*). Taking this value into account, calculate and add to the raw material the quantity of the ethanol/glycerol mixture of the appropriate concentration to produce, unless otherwise prescribed, a 1 in 20 glycerol macerate. Allow to macerate for at least 3 weeks, with sufficient shaking. Decant and strain under pressure if necessary. Allow the combined liquids to stand for 48 h and filter.

Potentisation

The 1st decimal dilution (D1) is made from:
— 1 part of the glycerol macerate;
— 9 parts of a water/ethanol/glycerol mixture of appropriate concentration.

The 2nd decimal dilution (D2) is made from:
— 1 part of the 1st decimal dilution;
— 9 parts of a water/ethanol/glycerol mixture of appropriate concentration.

Subsequent decimal dilutions are produced as stated for D2 or using another appropriate vehicle.

The 1st centesimal dilution (C1) is made from:
— 1 part of the glycerol macerate;
— 99 parts of a water/ethanol/glycerol mixture of appropriate concentration.

The 2nd centesimal dilution (C2) is made from:
— 1 part of the 1st centesimal dilution;
— 99 parts of a water/ethanol/glycerol mixture of appropriate concentration.

Subsequent centesimal dilutions are produced as stated for C2 or using another appropriate vehicle.

METHOD 2.2

METHODS 2.2.1, 2.2.2, 2.2.3, 2.2.4 (EQUIVALENT TO HAB 41a, 41b, 41c AND 41d: GL MOTHER TINCTURES AND LIQUID DILUTIONS THEREOF)

Method 2.2 is used for maceration of raw materials of animal origin in a glycerol solution containing sodium chloride. Pathological material is excluded.

Raw materials from freshly killed animals, parts or secretions thereof are used in Methods 2.2.1, 2.2.2 and 2.2.3. Lower animals are killed with carbon dioxide in a covered vessel. All animals are processed immediately after being killed.

Blood components from live horses are used in method 2.2.4.

Sample collection and/or pre-treatment

The raw materials used in Methods 2.2.1, 2.2.2 and 2.2.3 are finely minced before use, where appropriate.

The blood used in Method 2.2.4 is collected by a veterinarian. Blood obtained from animals killed by bleeding must not be used. Take 200 mL of this blood and add 15 IU of heparin sodium and 0.625 mL of a 9 g/kg solution of sodium chloride per millilitre. Separate the blood components by fractional centrifugation and resuspend each individual cell sediment in 1.1 mL of a 9 g/kg solution of sodium chloride. These cell suspensions are processed into the glycerol macerate.

Maceration

Mix 1 part of finely minced animal material, secretions or blood cell suspensions, according to the method used, with 5 parts of a sodium chloride solution of the appropriate concentration (see table 2371.-1) and 95 parts of glycerol. Allow to stand protected from light for at least 7 days, then decant. If necessary for Methods 2.2.1, 2.2.2 and 2.2.3, centrifuge before decanting, then filter the supernatant if necessary. The decanted liquid or the filtrate respectively is the glycerol macerate.

Any sediment present must be resuspended before processing the glycerol macerate.

Table 2371.-1

Methods 2.2.1 and 2.2.4	Method 2.2.2	Method 2.2.3
15 g/kg solution of sodium chloride in purified water	40 g/kg solution of sodium chloride in purified water	80 g/kg solution of sodium chloride in purified water

Vehicle

0.2 parts of sodium hydrogen carbonate and 8.8 parts of sodium chloride in 991 parts of water for injections or purified water as appropriate.

Potentisation

The glycerol macerate corresponds to the 2nd decimal dilution ('D2') or the 1st centesimal dilution (C1).

The 3rd decimal dilution (D3) is made from:
— 1 part of the 2nd decimal dilution;
— 9 parts of the appropriate vehicle.

Subsequent decimal dilutions are produced as stated for D3.

Where appropriate, the 4th decimal dilution (D4) is made from 1 part of the 3rd decimal dilution, 5.6 parts of the vehicle and 3.4 parts of water for injections.

The 2nd centesimal dilution (C2) is made from:
— 1 part of the 1st centesimal dilution;
— 99 parts of the appropriate vehicle.

Subsequent centesimal dilutions are produced as stated for C2.

3. LIQUID DILUTIONS

METHOD 3.1

Methods 3.1.1, 3.1.2 and 3.1.3 are used for dissolution of any suitable inorganic or organic starting material, for example minerals or venoms.

Unless otherwise specified, dissolve 1 part of the starting material in 9 parts (D1) or 99 parts (C1) of the liquid vehicle and succuss.

Where justified and authorised, in case of insufficient solubility of the starting material in the specified vehicle, directly produce the first possible dilution. For example, if the starting material is slightly soluble, dissolve 1 part of the starting material in 99 parts of the vehicle (C1 or 'D2' if to be used for further decimal dilutions).

METHODS 3.1.1, 3.1.2 (EQUIVALENT TO HAB 5a, 5b: SOLUTIONS, AQUEOUS SOLUTIONS)

Vehicles

The vehicles in Table 2371.-2 may be used.

Table 2371.-2

Method 3.1.1	Method 3.1.2
Anhydrous ethanol	Water for injections
Ethanol (96 per cent V/V) [ethanol (94 per cent m/m)]	Purified water
Ethanol (90 per cent V/V) [ethanol (86 per cent m/m)]	
Ethanol (80 per cent V/V) [ethanol (73 per cent m/m)]	
Ethanol (70 per cent V/V) [ethanol (62 per cent m/m)]	
Ethanol (50 per cent V/V) [ethanol (43 per cent m/m)]	
Ethanol (36 per cent V/V) [ethanol (30 per cent m/m)]	
Ethanol (18 per cent V/V) [ethanol (15 per cent m/m)]	
Purified water	
Glycerol (85 per cent)	

For Method 3.1.1, if ethanol (18 per cent V/V) [ethanol (15 per cent m/m)] is used, the starting material may be dissolved in 7.58 parts of purified water and the ethanol concentration adjusted by adding 1.42 parts of ethanol (96 per cent V/V) [ethanol (94 per cent m/m)] to the solution, for decimal dilutions. For centesimal dilutions, use 83.4 parts of purified water for 15.6 parts of ethanol (96 per cent V/V) [ethanol (94 per cent m/m)].

For Method 3.1.2, if the starting material is not stable and/or soluble in water, glycerol (85 per cent) may be added at a concentration of not more than 35 per cent of the vehicle, for potentisation up to D4.

Potentisation

Unless otherwise specified, the 2nd decimal dilution (D2) is made from:
— 1 part of the 1st decimal dilution (D1);
— 9 parts of ethanol (50 per cent V/V) [ethanol (43 per cent m/m)] for Method 3.1.1 or 9 parts of water for injections (or purified water, as appropriate) for Method 3.1.2.

Subsequent decimal dilutions are produced as stated for D2.

Unless otherwise specified, the 2nd centesimal dilution (C2) is made from:
— 1 part of the 1st centesimal dilution (C1);
— 99 parts of ethanol (50 per cent V/V) [ethanol (43 per cent m/m)] for Method 3.1.1 or 99 parts of water for injections (or purified water, as appropriate) for Method 3.1.2.

Subsequent centesimal dilutions are produced as stated for C2.

Additives

For Method 3.1.1, if a reaction such as precipitation is observed in the final dilution, the following additives may be used to enhance stability and/or solubility, unless otherwise specified:
— glacial acetic acid;
— concentrated hydrochloric acid;
— lactic acid;
— sodium hydroxide.

Where solutions or dilutions have been pH-adjusted, they must not be potentised further.

METHOD 3.1.3

Vehicles

Suitable vehicles, for example, ethanol of an appropriate concentration, glycerol or purified water may be used alone or combined.

Potentisation

Unless otherwise specified, the 2nd decimal dilution (D2) is made from:
— 1 part of the 1st decimal dilution (D1);
— 9 parts of the appropriate vehicle.

Subsequent decimal dilutions are produced as stated for D2.

Unless otherwise specified, the 2nd centesimal dilution (C2) is made from:
— 1 part of the 1st centesimal dilution (C1);
— 99 parts of the appropriate vehicle.

Subsequent centesimal dilutions are produced as stated for C2.

METHOD 3.2

Method 3.2 is generally used to produce liquid dilutions of triturations of substances that for the most part are sparingly soluble to practically insoluble.

METHODS 3.2.1, 3.2.2 (EQUIVALENT TO HAB 8a, 8b: LIQUID PREPARATIONS MADE FROM TRITURATIONS, AQUEOUS PREPARATIONS MADE FROM TRITURATIONS)

Preparations made according to Method 3.2.1 and Method 3.2.2 are produced from triturations D4, D5 and D6 or from triturations C4, C5 and C6, prepared according to method 4.1.1 by at least 2 potentisation steps.

Vehicles

The vehicles in Table 2371.-3 may be used.

Table 2371.-3

Method 3.2.1	Method 3.2.2
1st potentisation: Purified water	All potentisations: Water for injections Purified water
2nd potentisation: Ethanol (36 per cent V/V) [ethanol (30 per cent m/m)]	
Further potentisations: Ethanol (50 per cent V/V) [ethanol (43 per cent m/m)]	

Potentisation

For the first liquid potentisation, dissolve 1 part of the trituration in 9 parts (decimal dilutions) or 99 parts (centesimal dilutions) of the specified vehicle (see Table 2371.-3) and succuss. For further potentisations, proceed in the same manner with 1 part of the previous dilution.

The D6, D7, C6 and C7 dilutions produced by the above method are not to be used for the preparation of further dilutions.

METHOD 3.2.3

Preparations made according to Method 3.2.3 are produced from triturations D2 onwards and from triturations C1, C2, C3 and C4, prepared according to method 4.1.2.

Vehicles

Suitable vehicles such as ethanol of an appropriate concentration or purified water may be used.

Potentisation

Unless otherwise specified, the first liquid decimal dilution (Dn-1) is made from:
— 1 part of the decimal trituration Dn-2;
— 9 parts of purified water or of another suitable vehicle in appropriate proportions.

The following decimal dilution (Dn) is made from:
— 1 part of the first liquid decimal dilution Dn-1;
— 9 parts of a suitable vehicle.

Subsequent decimal dilutions are produced as stated for Dn.

Unless otherwise specified, the first liquid centesimal dilution (Cn-1) is made from:
— 1 part of the centesimal trituration Cn-2;
— 99 parts of purified water or of another suitable vehicle in appropriate proportions.

The following centesimal dilution (Cn) is made from:
— 1 part of the first liquid centesimal dilution Cn-1;
— 99 parts of a suitable vehicle.

Subsequent centesimal dilutions are produced as stated for Cn.

4. TRITURATIONS

METHOD 4.1

Method 4.1 is used for triturations, that is solid dilutions, of raw materials or of triturations prepared according to Methods 4.2.1 or 4.2.2. The duration and intensity of the trituration are such that homogeneity and potentisation are achieved.

Vehicle

Unless otherwise specified, lactose monohydrate is used.

METHOD 4.1.1 (EQUIVALENT TO HAB 6: TRITURATIONS)

Triturations are prepared manually or mechanically. Mechanical trituration must be used for quantities exceeding 1 kg. The resulting particle size of the raw material in the first decimal or centesimal dilution does not exceed 100 μm, unless otherwise prescribed in the individual monograph.

Ratios of raw material to vehicle

Decimal triturations	Centesimal triturations
The 1st decimal trituration (D1) is made from:	The 1st centesimal trituration (C1) is made from:
1 part of the raw material	1 part of the raw material
9 parts of the vehicle	99 parts of the vehicle
Subsequent decimal triturations (Dn) are produced as stated for D1, using 1 part of the previous trituration (Dn-1).	Subsequent centesimal triturations (Cn) are produced as stated for C1, using 1 part of the previous trituration (Cn-1).

Where fresh plant material is used, the quantity of vehicle added is such so as to obtain 10 parts of the trituration (decimal trituration) or 100 parts of the trituration (centesimal trituration) from 1 part of the raw material (replace the mass of water lost from the fresh plant by an equivalent amount of the vehicle). A suitable gentle drying process may need to be applied to the solid dilution.

Where justified and authorised, it may be necessary to directly produce a C1 or 'D2' if to be used for further decimal triturations as the first solid trituration, made from 1 part of raw material and 99 parts of vehicle.

Trituration

Unless otherwise justified and authorised, the method consists of dividing the vehicle into 3 equal parts and adding the raw material to the first part, then adding the second and third part of the vehicle, thoroughly triturating after each addition.

For mechanical trituration, use a machine allowing the requirements for particle size of the first decimal or centesimal solid trituration to be met. A machine fitted with a scraping device may be used to ensure even trituration. The time required to prepare one trituration is at least 1 h, unless otherwise justified and authorised.

For manual trituration, divide the vehicle into 3 equal parts and briefly triturate the first part in a porcelain mortar. Add the raw material, triturate the mixture for 6 min, scrape down for 4 min with an appropriate non-metallic device (for example, a porcelain spatula). Triturate for a further 6 min, scrape down again for a further 4 min, then add the second part of the vehicle and continue as above. Proceed in the same manner with the rest of the vehicle. The minimum time required for the whole process is thus 1 h. Carry out the whole process again for each subsequent solid dilution.

Triturations from D5 or C5 onwards may also be prepared by intense mechanical treatment by a suitable mixing machine as follows: add the solid trituration to one third of the vehicle and mix. Add the second third of the vehicle, mix and proceed in the same manner with the last third of the vehicle. The whole process lasts minimum 1 hour, unless otherwise justified and authorised.

In all cases, it is possible to change to a liquid medium from the 4th, 5th and 6th decimal or centesimal triturations, as described in Methods 3.2.1 and 3.2.2.

METHOD 4.1.2 (FRENCH PHARMACOPOEIA)

Trituration

Triturations are prepared as follows:

Decimal triturations

Reduce 1 part of the homoeopathic stock to a powder. Triturate carefully with a small quantity of the vehicle. Add the vehicle in small quantities until 9 parts of this vehicle have been used. The resulting trituration is the 1st decimal trituration (D1).

Triturate as described above 1 part of this trituration with 9 parts of the vehicle. The resulting trituration is the 2nd decimal trituration (D2).

In all cases, it is possible to change to a liquid medium after the 7th decimal trituration (D7) as described in Method 3.2.3.

Centesimal triturations

Proceed in the same manner but following a centesimal series.

In all cases, it is possible to change to a liquid medium after the 3rd centesimal trituration (C3) as described in Method 3.2.3.

METHOD 4.2

Method 4.2 is used for triturations, that is solid dilutions, of liquid preparations such as mother tinctures and solutions, their dilutions, mixtures and co-potentised mixtures.

Gradually impregnate the total amount of vehicle, gently dry the moist mixture, mill and sieve if necessary, then mix and triturate until homogeneity and potentisation are achieved. Trituration is further carried out as described for Method 4.1.1 or Method 4.1.2.

Vehicle

Unless otherwise specified, lactose monohydrate is used.

METHOD 4.2.1 (EQUIVALENT TO HAB 7: TRITURATIONS)

Ratios of starting material to vehicle

The quantity of vehicle added must always be such so as to obtain 10 parts of the trituration (decimal trituration) or 100 parts of the trituration (centesimal trituration) from the required number of parts of the liquid preparation (see Table 2371.-4), taking the mass of the dry residue into consideration. Where the dry residue is considered negligible, the quantity of vehicle added is 10 parts (decimal trituration) or 100 parts (centesimal trituration), for 1 part of the liquid preparation.

Table 2371.-4

Decimal triturations	Centesimal triturations
Mother tinctures prepared according to Methods 1.1.1, 1.1.3 and 1.1.4	
The 1st 'decimal' trituration (D1) is made from:	The 1st 'centesimal' trituration (C1) is made from:
2 parts of the mother tincture	2 parts of the mother tincture
maximum 10 parts of the vehicle, taking the mass of the dry residue into consideration	maximum 100 parts of the vehicle, taking the mass of the dry residue into consideration
Mother tinctures prepared according to Methods 1.1.2, 1.1.5, 1.1.6 and 1.1.7	
The 1st 'decimal' trituration (D1) is made from:	The 1st 'centesimal' trituration (C1) is made from:
3 parts of the mother tincture	3 parts of the mother tincture
maximum 10 parts of the vehicle, taking the mass of the dry residue into consideration	maximum 100 parts of the vehicle, taking the mass of the dry residue into consideration
Mother tinctures prepared according to Methods 1.1.8 and 1.1.9	
The mother tincture corresponds to the 1st decimal dilution (D1)	
The 2nd decimal trituration (D2) is made from:	The 1st 'centesimal' trituration (C1) is made from:
1 part of the mother tincture	10 parts of the mother tincture
maximum 10 parts of the vehicle, taking the mass of the dry residue into consideration	maximum 100 parts of the vehicle, taking the mass of the dry residue into consideration
Solutions prepared according to Method 3.1.1 or liquid dilutions, mixtures and co-potentised mixtures	
Decimal trituration n+1 (Dn+1) is made from:	Centesimal trituration n+1 (Cn+1) is made from:
1 part of the dilution (Dn)	1 part of the dilution (Cn)
maximum 10 parts of the vehicle, taking the mass of the dry residue into consideration	maximum 100 parts of the vehicle, taking the mass of the dry residue into consideration

METHOD 4.2.2

Ratios of starting material to vehicle

Mother tinctures prepared according to Methods 1.1.10 and 1.1.11	
The 1st decimal trituration (D1) is made from:	The 1st centesimal trituration (C1) is made from:
1 part of the mother tincture	1 part of the mother tincture
10 parts of the vehicle	100 parts of the vehicle

5. OTHER PREPARATIONS

METHOD 5.1

Method 5.1 is used for preparing homoeopathic preparations by co-potentising 2 or more stocks and/or dilutions thereof, where co-potentisation consists of mixing several stocks or dilutions of stocks then potentising them together in one or more potentisation steps.

METHODS 5.1.1, 5.1.2, 5.1.3 (EQUIVALENT TO HAB 40a, 40b, 40c: CO-POTENTISED MIXTURES)

The stocks and/or dilutions in Table 2371.-5 may be used.

Table 2371.-5

Method 5.1.1	Method 5.1.2	Method 5.1.3
Stocks	Aqueous preparations	Triturations
Solutions	Glycerol macerates and aqueous dilutions thereof	
Triturations	Triturations	
Liquid dilutions		
Mother tinctures whose method of production specifies a 1/10 (or 1/100) dilution		

Vehicles

The choice of the vehicle is determined by and must comply with any special requirement for the particular stock as well as the dosage form (see table Table 2371.-6).

Table 2371.-6

Method 5.1.1	Method 5.1.2	Method 5.1.3
Ethanol (96 per cent V/V [ethanol (94 per cent m/m)]	Water for injections	Lactose monohydrate
Ethanol (90 per cent V/V [ethanol (86 per cent m/m)]	Purified water	
Ethanol (80 per cent V/V [ethanol (73 per cent m/m)]	Sugar syrup (sucrose, purified water (64:36))	
Ethanol (70 per cent V/V [ethanol (62 per cent m/m)]		
Ethanol (50 per cent V/V [ethanol (43 per cent m/m)]		
Ethanol (36 per cent V/V [ethanol (30 per cent m/m)]		
Ethanol (18 per cent V/V [ethanol (15 per cent m/m)]		

For Method 5.1.1, when starting from a trituration and where justified, purified water is used for the 1st potentisation step.

For Method 5.1.2, when starting from a glycerol macerate containing sodium chloride, unless otherwise justified and authorised, the following vehicle is used: 0.2 parts of sodium hydrogen carbonate and 8.8 parts of sodium chloride in 991 parts of water for injections.

Potentisation

For each potentisation step, combine and succuss or triturate 1 part of the given mixture with 9 parts (decimal dilutions) or 99 parts (centesimal dilutions) of the appropriate vehicle.

METHOD 5.1.4

Vehicles

Ethanol of an appropriate concentration, purified water or lactose monohydrate may, for example, be used.

Potentisation

Potentisation may be performed as prescribed for Methods 5.1.1, 5.1.2 and 5.1.3, either on the last step or on several successive steps.

METHOD 5.1.5

Vehicle

Ethanol of an appropriate concentration, purified water or lactose monohydrate may, for example, be used.

Potentisation

For a co-potentisation of centesimal dilutions, each dilution (Cn-1) represents 1 per cent of the final product and the proportion of vehicle to be added is reduced by the proportion of the active substances [i.e. 100 per cent − (1 per cent × the number of active substances)]. The same procedure applies, in the appropriate proportions, when co-potentising decimal dilutions.

_____ *Ph Eur*

Mother Tinctures for Homoeopathic Preparations

(*Ph Eur monograph 2029*)

Ph Eur _____

DEFINITION

Mother tinctures for homoeopathic preparations are liquid preparations obtained by the solvent action of a suitable vehicle upon raw materials. The raw materials are usually in the fresh form but may be dried. Mother tinctures for homoeopathic preparations may also be obtained from plant juices, with or without the addition of a vehicle. For some preparations, the matter to be extracted may undergo a preliminary treatment.

PRODUCTION

Mother tinctures for homoeopathic preparations are prepared by maceration, digestion, infusion, decoction, fermentation or as described in the individual monographs, usually using alcohol of suitable concentration.

Mother tinctures for homoeopathic preparations are obtained using a fixed proportion of raw material to solvent, taking the moisture content of the raw material into account, unless otherwise justified and authorised.

If fresh plants are used, suitable procedures are used to ensure freshness. The competent authorities may require that the freshness is demonstrated by means of a suitable test.

Mother tinctures for homoeopathic preparations are usually clear. A slight sediment may form on standing and that is acceptable as long as the composition of the tincture is not changed significantly.

The manufacturing process is defined so that it is reproducible.

Production by maceration

Unless otherwise prescribed, reduce the matter to be extracted to pieces of suitable size, mix thoroughly and extract according to the prescribed extraction method with the prescribed extraction solvent. Allow to stand in a closed vessel for the prescribed time. The residue is separated from the extraction solvent and, if necessary, pressed out. In the latter case, the 2 liquids obtained are combined.

Adjustment of the contents

Adjustment of the content of constituents may be carried out if necessary, either by adding the extraction solvent of suitable concentration, or by adding another mother tincture for homoeopathic preparations of the vegetable or animal matter used for the preparation.

IDENTIFICATION

Where applicable, at least 1 chromatographic identification test is carried out.

TESTS

The limits in an individual monograph are set to include official methods of production. Specific limits will apply to each defined method of production.

If the test for relative density is carried out, the test for ethanol need not be carried out, and vice versa.

Relative density (*2.2.5*)

The mother tincture for homoeopathic preparations complies with the limits prescribed in the monograph.

Ethanol (*2.9.10*)

The ethanol content complies with that prescribed in the monograph.

Methanol and 2-propanol (*2.9.11*)

Maximum 0.05 per cent *V/V* of methanol and maximum 0.05 per cent *V/V* of 2-propanol, unless otherwise prescribed.

Dry residue (*2.8.16*)

Where applicable, the mother tincture for homoeopathic preparations complies with the limits prescribed in the monograph.

Pesticides (*2.8.13*)

Where applicable, the mother tincture for homoeopathic preparations complies with the test. This requirement is met if the herbal drug has been shown to comply with the test.

Justification is provided in cases where the test for pesticides is performed on the mother tincture, instead of on the herbal drug according to the requirements of the general monograph *Herbal drugs for homoeopathic preparations (2045)*. Limits will be set, taking into consideration the nature and the origin of the herbal drug. The dilution factor of the mother tincture and the limit of detection of the method are also taken into account when fixing these limits.

Heavy metals (*2.4.27*)

Justification is provided in cases where the test for heavy metals is performed on the mother tincture, instead of on the herbal drug according to the requirements of the general monograph *Herbal drugs for homoeopathic preparations (2045)*. Limits will be set, taking into consideration the nature and the origin of the herbal drug. The dilution factor of the mother tincture and the limit of detection of the method are also taken into account when fixing these limits.

If required by the competent authority, suitable limits for the content of other heavy metals such as arsenic or nickel may be defined.

ASSAY

Where applicable, an assay with quantitative limits is performed.

STORAGE

Protected from light. A maximum storage temperature may be specified.

LABELLING

The label states:
— that the product is a mother tincture for homoeopathic preparations (designated as 'TM' or 'Ø');
— the name of the raw material using the Latin title of the European Pharmacopoeia monograph where one exists;
— the method of preparation;
— the ethanol content or other solvent content, in per cent *V/V*, in the mother tincture;
— the ratio of raw material to mother tincture;
— where applicable, the storage conditions.

———————————————————— *Ph Eur*

Impregnated Homoeopathic Pillules

(*Ph Eur monograph 2079*)

Ph Eur ———————

DEFINITION

Preparations of solid consistency obtained from sucrose, lactose or other suitable excipients. They possess a suitable mechanical strength to resist handling without crumbling or breaking. Impregnated homoeopathic pillules are prepared by impregnation of *Pillules for homoeopathic preparations (2153)* with one or more liquid homoeopathic preparations. They are intended for sublingual or oral use.

PRODUCTION

Impregnation takes place using liquid preparations containing ethanol usually at a concentration of at least 68 per cent *V/V* (60 per cent *m/m*) in proportions of 1 mass part of liquid to 100 mass parts of pillules.

In the manufacture, packaging, storage and distribution of homoeopathic pillules, suitable measures are taken to ensure their microbiological quality; recommendations on this aspect are provided in chapter *5.1.4. Microbiological quality of non-sterile pharmaceutical preparations and substances for pharmaceutical use.*

CHARACTERS

Appearance
White, almost white or slightly coloured spheroids.

Solubility
Usually freely soluble in water.

TESTS

Microbial contamination
Unless otherwise justified, authorised and labelled, the pillules are intended for sublingual administration and the following acceptance criteria apply.

TAMC: acceptance criterion 10^2 CFU/g (*2.6.12*).

TYMC: acceptance criterion 10^1 CFU/g (*2.6.12*).

Absence of *Staphylococcus aureus* (*2.6.13*).

Absence of *Pseudomonas aeruginosa* (*2.6.13*).

———————————————————— *Ph Eur*

Pillules for Homoeopathic Preparations

(*Ph Eur monograph 2153*)

Ph Eur ———————

DEFINITION

Preparations of solid consistency obtained from sucrose, lactose or other suitable excipients. They possess a suitable mechanical strength to resist handling without crumbling or breaking. They are intended for impregnation or coating with one or more homoeopathic preparations. The impregnated pillules comply with the requirements of the monograph *Homoeopathic pillules, impregnated (2079)*.

PRODUCTION

In the manufacture, packaging, storage and distribution of pillules for homoeopathic preparations, suitable measures are taken to ensure their microbiological quality; recommendations on this aspect are provided in chapter *5.1.4. Microbiological quality of non-sterile pharmaceutical preparations and substances for pharmaceutical use.*

If a system of sizing is used, the indications in Table 2153.-1 are used.

Table 2153.-1. – *Classification of pillules according to their mass and size*

Category	Number of pillules for homoeopathic preparations	Mass (g)	Fineness (µm)
1	470 - 530	1.0	1000 - 1600
2	160 - 333	1.0	1400 - 2000
3	110 - 130	1.0	1800 - 2500
4	70 - 90	1.0	2000 - 2800
5	40 - 50	1.0	2500 - 3350
6	16 - 30	1.0	3150 - 4500
7	10	0.9 - 1.1	4000 - 5600
8	5	0.9 - 1.1	5600 - 6700
9	3	0.9 - 1.1	7100 - 8000
10	2	0.9 - 1.1	8000 - 9500

NOTE: for categories 7-10, the mass is obtained by weighing the specified number of pillules.

CHARACTERS

Appearance
White or almost white spheroids.

Solubility
Usually freely soluble in water.

IDENTIFICATION

The excipients used for the manufacture of pillules for homoeopathic preparations are identified by one or more suitable test(s).

TESTS

If the test for fineness is carried out, the test for uniformity of mass need not be carried out, and vice versa.

Uniformity of mass
Carry out the test using 20 pillules to constitute 1 unit. Weigh individually 20 units taken at random and determine the individual and average masses. Not more than 2 of the individual masses deviate from the average mass by more than 10 per cent and none deviate by more than 20 per cent.

Fineness (*2.9.35*)

Not less than 90 per cent m/m of the pillules are between the lower and upper limits of the corresponding category as indicated in Table 2153.-1.

Impregnation

Use an approved method. The average for the results is within a validated range.

Microbial contamination

TAMC: acceptance criterion 10^2 CFU/g (*2.6.12*).

TYMC: acceptance criterion 10^1 CFU/g (*2.6.12*).

Absence of *Staphylococcus aureus* (*2.6.13*).

Absence of *Pseudomonas aeruginosa* (*2.6.13*).

LABELLING

The label states:

— the composition of the pillules;

— where applicable, the size of the pillules.

Ph Eur

Apomorphine Hydrochloride for Homoeopathic Preparations

Apomorphinum Muriaticum for Homoeopathic Preparations

DEFINITION

Apomorphine Hydrochloride for Homoeopathic Preparations contains Apomorphine Hydrochloride Hemihydrate.

PRODUCTION OF STOCK

The first trituration of Apomorphine Hydrochloride for Homoeopathic Preparations is prepared using a suitable quantity of Lactose or Anhydrous Lactose as the vehicle and a validated trituration method that ensures homogeneity is achieved. The vehicle complies with the statement under Vehicles in the monograph for Homoeopathic Preparations.

Content of apomorphine hydrochloride, $C_{17}H_{17}NO_2,HCl$

The first decimal trituration contains 9.5% to 10.5% of $C_{17}H_{17}NO_2,HCl$ (dried substance).

CHARACTERISTICS

The first decimal trituration is a white powder.

IDENTIFICATION

Dissolve 2.5 g of the substance being examined without heating in *water* and dilute to 25 mL with the same solvent (solution S).

A. To 5 mL of solution S add a few millilitres of *sodium hydrogen carbonate solution* until a permanent, white precipitate is formed. The precipitate slowly becomes a greenish colour. Add 0.25 mL of *0.05M iodine* and shake. The precipitate becomes a greyish-green colour. Collect the precipitate. The precipitate dissolves in *ether* giving a purple solution, dissolves in *dichloromethane chloride* giving a violet-blue solution and dissolves in *alcohol* giving a blue solution.

B. To 2 mL of solution S add 0.1 mL of *nitric acid*, mix and filter. The filtrate yields reaction A characteristic of *chlorides*, Appendix VI.

C. Dissolve 0.25 g of the substance being examined in 5 mL of *water*. Add 5 mL of *ammonia* and heat in a water-bath at 80° for 10 minutes. A red colour develops.

ASSAY

Disperse 2.5 g of the substance being examined in a mixture of 5.0 mL of 0.01M *hydrochloric acid* and 50 mL of *ethanol*

(96%). Carry out the method for *potentiometric titration*, Appendix VIII B, using 0.1M *sodium hydroxide*. Measure the titrant between the first 2 points of inflexion. Each mL of 0.1M *sodium hydroxide* is equivalent to 30.38 mg of $C_{17}H_{17}NO_2,HCl$.

Arsenious Trioxide for Homoeopathic Preparations

(*Ph Eur monograph 1599*)

As_2O_3	197.8	*1327-53-3*

Ph Eur

DEFINITION

Content

99.5 per cent to 100.5 per cent of As_2O_3.

CHARACTERS

Appearance

White or almost white powder.

Solubility

Practically insoluble to sparingly soluble in water. It dissolves in solutions of alkali hydroxides and carbonates.

IDENTIFICATION

A. Dissolve 20 mg in 1 mL of *dilute hydrochloric acid R*, add 4 mL of *water R* and 0.1 mL of *sodium sulfide solution R*. The resulting yellow precipitate is soluble in *dilute ammonia R1*.

B. Dissolve 20 mg in 1 mL of *hydrochloric acid R1*, add 5 mL of *hypophosphorous reagent R* and heat for 15 min on a water-bath. A black precipitate develops.

TESTS

Appearance of solution

A 100 g/L solution in *dilute ammonia R1* is clear (*2.2.1*) and colourless (*2.2.2, Method II*).

Sulfides

Dissolve 1.0 g in 10.0 mL of *dilute sodium hydroxide solution R*. Add 0.05 mL of *lead acetate solution R*. Any colour in the test solution is not more intense than that in a standard prepared at the same time and in the same manner using a mixture of 10.0 mL of a 0.015 g/L solution of *sodium sulfide R* in *dilute sodium hydroxide solution R* and 0.05 mL of *lead acetate solution R* (20 ppm).

ASSAY

Dissolve 40.0 mg in a mixture of 10 mL of *water R* and 10 mL of *dilute sodium hydroxide solution R*. Add 10 mL of *dilute hydrochloric acid R* and 3 g of *sodium hydrogen carbonate R* and mix. Add 1 mL of *starch solution R* and titrate with *0.05 M iodine*.

1 mL of *0.05 M iodine* is equivalent to 4.946 mg of As_2O_3.

Ph Eur

Artemisia Cina for Homoeopathic Preparations

DEFINITION

Artemisia Cina for Homoeopathic Preparations is the dried, unexpanded flower heads of *Seriphidium cinum* (Berg ex Poljakov) Poljakov (Syn *Artemisia cina* Berg ex Poljakov) *Artemisia cina* O.C.Berg et C.F. Schmidt.

It contains not less than 1.0% of santonin ($C_{15}H_{18}O_3$) calculated with reference to the dried material.

IDENTIFICATION

A. The dried, slightly shiny capitula are conical to elongated-ovoid, 2 to 4 mm long and 1 to 2 mm wide, yellow-green to brownish and composed of 3 to 6 hermaphrodite florets enclosed in an involucre of 14 to 20 imbricated ovate to lanceolate bracts. Each bract has a distinct keel which is most pronounced in the ovate outer bracts near the base; the keel forms the midrib and it branches freely, the veinlets becoming contorted and frequently anastomising. The outer surface of the bracts is covered with glistening glandular hairs. The florets are about 1 mm long and 0.5 mm wide; the corolla is contracted at the base and divides at the apex into 5 short, triangular teeth.

B. Reduce to a powder and examine under a microscope using *chloral hydrate solution*. Abundant fragments of the involucral bracts in surface view are seen. Fragments from the margins are usually only one or two cells thick and are composed of very thin-walled, elongated cells; fragments from the central region of the bracts show polygonal, isodiametric epidermal cells with thickened and beaded walls; fairly numerous anomocytic stomata are present on the outer surface only. Very small cluster crystals of calcium oxalate may be present in the parenchymatous cells underlying the epidermis.

Groups of sclereids from the central region of the bracts show: individual cells varying in shape but usually considerably elongated; the ends are square or bluntly tapering or, occasionally, somewhat enlarged; the walls are strongly thickened and have scattered pits. Small groups of these sclereids are occasionally found attached to fragments of the epidermis of the bracts.

The unicellular covering trichomes are nearly always found detached; they are usually very thin-walled although slight thickening may occur in the basal region; some of these trichomes are very long and can be found in groups forming loosely felted, cottony masses. The typically labiate glandular trichomes are abundant on the bracts and are also found detached; each has a short, biseriate stalk, and a biseriate head of two or four cells around which the cuticle is raised to form a bladder-like covering.

The abundant pollen grains are fairly small, spherical, with three pores and three furrows; the exine is finely warted. A large number of immature pollen grains are present, forming elongated, closely packed masses.

C. Carry out the method for *thin-layer chromatography*, Appendix III A, using the following solutions.

(1) Add 10 mL of *ethanol* (90%) to 1 g of the coarsely powdered drug, stir for one hour and filter.

(2) 0.1% w/v each of *santonin* and *cineole* in *methanol*.

CHROMATOGRAPHIC CONDITIONS

(a) Use as the coating *silica gel H*.

(b) Use the mobile phase as described below.

(c) Apply 10 µL of each solution.

(d) Develop the plate to 10 cm.

(e) After removal of the plate, allow to dry in air, spray with *ethanolic phosphomolybdic acid solution*, heat at 100° to 105° for about 5 minutes and examine in daylight.

mobile phase

5 volumes of *glacial acetic acid*, 45 volumes of *hexane* and 50 volumes *ethyl acetate*.

SYSTEM SUITABILITY

The test is not valid unless the chromatogram obtained with solution (2) shows the grey-blue santonin band just between the lower third and middle third and the grey-blue cineole band in the upper third.

CONFIRMATION

The chromatogram obtained with solution (1) shows a grey-blue band below the band obtained for santonin in solution (2), a strong grey-blue band level with that of santonin in solution (2) and one or two grey-blue bands just above santonin; one or two grey-blue bands between the bands obtained for santonin and cineole in solution (2) and a strong grey-blue band level with the band obtained with cineole.

Top of the plate	
A grey-blue band	Cineole: a grey-blue band
1 or 2 a grey-blue bands	
1 or 2 grey-blue bands a grey-blue band a grey-blue band	Santonin: a grey-blue band
Solution (1)	**Solution (2)**

TESTS

Foreign matter

Not more than 5% of sections of stem and pieces of narrow-linear hairy leaves; not more than 2% of other foreign matter, Appendix XI D.

Ash

Not more than 11.0%, Appendix XI J, Method II.

Loss on drying

Not more than 10.0%, Appendix IX D.

ASSAY

Carry out the method for *liquid chromatography*, Appendix III D, using the following solutions.

(1) To 1.0 g of the powdered herbal drug add 50 mL of *methanol* and stir for 2hours. Filter the solution using a dry filter paper into a 100 mL volumetric flask, wash the filtrate with *methanol*, add the washings to the filtrate and dilute to 100 mL with *methanol* and mix. Weigh approximately 5 g (6.5 mL) of the solution and add 20 mL of *methanol* in a 50 mL volumetric flask and dilute to volume with *water*.

(2) 0.005% w/v of *santonin BPCRS* prepared by dissolving 100 mg *santonin BPCRS* in 100 ml *methanol* and diluting 5 mL of the resulting solution to 100 mL with the mobile phase.

(3) 0.005% w/v each of *santonin BPCRS* and *methyl 4-hydroxybenzoate* in the mobile phase.

CHROMATOGRAPHIC CONDITIONS

(a) Use a stainless steel column (15 cm × 4.6 mm) packed with *octadecylsilyl silica gel for chromatography* (5 μm) (Kromasil C18 is suitable) fitted with a stainless steel guard column packed with the same material.

(b) Use isocratic elution and the mobile phase described below.

(c) Use a flow rate of 1.0 mL per minute.

(d) Use a column temperature of 25°.

(e) Use a detection wavelength of 236 nm.

(f) Inject 10 μL of each solution.

MOBILE PHASE

Equal volumes of *methanol* and *water*.

SYSTEM SUITABILITY

The test is not valid unless, in the chromatogram obtained with solution (3), the *resolution factor* between the peaks due to *methyl 4-hydroxybenzoate* and *santonin* is not less than 2.0.

DETERMINATION OF CONTENT

Calculate the content of $C_{15}H_{18}O_3$ in the herbal drug using the declared content of $C_{15}H_{18}O_3$ in *santonin BPCRS* using the following expression:

$$\frac{A_1}{A_2} \times \frac{m_2}{V_2} \times \frac{V_1}{m_1} \times p \times \frac{100}{100-d}$$

A_1 =   area of the peak due to santonin in the chromatogram obtained with solution (1);

A_2 =   area of the peak due to santonin in the chromatogram obtained with solution (2);

m_1 =   weight of the herbal drug being examined in mg;

m_2 =   weight of *santonin BPCRS* in mg;

V_1 =   dilution volume of solution (1) in mL;

V_2 =   dilution volume of solution (2) in mL;

p =   percentage content of santonin ($C_{15}H_{18}O_3$) in *santonin BPCRS*;

d =   percentage loss on drying of the herbal drug being examined.

MOTHER TINCTURE

The mother tincture complies with the requirements stated under Mother Tinctures for Homoeopathic Preparations and with the following requirements.

DEFINITION

It contains not less than 0.1% of santonin ($C_{15}H_{18}O_3$).

PRODUCTION

The mother tincture of *Artemisia cina* is prepared from the powdered drug using *Method 1.1.8* described in the monograph for Methods of Preparation of Homoeopathic Stocks and Potentisation. Use 86% w/w (90% v/v) of *ethanol*.

CHARACTERISTICS

The mother tincture is a golden yellow to greenish liquid.

IDENTIFICATION

The mother tincture complies with Identification test C above using the mother tincture as solution (1).

TESTS

Ethanol

40% to 46% w/w (47% to 54% v/v), Appendix VIII F.

Dry residue

Not less than 1.8% w/w, Appendix XI P.

Relative density

0.835 to 0.855, Appendix V G.

ASSAY

Carry out the method for *liquid chromatography*, Appendix III D, as described for the herbal drug using as solution (1) the mother tincture.

DETERMINATION OF CONTENT

Calculate the content of $C_{15}H_{18}O_3$ in the mother tincture using the declared content of $C_{15}H_{18}O_3$ in *santonin BPCRS* using the following expression:

$$\frac{A_1}{A_2} \times \frac{m_2}{V_2} \times \frac{V_1}{m_1} \times p$$

A_1 =   area of the peak due to santonin in the chromatogram obtained with solution (1);

A_2 =   area of the peak due to santonin in the chromatogram obtained with solution (2);

m_1 =   weight of the herbal drug being examined in mg;

m_2 =   weight of *santonin BPCRS* in mg;

V_1 =   dilution volume of solution (1) in mL;

V_2 =   dilution volume of solution (2) in mL;

p =   percentage content of santonin ($C_{15}H_{18}O_3$) in *santonin BPCRS*.

Barium Chloride Dihydrate for Homoeopathic Preparations

(Ph Eur monograph 2142)

$BaCl_2,2H_2O$	244.3	*10326-27-9*

Ph Eur ⎯⎯⎯⎯⎯⎯⎯⎯⎯⎯⎯⎯⎯⎯⎯⎯⎯⎯⎯⎯⎯⎯⎯⎯

DEFINITION

Content

99.0 per cent to 101.0 per cent of $BaCl_2,2H_2O$.

CHARACTERS

Appearance

White or almost white, crystalline powder or colourless crystals.

Solubility

Freely soluble in water, very slightly soluble or practically insoluble in ethanol (96 per cent).

IDENTIFICATION

A. Dissolve 0.1 g in 1 mL of *water R*. Add 0.3 mL of *dilute sulfuric acid R*. A white precipitate is formed; it is insoluble in *dilute hydrochloric acid R* and in *dilute nitric acid R*.

B. It gives reaction (a) of chlorides *(2.3.1)*.

TESTS

Solution S

Dissolve 10.0 g in *water R* and dilute to 100 mL with the same solvent.

Appearance of solution

Solution S is clear *(2.2.1)* and colourless *(2.2.2, Method II)*.

Acidity or alkalinity

To 10 mL of solution S add 0.1 mL of *phenolphthalein solution R*. Not more than 0.2 mL of *0.01 M hydrochloric acid* or *0.01 M sodium hydroxide* is required to change the colour of the indicator.

Heavy metals *(2.4.8)*
Maximum 10 ppm.

12 mL of solution S complies with limit test A. Prepare the reference solution using *lead standard solution (1 ppm Pb) R*.

ASSAY
Dissolve 0.200 g in 100 mL of *water R*. Add 100 mL of *methanol R*, 10 mL of *concentrated ammonia R* and 2 mg of *phthalein purple R*. Titrate with *0.1 M sodium edetate* until the colour changes from violet to colourless.

1 mL of *0.1 M sodium edetate* is equivalent to 24.43 mg of $BaCl_2,2H_2O$.

_____ *Ph Eur*

Cadmium Sulfate Hydrate for Homoeopathic Preparations

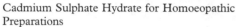

Cadmium Sulphate Hydrate for Homoeopathic Preparations

(Ph Eur monograph 2143)

| $CdSO_4,8/3H_2O$ | 256.5 | *10124-36-4* |

Ph Eur _____

DEFINITION
Content
98.0 per cent to 102.0 per cent (anhydrous substance).

CHARACTERS
Appearance
White or almost white, crystalline powder.

Solubility
Freely soluble in water, practically insoluble in ethanol (96 per cent).

IDENTIFICATION
A. It gives reaction (a) of sulfates *(2.3.1)*.

B. To 2 mL of solution S (see Tests) add 2 mL of *sodium sulfide solution R*. A yellow precipitate is formed.

TESTS
Solution S
Dissolve 5.0 g in *carbon dioxide-free water R* and dilute to 50 mL with the same solvent.

Appearance of solution
Solution S is clear *(2.2.1)* and colourless *(2.2.2, Method II)*.

Acidity or alkalinity
To 10 mL of solution S add 0.3 mL of *methyl orange solution R*. Not more than 0.5 mL of *0.01 M hydrochloric acid* or *0.01 M sodium hydroxide* is required to change the colour of the indicator.

Nitrates
Maximum 100 ppm.

Dissolve 1.0 g in *water R* and dilute to 20.0 mL with the same solvent. To 1.0 mL of this solution add 0.2 mL of a 10 g/L solution of *sulfanilic acid R* in *acetic acid R* and 0.2 mL of a recently prepared 3 g/L solution of *naphthylamine R* in *acetic acid R*. Add a turning of *zinc R*. A pink colour is produced within 5 min. It is not more intense than that of a mixture of 0.5 mL of *nitrate standard solution (10 ppm NO₃) R* and 0.5 mL of *water R*, prepared at the same time.

Zinc sulfate, alkaline-earth sulfates, rare-earth sulfates
Dissolve 1.0 g in 17 mL of *water R*. Add 0.5 mL of *hydrochloric acid R* and 1 g of *thioacetamide R*. Heat in a water-bath for 10 min. Dilute to 20.0 mL with *water R* and filter. Evaporate 10.0 mL of this solution to dryness in an oven. Ignite the residue at about 800 ± 50 °C to constant mass. The residue weighs a maximum of 2 mg.

Arsenic *(2.4.2, Method A)*
Maximum 2 ppm, determined on 5 mL of solution S.

Water *(2.5.12)*
16.0 per cent to 20.0 per cent, determined on 80 mg. Shake for 10 min before carrying out the determination.

ASSAY
Dissolve 0.200 g in 50 mL of *water R*. Add 10 mL of *ammonium chloride buffer solution pH 10.0 R* and 50 mg of *mordant black 11 triturate R1*. Titrate with *0.1 M sodium edetate* until the colour changes from red to green.

1 mL of *0.1 M sodium edetate* is equivalent to 20.85 mg of $CdSO_4$.

_____ *Ph Eur*

Calcium Iodide Tetrahydrate for Homoeopathic Preparations

(Ph Eur monograph 2144)

| $CaI_2,4H_2O$ | 366.0 | *13640-62-5* |

Ph Eur _____

DEFINITION
Content
97.0 per cent to 102.0 per cent of CaI_2 (anhydrous substance).

CHARACTERS
Appearance
White or almost white powder, very hygroscopic.

Solubility
Very soluble to freely soluble in water and in ethanol (96 per cent).

IDENTIFICATION
A. Solution S (see Tests) gives reaction (a) of calcium *(2.3.1)*.

B. Solution S (see Tests) gives reaction (b) of iodides *(2.3.1)*.

TESTS
Solution S
Dissolve 10.0 g in *distilled water R* and dilute to 100.0 mL with the same solvent.

Appearance of solution
Solution S is clear *(2.2.1)* and not more intensely coloured than reference solution GY₅ *(2.2.2, Method II)*.

Free iodine, iodates
To 5 mL of solution S add 2 mL of *methylene chloride R*. Shake and allow to stand. The organic layer is colourless *(2.2.2, Method I)* (free iodine). Add 0.2 mL of *dilute sulfuric acid R*. Shake and allow to stand. The organic layer remains colourless *(2.2.2, Method I)* (iodates).

Sulfates *(2.4.13)*
Maximum 150 ppm.

Dilute 10 mL of solution S to 15 mL with *distilled water R*.

Iron *(2.4.9)*
Maximum 10 ppm, determined on 10 mL of solution S.

Heavy metals (*2.4.8*)

Maximum 10 ppm.

12 mL of solution S complies with limit test A. Prepare the reference solution using *lead standard solution (1 ppm Pb) R*.

Water (*2.5.12*)

18.0 per cent to 22.0 per cent, determined on 0.100 g.

ASSAY

Dissolve 0.300 g in 50 mL of *water R*. Add 5 mL of *dilute nitric acid R* and 25.0 mL of *0.1 M silver nitrate*. Shake. Add 2 mL of *ferric ammonium sulfate solution R2* and titrate with *0.1 M ammonium thiocyanate* until the colour changes to reddish-yellow.

1 mL of *0.1 M silver nitrate* is equivalent to 14.70 mg of CaI_2.

STORAGE

In an airtight container.

_____ *Ph Eur*

Calcium Phosphate for Homoeopathic Preparations

Calcium Phosphoricum for Homoeopathic Preparations

DEFINITION

Calcium Phosphate for Homoeopathic Preparations contains Calcium Phosphate.

PRODUCTION OF STOCK

The first trituration of Calcium Phosphate for Homoeopathic Preparations is prepared using a suitable quantity of a vehicle, such as Lactose, Anhydrous Lactose or Sucrose, and a validated method for trituration that ensures homogeneity is achieved. The vehicle complies with the statement under Vehicles in the monograph for Homoeopathic Preparations.

Content of calcium Ca

The first decimal trituration contains 3.5% to 4.0% of Ca.

CHARACTERISTICS

The first decimal trituration is a white powder.

IDENTIFICATION

Wash 5 g of the first decimal trituration of the substance being examined with three 10-mL quantities of *water*. The dried residue complies with the following tests.

A. Dissolve 0.1 g of the dried residue in 5 mL of a 25% v/v solution of *nitric acid*. The resulting solution yields reaction B of *phosphates*, Appendix VI.

B. The dried residue yields reaction B characteristic of *calcium salts*, Appendix VI. Filter before adding *potassium ferrocyanide solution*.

C. The dried residue complies with the limits of the Assay.

D. If the preparation includes Lactose as the vehicle, it complies with the following test. Dissolve 0.25 g in 5 mL of *water*. Add 5 mL of *ammonia* and heat in a water-bath at 80° for 10 minutes. A red colour develops.

E. If the preparation includes Sucrose as the vehicle, it complies with the following test. Dissolve 5.0 g in *carbon dioxide-free water* and dilute to 10 mL with the same solvent. Dilute 1 mL of the solution to 100 mL with *water*. To 5 mL of the solution add 0.15 mL of freshly prepared *copper sulfate solution* and 2 mL of freshly prepared *dilute sodium hydroxide solution*. The solution is blue and clear and remains so after boiling. To the hot solution add 4 mL of *dilute hydrochloric*

acid and boil for 1 minute. Add 4 mL of *dilute sodium hydroxide solution*. An orange precipitate is formed immediately.

ASSAY

Dissolve 0.2 g of the residue in a mixture of 1.0 mL of hydrochloric acid R1 and 5 mL of water. Add 25.0 mL of 0.1M disodium edetate and dilute to 200 mL with water. Adjust to about pH 10 with concentrated ammonia. Add 10 mL of ammonia buffer pH 10.0 and a few milligrams of mordant black 11 triturate. Titrate the excess disodium edetate with 0.1M zinc sulfate until the colour changes from blue to violet. Each mL of 0.1M sodium hydroxide is equivalent to 4.008 mg of Ca.

Oriental Cashew for Homoeopathic Preparations

(*Ph Eur monograph 2094*)

Ph Eur _____

DEFINITION

Dried fruit of *Semecarpus anacardium* L. (*Anacardium orientale* L.).

Content

Minimum 6.0 per cent *m/m* of total phenol derivatives expressed as eugenol ($C_{10}H_{12}O_2$; M_r 164.2) (dried drug).

IDENTIFICATION

A. The dried fruit is oval and more or less heart-shaped; about 2 cm long, nearly 2 cm wide and 0.5 cm thick. Its surface is smooth, shiny and blackish. A transverse section shows a rather well developed, tough pericarp riddled with rather wide lacunae containing an abundant thick reddish-brown juice. The pericarp covers a white kernel under a reddish skin. The fruit may include the blackish, fleshy, wrinkled, cupuliferous receptacle.

B. Thin-layer chromatography (*2.2.27*).

Test solution   To 1.0 g of suitably cut drug, add 10 mL of *ethanol (90 per cent V/V) R*. Heat under reflux on a water-bath at 60 °C for 15 min. Allow to cool and filter.

Reference solution   Dissolve 5 mg of *gallic acid R* and 5 mg of *caffeic acid R* in *methanol R* and dilute to 10 mL with the same solvent.

Plate   TLC silica gel plate R.

Mobile phase   methanol R, toluene R (15:85 *V/V*).

Application   20 µL of the test solution and 10 µL of the reference solution, as bands.

Development   Over a path of 15 cm.

Drying   In air.

Detection   Spray with a solution containing 10 g/L of *diphenylboric acid aminoethyl ester R* and 50 g/L of *macrogol 400 R* in *methanol R*. Examine in ultraviolet light at 365 nm.

Results   See below the sequence of zones present in the chromatograms obtained with the reference solution and the test solution. Furthermore, other fainter zones may be present in the chromatogram obtained with the test solution.

Top of the plate	
	A greenish-blue fluorescent zone
———	———
	Several violet-blue fluorescent zones
	A yellow fluorescent zone
Caffeic acid: a violet-blue fluorescent zone	
———	———
Gallic acid: a violet-blue fluorescent zone	A violet-blue fluorescent zone (gallic acid)
Reference solution	**Test solution**

TESTS

Anacardium occidentale L.

Fruits of *Anacardium occidentale* L. are not present. These are up to 35 mm long, 30 mm large, 20 mm thick, light brown and distinctly kidney-shaped. The pericarp is smooth or slightly crinkled with dark marbling in places.

Loss on drying (2.2.32)

Maximum 12.0 per cent, determined on 1.000 g of the finely divided drug by drying in an oven at 105 °C for 2 h.

Total ash (2.4.16)

Maximum 5.0 per cent.

ASSAY

Total phenol derivatives

Absorption spectrophotometry (*2.2.25*).

Stock solution Place 4.500 g of the crushed drug in a flask. Add 200 mL of *ethanol (90 per cent V/V) R*. Boil in a water-bath under reflux for 4 h. Cool the flask. Quantitatively transfer into a volumetric flask. Dilute to 250.0 mL with *ethanol (90 per cent V/V) R*. Filter the liquid through a paper filter 125 mm in diameter. Discard the first 50 mL of the filtrate. Dilute 5.0 mL of filtrate to 50.0 mL with *ethanol (90 per cent V/V) R* and shake. Dilute 5.0 mL of this solution to 10.0 mL with *ethanol (90 per cent V/V) R* and shake.

Test solution To 2.0 mL of stock solution add 1.0 mL of *phosphomolybdotungstic reagent R* and 10 mL of *water R*, mix and dilute to 25.0 mL with a 290 g/L solution of *sodium carbonate R*. Wait exactly 3 min then filter the solution through a fibre-glass filter with a 1 μm mesh aperture, discarding the first 5 mL.

Reference solution Dissolve 80.0 mg of *eugenol R* in *ethanol (90 per cent V/V) R* and dilute to 250.0 mL with the same solvent. Dilute 5.0 mL of the solution to 25.0 mL with *ethanol (90 per cent V/V) R*. To 2.0 mL of this solution add 1.0 mL of *phosphomolybdotungstic reagent R* and 10 mL of *water R*, mix and dilute to 25.0 mL with a 290 g/L solution of *sodium carbonate R*. Wait exactly 3 min then filter the solution through a fibre-glass filter with a 1 μm mesh aperture, discarding the first 5 mL.

Measure the absorbance (*2.2.25*) of the test solution and the reference solution at 755 nm after 30 min using *water R* as compensation liquid.

Calculate the percentage content *m/m* of total phenol derivatives, expressed as eugenol, from the following expression:

$$\frac{A_1 \times m_2 \times 400}{A_2 \times m_1}$$

A_1 = absorbance of the test solution;
A_2 = absorbance of the reference solution;
m_1 = mass of the drug to be examined, in milligrams;
m_2 = mass of eugenol in the reference solution, in milligrams.

MOTHER TINCTURE

The mother tincture complies with the requirements of the general monograph on *Mother tinctures for homoeopathic preparations (2029)*.

DEFINITION

The mother tincture of oriental cashew is prepared by maceration using ethanol of a suitable concentration from the dried fruit of *Semecarpus anacardium* L. (*Anacardium orientale* L.).

Content
0.5 per cent *m/m* to 1.0 per cent *m/m* of total phenol derivatives expressed as eugenol.

CHARACTERS

Appearance
Yellowish-brown or reddish-brown liquid.

IDENTIFICATION

Thin-layer chromatography (*2.2.27*) as described under Identification B of the drug with the following modification.

Test solution The tincture to be examined.

Results See identification B for the drug.

TESTS

Relative density (*2.2.5*)
0.815 to 0.845.

Ethanol (*2.9.10*)
85 per cent *V/V* to 95 per cent *V/V*.

Dry residue (*2.8.16*)
Minimum 1.50 per cent *m/m*.

ASSAY

Total phenol derivatives
Absorption spectrophotometry (*2.2.25*) as described in the assay of the drug to be examined with the following modifications.

Stock solution Place 8.000 g of the mother tincture to be examined in a volumetric flask and dilute to 250.0 mL with *ethanol (90 per cent V/V) R*. Dilute 5.0 mL of this solution to 20.0 mL with *ethanol (90 per cent V/V) R*.

Test solution To 2.0 mL of stock solution add 1.0 mL of *phosphomolybdotungstic reagent R* and 10 mL of *water R*, mix and dilute to 25.0 mL with a 290 g/L solution of *sodium carbonate R*. Wait exactly 3 min then filter the solution through a fibre-glass filter with a 1 μm mesh aperture, discarding the first 5 mL.

Reference solution Dissolve 80.0 mg of *eugenol R* in *ethanol (90 per cent V/V) R* and dilute to 250.0 mL with the same solvent. Dilute 5.0 mL of the solution to 25.0 mL with *ethanol (90 per cent V/V) R*. To 2.0 mL of this solution add 1.0 mL of *phosphomolybdotungstic reagent R* and 10 mL of *water R*, mix and dilute to 25.0 mL with a 290 g/L solution of *sodium carbonate R*. Wait exactly 3 min then filter the solution through a fibre-glass filter with a 1 μm mesh aperture, discarding the first 5 mL.

Measure the absorbance (*2.2.25*) of the test solution and the reference solution at 755 nm after 30 min, using *water R* as compensation liquid.

Calculate the percentage content *m/m* of total phenol derivatives expressed as eugenol, using the following expression:

$$\frac{A_1 \times m_2 \times 80}{A_2 \times m_1}$$

A_1 = absorbance of the test solution;
A_2 = absorbance of the reference solution;
m_1 = mass of the mother tincture to be examined, in milligrams;
m_2 = mass of eugenol in the reference solution, in milligrams.

_____ *Ph Eur*

Cineraria Maritima for Homoeopathic Preparations

DEFINITION
Cineraria Maritima for Homoeopathic Preparations is the fresh aerial parts of *Cineraria maritima* L. harvested before flowering.

IDENTIFICATION
Plant Low growing, woody-based perennial 25 to 30 cm occasionally up to 100 cm high, with strong, white tomentose shoots up to 20 mm in diameter. The shoots are much branched and those bearing the flowers are elongated with some smaller leaves in the upper part; the shorter, non-flowering shoots remain compressed with the leaves forming a rosette at the top.

Leaves The leaves are alternate, up to 25 cm long and 12 cm wide, ovate or oblong-ovate, the lowest coarsely toothed, the upper ones deeply pinnatified or pinnate with 4 to 6 oblong to blunt, often 3 to 5 lobed, unequal segments. The under surface is covered with a dense white felt, the upper surface is green with scattered cottony hairs.

MOTHER TINCTURE

The mother tincture complies with the requirements stated under Mother Tinctures for Homoeopathic Preparations and with the following requirements.

PRODUCTION
The mother tincture of *Cineraria maritima* L. is prepared from the cut drug using *Method 1.1.7* described in the monograph for Methods of Preparation of Homoeopathic Stocks and Potentisation. Use 43% w/w (50% v/v) of *ethanol*.

CHARACTERISTICS
The mother tincture is a dark yellow, clear to slightly turbid liquid.

IDENTIFICATION
A. Carry out the method for *thin-layer chromatography*, Appendix III A, using the following solutions.

(1) Dilute 5 mL of the mother tincture with 15 mL of *water* and transfer to a cartridge containing *octadecyl-bonded silica sorbent* (a Sep-pak C18 cartridge is suitable) previously washed with 10 mL of *methanol* followed by 10 mL of *water*. Elute with 10 mL of *methanol*, evaporate the eluant and dissolve the residue in 0.5 mL of *methanol*.

(2) 0.05% w/v each of *hyperoside* and *rutin* and 0.01% w/v of *scopoletin* in *methanol*.

CHROMATOGRAPHIC CONDITIONS
(a) Use as the coating *silica gel F_{254}*.
(b) Use the mobile phase described below.
(c) Apply 30 µL of solution (1) and 10 µL of solution (2) as 10 mm bands.
(d) Develop the plate to 15 cm.
(e) After removal of the plate, dry in air and spray the plate with a 1% w/v solution of *diphenylboric acid aminoethyl ester* in *methanol* and then spray with a 5% w/v solution of *polyethylene glycol 400* in *methanol*. Heat at 100° to 105° for 5 minutes, allow to dry in air and examine immediately in *ultraviolet light (365 nm)*.

MOBILE PHASE
10 volumes of *water*, 10 volumes of *formic acid* and 80 volumes of *ethyl acetate*.

SYSTEM SUITABILITY
The test is not valid unless the chromatogram obtained with solution (2) shows three fluorescent bands: an orange fluorescent band with a low Rf value (rutin), an orange fluorescent band with an Rf value in the middle region (hyperoside) and a blue fluorescent band with an Rf value in the upper region (scopoletin).

CONFIRMATION
The chromatogram obtained with solution (1) shows an orange fluorescent band in a similar position to rutin, another fluorescent band above this orange band, another orange fluorescent band in a similar position to hyperoside with a green fluorescent band just below, one or two green fluorescent bands between the bands in similar positions to hyperoside and scopoletin, one blue-green fluorescent band in a similar position to scopoletin and one yellow-green to orange fluorescent band above the blue-green fluorescent band.

Top of the plate	
A yellow-green to orange band	
A blue-green band	Scopoletin: a blue band
An orange band	Hyperoside: an orange band
A green band	
A band	
An orange band	Rutin: an orange band
Solution (1)	Solution (2)

B. Carry out the method for *thin-layer chromatography*, Appendix III A, using the following solutions.

(1) Evaporate off the ethanol from 50 mL of the mother tincture. Make the residue alkaline with *dilute ammonia R1* and extract with three 20-mL quantities of *chloroform*. Evaporate the combined chloroform extracts to dryness and dissolve the residue in 1 mL of *ethanol (60%)*.

(2) 0.1% w/v of *reserpine* in *acetone*.

CHROMATOGRAPHIC CONDITIONS

(a) Use as the coating *silica gel F₂₅₄*.

(b) Use the mobile phase described below.

(c) Apply 30 μL of solution (1) and 20 μL of solution (2) as 10 mm bands.

(d) Develop the plate to 10 cm.

(e) After removal of the plate, dry in air and spray the plate with a 2% w/v solution of *dimethylaminobenzaldehyde* in *ethanol* and then spray with a solution of *sulfuric acid*. Heat at 100° to 105° for 5 minutes and examine in daylight.

MOBILE PHASE

10 volumes of *methanol* and 90 volumes of *chloroform*.

SYSTEM SUITABILITY

The test is not valid unless the chromatogram obtained with solution (2) shows one blue band with an Rf value of 0.80.

CONFIRMATION

The chromatogram obtained with solution (1) shows a series of violet bands between the line of application and Rf value 0.65, one pink band at Rf value 0.75 and one red band at Rf value 0.90.

Top of the plate	
A red band	Reserpine: a blue band
A pink band	
A series of violet bands between the line of application and Rf 0.65	
Solution (1)	Solution (2)

TESTS

Ethanol
25 to 35% w/w (31 to 42% v/v), Appendix VIII F.

Dry residue
Not less than 1.0%, determined on 2 mL, Appendix XI P.

Relative density
0.957 to 0.977, Appendix V G.

STORAGE

Cineraria Maritima for Homoeopathic Preparations should be protected from light.

Citrullus Colocynthis Fruit for Homoeopathic Preparations

DEFINITION

Citrullus Colocynthis Fruit for Homoeopathic Preparations is the dried, peeled fruits of *Citrullus colocynthis* (L.) Schrad. with the seeds removed.

IDENTIFICATION

A. The peeled fruits are spherical with a diameter of 5 to 10 cm, white to pale yellow and very light in texture, consisting mainly of soft, spongy tissue from the inner cupule and the placentae. The external surface is marked by spiral, flattish, knife marks where the peel has been removed. In cross section, three conspicuous fissures can be seen radiating from the centre and dividing the fruit into three parts. Each part contains two groups of seeds near the periphery, the remaining space being filled with pithy parenchyma. Each fruit contains 200 to 300 seeds. The inferior ovary is initially tripartite but as the placentae grow out from the centre towards the circumference, each divides into two, half curving backwards, and giving the appearance of a hexapartite ovary.

B. Reduce to a powder. The powder is pale yellowish-buff. Examine under a microscope using *chloral hydrate solution*. The powder shows abundant, large, partly lignified, thin-walled, finely pitted, usually fragmented parenchyma; smaller cells with slightly collenchymatous thickening and more distinct pitted circular to oval areas, lignified, spirally or annularly thickened vessels.

C. Carry out the method for *thin-layer chromatography*, Appendix III A, using the following solutions.

(1) Add 30 mL of 86% v/v *ethanol* to 3 g of the coarsely powdered drug and heat under reflux for 2 hours. Allow to cool and filter. Evaporate 20 mL of the filtrate to about 5 mL.

(2) 0.1% w/v each of *caffeine*, *coumarin* and *resorcinol* in *methanol*.

CHROMATOGRAPHIC CONDITIONS

(a) Use as the coating *silica gel F₂₅₄*.

(b) Use the mobile phase described below.

(c) Apply 20 μL of each solution.

(d) Develop the plate to 10 cm.

(e) Remove the plate, dry it in air and examine under *ultraviolet light (254 nm)*.

MOBILE PHASE

1 volume of 13.5M *ammonia*, 9 volumes of *methanol* and 90 volumes of *dichloromethane*.

SYSTEM SUITABILITY

The test is not valid unless the chromatogram obtained with solution (2) shows three clearly separated bands (approximate Rf values: resorcinol 0.31, caffeine 0.67 and coumarin 0.87).

CONFIRMATION

The chromatogram obtained with solution (1) shows two dark bands at Rf values of 0.08 and 0.1 respectively between the line of application and the band due to resorcinol, one dark band at an Rf value of 0.56 positioned between the band due to resorcinol and that due to caffeine, and one dark band at approximately Rf value of 0.78 positioned between the band due to caffeine and that due to coumarin. Other bands may be present.

TESTS

Foreign matter
Not more than 2.0% of the outer part of the pericarp; not more than 5.0% of seeds; not more than 2.0% of other foreign matter, Appendix XI D.

Loss on drying
When dried at 100° to 105° for 2 hours, loses not more than 22.0% of its weight. Use 1 g.

Total ash
Not more than 13.0%, Appendix XI J, Method II.

Top of the plate	
A dark band	Coumarin: a dark band
A dark band	Caffeine: a dark band
A dark band A dark band	Resorcinol: a dark band
Solution (1)	Solution (2)

MOTHER TINCTURE

The mother tincture complies with the requirements stated under Mother Tinctures for Homoeopathic Preparations and with the following requirements.

PRODUCTION

The mother tincture of *Citrullus colocynthis* (L.) Schrad. is prepared from the powdered drug using *Method 4a* described in the monograph for Methods of Preparation of Homoeopathic Stocks and Potentisation. Use 86% w/w (90% v/v) *ethanol.*

CHARACTERISTICS

The mother tincture is a light yellow to yellow liquid.

IDENTIFICATION

The mother tincture complies with Identification test C above using the mother tincture as solution (1).

TESTS

Ethanol
81% to 91% w/w (86% to 94% v/v), Appendix VIII F.

Dry residue
1.0% to 2.5% w/w, Appendix XI P.

Relative density
0.830 to 0.850, Appendix V G.

Cocculus Indicus for Homoeopathic Preparations

(*Anamirta Cocculus for Homoeopathic Preparations,* Ph Eur monograph 2486)

Ph Eur —————

DEFINITION

Dried, ripe fruit of *Anamirta paniculata* Colebr. (*A. cocculus* Wight et Arn.).

Content

Minimum 0.80 per cent of picrotoxinin ($C_{15}H_{16}O_6$; M_r 292.3) (dried drug).

IDENTIFICATION

First identification A, B, D.

Second identification A, B, C.

A. The fruits are dark greyish-brown or black, reniform sub-spherical, about 6-10 mm in diameter and 9-12 mm long; the outer surface is irregularly wrinkled with a ridge about 4-6 mm long running between the pale, circular scar left by the stalk and a small beak of the remains of the stigma. The pericarp is hard, about 1 mm thick and the inner surface is brownish-grey, hard and woody. Cut transversely, the fruit shows a single, cup-shaped seed into the hollow of which an ingrowth of the mesocarp and endocarp projects. Cut longitudinally, the endosperm shows the presence of 2 narrow cavities in each of which is enclosed 1 of the foliaceous cotyledons.

B. Microscopic examination (*2.8.23*). The powder (710) is brown. Examine under a microscope using *chloral hydrate solution R*. The powder shows brownish, thin-walled, elongated cells with brown granular contents; rather large vascular bundles; very thick lignified fibres; sclereids; large, thin-walled, cubic or polygonal cells containing fatty oil and large protein granules; cells containing small needle-shaped crystals and, in the largest cavities, prism crystals.

C. Thin-layer chromatography (*2.2.27*).

Test solution To 2.00 g of the powdered herbal drug (710) (*2.9.12*) add 20 mL of *ethanol (90 per cent V/V) R*, shake for 2 h and then centrifuge (1000 *g*). Use the supernatant.

Reference solution Dissolve 10 mg of *picrotin CRS* and 10 mg of *picrotoxinin CRS* in *ethanol (96 per cent) R* and dilute to 10 mL with the same solvent.

Plate TLC silica gel plate R (5-40 μm) [or *TLC silica gel plate R* (2-10 μm)].

Mobile phase *methanol R, ethyl acetate R, heptane R* (10:40:50 *V/V/V*).

Application 40 μL [or 10 μL], as bands of 20 mm [or 10 mm].

Development Over a path of 10 cm [or 6 cm].

Drying In air.

Detection Spray with *anisaldehyde solution R*, heat at 100-105 °C for 5-10 min and examine in daylight within 5-10 min.

Results See below the sequence of zones present in the chromatograms obtained with the reference solution and the test solution. Above the zone due to picrotoxinin, several pink or violet zones may also be visible in the chromatogram obtained with the test solution.

Top of the plate	
———	———
Picrotoxinin: a blue zone	A blue zone (picrotoxinin)
———	———
Picrotin: a blue zone	A blue zone (picrotin)
Reference solution	**Test solution**

D. Examine the chromatograms obtained in the assay.

Results The peaks due to picrotoxinin and picrotin in the chromatogram obtained with the test solution are similar in retention time to the corresponding peaks in the chromatogram obtained with the reference solution.

TESTS

Loss on drying (*2.2.32*)

Maximum 10.0 per cent, determined on 1.000 g of the powdered drug (710) (*2.9.12*) by drying in an oven at 105 °C for 2 h.

Total ash (*2.4.16*)

Maximum 6.0 per cent.

ASSAY

Liquid chromatography (*2.2.29*).

Test solution To 2.00 g of the powdered drug (710) (*2.9.12*) add 20.0 mL of *ethanol (90 per cent V/V) R*, shake for 2 h and then centrifuge at 1000 *g* for 5 min. Dilute 2.0 mL of the supernatant to 20.0 mL with the mobile phase and filter through a membrane filter (nominal pore size 0.45 μm).

Reference solution Dissolve 5.0 mg of *picrotin CRS* and 5.0 mg of *picrotoxinin CRS* in 10.0 mL of *acetonitrile R*. Dilute 2.0 mL of the solution to 20.0 mL with the mobile phase.

Column:
— *size*: l = 0.125 m, Ø = 4.0 mm;
— *stationary phase*: *octadecylsilyl silica gel for chromatography R* (5 μm).

Mobile phase *acetonitrile for chromatography R, water R* (30:70 *V/V*).

Flow rate 0.5 mL/min.

Detection Spectrophotometer at 200 nm.

Injection 10 μL.

Run time Twice the retention time of picrotoxinin CRS.

Retention time Picrotin = about 6 min; picrotoxinin = about 10 min.

System suitability Reference solution:
— *resolution*: minimum 2.0 between the peaks due to picrotin and picrotoxinin.

Calculate the percentage content of picrotoxinin using the following expression:

$$\frac{A_1 \times m_2 \times p \times 2}{A_2 \times m_1}$$

A_1 = area of the peak due to picrotoxinin in the chromatogram obtained with the test solution;

A_2 = area of the peak due to picrotoxinin in the chromatogram obtained with the reference solution;

m_1 = mass of the herbal drug to be examined to prepare the test solution, in grams;

m_2 = mass of *picrotoxinin CRS* used to prepare the reference solution, in grams;

p = assigned percentage content of picrotoxinin in *picrotoxinin CRS*.

MOTHER TINCTURE

The mother tincture complies with the requirements of the general monograph on *Mother tinctures for homeopathic preparations (2029)*.

DEFINITION

Content

0.07 per cent m/m to 0.15 per cent m/m of picrotoxinin ($C_{15}H_{16}O_6$).

PRODUCTION

The mother tincture is prepared from the dried, ripe fruit of *A. paniculata Colebr.* according to the following methods prescribed in the monograph *Methods of preparation of homoeopathic stocks and potentisation (2371)*:

— method 1.1.8 using the powdered herbal drug (710) (*2.9.12*) and *ethanol (90 per cent V/V) R*; use *ethanol (70 per cent V/V) R* to prepare the 4th decimal dilution and *ethanol (50 per cent V/V) R* for subsequent dilutions;
— method 1.1.10 using the crushed drug in fragments of about 2-3 mm, *ethanol (90 per cent V/V) R* and a maceration time of about 3 weeks.

CHARACTERS

Appearance

Yellow or dark yellow liquid.

IDENTIFICATION

A. Thin-layer chromatography (*2.2.27*) as described in identification test C of the herbal drug with the following modification.

Test solution The mother tincture to be examined.

B. Examine the chromatograms obtained in the assay.

Results The peaks due to picrotoxinin and picrotin in the chromatogram obtained with the test solution are similar in retention time to the corresponding peaks in the chromatogram obtained with the reference solution.

TESTS

Relative density (*2.2.5*)

0.830 to 0.845 (method 1.1.8).

Ethanol (*2.9.10*)

85 per cent *V/V* to 95 per cent *V/V* (method 1.1.10).

Dry residue (*2.8.16*)

Minimum 0.7 per cent.

ASSAY

Liquid chromatography (*2.2.29*) as described in the assay for the herbal drug with the following modification.

Test solution Dilute 0.500 g of the mother tincture to be examined to 10.0 mL with the mobile phase and filter using a membrane filtre (nominal pore size 0.45 μm).

Calculate the percentage content of picrotoxinin using the following expression:

$$\frac{A_1 \times m_2 \times p}{A_2 \times m_1 \times 10}$$

A_1 = area of the peak due to picrotoxinin in the chromatogram obtained with the test solution;

A_2 = area of the peak due to picrotoxinin in the chromatogram obtained with the reference solution;

m_1 = mass of the mother tincture to be examined used to prepare the test solution, in grams;

m_2 = mass of *picrotoxinin CRS* used to prepare the reference solution, in grams;

p = assigned percentage content of picrotoxinin in *picrotoxinin CRS*.

_____ Ph Eur

Copper for Homoeopathic Preparations

Copper for Homoeopathic Use

(*Ph Eur monograph 1610*)

| Cu | 63.5 | *7440-50-8* |

Ph Eur _____

DEFINITION

Content

99.0 per cent to 101.0 per cent of Cu.

CHARACTERS

Appearance

Reddish-brown powder.

Solubility

Practically insoluble in water, soluble in hydrochloric acid and in nitric acid, practically insoluble in alcohol.

IDENTIFICATION

A. To 2 mL of solution S (see Tests) add 0.5 mL of *potassium ferrocyanide solution R*. A reddish-brown precipitate is formed.

B. To 5 mL of solution S add 0.6 mL of *ammonia R*. A blue precipitate is formed. Add 2 mL of *ammonia R*.
The precipitate disappears; the solution has an intense blue colour.

TESTS

Solution S

Dissolve 2.0 g in 10 mL of *nitric acid R*. After nitrous fumes are no longer evolved, dilute to 60 mL with *distilled water R*.

Acidity or alkalinity

To 5.0 g add 20 mL of *carbon dioxide-free water R*. Boil for 1 min. Cool. Filter and dilute to 25.0 mL with *carbon dioxide free water R*. To 10 mL of the solution add 0.1 mL of *bromothymol blue solution R1*. Not more than 0.5 mL of *0.01 M hydrochloric acid* or *0.01 M sodium hydroxide* is required to change the colour of the indicator.

Chlorides (*2.4.4*)

Maximum 100 ppm.

15 mL of solution S complies with the limit test for chlorides.

Sulfates (*2.4.13*)

Maximum 300 ppm.

15 mL of solution S complies with the limit test for sulfates.

Iron

Maximum 50 ppm.

Atomic absorption spectrometry (*2.2.23, Method I*).

Test solution Dissolve 1.00 g in 5 mL of *nitric acid R* and dilute to 50.0 mL with *water R*.

Reference solutions Prepare the reference solutions using *iron standard solution (20 ppm Fe) R*, diluted as necessary with a 1 per cent *V/V* solution of *nitric acid R*.

Source Iron hollow-cathode lamp.

Wavelength 248.3 nm.

Flame Air-acetylene.

Lead

Maximum 100 ppm.

Atomic absorption spectrometry (*2.2.23, Method I*).

Test solution Use the test solution prepared for the test for iron.

Reference solutions Prepare the reference solutions using *lead standard solution (0.1 per cent Pb) R*, diluted as necessary with a 1 per cent *V/V* solution of *nitric acid R*.

Source Lead hollow-cathode lamp.

Wavelength 283.3 nm.

Flame Air-acetylene.

Zinc

Maximum 50 ppm.

Atomic absorption spectrometry (*2.2.23, Method I*).

Test solution Use the test solution prepared for the test for iron.

Reference solutions Prepare the reference solutions using *zinc standard solution (100 ppm Zn) R*, diluted as necessary with a 1 per cent *V/V* solution of *nitric acid R*.

Source Zinc hollow-cathode lamp.

Wavelength 213.9 nm.

Flame Air-acetylene.

ASSAY

Dissolve 0.100 g in 5 mL of *nitric acid R*. Heat to expel the nitrous fumes. Add 200 mL of *water R* and neutralise (*2.2.3*) with *dilute ammonia R1*. Add 1 g of *ammonium chloride R* and 3 mg of *murexide R*. Titrate with *0.1 M sodium edetate* until the colour changes from green to violet.

1 mL of *0.1 M sodium edetate* is equivalent to 6.354 mg of Cu.

_____ *Ph Eur*

Copper Acetate Monohydrate for Homoeopathic Preparations

(*Ph Eur monograph 2146*)

| Cu(C₂H₃O₂)2,H₂O | 199.7 | *6046-93-1* |

Formula: $Cu(C_2H_3O_2)_2,H_2O$ 199.7   *6046-93-1*

Ph Eur _____

DEFINITION

Content

99.0 per cent to 101.0 per cent of $Cu(C_2H_3O_2)_2,H_2O$.

CHARACTERS

Appearance

Greenish-blue crystals or green powder.

Solubility

Soluble in water, slightly soluble or very slightly soluble in ethanol (96 per cent).

IDENTIFICATION

A. It gives reaction (a) of acetates (*2.3.1*).

B. Dissolve 0.1 g in 10 mL of *water R* and add *dilute ammonia R1* dropwise. A dark blue colour is produced.

TESTS

Solution S

Dissolve 3.0 g in a mixture of 40 mL of *distilled water R* and 0.6 mL of *glacial acetic acid R*, with heating at 70 °C. Cool and dilute to 45 mL with *distilled water R*.

Appearance of solution

Solution S is clear (*2.2.1*).

Impurities not precipitating with hydrogen sulfide

Maximum 0.1 per cent, calculated as sulfates.

To 2.000 g add 92 mL of *water R* and 8.0 mL of *dilute sulfuric acid R*. Heat to 70 °C. Pass a current of *hydrogen sulfide R* until there is no longer precipitation of copper sulfide. Allow to cool and stand, then filter. Evaporate to dryness 50.0 mL of the filtrate in a crucible. Ignite the residue at about 600 ± 50 °C to constant mass.

Chlorides (*2.4.4*)

Maximum 50 ppm, determined on 15 mL of solution S.

Sulfates (*2.4.13*)

Maximum 150 ppm, determined on 15 mL of solution S.

Iron (*2.4.9*)

Maximum 20 ppm.

Dissolve 0.500 g in 10 mL of *water R*. Transfer to a separating funnel. Add 20 mL of *hydrochloric acid R1* and 10 mL of *methyl isobutyl ketone R*. Shake vigorously for 3 min. Allow to stand. Transfer the organic layer to a second separating funnel and add 10 mL of *water R*. Shake vigorously for 3 min. Allow to stand. The aqueous layer complies with the limit test for iron.

Nickel

Maximum 10 ppm.

To the residue obtained in the test for impurities not precipitating with hydrogen sulfide, add 2.0 mL of *hydrochloric acid R* and 1.0 mL of *sulfuric acid R*. Evaporate to dryness. Dissolve the residue in a mixture of 3.0 mL of *dilute sulfuric acid R* and 17.0 mL of *water R*. To 4.0 mL of this solution add 4.0 mL of *water R*, 5.0 mL of *bromine water R*, 7.0 mL of *dilute ammonia R1* and 3.0 mL of a 10 g/L solution of *dimethylglyoxime R* in *ethanol (90 per cent V/V) R*. This solution is not more intensely coloured within 1 min than a solution prepared as follows: mix 4.0 mL of a 1 ppm solution of nickel (Ni) prepared from *nickel standard solution (10 ppm Ni) R*, 4.0 mL of *water R* and 5.0 mL of *bromine water R*; carefully add 7.0 mL of *dilute ammonia R1* and 3.0 mL of a 10 g/L solution of *dimethylglyoxime R* in *ethanol (90 per cent V/V) R*.

ASSAY

Dissolve 0.400 g in *water R* and dilute to 50 mL with the same solvent. Add 6.0 mL of *glacial acetic acid R*, 10.0 g of *potassium iodide R* and 1 mL of *starch solution R*. Titrate with *0.1 M sodium thiosulfate*.

1 mL of *0.1 M sodium thiosulfate* is equivalent to 19.97 mg of $Cu(C_2H_3O_2)_2,H_2O$.

Ph Eur

Cydonia Oblonga for Homoeopathic Preparations

DEFINITION

Cydonia Oblonga for Homoeopathic Preparations is the seeds of *Cydonia oblonga* Mill.

IDENTIFICATION

The seeds are 6 to 7 mm long, reddish-brown to dark-brown, frequently cohering by a white mucilage appearing in flakes on the surface and in the spaces between the seeds; four-sided, one arched, one often distinctly ridged and two larger and flattened; pointed at one end, where the hilum occurs as a paler spot, obtuse at the other extremity, where the chalaza is situated. Cut transversely, the seed shows a very narrow endosperm surrounding two yellowish-white cotyledons.

TESTS

Total ash

Not more than 5%, Appendix XI J, Method II.

MOTHER TINCTURE

The mother tincture complies with the requirements stated under Mother Tinctures for Homoeopathic Preparations and with the following requirements.

PRODUCTION

The mother tincture of *Cydonia oblonga* Mill. is prepared from the powdered drug using *Method 1.1.8* described in the monograph for Methods of Preparation of Homoeopathic Stocks and Potentisation. Use *glycerol*.

CHARACTERISTICS

The mother tincture is a pale yellow, clear or slightly turbid viscous liquid.

IDENTIFICATION

Carry out the method for *thin-layer chromatography*, Appendix III A, using the following solutions.

(1) Dilute 5 mL of the mother tincture with 5 mL of *water*, mix thoroughly and transfer the diluted tincture to a cartridge containing *octadecyl-bonded silica sorbent* (a Sep-pak C18 cartridge is suitable) previously washed with 10 mL of *methanol* followed by 10 mL of *water*. Wash the cartridge with 15 mL of *water* and elute with 10 mL of *methanol*. Evaporate the eluant to dryness using a rotary evaporator. Dissolve the residue in 0.5 mL of *methanol*.

(2) 0.1% w/v of *hyperoside*, 0.1% w/v of *rutin* and 0.01% w/v of *scopoletin* in *methanol*.

CHROMATOGRAPHIC CONDITIONS

(a) Use as the coating *silica gel 60 F₂₅₄*.

(b) Use the mobile phase as described below.

(c) Apply 40 μL of solution (1) and 10 μL of solution (2), as 12 mm bands.

(d) Develop the plate to 15 cm.

(e) After removal of the plate, dry in air and spray the plate with a 1% w/v solution of *diphenylboric acid aminoethyl ester* in *methanol*, and then with a 5% w/v solution of *polyethylene glycol 400* in *methanol* and examine under *ultraviolet light (365 nm)*.

MOBILE PHASE

15 volumes of *anhydrous formic acid*, 15 volumes of *water* and 70 volumes of *ethyl acetate*.

SYSTEM SUITABILITY

The test is not valid unless the chromatogram obtained with solution (2) shows two clearly separated orange fluorescent bands and one blue fluorescent band at a higher Rf value. In order of increasing Rf value the bands are: rutin, hyperoside and scopoletin.

CONFIRMATION

The chromatogram obtained with solution (1) shows three yellow fluorescent bands in the lower third, a blue fluorescent band just below the rutin standard, a blue fluorescent band just below the hyperoside standard and a blue fluorescent band with the same Rf value of the scopoletin standard. Other bands may be present.

TEST

Refractive index

1.468 to 1.475, Appendix V E.

Top of the plate	
A blue band	Scopoletin: a blue band
A blue band	Hyperoside: an orange band
A blue band A yellow band A yellow band A yellow band	Rutin: an orange band
Solution (1)	Solution (2)

Garlic for Homoeopathic Preparations

(Ph Eur monograph 2023)

Ph Eur _____

DEFINITION

Fresh bulb of *Allium sativum L.*

CHARACTERS

It has a characteristic odour after cutting.

IDENTIFICATION

The bulb is generally 3 cm to 5 cm broad and almost spherical; the flat base bears the remnants of numerous short greyish-brown adventitious roots. The bulb consists of about 10 daughter bulbs (cloves) arranged roughly in a circle around a central axis. Individual daughter bulbs are 1 cm to 3 cm long, laterally compressed and convex on the dorsal side. Each daughter bulb has a tough, white or reddish skin around a fleshy tubular leaf, investing a more or less rounded elongated cone of leaf primordia and vegetative apex.

TESTS

Water *(2.2.13)*

Minimum 55.0 per cent, determined on 10.0 g of the finely cut drug, if performed to demonstrate the freshness of the drug.

MOTHER TINCTURE

The mother tincture complies with the requirements of the general monograph on *Mother tinctures for homoeopathic preparations (2029)*.

PRODUCTION

The mother tincture of *Allium sativum L.* is prepared by maceration of the cut drug using alcohol of a suitable concentration.

CHARACTERS

Appearance

Brownish-yellow liquid.

It has a peculiar and unpleasant aromatic odour.

IDENTIFICATION

A. To 2 mL of the mother tincture to be examined, add 0.2 mL of *dilute sodium hydroxide solution R*. A yellowish-white precipitate develops.

B. Thin-layer chromatography *(2.2.27)*.

Test solution   Extract 5 mL of the mother tincture to be examined with 2 quantities, each of 10 mL, of *ether R*. Combine the ether layers and dry over *anhydrous sodium sulfate R*. Filter and evaporate the filtrate in a water-bath at low temperature. Dissolve the residue in 0.4 mL of *methanol R*.

Reference solution   Dissolve 10 mg of *resorcinol R*, 10 mg of *thymol R* and 30 mg of *gallic acid R* in 10 mL of *methanol R*.

Plate   TLC silica gel F_{254} plate R.

Mobile phase   anhydrous formic acid R, toluene R, di-isopropyl ether R (10:40:50 *V/V/V*).

Application   40 µL of the test solution and 10 µL of the reference solution.

Development   Over a path of 10 cm.

Drying   In air.

Detection   Examine in ultraviolet light at 254 nm and identify gallic acid; spray with *anisaldehyde solution R*, heat to 105-110 °C for 5-10 min. Examine in daylight within 10 min.

Results   See below the sequence of the zones present in the chromatograms obtained with the reference solution and the test solution. Other zones may also be visible in the chromatogram obtained with the test solution.

Top of the plate	
	An intense reddish-violet zone
Thymol: an orange-red zone	An intense reddish-violet zone
	A violet zone
	A yellowish or greenish zone
_____	_____
Resorcinol: an intense orange-red zone	
_____	_____
Gallic acid: a yellow zone	A violet zone
(UV at 254 nm: a fluorescent quenching zone)	A greenish-yellow zone
	A violet zone may be present
Reference solution	**Test solution**

TESTS

Relative density *(2.2.5)*

0.885 to 0.960.

Ethanol *(2.9.10)*

50 per cent *V/V* to 70 per cent *V/V*.

Dry residue *(2.8.16)*

Minimum 4.0 per cent.

STORAGE

In an airtight container.

_____ *Ph Eur*

Hedera Helix for Homoeopathic Preparations

(*Ph Eur monograph 2092*)

Ph Eur

DEFINITION

Fresh, young, fully developed but not yet lignified branch of *Hedera helix* L., harvested immediately before or at the beginning of flowering.

IDENTIFICATION

The fresh, young branches of *Hedera helix* L. are thin and flexible, climbing; they cling to their support by stem-roots. The leaves are alternate, simple and petiolate. The petiole shows a cylindrical section. The upper surface of the leaves is glabrous and shiny, darker than the lower surface.
The lamina is usually divided into 3-5 more or less deeply cut lobes on sterile branches; it is oval, with a pointed apex on fertile branches. The inflorescences are arranged in a simple semi-globular corymb and grouped in terminal clusters. The pedicels of the umbel are covered in whitish hairs. Each flower shows 5 small teeth formed by the upper part of the sepals and 5 petals covered in very small inverted hairs.

TESTS

Foreign matter (*2.8.2*)
If required by the competent authority, maximum 5 per cent.

Loss on drying (*2.2.32*)
If required by the competent authority, minimum 50 per cent, determined on 5.0 g of the finely cut drug by drying in an oven at 105 °C for 2 h.

MOTHER TINCTURE

The mother tincture complies with the requirements of the general monograph on *Mother tinctures for homoeopathic preparations (2029)*.

PRODUCTION

The mother tincture of *Hedera helix* L. is prepared by maceration using ethanol of a suitable concentration.

Content

Minimum 0.15 per cent *m/m* of hederacoside C ($C_{59}H_{96}O_{26}$; M_r 1221).

CHARACTERS

Appearance
Dark greenish-brown liquid.

IDENTIFICATION

Thin-layer chromatography (*2.2.27*).

Test solution   The mother tincture to be examined.

Reference solution   Dissolve 1 mg of α-*hederin R* and 1 mg of *hederacoside C R* in *methanol R* and dilute to 2 mL with the same solvent.

Plate   *TLC silica gel plate R*.

Mobile phase   *glacial acetic acid R, water R, butanol R* (1:1:4 *V/V/V*).

Application   20 μL as bands.

Development   Over half of the plate.

Drying   In air.

Detection   Spray with a 10 per cent *V/V* solution of *sulfuric acid R* in *methanol R* and heat at 100-105 °C for 10 min. Examine in daylight.

Results   See below the sequence of the zones present in the chromatograms obtained with the reference solution and the test solution. Other faint zones may also be present in the chromatogram obtained with the test solution.

Top of the plate	
	A violet zone (α-hederin)
α-Hederin: a violet zone	
	A brown zone (hederacoside C)
Hederacoside C: a brown zone	
	A greyish-brown zone
	A yellow zone
Reference solution	**Test solution**

TESTS

Relative density (*2.2.5*)
0.890 to 0.925.

Ethanol (*2.9.10*)
60 per cent *V/V* to 70 per cent *V/V*.

Dry residue (*2.8.16*)
Minimum 2.0 per cent.

ASSAY

Liquid chromatography (*2.2.29*).

Test solution   In a 20.0 mL volumetric flask, dilute 3.000 g of the mother tincture to be examined to 20.0 mL with the mobile phase.

Reference solution   In a 50.0 mL volumetric flask, dissolve 20.0 mg of *hederacoside C R* in the mobile phase and dilute to 50.0 mL with the mobile phase.

Column:
— size: l = 0.25 m, Ø = 4 mm;
— stationary phase: *octadecylsilyl silica gel for chromatography R* (5 μm).

Mobile phase   Mix 35 volumes of *water R*, adjusted to pH 3 with *phosphoric acid R*, and 65 volumes of *methanol R*.

Flow rate   1 mL/min.

Detection   Spectrophotometer at 205 nm.

Injection   20 μL.

Retention time   Hederacoside C = about 8 min.

Calculate the percentage content *m/m* of hederacoside C using the following expression:

$$\frac{A_1 \times m_2 \times C \times 0.4}{A_2 \times m_1}$$

A_1 = area of the peak due to hederacoside C in the chromatogram obtained with the test solution;
A_2 = area of the peak due to hederacoside C in the chromatogram obtained with the reference solution;
m_1 = mass of the mother tincture in the test solution, in grams;
m_2 = mass of *hederacoside C R* in the reference solution, in grams;
C = percentage content of *hederacoside C R*.

Ph Eur

Honey Bee for Homoeopathic Preparations

(*Ph Eur monograph 2024*)

Ph Eur _____

DEFINITION
Live worker honey bee (*Apis mellifera* L.).

CHARACTERS
Characters described under Identification.

PRODUCTION
If the bee has been exposed to treatment to prevent or cure diseases, appropriate steps are taken to ensure that the levels of residues are as low as possible.

IDENTIFICATION
The body of a honey bee is about 15 mm long, black, with a silky sheen, and covered with red hairs with a touch of grey. The broad tibiae are without spines. The posterior margins of the segments and legs are brown, with gradual transition to orange-red. The claws are two-membered, the maxillary palps single-membered. On the hind legs are baskets or scoops invested with bristles. The wings have 3 complete cubital cells, with the radial cell twice as long as it is wide; the 3 cells on the lower margin and the 3 middle cells are closed. A duct connects the barbed sting with the poison sac.

MOTHER TINCTURE

The mother tincture complies with the requirements of the general monograph on *Mother tinctures for homoeopathic preparations (2029)*.

PRODUCTION
The mother tincture of *Apis mellifera* L. is prepared by maceration using alcohol of a suitable concentration.

CHARACTERS
Pale yellow liquid that may darken on storage.

IDENTIFICATION
Thin-layer chromatography (*2.2.27*).

Test solution   The mother tincture to be examined.

Reference solution   Dissolve 12 mg of *4-aminobutanoic acid R*, 12 mg of *leucine R* and 12 mg of *proline R* in 5 mL of *water R* and dilute to 50 mL with *alcohol R*.

Plate   TLC silica gel plate R.

Mobile phase   water R, ethanol R (17:63 *V/V*).

Application   20 μL, as bands.

Development   Over a path of 10 cm.

Drying   In air.

Detection   Spray with *ninhydrin solution R* and heat at 100-105 °C for 10 min; examine in daylight.

Results   See below the sequence of the zones present in the chromatograms obtained with the reference and test solutions. Other zones may also be visible.

TESTS
Relative density (*2.2.5*)
0.890 to 0.910.

Ethanol (*2.9.10*)
60 per cent *V/V* to 70 per cent *V/V*.

Dry residue (*2.8.16*)
Minimum 0.30 per cent.

_____ *Ph Eur*

Top of the plate	
	A pink zone
Leucine: a pink zone	A pink zone
	A pink zone
	A pink zone
Proline: an orange-yellow zone	An orange-yellow zone
4-Aminobutanoic acid: a pink zone	A pink zone
Reference solution	**Test solution**

Hydrastis Canadensis for Homoeopathic Preparations

(*Ph Eur monograph 2500*)

Ph Eur _____

The herbal drug complies with the requirements of the monograph *Goldenseal rhizome (1831)*.

MOTHER TINCTURE
The mother tincture complies with the requirements of the general monograph *Mother tinctures for homoeopathic preparations (2029)*.

DEFINITION
The mother tincture is prepared from the whole or cut, dried rhizome and roots of *Hydrastis canadensis* L.

Content:
— hydrastine ($C_{21}H_{21}NO_6$; M_r 383.4): 0.10 per cent to 0.40 per cent;
— berberine ($C_{20}H_{18}NO_4$; M_r 336.4): 0.20 per cent to 0.50 per cent.

PRODUCTION
The mother tincture is prepared by the following methods prescribed in the monograph *Methods of preparation of homoeopathic stocks and potentisation (2371)*:
— Method 1.1.8, using the powdered herbal drug (710) (*2.9.12*) and ethanol (70 per cent *V/V* [or ethanol (62 per cent *m/m*)];
— Method 1.1.10, using the fragmented herbal drug (pieces about 1 cm in diameter), ethanol (65 per cent *V/V*) and maceration for 3-5 weeks.

CHARACTERS
Appearance
Yellowish-brown liquid.

IDENTIFICATION
Thin-layer chromatography (*2.2.27*).

Test solution   The mother tincture to be examined.

Reference solution   Immediately before use, dissolve 5 mg of *hydrastine hydrochloride R* and 5 mg of *berberine chloride R* in 10 mL of *methanol R*.

Plate   TLC silica gel plate R (5-40 μm) [or TLC silica gel plate R (2-10 μm)].

Mobile phase   anhydrous formic acid R, water R, ethyl acetate R (10:10:80 *V/V/V*).

Application   20 μL [or 5 μL] as bands.

Development   Over a path of 15 cm [or 6 cm].

Drying   In air.

Detection   Examine in ultraviolet light at 365 nm.

Results   See below the sequence of fluorescent zones present in the chromatograms obtained with the reference solution and the test solution. Furthermore, other faint fluorescent zones may be present in the chromatogram obtained with the test solution.

Top of the plate	
Berberine: a bright yellow fluorescent zone	A bright yellow fluorescent zone (berberine)
Hydrastine: a deep blue fluorescent zone	A deep blue fluorescent zone (hydrastine)
Reference solution	Test solution

TESTS

Relative density *(2.2.5)*
0.890 to 0.905, where Method 1.1.8 is used.

Ethanol *(2.9.10)*
60 per cent *V/V* to 70 per cent *V/V*, where Method 1.1.10 is used.

Dry residue *(2.8.16)*
Minimum 1.2 per cent *m/m*.

ASSAY

Liquid chromatography *(2.2.29)*.

Test solution   Dilute about 1.000 g, accurately weighed, of the mother tincture to be examined to 20.0 mL with the mobile phase.

Reference solution   Immediately before use, dissolve 10.0 mg of *hydrastine hydrochloride CRS* and 10.0 mg of *berberine chloride CRS* in *methanol R* and dilute to 100.0 mL with the same solvent.

Column:
— *size*: l = 0.125 m, Ø = 4 mm;
— *stationary phase*: end-capped octadecylsilyl silica gel for chromatography *R* (5 μm).

Mobile phase   Dissolve 9.93 g of *potassium dihydrogen phosphate R* in 730 mL of *water R*, add 270 mL of *acetonitrile R* and mix.

Flow rate   1.2 mL/min.

Detection   Spectrophotometer at 235 nm.

Injection   10 μL.

Elution order   Hydrastine, berberine.

Identification of peaks   Use the chromatogram obtained with the reference solution to identify the peaks due to hydrastine and berberine.

System suitability   Reference solution:
— *resolution*: minimum 1.5 between the peaks due to hydrastine and berberine.

Calculate the percentage contents *m/m* of hydrastine using the following expression:

$$\frac{A_1 \times m_2 \times p}{A_2 \times m_1 \times 5} \times 0.913$$

Calculate the percentage contents *m/m* of berberine using the following expression:

$$\frac{A_1 \times m_2 \times p}{A_2 \times m_1 \times 5} \times 0.905$$

A_1 = area of the peak due to hydrastine or to berberine in the chromatogram obtained with the test solution;

A_2 = area of the peak due to hydrastine or to berberine in the chromatogram obtained with the reference solution;

m_1 = mass of the mother tincture to be examined used to prepare the test solution, in grams;

m_2 = mass of *hydrastine hydrochloride CRS* or mass of *berberine chloride CRS* used to prepare the reference solution, in grams;

p = percentage content of *hydrastine hydrochloride CRS* or percentage content of *berberine chloride CRS*.

Ph Eur

Hyoscyamus for Homoeopathic Preparations

(Ph Eur monograph 2091)

Ph Eur

DEFINITION

Whole, fresh flowering plant of *Hyoscyamus niger* L.

IDENTIFICATION

Hyoscyamus is an annual or biennial plant, with a well developed taproot. The robust, erect stem is hollow and subcylindrical and up to 80 cm long. The soft, viscid, dull dark-green leaves are densely pubescent on both surfaces, especially on the veins. The lower leaves are petiolate and are arranged in a rosette; the lower cauline leaves are semi-amplexicaul and the upper ones are completely amplexicaul. The lamina, up to 25 cm long, is oblong to ovate with 2 to 5 broadly dentate lobes on each side. The midrib is well developed. The secondary veins arise at a wide angle from the midrib and terminate in the apices of the lobes.
The flowering tops are densely pubescent and form a short drooping cluster. Each flower arises in the axils of a large bract. The gamosepalous calyx is covered with dense cotton-like hairs and has 5 triangular-ovate lobes, each ending in a short point that becomes spiny. The gamopetalous corolla, with 5 nearly equal lobes, is yellowish and with a delicate, brown to blackish-violet venation. The fruit, sometimes present at the base of the inflorescences, is a pyxis distinctly swollen at the base.

TESTS

Foreign matter *(2.8.2)*
If required by the competent authority, maximum 5 per cent.

Loss on drying *(2.2.32)*
If required by the competent authority, minimum 50 per cent, determined on 5.0 g of the finely cut drug by drying in an oven at 105 °C for 2 h.

***Hyoscyamus albus* L.**
The presence of middle and upper leaves with a petiole and of fruits barely swollen at the base indicates adulteration by *Hyoscyamus albus* L.

MOTHER TINCTURE

The mother tincture complies with the requirements of the general monograph on *Mother tinctures for homoeopathic preparations (2029)*.

PRODUCTION

The mother tincture of *Hyoscyamus niger* L. is prepared by maceration of the drug, using ethanol of a suitable concentration.

Content

0.002 per cent m/m to 0.01 per cent *m/m* of total alkaloids, expressed as hyoscyamine ($C_{17}H_{23}NO_3$; M_r 289.4).

CHARACTERS

Appearance

Dark greenish-brown liquid.

IDENTIFICATION

Thin-layer chromatography (*2.2.27*).

Test solution Evaporate 10 mL of the mother tincture to be examined in a water-bath at 40 °C, under reduced pressure. Take up the residue with 1 mL of *ammonia R*, and shake with 2 quantities, each of 10 mL, of *ether R*. Combine the ether layers, dry over *anhydrous sodium sulfate R* and filter. Evaporate on a water-bath and dissolve the residue in 0.50 mL of *methanol R*.

Reference solution (a) Dissolve 50 mg of *hyoscyamine sulfate R* in 10 mL of *methanol R* (solution A). Dissolve 15 mg of *hyoscine hydrobromide R* in 10 mL of *methanol R* (solution B). Mix 4 mL of solution A and 2 mL of solution B and dilute to 10 mL with *methanol R*.

Reference solution (b) Dissolve 20 mg of *atropine sulfate R* in *methanol R* and dilute to 10 mL with the same solvent.

Plate   TLC silica gel plate R.

Mobile phase   concentrated ammonia R, water R, acetone R (3:7:90 *V/V/V*).

Application   20 µL, as bands.

Development   Over a path of 10 cm.

Drying   At 100-105 °C for 15 min.

Detection A   Spray with *dilute potassium iodobismuthate solution R* until orange zones become visible. Examine in daylight.

Results A   See below the sequence of the zones present in the chromatograms obtained with the reference solutions and the test solution. Other faint zones may be present in the chromatogram obtained with the test solution.

Top of the plate		
Hyoscine: an orange zone		An orange zone (hyoscine)
———		———
Hyoscyamine: an orange zone	Atropine: an orange zone	A orange zone (hyoscyamine/atropine)
		———
———	———	Faint orange zones (line of application)
Reference solution (a)	**Reference solution (b)**	**Test solution**

Detection B   Subsequently spray with *sodium nitrite solution R* until the yellow background disappears. Examine in daylight after 15 min.

Results B   See test for atropine.

TESTS

Relative density (*2.2.5*)
0.930 to 0.960.

Atropine
Examine the chromatograms obtained in the test for identification.

Results   The zone due to hyoscyamine in the chromatogram obtained with the test solution changes from orange to reddish-brown but not to greyish-blue (atropine).

Ethanol (*2.9.10*)
40 per cent *V/V* to 50 per cent *V/V*.

Dry residue (*2.8.16*)
Minimum 1.2 per cent.

ASSAY

Evaporate 100.0 g of the mother tincture to be examined, at a low temperature under reduced pressure, until a residue of about 10 g is obtained. Quantitatively transfer the residue to a separating funnel using a few millilitres of *ethanol (70 per cent V/V) R*. Add 5 mL of *concentrated ammonia R* and 25 mL of *water R*. Extract with successive fractions of a mixture of 1 volume of *chloroform R* and 3 volumes of *peroxide-free ether R* until the alkaloids are completely extracted. Evaporate to dryness a few millilitres of the last organic fraction. Take up the residue in *0.25 M sulfuric acid* and verify the absence of alkaloids using *potassium tetraiodomercurate solution R*. Combine the organic layers and extract several times with *0.25 M sulfuric acid*. Separate the layers by centrifugation if necessary and transfer the acid layers to a second separating funnel. Make the acid layer alkaline with *ammonia R* and shake with at least 3 quantities, each of 30 mL, of *chloroform R*. Combine the chloroform layers, add 4 g of *anhydrous sodium sulfate R* and allow to stand for 30 min with occasional shaking. Decant the chloroform and wash the anhydrous sodium sulfate with 3 quantities, each of 10 mL, of *chloroform R*. Combine the chloroform fractions, evaporate to dryness on a water-bath and dry in an oven at 100-105 °C for 15 min. Dissolve the residue in a few millilitres of chloroform R, add 10.0 mL of *0.005 M sulfuric acid* and remove the chloroform by evaporation on a water-bath. Titrate the excess of acid with *0.01 M sodium hydroxide* using *methyl red mixed solution R* as indicator.

Calculate the percentage content *m/m* of total alkaloids, expressed as hyoscyamine, from the expression:

$$\frac{0.2894\,(10 - n)}{m}$$

n = volume of *0.01 M sodium hydroxide* used, in millilitres,
m = mass of the mother tincture used, in grams.

_____ *Ph Eur*

HOMOEOPATHIC PREPARATIONS

Hypericum for Homoeopathic Preparations

(Ph Eur monograph 2028)

Ph Eur _____

DEFINITION

Whole, fresh plant of *Hypericum perforatum* L., at the beginning of the flowering period.

IDENTIFICATION

The perennial plant consists of a spindle-shaped root and a branched rhizome, giving rise to long, decumbent runners. The cylindrical, erect stem is woody at the base, 0.2 m to 1 m long, branched in the upper part, with 2 raised longitudinal lines.

The leaves are opposite, sessile, exstipulate, oblong-oval and 15 mm to 30 mm long. The leaf margins show black glandular dots, and many small translucent oil glands are present on the entire surface and are visible by transmitted light.

The flowers are regular and form corymbose clusters at the apex of the stem. They have 5 green, lanceolate sepals with acuminate apices, and black oil glands near the entire margins; 5 orange-yellow petals, much longer than the sepals, with black oil glands near the terminal margins only; 3 staminal blades, each divided into many orange-yellow stamens and 3 carpels surmounted by red styles. Each petal is asymmetrically linear-ovate in shape, with one of the margin entire and the other dentate.

TESTS

Foreign matter *(2.8.2)*
Maximum 4 per cent of fruits and maximum 1 per cent of other foreign matter.

Loss on drying *(2.2.32)*
If performed to demonstrate the freshness of the drug, minimum 55 per cent, determined on 5.0 g of finely cut drug by drying in an oven at 105 °C.

MOTHER TINCTURE

The mother tincture complies with the requirements of the general monograph on *Mother tinctures for homoeopathic preparations (2029)*.

PRODUCTION

The mother tincture of *Hypericum perforatum* L. is prepared by maceration using alcohol of a suitable concentration.

CHARACTERS

Dark red to brownish red liquid.

IDENTIFICATION

Thin-layer chromatography *(2.2.27)*.

Test solution   The mother tincture to be examined.

Reference solution   Dissolve 5 mg of *rutin R*, 1 mg of *hypericin R* and 5 mg of *hyperoside R* in *methanol R* and dilute to 5 mL with the same solvent.

Plate   *TLC silica gel plate R.*

Mobile phase   *anhydrous formic acid R, water R, ethyl acetate R* (6:9:90 *V/V/V*).

Application   10 µL of the test solution and 5 µL of the reference solution, as 10 mm bands.

Development   Over a path of 10 cm.

Drying   At 100-105 °C for 10 min.

Detection   Spray with a 10 g/L solution of *diphenylboric acid aminoethyl ester R* in *methanol R* and then a 50 g/L solution of *macrogol 400 R* in *methanol R*. Examine the plates after 30 min in ultraviolet light at 365 nm.

Results   See below the sequence of the zones present in the chromatograms obtained with the reference solution and the test solution. In the chromatogram obtained with the test solution, the zone due to rutin may be weak or even absent. The chromatogram obtained with the test solution shows a group of zones that may be blue or yellow, with a R_F similar to that of the zone due to hyperoside in the chromatogram obtained with the reference solution. Other weak zones may also be visible.

Top of the plate	
	A yellow to blue zone
Hypericin: a red zone	2 red zones
————	————
	Several zones
	————
Hyperoside: a yellow to orange zone	Blue or yellow zones
Rutin: a yellow to orange zone	A yellow to orange zone
Reference solution	**Test solution**

TESTS

Relative density *(2.2.5)*
0.900 to 0.920.

Ethanol *(2.9.10)*
60 per cent *V/V* to 75 per cent *V/V*.

Dry residue *(2.8.16)*
Minimum 1.3 per cent.

_____ *Ph Eur*

Iron for Homoeopathic Preparations

Iron for Homoeopathic Use
(Ph Eur monograph 2026)

Fe	55.85	7439-89-6

Ph Eur _____

DEFINITION

Obtained by reduction or sublimation as a fine blackish-grey powder.

Content
97.5 per cent to 101.0 per cent.

CHARACTERS

Appearance
Fine, blackish-grey powder, without metallic lustre.

Solubility
Practically insoluble in water and in alcohol. It dissolves with heating in dilute mineral acids.

IDENTIFICATION

Dissolve 50 mg in 2 mL of *dilute sulfuric acid R* and dilute to 10 mL with *water R*. The solution gives reaction (a) of iron *(2.3.1)*.

TESTS

Solution S

To 10.0 g add 40 mL of *water R*. Boil for 1 min. Cool, filter and dilute to 50.0 mL with *water R*.

Alkalinity

To 10 mL of solution S add 0.1 mL of *bromothymol blue solution R1*. Not more than 0.1 mL of *0.01 M hydrochloric acid* is required to change the colour of the indicator to yellow.

Substances insoluble in hydrochloric acid

Dissolve 2.00 g in 40 mL of *hydrochloric acid R*. Heat on a water-bath. As soon as fumes are no longer evolved, filter through a sintered-glass filter (16) (*2.1.2*). Rinse with *water R*. Dry the residue in an oven at 100-105 °C for 1 h. The residue weighs a maximum of 20 mg (1.0 per cent).

Substances soluble in water

Evaporate 10.0 mL of solution S on a water-bath and dry at 100-105 °C for 1 h. The residue weighs a maximum of 2 mg (0.1 per cent).

Chlorides (*2.4.4*)

Maximum 50 ppm.

Dilute 5 mL of solution S to 15 mL with *water R*.
The solution complies with the limit test for chlorides.

Sulfides and phosphides

In a 100 mL conical flask carefully mix 1.0 g with 10 mL of *dilute hydrochloric acid R*. Within 30 s *lead acetate paper R* moistened with *water R* and placed over the mouth of the flask is not coloured more intensely than light brown by the resulting fumes.

Arsenic (*2.4.2*)

Maximum 5 ppm.

Boil 0.2 g in 25 mL of *dilute hydrochloric acid R* until completely dissolved. The solution complies with limit test A.

Copper

Maximum 50 ppm.

Atomic absorption spectrometry (*2.2.23, Method I*).

Test solution Dissolve 1.00 g in a mixture of 60 mL of *dilute hydrochloric acid R* and 10 mL of *dilute hydrogen peroxide solution R*. Reduce to a volume of 5 mL and dilute to 50.0 mL with *water R*.

Reference solutions Prepare the reference solutions using *copper standard solution (0.1 per cent Cu) R*, diluted as necessary with a 1 per cent *V/V* solution of *hydrochloric acid R*.

Source Copper hollow-cathode lamp.

Wavelength 324.8 nm.

Flame Air-acetylene.

Lead

Maximum 50 ppm.

Atomic absorption spectrometry (*2.2.23, Method I*).

Test solution In a separating funnel, place 20 mL of the test solution prepared for the test for copper. Add 25 mL of *lead-free hydrochloric acid R*. Stir with 3 quantities, each of 25 mL, of *di-isopropyl ether R*. Collect the aqueous layer. Add 0.10 g of *sodium sulfate decahydrate R*. Evaporate to dryness. Take up the residue with 1 mL of *lead-free nitric acid R* and dilute to 20 mL with *water R*.

Reference solutions Prepare the reference solutions using *lead standard solution (0.1 per cent Pb) R*, diluted as necessary with a 10 per cent *V/V* solution of *nitric acid R* containing 5 g/L of *sodium sulfate decahydrate R*.

Source Lead hollow-cathode lamp.

Wavelength 217 nm.

Flame Air-acetylene.

ASSAY

Stir for 10 min 0.100 g in a hot solution of 1.25 g of *copper sulfate R* in 20 mL of *water R* in a 100 mL conical flask with a ground-glass stopper. Filter rapidly and wash the filter. Combine the filtrate and the washings, acidify with *dilute sulfuric acid R* and titrate with *0.02 M potassium permanganate* until a pink colour is obtained.

1 mL of *0.02 M potassium permanganate* is equivalent to 5.585 mg of Fe.

LABELLING

The label indicates whether the iron for homoeopathic preparations is obtained by reduction or sublimation.

_____ *Ph Eur*

Hydrated Iron(III) Phosphate for Homoeopathic Preparations

$FePO_4, 4H_2O$ 222.8   *10045-86-0*
(anhydrous)

DEFINITION

Hydrated Iron(III) Phosphate for Homoeopathic Preparations contains hydrated iron(III) phosphate. It contains not less than 96.0% and not more than 106.5% of $FePO_4, 4H_2O$.

CHARACTERISTICS

A yellow to pale ochre powder.

Insoluble in *water;* soluble in dilute mineral acids.

IDENTIFICATION

Dissolve 0.5 g of the substance being examined in 5 mL of *dilute hydrochloric acid*, with warming. Dilute the resulting solution to 35 mL with *water* and filter if necessary (solution S).

A. Solution S yields reactions B and C characteristic of *iron and iron salts*, Appendix VI.

B. Solution S yields reaction B characteristic of *phosphates*, Appendix VI.

TESTS

Clarity of solution

Solution S is *clear*, Appendix IV A, Method II.

Chloride

To 0.05 g of the substance being examined add 1 mL of *dilute nitric acid*. Heat, dilute with 14 mL of *water* and filter. The filtrate complies with the *limit test for chlorides*, Appendix VII (0.1%).

Heavy metals

Dissolve 1.0 g of the substance being examined in 20 mL of *hydrochloric acid* if necessary with heating. Extract the solution using five 20-mL quantities of a mixture of 100 mL of freshly distilled *methyl isobutyl ketone* and 1 mL of *hydrochloric acid R1*. Allow to stand, separate the aqueous layer and evaporate to half its volume, allow to cool and dilute to 35 mL with *water*. Neutralise 7.5 mL of this solution to *litmus paper* using *dilute ammonia R1* and dilute to 15 mL with *water*. 12 mL of the resulting solution complies with *limit test heavy metals*, Appendix VII, Method A (70 ppm). Use *lead standard solution (1 ppm Pb)* to prepare the standard.

Loss on drying

When dried to constant weight at 200°, loses not less than 28% and not more than 33% of its weight, Appendix IX D. Use 1 g.

ASSAY

Dissolve 0.45 g in 3 mL of *hydrochloric acid R1* in an iodine flask, add 10 mL of *water* and 6.0 g of *potassium iodide,* close the flask and allow to stand protected from light for 30 minutes. Add 100 mL of *water* and 1 mL of *starch solution* and titrate with 0.1M *sodium thiosulfate VS.* Each mL of 0.1M *sodium thiosulfate VS* is equivalent to 22.29 mg of $FePO_4,4H_2O$.

PRODUCTION OF STOCK

The first decimal trituration of Hydrated Iron(III) Phosphate for Homoeopathic Preparations is prepared using a suitable quantity of Lactose or Anhydrous Lactose as the vehicle and a validated trituration method that ensures homogeneity is achieved. The vehicle complies with the statement under Vehicles in the monograph for Homoeopathic Preparations.

Content of hydrated iron(iii) phosphate FePO₄, 4H₂O

The first decimal trituration contains 9.0% to 11.0% of $FePO_4, 4H_2O$.

CHARACTERISTICS

The first decimal trituration is a yellowish powder.

IDENTIFICATION

Dissolve, with warming, 1.5 g of the first decimal trituration in a mixture of 1.5 mL of *dilute hydrochloric acid* and 9 mL of *water* (solution S1).

A. Solution S1 yields reactions B and C characteristic of *iron and iron salts,* Appendix VI.

B. Solution S1 yields reaction B characteristic of *phosphates,* Appendix VI.

C. Dissolve 0.25 g of the substance being examined in 5 mL of *water.* Add 5 mL of *ammonia* and heat in a water-bath at 80° for 10 minutes. A red colour develops.

ASSAY

Dissolve 4.0 g of the first decimal trituration in 3 mL of *hydrochloric acid R1* in an iodine flask, add 10 mL of *water* and 8.0 g of *potassium iodide,* close the flask and allow to stand protected from light for 30 minutes. Add 100 mL of *water* and 1 mL of *starch solution* and titrate with 0.1M *sodium thiosulfate VS.* Each mL of 0.1M *sodium thiosulfate VS* is equivalent to 22.29 mg of $FePO_4,4H_2O$.

STORAGE

Hydrated Iron(III) Phosphate for Homoeopathic Preparations should be protected from light.

Hydrated Iron(ii) and Iron(iii) Phosphate for Homoeopathic Preparations

DEFINITION

Hydrated Iron(II) and Iron(III) Phosphate for Homoeopathic Preparations contains a mixture of hydrated iron(II) phosphate and iron(III) phosphate and some hydrated oxides of iron. It contains not less than 16.0% of Fe^{2+}, equivalent to not less than 47.9% of $Fe_3(PO_4)_2,8H_2O$.

CHARACTERISTICS

A slate blue amorphous powder.

Insoluble in *water;* soluble in *hydrochloric acid.*

IDENTIFICATION

Dissolve 0.5 g in 5 mL of *dilute hydrochloric acid* with warming. Dilute the resulting solution to 35 mL with *water* and filter if necessary (solution S).

A. Solution S yields the reactions characteristic of *iron and iron salts,* Appendix VI.

B. Solution S yields the reactions characteristic of *phosphates,* Appendix VI.

TESTS

Heavy metals

Dissolve 1.0 g of the substance being examined in 20 mL of *hydrochloric acid.* Extract the solution using five 20-mL quantities of a mixture of 100 mL of freshly distilled *methyl isobutyl ketone* with 1 mL of *hydrochloric acid R1.* Allow to stand, separate the aqueous layer and evaporate to half its volume, allow to cool and dilute to 35 mL with *water.* Neutralise 7.5 mL of this solution to *litmus paper* using *dilute ammonia R1* and dilute to 15 mL with *water.* 12 mL of the resulting solution complies with *limit test A for heavy metals,* Appendix VII (70 ppm). Use *lead standard solution (1 ppm Pb)* to prepare the standard.

Sulfates

Dissolve 0.25 g of the substance being examined in *water.* Add 3 mL of *dilute hydrochloric acid* and dilute to 15 mL with *water.* The resulting solution complies with the *limit test for sulfates,* Appendix VII.

ASSAY

Dissolve 0.3 g of the substance being examined in 3 mL of *orthophosphoric acid* and 10 mL of a 14% v/v solution of *sulfuric acid* in *water.* Add 100 mL of *water* and titrate with 0.1M *potassium permanganate.* Each mL of 0.1M *potassium permanganate VS* is equivalent to 27.925 mg of Fe^{2+}.

PRODUCTION OF STOCK

The first decimal trituration of Hydrated Iron(II) and Iron(III) Phosphate for Homoeopathic Preparations is prepared using a suitable quantity of Lactose or Anhydrous Lactose as the vehicle and a validated trituration method that ensures homogeneity is achieved. The vehicle complies with the statement under Vehicles in the monograph for Homoeopathic Preparations.

Content of hydrated iron(ii) and iron(iii) phosphate

The first decimal trituration contains 4.5% to 5.0% of $Fe_3(PO_4)_2, 8H_2O$.

CHARACTERISTICS

The first decimal trituration is a light grey powder.

IDENTIFICATION

A. Yields the reactions characteristic of *iron and iron salts,* Appendix VI.

B. Yields the reactions characteristic of *phosphates,* Appendix VI.

C. Dissolve 0.25 g in 5 mL of *water.* Add 5 mL of *ammonia* and heat in a water-bath at 80° for 10 minutes. A red colour develops.

ASSAY

Dissolve 3.0 g of the first decimal trituration in 3 mL of *orthophosphoric acid* and 10 mL of a 14% v/v solution of *sulfuric acid* in *water.* Add 100 mL of *water* and titrate with 0.1M *potassium permanganate.* Each mL of 0.1M *potassium permanganate VS* is equivalent to 27.925 mg of Fe^{2+}.

STORAGE

Hydrated Iron(II) and Iron(III) Phosphate for Homoeopathic Preparations should be protected from light.

Medicago Sativa for Homoeopathic Preparations

DEFINITION

Medicago Sativa for Homoeopathic Preparations is the fresh whole flowering plant of *Medicago sativa* L.

IDENTIFICATION

Plant A herbaceous perennial, reaching up to 100 cm.

Leaves Alternate, petiolate, trifoliolate, leaflets mucronate, approximately 2 cm long, 1 cm broad, typically oblanceolate or oblong, with a toothed or entire margin, glabrous on the upper surface and sparsely pubescent on the lower surface; stipules lanceolate, up to 1 cm long, toothed to entire.

Stems 4-angled, branching, glabrous to pubescent.

Flowers Compact, axillary, racemes of up to 40 flowers, peduncle up to 3 cm long, typically pubescent; corolla papilionaceous, up to 1 cm long, 5 mm broad, purple to whitish; calyx tube approximately 5 mm in length, 2 mm in diameter, 5-lobed, typically glabrous, lobes equal or subequal, up to 4 mm long.

MOTHER TINCTURE

The mother tincture complies with the requirements stated under Mother Tinctures for Homoeopathic Preparations and with the following requirements.

PRODUCTION

The mother tincture of Medicago sativa *L.* is prepared from the herbal drug using *method 1.1.5* described in the monograph for Methods of Preparation of Homoeopathic Stocks and Potentisation. Use 86% w/w (90% v/v) of *ethanol.*

CHARACTERISTICS

The mother tincture is a greenish-brown liquid.

IDENTIFICATION

Carry out the method for *thin-layer chromatography*, Appendix III A, using the following solutions.

(1) The mother tincture.

(2) 0.1% w/v *coumarin BPCRS* and 0.05% w/v of *formononetin BPCRS* in *methanol.*

CHROMATOGRAPHIC CONDITIONS

(a) Use as the coating *silica gel 60 F$_{254}$ (*Merck silica gel 60 precoated plates are suitable).

(b) Use the mobile phase described below.

(c) Apply 10 µL of each solution as 3 mm bands.

(d) Develop the plate to 15 cm.

(e) After removal of the plate dry in air and examine under *ultra-violet light (365 nm)*.

(f) Spray the plate with *anisaldehyde solution* and heat at 105° for 5 minutes and examine under *ultra-violet light (365 nm)*.

MOBILE PHASE

10 volumes of *methanol* and 90 volumes of *toluene*.

SYSTEM SUITABILITY

The test is not valid unless, in the chromatogram obtained with solution (2), two clearly separated bands are observed under *ultra-violet light (365 nm)* before and after spraying with *anisaldehyde solution*.

CONFIRMATION

Under ultra-violet light, the chromatogram obtained with solution (1) shows the following fluorescent bands: one blue or pink fluorescent band close to the origin, followed by a blue or pink fluorescent band and then a blue band below the band obtained for formononetin in solution (2), followed by one or two blue bands approximately level with formononetin

and a red band between the bands obtained for formononetin and coumarin in solution (2). Other bands may be present in the chromatogram obtained with solution (1).

Ultraviolet light (365 nm)

Top of the plate	
	Coumarin: a turquoise blue fluorescent band
Red fluorescent band	
One or two blue fluorescent bands	Formononetin: a turquoise blue fluorescent band with slight tailing
Blue fluorescent band	
Blue or pink fluorescent band	
Blue or pink fluorescent band	
Solution (1)	**Solution (2)**

The chromatogram obtained with solution (1) sprayed with the anisaldehyde solution shows the following fluorescent bands: a faint blue band close to the origin, followed by a faint purple or blue fluorescent band and a blue band below the band obtained for formononetin in solution (2), followed by three yellow to orange bands between the bands obtained for formononetin and coumarin in solution (2) and an orange band between the band obtained for coumarin and the solvent front. Other bands may be present in the chromatogram obtained with solution (1).

Anisaldehyde solution spray and ultraviolet light (365 nm)

Top of the plate	
Orange fluorescent band	
	Coumarin: a faint indigo blue fluorescent band
Yellow orange fluorescent band	
Faint orange fluorescent band	
Orange fluorescent band	Formononetin: a yellow fluorescent band
Blue fluorescent band	
Faint purple or blue fluorescent band	
Faint blue band	
Solution (1)	**Solution (2)**

CHARACTERISTICS

The mother tincture is a greenish-brown liquid.

TESTS

Ethanol
55% to 65% w/w (63% to 72% v/v), Appendix VIII F.

Dry residue
Not less than 1.0% w/w, Appendix XI P.

Relative density
0.880 to 0.950, Appendix V G.

Potassium Dichromate for Homoeopathic Preparations

(*Ph Eur monograph 2501*)

K$_2$Cr$_2$O$_7$	294.2	7778-50-9

Ph Eur

DEFINITION

Content
99.0 per cent to 101.0 per cent of K$_2$Cr$_2$O$_7$.

CHARACTERS

Appearance
Orange crystals.

Solubility
Freely soluble in water, practically insoluble in ethanol (96 per cent).

IDENTIFICATION

A. It gives reaction (b) of potassium (*2.3.1*).

B. Dissolve 10 mg in 5 mL of *water R*. Add 0.25 mL of *dilute sulfuric acid R*, 0.5 mL of *strong hydrogen peroxide solution R* and 1 mL of *ether R*. Shake. The upper layer is blue.

TESTS

Solution S1
Dissolve 5.0 g in *distilled water R* and dilute to 50.0 mL with the same solvent.

Solution S2
To 20.0 mL of solution S1 add 20 mL of *hydrochloric acid R* and 50 mL of *tributyl phosphate R*. Stir for 2 min. Remove the lower layer and shake it with 10 mL of *ether R*. Evaporate the lower layer to dryness under reduced pressure. Dissolve the residue in 10 mL of *distilled water R*. Add *dilute ammonia R1* until the solution is neutral to *blue litmus paper R* and dilute to 20.0 mL with *distilled water R*.

Appearance of solution
Solution S1 is clear (*2.2.1*).

Calcium (*2.4.3*)
Maximum 500 ppm.

Dilute 2.0 mL of solution S2 to 15 mL with *distilled water R*.

Chlorides (*2.4.4*)
Maximum 50 ppm.

Dissolve 1.0 g in 15 mL of *dilute nitric acid R*. Use 1 mL of *nitric acid R* instead of the prescribed *dilute nitric acid R*.

Sulfates (*2.4.13*)
Maximum 150 ppm.

Dilute 10 mL of solution S2 to 15 mL with *distilled water R*.

ASSAY

Dissolve 0.100 g in 25 mL of *water R*. Add 2 g of *potassium iodide R* and 25 mL of *dilute sulfuric acid R*. Allow to stand in the dark for 10 min. Add 150 mL of *water R*. Titrate with *0.1 M sodium thiosulfate* until the colour changes from blue to green, adding 1 mL of *starch solution R* near the end of the titration.

1 mL of *0.1 M sodium thiosulfate* is equivalent to 4.903 mg of K$_2$Cr$_2$O$_7$.

Ph Eur

Prunus Spinosa Fruit for Homoeopathic Preparations

DEFINITION

Prunus Spinosa Fruit for Homoeopathic Preparations is the fresh ripe fruit of *Prunus spinosa* L.

IDENTIFICATION

The ripe fruit is nearly a globose drupe, 8 to 15 mm in diameter, bluish-black with a blue-grey bloom. The dense green pulp surrounds a hard, spherical to ovoid and flattened stone, 6 to 9 mm long, 6 to 8 mm wide and 4 to 6 mm thick. The stone bulges slightly and has a sharp edge.

MOTHER TINCTURE

The mother tincture complies with the requirements stated under Mother Tinctures for Homoeopathic Preparations and with the following requirements.

PRODUCTION

The mother tincture of *Prunus spinosa* L. is prepared from the herbal drug using *Method 1.1.7* described in the monograph for Methods of Preparation of Homoeopathic Stocks and Potentisation. Use 43% w/w (50% v/v) of *ethanol*.

CHARACTERISTICS

The mother tincture is a purple-red to red, clear to slightly turbid liquid.

IDENTIFICATION

Carry out the method for *thin-layer chromatography*, Appendix III A, using the following solutions.

(1) Centrifuge 10 mL of the mother tincture at about 3000 rpm for 5 minutes. Precondition a cartridge containing octadecyl-bonded silica sorbent (a Sep-pak C18 cartridge is suitable) with 10 mL of *methanol* followed by 10 mL of *water*. Apply 4.5 mL of the clear supernatant to the column, wash with 5 mL *water* and elute with 5 mL of *methanol*. Evaporate the eluant on a rotary evaporator at 50°. Dissolve the residue in 1 mL of *methanol*.

(2) 0.025% w/v of *chlorogenic acid* and 0.005% w/v of *scopoletin* in *methanol*.

CHROMATOGRAPHIC CONDITIONS

(a) Use as the coating *silica gel F$_{254}$*.

(b) Use the mobile phase described below.

(c) Apply 40 µL of each solution as 12 mm bands.

(d) Develop the plate to 15 cm.

(e) After removal of the plate, dry it in air and spray with a 1% w/v solution of *diphenylboric acid aminoethyl ester* in *methanol*, followed by a 5% w/v solution of *polyethylene glycol 400* in *methanol* and examine under *ultraviolet light (365 nm)*.

MOBILE PHASE

15 volumes of *anhydrous formic acid*, 15 volumes of *water* and 70 volumes of *ethyl acetate*.

SYSTEM SUITABILITY

The test is not valid unless the chromatogram obtained with solution (2) shows a yellow-green fluorescent band (chlorogenic acid) in the middle third of the plate and a blue fluorescent band (scopoletin) in the upper third of the plate.

CONFIRMATION

The chromatogram obtained with solution (1) shows at least one orange fluorescent band below chlorogenic acid, one yellow-green fluorescent band with the Rf of chlorogenic acid and one orange fluorescent band below scopoletin.

In addition the following bands may be present: a blue fluorescent band with the same Rf as scopoletin and an orange fluorescent band with an Rf slightly higher than that of scopoletin. Two or more orange fluorescent bands may be present between the two standards.

Top of the plate	
	Scopoletin: a blue band
Orange band	
A yellow-green band	Chlorogenic acid: a yellow-green band
Orange band	
Solution (1)	Solution (2)

TESTS

Ethanol
24 to 34% w/w (29.3 to 40.8% v/v), Appendix VIII F.

Dry residue
Not less than 3.5% w/w, Appendix XI P.

Relative density
0.955 to 0.995, Appendix V G.

Common Stinging Nettle for Homoeopathic Preparations

(*Ph Eur monograph 2030*)

Ph Eur _____

DEFINITION
Whole, fresh, flowering plant of Urtica dioica L.

CHARACTERS
The plant causes an itching, burning sensation on the skin.

IDENTIFICATION
A. Common stinging nettle is perennial. The taproot sends out creeping subterranean rhizomes, more or less 4-angled in transverse section, from which extend adventious secondary roots and very numerous brownish hairy rootlets. The stipes are erect, generally unbranched, 3-5 mm in diameter and 0.3-1.5 m high, rarely up to 2.5 m high, 4-angled, greyish-green and covered in short hairs and stinging hairs.

The decussate leaves are 30-150 mm long and 20-80 mm wide. The petiole is hispid and usually slightly less than one-third the length of the lamina. The leaf blade is ovate, acuminate, cordate or rounded at the base, and coarsely dentate; the apical tooth is distinctly larger than the lateral teeth. The upper side of the leaves is dark green and usually matt, both sides bear short serried hairs intermingled with long stinging hairs. The 2 stipules are linear-subulate and free. The inflorescences growing from the leaf axils are complex, the flowers unisexual, and, particularly in male plants, generally distinctly longer than the petiole. After shedding their pollen, male inflorescences are erect at an oblique angle or horizontal; female inflorescences are pendent when the fruit is ripe. All flowers have long stalks. The perianth of the male flowers is divided half-way down into equal green lobes, widest at their base, with short bristles and stinging hairs at the margins. The stamens are equal and opposite to the perianth segments, each with a long, whitish filament that curves inwards before pollen is shed and spreads out afterwards. The ovary is rudimentary, button or cup-shaped. The perianth of the female flowers is downy or bristly on the outside and consists of outer, and 2 inner segments; the inner segments are about twice the length of the outer ones. The hypogynous, ovate, unilocular ovary bears a large capitate stigma with a brush-like shock of hair. As the one-seeded fruit grows ripe, the 2 inner segments of the perianth fold around it like wings.

B. It complies with the test for *Urtica urens* (see Tests).

TESTS
Urtica urens
The margin of the lamina is not serrate with teeth twice as long as wide. The clusters of flowers in the axils are longer than the petiole of the leaf. Unisexual, apetalous flowers are not together on the same plant and in the same cluster.

Foreign matter (*2.8.2*)
Maximum 5 per cent.

Loss on drying (*2.2.32*)
Minimum 65.0 per cent, determined on 5.0 g of finely cut drug by drying in an oven at 105 °C for 2 h, if performed to demonstrate the freshness of the drug.

MOTHER TINCTURE

The mother tincture complies with the requirements of the general monograph on *Mother tinctures for homoeopathic preparations (2029)*.

PRODUCTION
The mother tincture of *Urtica dioica* L. is prepared by maceration using alcohol of a suitable concentration.

CHARACTERS
Appearance
Greenish-brown or orange-brown liquid.

IDENTIFICATION
Thin-layer chromatography (*2.2.27*).

Test solution   The mother tincture to be examined.

Reference solution   Dissolve 10 mg of *phenylalanine R* and 10 mg of *serine R* in a mixture of equal volumes of *methanol R* and *water R* and dilute to 10 mL with the same mixture of solvents.

Plate   *TLC silica gel plate R.*

Mobile phase glacial acetic acid *R*, water *R*, acetone *R*, butanol *R* (10:20:35:35 *V/V/V/V*).

Application 20 µL, as bands.

Development Over a path of 10 cm.

Drying In air.

Detection Spray with a 1 g/L solution of *ninhydrin R* in *alcohol R*. Heat the plate at 105-110 °C for 5-10 min then examine in daylight within 10 min.

Results See below the sequence of the zones present in the chromatograms obtained with the reference solution and the test solution.

Top of the plate	
Phenylalanine: a violet to reddish-brown zone	
	4 red to violet zones
Serine: a reddish-violet zone	A violet zone
	A violet zone
Reference solution	**Test solution**

TESTS

Relative density (*2.2.5*)
0.930 to 0.950.

Ethanol (*2.9.10*)
40 per cent *V/V* to 56 per cent *V/V*.

Methanol (*2.9.11*)
Maximum 0.10 per cent *V/V*.

Dry residue (*2.8.16*)
Minimum 1.1 per cent.

————————————————— *Ph Eur*

Saffron for Homoeopathic Preparations

Saffron for Homoeopathic Use

(*Ph Eur monograph 1624*)

Ph Eur ————

DEFINITION

Dried stigmas of *Crocus sativus* L. usually joined by the base to a short style.

CHARACTERS

Characteristic, aromatic odour.

IDENTIFICATION

A. The dark brick-red stigmas, when dry, are 20 mm to 40 mm long and after soaking with water, about 35 mm to 50 mm long. The tubes, gradually widening at the top, are incised on one side, the upper margin is open and finely crenated. The style connecting the 3 stigmas is pale yellow and not more than 5 mm long.

B. Examine under a microscope using *chloral hydrate solution R*. It shows the following diagnostic characters: elongated epidermal cells, frequently with a short, central papilla; in water they release a yellow colouring matter; the upper border of the stigma has finger-shaped papillae, up to 150 µm long; between them are single, globular pollen grains, about 100 µm wide, with a finely pitted exine,

vascular bundles with small spirally thickened vessels and no fibres.

C. Carefully crush pieces of the drug to coarse particles and moisten with 0.2 mL of *phosphomolybdic acid solution R*. The particles turn blue within 1-2 min or they have a blue areole around them.

D. Examine by thin-layer chromatography (*2.2.27*).

Test solution Carefully crush 0.1 g of the drug with a glass rod and moisten with 0.2 mL of *water R*. After 3 min add 5 mL of *methanol R*, allow to stand for 20 min, protected from light, and filter through a plug of glass wool.

Reference solution Dissolve 5 mg of *naphthol yellow R* in 5 mL of *methanol R* and add a solution of 5 mg of *Sudan red G R* in 5 mL of *methylene chloride R*.

Plate TLC silica gel F$_{254}$ plate *R*.

Mobile phase water *R*, 2-propanol *R*, ethyl acetate *R* (10:25:65 *V/V/V*).

Application 10 µL of the test solution and 5 µL of the reference solution as bands.

Development Over a path of 10 cm.

Drying In air.

Detection Examine in daylight.

Results See below the sequence of the zones present in the chromatograms obtained with the reference and test solutions.

Top of the plate	
A red zone	
A yellow zone	
	2 yellow zones
	An intense yellow zone (crocine)
Reference solution	**Test solution**

Detection In ultraviolet light at 254 nm.

Results See below the sequence of the zones present in the chromatograms obtained with the reference and test solutions.

Top of the plate	
A red zone	1 or 2 quenching zones
A yellow zone	A quenching zone
Reference solution	**Test solution**

Detection Spray with *anisaldehyde solution R* and examine in daylight while heating at 100-105 °C for 5-10 min.

Results See below the sequence of the zones present in the chromatograms obtained with the reference and test solutions.

Top of the plate	
A red zone	1 or 2 red to reddish-violet zones
A blue to bluish-green zone	A red to reddish-violet zone
	2 blue to bluish-green zones
	An intense blue to bluish-green zone (crocine)
Reference solution	**Test solution**

E. Dilute 0.1 mL of the test solution (see Identification test D) with 1 mL of *methanol R*. Deposit 0.1 mL of this solution on a filter paper, allow to dry and spray with a 10 g/L solution of *diphenylboric acid aminoethyl ester R* in *methanol R*. Examine in ultraviolet light at 365 nm. The spot shows an intense orange-yellow fluorescence.

TESTS

Colouring intensity
Introduce 0.10 g into a 5 mL volumetric flask and add to 5.0 mL with *distilled water R*. Close the flask and shake every 30 min for 8 h. Then allow to stand for 16 h. Dilute 1.0 mL to 500.0 mL with *distilled water R*. The absorbance (*2.2.25*) measured at 440 nm using *distilled water R* as the compensation liquid, is not less than 0.44.

Foreign matter
Examine the drug microscopically. No parts with rough walls, no crystals and no pollen grains containing 3 germinal pores are present.

Loss on drying (*2.2.32*)
Maximum 10.0 per cent, determined on 0.200 g by drying in an oven at 105 °C.

Total ash (*2.4.16*)
Maximum 7.0 per cent, determined on the residue obtained in the test for loss on drying.

———————————————————— Ph Eur

Sodium Tetrachloroaurate Dihydrate for Homoeopathic Preparations

(*Ph Eur monograph 2141*)

$Na[AuCl_4],2H_2O$ 397.8

Ph Eur ————————————————————

DEFINITION
Sodium tetrachloroaurate(1-) dihydrate.

Content
97.0 per cent to 101.0 per cent of $Na[AuCl_4],2H_2O$.

CHARACTERS

Appearance
Orange-yellow, hygroscopic powder or crystals.

Solubility
Very soluble or freely soluble in water and in ethanol (96 per cent).

IDENTIFICATION
A. Dissolve 20 mg in 2.0 mL of *0.1 M nitric acid*. Add 0.1 g of *oxalic acid R* and boil in a water-bath for 1 h. A deposit of metallic gold is formed.

B. Solution S (see Tests) gives reaction (a) of chlorides (*2.3.1*).

C. Solution S gives reaction (b) of sodium (*2.3.1*).

TESTS

Solution S
Ignite 0.20 g in a porcelain crucible at 600 °C ± 50 °C for 30 min. Allow to cool and extract with 3 mL of *water R*, heating if necessary. Use the supernatant.

Free hydrochloric acid
When a glass rod impregnated with *concentrated ammonia R* is held close to the substance to be examined, no white fumes are produced.

Nitrates
Maximum 200 ppm.

Dissolve 0.20 g in 10 mL of *nitrate-free water R*. Add 0.2 g of *oxalic acid R*. Heat the solution on a water-bath for 30 min, allow to cool and filter. Rinse the filter with *nitrate-free water R* and dilute the filtrate to 20 mL with the same solvent. To 1.0 mL of the solution obtained add 4.0 mL of *nitrate-free water R*, 0.4 mL of a 100 g/L solution of *potassium chloride R*, 0.1 mL of *diphenylamine solution R* and, dropwise with shaking, 5 mL of *nitrogen-free sulfuric acid R*. Transfer the tube to a water-bath at 50 °C. After 15 min, any blue colour in the solution is not more intense than that in a reference solution prepared at the same time in the same manner using a mixture of 0.2 mL of *nitrate standard solution (10 ppm NO₃) R* and 4.8 mL of *nitrate-free water R*.

Heavy metals (*2.4.8*)
Maximum 100 ppm.

Dissolve 0.20 g in 15 mL of *water R*. Add 0.25 g of *hydrazine sulfate R*. Heat the solution on a water-bath for 30 min, allow to cool and filter. Rinse the filter with *water R* and dilute the filtrate to 20 mL with the same solvent. 12 mL of the solution complies with test A. Prepare the reference solution using *lead standard solution (1 ppm Pb) R*.

ASSAY
Dissolve 40.0 mg in 10 mL of *potassium iodide solution R*. Allow to stand for 5 min. Titrate with *0.01 M sodium thiosulfate* until decolourised. Shortly before reaching the endpoint, add 0.5 mL of *starch solution R*.

1 mL of *0.01 M sodium thiosulfate* is equivalent to 1.989 mg of $Na[AuCl_4],2H_2O$.

STORAGE
In an airtight container, protected from light.

———————————————————— Ph Eur

Sulfur for Homoeopathic Preparations

(*Ph Eur monograph 2515*)

S   32.07   *7704-34-9*

Ph Eur ————————————————————

DEFINITION
Obtained by sublimation.

Content
99.0 per cent to 101.0 per cent.

CHARACTERS

Appearance
Yellow powder.

Solubility
Practically insoluble in water, soluble in carbon disulfide, slightly soluble in vegetable oils.

mp
About 120 °C.

IDENTIFICATION
A. Heated in the presence of air, it burns with a blue flame, emitting sulfur dioxide, which changes the colour of moistened *blue litmus paper R* to red.

B. Heat 0.1 g with 0.5 mL of *bromine water R* until decolourised. Add 5 mL of *water R* and filter. The solution gives reaction (a) of sulfates (*2.3.1*).

TESTS

Solution S

To 5.0 g add 50 mL of *carbon dioxide-free water R* prepared from *distilled water R*. Allow to stand for 30 min with frequent shaking and filter.

Appearance of solution

Solution S is colourless (*2.2.2, Method II*).

Odour (*2.3.4*)

It has no perceptible odour of hydrogen sulfide.

Acidity or alkalinity

To 5 mL of solution S add 0.1 mL of *phenolphthalein solution R1*. The solution is colourless. Add 0.2 mL of *0.01 M sodium hydroxide*. The solution is red. Add 0.3 mL of *0.01 M hydrochloric acid*. The solution is colourless. Add 0.15 mL of *methyl red solution R*. The solution is orange-red.

Chlorides (*2.4.4*)

Maximum 100 ppm.

Dilute 5 mL of solution S to 15 mL with *water R*.

Sulfates (*2.4.13*)

Maximum 100 ppm, determined on solution S.

Sulfides

To 10 mL of solution S add 2 mL of *buffer solution pH 3.5 R* and 1 mL of a freshly prepared 1.6 g/L solution of *lead nitrate R* in *carbon dioxide-free water R*. Shake. After 1 min any colour in the solution is not more intense than that in a reference solution prepared at the same time using 1 mL of *lead standard solution (10 ppm Pb) R*, 9 mL of *carbon dioxide-free water R*, 2 mL of *buffer solution pH 3.5 R* and 1.2 mL of *thioacetamide reagent R*.

Arsenic (*2.4.2, Method B*)

Maximum 8 ppm.

Shake 2.5 g with 50 mL of *dilute ammonia R1* for 1 h and filter. Evaporate 25 mL of the filtrate to dryness. Add 2 mL of *water R* and 3 mL of *nitric acid R* to the residue and evaporate to dryness. The residue complies with the test. Prepare the standard using 1 mL of *arsenic standard solution (10 ppm As) R*.

Sulfated ash (*2.4.14*)

Maximum 0.2 per cent, determined on 1.0 g.

ASSAY

Carry out the oxygen-flask method (*2.5.10*), using 60.0 mg in a 1000 mL combustion flask with a teflon joint. Absorb the combustion products in a mixture of 5 mL of *dilute hydrogen peroxide solution R* and 10 mL of *water R*. Heat to boiling, boil gently for 2 min and cool. Using 0.2 mL of *phenolphthalein solution R* as indicator, titrate with *0.1 M sodium hydroxide* until the colour changes from colourless to red. Carry out a blank titration under the same conditions.

1 mL of *0.1 M sodium hydroxide* is equivalent to 1.603 mg of S.

STORAGE

Protected from light.

_____ *Ph Eur*

Symphytum Officinale Root for Homoeopathic Preparations

DEFINITION

Symphytum Officinale Root for Homoeopathic Preparations is the fresh root of *Symphytum officinale* L.

IDENTIFICATION

The strong, spirally-formed rootstock with a smooth, black-brown cortex, subdivides at the base. It is about 5 to 8 cm in diameter and 17 to 30 cm long, surmounted by several tops, close together, consisting of the black residues of the previous year's rosettes of leaves between the current year's new growths. A ring of 10 to 15 horizontally-running, secondary, glabrous smooth roots grows from the base of the rosettes, the roots often reaching a length of more than 50 cm and a diameter of approximately 1.5 cm. The middle portion of the rootstock, which is more or less glabrous, branches at the lower end into several clearly separated, straight downwards pointing, smooth roots, each about 1.5 cm thick and bearing a few secondary rootlets 1 to 2 cm long.

The rootstock and the thick secondary roots are non-lignified, succulent and break off easily. In the yellowish-white, glassy, slightly differentiated cross section, there is a very thin, black rhizodermis, and an easily detachable layer of cortex, 5-8 mm thick. Within this is a single dark pigmented vascular ring. The cut surface and particularly the richly exuding mucilagenous substance turn yellow to red-brown on exposure.

TESTS

Foreign matter

Not more than 2%, Appendix XI D.

MOTHER TINCTURE

The mother tincture complies with the requirements stated under Mother Tinctures for Homoeopathic Preparations and with the following requirements.

PRODUCTION

The mother tincture of *Symphytum officinale* L., is prepared from the herbal drug using *Method 1.1.3* described in the monograph for Methods of Preparation of Homoeopathic Stocks and Potentisation. Use 86% w/w (90% v/v) of *ethanol*.

CHARACTERISTICS

The mother tincture is a brown liquid.

IDENTIFICATION

Carry out the method for *thin-layer chromatography*, Appendix III A, using the following solutions.

(1) The mother tincture.

(2) 0.1% w/v of *allantoin* in *ethanol (45%)*.

CHROMATOGRAPHIC CONDITIONS

(a) Use as the coating *silica gel*.

(b) Use the mobile phase as described below.

(c) Apply 20 µL of solution (1) and 10 µL of solution (2) as 10 mm bands.

(d) Develop the plate to 10 cm.

(e) After removal of the plate, dry in air and examine under *ultraviolet light (365 nm)*.

(f) Spray the plate with a 5% w/v solution of *dimethylaminobenzaldehyde* in *hydrochloric acid* and examine in daylight.

MOBILE PHASE

10 volumes of *anhydrous formic acid,* 10 volumes of *water* and 80 volumes of *ethyl acetate.*

SYSTEM SUITABILITY

The test is not valid unless under *ultraviolet light (365 nm)* the chromatogram of solution (1) shows two bluish fluorescent bands at Rf 0.25 and Rf 0.55 and one light-green fluorescent band at the solvent front.

CONFIRMATION

After spraying, the chromatogram obtained with solution (2) shows the yellow allantoin band at Rf 0.35.

The chromatogram obtained with solution (1) shows one yellow band with the same Rf of 0.35 as that for allantoin.

TESTS
Ethanol
35 to 45% w/w (42 to 53% v/v), Appendix VIII F.

Dry residue
Not less than 1.5% w/w, Appendix XI P.

Relative density
0.920 to 0.970, Appendix V G.

Symphytum Officinale Root for Ethanol Decoction for Homoeopathic Preparations

DEFINITION
Symphytum Officinale Root for Ethanol Decoction for Homoeopathic Preparations is the fresh root of *Symphytum officinale* L.

IDENTIFICATION
The strong, spirally-formed rootstock with a smooth, black-brown cortex, subdivides at the base. It is about 5 to 8 cm in diameter and 17 to 30 cm long, surmounted by several tops, close together, consisting of the black residues of the previous year's rosettes of leaves between the current year's new growths. A ring of 10 to 15 horizontally-running, secondary, glabrous smooth roots, grows from the base of the rosettes, the roots often reaching a length of more than 50 cm and a diameter of approximately 1.5 cm. The middle portion of the rootstock, which is more or less glabrous, branches at the lower end into several clearly separated, straight downwards pointing, smooth roots, each about 1.5 cm thick and bearing a few secondary rootlets 1 to 2 cm long.

The rootstock and the thick secondary roots are non-lignified, succulent and break off easily. In the yellowish-white, glassy, slightly differentiated cross section, there is a very thin, black rhizodermis, and an easily detachable layer of cortex, 5-8 mm thick. Within this is a single dark pigmented vascular ring. The cut surface and particularly the richly exuding mucilagenous substance turn yellow to red-brown on exposure.

MOTHER TINCTURE

The mother tincture complies with the requirements stated under Mother Tinctures for Homoeopathic Preparations and with the following requirements.

PRODUCTION
The mother tincture of *Symphytum officinale* L. is prepared by decoction of the herbal drug using 43% w/w (50% v/v) of *ethanol.*

CHARACTERISTICS
The mother tincture is a brown liquid.

IDENTIFICATION
Carry out the method for *thin-layer chromatography,* Appendix III A, using the following solutions.

(1) The mother tincture.

(2) 0.1% w/v of *allantoin* in *ethanol (45%).*

CHROMATOGRAPHIC CONDITIONS

(a) Use as the coating *silica gel.*

(b) Use the mobile phase as described below.

(c) Apply 20 µL of solution (1) and 10 µL of solution (2) as 10 mm bands.

(d) Develop the plate to 10 cm.

(e) After removal of the plate, dry it in air and examine under *ultraviolet light (365 nm).*

(f) Spray the plate with a 5% w/v solution of *dimethylaminobenzaldehyde* in *hydrochloric acid* and examine in daylight.

MOBILE PHASE

10 volumes of *anhydrous formic acid,* 10 volumes of *water* and 80 volumes of *ethyl acetate.*

SYSTEM SUITABILITY

The test is not valid unless under *ultraviolet light (365 nm),* the chromatogram obtained with solution (1) shows two bluish fluorescent bands at Rf value of 0.25 and Rf value of 0.55 and one light-green fluorescent band at the solvent front.

CONFIRMATION

After spraying, the chromatogram obtained with solution (1) shows a yellow band at Rf value of 0.35 corresponding in position and colour to that obtained with solution (2).

TESTS
Ethanol
25 to 35% w/w (31 to 42% v/v), Appendix VIII F.

Dry residue
Not less than 3.0% w/w, Appendix XI P.

Relative density
0.973 to 0.982, Appendix V G.

Toxicodendron Quercifolium for Homoeopathic Preparations

Rhus Toxicodendron for Homoeopathic Preparations

DEFINITION
Toxicodendron Quercifolium for Homoeopathic Preparations is the fresh, young, not yet lignified shoots, with leaves, of *Toxicodendron quercifolium* (Michx.) Greene.

CAUTION The shoots contain a yellowish-white milky sap that is a strong cutaneous irritant and darkens the skin. Contact with the skin and mucous membranes is to be avoided.

IDENTIFICATION
Shoots The thin shoots have a downy to cottony indumentum and may bear at their ends, and in the axils of the alternate leaves, pointed buds covered in brown, woolly hairs.

Leaves Dark green on the upper surface, lighter green on the lower surface and have scattered hairs, more numerous on the veins; they are tripinnate with petioles 15 to 20 cm long.

The leaflets are ovate to slightly rhombic and of varying size, the middle leaflet being the largest, up to 20 cm long and 11 cm wide with long petiolule; the two lateral leaflets are smaller, up to 16 cm long and 9 cm wide with short petiolules. The margins of the laminae may be entire or broadly dentate with up to 3 or more short triangular lobes on each side, particularly in the apical region of the middle leaflets; on the lateral leaflets the margin is frequently asymmetrical with the lobes on one side only; all the leaflets are cuneate at the base and acute at the apex.

MOTHER TINCTURE

The mother tincture complies with the requirements stated under Mother Tinctures for Homoeopathic Preparations and with the following requirements.

DEFINITION

It contains not less than 0.1% w/w of total flavonoids expressed as quercitrin ($C_{21}H_{20}O_{11}$).

PRODUCTION

The mother tincture of *Toxicodendron quercifolium* (Michx.) Greene is prepared from the herbal drug using *Method 1.1.3* described in the monograph for Methods of Preparation of Homoeopathic Stocks and Potentisation. Use 86% w/w (90% v/v) of *ethanol*.

CHARACTERISTICS

The mother tincture is a yellowish-brown to reddish-brown liquid.

IDENTIFICATION

A. To 1 mL of the mother tincture add 1 granule of *zinc*, a few turnings of *magnesium* and 1 mL of *hydrochloric acid*. A dark red colour is produced which can be extracted with tert-*pentyl alcohol*.

B. Carry out the method for *thin-layer chromatography*, Appendix III A, using the following solutions.

(1) Use the mother tincture.

(2) Dissolve 20 mg of *arbutin* and 10 mg of *gallic acid* in 10 mL of *methanol*.

CHROMATOGRAPHIC CONDITIONS

(a) Use as the coating *silica gel*.

(b) Use the mobile phase as described below.

(c) Apply 10 µL of each solution as bands.

(d) Develop the plate to 10 cm.

(e) Remove the plate, dry in air, spray with a 0.5% w/v solution of *fast blue B salt* in *water*, dry briefly and spray with 0.1M *alcoholic sodium hydroxide*. Examine in daylight.

MOBILE PHASE

10 volumes of *anhydrous formic acid*, 10 volumes of *water* and 80 volumes of *ethyl acetate*.

SYSTEM SUITABILITY

The test is not valid unless the chromatogram obtained with solution (2) shows two well separated bands.

CONFIRMATION

The chromatogram obtained with solution (1) shows the following reddish-brown bands: two or three bands, which lie close together at a position between those obtained for arbutin and gallic acid in solution (2) and two further pronounced bands at about the same level as that obtained for gallic acid in solution (2). Other bands may be present in the chromatogram obtained with solution (1).

Top of the plate	
A reddish-brown band A reddish-brown band	Gallic acid: a reddish-brown band
2 or 3 closely positioned reddish-brown bands	
	Arbutin: a reddish-brown band
Solution (1)	**Solution (2)**

TESTS

Ethanol

36% to 46% w/w (43% to 54% v/v), Appendix VIII F.

Dry residue

Not less than 3.5% w/w, Appendix XI P.

Relative density

0.945 to 0.965, Appendix V G.

Urushiols

Carry out the method for *liquid chromatography*, Appendix III D, using the following solutions.

(1) Evaporate 10.00 g of the mother tincture to dryness using a rotary evaporator at a temperature not exceeding 40°. Add 10 mL *water* to the residue and mix with the aid of ultrasound for 20 minutes. Add 10 mL of *heptane* and shake vigorously for 15 minutes. Allow to separate, remove and retain the heptane layer avoiding any suspended particles. Perform the extraction twice more on the aqueous phase, then discard the remaining aqueous layer and rinse the flask with 10 mL of *heptane*. Combine the extracts and washings and filter through *anhydrous sodium sulfate* and evaporate the filtrate to dryness using a rotary evaporator at a temperature not exceeding 40°. Dissolve the residue in 2.0 mL of *methanol*.

(2) To 0.5 mL of a 0.175% w/v solution of *4-dodecylresorcinol* in *methanol* add 0.5 mL of a solution containing 0.1% w/v each of *urushiol I* and *urushiol II* in *methanol* and dilute to 5 mL with *methanol*.

(3) Dilute 1 volume of solution (2) to 20 volumes with *methanol*.

(4) 0.00025% w/v of *4-dodecylresorcinol* in *methanol*.

CHROMATOGRAPHIC CONDITIONS

(a) Use a stainless steel column (25 cm × 4.6 mm) packed with *octadecylsilyl silica gel for chromatography* (5 µm) (Waters Symmetry C18 is suitable).

(b) Use gradient elution and the mobile phase described below.

(c) Use a flow rate of 1 mL per minute.

(d) Use a column temperature of 30°.

(e) Use a detection wavelength of 276 nm.

(f) Inject 20 µL of each solution.

MOBILE PHASE

Mobile phase A   0.2% v/v *orthophosphoric acid*.

Mobile phase B   methanol.

Time (Minutes)	Mobile phase A (% v/v)	Mobile phase B (% v/v)	Comment
0-2	20	80	isocratic
2-82	20→0	80→100	linear gradient
82-83	0→20	100→80	linear gradient
83-100	20	80	re-equilibration

When the chromatograms are recorded under the prescribed conditions the relative retentions with reference to 4-dodecylresorcinol (retention time about 27 minutes) are urushiol I about 2.0 and urushiol II about 2.4. The relative retention of urushiol I to urushiol II is about 0.8.

SYSTEM SUITABILITY

The test is not valid unless, in the chromatogram obtained with solution (2), the *column efficiency*, determined using the peak due to 4-dodecyl resorcinol, is not less than 20,000 theoretical plates, and

in the chromatogram obtained with solution (3) the *signal-to-noise ratio* of the peaks due to urushiol I and urushiol II is at least 10.

LIMITS

Calculate the percentage w/w content of urushiols in solution (1), expressed as 4-dodecylresorcinol, using the following expression:

$$\frac{A_1 \times c_2 \times p \times 1.20}{A_2 \times c_1 \times 100}$$

A_1 = sum of the peak areas due to urushiols in the chromatogram obtained with solution (1);

A_2 = area of the peak due to 4-dodecylresorcinol in the chromatogram obtained with solution (2);

c_1 = concentration of the mother tincture sample in solution (1) in % w/v;

c_2 = concentration of 4-dodecylresorcinol in solution (2) in % w/v;

p = percentage content of 4-dodecylresorcinol in *4-dodecylresorcinol*;

1.20 = average molar mass ratio of urushiol I and II to *4-dodecylresorcinol*.

In the chromatogram obtained with solution (1):

The total content of urushiols, expressed as 4-dodecylresorcinol, is not more than 0.05%.

Disregard any peak:

with an area less than the area of the peak due to 4-dodecyl resorcinol in solution (4) (0.00005%);

with a retention time less than 0.25 times that of the peak due to 4-dodecylresorcinol, or with a retention time greater than the peak due to urushiol II in the chromatogram obtained with solution (2).

ASSAY

Carry out the method for *liquid chromatography*, Appendix III D, using the following solutions in 50 volumes of *methanol* and 50 volumes of *water*.

(1) 10% w/v of the mother tincture.

(2) 0.018% w/v each of *isoquercitrin* and *quercitrin BPCRS*.

(3) 0.0000018% w/v of *quercitrin BPCRS*.

CHROMATOGRAPHIC CONDITIONS

(a) Use a stainless steel column (25 cm × 4.6 mm) packed with *octadecylsilyl silica gel for chromatography* (5 μm) (Waters Symmetry C18 is suitable).

(b) Use gradient elution and the mobile phase described below.

(c) Use a flow rate of 1 mL per minute.

(d) Use an ambient column temperature.

(e) Use a detection wavelength of 340 nm.

(f) Inject 20 μL of each solution.

MOBILE PHASE

Mobile phase A   *water* adjusted to pH to 2.3 with *orthophosphoric acid*.

Mobile phase B   *acetonitrile*.

Time (Minutes)	Mobile phase A (% v/v)	Mobile phase B (% v/v)	Comment
0-2	95	5	isocratic
2-18	95→87	5→13	linear gradient
18-32	87→74	13→26	linear gradient
32-42	74	26	isocratic
42-43	74→95	26→5	linear gradient
43-60	95	5	re-equilibration

When the chromatograms are recorded using the prescribed conditions, the retention time of isoquercitrin is about 31 minutes and that of quercitrin is about 34 minutes, the relative retention is about 0.9.

SYSTEM SUITABILITY

The test is not valid unless, in the chromatogram obtained with solution (2):

the *symmetry factor* for both isoquercitrin and quercitrin is not less than 0.8 and not more than 1.2;

the number of theoretical plates with respect to isoquercitrin is at least 200,000.

DETERMINATION OF CONTENT

Calculate the content of total flavonoids, expressed as quercitrin from the chromatograms obtained and using the declared content of $C_{21}H_{20}O_{11}$ in *quercitrin BPCRS* and the following expression. Disregard any peak with an area less than that in solution (3).

$$\frac{A_1 \times c_2 \times p}{A_2 \times c_1}$$

A_1 = Sum of the peak areas due to quercitrin and flavonoids in the chromatogram obtained with solution (1);

A_2 = area of the peak due to quercitrin in the chromatogram obtained with solution (2);

c_1 = concentration of the mother tincture sample in solution (1) in % w/v;

c_2 = concentration of *quercitrin BPCRS* in solution (2) in % w/v;

p = percentage content of quercitrin in *quercitrin BPCRS*.

Urtica Urens Herb for Homoeopathic Preparations

DEFINITION

Urtica Urens Herb for Homoeopathic Preparations is the fresh leaves and flowers of *Urtica urens* L.

CHARACTERISTICS

The plant produces an itchy, burning sensation.

IDENTIFICATION

Plant Annual.

Leaves Decussate with diffusely haired petiole, which in the lower leaves is mostly as long as the lamina; ovate to elliptic, 1 to 5 cm long and 1 to 4 cm wide lamina with incised serrated leaf margin, blunt to cuneate at the base, acuminate towards the apex. The leaves are dark-green on the upper surface, slightly shiny and paler green on the lower surface; prominent stinging hairs occur scattered all over the upper surface, on the lower surface they occur mostly over the veins. The two stipules on each side are lanceolate and the margins are entire.

Flowers The complicated inflorescences consist mainly of female flowers and only a few male flowers; they arise from the leaf axils and are about 1.5 to 2 cm long and usually shorter than the leaf petioles. The perigonium of the male flowers is split into four pale green lobes of equal size; each one of the four stamens situated in front of one of the perigonium lobes and has a long filament which at first is incurved and then widens out before the anther releases the pollen. The perigonium of the female flowers consists of two outer, short, bract-like segments and two longer, inner ones, all with ciliated margins and scattered hairs over the surfaces; the superior ovary is ovoid with a short style and a conspicuous, brushlike stigma. The ripe fruits are monospermic and enclosed by the two inner segments of the perigonium.

TESTS

Urtica dioica

The plant is dioecious as follows:

the male and female flowers occur on separate plants;

the inflorescences are longer than the leaf petioles;

the leaves, especially those on the lower part of the stem, are longer than their petioles.

MOTHER TINCTURE

The mother tincture complies with the requirements stated under Mother Tinctures for Homoeopathic Preparations and with the following requirements.

PRODUCTION

The mother tincture of *Urtica urens* L., is prepared from the herbal drug using *Method 2b* described in the monograph for Methods of Preparation of Homoeopathic Stocks and Potentisation. Use 62% w/w (70% v/v) of *ethanol*.

CHARACTERISTICS

The mother tincture is a green to brownish-green liquid.

IDENTIFICATION

A. To 1 mL of *potassium hydroxide solution* add 1 mL of the mother tincture and heat to boiling. *Red litmus paper* held over the mouth of the test tube turns blue.

B. Add 1 mL of *hydrochloric acid* and a few crystals of *resorcinol* to 1 mL of the mother tincture. Heat to boiling. A red colour is produced.

C. Carry out the method for *thin-layer chromatography*, Appendix III A, using the following solutions.

(1) The mother tincture.

(2) Dissolve 10 mg of *leucine* and 10 mg of *threonine* in 10 mL of 50% v/v *ethanol*.

CHROMATOGRAPHIC CONDITIONS

(a) Use as the coating *silica gel G*.

(b) Use the mobile phase described below.

(c) Apply 20 μL of each solution as bands.

(d) Develop the plate to 15 cm.

(e) After removal of the plate, dry in a current of warm air or in an oven at 100° to 105°. Spray the chromatogram with a 0.5% w/v solution of *ninhydrin* in *butan-1-ol*. Heat for 10 minutes at 100° to 105° and examine in daylight.

MOBILE PHASE

10 volumes of *glacial acetic acid*, 20 volumes of *water*, 35 volumes of *acetone* and 35 volumes of *butan-1-ol*.

SYSTEM SUITABILITY

The test is not valid unless the chromatogram obtained with the solution (2) shows two clearly separated coloured zones due to threonine (reddish pink) in the lower region and leucine (pink) in the middle region.

CONFIRMATION

The chromatogram obtained with solution (1) shows a pink spot (which may be separated into two spots) corresponding to leucine. A reddish pink spot occurs in the lower region corresponding to threonine. Between the spots corresponding to threonine and leucine there is an orange pink spot and a pink spot present, in order of increasing Rf value. Several spots are present below the spot corresponding to threonine.

Top of the plate	
A pink band (may be two bands)	Leucine: a pink band
A pink band An orange-pink band	
A reddish-pink band	Threonine: a reddish-pink band
Several bands may be observed	
Solution (1)	Solution (2)

TESTS

Ethanol

25% to 35% w/w (30% to 42% v/v), Appendix VIII F.

Dry residue

Not less than 1.0% w/w, Appendix XI P.

Relative density

0.956 to 0.968, Appendix V G.

Monographs

Blood-related Products

BLOOD-RELATED PRODUCTS

Anticoagulant and Preservative Solutions for Blood

(Anticoagulant and Preservative Solutions for Human Blood, Ph Eur monograph 0209)

Ph Eur _____

DEFINITION

Anticoagulant and preservative solutions for human blood are sterile and pyrogen-free solutions prepared with water for injections, filtered, distributed in the final containers and sterilised. The content of sodium citrate ($C_6H_5Na_3O_7,2H_2O$), glucose monohydrate ($C_6H_{12}O_6,H_2O$) or anhydrous glucose ($C_6H_{12}O_6$) and sodium dihydrogen phosphate dihydrate ($NaH_2PO_4,2H_2O$) is not less than 95.0 per cent and not more than 105.0 per cent of that stated in the formulae below. The content of citric acid monohydrate ($C_6H_8O_7,H_2O$) or anhydrous citric acid ($C_6H_8O_7$) is not less than 90.0 per cent and not more than 110.0 per cent of that stated in the formulae below. Subject to agreement by the competent authority, other substances, such as red-cell preservatives, may be included in the formula provided that their name and concentration are stated on the label.

Anticoagulant and preservative solutions for human blood are presented in airtight, tamper-proof containers of glass (*3.2.1*) or plastic (*3.2.3*).

ANTICOAGULANT ACID-CITRATE-GLUCOSE SOLUTIONS (ACD)

	A	B
Sodium citrate (0412)	22.0 g	13.2 g
Citric acid monohydrate (0456)	8.0 g	4.8 g
or *Citric acid, anhydrous (0455)*	7.3 g	4.4 g
Glucose monohydrate (0178)˙	24.5 g	14.7 g
or *Glucose, anhydrous (0177)*˙	22.3 g	13.4 g
Water for injections (0169) to	1000.0 mL	1000.0 mL
Volume to be used per 100 mL of blood	15.0 mL	25.0 mL

˙The competent authority may require that the substances comply with the test for pyrogens given in the monographs on *Glucose monohydrate (0178)* and *Glucose, anhydrous (0177)*, respectively.

CHARACTERS

A colourless or faintly yellow, clear liquid, practically free from particles.

IDENTIFICATION

A. Examine by thin-layer chromatography (*2.2.27*), using *silica gel G R* as the coating substance.

Test solution Dilute 2 mL of the solution to be examined (for formula A) or 3 mL (for formula B) to 100 mL with a mixture of 2 volumes of *water R* and 3 volumes of *methanol R*.

Reference solution (a) Dissolve 10 mg of *glucose CRS* in a mixture of 2 volumes of *water R* and 3 volumes of *methanol R* and dilute to 20 mL with the same mixture of solvents.

Reference solution (b) Dissolve 10 mg each of *glucose CRS*, *lactose CRS*, *fructose CRS* and *sucrose CRS* in a mixture of

2 volumes of *water R* and 3 volumes of *methanol R* and dilute to 20 mL with the same mixture of solvents.

Apply separately to the plate 2 μL of each solution and thoroughly dry the points of application. Develop over a path of 15 cm using a mixture of 10 volumes of *water R*, 15 volumes of *methanol R*, 25 volumes of *anhydrous acetic acid R* and 50 volumes of *ethylene chloride R*. The volumes of solvents have to be measured accurately since a slight excess of water produces cloudiness. Dry the plate in a current of warm air. Repeat the development immediately, after renewing the mobile phase. Dry the plate in a current of warm air and spray evenly with a solution of 0.5 g of *thymol R* in a mixture of 5 mL of *sulfuric acid R* and 95 mL of *alcohol R*. Heat at 130 °C for 10 min. The principal spot in the chromatogram obtained with the test solution is similar in position, colour and size to the principal spot in the chromatogram obtained with reference solution (a). The test is not valid unless the chromatogram obtained with reference solution (b) shows 4 clearly separated spots.

B. To 2 mL add 5 mL of *cupri-citric solution R*. Heat to boiling. An orange precipitate is formed and the solution becomes yellow.

C. To 2 mL (for formula A) add 3 mL of *water R* or to 4 mL (for formula B) add 1 mL of *water R*. The solution gives the reaction of citrates (*2.3.1*).

D. 0.5 mL gives reaction (b) of sodium (*2.3.1*).

TESTS
pH (*2.2.3*)

The pH of the solution to be examined is 4.7 to 5.3.

Hydroxymethylfurfural

To 2.0 mL add 5.0 mL of a 100 g/L solution of *p-toluidine R* in *2-propanol R* containing 10 per cent *V/V* of *glacial acetic acid R* and 1.0 mL of a 5 g/L solution of *barbituric acid R*. The absorbance (*2.2.25*), determined at 550 nm after allowing the mixture to stand for 2 min to 3 min, is not greater than that of a standard prepared at the same time in the same manner using 2.0 mL of a solution containing 5 ppm of *hydroxymethylfurfural R* for formula A or 3 ppm of *hydroxymethylfurfural R* for formula B.

Sterility (*2.6.1*)

They comply with the test for sterility.

Pyrogens (*2.6.8*)

They comply with the test for pyrogens. Dilute with a pyrogen-free, 9 g/L solution of *sodium chloride R* to obtain a solution containing approximately 5 g/L of sodium citrate. Inject 10 mL of the diluted solution per kilogram of the rabbit's mass.

ASSAY
Citric acid

To 10.0 mL (for formula A) or to 20.0 mL (for formula B) add 0.1 mL of *phenolphthalein solution R1*. Titrate with *0.2 M sodium hydroxide* until a pink colour is obtained.

1 mL of *0.2 M sodium hydroxide* is equivalent to 14.01 mg of $C_6H_8O_7,H_2O$ or to 12.81 mg of $C_6H_8O_7$.

Sodium citrate

Prepare a chromatography column 0.10 m long and 10 mm in internal diameter and filled with *strongly acidic ion-exchange resin R* (300 μm to 840 μm). Maintain a 1 cm layer of liquid above the resin at all times. Wash the column with 50 mL of de-ionised *water R* at a flow rate of 12-14 mL/min.

Dilute 10.0 mL of the solution to be examined (for formula A) or 15.0 mL (for formula B) to about 40 mL with de-ionised *water R* in a beaker and transfer to the column reservoir, washing the beaker 3 times with a few millilitres of de-ionised *water R*. Allow the solution to run through the column at a flow rate of 12-14 mL/min and collect the eluate. Wash the column with 2 quantities, each of 30 mL, and with one quantity of 50 mL, of de-ionised *water R*. The column can be used for 3 successive determinations before regeneration with 3 times its volume of *dilute hydrochloric acid R*. Titrate the combined eluate and washings (about 150 mL) with *0.2 M sodium hydroxide*, using 0.1 mL of *phenolphthalein solution R1* as indicator.

Calculate the content of sodium citrate in grams per litre from the following expressions:

For formula A:

$$1.961n - 1.40C$$

or

$$1.961n - 1.53C'$$

For formula B:

$$1.307n - 1.40C$$

or

$$1.307n - 1.53C'$$

n = number of millilitres of *0.2 M sodium hydroxide* used in the titration,

C = content of citric acid monohydrate in grams per litre determined as prescribed above,

C' = content of anhydrous citric acid in grams per litre determined as prescribed above.

Reducing sugars

Dilute 5.0 mL (for formula A) or 10.0 mL (for formula B) to 100.0 mL with *water R*. Introduce 25.0 mL of the solution into a 250 mL conical flask with ground-glass neck and add 25.0 mL of *cupri-citric solution R1*. Add a few pieces of porous material, attach a reflux condenser, heat so that boiling begins within 2 min and boil for exactly 10 min. Cool and add 3 g of *potassium iodide R* dissolved in 3 mL of *water R*. Add 25 mL of a 25 per cent *m/m* solution of *sulfuric acid R* with caution and in small quantities. Titrate with *0.1 M sodium thiosulfate* using 0.5 mL of *starch solution R*, added towards the end of the titration, as indicator (n_1 mL). Carry out a blank titration using 25.0 mL of *water R* (n_2 mL).

Calculate the content of reducing sugars as anhydrous glucose or as glucose monohydrate, as appropriate, from Table 0209.-1.

Table 0209.-1

Volume of *0.1 M* sodium thiosulfate (n_2-n_1 mL)	Anhydrous glucose in milligrams	Glucose mono-hydrate in milligrams
8	19.8	21.6
9	22.4	24.5
10	25.0	27.2
11	27.6	30.2
12	30.3	33.1
13	33.0	36.1
14	35.7	39.0
15	38.3	42.1
16	41.3	45.2

STORAGE

Store in an airtight, tamper-proof container, protected from light.

LABELLING

The label states:

— the composition and volume of the solution,

— the maximum amount of blood to be collected in the container.

ANTICOAGULANT CITRATE-PHOSPHATE-GLUCOSE SOLUTION (CPD)

Sodium citrate (0412)	26.3 g
Citric acid monohydrate (0456)	3.27 g
or Citric acid, anhydrous (0455)	2.99 g
Glucose monohydrate (0178)*	25.5 g
or Glucose, anhydrous (0177)*	23.2 g
Sodium dihydrogen phosphate dihydrate (0194)	2.51 g
Water for injections (0169) to	1000.0 mL
Volume to be used per 100 mL of blood	14.0 mL

*The competent authority may require that the substances comply with the test for pyrogens given in the monographs on *Glucose monohydrate (0178)* and *Glucose, anhydrous (0177)*, respectively.

CHARACTERS

A colourless or faintly yellow, clear liquid, practically free from particles.

IDENTIFICATION

A. Examine by thin-layer chromatography (*2.2.27*), using *silica gel G R* as the coating substance.

Test solution Dilute 2 mL of the solution to be examined to 100 mL with a mixture of 2 volumes of *water R* and 3 volumes of *methanol R*.

Reference solution (a) Dissolve 10 mg of *glucose CRS* in a mixture of 2 volumes of *water R* and 3 volumes of *methanol R* and dilute to 20 mL with the same mixture of solvents.

Reference solution (b) Dissolve 10 mg each of *glucose CRS*, *lactose CRS*, *fructose CRS* and *sucrose CRS* in a mixture of 2 volumes of *water R* and 3 volumes of *methanol R* and dilute to 20 mL with the same mixture of solvents.

Apply separately to the plate 2 μL of each solution and thoroughly dry the starting points. Develop over a path of 15 cm using a mixture of 10 volumes of *water R*, 15 volumes of *methanol R*, 25 volumes of *anhydrous acetic acid R* and 50 volumes of *ethylene chloride R*. The volumes of solvents have to be measured accurately since a slight excess of water produces cloudiness. Dry the plate in a current of warm air. Repeat the development immediately, after renewing the mobile phase. Dry the plate in a current of warm air and spray evenly with a solution of 0.5 g of *thymol R* in a mixture of 5 mL of *sulfuric acid R* and 95 mL of *alcohol R*. Heat at 130 °C for 10 min. The principal spot in the chromatogram obtained with the test solution is similar in position, colour and size to the principal spot in the chromatogram obtained with reference solution (a). The test is not valid unless the chromatogram obtained with reference solution (b) shows 4 clearly separated spots.

B. To 2 mL add 5 mL of *cupri-citric solution R*. Heat to boiling. An orange precipitate is formed and the solution becomes yellow.

C. To 2 mL add 3 mL of *water R*. The solution gives the reaction of citrates (*2.3.1*).

D. 1 mL gives reaction (b) of phosphates (*2.3.1*).

E. 0.5 mL gives reaction (b) of sodium (*2.3.1*).

TESTS

pH (2.2.3)

The pH of the solution is 5.3 to 5.9.

Hydroxymethylfurfural

To 2.0 mL add 5.0 mL of a 100 g/L solution of *p-toluidine R* in *2-propanol R* containing 10 per cent *V/V* of *glacial acetic acid R* and 1.0 mL of a 5 g/L solution of *barbituric acid R*. The absorbance (2.2.25), determined at 550 nm after allowing the mixture to stand for 2 min to 3 min, is not greater than that of a standard prepared at the same time in the same manner using 2.0 mL of a solution containing 5 ppm of *hydroxymethylfurfural R*.

Sterility (2.6.1)

They comply with the test for sterility.

Pyrogens (2.6.8)

They comply with the test for pyrogens. Dilute with a pyrogen-free, 9 g/L solution of *sodium chloride R* to obtain a solution containing approximately 5 g/L of sodium citrate. Inject 10 mL of the diluted solution per kilogram of the rabbit's mass.

ASSAY

Sodium dihydrogen phosphate

Dilute 10.0 mL to 100.0 mL with *water R*. To 10.0 mL of this solution add 10.0 mL of *nitro-vanado-molybdic reagent R*. Mix and allow to stand at 20 °C to 25 °C for 30 min. At the same time and in the same manner, prepare a reference solution using 10.0 mL of a standard solution containing 0.219 g of *potassium dihydrogen phosphate R* per litre. Measure the absorbance (2.2.25) of the 2 solutions at 450 nm using as the compensation liquid a solution prepared in the same manner using 10 mL of *water R*. Calculate the content of sodium dihydrogen phosphate dihydrate (P) in grams per litre from the expression:

$$\frac{11.46 \times C \times A_1}{A_2}$$

C = concentration of *potassium dihydrogen phosphate R* in the standard solution in grams per litre,

A_1 = absorbance of the test solution,

A_2 = absorbance of the reference solution.

Citric acid

To 20.0 mL add 0.1 mL of *phenolphthalein solution R1* and titrate with *0.2 M sodium hydroxide*.

Calculate the content of citric acid monohydrate (C), or anhydrous citric acid (C'), in grams per litre from the equations:

$$C = 0.7005n - 0.4490P$$

$$C' = 0.6404n - 0.4105P$$

n = number of millilitres of *0.2 M sodium hydroxide* used in the titration,

P = content of sodium dihydrogen phosphate dihydrate in grams per litre determined as prescribed above.

Sodium citrate

Prepare a chromatography column 0.10 m long and 10 mm in internal diameter and filled with *strongly acidic ion-exchange resin R* (300 μm to 840 μm). Maintain a 1 cm layer of liquid above the resin at all times. Wash the column with 50 mL of de-ionised *water R* at a flow rate of 12-14 mL/min.

Dilute 10.0 mL of the solution to be examined to about 40 mL with de-ionised *water R* in a beaker and transfer to the column reservoir, washing the beaker 3 times with a few millilitres of de-ionised *water R*. Allow the solution to run through the column at a flow rate of 12-14 mL/min and collect the eluate. Wash the column with 2 quantities, each of 30 mL, and with one quantity of 50 mL, of de-ionised *water R*. The column can be used for 3 successive determinations before regeneration with 3 times its volume of *dilute hydrochloric acid R*. Titrate the combined eluate and washings (about 150 mL) with *0.2 M sodium hydroxide*, using 0.1 mL of *phenolphthalein solution R1* as indicator.

Calculate the content of sodium citrate in grams per litre from the following expressions:

$$1.961n - 1.257P - 1.40C$$

$$1.961n - 1.257P - 1.53C'$$

n = number of millilitres *of 0.2 M sodium hydroxide* used in the titration,

P = content of sodium dihydrogen phosphate dihydrate in grams per litre determined as prescribed above,

C = content of citric acid monohydrate in grams per litre determined as prescribed above

C' = content of anhydrous citric acid in grams per litre determined as prescribed above.

Reducing sugars

Dilute 5.0 mL to 100.0 mL with *water R*. Introduce 25.0 mL of the solution into a 250 mL conical flask with ground-glass neck and add 25.0 mL of *cupri-citric solution R1*. Add a few pieces of porous material, attach a reflux condenser, heat so that boiling begins within 2 min and boil for exactly 10 min. Cool and add 3 g of *potassium iodide R* dissolved in 3 mL of *water R*. Add 25 mL of a 25 per cent *m/m* solution of *sulfuric acid R* with caution and in small quantities. Titrate with *0.1 M sodium thiosulfate* using 0.5 mL of *starch solution R*, added towards the end of the titration, as indicator (n_1 mL). Carry out a blank titration using 25.0 mL of *water R* (n_2 mL).

Calculate the content of reducing sugars as anhydrous glucose or as glucose monohydrate, as appropriate, from Table 0209.-1.

STORAGE

Store in an airtight, tamper-proof container, protected from light.

LABELLING

The label states:

— the composition and volume of the solution,

— the maximum amount of blood to be collected in the container.

Ph Eur

Plasma for Fractionation

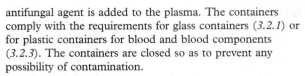

*(Human Plasma for Fractionation,
Ph Eur monograph 0853)*

Ph Eur

DEFINITION

Liquid part of human blood remaining after separation of the cellular elements from blood collected in a receptacle containing an anticoagulant, or separated by continuous filtration or centrifugation of anticoagulated blood in an apheresis procedure; it is intended for the manufacture of plasma-derived products.

PRODUCTION

DONORS

Only a carefully selected, healthy donor who, as far as can be ascertained after medical examination, laboratory blood tests and a study of the donor's medical history, is free from detectable agents of infection transmissible by plasma-derived products may be used. Recommendations in this field are made by the Council of Europe [*Recommendation No. R (95) 15 on the preparation, use and quality assurance of blood components*, or subsequent revision]; a directive of the European Union also deals with the matter: *Commission Directive 2004/33/EC of 22 March 2004 implementing Directive 2002/98/EC of the European Parliament and of the Council as regards certain technical requirements for blood and blood components.*

Immunisation of donors

Immunisation of donors to obtain immunoglobulins with specific activities may be carried out when sufficient supplies of material of suitable quality cannot be obtained from naturally immunised donors. Recommendations for such immunisations are formulated by the World Health Organization (*Requirements for the collection, processing and quality control of blood, blood components and plasma derivatives*, WHO Technical Report Series, No. 840, 1994 or subsequent revision).

Records

Records of donors and donations made are kept in such a way that, while maintaining the required degree of confidentiality concerning the donor's identity, the origin of each donation in a plasma pool and the results of the corresponding acceptance procedures and laboratory tests can be traced.

Laboratory tests

Laboratory tests are carried out for each donation to detect the following viral markers:

1. antibodies against human immunodeficiency virus 1 (anti-HIV-1);

2. antibodies against human immunodeficiency virus 2 (anti-HIV-2);

3. hepatitis B surface antigen (HBsAg);

4. antibodies against hepatitis C virus (anti-HCV).

The test methods used are of suitable sensitivity and specificity and comply with the regulations in force. If a repeat-reactive result is found in any of these tests, the donation is not accepted.

INDIVIDUAL PLASMA UNITS

The plasma is prepared by a method that removes cells and cell debris as completely as possible. Whether prepared from whole blood or by plasmapheresis, the plasma is separated from the cells by a method designed to prevent the introduction of micro-organisms. No antibacterial or antifungal agent is added to the plasma. The containers comply with the requirements for glass containers (*3.2.1*) or for plastic containers for blood and blood components (*3.2.3*). The containers are closed so as to prevent any possibility of contamination.

If 2 or more units are pooled prior to freezing, the operations are carried out using sterile connecting devices or under aseptic conditions and using containers that have not previously been used.

When obtained by plasmapheresis or from whole blood (after separation from cellular elements), plasma intended for the recovery of proteins that are labile in plasma is frozen within 24 h of collection by cooling rapidly in conditions validated to ensure that a temperature of −25 °C or below is attained at the core of each plasma unit within 12 h of placing in the freezing apparatus.

When obtained by plasmapheresis, plasma intended solely for the recovery of proteins that are not labile in plasma is frozen by cooling rapidly in a chamber at −20 °C or below as soon as possible and at the latest within 24 h of collection.

When obtained from whole blood, plasma intended solely for the recovery of proteins that are not labile in plasma is separated from cellular elements and frozen in a chamber at −20 °C or below as soon as possible and at the latest within 72 h of collection.

It is not intended that the determination of total protein and human coagulation factor VIII shown below be carried out on each unit of plasma. They are rather given as guidelines for good manufacturing practice, the test for human coagulation factor VIII being relevant for plasma intended for use in the preparation of concentrates of labile proteins.

The total protein content of a unit of plasma depends on the serum protein content of the donor and the degree of dilution inherent in the donation procedure. When plasma is obtained from a suitable donor and using the intended proportion of anticoagulant solution, a total protein content complying with the limit of 50 g/L is obtained. If a volume of blood or plasma smaller than intended is collected into the anticoagulant solution, the resulting plasma is not necessarily unsuitable for pooling for fractionation. The aim of good manufacturing practice must be to achieve the prescribed limit for all normal donations.

Preservation of human coagulation factor VIII in the donation depends on the collection procedure and the subsequent handling of the blood and plasma. With good practice, 0.7 IU/mL can usually be achieved, but units of plasma with a lower activity may still be suitable for use in the production of coagulation factor concentrates. The aim of good manufacturing practice is to conserve labile proteins as much as possible.

Total protein

Carry out the test using a pool of not fewer than 10 units. Dilute an appropriate volume of the preparation with a 9 g/L solution of *sodium chloride R* to obtain a solution containing about 15 mg of protein in 2 mL. To 2.0 mL of this solution in a round-bottomed centrifuge tube, add 2 mL of a 75 g/L solution of *sodium molybdate R* and 2 mL of a mixture of 1 volume of *nitrogen-free sulfuric acid R* and 30 volumes of *water R*. Shake, centrifuge for 5 min, decant the supernatant and allow the inverted tube to drain on filter paper. Determine the nitrogen in the residue by the method of sulfuric acid digestion (*2.5.9*) and calculate the protein content by multiplying the quantity of nitrogen by 6.25. The total protein content is not less than 50 g/L.

Human coagulation factor VIII (*2.7.4*)

Carry out the test using a pool of not fewer than 10 units. Thaw the samples to be examined, if necessary, at 37 °C. Carry out the assay using a reference plasma calibrated against the International Standard for human coagulation factor VIII in plasma. The activity is not less than 0.7 IU/mL.

STORAGE AND TRANSPORT

Frozen plasma is stored and transported in conditions designed to maintain the temperature at or below −20 °C; for accidental reasons, the storage temperature may rise above −20 °C on one or more occasions during storage and transport but the plasma is nevertheless considered suitable for fractionation if all the following conditions are fulfilled:

— the total period of time during which the temperature exceeds −20 °C does not exceed 72 h;

— the temperature does not exceed −15 °C on more than 1 occasion;

— the temperature at no time exceeds −5 °C.

POOLED PLASMA

During the manufacture of plasma products, the first homogeneous pool of plasma (for example, after removal of cryoprecipitate) is tested for HBsAg and for HIV antibodies using test methods of suitable sensitivity and specificity; the pool must give negative results in these tests.

The plasma pool is also tested for hepatitis C virus RNA using a validated nucleic acid amplification technique (*2.6.21*). A positive control with 100 IU/mL of hepatitis C virus RNA and, to test for inhibitors, an internal control prepared by addition of a suitable marker to a sample of the plasma pool are included in the test. The test is invalid if the positive control is non-reactive or if the result obtained with the internal control indicates the presence of inhibitors. The plasma pool complies with the test if it is found non-reactive for hepatitis C virus RNA.

Hepatitis C virus RNA for NAT testing BRP is suitable for use as a positive control.

CHARACTERS

Before freezing: clear or slightly turbid liquid without visible signs of haemolysis; it may vary in colour from light yellow to green.

LABELLING

The label enables each individual unit to be traced to a specific donor.

_____ *Ph Eur*

Plasma (Pooled and Treated for Virus Inactivation)

(*Human Plasma (Pooled and Treated for Virus Inactivation), Ph Eur monograph 1646*)

Ph Eur _____

DEFINITION

Human plasma (pooled and treated for virus inactivation) is a frozen or freeze-dried, sterile, non-pyrogenic preparation obtained from human plasma derived from donors belonging to the same ABO blood group. The preparation is thawed or reconstituted before use to give a solution for infusion.

The human plasma used complies with the monograph *Human plasma for fractionation (0853)*.

PRODUCTION

The units of plasma to be used are cooled to −30 °C or lower within 6 h of separation of cells and always within 24 h of collection.

The pool is prepared by mixing units of plasma belonging to the same ABO blood group.

The pool of plasma is tested for hepatitis B surface antigen (HBsAg) and for HIV antibodies using test methods of suitable sensitivity and specificity; the pool must give negative results in these tests.

Hepatitis A virus RNA

The plasma pool is tested using a validated nucleic acid amplification technique (*2.6.21*). A positive control with 1.0 × 10² IU of hepatitis A virus RNA per millilitre and, to test for inhibitors, an internal control prepared by addition of a suitable marker to a sample of the plasma pool are included in the test. The test is invalid if the positive control is non-reactive or if the result obtained with the internal control indicates the presence of inhibitors. The pool complies with the test if it is found non-reactive for hepatitis A virus RNA.

Hepatitis C virus RNA

The plasma pool is tested using a validated nucleic acid amplification technique (*2.6.21*). A positive control with 1.0 × 10² IU of hepatitis C virus RNA per millilitre and, to test for inhibitors, an internal control prepared by addition of a suitable marker to a sample of the plasma pool are included in the test. The test is invalid if the positive control is non-reactive or if the result obtained with the internal control indicates the presence of inhibitors. The pool complies with the test if it is found non-reactive for hepatitis C virus RNA.

Hepatitis C virus RNA for NAT testing BRP is suitable for use as a positive control.

To limit the potential burden of B19 virus in plasma pools, the plasma pool is also tested for B19 virus using a validated nucleic acid amplification technique (*2.6.21*).

B19 virus DNA

The plasma pool contains not more than 10.0 IU/µL.

A positive control with 10.0 IU of B19 virus DNA per microlitre and, to test for inhibitors, an internal control prepared by addition of a suitable marker to a sample of the plasma pool are included in the test. The test is invalid if the positive control is non-reactive or if the result obtained with the internal control indicates the presence of inhibitors.

B19 virus DNA for NAT testing BRP is suitable for use as a positive control.

The method of preparation is designed to minimise activation of any coagulation factor (to minimise potential thrombogenicity) and includes a step or steps that have been shown to inactivate known agents of infection; if substances are used for the inactivation of viruses during production, the subsequent purification procedure must be validated to demonstrate that the concentration of these substances is reduced to a suitable level and that any residues are such as not to compromise the safety of the preparation for patients.

Inactivation process

The solvent-detergent process, which is one of the methods used to inactivate enveloped viruses, uses treatment with a combination of tributyl phosphate and octoxinol 10; these reagents are subsequently removed by oil extraction or by solid phase extraction so that the amount in the final product is less than 2 µg/mL for tributyl phosphate and less than 5 µg/mL for octoxinol 10.

No antimicrobial preservative is added.

The solution is passed through a bacteria-retentive filter, distributed aseptically into the final containers and immediately frozen; it may subsequently be freeze-dried.

Plastic containers comply with the requirements for sterile plastic containers for human blood and blood components *(3.2.3)*.

Glass containers comply with the requirements for glass containers for pharmaceutical use *(3.2.1)*.

CHARACTERS

Frozen preparation: clear or slightly opalescent liquid, free from solid and gelatinous particles after thawing.

Freeze-dried preparation: almost white or slightly yellow powder or friable solid.

Thaw or reconstitute the preparation to be examined as stated on the label immediately before carrying out the identification, tests and assay.

IDENTIFICATION

A. Examine by electrophoresis *(2.2.31)* comparing with normal human plasma. The electropherograms show the same bands.

B. It complies with the test for anti-A and anti-B haemagglutinins (see Tests).

TESTS

pH *(2.2.3)*
6.5 to 7.6.

Osmolality *(2.2.35)*
Minimum 240 mosmol/kg.

Total protein
Minimum 45 g/L.

Dilute if necessary with a 9 g/L solution of *sodium chloride R* to obtain a protein concentration of about 7.5 mg/mL. Place 2.0 mL of this solution in a round-bottomed centrifuge tube and add 2 mL of a 75 g/L solution of *sodium molybdate R* and 2 mL of a mixture of 1 volume of *nitrogen-free sulfuric acid R* and 30 volumes of *water R*. Shake, centrifuge for 5 min, decant the supernatant and allow the inverted tube to drain on filter paper. Determine the nitrogen in the residue by the method of sulfuric acid digestion *(2.5.9)* and calculate the quantity of protein by multiplying the result by 6.25.

Activated coagulation factors *(2.6.22)*
It complies with the test for activated coagulation factors. Carry out the test with 0.1 mL of the preparation to be examined instead of 10-fold and 100-fold dilutions. The coagulation time for the preparation to be examined is not less than 150 s.

Anti-A and anti-B haemagglutinins *(2.6.20, Method A)*
The presence of haemagglutinins (anti-A or anti-B) corresponds to the blood group stated on the label.

Hepatitis A virus antibodies
Minimum 1.0 IU/mL, determined by a suitable immunochemical method *(2.7.1)*.

Human hepatitis A immunoglobulin BRP is suitable for use as a reference preparation.

Irregular erythrocyte antibodies
The preparation to be examined does not show the presence of irregular erythrocyte antibodies when examined without dilution by an indirect antiglobulin test.

Citrate
Liquid chromatography *(2.2.29)*.

Test solution Dilute the preparation to be examined with an equal volume of a 9 g/L solution of *sodium chloride R*. Filter the solution using a filter with 0.45 μm pores.

Reference solution Dissolve 0.300 g of *sodium citrate R* in *water R* and dilute to 100.0 mL with the same solvent.

Column:
— *size*: l = 0.3 m, Ø = 7.8 mm;
— *stationary phase*: cation exchange resin R (9 μm).

Mobile phase 0.51 g/L solution of *sulfuric acid R*.

Flow rate 0.5 mL/min.

Detection Spectrophotometer at 215 nm.

Equilibration 15 min.

Injection 10 μL.

Retention time Citrate = about 10 min.

Limit:
— *citrate*: maximum 25 mmol/L.

Calcium
Maximum 5.0 mmol/L.

Atomic absorption spectrometry *(2.2.23, Method I)*.

Source Calcium hollow-cathode lamp using a transmission band preferably of 0.5 nm.

Wavelength 622 nm.

Atomisation device Air-acetylene or acetylene-propane flame.

Potassium
Maximum 5.0 mmol/L.

Atomic emission spectrometry *(2.2.22, Method I)*.

Wavelength 766.5 nm.

Sodium
Maximum 200 mmol/L.

Atomic emission spectrometry *(2.2.22, Method I)*.

Wavelength 589 nm.

Water
Determined by a suitable method, such as the semi-micro determination of water *(2.5.12)*, loss on drying *(2.2.32)* or near-infrared spectrometry *(2.2.40)*, the water content is within the limits approved by the competent authority (freeze-dried product).

Sterility *(2.6.1)*
It complies with the test.

Pyrogens *(2.6.8)* **or Bacterial endotoxins** *(2.6.14)*
It complies with the test for pyrogens or, preferably and where justified and authorised, with a validated *in vitro* test such as the bacterial endotoxin test.

For the pyrogen test, inject 3 mL per kilogram of the rabbit's mass.

Where the bacterial endotoxin test is used, the preparation to be examined contains less than 0.1 IU of endotoxin per millilitre.

ASSAY

Assay of human coagulation factor VIII *(2.7.4)*
Use a reference plasma calibrated against the International Standard for blood coagulation factor VIII in plasma.

The estimated potency is not less than 0.5 IU/mL.
The confidence limits (P = 0.95) are not less than 80 per cent and not more than 120 per cent of the estimated potency.

Assay of human coagulation factor V
Carry out the assay of human coagulation factor V described below using a reference plasma calibrated against the

International Standard for blood coagulation factor V in plasma.

Using *imidazole buffer solution pH 7.3 R*, prepare at least 3 twofold dilutions of the preparation to be examined, preferably in duplicate, from 1 in 10 to 1 in 40. Test each dilution as follows: mix 1 volume of *plasma substrate deficient in factor V R*, 1 volume of the dilution to be examined, 1 volume of *thromboplastin R* and 1 volume of a 3.5 g/L solution of *calcium chloride R*; measure the coagulation times, i.e. the interval between the moment at which the calcium chloride solution is added and the 1st indication of the formation of fibrin, which may be observed visually or by means of a suitable apparatus.

In the same manner, determine the coagulation time of 4 twofold dilutions (1 in 10 to 1 in 80) of human normal plasma in *imidazole buffer solution pH 7.3 R*.

Check the validity of the assay and calculate the potency of the test preparation by the usual statistical methods (for example, *5.3*).

The estimated potency is not less than 0.5 IU/mL. The confidence limits (*P* = 0.95) are not less than 80 per cent and not more than 120 per cent of the estimated potency.

Assay of human coagulation factor XI (*2.7.22*)
Use a reference plasma calibrated against the International Standard for blood coagulation factor XI in plasma.

The estimated potency is not less than 0.5 IU/mL. The confidence limits (*P* = 0.95) are not less than 80 per cent and not more than 125 per cent of the estimated potency.

Assay of human protein C (*2.7.30*)
Use a reference plasma calibrated against the International Standard for human protein C in plasma.

The estimated potency is not less than 0.7 IU/mL. The confidence limits (*P* = 0.95) are not less than 80 per cent and not more than 120 per cent of the estimated potency.

Assay of human protein S (*2.7.31*)
Use a reference plasma calibrated against the International Standard for human protein S in plasma.

The estimated potency is within the limits approved for the particular product. The confidence limits (*P* = 0.95) are not less than 80 per cent and not more than 120 per cent of the estimated potency.

Assay of human plasmin inhibitor (*2.7.25*) (α_2-antiplasmin)
Use a reference plasma calibrated against human normal plasma.

1 unit of human plasmin inhibitor is equal to the activity of 1 mL of human normal plasma. Human normal plasma is prepared by pooling plasma units from not fewer than 30 donors and storing at −30 °C or lower.

The estimated potency is not less than 0.2 units/mL. The confidence limits (*P* = 0.95) are not less than 80 per cent and not more than 120 per cent of the estimated potency.

Activated partial thromboplastin time (APTT)
Use an apparatus suitable for measurement of coagulation times or perform the assay with incubation tubes maintained in a water-bath at 37 °C. Place in each tube 0.1 mL of the preparation to be examined and 0.1 mL of a suitable APTT reagent (containing phospholipid and contact activator), both previously heated to 37 °C, and incubate the mixture for a recommended time at 37 °C. To each tube add 0.1 mL of a 3.7 g/L solution of *calcium chloride R* previously heated to 37 °C. Using a timer, measure the coagulation time, i.e. the interval between the moment of the addition of the calcium chloride and the 1st indication of the formation of fibrin, which may be observed visually or by means of a suitable apparatus. The volumes given above may be adapted to the APTT reagent and apparatus used. The coagulation time complies with the agreed specification for the product.

LABELLING
The label states:
— the ABO blood group;
— the method used for virus inactivation.

Ph Eur

Albumin Solution

Albumin; Human Albumin

(*Human Albumin Solution, Ph Eur monograph 0255*)

Ph Eur

DEFINITION
Sterile liquid preparation of a plasma protein fraction containing human albumin. It is obtained from plasma that complies with the monograph *Human plasma for fractionation (0853)*. The preparation may contain excipients such as sodium caprylate (sodium octanoate) or *N*-acetyltryptophan or a combination of the two.

PRODUCTION
Separation of the albumin is carried out under controlled conditions, particularly of pH, ionic strength and temperature so that in the final product not less than 95 per cent of the total protein is albumin. Human albumin solution is prepared as a concentrated solution containing 150-250 g/L of total protein or as an isotonic solution containing 35-50 g/L of total protein. No antimicrobial preservative or antibiotic is added. The solution is passed through a bacteria-retentive filter and distributed aseptically into sterile containers which are then closed so as to prevent contamination. The solution in its final container is heated to 60 ± 1.0 °C and maintained at this temperature for not less than 10 h. The containers are then incubated at 30-32 °C for not less than 14 days or at 20-25 °C for not less than 4 weeks and examined visually for evidence of microbial contamination.

CHARACTERS
Appearance
Clear, slightly viscous liquid, almost colourless, yellow, amber or green.

IDENTIFICATION
Examine by a suitable immunoelectrophoresis technique. Using antiserum to normal human serum, compare normal human serum and the preparation to be examined, both diluted to contain 10 g/L of protein. The main component of the preparation to be examined corresponds to the main component of normal human serum. The preparation may show the presence of small quantities of other plasma proteins.

TESTS
pH (*2.2.3*)
6.7 to 7.3.

Dilute the preparation to be examined with a 9 g/L solution of *sodium chloride R* to obtain a solution containing 10 g/L of protein.

Total protein

If necessary, dilute an accurately measured volume of the preparation to be examined with a 9 g/L solution of *sodium chloride R* to obtain a solution containing about 15 mg of protein in 2 mL. To 2.0 mL of this solution in a round-bottomed centrifuge tube add 2 mL of a 75 g/L solution of *sodium molybdate R* and 2 mL of a mixture of 1 volume of *nitrogen-free sulfuric acid R* and 30 volumes of *water R*. Shake, centrifuge for 5 min, decant the supernatant and allow the inverted tube to drain on filter paper. Determine the nitrogen in the residue by the method of sulfuric acid digestion (*2.5.9*) and calculate the quantity of protein by multiplying by 6.25. The protein content is not less than 95 per cent and not more than 105 per cent of the stated content.

Protein composition

Zone electrophoresis (*2.2.31*).

Use strips of suitable cellulose acetate gel or agarose gel as the supporting medium and *barbital buffer solution pH 8.6 R1* as the electrolyte solution.

If cellulose acetate is the supporting material, the method described below can be used. If agarose gels are used, and because they are normally part of an automated system, the manufacturer's instructions are followed instead.

Test solution Dilute the preparation to be examined with a 9 g/L solution of *sodium chloride R* to a protein concentration of 20 g/L.

Reference solution Dilute *human albumin for electrophoresis BRP* with a 9 g/L solution of *sodium chloride R* to a protein concentration of 20 g/L.

To a strip apply 2.5 μL of the test solution as a 10 mm band or apply 0.25 μL per millimetre if a narrower strip is used. To another strip, apply in the same manner the same volume of the reference solution. Apply a suitable electric field such that the most rapid band migrates at least 30 mm. Treat the strips with *amido black 10B solution R* for 5 min. Decolorise with a mixture of 10 volumes of *glacial acetic acid R* and 90 volumes of *methanol R* until the background is just free of colour. Develop the transparency of the strips with a mixture of 19 volumes of *glacial acetic acid R* and 81 volumes of *methanol R*. Measure the absorbance of the bands at 600 nm in an instrument having a linear response over the range of measurement. Calculate the result as the mean of 3 measurements of each strip.

System suitability In the electropherogram obtained with the reference solution on cellulose acetate or on agarose gels, the proportion of protein in the principal band is within the limits stated in the leaflet accompanying the reference preparation.

Results In the electropherogram obtained with the test solution on cellulose acetate or on agarose gels, not more than 5 per cent of the protein has a mobility different from that of the principal band.

Molecular-size distribution

Size exclusion chromatography (*2.2.30*).

Test solution Dilute the preparation to be examined with a 9 g/L solution of *sodium chloride R* to a concentration suitable for the chromatographic system used. A concentration in the range of 4-12 g/L and injection of 50-600 μg of protein are usually suitable.

Column:
— size: l = 0.6 m, Ø = 7.5 mm, or l = 0.3 m, Ø = 7.8 mm;

— *stationary phase*: *hydrophilic silica gel for chromatography R*, of a grade suitable for fractionation of globular proteins with relative molecular masses in the range 10 000 to 500 000.

Mobile phase Dissolve 4.873 g of *disodium hydrogen phosphate dihydrate R*, 1.741 g of *sodium dihydrogen phosphate monohydrate R*, 11.688 g of *sodium chloride R* and 50 mg of *sodium azide R* in 1 L of *water R*.

Flow rate 0.5 mL/min.

Detection Spectrophotometer at 280 nm.

The peak due to polymers and aggregates is located in the part of the chromatogram representing the void volume. Disregard the peak due to the stabiliser. The area of the peak due to polymers and aggregates is not greater than 10 per cent of the total area of the chromatogram. This represents not more than 5 per cent when expressed in percentage of protein considering the difference in response factor between the albumin monomer and the polymers and aggregates.

Haem

Dilute the preparation to be examined using a 9 g/L solution of *sodium chloride R* to obtain a solution containing 10 g/L of protein. The absorbance (*2.2.25*) of the solution measured at 403 nm using *water R* as the compensation liquid is not greater than 0.15.

Prekallikrein activator (*2.6.15*)

Maximum 35 IU/mL.

Aluminium

Maximum 200 μg/L.

Atomic absorption spectrometry (*2.2.23, Method I or II*).

Use a furnace as atomic generator.

Use plastic containers for preparation of the solutions and use plastic equipment where possible. Wash glassware (or equipment) in nitric acid (200 g/L HNO₃) before use.

Test solution Use the preparation to be examined, diluted if necessary.

Reference solutions Prepare at least 3 reference solutions in a range spanning the expected aluminium concentration of the preparation to be examined, for example by diluting *aluminium standard solution (10 ppm Al) R* with a 1 g/L solution of *octoxinol 10 R*.

Monitor solution Add *aluminium standard solution (10 ppm Al) R* or a suitable certified reference material to the test solution in a sufficient amount to increase the aluminium concentration by 20 μg/L.

Blank solution 1 g/L solution of *octoxinol 10 R*.

Wavelength 309.3 nm or other suitable wavelength.

Slit width 0.5 nm.

Tube Pyrolytically coated, with integrated platform.

Background corrector Off.

Atomisation device Furnace; fire between readings.

The operating conditions in Table 0255.-1 are cited as an example of conditions found suitable for a given apparatus; they may be modified to obtain optimum conditions.

Injection Each of the following solutions 3 times: blank solution, reference solutions, test solution and monitor solution.

System suitability:
— the recovery of aluminium added in preparation of the monitor solution is within the range 80-120 per cent.

Prepare a calibration curve from the mean of the readings obtained with the reference solutions and determine the

Table 0255.-1. – *Operating conditions found suitable, cited as an example*

Step	Final temperature (°C)	Ramp time (s)	Hold time (s)	Gas
1	120	10	80	argon
2	200	5	20	argon
3	650	5	10	argon
4	1300	5	10	argon
5	1300	1	10	no gas
6	2500	0.7	4	no gas
7	2600	0.5	3	argon
8	20	12.9	3	no gas

aluminium content of the preparation to be examined using the calibration curve.

Potassium

Maximum 0.05 mmol of K per gram of protein.

Atomic emission spectrometry (*2.2.22, Method I*).

Wavelength   766.5 nm.

Sodium

Maximum 160 mmol/L and 95 per cent to 105 per cent of the content of Na stated on the label.

Atomic emission spectrometry (*2.2.22, Method I*).

Wavelength   589 nm.

Sterility (*2.6.1*)

It complies with the test.

Pyrogens (*2.6.8*) or Bacterial endotoxins (*2.6.14*)

It complies with the test for pyrogens or, preferably and where justified and authorised, with a validated in vitro test such as the bacterial endotoxin test.

For the pyrogen test, for a solution with a protein content of 35-50 g/L, inject 10 mL per kilogram of the rabbit's mass; for a solution with a protein content of 150-250 g/L, inject 5 mL per kilogram of the rabbit's mass.

Where the bacterial endotoxin test is used, the preparation to be examined contains less than 0.5 IU of endotoxin per millilitre for solutions with a protein content not greater than 50 g/L, less than 1.3 IU of endotoxin per millilitre for solutions with a protein content greater than 50 g/L but not greater than 200 g/L, and less than 1.7 IU of endotoxin per millilitre for solutions with a protein content greater than 200 g/L but not greater than 250 g/L.

STORAGE

Protected from light.

LABELLING

The label states:
— the name of the preparation;
— the volume of the preparation;
— the content of protein expressed in grams per litre;
— the content of sodium expressed in millimoles per litre;
— that the product is not to be used if it is cloudy or if a deposit has formed;
— the name and quantity of any added substance

_____ *Ph Eur*

Antithrombin III Concentrate

(*Human Antithrombin III Concentrate,
Ph Eur monograph 0878*)

Action and use

Anticoagulant factor.

Ph Eur _____

DEFINITION

Sterile, freeze-dried preparation of a plasma glycoprotein fraction that inactivates thrombin in the presence of an excess of heparin. It is obtained from human plasma that complies with the monograph on *Human plasma for fractionation (0853)*. The preparation may contain excipients such as stabilisers.

When reconstituted in the volume of solvent stated on the label, the potency is not less than 25 IU of antithrombin III per millilitre.

PRODUCTION

The method of preparation is designed to maintain functional integrity of antithrombin III. It includes a step or steps that have been shown to remove or to inactivate known agents of infection; if substances are used for inactivation of viruses during production, the subsequent purification procedure must be validated to demonstrate that the concentration of these substances is reduced to a suitable level and any residues are such as not to compromise the safety of the preparation for patients.

The specific activity is not less than 3 IU of antithrombin III per milligram of total protein, excluding albumin.

The antithrombin III is purified and concentrated. No antimicrobial preservative or antibiotic is added. The antithrombin III concentrate is passed through a bacteria-retentive filter, distributed aseptically into its final, sterile containers and immediately frozen. It is then freeze-dried and the containers are closed under vacuum or in an atmosphere of inert gas.

It shall be demonstrated that the manufacturing process yields a product with a consistent fraction of antithrombin III able to bind to heparin. It is evaluated by a suitable analytical procedure which is determined during process development, such as:

Heparin-binding fraction   Examine by agarose gel electrophoresis (*2.2.31*). Prepare a 10 g/L solution of *agarose for electrophoresis R* containing 15 IU of *heparin R* per millilitre in *barbital buffer solution Ph 8.4 R*. Pour 5 mL of this solution onto a glass plate 5 cm square. Cool at 4 °C for 30 min. Cut 2 wells 2 mm in diameter 1 cm and 4 cm from the side of the plate and 1 cm from the cathode. Introduce into one well 5 µL of the preparation to be examined, diluted to an activity of about 1 IU of antithrombin III per millilitre. Introduce into the other well 5 µL of a solution of a marker dye such as *bromophenol blue R*. Allow the electrophoresis to proceed at 4 °C, using a constant electric field of 7 V/cm, until the dye reaches the anode.

Cut across the agarose gel 1.5 cm from that side of the plate on which the preparation to be examined was applied and remove the larger portion of the gel leaving a band 1.5 cm wide containing the material to be examined. Replace the removed portion with an even layer consisting of 3.5 mL of a 10 g/L solution of *agarose for electrophoresis R* in barbital buffer solution pH 8.4 R, containing a rabbit anti-human antithrombin III antiserum at a suitable concentration, previously determined, to give adequate peak heights of at least 1.5 cm. Place the plate with the original gel at the cathode so that a 2nd electrophoretic migration can occur at right angles to the 1st. Allow this 2nd electrophoresis to proceed using a constant electric field of 2 V/cm for 16 h. Cover the plates with filter paper and several layers of thick lint soaked in a 9 g/L solution of *sodium chloride R* and compress for 2 h, renewing the saline several times. Rinse with *water R*, dry the plates and stain with *acid blue 92 solution R*.

Calculate the fraction of antithrombin III bound to heparin, which is the peak closest to the anode, with respect to the total amount of antithrombin III, by measuring the area defined by the 2 precipitation peaks.

The fraction of antithrombin III able to bind to heparin is not less than 60 per cent.

CHARACTERS
Appearance
White or almost white, hygroscopic, friable solid or powder.

Reconstitute the preparation to be examined as stated on the label immediately before carrying out the identification, tests (except those for solubility, total protein and water) and assay.

IDENTIFICATION
It complies with the limits of the assay.

TESTS
Solubility
To a container of the preparation to be examined add the volume of liquid stated on the label at the recommended temperature. The preparation dissolves completely under gentle swirling within 10 min in the volume of the solvent stated on the label, forming a clear or slightly turbid, colourless or almost colourless solution.

pH (2.2.3)
6.0 to 7.5.

Osmolality (2.2.35)
Minimum 240 mosmol/kg.

Total protein
If necessary, dilute an accurately measured volume of the reconstituted preparation to obtain a solution containing about 15 mg of protein in 2 mL. To 2.0 mL of the solution in a round-bottomed centrifuge tube add 2 mL of a 75 g/L solution of *sodium molybdate R* and 2 mL of a mixture of 1 volume of *nitrogen-free sulfuric acid R* and 30 volumes of *water R*. Shake, centrifuge for 5 min, decant the supernatant and allow the inverted tube to drain on filter paper. Determine the nitrogen in the residue by the method of sulfuric acid digestion (2.5.9) and calculate the amount of protein by multiplying the result by 6.25.

Heparin (2.7.5)
Maximum 0.1 IU of heparin per International Unit of antithrombin III.

It is necessary to validate the method for assay of heparin for each preparation to be examined to allow for interference by antithrombin III.

Water
Determined by a suitable method, such as semi-micro determination of water (2.5.12), loss on drying (2.2.32) or near-infrared spectrophotometry (2.2.40), the water content is within the limits approved by the competent authority.

Sterility (2.6.1)
It complies with the test.

Pyrogens (2.6.8) or Bacterial endotoxins (2.6.14)
It complies with the test for pyrogens or, preferably and where justified and authorised, with a validated in vitro test such as the bacterial endotoxin test.

For the pyrogen test, inject per kilogram of the rabbit's mass a volume equivalent to 50 IU of antithrombin III.

Where the bacterial endotoxin test is used, the preparation to be examined contains less than 0.1 IU of endotoxin per International Unit of antithrombin III.

ASSAY
Human antithrombin III (2.7.17)
The estimated potency is not less than 80 per cent and not more than 120 per cent of the stated potency.
The confidence limits ($P = 0.95$) are not less than 90 per cent and not more than 110 per cent of the estimated potency.

STORAGE
Protected from light, in an airtight container.

LABELLING
The label states:
— the number of International Units of antithrombin III in the container;
— the name and volume of the liquid to be used for reconstitution;
— where applicable, the amount of albumin added as a stabiliser.

———————————————— Ph Eur

Dried Factor VII Fraction

(Human Coagulation Factor VII, Ph Eur monograph 1224)

Action and use
Coagulation factor VII substitute.

Ph Eur ————————————————

DEFINITION
Sterile, liquid or freeze-dried preparation of a plasma protein fraction containing the single-chain glycoprotein human coagulation factor VII and may also contain small amounts of the activated form, the 2-chain derivative human coagulation factor VIIa. It may also contain human coagulation factors II, IX and X, protein C and protein S. It is obtained from human plasma that complies with the monograph on *Human plasma for fractionation (0853)*.
The preparation may contain excipients such as stabilisers, heparin and antithrombin.

The potency of the preparation, reconstituted as stated on the label, is not less than 15 IU of human coagulation factor VII per millilitre.

PRODUCTION
GENERAL PROVISIONS
The method of preparation is designed to maintain functional integrity of human coagulation factor VII and to minimise activation of any coagulation factor (to minimise potential thrombogenicity). It includes a step or steps that have been shown to remove or to inactivate known agents of infection; if substances are used for inactivation of viruses during production, the subsequent purification procedure must be validated to demonstrate that the concentration of these substances is reduced to a suitable level and that any

residues are such as not to compromise the safety of the preparation for patients.

The specific activity is not less than 2 IU of human coagulation factor VII per milligram of total protein, before the addition of any protein stabiliser.

The human coagulation factor VII fraction is dissolved in a suitable liquid. No antimicrobial preservative or antibiotic is added. The solution is passed through a bacteria-retentive filter, distributed aseptically into the final containers and immediately frozen. It is subsequently freeze-dried and the containers are closed under vacuum or under an inert gas.

CONSISTENCY OF THE METHOD OF PRODUCTION

It shall be demonstrated that the manufacturing process yields a product with consistent activities of human coagulation factors II, IX and X, expressed in International Units relative to the activity of human coagulation factor VII. This is evaluated by suitable analytical procedure(s) that is (are) determined during process development.

It shall be demonstrated that the manufacturing process yields a product with a consistent activity of human coagulation factor VIIa. This is evaluated by suitable analytical procedure(s) that is (are) determined during process development.

Activity of human coagulation factor VIIa

It may be determined, for example, using a recombinant soluble tissue factor that does not activate human coagulation factor VII but possesses a cofactor function specific for human coagulation factor VIIa; after incubation of a mixture of the recombinant soluble tissue factor with phospholipids reagent and the dilution of the test sample in human coagulation factor VII-deficient plasma, calcium chloride is added and the clotting time determined; the clotting time is inversely related to the human coagulation factor VIIa activity of the test sample.

CHARACTERS

Appearance

White or almost white, pale yellow, green or blue, hygroscopic powder or friable solid.

Reconstitute the preparation to be examined as stated on the label immediately before carrying out the identification, tests (except those for solubility and water) and assay.

IDENTIFICATION

It complies with the limits of the assay.

TESTS

Solubility

To a container of the preparation to be examined add the volume of liquid stated on the label at the recommended temperature. The preparation dissolves completely with gentle swirling within 10 min, giving a clear or slightly opalescent solution that may be coloured.

pH (*2.2.3*)

6.5 to 7.5.

Osmolality (*2.2.35*)

Minimum 240 mosmol/kg.

Total protein

If necessary, dilute an accurately measured volume of the reconstituted preparation with a 9 g/L solution of *sodium chloride R* to obtain a solution containing about 15 mg of protein in 2 mL. To 2.0 mL of the solution in a round-bottomed centrifuge tube, add 2 mL of a 75 g/L solution of *sodium molybdate R* and 2 mL of a mixture of 1 volume of *nitrogen-free sulfuric acid R* and 30 volumes of *water R*. Shake, centrifuge for 5 min, decant the supernatant and allow the

inverted tube to drain on filter paper. Determine the nitrogen in the residue by the method of sulfuric acid digestion (*2.5.9*) and calculate the amount of protein by multiplying the result by 6.25.

Activated coagulation factors (*2.6.22*)

For each of the dilutions, the coagulation time is not less than 150 s.

Heparin (*2.7.12*)

If heparin has been added, the preparation to be examined contains not more than the amount of heparin stated on the label and in any case not more than 0.5 IU of heparin per International Unit of human coagulation factor VII.

Thrombin

If the preparation to be examined contains heparin, determine the amount present as described in the test for heparin and neutralise the heparin by addition of *protamine sulfate R* (10 µg of protamine sulfate neutralises 1 IU of heparin). In each of 2 test-tubes, mix equal volumes of the reconstituted preparation and of a 3 g/L solution of *fibrinogen R*. Keep one of the tubes at 37 °C for 6 h and the other at room temperature for 24 h. In a 3rd tube, mix equal volumes of the fibrinogen solution and of a solution of *human thrombin R* (1 IU/mL) and place the tube in a water-bath at 37 °C. No coagulation occurs in the tubes containing the preparation to be examined. Coagulation occurs within 30 s in the tube containing thrombin.

Human coagulation factor II (*2.7.18*)

The estimated content is not more than 125 per cent of the stated content. The confidence limits ($P = 0.95$) are not less than 90 per cent and not more than 111 per cent of the estimated potency.

Human coagulation factor IX (*2.7.11*)

The estimated content is not more than 125 per cent of the stated content. The confidence limits ($P = 0.95$) are not less than 80 per cent and not more than 125 per cent of the estimated potency.

Human coagulation factor X (*2.7.19*)

The estimated content is not more than 125 per cent of the stated content. The confidence limits ($P = 0.95$) are not less than 90 per cent and not more than 111 per cent of the estimated potency.

Water

Determined by a suitable method, such as the semi-micro determination of water (*2.5.12*), loss on drying (*2.2.32*) or near-infrared spectrometry (*2.2.40*), the water content is within the limits approved by the competent authority.

Sterility (*2.6.1*)

It complies with the test.

Pyrogens (*2.6.8*) or Bacterial endotoxins (*2.6.14*)

It complies with the test for pyrogens or, preferably and where justified and authorised, with a validated *in vitro* test such as the test for bacterial endotoxins.

For the pyrogen test, inject per kilogram of the rabbit's mass a volume equivalent to not less than 30 IU of human coagulation factor VII.

Where the test for bacterial endotoxins is used, the preparation to be examined contains less than 0.1 IU of endotoxin per International Unit of human coagulation factor VII.

ASSAY

Human coagulation factor VII (*2.7.10*). The estimated potency is not less than 80 per cent and not more than 125 per cent of the stated potency. The confidence limits

($P = 0.95$) are not less than 80 per cent and not more than 125 per cent of the estimated potency.

STORAGE
In an airtight container, protected from light.

LABELLING
The label states:
— the number of International Units of human coagulation factor VII per container;
— the maximum content of human coagulation factor II, human coagulation factor IX and human coagulation factor X per container, in International Units;
— the amount of protein per container;
— the name and quantity of any added substances, including, where applicable, heparin;
— the name and volume of the liquid to be used for reconstitution;
— that the transmission of infectious agents cannot be totally excluded when medicinal products prepared from human blood or plasma are administered.

Ph Eur

Dried Factor VIII (rDNA)

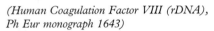

(Human Coagulation Factor VIII (rDNA), Ph Eur monograph 1643)

Action and use
Coagulation factor VIII substitute.

Ph Eur

DEFINITION
Human coagulation factor VIII (rDNA) is a freeze-dried preparation of glycoproteins having the same activity as coagulation factor VIII in human plasma. It acts as a cofactor of the activation of factor X in the presence of factor IXa, phospholipids and calcium ions.

Human coagulation factor VIII circulates in plasma mainly as a two-chain glycosylated protein with 1 heavy (relative molecular mass of about 200 000) and 1 light (relative molecular mass 80 000) chain held together by divalent metal ions. Human coagulation factor VIII (rDNA) is prepared as full-length factor VIII (octocog alfa), or as a shortened two-chain structure (relative molecular mass 90 000 and 80 000), in which the B-domain has been deleted from the heavy chain (moroctocog alfa).

Full-length human rDNA coagulation factor VIII contains 25 potential *N*-glycosylation sites, 19 in the B domain of the heavy chain, 3 in the remaining part of the heavy chain (relative molecular mass 90 000) and 3 in the light chain (relative molecular mass 80 000). The different products are characterised by their molecular size and post-translational modification and/or other modifications.

PRODUCTION
Human coagulation factor VIII (rDNA) is produced by recombinant DNA technology in mammalian cell culture. It is produced under conditions designed to minimise microbial contamination.

Purified bulk factor VIII (rDNA) may contain added human albumin and/or other stabilising agents, as well as other auxiliary substances to provide, for example, correct pH and osmolality.

The specific activity is not less than 2000 IU of factor VIII:C per milligram of total protein before the addition of any protein stabiliser, and varies depending on purity and the type of modification of molecular structure of factor VIII.

The quality of the bulk preparation is controlled using one or more manufacturer's reference preparations as reference.

MANUFACTURER'S REFERENCE PREPARATIONS
During development, reference preparations are established for subsequent verification of batch consistency during production, and for control of bulk and final preparation. They are derived from representative batches of purified bulk factor VIII (rDNA) that are extensively characterised by tests including those described below and whose procoagulant and other relevant functional properties have been ascertained and compared, wherever possible, with the International Standard for factor VIII concentrate. The reference preparations are suitably characterised for their intended purpose and are stored in suitably sized aliquots under conditions ensuring their stability.

PURIFIED BULK FACTOR VIII (rDNA)
The purified bulk complies with a suitable combination of the following tests for characterisation of integrity of the factor VIII (rDNA). Where any substance added during preparation of the purified bulk interferes with a test, the test is carried out before addition of that substance. Where applicable, the characterisation tests may alternatively be carried out on the finished product.

Specific biological activity or ratio of factor VIII activity to factor VIII antigen
Carry out the assay of human coagulation factor VIII (*2.7.4*). The protein content, or where a protein stabiliser is present, the factor VIII antigen content, is determined by a suitable method and the specific biological activity or the ratio of factor VIII activity to factor VIII antigen is calculated.

Protein composition
The protein composition is determined by a selection of appropriate characterisation techniques which may include peptide mapping, Western blots, HPLC, gel electrophoresis, capillary electrophoresis, mass spectrometry or other techniques to monitor integrity and purity. The protein composition is comparable to that of the manufacturer's reference preparation.

Molecular size distribution
Using size-exclusion chromatography (*2.2.30*), the molecular size distribution is comparable to that of the manufacturer's reference preparation.

Peptide mapping (*2.2.55*)
There is no significant difference between the test protein and the manufacturer's reference preparation.

Carbohydrates/sialic acid
To monitor batch-to-batch consistency, the monosaccharide content and the degree of sialylation or the oligosaccharide profile are monitored and correspond to those of the manufacturer's reference preparation.

FINAL LOT
It complies with the requirements under Identification, Tests and Assay.

Excipients
80 per cent to 120 per cent of the stated content, determined by a suitable method, where applicable.

CHARACTERS
Appearance
White or slightly yellow powder or friable mass.

IDENTIFICATION

A. It complies with the limits of the assay.

B. The distribution of characteristic peptide bands corresponds with that of the manufacturer's reference preparation (SDS-PAGE or Western blot).

TESTS

Reconstitute the preparation as stated on the label immediately before carrying out the tests (except those for solubility and water) and assay.

Solubility

It dissolves within 5 min at 20-25 °C, giving a clear or slightly opalescent solution.

pH (*2.2.3*)

6.5 to 7.5.

Osmolality (*2.2.35*)

Minimum 240 mosmol/kg.

Water

Determined by a suitable method, such as the semi-micro determination of water (*2.5.12*), loss on drying (*2.2.32*) or near infrared spectrophotometry (*2.2.40*), the water content is within the limits approved by the competent authority.

Sterility (*2.6.1*)

It complies with the test for sterility.

Bacterial endotoxins (*2.6.14*)

Less than 3 IU in the volume that contains 100 IU of factor VIII activity.

ASSAY

Carry out the assay of human coagulation factor VIII (*2.7.4*).

The estimated potency is not less than 80 per cent and not more than 125 per cent of the stated potency.

The confidence limits ($P = 0.95$) are not less than 80 per cent and not more than 120 per cent of the estimated potency.

STORAGE

Protected from light.

LABELLING

The label states:

— the factor VIII content in International Units,

— the name and amount of any excipient,

— the composition and volume of the liquid to be used for reconstitution.

_____ *Ph Eur*

Dried Factor VIII Fraction

(*Human Coagulation Factor VIII,
Ph Eur monograph 0275*)

Action and use

Coagulation factor VIII substitute.

Ph Eur _____

DEFINITION

Sterile, freeze-dried preparation of a plasma protein fraction containing the glycoprotein human coagulation factor VIII together with varying amounts of human von Willebrand factor, depending on the method of preparation. It is prepared from human plasma that complies with the monograph on *Human plasma for fractionation (0853)*.

The preparation may contain excipients such as stabilisers.

The potency of the preparation, reconstituted as stated on the label, is not less than 20 IU of factor VIII:C per millilitre.

PRODUCTION

GENERAL PROVISIONS

The method of preparation is designed to maintain functional integrity of human coagulation factor VIII and to minimise potential neoantigenicity. It includes a step or steps that have been shown to remove or to inactivate known agents of infection; if substances are used for the inactivation of viruses, the subsequent purification procedure must be validated to demonstrate that the concentration of these substances is reduced to a suitable level and that any residues are such as not to compromise the safety of the preparation for patients.

The specific activity is not less than 1 IU of factor VIII:C per milligram of total protein before the addition of any protein stabiliser.

The human coagulation factor VIII fraction is dissolved in a suitable liquid. No antimicrobial preservative or antibiotic is added. The solution is passed through a bacteria-retentive filter, distributed aseptically into the final containers and immediately frozen. It is subsequently freeze-dried and the containers are closed under vacuum or under an inert gas.

CONSISTENCY OF THE METHOD OF PRODUCTION

Products stated to have human von Willebrand factor activity (products intended for treatment of von Willebrand's disease). It shall be demonstrated by suitable analytical procedures determined during process development that the manufacturing process yields a product with a consistent composition with respect to human von Willebrand factor. This composition may be characterised in a number of ways. For example, the distribution of the different human von Willebrand factor multimers may be determined by sodium dodecyl sulfate (SDS) agarose gel electrophoresis (about 1 per cent agarose) with or without Western blot analysis, using a normal human plasma pool as reference. Visualisation of the multimeric pattern may be performed using, for example, an immunoenzymatic technique and quantitative evaluation may be carried out by densitometric analysis.

Products that show flakes or particles after reconstitution for use. If a few small flakes or particles remain when the preparation is reconstituted, it shall be demonstrated during validation studies that the potency is not significantly affected after passage of the preparation through the filter provided.

CHARACTERS

Appearance

White or pale yellow, hygroscopic powder or friable solid.

Reconstitute the preparation to be examined as stated on the label immediately before carrying out the identification, tests (except those for solubility and water) and assay.

IDENTIFICATION

It complies with the limits of the assay.

TESTS

Solubility

To a container of the preparation to be examined, add the volume of the liquid stated on the label at the recommended temperature. The preparation dissolves completely with gentle swirling within 10 min, giving a clear or slightly opalescent, colourless or slightly yellow solution.

Where the label states that the product may show a few small flakes or particles after reconstitution, reconstitute the preparation as described on the label and pass it through the filter provided: the filtered solution is clear or slightly opalescent.

pH *(2.2.3)*
6.5 to 7.5.

Osmolality *(2.2.35)*
Minimum 240 mosmol/kg.

Total protein
If necessary, dilute an accurately measured volume of the reconstituted preparation with a 9 g/L solution of *sodium chloride R* to obtain a protein concentration of about 7.5 mg/mL. Place 2.0 mL of this solution in a round-bottomed centrifuge tube and add 2 mL of a 75 g/L solution of *sodium molybdate R* and 2 mL of a mixture of 1 volume of *nitrogen-free sulfuric acid R* and 30 volumes of *water R*. Shake, centrifuge for 5 min, decant the supernatant and allow the inverted tube to drain on filter paper. Determine the nitrogen in the residue by the method of sulfuric acid digestion *(2.5.9)* and calculate the amount of protein by multiplying the result by 6.25. *For some products, especially those without a protein stabiliser such as albumin, this method may not be applicable and another validated method for protein determination must therefore be performed.*

Anti-A and anti-B haemagglutinins *(2.6.20, Method A)*
The 1 to 64 dilution does not show agglutination. Dilute the reconstituted preparation with a 9 g/L solution of *sodium chloride R* to contain 3 IU of factor VIII:C per millilitre.

Water
Determined by a suitable method, such as semi-micro determination of water *(2.5.12)*, loss on drying *(2.2.32)* or near-infrared spectrophotometry *(2.2.40)*, the water content is within the limits approved by the competent authority.

Sterility *(2.6.1)*
It complies with the test.

Pyrogens *(2.6.8)* **or Bacterial endotoxins** *(2.6.14)*
It complies with the test for pyrogens or, preferably and where justified and authorised, with a validated *in vitro* test such as the test for bacterial endotoxins.

For the pyrogen test, inject per kilogram of the rabbit's mass a volume equivalent to not less than 50 IU of factor VIII:C.

Where the test for bacterial endotoxins is used, the preparation to be examined contains less than 0.03 IU of endotoxin per International Unit of factor VIII:C.

ASSAY

Human coagulation factor VIII *(2.7.4)*
The estimated potency is not less than 80 per cent and not more than 120 per cent of the stated potency.
The confidence limits $(P = 0.95)$ are not less than 80 per cent and not more than 120 per cent of the estimated potency.

Human von Willebrand factor *(2.7.21)*
If preparations are intended for the treatment of von Willebrand's disease, the estimated potency is not less than 60 per cent and not more than 140 per cent of the stated potency.

Pending the availability of an International Standard for human von Willebrand factor concentrate calibrated for use in the collagen-binding assay, only the ristocetin cofactor assay may be used.

STORAGE
In an airtight container, protected from light.

LABELLING
The label states:

— the number of International Units of factor VIII:C and, where applicable, of human von Willebrand factor in the container;
— the amount of protein in the container;
— the name and quantity of any added substance;
— the name and volume of the liquid to be used for reconstitution;
— where applicable, that the preparation may show the presence of a few small flakes or particles after reconstitution;
— that the transmission of infectious agents cannot be totally excluded when medicinal products prepared from human blood or plasma are administered.

Ph Eur

Dried Factor IX Fraction

(Human Coagulation Factor IX, Ph Eur monograph 1223)

Action and use
Coagulation factor IX substitute.

Ph Eur

DEFINITION
Sterile freeze-dried preparation of a plasma protein fraction containing coagulation factor IX. It is obtained from human plasma that complies with the monograph on *Human plasma for fractionation (0853)*, by a method that effectively separates human coagulation factor IX from other prothrombin complex factors (human coagulation factors II, VII and X). The preparation may contain excipients such stabilisers, heparin and antithrombin.

The potency of the preparation, reconstituted as stated on the label, is not less than 20 IU of human coagulation factor IX per millilitre.

PRODUCTION

GENERAL PROVISIONS
The method of preparation is designed to maintain functional integrity of human coagulation factor IX and to minimise activation of any coagulation factor (to minimise potential thrombogenicity). It includes a step or steps that have been shown to remove or to inactivate known agents of infection; if substances are used for inactivation of viruses during production, the subsequent purification procedure must be validated to demonstrate that the concentration of these substances is reduced to a suitable level and that any residues are such as not to compromise the safety of the preparation for patients.

The specific activity is not less than 50 IU of human coagulation factor IX per milligram of total protein, before the addition of any protein stabiliser.

The human coagulation factor IX fraction is dissolved in a suitable liquid. No antimicrobial preservative or antibiotic is added. The solution is passed through a bacteria-retentive filter, distributed aseptically into the final containers and immediately frozen. It is subsequently freeze-dried and the containers are closed under vacuum or under an inert gas.

CONSISTENCY OF THE METHOD OF PRODUCTION
It shall be demonstrated that the manufacturing process yields a product having a consistent composition. This is evaluated by suitable analytical procedures that are

determined during process development and that normally include:
— assay of human coagulation factor IX;
— determination of activated coagulation factors;
— determination of activities of human coagulation factors II, VII and X, which shall be shown to be not more than 5 per cent of the activity of human coagulation factor IX.

CHARACTERS
Appearance
White or pale yellow, hygroscopic powder or friable solid.

Reconstitute the preparation to be examined as stated on the label immediately before carrying out the identification, tests (except those for solubility and water) and assay.

IDENTIFICATION
It complies with the limits of the assay.

TESTS
Solubility
To a container of the preparation to be examined add the volume of the liquid stated on the label at the recommended temperature. The preparation dissolves completely with gentle swirling within 10 min, giving a clear or slightly opalescent, colourless solution.

pH (2.2.3)
6.5 to 7.5.

Osmolality (2.2.35)
Minimum 240 mosmol/kg.

Total protein
If necessary, dilute an accurately measured volume of the reconstituted preparation with a 9 g/L solution of *sodium chloride R* to obtain a solution containing about 15 mg of protein in 2 mL. To 2.0 mL of the solution in a round-bottomed centrifuge tube, add 2 mL of a 75 g/L solution of *sodium molybdate R* and 2 mL of a mixture of 1 volume of *nitrogen-free sulfuric acid R* and 30 volumes of *water R*. Shake, centrifuge for 5 min, decant the supernatant and allow the inverted tube to drain on filter paper. Determine the nitrogen in the residue by the method of sulfuric acid digestion (2.5.9) and calculate the amount of protein by multiplying the result by 6.25. *For some products, especially those without a protein stabiliser such as albumin, this method may not be applicable. Another validated method for protein determination must therefore be performed.*

Activated coagulation factors (2.6.22)
If necessary, dilute the reconstituted preparation to contain 20 IU of human coagulation factor IX per millilitre. For each of the dilutions, the coagulation time is not less than 150 s.

Heparin (2.7.12)
If heparin has been added, the preparation to be examined contains not more than the amount of heparin stated on the label and in all cases not more than 0.5 IU of heparin per International Unit of human coagulation factor IX.

Water
Determined by a suitable method, such as semi-micro determination of water (2.5.12), loss on drying (2.2.32) or near-infrared spectrophotometry (2.2.40), the water content is within the limits approved by the competent authority.

Sterility (2.6.1)
It complies with the test.

Pyrogens (2.6.8) or Bacterial endotoxins (2.6.14)
It complies with the test for pyrogens or, preferably and where justified and authorised, with a validated *in vitro* test such as the test for bacterial endotoxins.

For the pyrogen test, inject per kilogram of the rabbit's mass a volume equivalent to not less than 50 IU of human coagulation factor IX.

Where the test for bacterial endotoxins is used, the preparation to be examined contains less than 0.03 IU of endotoxin per International Unit of human coagulation factor IX.

ASSAY
Human coagulation factor IX (2.7.11). The estimated potency is not less than 80 per cent and not more than 125 per cent of the stated potency. The confidence limits (P = 0.95) are not less than 80 per cent and not more than 125 per cent of the estimated potency.

STORAGE
In an airtight container, protected from light.

LABELLING
The label states:
— the number of International Units of human coagulation factor IX per container;
— the amount of protein per container;
— the name and quantity of any added substances including, where applicable, heparin;
— the name and volume of the liquid to be used for reconstitution;
— that the transmission of infectious agents cannot be totally excluded when medicinal products prepared from human blood or plasma are administered.

_____ Ph Eur

Dried Factor XI Fraction

(Human Coagulation Factor XI, Ph Eur monograph 1644)

Action and use
Coagulation factor XI substitute.

Ph Eur _____

DEFINITION
Sterile plasma protein fraction containing coagulation factor XI. It is prepared from *Human plasma for fractionation (0853)*. The preparation may contain excipients such as heparin, C_1-esterase inhibitor and antithrombin III.

The potency of the preparation, reconstituted as stated on the label, is not less than 50 units per millilitre.

PRODUCTION
The method of preparation is designed to maintain functional integrity of human coagulation factor XI and to minimise activation of any coagulation factor (to minimise potential thrombogenicity). It includes a step or steps that have been shown to remove or to inactivate known agents of infection; if substances are used for inactivation of viruses during production, the subsequent purification procedure must be validated to demonstrate that the concentration of these substances is reduced to a suitable level and any residues are such as not to compromise the safety of the preparation for patients.

After preparation, the factor XI fraction is dissolved in a suitable liquid. No antimicrobial preservative or antibiotic is added. The solution is distributed into the final containers and immediately frozen. It is subsequently freeze-dried and the containers are closed under vacuum or under inert gas.

CHARACTERS

Appearance

White or almost white powder or friable solid.

Reconstitute the preparation to be examined as stated on the label immediately before carrying out the identification, tests (except those for solubility and water) and assay.

IDENTIFICATION

It complies with the limits of the assay.

TESTS

Solubility

To a container of the preparation to be examined, add the volume of liquid stated on the label at room temperature. The preparation dissolves completely with gentle swirling within 10 min.

pH *(2.2.3)*

6.8 to 7.4.

Osmolality *(2.2.35)*

Minimum 240 mosmol/kg.

Total protein

If necessary, dilute an accurately measured volume of the preparation to be examined with a 9 g/L solution of *sodium chloride R* to obtain a protein concentration of about 7.5 mg/mL. Place 2.0 mL of this solution in a round-bottomed centrifuge tube and add 2 mL of a 75 g/L solution of *sodium molybdate R* and 2 mL of a mixture of 1 volume of *nitrogen-free sulfuric acid R* and 30 volumes of *water R*. Shake, centrifuge for 5 min, decant the supernatant and allow the inverted tube to drain on filter paper. Determine the nitrogen in the residue by the method of sulfuric acid digestion *(2.5.9)* and calculate the amount of protein by multiplying the result by 6.25.

Activated coagulation factors *(2.6.22)*

For each of the dilutions, the coagulation time is not less than 150 s.

Heparin *(2.7.12)*

If heparin has been added, the preparation to be examined contains not more than the amount of heparin stated on the label and in all cases not more than 0.5 IU of heparin per unit of factor XI.

Antithrombin III *(2.7.17)*

If antithrombin III has been added, the preparation to be examined contains not more than the amount of antithrombin III stated on the label.

C_1-esterase inhibitor

If C_1-esterase inhibitor has been added, the preparation to be examined contains not more than the amount of C_1-esterase inhibitor stated on the label.

The C_1-esterase inhibitor content of the preparation to be examined is determined by comparing its ability to inhibit C_1-esterase with the same ability of a reference preparation consisting of human normal plasma. 1 unit of C_1-esterase is equal to the activity of 1 mL of human normal plasma. Varying quantities of the preparation to be examined are mixed with an excess of C_1-esterase and the remaining C_1-esterase activity is determined using a suitable chromogenic substrate.

Method Reconstitute the preparation as stated on the label. Prepare an appropriate series of 3 or 4 independent dilutions from 1 unit/mL of factor XI, for both the preparation to be examined and the reference preparation, using a solution containing 9 g/L of *sodium chloride R* and either 10 g/L of *human albumin R* or 10 g/L of *bovine albumin R*. Warm all solutions to 37 °C in a water-bath for 1-2 min before use.

Place a suitable amount of C_1-esterase solution in tubes or in microtitre plate wells and incubate at 37 °C. Add a suitable amount of one of the dilutions of the reference preparation or of the preparation to be examined and incubate at 37 °C for 5 min. Add a suitable amount of a suitable chromogenic substrate such as methoxycarbonyl-L-lysyl(ε-benzyloxycarbonyl)-glycyl-L-arginine 4-nitroanilide. Read the rate of increase of absorbance (ΔA/min) at 405 nm. Carry out a blank test using *tris(hydroxymethyl)aminomethane sodium chloride buffer solution pH 7.4 R* instead of the C_1-esterase and the substrate.

Calculate the C_1-esterase inhibitor content using the usual statistical methods (for example, *5.3*).

Anti-A and anti-B haemagglutinins *(2.6.20, Method A)*

The 1 to 64 dilution does not show agglutination.

Water

Determined by a suitable method, such as the semi-micro determination of water *(2.5.12)*, loss on drying *(2.2.32)* or near-infrared spectrophotometry *(2.2.40)*, the water content is within the limits approved by the competent authority.

Sterility *(2.6.1)*

It complies with the test.

Pyrogens *(2.6.8)* or Bacterial endotoxins *(2.6.14)*

It complies with the test for pyrogens or, preferably and where justified and authorised, with a validated *in vitro* test such as the bacterial endotoxin test.

For the pyrogen test, inject per kilogram of the rabbit's mass a volume equivalent to 100 IU of factor XI.

Where the bacterial endotoxin test is used, the preparation to be examined contains less than 0.1 IU of endotoxin per International Unit of factor XI.

ASSAY

Carry out the assay of human coagulation factor XI *(2.7.22)*.

The estimated potency is not less than 80 per cent and not more than 120 per cent of the stated potency.

The confidence limits ($P = 0.95$) are not less than 80 per cent and not more than 125 per cent of the estimated potency.

STORAGE

Protected from light, at a temperature of 2 °C to 8 °C.

LABELLING

The label states:

— the number of units per container;
— the maximum amount of protein per container;
— where applicable, the amount of heparin per container;
— where applicable, the amount of antithrombin III per container;
— where applicable, the amount of C_1-esterase inhibitor per container;
— the name and volume of the liquid to be used for reconstitution.

Ph Eur

Dried Prothrombin Complex

(*Human Prothrombin Complex,*
Ph Eur monograph 0554)

Action and use
Coagulation factor IX substitute. Preparations with appropriate activity may be used to correct deficiencies of coagulation factors II or X.

Ph Eur _____

DEFINITION
Sterile plasma protein fraction containing human coagulation factor IX together with variable amounts of human coagulation factors II, VII and X; the presence and proportion of these additional factors depends on the method of fractionation. It is obtained from human plasma that complies with the monograph on *Human plasma for fractionation (0853)*. The preparation may contain excipients such as stabilisers, heparin and antithrombin.

The potency of the preparation, reconstituted as stated on the label, is not less than 20 IU of human coagulation factor IX per millilitre.

If the content of any of the factors is stated as a single value, the estimated potency is not less than 80 per cent and not more than 125 per cent of the stated potency; if the content of any of the factors is stated as a range, the estimated potency is not less than the lower limit and not greater than the upper limit of the stated range.

PRODUCTION
The method of preparation is designed to maintain functional integrity of the relevant coagulation factors it contains and to minimise activation of any coagulation factor (to minimise potential thrombogenicity). It includes a step or steps that have been shown to remove or to inactivate known agents of infection; if substances are used for inactivation of viruses during production, the subsequent purification procedure must be validated to demonstrate that the concentration of these substances is reduced to a suitable level and that any residues are such as not to compromise the safety of the preparation for patients.

The specific activity is not less than 0.6 IU of human coagulation factor IX per milligram of total protein, before the addition of any protein stabiliser.

The prothrombin complex fraction is dissolved in a suitable liquid. No antimicrobial preservative or antibiotic is added. The solution is passed through a bacteria-retentive filter, distributed aseptically into the final containers and immediately frozen. It is subsequently freeze-dried and the containers are closed under vacuum or under an inert gas.

CHARACTERS
Appearance
White or slightly coloured, very hygroscopic powder or friable solid.

Reconstitute the preparation to be examined as stated on the label immediately before carrying out the identification, tests (except those for solubility and water) and assay.

IDENTIFICATION
It complies with the limits of the assays for human coagulation factors IX and II and, where applicable, those for human coagulation factors VII and X.

TESTS
Solubility
To a container of the preparation to be examined add the volume of the liquid stated on the label at the recommended temperature. The preparation dissolves completely with gentle swirling within 10 min, giving a clear solution that may be coloured.

pH (*2.2.3*)
6.5 to 7.5.

Osmolality (*2.2.35*)
Minimum 240 mosmol/kg.

Total protein
If necessary, dilute an accurately measured volume of the reconstituted preparation with a 9 g/L solution of *sodium chloride R* to obtain a solution containing about 15 mg of protein in 2 mL. To 2.0 mL of the solution in a round-bottomed centrifuge tube add 2 mL of a 75 g/L solution of *sodium molybdate R* and 2 mL of a mixture of 1 volume of *nitrogen-free sulfuric acid R* and 30 volumes of *water R*. Shake, centrifuge for 5 min, decant the supernatant and allow the inverted tube to drain on filter paper. Determine the nitrogen in the residue by the method of sulfuric acid digestion (*2.5.9*) and calculate the amount of protein by multiplying the result by 6.25.

Activated coagulation factors (*2.6.22*)
If necessary, dilute the reconstituted preparation to contain 20 IU of human coagulation factor IX per millilitre. For each of the dilutions, the coagulation time is not less than 150 s.

Heparin (*2.7.12*)
If heparin has been added during preparation, the preparation to be examined contains not more than the amount of heparin stated on the label and in all cases not more than 0.5 IU of heparin per International Unit of human coagulation factor IX.

Thrombin
If the preparation to be examined contains heparin, determine the amount present as described in the test for heparin and neutralise it by addition of *protamine sulfate R* (10 µg of protamine sulfate neutralises 1 IU of heparin). In each of 2 test-tubes, mix equal volumes of the reconstituted preparation and of a 3 g/L solution of *fibrinogen R*. Keep one of the tubes at 37 °C for 6 h and the other at room temperature for 24 h. In a 3rd tube, mix equal volumes of the fibrinogen solution and of a solution of *human thrombin R* (1 IU/mL) and place the tube in a water-bath at 37 °C. No coagulation occurs in the tubes containing the preparation to be examined. Coagulation occurs within 30 s in the tube containing thrombin.

Water
Determined by a suitable method, such as semi-micro determination of water (*2.5.12*), loss on drying (*2.2.32*) or near-infrared spectrometry (*2.2.40*), the water content is within the limits approved by the competent authority.

Sterility (*2.6.1*)
It complies with the test.

Pyrogens (*2.6.8*) **or Bacterial endotoxins** (*2.6.14*)
It complies with the test for pyrogens or, preferably and where justified and authorised, with a validated in vitro test such as the bacterial endotoxin test.

For the pyrogen test, inject per kilogram of the rabbit's mass a volume equivalent to not less than 30 IU of human coagulation factor IX.

Where the bacterial endotoxin test is used, the preparation to be examined contains less than 0.05 IU of endotoxin per International Unit of human coagulation factor IX.

ASSAY

Human coagulation factor IX (*2.7.11*)

The estimated potency is not less than 80 per cent and not more than 125 per cent of the stated potency.

The confidence interval ($P = 0.95$) is not greater than 80 per cent to 125 per cent of the estimated potency.

Human coagulation factor II (*2.7.18*)

The estimated potency is not less than 80 per cent and not more than 125 per cent of the stated potency.

The confidence interval ($P = 0.95$) is not greater than 90 per cent to 111 per cent of the estimated potency.

The estimated human coagulation factor II potency is not less than 70 per cent and not more than 165 per cent of the estimated human coagulation factor IX potency.

Human coagulation factor VII (*2.7.10*)

If the label states that the preparation contains human coagulation factor VII, the estimated potency is not less than 80 per cent and not more than 125 per cent of the stated potency. The confidence interval ($P = 0.95$) is not greater than 80 per cent to 125 per cent of the estimated potency.

Human coagulation factor X (*2.7.19*)

If the label states that the preparation contains human coagulation factor X, the estimated potency is not less than 80 per cent and not more than 125 per cent of the stated potency. The confidence interval ($P = 0.95$) is not greater than 90 per cent to 111 per cent of the estimated potency.

STORAGE

In an airtight container, protected from light.

LABELLING

The label states:

— the number of International Units of human coagulation factor IX, and the number or range of International Units of human coagulation factor II per container;
— where applicable, the number or range of International Units of human coagulation factor VII and human coagulation factor X per container;
— the amount of protein per container;
— the name and quantity of any added substances, including, where applicable, heparin and antithrombin;
— the name and quantity of the liquid to be used for reconstitution;
— that the transmission of infectious agents cannot be totally excluded when medicinal products prepared from human blood or plasma are administered.

———————————————————— Ph Eur

Dried Fibrinogen

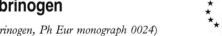

(*Human Fibrinogen, Ph Eur monograph 0024*)

Ph Eur —————————————————————

DEFINITION

Sterile, freeze-dried preparation of a plasma protein fraction containing the soluble constituent of human plasma that is transformed to fibrin on the addition of thrombin. It is obtained from human plasma that complies with the monograph on *Human plasma for fractionation (0853)*.

The preparation may contain excipients such as salts, buffers and stabilisers.

When reconstituted as stated on the label, the solution contains not less than 10 g/L of fibrinogen.

PRODUCTION

The method of preparation is designed to maintain functional integrity of human fibrinogen. It includes a step or steps that have been shown to remove or to inactivate known agents of infection; if substances are used for inactivation of viruses during production, the subsequent purification procedure must be validated to demonstrate that the concentration of these substances is reduced to a suitable level and any residues are such as not to compromise the safety of the preparation for patients.

The specific activity (fibrinogen content with respect to total protein content) is not less than 80 per cent before addition of any protein stabiliser. The fibrinogen content is determined by a suitable method such as that described under Assay, and the total protein content is determined by a suitable method such as that described under Total protein in *Human albumin solution (0255)*. Albumin may also be obtained with fibrinogen during fractionation, in which case a specific determination of albumin is carried out by a suitable immunochemical method (*2.7.1*) and the quantity of albumin determined is subtracted from the total protein content for the calculation of the specific activity.

The protein fraction is dissolved in a suitable liquid. No antimicrobial preservative or antibiotic is added. The solution is passed through a bacteria-retentive filter, distributed aseptically into the final containers and immediately frozen. It is subsequently freeze-dried and the containers are closed under vacuum or under an inert gas.

CHARACTERS

Appearance

White or pale yellow, hygroscopic powder or friable solid.

Reconstitute the preparation to be examined as stated on the label immediately before carrying out the identification, tests (except those for solubility and water) and assay.

IDENTIFICATION

It complies with the limits of the assay.

TESTS

Solubility

To a container of the preparation to be examined add the volume of liquid stated on the label at the recommended temperature. The preparation dissolves within 30 min at 20-25 °C, forming an almost colourless, slightly opalescent solution.

pH (*2.2.3*)

6.5 to 7.5.

Osmolality (*2.2.35*)

Minimum 240 mosmol/kg.

Stability of solution

No gel formation appears at 20-25 °C within 60 min following reconstitution.

Water

Determined by a suitable method, such as semi-micro determination of water (*2.5.12*), loss on drying (*2.2.32*) or near-infrared spectrophotometry (*2.2.40*), the water content is within the limits approved by the competent authority.

Sterility (*2.6.1*)

It complies with the test.

Pyrogens (*2.6.8*) **or Bacterial endotoxins** (*2.6.14*)
It complies with the test for pyrogens or, preferably and where justified and authorised, with a validated *in vitro* test such as the test for bacterial endotoxins.

For the pyrogen test, inject per kilogram of the rabbit's mass a volume equivalent to not less than 30 mg of fibrinogen.

Where the test for bacterial endotoxins is used, the preparation to be examined contains less than 0.03 IU of endotoxin per milligram of fibrinogen.

ASSAY
Mix 0.2 mL of the reconstituted preparation with 2 mL of a suitable buffer solution (pH 6.6-6.8) containing sufficient thrombin (approximately 3 IU/mL) and calcium (0.05 mol/L). Maintain at 37 °C for 20 min, separate the precipitate by centrifugation (5000 *g*, 20 min) and wash thoroughly with a 9 g/L solution of *sodium chloride R*. Determine the nitrogen content by sulfuric acid digestion (*2.5.9*) and calculate the fibrinogen (clottable protein) content by multiplying the result by 6.0. The content is not less than 70 per cent and not more than 130 per cent of the stated content of fibrinogen.

STORAGE
In an airtight container, protected from light.

LABELLING
The label states:
— the content of fibrinogen in the container;
— the name and volume of the liquid to be used for reconstitution;
— where applicable, the name and amount of protein stabiliser added in the preparation.

_____ *Ph Eur*

Fibrin Sealant Kit

(*Ph Eur monograph 0903*)

Ph Eur _____

DEFINITION
Sterile, freeze-dried, frozen or liquid preparation of plasma protein fractions containing essentially 2 components, namely fibrinogen concentrate (component 1), a protein fraction containing human fibrinogen, and a preparation containing human thrombin (component 2). A fibrin clot is rapidly formed when the 2 thawed or reconstituted components are mixed. Other ingredients (for example, human coagulation factor XIII, a fibrinolysis inhibitor or calcium ions) and stabilisers (for example, *Human albumin solution (0255)*) may be added.

Human constituents are obtained from plasma that complies with the monograph on *Human plasma for fractionation (0853)*.

When thawed or reconstituted as stated on the label, component 1 contains not less than 40 g/L of clottable protein; the thrombin activity of component 2 varies over a wide range (approximately 4-1000 IU/mL).

PRODUCTION
The method of preparation is designed to maintain functional integrity of the components. It includes a step or steps that have been shown to remove or to inactivate known agents of infection; if substances are used for inactivation of viruses during production, the subsequent purification procedure must be validated to demonstrate that the concentration of these substances is reduced to a suitable level and any residues are such as not to compromise the safety of the preparation for patients.

The constituents or mixtures of constituents are dissolved in a suitable liquid. No antimicrobial preservative or antibiotic is added. Constituents or mixtures of constituents are passed through a bacteria-retentive filter and distributed aseptically into sterile containers. Containers of freeze-dried constituents are closed under vacuum or filled with a suitable inert gas, such as oxygen-free nitrogen, before being closed.

If the human coagulation factor XIII content in component 1 is greater than 10 units/mL, the assay of human coagulation factor XIII is carried out.

CHARACTERS
Appearance:
— *freeze-dried constituents*: white or pale yellow, hygroscopic powder or friable solid,
— *frozen constituents*: colourless or pale yellow, opaque solid,
— *liquid constituents*: colourless or pale yellow liquid.

For the freeze-dried or frozen constituents, reconstitute or thaw as stated on the label immediately before carrying out the identification and the tests, except those for solubility and water.

COMPONENT 1 (FIBRINOGEN CONCENTRATE)

IDENTIFICATION
A. It complies with the limits of the assay of fibrinogen.

B. It complies with the limits of the assay of human coagulation factor XIII (where applicable).

TESTS
Solubility
Freeze-dried concentrates dissolve within 20 min in the volume of liquid and at the temperature stated on the label, forming an almost colourless, clear or slightly turbid solution.

pH (*2.2.3*)
6.5 to 8.0.

Stability of solution
No gel formation appears at room temperature during 120 min following thawing or reconstitution.

Water
Determined by a suitable method, such as semi-micro determination of water (*2.5.12*), loss on drying (*2.2.32*) or near-infrared spectrophotometry (*2.2.40*), the water content is within the limits approved by the competent authority.

Sterility (*2.6.1*)
It complies with the test.

ASSAY
Fibrinogen (clottable protein)
Mix 0.2 mL of the reconstituted concentrate with 2 mL of a suitable buffer solution (pH 6.6-7.4) containing sufficient *human thrombin R* (approximately 3 IU/mL) and calcium (0.05 mol/L). Maintain at 37 °C for 20 min, separate the precipitate by centrifugation at 5000 *g* for 20 min, wash thoroughly with a 9 g/L solution of *sodium chloride R* and determine the protein as nitrogen by sulfuric acid digestion (*2.5.9*). Calculate the clottable protein content by multiplying the result by 6.0. The estimated content in milligrams of clottable protein is not less than 70 per cent and not more than 130 per cent of the stated content. If for a particular preparation this method cannot be applied, use another validated method for determination of fibrinogen.

Human coagulation factor XIII
Where the label indicates that the human coagulation factor XIII potency is greater than 10 units/mL, the estimated

potency is not less than 80 per cent and not more than 120 per cent of the stated potency.

Make at least 3 suitable dilutions of thawed or reconstituted concentrate and of human normal plasma (reference preparation) using human coagulation factor XIII-deficient plasma or another suitable diluent. Add to each dilution suitable amounts of the following reagents:

— activator reagent, containing bovine or human thrombin, a suitable buffer, calcium chloride and a suitable inhibitor such as Gly-Pro-Arg-Pro-Ala-NH$_2$ which inhibits clotting of the sample but does not prevent human coagulation factor XIII activation by thrombin;

— detection reagent, containing a suitable factor XIIIa-specific peptide substrate, such as Leu-Gly-Pro-Gly-Glu-Ser-Lys-Val-Ile-Gly-NH$_2$ and glycine ethyl ester as 2nd substrate in a suitable buffer solution;

— NADH reagent, containing glutamate dehydrogenase, α-ketoglutarate and NADH in a suitable buffer solution.

After mixing, the absorbance changes (ΔA/min) are measured at a wavelength of 340 nm, after the linear phase of the reaction is reached.

1 unit of human coagulation factor XIII is equal to the potency of 1 mL of human normal plasma.

Calculate the potency of the test preparation by the usual statistical methods (*5.3, for example*). The confidence limits ($P = 0.95$) are not less than 80 per cent and not more than 125 per cent of the estimated potency.

COMPONENT 2 (THROMBIN PREPARATION)

IDENTIFICATION

It complies with the limits of the assay of thrombin.

TESTS

Solubility

Freeze-dried preparations dissolve within 5 min in the volume of liquid stated on the label, forming a colourless, clear or slightly turbid solution.

pH (*2.2.3*)

5.0 to 8.0.

Water

Determined by a suitable method, such as semi-micro determination of water (*2.5.12*), loss on drying (*2.2.32*) or near-infrared spectrophotometry (*2.2.40*), the water content is within the limits approved by the competent authority.

Sterility (*2.6.1*)

It complies with the test.

ASSAY

Thrombin

If necessary, dilute the reconstituted preparation to be examined to approximately 2-20 IU of thrombin per millilitre using as diluent a suitable buffer solution (pH 7.3-7.5), such as *imidazole buffer solution pH 7.3 R* containing 10 g/L of *human albumin R* or *bovine albumin R*. To a suitable volume of the dilution, add a suitable volume of fibrinogen solution (1 g/L of clottable protein) warmed to 37 °C and start measurement of the clotting time immediately. Repeat the procedure with each of at least 3 dilutions, in the range stated above, of a reference preparation of thrombin, calibrated in International Units.

Calculate the activity of the test preparation by the usual statistical methods (*5.3, for example*). The estimated activity is not less than 80 per cent and not more than 125 per cent of the stated activity. The confidence limits ($P = 0.95$) are not less than 80 per cent and not more than 125 per cent of the estimated activity.

STORAGE

Protected from light and, for freeze-dried components, in an airtight container.

LABELLING

The label states:

— the amount of fibrinogen (milligrams of clottable protein), thrombin (International Units) per container, and of human coagulation factor XIII, if the latter is greater than 10 units/mL,

— where applicable, the name and volume of liquid to be used to reconstitute the components.

—————————————————— Ph Eur

Human Haematopoietic Stem Cells

(*Ph Eur monograph 2323*)

Ph Eur —————————————————————————

This monograph provides a standard for the preparation and control of human haematopoietic stem cells for use in therapy. It does not exclude the use of alternative preparation and control methods that are acceptable to the competent authority.

DEFINITION

Human haematopoietic stem cells are primitive multipotent cells capable of self-renewal as well as differentiation and maturation into all haematopoietic lineages. They are found in small numbers in bone marrow, in the mononuclear cell fraction of circulating blood and in umbilical cord blood. The preparation also contains haematopoietic progenitor cells, which are capable of differentiation but not self-renewal. The numbers of haematopoietic stem cells and haematopoietic progenitor cells are correlated.

This monograph applies to haematopoietic stem cells that have not undergone expansion or genetic modification, and that are intended to provide a successful engraftment leading to a permanent restoration of all lineages of blood cell production to a sufficient level and function in a recipient whose haematopoiesis has been compromised by, for example, disease or high doses of chemotherapy and/or radiation therapy, or has to be replaced in certain congenital diseases. The infused haematopoietic stem cells can originate from the recipient (autologous) or from another individual (allogeneic).

Haematopoietic stem cells are recognised by their ability to reconstitute human haematopoiesis *in vivo*. They also have the capacity to differentiate into colony-forming cells, which are able to give rise to colonies in the presence of various growth factors. The membrane marker CD34 is commonly used for the successful isolation/purification of haematopoietic stem cells from crude preparations and as an indicator of haematopoietic stem cell content in routine quality control.

PRODUCTION

DONORS

Where allogeneic cells are used, they are derived from carefully selected donors in accordance with donor selection criteria. Directive 2004/23/EC of the European Union deals with the criteria for donor selection.

COLLECTION

Peripheral blood stem cells These are collected by cytapheresis after mobilisation from the bone marrow by administration of growth factors and/or treatment of autologous donors with cytotoxic substances. The cells may be processed to select a population of interest and may be cryopreserved.

Bone marrow Bone marrow is harvested by aspirating the cells from the cavities of hollow bones, then removing bone fragments by filtration and, if necessary, separating the buffy coat cells after centrifugation or with commercial kits based on the cytapheresis principle. The cells may be processed to select a population of interest and may be cryopreserved.

Umbilical cord blood Placental blood haematopoietic cells are collected from placentae via the vein of the umbilical cord. The cells are then cryopreserved.

CRYOPRESERVATION

Cryopreservation allows storage for long periods. The cells are suspended in a validated medium containing a suitable cryoprotectant (for example, dimethyl sulfoxide) and macromolecules (for example, autologous plasma/albumin) and are frozen in cryobags in a manner designed to maintain viability of the cells by controlled cooling according to a validated method. They are stored at a temperature of $- 140$ °C or lower. Where cryobags are stored under other conditions of temperature and duration, the functionality of the preparation must be validated. Cryobags from donors that test positive for any infectious disease marker must be stored in such a way as to avoid cross-contamination.

SUBSTANCES USED IN PRODUCTION

The quality of substances used in production may be critical with respect to the quality, safety and efficacy of the final product, particularly for substances of biological origin. This is of particular importance for:
— proteins, including enzymes and antibodies;
— cryopreservation reagents;
— purification reagents.

Quality assurance

All substances must be produced within a recognised quality management system using suitable production facilities.

Quality specifications

A suitable quality specification must be presented for each substance, including notably:
— identity;
— potency (where applicable);
— purity;
— determination of bacterial endotoxins (*2.6.14*) (where applicable);
— microbiological quality (total viable count, tests for specified micro-organisms);
— sterility (*2.6.1*) (where applicable).

Viral safety

The requirements of chapter *5.1.7* apply.

Transmissible spongiform encephalopathies

A risk assessment of the product with respect to transmissible spongiform encephalopathies is carried out, and suitable measures are taken to minimise any such risk (*5.2.8*).

Water

Water used in the preparation of cellular products complies with the relevant monograph (*Water for injections (0169)*, *Water, highly purified (1927)*, *Purified water (0008)*). Water incorporated into the final product complies with the section on Water for injections in bulk in the monograph *Water for injections (0169)*, and in addition is sterile.

TESTS

Target specifications are established for the different tests, but these are not used as rigid acceptance criteria.

Tests carried out include the following (further tests, such as purging, cell depletion, allogeneic application, may be necessary depending on any treatment applied to the cells and on the intended recipient):

Nucleated cell count (*2.7.29*).

Viability (*2.7.29*)
Viability is assessed for products that are not infused within 24 h of collection.

CD34+ cell count
For peripheral blood stem cells, CD34+ cell count is determined using a validated automated apparatus to analyse cells labelled with anti-CD34 antibodies. The apparatus and method employed must be able to determine the number of CD34+ cells with a sensitivity, accuracy and reproducibility comparable with those of immunophenotyping (*2.7.23*), where cells are labelled using anti-CD34 and anti-CD45 antibodies conjugated to a fluorochrome and analysed by flow cytometry (*2.7.24*).

Colony-forming cell (CFC) assay (*2.7.28*)
Proliferative capacity is established by a suitable assay. The test is not necessarily carried out on each unit. The correlation between the dose of CD34 and the number of CFCs in a given situation (pathology, packaging, mobilisation) is determined. The CFC assay is carried out periodically; whenever a change that could affect the quality of CD34+ cells is made to the protocol for packaging or mobilisation, it is carried out on a suitable number of units.

Microbiological control
Examine as prescribed in general method *2.6.27*.
Microbiological control of cellular products. Where justified, the product may be released before completion of the test.

_____ *Ph Eur*

Normal Immunoglobulin

Normal Immunoglobulin Injection
(*Human Normal Immunoglobulin, Ph Eur monograph 0338*)

Ph Eur _____

DEFINITION

Human normal immunoglobulin is a sterile liquid or freeze-dried preparation containing immunoglobulins, mainly immunoglobulin G (IgG). Other proteins may be present. Human normal immunoglobulin contains the IgG antibodies of normal subjects. It is intended for intramuscular or subcutaneous administration. The preparation may contain excipients such as stabilisers. Multidose preparations contain an antimicrobial preservative.

Human normal immunoglobulin is obtained from plasma that complies with the requirements of the monograph *Human plasma for fractionation (0853)*.

PRODUCTION

The method of preparation includes a step or steps that have been shown to remove or to inactivate known agents of infection; if substances are used for inactivation of viruses, it shall have been shown that any residues present in the final product have no adverse effects on the patients treated with the immunoglobulin.

For preparations intended for subcutaneous administration, the method of preparation also includes a step or steps that have been shown to remove thrombosis-generating agents. Emphasis is given to the identification of activated coagulation factors and their zymogens and process steps that may cause their activation. Consideration is also to be given to other procoagulant agents that could be introduced by the manufacturing process.

The product shall have been shown, by suitable tests in animals and evaluation during clinical trials, to be well tolerated when administered intramuscularly or subcutaneously. Any antimicrobial preservative or stabilising agent used shall have been shown to have no deleterious effect on the final product in the amount present.

Human normal immunoglobulin is prepared from pooled material from at least 1000 donors by a method that has been shown to yield a product that:
— does not transmit infection;
— at a protein concentration of 160 g/L, contains antibodies for at least 2 of which (1 viral and 1 bacterial) an International Standard or Reference Preparation is available, the concentration of such antibodies being at least 10 times that in the initial pooled material;
— has a defined distribution of IgG subclasses;
— complies with the test for Fc function of immunoglobulin (2.7.9), if the preparation is intended for subcutaneous administration.

Human normal immunoglobulin is prepared as a stabilised solution, for example in a 9 g/L solution of sodium chloride, a 22.5 g/L solution of glycine or, if the preparation is to be freeze-dried, a 60 g/L solution of glycine. No antibiotic is added to the plasma used. Single-dose preparations do not contain an antimicrobial preservative. The solution is passed through a bacteria-retentive filter. The preparation may subsequently be freeze-dried and the containers closed under vacuum or under an inert gas. The stability of the preparation is demonstrated by suitable tests carried out during development studies.

CHARACTERS
Appearance:
— *liquid preparation*: clear and colourless or pale-yellow or light-brown; during storage it may show formation of slight turbidity or a small amount of particulate matter.
— *freeze-dried preparation*: powder or solid, friable mass, hygroscopic, white or slightly yellow.

For the freeze-dried preparation, reconstitute as stated on the label immediately before carrying out the identification and the tests, except those for solubility and water.

IDENTIFICATION
Examine by a suitable immunoelectrophoresis technique. Using antiserum to normal human serum, compare normal human serum and the preparation to be examined, both diluted to a protein concentration of 10 g/L. The main component of the preparation to be examined corresponds to the IgG component of normal human serum. The solution may show the presence of small quantities of other plasma proteins.

TESTS
Solubility
For the freeze-dried preparation, to a container of the preparation to be examined add the volume of the liquid stated on the label at the recommended temperature. The preparation dissolves completely within 20 min at 20-25 °C.

pH (2.2.3)
5.0 to 7.2.

Dilute the preparation to be examined with a 9 g/L solution of *sodium chloride R* to a protein concentration of 10 g/L.

Total protein
The preparation has a protein concentration of not less than 100 g/L and not more than 180 g/L and contains not less than 90 per cent and not more than 110 per cent of the quantity of protein stated on the label.

Dilute the preparation to be examined with a 9 g/L solution of *sodium chloride R* to obtain a solution containing about 15 mg of protein in 2 mL. To 2.0 mL of this solution in a round-bottomed centrifuge tube add 2 mL of a 75 g/L solution of *sodium molybdate R* and 2 mL of a mixture of 1 volume of *nitrogen-free sulfuric acid R* and 30 volumes of *water R*. Shake, centrifuge for 5 min, decant the supernatant liquid and allow the inverted tube to drain on filter paper. Determine the nitrogen in the residue by the method of sulfuric acid digestion (2.5.9) and calculate the content of protein by multiplying the result by 6.25.

Protein composition
Examine by zone electrophoresis (2.2.31).

Use strips of suitable cellulose acetate gel or suitable agarose gel as the supporting medium and *barbital buffer solution pH 8.6 R1* as the electrolyte solution.

If cellulose acetate is the supporting material, the method described below can be used. If agarose gels are used, and because they are normally part of an automated system, the manufacturer's instructions are followed instead.

Test solution Dilute the preparation to be examined with a 9 g/L solution of *sodium chloride R* to a protein concentration of 50 g/L.

Reference solution Reconstitute *human immunoglobulin for electrophoresis BRP* and dilute with a 9 g/L solution of *sodium chloride R* to a protein concentration of 50 g/L.

To a strip apply 2.5 µL of the test solution as a 10 mm band or apply 0.25 µL per millimetre if a narrower strip is used. To another strip apply in the same manner the same volume of the reference solution. Apply a suitable electric field such that the albumin band of normal human serum applied on a control strip migrates at least 30 mm. Stain the strip with *amido black 10B solution R* for 5 min. Decolourise with a mixture of 10 volumes of *glacial acetic acid R* and 90 volumes of *methanol R* so that the background is just free of colour. Develop the transparency of the strips with a mixture of 19 volumes of *glacial acetic acid R* and 81 volumes of *methanol R*. Measure the absorbance of the bands at 600 nm in an instrument having a linear response over the range of measurement. Calculate the result as the mean of 3 measurements of each strip.

System suitability In the electropherogram obtained with the reference solution, the proportion of protein in the principal band is within the limits stated in the leaflet accompanying the reference preparation.

Results In the electropherogram obtained with the test solution, not more than 10 per cent of protein has a mobility different from that of the principal band.

Distribution of molecular size
Size exclusion chromatography (2.2.30).

Test solution Dilute the preparation to be examined with a 9 g/L solution of *sodium chloride R* to a concentration suitable for the chromatographic system used. A concentration in the range of 4-12 g/L and injection of 50-600 µg of protein are usually suitable.

Reference solution Dilute *human immunoglobulin (molecular size) BRP* with a 9 g/L solution of *sodium chloride R* to the same protein concentration as the test solution.

Column:
— *size:* l = 0.6 m, Ø = 7.5 mm, or l = 0.3 m, Ø = 7.8 mm;
— *stationary phase:* hydrophilic silica gel for chromatography R, of a grade suitable for fractionation of globular proteins with relative molecular masses in the range 10 000 to 500 000.

Mobile phase   Dissolve 4.873 g of *disodium hydrogen phosphate dihydrate R*, 1.741 g of *sodium dihydrogen phosphate monohydrate R*, 11.688 g of *sodium chloride R* and 50 mg of *sodium azide R* in 1 L of *water R*.

Flow rate   0.5 mL/min.

Detection   Spectrophotometer at 280 nm.

In the chromatogram obtained with the reference solution, the principal peak corresponds to the IgG monomer and there is a peak corresponding to the dimer with a relative retention to the principal peak of about 0.85. Identify the peaks in the chromatogram obtained with the test solution by comparison with the chromatogram obtained with the reference solution; any peak with a retention time less than that of the dimer corresponds to polymers and aggregates.

Results   In the chromatogram obtained with the test solution:
— *retention time*: for the monomer and for the dimer, the retention time relative to the corresponding peak in the chromatogram obtained with the reference solution is 1 ± 0.02;
— *peak area*: the sum of the peak areas of the monomer and the dimer represent not less than 85 per cent of the total area of the chromatogram and the sum of the peak areas of polymers and aggregates represents not more than 10 per cent of the total area of the chromatogram.

Anti-A and anti-B haemagglutinins (*2.6.20, method B*)
If human normal immunoglobulin is intended for subcutaneous administration, it complies with the test.

Anti-D antibodies (*2.6.26*)
If human normal immunoglobulin is intended for subcutaneous administration, it complies with the test.

Antibody to hepatitis B surface antigen
Minimum 0.5 IU per gram of immunoglobulin, determined by a suitable immunochemical method (*2.7.1*).

Antibody to hepatitis A virus
If intended for use in the prophylaxis of hepatitis A, it complies with the following additional requirement.

Determine the antibody content by comparison with a reference preparation calibrated in International Units, using an immunoassay of suitable sensitivity and specificity (*2.7.1*).

The International Unit is the activity contained in a stated amount of the International Standard for anti-hepatitis A immunoglobulin. The equivalence in International Units of the International Standard is stated by the World Health Organization.

Human hepatitis A immunoglobulin BRP is calibrated in International Units by comparison with the International Standard.

The stated potency is not less than 100 IU/mL.
The estimated potency is not less than the stated potency. The confidence limits (*P* = 0.95) are not less than 80 per cent and not more than 125 per cent of the estimated potency.

Immunoglobulin A
As determined by a suitable immunochemical method (*2.7.1*), the content of immunoglobulin A is not greater than the maximum content stated on the label.

Water
Determined by a suitable method, such as the semi-micro determination of water (*2.5.12*), loss on drying (*2.2.32*) or near infrared spectrophotometry (*2.2.40*), the water content is within the limits approved by the competent authority.

Sterility (*2.6.1*)
It complies with the test for sterility.

Pyrogens (*2.6.8*) **or Bacterial endotoxins** (*2.6.14*)
It complies with the test for pyrogens or, preferably and where justified and authorised, with a validated in vitro test such as the bacterial endotoxin test.

For the pyrogen test, inject 1 mL per kilogram of the rabbit's mass.

Where the bacterial endotoxin test is used, the product contains less than 5 IU of endotoxin per millilitre.

STORAGE
Liquid preparation   In a colourless glass container, protected from light.

Freeze-dried preparation   In an airtight, colourless glass container, protected from light.

LABELLING
The label states:
— for liquid preparations, the volume of the preparation in the container and the protein content expressed in grams per litre;
— for freeze-dried preparations, the quantity of protein in the container;
— the route of administration;
— for freeze-dried preparations, the name or composition and the volume of the reconstituting liquid to be added;
— the distribution of subclasses of IgG present in the preparation;
— where applicable, that the preparation is suitable for use in the prophylaxis of hepatitis A infection;
— where applicable, the anti-hepatitis A virus activity in International Units per millilitre;
— where applicable, the name and amount of antimicrobial preservative in the preparation;
— the maximum content of immunoglobulin A.

_____ *Ph Eur*

Normal Immunoglobulin for Intravenous Use

(*Human Normal Immunoglobulin for Intravenous Administration, Ph Eur monograph 0918*)

Ph Eur _____

DEFINITION
Human normal immunoglobulin for intravenous administration is a sterile liquid or freeze-dried preparation containing immunoglobulins, mainly immunoglobulin G (IgG). Other proteins may be present. Human normal immunoglobulin for intravenous administration contains the IgG antibodies of normal subjects. This monograph does not apply to products intentionally prepared to contain fragments or chemically modified IgG.

Human normal immunoglobulin for intravenous administration is obtained from plasma that complies with the requirements of the monograph *Human plasma for fractionation (0853)*. The preparation may contain excipients such as stabilisers.

PRODUCTION

The method of preparation includes a step or steps that have been shown to remove or to inactivate known agents of infection; if substances are used for inactivation of viruses, it shall have been shown that any residues present in the final product have no adverse effects on the patients treated with the immunoglobulin. The method of preparation also includes a step or steps that have been shown to remove thrombosis-generating agents. Emphasis is given to the identification of activated coagulation factors and their zymogens and process steps that may cause their activation. Consideration is also to be given to other procoagulant agents that could be introduced by the manufacturing process.

The product shall have been shown, by suitable tests in animals and evaluation during clinical trials, to be well tolerated when administered intravenously.

Human normal immunoglobulin for intravenous administration is prepared from pooled material from not fewer than 1000 donors by a method that has been shown to yield a product that:
— does not transmit infection;
— at an immunoglobulin concentration of 50 g/L, contains antibodies for at least 2 of which (1 viral and 1 bacterial) an International Standard or Reference Preparation is available, the concentration of such antibodies being at least 3 times that in the initial pooled material;
— has a defined distribution of immunoglobulin G subclasses;
— complies with the test for Fc function of immunoglobulin (2.7.9);
— does not exhibit thrombogenic (procoagulant) activity.

Human normal immunoglobulin for intravenous administration is prepared as a stabilised solution or as a freeze-dried preparation. In both cases the preparation is passed through a bacteria-retentive filter. The preparation may subsequently be freeze-dried and the containers closed under vacuum or under an inert gas. No antibiotic is added to the plasma used. No antimicrobial preservative is added either during fractionation or at the stage of the final bulk solution.

The stability of the preparation is demonstrated by suitable tests carried out during development studies.

CHARACTERS

Appearance:
— *liquid preparation*: clear or slightly opalescent and colourless or pale yellow liquid;
— *freeze-dried preparation*: hygroscopic, white or slightly yellow powder or solid friable mass.

For the freeze-dried preparation, reconstitute as stated on the label immediately before carrying out the identification and the tests, except those for solubility and water.

IDENTIFICATION

Examine by a suitable immunoelectrophoresis technique. Using antiserum to normal human serum, compare normal human serum and the preparation to be examined, both diluted to contain 10 g/L of protein. The main component of the preparation to be examined corresponds to the IgG component of normal human serum. The preparation to be examined may show the presence of small quantities of other plasma proteins; if human albumin has been added as a stabiliser, it may be seen as a major component.

TESTS

Solubility

For the freeze-dried preparation, add to the container the volume of the liquid stated on the label at the recommended temperature. The preparation dissolves completely within 30 min at 20-25 °C.

pH (2.2.3)

4.0 to 7.4.

Dilute the preparation to be examined with a 9 g/L solution of *sodium chloride R* to obtain a solution containing 10 g/L of protein.

Osmolality (2.2.35)

Minimum 240 mosmol/kg.

Total protein

The preparation contains not less than 30 g/L and between 90 per cent and 110 per cent of the quantity of protein stated on the label.

Dilute the preparation to be examined with a 9 g/L solution of *sodium chloride R* to obtain a solution containing about 15 mg of protein in 2 mL. To 2.0 mL of this solution in a round-bottomed centrifuge tube add 2 mL of a 75 g/L solution of *sodium molybdate R* and 2 mL of a mixture of 1 volume of *nitrogen-free sulfuric acid R* and 30 volumes of *water R*. Shake, centrifuge for 5 min, decant the supernatant liquid and allow the inverted tube to drain on filter paper. Determine the nitrogen in the centrifugation residue by the method of sulfuric acid digestion (2.5.9) and calculate the content of protein by multiplying the result by 6.25.

Protein composition

Zone electrophoresis (2.2.31).

Use strips of suitable cellulose acetate gel or suitable agarose gel as the supporting medium and *barbital buffer solution pH 8.6 R1* as the electrolyte solution.

If cellulose acetate is the supporting material, the method described below can be used. If agarose gels are used, and because they are normally part of an automated system, the manufacturer's instructions are followed instead.

Test solution   Dilute the preparation to be examined with a 9 g/L solution of *sodium chloride R* to an immunoglobulin concentration of 30 g/L.

Reference solution   Reconstitute *human immunoglobulin for electrophoresis BRP* and dilute with a 9 g/L solution of *sodium chloride R* to a protein concentration of 30 g/L.

To a strip apply 4.0 μL of the test solution as a 10 mm band or apply 0.4 μL per millimetre if a narrower strip is used. To another strip apply in the same manner the same volume of the reference solution. Apply a suitable electric field such that the albumin band of normal human serum applied on a control strip migrates at least 30 mm. Stain the strips with *amido black 10B solution R* for 5 min. Decolourise with a mixture of 10 volumes of *glacial acetic acid R* and 90 volumes of *methanol R* so that the background is just free of colour. Develop the transparency of the strips with a mixture of 19 volumes of *glacial acetic acid R* and 81 volumes of *methanol R*. Measure the absorbance of the bands at 600 nm in an instrument having a linear response over the range of measurement. Calculate the result as the mean of 3 measurements of each strip.

System suitability   In the electropherogram obtained with the reference solution, the proportion of protein in the principal band is within the limits stated in the leaflet accompanying the reference preparation.

Results In the electropherogram obtained with the test solution, not more than 5 per cent of protein has a mobility different from that of the principal band. This limit is not applicable if albumin has been added to the preparation as a stabiliser; for such preparations, a test for protein composition is carried out during manufacture before addition of the stabiliser.

Molecular size distribution
Size exclusion chromatography (*2.2.30*).

Test solution Dilute the preparation to be examined with a 9 g/L solution of *sodium chloride R* to a concentration suitable for the chromatographic system used. A concentration in the range of 4-12 g/L and injection of 50-600 µg of protein are usually suitable.

Reference solution Dilute *human immunoglobulin (molecular size) BRP* with a 9 g/L solution of *sodium chloride R* to the same protein concentration as the test solution.

Column:
— *size: l* = 0.6 m, Ø = 7.5 mm, or l = 0.3 m, Ø = 7.8 mm;
— *stationary phase: hydrophilic silica gel for chromatography R* of a grade suitable for fractionation of globular proteins with relative molecular masses in the range 10 000 to 500 000.

Mobile phase Dissolve 4.873 g of *disodium hydrogen phosphate dihydrate R*, 1.741 g of *sodium dihydrogen phosphate monohydrate R*, 11.688 g of *sodium chloride R* and 50 mg of *sodium azide R* in 1 L of *water R*.

Flow rate 0.5 mL/min.

Detection Spectrophotometer at 280 nm.

Identification of peaks In the chromatogram obtained with the reference solution, the principal peak corresponds to the IgG monomer and there is a peak corresponding to the dimer with a relative retention to the principal peak of about 0.85; identify the peaks in the chromatogram obtained with the test solution by comparison with the chromatogram obtained with the reference solution; any peak with a retention time shorter than that of the dimer corresponds to polymers and aggregates.

Results In the chromatogram obtained with the test solution:
— *retention time*: for the monomer and for the dimer, the retention time relative to the corresponding peak in the chromatogram obtained with the reference solution is 1 ± 0.02;
— *peak area*: the sum of the peak areas of the monomer and the dimer represent not less than 90 per cent of the total area of the chromatogram and the sum of the peak areas of polymers and aggregates represents not more than 3 per cent of the total area of the chromatogram. This requirement does not apply to products where albumin has been added as a stabiliser; for products stabilised with albumin, a test for distribution of molecular size is carried out during manufacture before addition of the stabiliser.

Anticomplementary activity (*2.6.17*)
The consumption of complement is not greater than 50 per cent (1 CH$_{50}$ per milligram of immunoglobulin).

Prekallikrein activator (*2.6.15*)
Maximum 35 IU/mL, calculated with reference to a dilution of the preparation to be examined containing 30 g/L of immunoglobulin.

Anti-A and anti-B haemagglutinins (*2.6.20, method B*)
It complies with the test for anti-A and anti-B haemagglutinins (direct method).

Anti-D antibodies (*2.6.26*)
It complies with the test for anti-D antibodies in human immunoglobulin.

Antibody to hepatitis B surface antigen
Minimum 0.5 IU per gram of immunoglobulin, determined by a suitable immunochemical method (*2.7.1*).

Immunoglobulin A
As determined by a suitable immunochemical method (*2.7.1*), the content of immunoglobulin A is not greater than the maximum content stated on the label.

Water
Determined by a suitable method, such as the semi-micro determination of water (*2.5.12*), loss on drying (*2.2.32*) or near-infrared spectrophotometry (*2.2.40*), the water content is within the limits approved by the competent authority.

Sterility (*2.6.1*)
It complies with the test.

Pyrogens (*2.6.8*) or Bacterial endotoxins (*2.6.14*)
It complies with the test for pyrogens or, preferably and where justified and authorised, with a validated *in vitro* test such as the bacterial endotoxin test.

For the pyrogen test, inject per kilogram of the rabbit's mass a volume equivalent to 0.5 g of immunoglobulin, but not more than 10 mL per kilogram of the rabbit's mass.

Where the bacterial endotoxin test is used, the preparation to be examined contains less than 0.5 IU of endotoxin per millilitre for solutions with a protein content not greater than 50 g/L, and less than 1.0 IU of endotoxin per millilitre for solutions with a protein content greater than 50 g/L but not greater than 100 g/L.

STORAGE
Liquid preparation In a colourless glass container, protected from light, at the temperature stated on the label.

Freeze-dried preparation In an airtight colourless glass container, protected from light, at a temperature not exceeding 25 °C.

LABELLING
The label states:
— for liquid preparations, the volume of the preparation in the container and the protein content expressed in grams per litre;
— for freeze-dried preparations, the quantity of protein in the container;
— the amount of immunoglobulin in the container;
— the route of administration;
— for freeze-dried preparations, the name or composition and the volume of the reconstituting liquid to be added;
— the distribution of subclasses of immunoglobulin G present in the preparation;
— where applicable, the amount of albumin added as a stabiliser;
— the maximum content of immunoglobulin A.

Ph Eur

Anti-D (Rh₀) Immunoglobulin

(Human Anti-D Immunoglobulin,
Ph Eur monograph 0557)

Ph Eur _____

DEFINITION

Sterile liquid or freeze-dried preparation containing immunoglobulins, mainly immunoglobulin G.
The preparation is intended for intramuscular administration. It contains specific antibodies against erythrocyte D-antigen and may also contain small quantities of other blood-group antibodies. *Human normal immunoglobulin (0338)* and/or *Human albumin solution (0255)* may be added.

It complies with the monograph *Human normal immunoglobulin (0338)*, except for the minimum number of donors and the minimum total protein content.

The test for anti-D antibodies *(2.6.26)* prescribed in the monograph *Human normal immunoglobulin (0338)* is not carried out, since it is replaced by the assay of human anti-D immunoglobulin *(2.7.13)* as prescribed below under Potency.

For products prepared by a method that eliminates immunoglobulins with specificities other than anti-D, where authorised, the test for antibodies to hepatitis B surface antigen is not required.

PRODUCTION

Human anti-D immunoglobulin is preferably obtained from the plasma of donors with a sufficient titre of previously acquired anti-D antibodies. Where necessary, in order to ensure an adequate supply of human anti-D immunoglobulin, it is obtained from plasma derived from donors immunised with D-positive erythrocytes that are compatible in relevant blood group systems in order to avoid formation of undesirable antibodies.

ERYTHROCYTE DONORS

Erythrocyte donors comply with the requirements for donors prescribed in the monograph *Human plasma for fractionation (0853)*.

IMMUNISATION

Immunisation of the plasma donor is carried out under proper medical supervision. Recommendations concerning donor immunisation, including testing of erythrocyte donors, have been formulated by the World Health Organization *(Requirements for the collection, processing and quality control of blood, blood components and plasma derivatives*, WHO Technical Report Series, No. 840, 1994 or subsequent revision).

POOLED PLASMA

To limit the potential B19 virus burden in plasma pools used for the manufacture of anti-D immunoglobulin, the plasma pool is tested for B19 virus using validated nucleic acid amplification techniques *(2.6.21)*.

B19 virus DNA

Maximum 10.0 IU/μL.

A positive control with 10.0 IU of B19 virus DNA per microlitre and, to test for inhibitors, an internal control prepared by addition of a suitable marker to a sample of the plasma pool are included in the test. The test is invalid if the positive control is non-reactive or if the result obtained with the internal control indicates the presence of inhibitors.

B19 virus DNA for NAT testing BRP is suitable for use as a positive control.

If *Human normal immunoglobulin (0338)* and/or *Human albumin solution (0255)* are added to the preparation, the plasma pool or pools from which they are derived comply with the above requirement for B19 virus DNA.

POTENCY

Human anti-D immunoglobulin *(2.7.13, Method A)*
The estimated potency is not less than 90 per cent of the stated potency. The confidence limits *(P = 0.95)* are not less than 80 per cent and not more than 120 per cent of the estimated potency.

Method B or C *(2.7.13)* may be used for potency determination if a satisfactory correlation with the results obtained by Method A has been established for the particular product.

STORAGE

See *Human normal immunoglobulin (0338)*.

LABELLING

See *Human normal immunoglobulin (0338)*.

The label states the number of International Units per container.

_____ *Ph Eur*

Anti-D Immunoglobulin for Intravenous Use

(Human Anti-D Immunoglobulin for Intravenous Administration, Ph Eur monograph 1527)

Ph Eur _____

DEFINITION

Sterile liquid or freeze-dried preparation containing immunoglobulins, mainly immunoglobulin G. It contains specific antibodies against erythrocyte D-antigen and may also contain small quantities of other blood-group antibodies. *Human normal immunoglobulin for intravenous administration (0918)* and/or *Human albumin solution (0255)* may be added.

It complies with the monograph *Human normal immunoglobulin for intravenous administration (0918)*, except for the minimum number of donors, the minimum total protein content, the limit for osmolality and the limit for prekallikrein activator.

The test for anti-D antibodies *(2.6.26)* prescribed in the monograph *Human normal immunoglobulin for intravenous administration (0918)* is not carried out, since it is replaced by the assay of human anti-D immunoglobulin *(2.7.13)* as prescribed below under Potency.

For products prepared by a method that eliminates immunoglobulins with specificities other than anti-D, where authorised, the test for antibodies to hepatitis B surface antigen is not required; a suitable test for Fc function is carried out instead of that described in general chapter *2.7.9*, which is not applicable to such a product.

PRODUCTION

Human anti-D immunoglobulin is preferably obtained from the plasma of donors with a sufficient titre of previously acquired anti-D antibodies. Where necessary, in order to ensure an adequate supply of human anti-D immunoglobulin, it is obtained from plasma derived from donors immunised with D-positive erythrocytes that are compatible in relevant blood group systems in order to avoid formation of undesirable antibodies.

ERYTHROCYTE DONORS

Erythrocyte donors comply with the requirements for donors prescribed in the monograph *Human plasma for fractionation (0853)*.

IMMUNISATION

Immunisation of the plasma donor is carried out under proper medical supervision. Recommendations concerning donor immunisation, including testing of erythrocyte donors, have been formulated by the World Health Organization (*Requirements for the collection, processing and quality control of blood, blood components and plasma derivatives*, WHO Technical Report Series, No. 840, 1994 or subsequent revision).

POOLED PLASMA

To limit the potential B19 virus burden in plasma pools used for the manufacture of anti-D immunoglobulin, the plasma pool is tested for B19 virus using validated nucleic acid amplification techniques (*2.6.21*).

B19 virus DNA

Maximum 10.0 IU/µL.

A positive control with 10.0 IU of B19 virus DNA per microlitre and, to test for inhibitors, an internal control prepared by addition of a suitable marker to a sample of the plasma pool are included in the test. The test is invalid if the positive control is non-reactive or if the result obtained with the internal control indicates the presence of inhibitors.

B19 virus DNA for NAT testing BRP is suitable for use as a positive control.

If *Human normal immunoglobulin for intravenous administration (0918)* and/or *Human albumin solution (0255)* are added to the preparation, the plasma pool or pools from which they are derived comply with the above requirement for B19 virus DNA.

ASSAY

Human anti-D immunoglobulin (*2.7.13, Method A*)

The estimated potency is not less than 90 per cent of the stated potency. The confidence limits ($P = 0.95$) are not less than 80 per cent and not more than 120 per cent of the estimated potency.

Method B or C (*2.7.13*) may be used for potency determination if a satisfactory correlation with the results obtained by Method A has been established for the particular product.

STORAGE

See *Human normal immunoglobulin for intravenous administration (0918)*.

LABELLING

See *Human normal immunoglobulin for intravenous administration (0918)*.

The label states the number of International Units per container.

Ph Eur

Hepatitis A Immunoglobulin

(*Human Hepatitis A Immunoglobulin,
Ph Eur monograph 0769*)

Ph Eur

DEFINITION

Sterile liquid or freeze-dried preparation containing immunoglobulins, mainly immunoglobulin G.
The preparation is intended for intramuscular administration. It is obtained from plasma from selected donors having antibodies against hepatitis A virus. *Human normal immunoglobulin (0338)* may be added.

It complies with the monograph on *Human normal immunoglobulin (0338)*, except for the minimum number of donors and the minimum total protein content.

POTENCY

The potency is determined by comparing the antibody titre of the immunoglobulin to be examined with that of a reference preparation calibrated in International Units, using an immunoassay of suitable sensitivity and specificity (*2.7.1*).

The International Unit is the activity contained in a stated amount of the International Standard for anti-hepatitis A immunoglobulin. The equivalence in International Units of the International Standard is stated by the World Health Organization.

Human hepatitis A immunoglobulin BRP is calibrated in International Units by comparison with the International Standard.

The stated potency is not less than 600 IU/mL.
The estimated potency is not less than the stated potency.
The confidence limits ($P = 0.95$) are not less than 80 per cent and not more than 125 per cent of the estimated potency.

STORAGE

See *Human normal immunoglobulin (0338)*.

LABELLING

See *Human normal immunoglobulin (0338)*.

The label states the number of International Units per container.

Ph Eur

Hepatitis B Immunoglobulin

(*Human Hepatitis B Immunoglobulin,
Ph Eur monograph 0722*)

Ph Eur

DEFINITION

Sterile liquid or freeze-dried preparation containing immunoglobulins, mainly immunoglobulin G.
The preparation is intended for intramuscular administration. It is obtained from plasma from selected and/or immunised donors having antibodies against hepatitis B surface antigen. *Human normal immunoglobulin (0338)* may be added.

It complies with the monograph on *Human normal immunoglobulin (0338)*, except for the minimum number of donors and the minimum total protein content.

POTENCY

The potency is determined by comparing the antibody titre of the immunoglobulin to be examined with that of a reference preparation calibrated in International Units, using an immunoassay of suitable sensitivity and specificity (*2.7.1*).

The International Unit is the activity contained in a stated amount of the International Reference Preparation of hepatitis B immunoglobulin. The equivalence in International Units of the International Reference Preparation is stated by the World Health Organization.

The stated potency is not less than 100 IU/mL. The estimated potency is not less than the stated potency. The confidence limits (P = 0.95) are not less than 80 per cent and not more than 125 per cent of the estimated potency.

STORAGE

See *Human normal immunoglobulin (0338)*.

LABELLING

See *Human normal immunoglobulin (0338)*.

The label states the number of International Units per container.

———————————————————— *Ph Eur*

Hepatitis B Immunoglobulin for Intravenous Use

(*Human Hepatitis B Immunoglobulin for Intravenous Administration, Ph Eur monograph 1016*)

Ph Eur ———————————————————

DEFINITION

Sterile liquid or freeze-dried preparation containing immunoglobulins, mainly immunoglobulin G. It is obtained from plasma from selected and/or immunised donors having antibodies against hepatitis B surface antigen. *Human normal immunoglobulin for intravenous administration (0918)* may be added.

It complies with the monograph *Human normal immunoglobulin for intravenous administration (0918)*, except for the minimum number of donors, the minimum total protein content and the limit for osmolality.

POTENCY

The potency is determined by comparing the antibody titre of the immunoglobulin to be examined with that of a reference preparation calibrated in International Units, using an immunoassay (*2.7.1*) of suitable sensitivity and specificity.

The International Unit is the activity contained in a stated amount of the International Reference Preparation of hepatitis B immunoglobulin. The equivalence in International Units of the International Reference Preparation is stated by the World Health Organization.

The stated potency is not less than 50 IU/mL. The estimated potency is not less than the stated potency. The confidence limits (*P* = 0.95) are not less than 80 per cent and not more than 125 per cent of the estimated potency.

STORAGE

See *Human normal immunoglobulin for intravenous administration (0918)*.

LABELLING

See *Human normal immunoglobulin for intravenous administration (0918)*.

The label states the minimum number of International Units of hepatitis B immunoglobulin per container.

———————————————————— *Ph Eur*

Measles Immunoglobulin

(*Human Measles Immunoglobulin, Ph Eur monograph 0397*)

Ph Eur ———————————————————

DEFINITION

Sterile liquid or freeze-dried preparation containing immunoglobulins, mainly immunoglobulin G.
The preparation is intended for intramuscular administration. It is obtained from plasma containing specific antibodies against measles virus. *Human normal immunoglobulin (0338)* may be added.

It complies with the monograph on *Human normal immunoglobulin (0338)*, except for the minimum number of donors and the minimum total protein content.

POTENCY

The potency of the liquid preparation and of the freeze-dried preparation after reconstitution as stated on the label is not less than 50 IU per millilitre of neutralising antibody against measles virus.

The potency is determined by comparing the antibody titre of the immunoglobulin to be examined with that of a reference preparation calibrated in International Units, using a challenge dose of measles virus in a suitable cell culture system. A method of equal sensitivity and precision may be used providing that the competent authority is satisfied that it correlates with neutralising activity for the measles virus by comparison with the reference preparation.

The International Unit is the specific neutralising activity for measles virus contained in a stated amount of the International Standard for human anti-measles serum.
The equivalence in International Units of the International Reference Preparation is stated by the World Health Organization.

Method

Prepare serial 2-fold dilutions of the immunoglobulin to be examined and of the reference preparation. Mix each dilution with an equal volume of a suspension of measles virus containing about 100 $CCID_{50}$ in 0.1 mL and incubate protected from light at 37 °C for 2 h. Using not fewer than 6 cell cultures per mixture, inoculate 0.2 mL of each mixture into each of the cell cultures allocated to that mixture and incubate for not less than 10 days. Examine the cultures for viral activity and compare the dilution containing the smallest quantity of the immunoglobulin which neutralises the virus with that of the corresponding dilution of the reference preparation.

Calculate the potency of the immunoglobulin to be examined in International Units per millilitre of neutralising antibody against measles virus.

STORAGE

See *Human normal immunoglobulin (0338)*.

LABELLING

See *Human normal immunoglobulin (0338)*.

The label states the number of International Units per container.

———————————————————— *Ph Eur*

Human α-1-proteinase Inhibitor

(Ph Eur monograph 2387)

Ph Eur _____

DEFINITION

Human α-1-proteinase inhibitor is a plasma protein fraction containing mainly human α-1-proteinase inhibitor (also known as human α-1-antitrypsin or α-1-antiproteinase). Human α-1-proteinase inhibitor is a glycoprotein existing in isoforms with different isoelectric points and is the most abundant multifunctional serine proteinase inhibitor in human plasma. It is obtained from human plasma that complies with the monograph *Human plasma for fractionation (0853)*, using a suitable fractionation process and further purification steps. Other plasma proteins may be present.

PRODUCTION

GENERAL PROVISIONS

The method of preparation includes steps that have been shown to remove or to inactivate known agents of infection. The subsequent purification procedure must be validated to demonstrate that the concentration of any substances used for inactivation of viruses during production is reduced to a suitable level and that any residues are such as not to compromise the safety of the preparation for patients.

The specific activity is not less than 0.35 mg of active human α-1-proteinase inhibitor per milligram of total protein. Ratio of human α-1 proteinase inhibitor activity to human α-1-proteinase inhibitor antigen is not less than 0.7.

Buffering and other auxiliary substances such as a stabiliser may be included. No antimicrobial preservative is added. The solution is passed through a bacteria-retentive filter and distributed aseptically into the final containers. The product may be freeze-dried.

CONSISTENCY OF THE METHOD OF PRODUCTION

The consistency of the method of production, including demonstration that the manufacturing process yields a product with a consistent composition and maintains the functional integrity of human α-1-proteinase inhibitor, is evaluated by suitable analytical procedures that are determined during process development, and which include:
— assay of human α-1-proteinase inhibitor activity;
— determination of specific human α-1-proteinase inhibitor activity, expressed as the ratio of active human α-1-proteinase inhibitor to total protein;
— characterisation of isoform composition and protein structure by suitable methods such as isoelectric focusing (2.2.54), spectrometric methods (for example, mass spectrometry) or capillary electrophoresis (2.2.47);
— determination of the ratio of human α-1-proteinase inhibitor activity to human α-1-proteinase inhibitor antigen;
— characterisation of accompanying plasma proteins that might be present, by a set of suitable methods such as SDS-PAGE, cellulose acetate electrophoresis or capillary zone electrophoresis (2.2.31) and quantitative determination of relevant accompanying plasma proteins;
— determination of molecular-size distribution, used to quantify the polymeric forms of human α-1-proteinase inhibitor; consideration is given to the potential presence of accompanying proteins that might affect the results.

CHARACTERS

Appearance

Freeze-dried products are hygroscopic, white or pale yellow or pale brown powders or friable solids; liquid products are clear or slightly opalescent, colourless or pale yellow or pale green or pale brown.

If the preparation to be examined is freeze-dried, reconstitute it as stated on the label immediately before carrying out the identification, tests (except those for solubility and water) and assay.

IDENTIFICATION

The assay of human α-1-proteinase inhibitor activity serves to identify the preparation.

TESTS

pH *(2.2.3)*
6.5 to 7.8.

Solubility

To a container of the preparation to be examined add the volume of the liquid stated on the label at room temperature. The preparation dissolves completely when reconstituted according to the instructions for use, giving a clear, colourless or pale green or pale yellow or pale brown solution.

Osmolality *(2.2.35)*
Minimum 210 mosmol/kg.

Total protein

Dilute the preparation to be examined with a 9 g/L solution of *sodium chloride R* to obtain a solution containing about 15 mg of protein in 2 mL. To 2.0 mL of this solution in a round-bottomed centrifuge tube add 2 mL of a 75 g/L solution of *sodium molybdate R* and 2 mL of a mixture of 1 volume of *nitrogen-free sulfuric acid R* and 30 volumes of *water R*. Shake, centrifuge for 5 min, decant the supernatant and allow the inverted tube to drain on filter paper. Determine the nitrogen in the residue by the method of sulfuric acid digestion (2.5.9) and calculate the protein content by multiplying by 6.25.

Water

Determined by a suitable method, such as the semi-micro determination of water (2.5.12), loss on drying (2.2.32) or near-infrared spectrophotometry (2.2.40), the water content is within the limits approved by the competent authority.

Sterility *(2.6.1)*
It complies with the test.

Pyrogens *(2.6.8)*
It complies with the test. Inject per kilogram of the rabbit's mass a volume equivalent to not less than 60 mg of human α-1-proteinase inhibitor.

ASSAY

Carry out the assay of human α-1-proteinase inhibitor (2.7.32). The estimated potency is not less than 80 per cent and not more than 120 per cent of the stated potency. The confidence limits ($P = 0.95$) are not less than 80 per cent and not more than 120 per cent of the estimated potency.

STORAGE

Unless otherwise justified and authorised, in an airtight and sterile container, at a temperature not exceeding 25 °C.

LABELLING

The label states:
— the potency of active (functional) human α-1-proteinase inhibitor per container;
— the name and quantity of any added substances;
— the quantity of protein per container;
— where applicable, the name and volume of the liquid to be used for reconstitution;

— that the transmission of infectious agents cannot be totally excluded when medicinal products prepared from human blood or plasma are administered.

Ph Eur

Rabies Immunoglobulin

(*Human Rabies Immunoglobulin,
Ph Eur monograph 0723*)

Ph Eur

DEFINITION

Sterile liquid or freeze-dried preparation containing immunoglobulins, mainly immunoglobulin G.

The preparation is intended for intramuscular administration. It is obtained from plasma from donors immunised against rabies. It contains specific antibodies neutralising the rabies virus. *Human normal immunoglobulin (0338)* may be added.

It complies with the monograph on *Human normal immunoglobulin (0338)*, except for the minimum number of donors and the minimum total protein content.

POTENCY

The potency is determined by comparing the dose of immunoglobulin required to neutralise the infectivity of a rabies virus suspension with the dose of a reference preparation, calibrated in International Units, required to produce the same degree of neutralisation (*2.7.1*). The test is performed in sensitive cell cultures and the presence of unneutralised virus is revealed by immunofluorescence.

The International Unit is the specific neutralising activity for rabies virus in a stated amount of the International Standard for anti-rabies immunoglobulin. The equivalence in International Units of the International Standard is stated by the World Health Organization.

Human rabies immunoglobulin BRP is calibrated in International Units by comparison with the International Standard.

Method

Carry out the test in suitable sensitive cells. It is usual to use the BHK-21 cell line, grown in the medium described below, between the 18th and 30th passage levels counted from the ATCC seed lot. Harvest the cells after 2 to 4 days of growth, treat with trypsin and prepare a suspension containing 500 000 cells per millilitre (cell suspension). 10 min before using this suspension add 10 µg of *diethylamino-ethyldextran R* per millilitre, if necessary, to increase the sensitivity of the cells.

Use a fixed virus strain grown in sensitive cells, such as the CVS strain of rabies virus adapted to growth in the BHK-21 cell line (seed virus suspension). Estimate the titre of the seed virus suspension as follows.

Prepare a series of dilutions of the viral suspension. In the chambers of cell-culture slides (8 chambers per slide), place 0.1 mL of each dilution and 0.1 mL of medium and add 0.2 mL of the cell suspension. Incubate in an atmosphere of carbon dioxide at 37 °C for 24 h. Carry out fixation, immunofluorescence staining and evaluation as described below. Determine the end-point titre of the seed virus suspension and prepare the working virus dilution corresponding to 100 $CCID_{50}$ per 0.1 mL.

For each assay, check the amount of virus used by performing a control titration: from the dilution corresponding to 100 $CCID_{50}$ per 0.1 mL, make 3 tenfold dilutions. Add 0.1 mL of each dilution to 4 chambers containing 0.1 mL of medium and add 0.2 mL of the cell suspension. The test is not valid unless the titre lies between 30 $CCID_{50}$ and 300 $CCID_{50}$.

Dilute the reference preparation to a concentration of 2 IU/mL using non-supplemented culture medium (stock reference dilution, stored below −80 °C). Prepare 2 suitable predilutions (1:8 and 1:10) of the stock reference dilution so that the dilution of the reference preparation that reduces the number of fluorescent fields by 50 per cent lies within the 4 dilutions of the cell-culture slide. Add 0.1 mL of the medium to each chamber, except the first in each of 2 rows, to which add respectively 0.2 mL of the 2 predilutions of the stock reference dilution transferring successively 0.1 mL to the other chambers.

Dilute the preparation to be examined 1 in 100 using non-supplemented medium (stock immunoglobulin dilution) – to reduce to a minimum errors due to viscosity of the undiluted preparation – and make 3 suitable predilutions so that the dilution of the preparation to be examined that reduces the number of fluorescent fields by 50 per cent lies within the 4 dilutions of the cell-culture slide. Add 0.1 mL of the medium to all the chambers except the first in each of 3 rows, to which add respectively 0.2 mL of the 3 predilutions of the stock immunoglobulin dilution. Prepare a series of 2-fold dilutions transferring successively 0.1 mL to the other chambers.

To all the chambers containing the dilutions of the reference preparation and the dilutions of the preparation to be examined, add 0.1 mL of the virus suspension corresponding to 100 $CCID_{50}$ per 0.1 mL (working virus dilution), shake manually, allow to stand in an atmosphere of carbon dioxide at 37 °C for 90 min, add 0.2 mL of the cell suspension, shake manually and allow to stand in an atmosphere of carbon dioxide at 37 °C for 24 h.

After 24 h, discard the medium and remove the plastic walls. Wash the cell monolayer with *phosphate buffered saline pH 7.4 R* and then with a mixture of 20 volumes of *water R* and 80 volumes of *acetone R* and fix in a mixture of 20 volumes of *water R* and 80 volumes of *acetone R* at −20 °C for 3 min. Spread on the slides *fluorescein-conjugated rabies antiserum R* ready for use. Allow to stand in an atmosphere with a high level of moisture at 37 °C for 30 min. Wash with *phosphate buffered saline pH 7.4 R* and dry. Examine 20 fields in each chamber at a magnification of 250 ×, using a microscope equipped for fluorescence readings. Note the number of fields with at least 1 fluorescent cell. Check the test dose used in the virus titration slide and determine the dilution of the reference preparation and the dilution of the preparation to be examined that reduce the number of fluorescent fields by 50 per cent, calculating the 2 or 3 dilutions together using probit analysis. The test is not valid unless the statistical analysis shows a significant slope of the dose-response curve and no evidence of deviation from linearity or parallelism.

The stated potency is not less than 150 IU/mL.

The estimated potency is not less than the stated potency and is not greater than twice the stated potency.

The confidence limits ($P = 0.95$) are not less than 80 per cent and not more than 125 per cent of the estimated potency.

CULTURE MEDIUM FOR GROWTH OF BHK-21 CELLS

Commercially available media that have a slightly different composition from that shown below may also be used.

Sodium chloride	6.4 g
Potassium chloride	0.40 g
Calcium chloride, anhydrous	0.20 g
Magnesium sulfate, heptahydrate	0.20 g
Sodium dihydrogen phosphate, monohydrate	0.124 g
Glucose monohydrate	4.5 g
Ferric nitrate, nonahydrate	0.10 mg
L-Arginine hydrochloride	42.0 mg
L-Cystine	24.0 mg
L-Histidine	16.0 mg
L-Isoleucine	52.0 mg
L-Leucine	52.0 mg
L-Lysine hydrochloride	74.0 mg
L-Phenylalanine	33.0 mg
L-Threonine	48.0 mg
L-Tryptophan	8.0 mg
L-Tyrosine	36.0 mg
L-Valine	47.0 mg
L-Methionine	15.0 mg
L-Glutamine	0.292 g
i-Inositol	3.60 mg
Choline chloride	2.0 mg
Folic acid	2.0 mg
Nicotinamide	2.0 mg
Calcium pantothenate	2.0 mg
Pyridoxal hydrochloride	2.0 mg
Thiamine hydrochloride	2.0 mg
Riboflavine	0.2 mg
Phenol red	15.0 mg
Sodium hydrogen carbonate	2.75 g
Water	to 1000 mL

The medium is supplemented with:

Foetal calf serum (heated at 56 °C for 30 min)	10 per cent
Tryptose phosphate broth	10 per cent
Benzylpenicillin sodium	60 mg/L
Streptomycin	0.1 g/L

STORAGE

See *Human normal immunoglobulin (0338)*.

LABELLING

See *Human normal immunoglobulin (0338)*.

The label states the number of International Units per container.

_____ Ph Eur

Rubella Immunoglobulin

(*Human Rubella Immunoglobulin,*
Ph Eur monograph 0617)

Ph Eur _____

DEFINITION

Sterile liquid or freeze-dried preparation containing immunoglobulins, mainly immunoglobulin G.
The preparation is intended for intramuscular administration.
It is obtained from plasma containing specific antibodies against rubella virus. *Human normal immunoglobulin (0338)* may be added.

It complies with the monograph on *Human normal immunoglobulin (0338)*, except for the minimum number of donors and the minimum total protein content.

POTENCY

The potency is determined by comparing the activity of the preparation to be examined in a suitable haemagglutination-inhibition test with that of a reference preparation calibrated in International Units.

The International Unit is the activity contained in a stated amount of the International Standard for anti-rubella immunoglobulin. The equivalence in International Units of the International Reference Preparation is stated by the World Health Organization.

The estimated potency is not less than 4500 IU/mL.
The confidence limits ($P = 0.95$) of the estimated potency are not less than 50 per cent and not more than 200 per cent of the stated potency.

STORAGE

See *Human normal immunoglobulin (0338)*.

LABELLING

See *Human normal immunoglobulin (0338)*.

The label states the number of International Units per millilitre.

_____ Ph Eur

Tetanus Immunoglobulin

(*Human Tetanus Immunoglobulin,*
Ph Eur monograph 0398)

Ph Eur _____

DEFINITION

Sterile liquid or freeze-dried preparation containing immunoglobulins, mainly immunoglobulin G.
The preparation is intended for intramuscular administration.
It is obtained from plasma containing specific antibodies against the toxin of *Clostridium tetani*. *Human normal immunoglobulin (0338)* may be added.

It complies with the monograph *Human normal immunoglobulin (0338)*, except for the minimum number of donors and the minimum total protein content.

PRODUCTION

During development, a satisfactory relationship shall be established between the potency determined by immunoassay as described under Potency and that determined by means of the following test for toxin-neutralising capacity in mice.

Toxin-neutralising capacity in mice The potency is determined by comparing the quantity necessary to protect mice against the paralytic effects of a fixed quantity of tetanus toxin with the quantity of a reference preparation of human tetanus immunoglobulin, calibrated in International Units, necessary to give the same protection.

The International Unit of antitoxin is the specific neutralising activity for tetanus toxin contained in a stated amount of the International Standard, which consists of freeze-dried human immunoglobulin. The equivalence in International Units of the International Standard is stated by the World Health Organization.

Human tetanus immunoglobulin BRP is calibrated in International Units by comparison with the International Standard.

Method

Selection of animals   Use mice weighing 16-20 g.

Preparation of the test toxin   Prepare the test toxin by a suitable method from the sterile filtrate of a culture in liquid medium of *C. tetani*. The 2 methods shown below are given as examples and any other suitable method may be used.

(1) To the filtrate of an approximately 9-day culture, add 1-2 volumes of *glycerol R* and store the mixture in the liquid state at a temperature slightly below 0 °C.

(2) Precipitate the toxin by addition to the filtrate of *ammonium sulfate R*, dry the precipitate *in vacuo* over *diphosphorus pentoxide R*, reduce to a powder and store dry, either in sealed ampoules or *in vacuo* over *diphosphorus pentoxide R*.

Determination of test dose of toxin (Lp/10 dose)   Prepare a solution of the reference preparation in a suitable liquid such that it contains 0.5 IU of antitoxin per millilitre. If the test toxin is stored dry, reconstitute it using a suitable liquid. Prepare mixtures of the solution of the reference preparation and the test toxin such that each contains 2.0 mL of the solution of the reference preparation, one of a graded series of volumes of the test toxin and sufficient of a suitable liquid to bring the volume to 5.0 mL. Allow the mixtures to stand, protected from light, for 60 min. Using 6 mice for each mixture, inject a dose of 0.5 mL subcutaneously into each mouse. Observe the mice for 96 h. Mice that become paralysed may be euthanised. The test dose of toxin is the quantity in 0.5 mL of the mixture made with the smallest amount of toxin capable of causing, despite partial neutralisation by the reference preparation, paralysis in all 6 mice injected with the mixture, within the observation period.

Determination of potency of the immunoglobulin   Prepare a solution of the reference preparation in a suitable liquid such that it contains 0.5 IU of antitoxin per millilitre. Prepare a solution of the test toxin in a suitable liquid such that it contains 5 test doses per millilitre. Prepare mixtures of the solution of the test toxin and the immunoglobulin to be examined such that each contains 2.0 mL of the solution of the test toxin, one of a graded series of volumes of the immunoglobulin to be examined and sufficient of a suitable liquid to bring the total volume to 5.0 mL. Also prepare mixtures of the solution of the test toxin and the solution of the reference preparation such that each contains 2.0 mL of the solution of the test toxin, one of a graded series of volumes of the solution of the reference preparation centred on that volume (2.0 mL) that contains 1 IU and sufficient of a suitable liquid to bring the total volume to 5.0 mL. Allow the mixtures to stand, protected from light, for 60 min. Using 6 mice for each mixture, inject subcutaneously a dose of 0.5 mL into each mouse. Observe the mice for 96 h. Mice that become paralysed may be euthanised. The mixture that contains the largest volume of immunoglobulin that fails to protect the mice from paralysis contains 1 IU. This quantity is used to calculate the potency of the immunoglobulin in International Units per millilitre.

The test is not valid unless all the mice injected with mixtures containing 2.0 mL or less of the solution of reference preparation show paralysis and all those injected with mixtures containing more do not.

POTENCY

The potency is determined by comparing the antibody titre of the preparation to be examined with that of a reference preparation calibrated in International Units, using suitable immunochemical methods (*2.7.1*) such as enzyme-linked immunosorbent assay (ELISA) or toxoid inhibition assay (TIA).

The International Unit is the activity contained in a stated amount of the International Standard for anti-tetanus immunoglobulin. The equivalence in International Units of the International Standard is stated by the World Health Organization.

Human tetanus immunoglobulin BRP is calibrated in International Units and is suitable for use as a reference preparation.

The stated potency is not less than 100 IU/mL of tetanus antitoxin. The estimated potency is not less than the stated potency. The confidence limits ($P = 0.95$) are not less than 80 per cent and not more than 125 per cent of the estimated potency.

The description of methods A and B below are provided as examples.

Method A: direct enzyme immunoassay

The amount of tetanus immunoglobulin bound to tetanus toxoid, which is coated to a microtitre plate, is determined by means of a peroxidase-conjugated polyclonal anti-human IgG antibody.

Materials

— *Phosphate-buffered saline pH 7.1 (PBS)*. Dissolve 0.2 g of *potassium chloride R*, 0.2 g of *potassium dihydrogen phosphate R*, 1.15 g of *anhydrous disodium hydrogen phosphate R* and 8.0 g of *sodium chloride R* in *water R* and adjust the pH (*2.2.3*) if necessary. Dilute to 1000 mL with *water R*.

— *PBS-T* PBS containing 0.05 per cent *V/V* of *polysorbate 20 R*.

— *Carbonate buffer pH 9.6*. Dissolve 1.4 g of *anhydrous sodium carbonate R* and 3.0 g of *sodium hydrogen carbonate R* in *water R* and adjust the pH (*2.2.3*) if necessary. Dilute to 1000 mL with *water R*.

— *Tetanus toxoid* Purified and chemically inactivated tetanus toxin.

— *Microtitre plate* Use a flat-bottomed microtitre plate with high protein-binding capacity.

Method

Distribute 100 μL of a 0.2 Lf/mL solution of tetanus toxoid in carbonate buffer pH 9.6 into each of the wells of the microtitre plate. Incubate at 4 °C for approximately 18 h. Wash the plate 5 times with PBS-T. To block unbound binding sites add 200 μL of PBS containing 5 g/L of *bovine albumin R* to each of the wells and incubate for 1 h at 37 °C on a plate shaker set at 120 r/min. Wash 5 times with PBS-T.

Reconstitute the reference preparation and the preparation to be examined according to the instructions. For each preparation, prepare 2 independent predilutions of 0.004 IU/mL in PBS by applying several dilution steps. Using PBS, prepare from each predilution 5 serial dilutions with a dilution factor of 1.5 resulting in a dilution series of 6 dilutions in the range of 0.0005-0.004 IU/mL. Depending on the reagents used, a small modification of the dilution series might be necessary to meet the conditions of the statistical model used.

Apply 100 μL of each of the samples of the dilution series to the plate. Incubate for 2 h at 37 °C on a plate shaker set at 120 r/min and wash the plate 5 times with PBS-T. Apply 100 μL of a peroxidase-conjugated anti-human IgG antibody diluted to a suitable concentration with PBS-T containing 5 g/L of *bovine albumin R* to each of the wells and incubate for 1 h at 37 °C on a plate shaker set at 120 r/min. Wash the plate 5 times with PBS-T and apply 100 µL of a suitable 3,3',5,5'-tetramethylbenzidine (TMB) substrate to each of the wells and incubate at room temperature for 10 min in the dark. To stop the reaction, add 100 µL of a 196.2 g/L solution of *sulfuric acid R* to each of the wells. Measure the absorbances at 450 nm and at the reference wavelength of 630 nm. Calculate the potencies of the preparations by the usual statistical methods (*5.3*).

Method B: indirect determination by toxoid-binding inhibition assay

The amount of unbound toxoid in a mixture of toxoid and tetanus immunoglobulin is determined by an enzyme immunoassay and is inversely proportional to the amount of tetanus immunoglobulin present. The method is performed over 2 consecutive days.

Materials
— *Phosphate-buffered saline pH 7.1 (PBS)* See under Method A.
— *PBS-T* See under Method A.
— *Carbonate buffer pH 9.6* See under Method A.
— *Tetanus toxoid* See under Method A.
— *Mab* Mouse monoclonal tetanus toxoid antibody. Use according to the instructions. Prepare a suitable dilution of Mab, e.g. 1/5000, in PBS.
— *Peroxidase-conjugated antibody* Peroxidase-conjugated anti-mouse IgG (H+L) antibody, affinity-purified F(ab)2 fragment without cross-reactivity to human serum proteins. Use according to the instructions. Prepare a suitable dilution of the peroxidase-conjugated antibody in PBS-T containing 5 g/L of *bovine albumin R*.
— *Microtitre plate* Use a round-bottomed microtitre plate with medium protein-binding capacity.
— *ELISA plate* Use a flat-bottomed microtitre plate with high protein-binding capacity.

Method

Day 1

To block the protein-binding sites of the microtitre plate, add 200 µL of PBS containing 5 g/L of *bovine albumin R* to each of the wells of the microtitre plate and incubate for 1 h at 37 °C on a plate shaker set at 120 r/min. Wash the plate 5 times with PBS-T.

Reconstitute the reference preparation and the preparation to be examined according to the instructions. For each preparation, prepare 2 independent predilutions of 0.4 IU/mL in PBS by applying several dilution steps. Prepare from each predilution a dilution series of dilutions containing 0.04 IU/mL, 0.10 IU/mL, 0.12 IU/mL, 0.14 IU/mL, 0.16 IU/mL, 0.18 IU/mL and 0.20 IU/mL. Prepare each dilution directly from the 0.4 IU/mL predilution.

Transfer 100 µL of each dilution of the dilution series to a well of the blocked plate and add 50 µL of a 0.2 Lf/mL solution of tetanus toxoid in carbonate buffer pH 9.6 into each of the wells. Incubate for approximately 18 h at 37 °C on a plate shaker set at 120 r/min.

To coat the ELISA plate, distribute 100 µL of a solution of a human tetanus immunoglobulin diluted to 1 IU/mL in carbonate buffer pH 9.6 into each of the wells of the ELISA plate. Incubate for approximately 18 h at 37 °C on a plate shaker set at 120 r/min.

Day 2

Wash the coated ELISA plate 5 times with PBS-T. To block unbound binding sites add 200 µL of PBS containing 5 g/L of *bovine albumin R* to each of the wells and incubate for 1 h at 37 °C on a plate shaker set at 120 r/min. Wash the plate 5 times with PBS-T. Transfer 100 µL of each mixture of toxoid and tetanus immunoglobulin from the microtitre plate to the coated ELISA plate and incubate for 2 hours at 37 °C on a plate shaker set at 120 r/min. Wash the plate 5 times with PBS-T. Add 100 µL of diluted Mab to each of the wells, incubate the plate for 1 h at 37 °C on a plate shaker set at 120 r/min and wash the plate 5 times with PBS-T. Add 100 µL of the diluted peroxidase-conjugated antibody to each of the wells, incubate the plate for 1 h at 37 °C on a plate shaker set at 120 r/min and wash the plate 5 times with PBS-T. Apply 100 µL of a suitable 3,3',5,5'-tetramethylbenzidine (TMB) substrate to each of the wells and incubate at room temperature for 10 min in the dark. To stop the reaction, add 100 µL of a 196.2 g/L solution of *sulfuric acid R* to each of the wells. Measure the absorbances at 450 nm and at the reference wavelength of 630 nm. Calculate the potencies of the preparations by the usual statistical methods (*5.3*).

STORAGE

See *Human normal immunoglobulin (0338)*.

LABELLING

See *Human normal immunoglobulin (0338)*.

The label states the number of International Units per container.

Ph Eur

Varicella Immunoglobulin

(Human Varicella Immunoglobulin, Ph Eur monograph 0724)

Ph Eur

DEFINITION

Sterile liquid or freeze-dried preparation containing immunoglobulins, mainly immunoglobulin G.
The preparation is intended for intramuscular administration. It is obtained from plasma from selected donors having antibodies against *Herpesvirus varicellae*. *Human normal immunoglobulin (0338)* may be added.

It complies with the monograph on *Human normal immunoglobulin (0338)* except for the minimum number of donors, the minimum total protein content and, where authorised, the test for antibody to hepatitis B surface antigen.

POTENCY

The potency is determined by comparing the antibody titre of the immunoglobulin to be examined with that of a reference preparation calibrated in International Units, using an immunoassay of suitable sensitivity and specificity (*2.7.1*).

The International Unit is the activity contained in a stated amount of the International Standard for anti varicella-zoster. The equivalence in International Units of the International Standard is stated by the World Health Organization.

The stated potency is not less than 100 IU/mL.
The estimated potency is not less than the stated potency. The confidence limits (*P* = 0.95) are not less than 80 per cent and not more than 125 per cent of the estimated potency.

STORAGE

See *Human normal immunoglobulin (0338)*.

LABELLING

See *Human normal immunoglobulin (0338)*.

The label states the number of International Units per container.

_____ Ph Eur

Varicella Immunoglobulin for Intravenous Use

(Human Varicella Immunoglobulin for Intravenous Administration, Ph Eur monograph 1528)

Ph Eur _____

DEFINITION

Sterile liquid or freeze-dried preparation containing immunoglobulins, mainly immunoglobulin G. It is obtained from plasma from selected donors having antibodies against human herpesvirus 3 (varicella-zoster virus 1). *Human normal immunoglobulin for intravenous administration (0918)* may be added.

It complies with the monograph on *Human normal immunoglobulin for intravenous administration (0918)*, except for the minimum number of donors, the minimum total protein content and the limit for osmolality.

POTENCY

The potency is determined by comparing the antibody titre of the immunoglobulin to be examined with that of a reference preparation calibrated in International Units, using an immunoassay of suitable sensitivity and specificity (2.7.1).

The International Unit is the activity contained in a stated amount of the International Standard for anti varicella-zoster immunoglobulin. The equivalence in International Units of the International Standard is stated by the World Health Organization.

The stated potency is not less than 25 IU/mL. The estimated potency is not less than the stated potency. The confidence limits ($P = 0.95$) are not less than 80 per cent and not more than 125 per cent of the estimated potency.

STORAGE

See *Human normal immunoglobulin for intravenous administration (0918)*.

LABELLING

See *Human normal immunoglobulin for intravenous administration (0918)*.

The label states the number of International Units per container.

_____ Ph Eur

von Willebrand Factor

(Human von Willebrand factor, Ph Eur monograph 2298)

Ph Eur _____

DEFINITION

Sterile, freeze-dried preparation of a plasma protein fraction containing the glycoprotein human von Willebrand factor with varying amounts of human coagulation factor VIII, depending on the method of preparation. It is prepared from human plasma that complies with the monograph on *Human*

plasma for fractionation (0853). The preparation may contain excipients such as stabilisers.

This monograph applies to preparations formulated according to the human von Willebrand factor activity.

The potency of the preparation, reconstituted as stated on the label, is not less than 20 IU of human von Willebrand factor per millilitre.

PRODUCTION

GENERAL PROVISIONS

The method of preparation is designed to maintain functional integrity of human von Willebrand factor. It includes steps that have been shown to remove or to inactivate known agents of infection; if substances are used for the inactivation of viruses, the subsequent purification procedure must be validated to demonstrate that the concentration of these substances is reduced to a suitable level and that any residues are such as not to compromise the safety of the preparation for patients.

The specific activity is not less than 1 IU of human von Willebrand factor per milligram of total protein, before the addition of any protein stabiliser.

The human von Willebrand factor fraction is dissolved in a suitable liquid. No antimicrobial preservative or antibiotic is added. The solution is passed through a bacteria-retentive filter, distributed aseptically into the final containers and immediately frozen. It is subsequently freeze-dried and the containers are closed under vacuum or under an inert gas.

CONSISTENCY OF THE METHOD OF PRODUCTION

It shall be demonstrated that the manufacturing process yields a product having a consistent composition with respect to human von Willebrand factor, human coagulation factor VIII and the proportions of human von Willebrand factor and human coagulation factor VIII. This is evaluated by suitable analytical procedures that are determined during process development, and that include the following checks:

Human von Willebrand factor multimers
The distribution of the different human von Willebrand factor multimers is determined by a suitable method such as sodium dodecyl sulfate (SDS) agarose gel electrophoresis with or without Western blot analysis, using a suitable normal human plasma as standard. Visualisation of the multimeric pattern may be performed using, for example, an immunoenzymatic technique and quantitative evaluation may be carried out by densitometric analysis.

Human von Willebrand factor activity (2.7.21)
The human von Willebrand factor activity is estimated by determining the ristocetin cofactor activity and by one or more other suitable assays such as determination of collagen-binding activity using a suitable reference preparation.

Human von Willebrand factor activity/antigen ratio
Consistency of the manufacturing process with respect to the ratio of human von Willebrand factor activity to human von Willebrand factor antigen content is demonstrated.

Products that show particles after reconstitution If a few particles remain when the preparation is reconstituted, it shall be demonstrated during validation studies that the potency is not significantly affected after passage of the preparation through the filter to be provided with the preparation.

CHARACTERS
Appearance
Hygroscopic, white or pale yellow, powder or friable solid.

Reconstitute the preparation to be examined as stated on the label immediately before carrying out the identification, tests (except those for solubility and water) and assay.

IDENTIFICATION
It complies with the limits of the assay.

TESTS
Solubility
To a container of the preparation to be examined, add the volume of the liquid stated on the label at the recommended temperature. The preparation dissolves completely with gentle swirling within 10 min, forming a clear or slightly opalescent, colourless or slightly yellow solution.

In addition, where the label states that the product may show a few particles after reconstitution, reconstitute the preparation as described on the label and pass it through the filter provided: the filtered solution is clear or slightly opalescent.

pH (*2.2.3*)
6.5 to 7.5.

Osmolality (*2.2.35*)
Minimum 240 mosmol/kg.

Total protein
If necessary, dilute an accurately measured volume of the reconstituted preparation with a 9 g/L solution of *sodium chloride R* to obtain a protein concentration of about 7.5 mg/mL. Place 2.0 mL of this solution in a round-bottomed centrifuge tube and add 2 mL of a 75 g/L solution of *sodium molybdate R* and 2 mL of a mixture of 1 volume of *nitrogen-free sulfuric acid R* and 30 volumes of *water R*. Shake, centrifuge for 5 min, decant the supernatant and allow the inverted tube to drain on filter paper. Determine the nitrogen in the residue by the method of sulfuric acid digestion (*2.5.9*) and calculate the amount of protein by multiplying the result by 6.25. *For some products, especially those without a protein stabiliser, this method may not be applicable. Another validated method for protein determination must therefore be performed.*

Anti-A and anti-B haemagglutinins (*2.6.20, Method A*)
The 1 to 64 dilution does not show agglutination. Dilute the reconstituted preparation with a 9 g/L solution of *sodium chloride R* to contain 6 IU of human von Willebrand factor activity per millilitre.

Water
Determined by a suitable method, such as semi-micro determination of water (*2.5.12*), loss on drying (*2.2.32*) or near-infrared spectrophotometry (*2.2.40*), the water content is within the limits approved by the competent authority.

Sterility (*2.6.1*)
It complies with the test.

Pyrogens (*2.6.8*) or Bacterial endotoxins (*2.6.14*)
It complies with the test for pyrogens or, preferably and where justified and authorised, with a validated in *vitro test* such as the test for bacterial endotoxins.

For the pyrogen test, inject per kilogram of the rabbit's mass a volume equivalent to not less than 100 IU of human von Willebrand factor.

Where the test for bacterial endotoxins is used, the preparation to be examined contains less than 0.05 IU of endotoxin per International Unit of human von Willebrand factor.

ASSAY
Human von Willebrand factor (*2.7.21*)
The estimated potency is not less than 80 per cent and not more than 120 per cent of the stated potency. The confidence limits ($P = 0.95$) are not less than 80 per cent and not more than 120 per cent of the estimated potency.

Pending the availability of an International Standard for human von Willebrand factor concentrate calibrated for use in the collagen-binding assay, only the ristocetin cofactor assay may be used.

Human coagulation factor VIII (*2.7.4*)
The assay is carried out where the human coagulation factor VIII content is greater than 10 IU of human coagulation factor VIII per 100 IU of human von Willebrand factor activity. The estimated potency is not less than 60 per cent and not more than 140 per cent of the stated potency. The confidence limits ($P = 0.95$) are not less than 80 per cent and not more than 120 per cent of the estimated potency.

STORAGE
In an airtight container, protected from light.

LABELLING
The label states:
— the number of International Units of human von Willebrand factor in the container;
— the number of International Units of human coagulation factor VIII in the container, or that the content of human coagulation factor VIII is less than or equal to 10 IU of human coagulation factor VIII per 100 IU of human von Willebrand factor activity;
— the amount of protein in the container;
— the name and quantity of any added substance;
— the name and volume of the liquid to be used for reconstitution;
— where applicable, that the preparation may show the presence of a few particles after reconstitution;
— that the transmission of infectious agents cannot be totally excluded when medicinal products prepared from human blood or plasma are administered.

_____ *Ph Eur*

Monographs

Immunological Products

Monoclonal Antibodies for Human Use

(Ph Eur monograph 2031)

Monoclonal Antibodies for Human Use comply with the requirements of the European Pharmacopoeia. These requirements are reproduced below.

The requirements of the monograph for Immunosera do not necessarily apply to the monograph for Monoclonal Antibodies for Human Use.

Ph Eur _____

DEFINITION

Monoclonal antibodies for human use are preparations of an immunoglobulin or a fragment of an immunoglobulin, for example, F(ab′)2, with defined specificity, produced by a single clone of cells. They may be conjugated to other substances, including for radiolabelling.

They can be obtained from immortalised B lymphocytes that are cloned and expanded as continuous cell lines or from rDNA-engineered cell lines.

Examined under suitable conditions of visibility, they are practically free from particles.

Currently available rDNA-engineered antibodies include the following antibodies.

Chimeric monoclonal antibodies   The variable heavy- and light-chain domains of a human antibody are replaced by those of a non-human species that possess the desired antigen specificity.

Humanised monoclonal antibodies   The 3 short hypervariable sequences (the complementarity-determining regions) of non-human variable domains for each chain are engineered into the variable domain framework of a human antibody; other sequence changes may be made to improve antigen binding.

Recombinant human monoclonal antibodies   The variable heavy- and light-chain domains of a human antibody are combined with the constant region of a human antibody.

Monoclonal antibodies obtained from cell lines modified by recombinant DNA technology also comply with the requirements of the monograph *Products of recombinant DNA technology (0784)*.

This monograph applies to monoclonal antibodies, including conjugates, for therapeutic and prophylactic use and for use as in vivo diagnostics. It does not apply to monoclonal antibodies used as reagents in the manufacture of medicinal products. Nor does it apply to monoclonal antibodies produced in ascites, for which requirements are decided by the competent authority.

PRODUCTION

GENERAL PROVISIONS

Production is based on a seed-lot system using a master cell bank and, if applicable, a working cell bank derived from the cloned cells. The production method is validated during development studies in order to prevent transmission of infectious agents by the final product. All biological materials and cells used in the production are characterised and are in compliance with chapter *5.2.8. Minimising the risk of transmitting animal spongiform encephalopathy agents via human and veterinary medicinal products*. Where monoclonal antibodies for human use are manufactured using materials of human or animal origin, the requirements of chapter *5.1.7. Viral safety* also apply. Where an immunogen is used, it is characterised and the method of immunisation is documented.

Process validation

During development studies, the production method is validated for the following aspects:
— consistency of the production process including cell-culture/fermentation, purification and, where applicable, fragmentation method;
— removal or inactivation of infectious agents;
— adequate removal of product- and process-related impurities (for example, host-cell protein and DNA, protein A, antibiotics, cell-culture components);
— specificity and biological activity of the monoclonal antibody;
— absence of non-endotoxin pyrogens, where applicable;
— reusability of purification components (for example, column material), limits or acceptance criteria being set as a function of the validation;
— methods used for conjugation, where applicable.

Product characterisation

The product is characterised to obtain adequate information including: structural integrity, isotype, amino-acid sequence, secondary structure, carbohydrate moiety, disulfide bridges, conformation, specificity, affinity, biological activity and heterogeneity (characterisation of isoforms).

A battery of suitable analytical techniques is used including chemical, physical, immunochemical and biological tests (for example, peptide mapping, *N*- and *C*-terminal amino-acid sequencing, mass spectrometry, chromatographic, electrophoretic and spectroscopic techniques). Additional tests are performed to obtain information on cross-reactivity with human tissues.

For those products that are modified by fragmentation or conjugation, the influence of the methods used on the antibody is characterised.

Process intermediates

Where process intermediates are stored, an expiry date or a storage period justified by stability data is established for each.

Biological assay

The biological assay is chosen in terms of its correlation with the intended mode of action of the monoclonal antibody.

Reference preparation

A batch shown to be stable and shown to be suitable in clinical trials, or a batch representative thereof, is used as a reference preparation for the identification, tests and assay. The reference preparation is appropriately characterised as defined under Product characterisation, except that it is not necessary to examine cross-reactivity for each batch of reference preparation.

Definition of a batch

Definition of a batch is required throughout the process.

SOURCE CELLS

Source cells include fusion partners, lymphocytes, myeloma cells, feeder cells and host cells for the expression of the recombinant monoclonal antibody.

The origin and characteristics of the parental cell are documented, including information on the health of the donors, and on the fusion partner used (for example, myeloma cell line, human lymphoblastoid B-cell line).

Wherever possible, source cells undergo suitable screening for extraneous agents and endogenous agents. The choice of viruses for the tests is dependent on the species and tissue of origin.

CELL LINE PRODUCING THE MONOCLONAL ANTIBODY

The suitability of the cell line producing the monoclonal antibody is demonstrated by:

— documentation on the history of the cell line including description of the cell fusion, immortalisation or transfection and cloning procedure;

— characterisation of the cell line (for example, phenotype, isoenzyme analysis, immunochemical markers and cytogenetic markers);

— characterisation of relevant features of the antibody;

— consistency of critical quality attributes for the antibody up to or beyond the population doubling level or generation number used for routine production;

— for recombinant DNA products, consistency of the coding sequence of the expression construct in cells cultivated to the limit of *in vitro* cell age for production use or beyond, by either nucleic acid testing or product analysis.

CELL BANKS

The master cell bank is a homogeneous suspension of the cell line producing the monoclonal antibody, distributed in equal volumes in a single operation into individual containers for storage.

A working cell bank is a homogeneous suspension of the cell material derived from the master cell bank at a finite passage level, distributed in equal volumes in a single operation into individual containers for storage.

Post-production cells are cells cultured up to or beyond the population doubling level or generation number used for routine production.

The following tests are performed on the master cell bank: viability, identity, absence of bacterial, fungal and mycoplasmal contamination, characterisation of the monoclonal antibody produced. Adventitious viral contamination is tested with a suitable range of *in vivo* and in *vitro* tests. Retrovirus and other endogenous viral contamination is tested using a suitable range of *in vitro* tests.

The following tests are performed on the working cell bank: viability, identity, absence of bacterial, fungal and mycoplasmal contamination. Adventitious viral contamination is tested with a suitable range of *in vivo* and *in vitro* tests. For the first working cell bank, these tests are performed on post-production cells, generated from that working cell bank; for working cell banks subsequent to the first working cell bank, a single *in vitro* and in vivo test can be done either directly on the working cell bank or on post-production cells.

For the master cell bank and working cell bank, tests for specific viruses are carried out when potentially contaminated biological material has been used during preparation of the cell banks, taking into account the species of origin of this material. This may not be necessary when this material is inactivated using validated procedures.

The following tests are performed on the post-production cells: absence of bacterial, fungal and mycoplasmal contamination. Adventitious viral contamination is tested with a suitable range of *in vivo* and *in vitro* tests. Retrovirus and other endogenous viral contamination is tested using a suitable range of in vitro tests.

CULTURE AND HARVEST

Production at finite passage level (single harvest)

Cells are cultivated up to a defined maximum number of passages or population doublings, or up to a fixed harvest time (in accordance with the stability of the cell line). Product is harvested in a single operation.

Continuous-culture production (multiple harvest)

Cells are continuously cultivated for a defined period (in accordance with the stability of the system and production consistency). Monitoring is necessary throughout the life of the culture; the required frequency and type of monitoring will depend on the nature of the production system.

Each harvest is tested for antibody content, bioburden, endotoxin and mycoplasmas. General or specific tests for adventitious viruses are carried out at a suitable stage depending on the nature of the manufacturing process and the materials used. For processes using production at finite passage level (single harvest), at least 3 harvests are tested for adventitious viruses using a suitable range of *in vitro* methods.

The acceptance criteria for harvests for further processing are clearly defined and linked to the schedule of monitoring applied. If any adventitious viruses are detected, the process is carefully investigated to determine the cause of the contamination and the harvest is not further processed. Harvests in which an endogenous virus has been detected are not used for purification unless an appropriate action plan has been defined to prevent transmission of infectious agents.

PURIFICATION

Harvests or intermediate pools may be pooled before further processing. The purification process includes steps that remove and/or inactivate non-enveloped and enveloped viruses. A validated purification process, for which removal and/or inactivation of infectious agents and removal of product- and process-related impurities has been demonstrated, is used. Defined steps of the process lead to a purified monoclonal antibody (active substance) of consistent quality and biological activity.

ACTIVE SUBSTANCE

The test programme for the active substance depends on the validation of the process, on demonstration of consistency and on the expected level of product- and process-related impurities. The active substance is tested for appearance, identity, bioburden and bacterial endotoxins, product-related substances, product- and process-related impurities including tests for host-cell-derived proteins and host-cell- and vector-derived DNA, as well as structural integrity, protein content and biological activity by suitable analytical methods, comparing with the reference preparation where necessary. When the active substance is a conjugated or transformed antibody, appropriate tests must be performed before and after the antibody conjugation/modification.

If storage of intermediates is intended, adequate stability of these preparations and its impact on quality or shelf-life of the finished product are evaluated.

FINAL BULK

One or more batches of active substance may be combined to produce the final bulk. Suitable stabilisers and other excipients may be added during preparation of the final bulk.

The final bulk must be stored under validated conditions with respect to bioburden and stability.

FINAL LOT

The final bulk is sterile-filtered and distributed under aseptic conditions into sterile containers, which may subsequently be freeze-dried.

As part of the in-process control each container (vial, syringe or ampoule) is inspected after filling to eliminate containers that contain visible particles. During development of the product it must be demonstrated that either the process will not generate visible proteinaceous particles in the final lot or such particles are reduced to a low level as justified and authorised.

CHARACTERS

Liquid preparations are clear or slightly opalescent, colourless or slightly coloured liquids. Freeze-dried products are white or slightly coloured powders or solid friable masses. After reconstitution they show the same characteristics as liquid preparations.

IDENTIFICATION

The identity is established by suitable validated methods comparing the product with the reference preparation, where appropriate. The assay also contributes to identification.

TESTS

Appearance

Liquid or reconstituted freeze-dried preparations comply with the limits approved for the particular product with regard to degree of opalescence (*2.2.1*) and degree of coloration (*2.2.2*). They are without visible particles, unless otherwise justified and authorised.

Solubility

Freeze-dried preparations dissolve completely in the prescribed volume of reconstituting liquid, within a defined time, as approved for the particular product.

pH (*2.2.3*)

It complies with the limits approved for the particular product.

Osmolality (*2.2.35*)

Minimum 240 mosmol/kg, unless otherwise justified and authorised.

Extractable volume (*2.9.17*)

It complies with the test for extractable volume.

Total protein (*2.5.33*)

It complies with the limits approved for the particular product.

Molecular-size distribution

Molecular-size distribution is determined by a suitable method, for example size-exclusion chromatography (*2.2.30*). It complies with the limits approved for the particular product.

Molecular identity and structural integrity

Depending on the nature of the monoclonal antibody, its microheterogeneity and isoforms, a number of different tests can be used to demonstrate molecular identity and structural integrity. These tests may include peptide mapping, isoelectric focusing, ion-exchange chromatography, hydrophobic interaction chromatography, oligosaccharide mapping, monosaccharide content and mass spectrometry.

Purity

Tests for process- and product-related impurities are carried out by suitable validated methods. Provided that tests for process-related impurities have been carried out on the active substance or on the final bulk with satisfactory results, they may be omitted on the final lot.

Stabiliser

Where applicable, it complies with the limits approved for the particular product.

Water (*2.5.12*)

Freeze-dried products comply with the limits approved for the particular product.

Sterility (*2.6.1*)

It complies with the test for sterility.

Bacterial endotoxins (*2.6.14*)

It complies with the limits approved for the particular product.

Tests applied to modified antibodies

Suitable tests are carried out depending on the type of modification.

ASSAY

Carry out a suitable biological assay compared to the reference preparation. Design of the assay and calculation of the results are made according to the usual principles (for example, 5.3).

STORAGE

As stated on the label.

Expiry date   The expiry date is calculated from the date of sterile filtration, the date of filling (for liquid preparations) or the date of freeze-drying (where applicable).

LABELLING

The label states:
— the number of units per millilitre, where applicable;
— the quantity of protein per container;
— the quantity of monoclonal antibody in the container;
— for liquid preparations, the volume of the preparation in the container;
— for freeze-dried preparations:
    — the name and the volume of the reconstitution liquid to be added;
    — the period of time within which the monoclonal antibody is to be used after reconstitution;
— the dilution to be made before use of the product, where applicable.

_____ *Ph Eur*

Immunosera

Antisera

(*Immunosera for Human Use, Animal, Ph Eur monograph 0084*)

Immunosera comply with the requirements of the European Pharmacopoeia monograph for Immunosera for Human Use, Animal. These requirements are reproduced below.

Ph Eur _____

DEFINITION

Animal immunosera for human use are liquid or freeze-dried preparations containing purified immunoglobulins or immunoglobulin fragments obtained from serum or plasma of immunised animals of different species.

The immunoglobulins or immunoglobulin fragments have the power of specifically neutralising or binding to the antigen used for immunisation. The antigens include microbial or other toxins, human antigens, suspensions of bacterial and viral antigens and venoms of snakes, scorpions and spiders. The preparation is intended for intravenous or intramuscular administration, after dilution where applicable.

PRODUCTION

GENERAL PROVISIONS

The production method shall have been shown to yield consistently immunosera of acceptable safety, potency in man and stability.

Any reagent of biological origin used in the production of immunosera shall be free of contamination with bacteria, fungi and viruses. The general requirements of chapter *5.1.7*.

Viral safety apply to the manufacture of animal immunosera for human use, in conjunction with the more specific requirements relating to viral safety in this monograph. The method of preparation includes a step or steps that have been shown to remove or inactivate known agents of infection.

Methods used for production are validated, effective, reproducible and do not impair the biological activity of the product.

The production method is validated to demonstrate that the product, if tested, would comply with the test for abnormal toxicity for immunosera and vaccines for human use (*2.6.9*).

Reference preparation A batch shown to be suitable in clinical trials, or a batch representative thereof, is used as the reference preparation for the tests for high molecular mass proteins and purity.

ANIMALS

The animals used are of a species approved by the competent authority, are healthy and are exclusively reserved for production of immunoserum. They are tested and shown to be free from a defined list of infectious agents.

The introduction of animals into a closed herd follows specified procedures, including definition of quarantine measures. Where appropriate, additional specific agents are considered depending on the geographical localisation of the establishment used for the breeding and production of the animals. The feed originates from a controlled source and no animal proteins are added. The suppliers of animals are certified by the competent authority.

If the animals are treated with antibiotics, a suitable withdrawal period is allowed before collection of blood or plasma. The animals are not treated with penicillin antibiotics. If a live vaccine is administered, a suitable waiting period is imposed between vaccination and collection of serum or plasma for immunoserum production.

IMMUNISATION

The antigens used are identified and characterised, where appropriate; where relevant, they are shown to be free from extraneous infectious agents. They are identified by their names and a batch number; information on the source and preparation are recorded.

The selected animals are isolated for at least 1 week before being immunised according to a defined schedule, with booster injections at suitable intervals. Adjuvants may be used.

Animals are kept under general health surveillance and specific antibody production is controlled at each cycle of immunisation.

Animals are thoroughly examined before collection of blood or plasma. If an animal shows any pathological lesion not related to the immunisation process, it is not used, nor are any other of the animals in the group concerned, unless it is evident that their use will not impair the safety of the product.

COLLECTION OF BLOOD OR PLASMA

Collection of blood is made by venepuncture or plasmapheresis. The puncture area is shaved, cleaned and disinfected. The animals may be anaesthetised under conditions that do not influence the quality of the product. Unless otherwise prescribed, an antimicrobial preservative may be added. The blood or plasma is collected in such a manner as to maintain sterility of the product. The blood or plasma collection is conducted at a site separate from the area where the animals are kept or bred and the area where

the immunoserum is purified. If the serum or plasma is stored before further processing, precautions are taken to avoid microbial contamination.

Several single plasma or serum samples may be pooled before purification. The single or pooled samples are tested before purification for the following tests.

Tests for contaminating viruses

If an antimicrobial preservative is added, it must be neutralised before carrying out the tests, or the tests are carried out on a sample taken before addition of the antimicrobial preservative. Each pool is tested for contaminating viruses by suitable *in vitro* tests.

Each pool is tested for viruses by inoculation to cell cultures capable of detecting a wide range of viruses relevant for the particular product.

Potency

Carry out a biological assay as indicated in the monograph and express the result in International Units per millilitre, where applicable. A validated in vitro method may also be used.

Protein content

Dilute the product to be examined with a 9 g/L solution of *sodium chloride R* to obtain a solution containing about 15 mg of protein in 2 mL. To 2 mL of this solution in a round-bottomed centrifuge tube add 2 mL of a 75 g/L solution of *sodium molybdate R* and 2 mL of a mixture of 1 volume of *nitrogen-free sulfuric acid R* and 30 volumes of *water R*. Shake, centrifuge for 5 min, decant the supernatant liquid and allow the inverted tube to drain on filter paper. Determine the nitrogen in the residue by the method of sulfuric acid digestion (*2.5.9*) and calculate the content of protein by multiplying by 6.25. The protein content is within approved limits.

PURIFICATION AND VIRAL INACTIVATION

The immunoglobulins are concentrated and purified by fractional precipitation, chromatography, immunoadsorption or by other chemical or physical methods. They may be processed further by enzyme treatment. The methods are selected and validated to avoid contamination at all steps of processing and to avoid formation of protein aggregates that affect the immunobiological characteristics of the product. For products intended to consist of immunoglobulin fragments, the methods are validated to guarantee total fragmentation. The methods of purification used are such that they do not generate additional components that compromise the quality and the safety of the product.

Unless otherwise justified and authorised, validated procedures are applied for removal and/or inactivation of viruses. The procedures are selected to avoid the formation of polymers or aggregates and, unless the product is intended to consist of Fab' fragments, to minimise the splitting of F(ab')2 into Fab' fragments.

After purification and treatment for removal and/or inactivation of viruses, a stabiliser may be added to the intermediate product, which may be stored for a period defined in light of stability data.

Only an intermediate product that complies with the following requirements may be used in the preparation of the final bulk.

Purity

Examine by non-reducing polyacrylamide gel electrophoresis (*2.2.31*), by comparison with the reference preparation. The bands are compared in intensity and no additional bands are found.

IMMUNOLOGICAL PRODUCTS

FINAL BULK

The final bulk is prepared from a single intermediate product or from a pool of intermediate products obtained from animals of the same species. Intermediate products with different specificities may be pooled.

An antimicrobial preservative and a stabiliser may be added. If an antimicrobial preservative has been added to the blood or plasma, the same substance is used as the antimicrobial preservative in the final bulk.

Only a final bulk that complies with the following requirements may be used in the preparation of the final lot.

Antimicrobial preservative

Where applicable, determine the amount of antimicrobial preservative by a suitable physico-chemical method. It contains not less than 85 per cent and not more than 115 per cent of the amount stated on the label.

Sterility (*2.6.1*)

It complies with the test for sterility.

FINAL LOT

The final bulk of immunoserum is distributed aseptically into sterile, tamper-proof containers. The containers are closed so as to prevent contamination.

Only a final lot that complies with the requirements prescribed below under Identification, Tests and Assay may be released for use. Provided that the tests for osmolality, protein content, molecular-size distribution, antimicrobial preservative, stabiliser, purity, foreign proteins and albumin and the assay have been carried out with satisfactory results on the final bulk, they may be omitted on the final lot.

Reconstitute the preparation to be examined as stated on the label immediately before carrying out the identification, tests (except those for solubility and water) and assay.

IDENTIFICATION

The identity is established by immunological tests and, where necessary, by determination of biological activity. The assay may also serve for identification.

CHARACTERS

Immunosera are clear to opalescent and colourless to very faintly yellow liquids. They are free from turbidity. Freeze-dried products are white or slightly yellow powders or solid friable masses. After reconstitution they show the same characteristics as liquid preparations.

TESTS

Solubility

To a container of the preparation to be examined, add the volume of the liquid for reconstitution stated on the label. The preparation dissolves completely within the time stated on the label.

Extractable volume (*2.9.17*)

It complies with the requirement for extractable volume.

pH (*2.2.3*)

The pH is within the limits approved for the particular product.

Osmolality (*2.2.35*)

Minimum 240 mosmol/kg after dilution, where applicable.

Protein content

90 per cent to 110 per cent of the amount stated on the label, and, unless otherwise justified and authorised, not more than 100 g/L.

Dilute the preparation to be examined with a 9 g/L solution of *sodium chloride R* to obtain a solution containing about 15 mg of protein in 2 mL. To 2 mL of this solution in a round-bottomed centrifuge tube add 2 mL of a 75 g/L solution of *sodium molybdate R* and 2 mL of a mixture of 1 volume of *nitrogen-free sulfuric acid R* and 30 volumes of *water R*. Shake, centrifuge for 5 min, decant the supernatant liquid and allow the inverted tube to drain on filter paper. Determine the nitrogen in the residue by the method of sulfuric acid digestion (*2.5.9*) and calculate the content of protein by multiplying by 6.25.

Molecular-size distribution

Examine by liquid chromatography (*2.2.29* or *2.2.30*). It complies with the specification approved for the particular product.

Antimicrobial preservative

Where applicable, determine the amount of antimicrobial preservative by a suitable physicochemical method. The amount is not less than the minimum amount shown to be effective and is not greater than 115 per cent of that stated on the label.

Phenol (*2.5.15*)

Maximum 2.5 g/L for preparations containing phenol.

Stabiliser

Determine the amount of stabiliser by a suitable physico-chemical method. The preparation contains not less than 80 per cent and not more than 120 per cent of the quantity stated on the label.

Purity

Examine by non-reducing polyacrylamide gel electrophoresis (*2.2.31*), by comparison with the reference preparation. No additional bands are found for the preparation to be examined.

Foreign proteins

When examined by precipitation tests with specific antisera, only protein from the declared animal species is shown to be present, unless otherwise prescribed, for example where material of human origin is used during production.

Albumin

Unless otherwise prescribed in the monograph, when examined electrophoretically, the content of albumin is not greater than the limit approved for the particular product and, in any case, is not greater than 3 per cent.

Water (*2.5.12*)

Maximum 3 per cent.

Sterility (*2.6.1*)

It complies with the test for sterility.

Pyrogens (*2.6.8*)

Unless otherwise justified and authorised, it complies with the test for pyrogens. Unless otherwise prescribed, inject 1 mL per kilogram of the rabbit's body mass.

ASSAY

Carry out a biological assay as indicated in the monograph and express the result in International Units per millilitre, where appropriate. A validated *in vitro* method may also be used.

STORAGE

Protected from light, at the temperature stated on the label. Do not allow liquid preparations to freeze.

Expiry date   The expiry date is calculated from the beginning of the assay.

LABELLING

The label states:

— the number of International Units per millilitre, where applicable;

— the amount of protein per container;
— for freeze-dried preparations:
  — the name and volume of the reconstituting liquid to be added;
  — that the immunoserum is to be used immediately after reconstitution;
  — the time required for complete dissolution;
— the route of administration;
— the storage conditions;
— the expiry date, except for containers of less than 1 mL which are individually packed; the expiry date may be omitted from the label on the container, provided it is shown on the package and the label on the package states that the container must be kept in the package until required for use;
— the animal species of origin;
— the name and amount of any antimicrobial preservative, any stabiliser and any other excipient.

Ph Eur

Anti-T Lymphocyte Immunoglobulin for Human Use, Animal

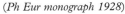

(*Ph Eur monograph 1928*)

Ph Eur

DEFINITION

Sterile liquid or freeze-dried preparation containing immunoglobulins, obtained from serum or plasma of animals, mainly rabbits or horses, immunised with human lymphocytic antigens.

The immunoglobulin has the property of diminishing the number and function of immunocompetent cells, in particular T-lymphocytes. The preparation contains principally immunoglobulin G. It may contain antibodies against other lymphocyte subpopulations and against other cells. The preparation is intended for intravenous administration, after dilution with a suitable diluent where applicable. The preparation may contain excipients such as stabilisers.

Applicable provisions of the monograph on *Immunosera for human use, animal (0084)* are stated below.

PRODUCTION

GENERAL PROVISIONS

The production method has been shown to yield consistently immunoglobulins of acceptable safety, potency in man and stability.

Any reagent of biological origin used in production shall be free of contamination with bacteria, fungi and viruses.
The method of preparation includes a step or steps that have been shown to remove or inactivate known agents of infection.

During development studies, it shall be demonstrated that the production method yields a product that:
— does not transmit infectious agents,
— is characterised by a defined pattern of immunological activity, notably: antigen binding, complement-dependent and independent cytotoxicity, cytokine release, induction of T-cell activation, cell death,
— does not contain antibodies that cross-react with human tissues to a degree that would impair clinical safety,

— has a defined maximum content of anti-thrombocyte antibody activity,
— has a defined maximum content of haemoglobin.

The product has been shown, by suitable tests in animals and evaluation during clinical trials, to be well tolerated.

Reference preparation   A batch shown to be suitable for checking the validity of the assay and whose efficacy has been demonstrated in clinical trials, or a batch representative thereof.

ANIMALS

The animals used are of a species approved by the competent authority, are healthy and exclusively reserved for production of anti-T lymphocyte immunoglobulin. They are tested and shown to be free from a defined list of infectious agents. The introduction of animals into a closed herd follows specified procedures, including definition of quarantine measures. Where appropriate, tests for additional specific agents are considered depending on the geographical localisation of the establishment used for the breeding and production of the animals. The feed originates from a controlled source and no animal proteins are added. The suppliers of animals are certified by the competent authority.

If the animals are treated with antibiotics, a suitable withdrawal period is allowed before collection of blood or plasma. The animals are not treated with penicillin antibiotics. If a live vaccine is administered, a suitable waiting period is imposed between vaccination and collection of serum or plasma for immunoglobulin production.

The species, origin and identification number of the animals are specified.

IMMUNISATION

The antigens used are identified and characterised, where appropriate. They are identified by their names and a batch number; information on the source and preparation are recorded.

The selected animals are isolated for at least 1 week before being immunised according to a defined schedule with booster injections at suitable intervals. Adjuvants may be used.

Animals are kept under general health surveillance and specific antibody production is controlled at each cycle of immunisation.

Animals are thoroughly examined before collection of blood or plasma. If an animal shows any pathological lesion not related to the immunisation process, it is not used, nor are any other of the animals in the group concerned, unless it is evident that their use will not impair the safety of the product.

Human antigens such as continuously growing T-lymphocyte cell lines or thymocytes are used to immunise the animals. Cells may be subjected to a sorting procedure.
The immunising antigens are shown to be free from infectious agents by validated methods for relevant blood-borne pathogens, notably hepatitis B virus (HBV), hepatitis C virus (HCV) and human immunodeficiency virus (HIV) and other relevant adventitious agents originating from the preparation of the antigen. The cells used comply with defined requirements for purity of the cell population and freedom from adventitious agents.

COLLECTION OF BLOOD OR PLASMA

Collection of blood is made by venepuncture or plasmapheresis. The puncture area is shaved, cleaned and disinfected. The animals may be anaesthetised under conditions that do not influence the quality of the product.

No antimicrobial preservative is added to the plasma and serum samples. The blood or plasma is collected in such a manner as to maintain sterility of the product. The blood or plasma collection is conducted at a site separate from the area where the animals are kept or bred and the area where the immunoglobulin is purified. If the serum or plasma is stored before further processing, precautions are taken to avoid microbial contamination.

Several single plasma or serum samples may be pooled before purification. The single or pooled samples are tested before purification for the following tests.

Tests for contaminating viruses

Each pool is tested for contaminating viruses by suitable *in vitro* tests including inoculation to cell cultures capable of detecting a wide range of viruses relevant for the particular product. Where applicable, *in vitro* tests for contaminating viruses are carried out on the adsorbed pool, after the last production stage that may introduce viral contaminants.

PURIFICATION AND VIRAL INACTIVATION

The immunoglobulins are concentrated and purified by fractional precipitation, chromatography, immuno-adsorption or by other suitable chemical or physical methods.

The methods are selected and validated to avoid contamination at all steps of processing and to avoid formation of protein aggregates that effect immunobiological characteristics of the product.

Unless otherwise justified and authorised, validated procedures are applied for removal and/or inactivation of viruses.

After purification and treatment for removal and/or inactivation of viruses, a stabiliser may be added to the intermediate product, which may be stored for a period defined in the light of stability data.

Only an intermediate product that complies with the following requirements may be used in the preparation of the final bulk.

If the method of preparation includes a step for adsorption of cross-reacting anti-human antibodies using material from human tissues and/or red blood cells, the human materials are submitted to a validated procedure for inactivation of infectious agents, unless otherwise justified and authorised. If erythrocytes are used for adsorption, the donors for such materials comply with the requirements for donors of blood and plasma of the monograph on *Human plasma for fractionation (0853)*. If other human material is used, it is shown by validated methods to be free from relevant blood-borne pathogens, notably HBV, HCV and HIV. If substances are used for inactivation or removal of viruses, it shall have been shown that any residues present in the final product have no adverse effects on the patients treated with the anti-T lymphocyte immunoglobulin.

FINAL BULK

The final bulk is prepared from a single intermediate product or from a pool of intermediate products obtained from animals of the same species. No antimicrobial preservative is added either during the manufacturing procedure or for preparation of the final bulk solution. During manufacturing, the solution is passed through a bacteria-retentive filter.

FINAL LOT

The final bulk of anti-T-lymphocyte immunoglobulin is distributed aseptically into sterile, tamper-proof containers. The containers are closed as to prevent contamination.

Only a final lot that complies with the requirements prescribed below under Identification, Tests and Assay may be released for use.

CHARACTERS

Appearance:

— *liquid preparation*: clear or slightly opalescent, colourless or pale yellow liquid;

— *freeze-dried preparation*: white or slightly yellow powder or solid friable mass, which after reconstitution gives a liquid preparation corresponding to the description above.

IDENTIFICATION

A. Using a suitable range of species-specific antisera, carry out precipitation tests on the preparation to be examined. It is recommended that the test be carried out using antisera specific to the plasma proteins of each species of domestic animal commonly used in the preparation of materials of biological origin in the country concerned and antisera specific to human plasma proteins. The preparation is shown to contain proteins originating from the animal used for the anti-T lymphocyte immunoglobulin production.

B. Examine by a suitable immunoelectrophoresis technique. Using antiserum to normal serum of the animal used for production, compare this serum and the preparation to be examined, both diluted to a concentration that will allow a clear gammaglobulin precipitation arc to be obtained on the gel. The main component of the preparation to be examined corresponds to the IgG component of normal serum of the animal used for production.

C. The preparation complies with the assay.

TESTS

Solubility

For the freeze-dried preparation, to a container add the volume of the liquid stated on the label. The preparation dissolves completely within the time stated on the label.

Extractable volume (2.9.17)

It complies with the requirement for extractable volume.

pH (2.2.3)

The pH is within the limits approved for the particular product.

Osmolality (2.2.35)

Minimum 240 mosmol/kg after dilution, where applicable.

Total protein (2.5.33)

90 per cent to 110 per cent of the amount stated on the label.

Stabiliser

Determine the amount of stabiliser by a suitable physico-chemical method. The preparation contains not less than 80 per cent and not more than 120 per cent of the quantity stated on the label.

Distribution of molecular size

Size-exclusion chromatography (2.2.30).

Test solution Dilute the preparation to be examined with a 9 g/L solution of *sodium chloride R* to a concentration suitable for the chromatographic system used. A concentration in the range 2-20 g/L is usually suitable.

Reference solution Dilute *human immunoglobulin (molecular size) BRP* with a 9 g/L solution of sodium chloride R to the same protein concentration as the test solution.

Column:

— *size*: l = 0.6 m, Ø = 7.5 mm,

— *stationary phase*: *silica gel for size-exclusion chromatography R*, a grade suitable for fractionation of

IMMUNOLOGICAL PRODUCTS

globular proteins in the molecular mass range of 20 000 to 200 000.

Mobile phase   Dissolve 4.873 g of *disodium hydrogen phosphate dihydrate R*, 1.741 g of *sodium dihydrogen phosphate monohydrate R* and 11.688 g of *sodium chloride R* in 1 litre of *water R*.

Flow rate   0.5 mL/min.

Detection   Spectrophotometer at 280 nm.

Injection   50-600 µg of protein.

Retention time   Identify the peaks in the chromatogram obtained with the test solution by comparison with the chromatogram obtained with the reference solution; any peak with a retention time shorter than that of dimer corresponds to polymers and aggregates.

System suitability:
— *reference solution*: the principal peak corresponds to IgG monomer and there is a peak corresponding to dimer with a retention time relative to monomer of 0.85 ± 0.05,
— *test solution*: the relative retentions of monomer and dimer are 1 ± 0.05 with reference to the corresponding peaks in the chromatogram obtained with the reference solution.

Limits:
— *total monomer and dimer*: at least 95 per cent of the total area of the peaks;
— *total polymers and aggregates*: maximum 5 per cent of the total area of the peaks.

Purity
Polyacrylamide gel electrophoresis (*2.2.31*), under non-reducing and reducing conditions.

Resolving gel   Non-reducing conditions: 8 per cent acrylamide; reducing conditions: 12 per cent acrylamide.

Test solution   Dilute the preparation to be examined to a protein concentration of 0.5-2 mg/mL.

Reference solution   Dilute the reference preparation to the same protein concentration as the test solution.

Application   10 µL.

Detection   Coomassie staining.

Results   Compared with the electropherogram of the reference solution, no additional bands are found in the electropherogram of the test solution.

Anti-A and anti-B haemagglutinins (*2.6.20, Method A*)
The 1 to 64 dilution does not show agglutination.

Where applicable, dilute the preparation to be examined as prescribed for use before preparing the dilutions for the test.

Haemolysins
Prepare a 1 to 64 dilution of the preparation to be examined, diluted if necessary as stated on the label. Take 6 aliquots of the 1 to 64 dilution. To 1 volume of 3 of the aliquots, add 1 volume of a 10 per cent *V/V* suspension of group A1, group B and group O erythrocytes in a 9 g/L solution of *sodium chloride R*, respectively. To 1 volume of the remaining 3 aliquots, add 1 volume of a 10 per cent *V/V* suspension of group A1, group B and group O erythrocytes in a 9 g/L solution of *sodium chloride R*, respectively, and to each aliquot 1 volume of fresh group AB serum (as a source of complement). Mix and incubate at 37 °C for 1 h. Examine the supernatant liquids for haemolysis. No signs of haemolysis are present.

Thrombocyte antibodies
Examined by a suitable method, the level of thrombocyte antibodies is shown to be below that approved for the specific product.

Water (*2.5.12*)
Maximum 3 per cent.

Sterility (*2.6.1*)
It complies with the test.

Pyrogens (*2.6.8*)
Unless otherwise justified and authorised, it complies with the test for pyrogens. Unless otherwise prescribed, inject 1 mL per kilogram of the rabbit's body mass.

ASSAY
The biological activity is determined by measuring the complement-dependent cytotoxicity on target cells. Flow cytometry is performed with read-out of dead cells stained using propidium iodide. The activity is expressed as the concentration of anti-T lymphocyte immunoglobulin in milligrams per millilitre which mediates 50 per cent cytotoxicity.

Lymphocyte separation medium   Commercial separation media with low viscosity and a density of 1.077 g/mL.

Complement   Commercial complement is suitable.

Buffered salt solution pH 7.2   Dissolve 8.0 g of *sodium chloride R*, 0.2 g of *potassium chloride R*, 3.18 g of *disodium hydrogen phosphate R* and 0.2 g of *potassium dihydrogen phosphate R* in *water R* and dilute to 1000.0 mL with the same solvent.

Buffer solution for flow cytometry   Add 40 mL of 0.1 per cent *V/V* sodium azide R and 10 mL of foetal calf serum to 440 mL of buffered salt solution pH 7.2. The foetal calf serum is inactivated at 56 °C for 30 min prior to use. Store at 4 °C.

Propidium iodide solution   Dissolve *propidium iodide R* in buffered salt solution pH 7.2, to a concentration of 1 mg/mL. Store this stock solution at 2-8 °C and use within 1 month. For the assay, dilute this solution with buffer solution for flow cytometry, to obtain a concentration of 5 µg/mL. Store at 2-8 °C and use within 3 h.

Microtitre plates   Plates used to prepare immunoglobulin dilutions are U- or V-bottomed polystyrene or poly(vinyl chloride) plates without surface treatment.

Micronic tubes   Suitable for flow cytometry measurement.

Cell suspension   Collect blood in anticoagulant from at least one healthy donor. Immediately isolate the peripheral blood mononuclear cells (PBMC) by gradient centrifugation in lymphocyte separation medium so that the PBMC form a visible clean interface between the plasma and the separation medium. Collect the layer containing the cells and dispense into centrifuge tubes containing buffered salt solution pH 7.2. Centrifuge at 400 *g* at 2-8 °C for 10 min. Discard the supernatant. Suspend the cell pellet in buffer solution for flow cytometry. Repeat the centrifugation and resuspension procedure of the cells twice. After the third centrifugation, resuspend the cell pellet in 1 mL of buffer solution for flow cytometry. Determine the number and vitality of the cells using a haemocytometer. Cell viability of at least 90 per cent is required. Adjust the cell number to 7 × 10^6/mL by adding buffer solution for flow cytometry. Store the cell suspension at 4 °C and use within 12 h.

If necessary, the first PBMC pellet may be resuspended in buffered salt solution pH 7.2 containing 20 per cent foetal calf serum and stored overnight at 2 °C. Centrifuge at 400 *g* at 2-8 °C for 10 min. Discard the supernatant. Suspend the cell pellet in buffer solution for flow cytometry. Determine the number and vitality of the cells using a haemocytometer. Cell viability of at least 90 per cent is required. Adjust the cell number to 7×10^6/mL by adding buffer solution for flow cytometry.

It is also possible for cells to be immediately frozen and stored in nitrogen using the following method.

Buffer solution for freezing   To 20 mL of cell culture medium, add 25 mL of foetal calf serum and 5 mL of dimethyl sulfoxide (DMSO). Store this solution at 2-8 °C and use within 3 h.

20×10^6 cells per ampoule are frozen. These ampoules are stored in liquid nitrogen.

Buffer solution for thawing   To 450 mL of cell culture medium, add 50 mL of foetal calf serum. Store this solution at 2-8 °C and use within 3 h.

Each ampoule is thawed in a water-bath at 37 °C with shaking. Cell suspension is repeated in a buffer solution for thawing. Centrifuge at 200 g at 2-8 °C for 10 min. Discard the supernatant. Suspend the cell pellet in buffer solution for flow cytometry. Repeat the procedure for centrifugation and resuspension of cells once. After the second centrifugation, resuspend the cells pellet in 1 mL of buffer solution for flow cytometry. Determine the number and vitality of the cells using a haemocytometer. Cell viability of at least 90 per cent is required. Adjust the cell number to 7×10^6/mL by adding buffer solution for flow cytometry. Store the cell suspension at 4 °C and use within 3 h.

Test solutions   For freeze-dried preparations, reconstitute as stated on the label. Prepare 3 independent series of not fewer than 7 dilutions using buffer solution for flow cytometry as diluent.

Reference solutions   For freeze-dried preparations, reconstitute according to the instructions for use. Prepare 3 independent dilution series of not fewer than 7 dilutions using buffer solution for flow cytometry as diluent.

Distribute 75 µL of each of the dilutions of the test solution or reference solution to each of a series of wells of a microtitre plate. Add 25 µL of the cell suspension of PBMC into each well. Add 25 µL of rabbit complement to each of the wells. Incubate at 37 °C for 30 min.

Centrifuge the plates at 200 *g* at 4 °C for 8 min, discard the supernatant and keep the plate on ice. Preparation for flow cytometry measurement is done step-wise by using a certain number of wells in order to allow labelling with *propidium iodide R* solution and measurement within a defined time period. Resuspend carefully the cell pellet of a certain number of wells with 200 µL of propidium iodide solution. Transfer the suspension into tubes. Incubate at 25 °C for 10 min then place immediately on ice.

Proceed with fluorescence measurement in a flow cytometer. Define a region including all propidium iodide-positive cells on the basis of Forward-Scattered, light (FSC) and flourescence (FL2 or FL3 for propidium iodide). Measure the percentage of propidium iodide-positive cells, without gating but excluding debris. Analyse at least 3000 cells for each of the test and reference solutions.

Use the percentages of dead cells to estimate the potency as the concentration in milligrams per millilitre of the preparation to be examined necessary to induce 50 per cent of cytotoxicity by fitting a sigmoidal dose response curve to the data obtained with the test and the reference preparations and by using a 4-parameter logistic model (see, for example, chapter *5.3*) and suitable software. The test is not valid unless the percentage of propidium iodide-positive cells at the lower asymptote of the curve is less then 15 per cent and the percentage of propidium iodide-positive cells at the upper asymptote of the curve is at least 80 per cent.

The estimated activity is 70 per cent to 130 per cent of the activity approved for the particular product.

The confidence limits ($P = 0.95$) are not less than 80 per cent and not more than 125 per cent of the estimated potency.

STORAGE
Protected from light at the temperature stated on the label.

Expiry date   The expiry date is calculated from the beginning of the assay.

LABELLING
The label states:
— for liquid preparations, the volume of the preparation in the container and the protein content,
— for freeze-dried preparations:
   — the name and the volume of the reconstitution liquid to be added,
   — the quantity of protein in the container,
   — that the immunoserum is to be used immediately after reconstitution,
   — the time required for complete dissolution,
— the animal species of origin,
— the name and amount of stabiliser, where applicable,
— the dilution to be made before use of the product.

_____ *Ph Eur*

Botulinum Antitoxin

(Ph Eur monograph 0085)

The label may state 'Bot/Ser' followed by a letter or letters indicating the type or types present.

When Mixed Botulinum Antitoxin or Botulinum Antitoxin is prescribed or demanded and the types to be present are not stated, Botulinum Antitoxin prepared from types A, B and E shall be dispensed or supplied.

Ph Eur _____

DEFINITION
Botulinum antitoxin is a preparation containing antitoxic globulins that have the power of specifically neutralising the toxins formed by *Clostridium botulinum* type A, type B or type E, or any mixture of these types.

PRODUCTION
It is obtained by fractionation from the serum of horses, or other mammals, that have been immunised against *Cl. botulinum* type A, type B and type E toxins.

IDENTIFICATION
It specifically neutralises the types of *Cl. botulinum toxins* stated on the label, rendering them harmless to susceptible animals.

POTENCY
Not less than 500 IU of antitoxin per millilitre for each of types A and B and not less than 50 IU of antitoxin per millilitre for type E.

The potency of botulinum antitoxin is determined by comparing the dose necessary to protect mice against the lethal effects of a fixed dose of botulinum toxin with the quantity of the standard preparation of botulinum antitoxin necessary to give the same protection. For this comparison a reference preparation of each type of botulinum antitoxin, calibrated in International Units, and suitable preparations of botulinum toxins, for use as test toxins, are required. The potency of each test toxin is determined in relation to the specific reference preparation; the potency of the botulinum antitoxin to be examined is determined in relation to the potency of the test toxins by the same method.

International Units of the antitoxin are the specific neutralising activity for botulinum toxin type A, type B and type E contained in stated amounts of the International Standards which consist of dried immune horse sera of types A, B and E. The equivalence in International Units of the International Standard is stated from time to time by the World Health Organisation.

Selection of animals   Use mice having body masses such that the difference between the lightest and the heaviest does not exceed 5 g.

Preparation of test toxins   *CAUTION: Botulinum toxin is extremely toxic: exceptional care must be taken in any procedure in which it is employed.* Prepare type A, B and E toxins from sterile filtrates of approximately 7-day cultures in liquid medium of *Cl. botulinum* types A, B and E. To the filtrates, add 2 volumes of glycerol, concentrate, if necessary, by dialysis against glycerol and store at or slightly below 0 °C.

Selection of test toxins   Select toxins of each type for use as test toxins by determining for mice the L+/10 dose and the LD$_{50}$, the observation period being 96 h. The test toxins contain at least 1000 LD$_{50}$ in an L+/10 dose.

Determination of test doses of the toxins (L+/10 dose)   Prepare solutions of the reference preparations in a suitable liquid such that each contains 0.25 IU of antitoxin per millilitre. Using each solution in turn, determine the test dose of the corresponding test toxin.

Prepare mixtures of the solution of the reference preparation and the test toxin such that each contains 2.0 mL of the solution of the reference preparation, one of a graded series of volumes of the test toxin and sufficient of a suitable liquid to bring the total volume to 5.0 mL. Allow the mixtures to stand at room temperature, protected from light, for 60 min. Using four mice for each mixture, inject a dose of 1.0 mL intraperitoneally into each mouse. Observe the mice for 96 h.

The test dose of toxin is the quantity in 1.0 mL of the mixture made with the smallest amount of toxin capable of causing, despite partial neutralisation by the reference preparation, the death of all four mice injected with the mixture within the observation period.

Determination of potency of the antitoxin   Prepare solutions of each reference preparation in a suitable liquid such that each contains 0.25 IU of antitoxin per millilitre.

Prepare solutions of each test toxin in a suitable liquid such that each contains 2.5 test doses per millilitre.

Using each toxin solution and the corresponding reference preparation in turn, determine the potency of the antitoxin. Prepare mixtures of the solution of the test toxin and the antitoxin to be examined such that each contains 2.0 mL of the solution of the test toxin, one of a graded series of volumes of the antitoxin to be examined, and sufficient of a suitable liquid to bring the total volume to 5.0 mL. Also prepare mixtures of the solution of the test toxin and the solution of the reference preparation such that each contains 2.0 mL of the solution of the test toxin, one of a graded series of volumes of the solution of the reference preparation centred on that volume (2.0 mL) that contains 0.5 IU, and sufficient of a suitable liquid to bring the total volume to 5.0 mL. Allow the mixtures to stand at room temperature,

protected from light, for 60 min. Using four mice for each mixture, inject a dose of 1.0 mL intraperitoneally into each mouse. Observe the mice for 96 h.

The mixture that contains the largest volume of antitoxin that fails to protect the mice from death contains 0.5 IU. This quantity is used to calculate the potency of the antitoxin in International Units per millilitre.

The test is not valid unless all the mice injected with mixtures containing 2.0 mL or less of the solution of the reference preparation die and all those injected with mixtures containing more survive.

LABELLING
The label states the types of *Cl. botulinum* toxin neutralised by the preparation.

Ph Eur

Diphtheria Antitoxin

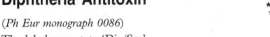

(Ph Eur monograph 0086)
The label may state 'Dip/Ser'.

Ph Eur —————————————————————

DEFINITION
Diphtheria antitoxin is a preparation containing antitoxic globulins that have the power of specifically neutralising the toxin formed by *Corynebacterium diphtheriae*.

PRODUCTION
It is obtained by fractionation from the serum of horses, or other mammals, that have been immunised against diphtheria toxin.

IDENTIFICATION
It specifically neutralises the toxin formed by *C. diphtheriae*, rendering it harmless to susceptible animals.

ASSAY
Not less than 1000 IU of antitoxin per millilitre for antitoxin obtained from horse serum. Not less than 500 IU of antitoxin per millilitre for antitoxin obtained from the serum of other mammals.

The potency of diphtheria antitoxin is determined by comparing the dose necessary to protect guinea-pigs or rabbits against the erythrogenic effects of a fixed dose of diphtheria toxin with the quantity of the standard preparation of diphtheria antitoxin necessary to give the same protection. For this comparison a reference preparation of diphtheria antitoxin, calibrated in International Units, and a suitable preparation of diphtheria toxin, for use as a test toxin, are required. The potency of the test toxin is determined in relation to the reference preparation; the potency of the diphtheria antitoxin to be examined is determined in relation to the potency of the test toxin by the same method.

The International Unit of antitoxin is the specific neutralising activity for diphtheria toxin contained in a stated amount of the International Standard, which consists of a quantity of dried immune horse serum. The equivalence in International Units of the International Standard is stated by the World Health Organisation.

Preparation of test toxin   Prepare diphtheria toxin from cultures of *C. diphtheriae* in a liquid medium. Filter the culture to obtain a sterile toxic filtrate and store at 4 °C.

Selection of test toxin   Select a toxin for use as a test toxin by determining for guinea-pigs or rabbits the lr/100 dose and the minimal reacting dose, the observation period being 48 h.

IMMUNOLOGICAL PRODUCTS

The test toxin has at least 200 minimal reacting doses in the lr/100 dose.

Minimal reacting dose   This is the smallest quantity of toxin which, when injected intracutaneously into guinea-pigs or rabbits, causes a small, characteristic reaction at the site of injection within 48 h.

The test toxin is allowed to stand for some months before being used for the assay of antitoxin. During this time its toxicity declines and the lr/100 dose may be increased. Determine the minimal reacting dose and the lr/100 dose at frequent intervals. When experiment shows that the lr/100 dose is constant, the test toxin is ready for use and may be used for a long period. Store the test toxin in the dark at 0 °C to 5 °C. Maintain its sterility by the addition of toluene or other antimicrobial preservative that does not cause a rapid decline in specific toxicity.

Determination of test dose of toxin (lr/100 dose)   Prepare a solution of the reference preparation in a suitable liquid such that it contains 0.1 IU of antitoxin per millilitre.

Prepare mixtures of the solution of the reference preparation and of the test toxin such that each contains 1.0 mL of the solution of the reference preparation, one of a graded series of volumes of the test toxin and sufficient of a suitable liquid to bring the total volume to 2.0 mL. Allow the mixtures to stand at room temperature, protected from light, for 15 min to 60 min. Using two animals for each mixture, inject a dose of 0.2 mL intracutaneously into the shaven or depilated flanks of each animal. Observe the animals for 48 h.

The test dose of toxin is the quantity in 0.2 mL of the mixture made with the smallest amount of toxin capable of causing, despite partial neutralisation by the reference preparation, a small but characteristic erythematous lesion at the site of injection.

Determination of potency of the antitoxin   Prepare a solution of the reference preparation in a suitable liquid such that it contains 0.125 IU of antitoxin per millilitre.

Prepare a solution of the test toxin in a suitable liquid such that it contains 12.5 test doses per millilitre.

Prepare mixtures of the solution of the test toxin and of the antitoxin to be examined such that each contains 0.8 mL of the solution of the test toxin, one of a graded series of volumes of the antitoxin to be examined and sufficient of a suitable liquid to bring the total volume to 2.0 mL. Also prepare mixtures of the solution of the test toxin and the solution of the reference preparation such that each contains 0.8 mL of the solution of the test toxin, one of a graded series of volumes of the solution of the reference preparation centred on that volume (0.8 mL) that contains 0.1 IU and sufficient of a suitable liquid to bring the total volume to 2.0 mL. Allow the mixtures to stand at room temperature, protected from light, for 15 min to 60 min. Using two animals for each mixture, inject a dose of 0.2 mL intracutaneously into the shaven or depilated flanks of each animal. Observe the animals for 48 h.

The mixture that contains the largest volume of antitoxin that fails to protect the guinea-pigs from the erythematous effects of the toxin contains 0.1 IU. This quantity is used to calculate the potency of the antitoxin in International Units per millilitre.

The test is not valid unless all the sites injected with mixtures containing 0.8 mL or less of the solution of the reference preparation show erythematous lesions and at all those injected with mixtures containing more there are no lesions.

———————————————————————————————— *Ph Eur*

European Viper Venom Antiserum

(Ph Eur monograph 0145)

The only poisonous snake native to the British Isles is the adder or common viper, *Vipera berus*. In a geographical region where other species of snake (including elapids) are found, antisera able to neutralise the venoms of the species of snake indigenous to the region should be used. When the preparation is intended to neutralise the venom or venoms of one or more snakes other than vipers, the title Snake Venom Antiserum is used.

Ph Eur ————————————————————————————————

DEFINITION

European viper venom antiserum is a preparation containing antitoxic globulins that have the power of neutralising the venom of one or more species of viper. The globulins are obtained by fractionation of the serum of animals that have been immunised against the venom or venoms.

IDENTIFICATION

It neutralises the venom of *Vipera ammodytes*, or *Vipera aspis*, or *Vipera berus*, or *Vipera ursinii* or the mixture of these venoms stated on the label, rendering them harmless to susceptible animals.

ASSAY

Each millilitre of the preparation to be examined contains sufficient antitoxic globulins to neutralise not less than 100 mouse LD_{50} of *Vipera ammodytes* venom or *Vipera aspis* venom and not less than 50 mouse LD_{50} of the venoms of other species of viper.

The potency of European viper venom antiserum is determined by estimating the dose necessary to protect mice against the lethal effects of a fixed dose of venom of the relevant species of viper.

Selection of test venoms   Use venoms which have the normal physicochemical, toxicological and immunological characteristics of venoms from the particular species of vipers. They are preferably freeze-dried and stored in the dark at 5 ± 3 °C.

Select a venom for use as a test venom by determining the LD_{50} for mice, the observation period being 48 h.

Determination of the test dose of venom   Prepare graded dilutions of the reconstituted venom in a 9 g/L solution of *sodium chloride R* or other isotonic diluent in such a manner that the middle dilution contains in 0.25 mL the dose expected to be the LD_{50}. Dilute with an equal volume of the same diluent. Using at least four mice, each weighing 18 g to 20 g, for each dilution, inject 0.5 mL intravenously into each mouse. Observe the mice for 48 h and record the number of deaths. Calculate the LD_{50} using the usual statistical methods.

Determination of the potency of the antiserum to be examined   Dilute the reconstituted test venom so that 0.25 mL contains the test dose of 5 LD_{50} (test venom solution).

Prepare serial dilutions of the antiserum to be examined in a 9 g/L solution of *sodium chloride R* or other isotonic diluent, the dilution factor being 1.5 to 2.5. Use a sufficient number and range of dilutions to enable a mortality curve between 20 per cent and 80 per cent mortality to be established and to permit an estimation of the statistical variation.

Prepare mixtures such that 5 mL of each mixture contains 2.5 mL of one of the dilutions of the antiserum to be examined and 2.5 mL of the test venom solution. Allow the

IMMUNOLOGICAL PRODUCTS

mixtures to stand in a water-bath at 37 °C for 30 min. Using not fewer than six mice, each weighing 18 g to 20 g, for each mixture, inject 0.5 mL intravenously into each mouse. Observe the mice for 48 h and record the number of deaths. Calculate the PD_{50}, using the usual statistical methods.

At the same time verify the number of LD_{50} in the test dose of venom, using the method described above. Calculate the potency of the antiserum using the following expression:

$$\frac{(T_v - 1)}{PD_{50}}$$

T_v = number of LD_{50} in the test dose of venom.

In each mouse dose of the venom-antiserum mixture at the end point there is one LD_{50} of venom remaining unneutralised by the antiserum and it is this unneutralised venom that is responsible for the deaths of 50 per cent of the mice inoculated with the mixture. The amount of venom neutralised by the antiserum is thus one LD_{50} less than the total amount contained in each mouse dose. Therefore, as the potency of the antiserum is defined in terms of the number of LD_{50} of venom that are neutralised. rather than the number of LD_{50} in each mouse dose, the expression required in the calculation of potency is $T_v - 1$ rather than T_v.

Alternatively, the quantity of test venom in milligrams that is neutralised by 1 mL or some other defined volume of the antiserum to be examined may be calculated.

LABELLING

The label states the venom or venoms against which the antiserum is effective.

CAUTION   Because of the allergenic properties of viper venoms, inhalation of venom dust should be avoided by suitable precautions.

——————————————————————— Ph Eur

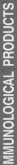

Gas-gangrene Antitoxin (Novyi)

Gas-gangrene Antitoxin (Oedematiens)

(*Ph Eur monograph 0087*)

The label may state 'Nov/Ser'.

Preparation
Mixed Gas-gangrene Antitoxin

Ph Eur _____

DEFINITION

Gas-gangrene antitoxin (novyi) is a preparation containing antitoxic globulins that have the power of neutralising the alpha toxin formed by *Clostridium novyi* (Former nomenclature: *Clostridium oedematiens*). It is obtained by fractionation from the serum of horses, or other mammals, that have been immunised against *Cl. novyi* alpha toxin.

IDENTIFICATION

It specifically neutralises the alpha toxin formed by *Cl. novyi*, rendering it harmless to susceptible animals.

ASSAY

Not less than 3750 IU of antitoxin per millilitre.

The potency of gas-gangrene antitoxin (novyi) is determined by comparing the dose necessary to protect mice or other suitable animals against the lethal effects of a fixed dose of *Cl. novyi* toxin with the quantity of the standard preparation of gas-gangrene antitoxin (novyi) necessary to give the same protection. For this comparison a reference preparation of gas-gangrene antitoxin (novyi), calibrated in International Units, and a suitable preparation of *Cl. novyi* toxin for use as a test toxin are required. The potency of the test toxin is determined in relation to the reference preparation; the potency of the gas-gangrene antitoxin (novyi) to be examined is determined in relation to the potency of the test toxin by the same method.

The International Unit of antitoxin is the specific neutralising activity for *Cl. novyi* toxin contained in a stated amount of the International Standard, which consists of a quantity of dried immune horse serum. The equivalence in International Units of the International Standard is stated by the World Health Organisation.

Selection of animals   Use mice having body masses such that the difference between the lightest and the heaviest does not exceed 5 g.

Preparation of test toxin   Prepare the test toxin from a sterile filtrate of an approximately 5-day culture in liquid medium of *Cl. novyi*. Treat the filtrate with *ammonium sulfate R*, collect the precipitate, which contains the toxin, dry *in vacuo* over *diphosphorus pentoxide R*, powder and store dry.

Selection of test toxin   Select a toxin for use as a test toxin by determining for mice the L+ dose and the LD_{50}, the observation period being 72 h. The test toxin has an L+ dose of 0.5 mg or less and contains not less than 25 LD_{50} in each L+ dose.

Determination of test dose of toxin (L+ dose)   Prepare a solution of the reference preparation in a suitable liquid such that it contains 12.5 IU of antitoxin per millilitre.

Prepare a solution of the test toxin in a suitable liquid such that 1 mL contains a precisely known amount such as 10 mg.

Prepare mixtures of the solution of the reference preparation and the solution of the test toxin such that each contains 0.8 mL of the solution of the reference preparation, one of a graded series of volumes of the solution of the test toxin and sufficient of a suitable liquid to bring the total volume to 2.0 mL. Allow the mixtures to stand at room temperature, protected from light, for 60 min. Using six mice for each mixture, inject a dose of 0.2 mL intramuscularly into each mouse. Observe the mice for 72 h.

The test dose of toxin is the quantity in 0.2 mL of the mixture made with the smallest amount of toxin capable of causing, despite partial neutralisation by the reference preparation, the death of all six mice injected with the mixture within the observation period.

Determination of potency of the antitoxin   Prepare a solution of the reference preparation in a suitable liquid such that it contains 12.5 IU of antitoxin per millilitre.

Prepare a solution of the test toxin in a suitable liquid such that it contains 12.5 test doses per millilitre.

Prepare mixtures of the solution of the test toxin and the antitoxin to be examined such that each contains 0.8 mL of the solution of the test toxin, one of a graded series of volumes of the antitoxin to be examined and sufficient of a suitable liquid to bring the total volume to 2.0 mL. Also prepare mixtures of the solution of the test toxin and the solution of the reference preparation such that each contains 0.8 mL of the solution of the test toxin, one of a graded series of volumes of the solution of the reference preparation centred on that volume (0.8 mL) that contains 10 IU and sufficient of a suitable liquid to bring the total volume to

2.0 mL. Allow the mixtures to stand at room temperature, protected from light, for 60 min. Using six mice for each mixture, inject a dose of 0.2 mL intramuscularly into each mouse. Observe the mice for 72 h.

The mixture that contains the largest volume of antitoxin that fails to protect the mice from death contains 10 IU. This quantity is used to calculate the potency of the antitoxin in International Units per millilitre.

The test is not valid unless all the mice injected with mixtures containing 0.8 mL or less of the solution of the reference preparation die and all those injected with mixtures containing a larger volume survive.

Ph Eur

Gas-gangrene Antitoxin (Perfringens)

(*Ph Eur monograph 0088*)

The label may state 'Perf/Ser'.

Preparation

Mixed Gas-gangrene Antitoxin

Ph Eur

DEFINITION

Gas-gangrene antitoxin (perfringens) is a preparation containing antitoxic globulins that have the power of specifically neutralising the alpha toxin formed by *Clostridium perfringens*. It is obtained by fractionation from the serum of horses, or other mammals, that have been immunised against *Cl. perfringens* alpha toxin.

IDENTIFICATION

It specifically neutralises the alpha toxin formed by *Cl. perfringens*, rendering it harmless to susceptible animals.

ASSAY

Not less than 1500 IU of antitoxin per millilitre.

The potency of gas-gangrene antitoxin (perfringens) is determined by comparing the dose necessary to protect mice or other suitable animals against the lethal effects of a fixed dose of *Cl. perfringens* toxin with the quantity of the standard preparation of gas-gangrene antitoxin (perfringens) necessary to give the same protection. For this comparison a reference preparation of gas-gangrene antitoxin (perfringens), calibrated in International Units, and a suitable preparation of *Cl. perfringens* toxin for use as a test toxin are required. The potency of the test toxin is determined in relation to the reference preparation; the potency of the gas-gangrene antitoxin (perfringens) to be examined is determined in relation to the potency of the test toxin by the same method.

The International Unit of antitoxin is the specific neutralising activity for *Cl. perfringens* toxin contained in a stated amount of the International Standard, which consists of a quantity of dried immune horse serum. The equivalence in International Units of the International Standard is stated by the World Health Organisation.

Selection of animals   Use mice having body masses such that the difference between the lightest and the heaviest does not exceed 5 g.

Preparation of test toxin   Prepare the test toxin from a sterile filtrate of an approximately 5-day culture in liquid medium of *Cl. perfringens*. Treat the filtrate with *ammonium sulfate R*, collect the precipitate, which contains the toxin, dry *in vacuo* over *diphosphorus pentoxide R*, powder and store dry.

Selection of test toxin   Select a toxin for use as a test toxin by determining for mice the L+ dose and the LD$_{50}$, the observation period being 48 h. The test toxin has an L+ dose of 4 mg or less and contains not less than 20 LD$_{50}$ in each L+ dose.

Determination of test dose of toxin (L+ dose)   Prepare a solution of the reference preparation in a suitable liquid such that it contains 5 IU of antitoxin per millilitre.

Prepare a solution of the test toxin in a suitable liquid such that 1 mL contains a precisely known amount such as 10 mg.

Prepare mixtures of the solution of the reference preparation and the solution of the test toxin such that each contains 2.0 mL of the solution of the reference preparation, one of a graded series of volumes of the solution of the test toxin and sufficient of a suitable liquid to bring the total volume to 5.0 mL. Allow the mixtures to stand at room temperature, protected from light, for 60 min. Using six mice for each mixture, inject a dose of 0.5 mL intravenously into each mouse. Observe the mice for 48 h.

The test dose of toxin is the quantity in 0.5 mL of the mixture made with the smallest amount of toxin capable of causing, despite partial neutralisation by the reference preparation, the death of all six mice injected with the mixture within the observation period.

Determination of potency of the antitoxin   Prepare a solution of the reference preparation in a suitable liquid such that it contains 5 IU of antitoxin per millilitre.

Prepare a solution of the test toxin in a suitable liquid such that it contains five test doses per millilitre.

Prepare mixtures of the solution of the test toxin and the antitoxin to be examined such that each contains 2.0 mL of the solution of the test toxin, one of a graded series of volumes of the antitoxin to be examined and sufficient of a suitable liquid to bring the total volume to 5.0 mL. Also prepare mixtures of the solution of the test toxin and the solution of the reference preparation such that each contains 2.0 mL of the solution of the test toxin, one of a graded series of volumes of the solution of the reference preparation centred on that volume (2.0 mL) that contains 10 IU and sufficient of a suitable liquid to bring the total volume to 5.0 mL. Allow the mixtures to stand at room temperature, protected from light, for 60 min. Using six mice for each mixture, inject a dose of 0.5 mL intravenously into each mouse. Observe the mice for 48 h.

The mixture that contains the largest volume of antitoxin that fails to protect the mice from death contains 10 IU. This quantity is used to calculate the potency of the antitoxin in International Units per millilitre.

The test is not valid unless all the mice injected with mixtures containing 2.0 mL or less of the solution of the reference preparation die and all those injected with mixtures containing a larger volume survive.

Ph Eur

IMMUNOLOGICAL PRODUCTS

Gas-gangrene Antitoxin (Septicum)

(*Ph Eur monograph 0089*)

The label may state 'Sep/Ser'.

Preparation

Mixed Gas-gangrene Antitoxin

Ph Eur ⎯⎯⎯⎯⎯⎯⎯⎯⎯⎯⎯⎯⎯

DEFINITION

Gas-gangrene antitoxin (septicum) is a preparation containing antitoxic globulins that have the power of specifically neutralising the alpha toxin formed by *Clostridium septicum*. It is obtained by fractionation from the serum of horses, or other mammals, that have been immunised against *Cl. septicum* alpha toxin.

IDENTIFICATION

It specifically neutralises the alpha toxin formed by *Cl. septicum*, rendering it harmless to susceptible animals.

ASSAY

Not less than 1500 IU of antitoxin per millilitre.

The potency of gas-gangrene antitoxin (septicum) is determined by comparing the dose necessary to protect mice or other suitable animals against the lethal effects of a fixed dose of *Cl. septicum* toxin with the quantity of the standard preparation of gas-gangrene antitoxin (septicum) necessary to give the same protection. For this comparison a reference preparation of gas-gangrene antitoxin (septicum), calibrated in International Units, and a suitable preparation of *Cl. septicum* toxin for use as a test toxin are required.

The potency of the test toxin is determined in relation to the reference preparation; the potency of the gas-gangrene antitoxin (septicum) to be examined is determined in relation to the potency of the test toxin by the same method.

The International Unit of antitoxin is the specific neutralising activity for *Cl. septicum* toxin contained in a stated amount of the International Standard, which consists of a quantity of dried immune horse serum. The equivalence in International Units of the International Standard is stated by the World Health Organisation.

Selection of animals Use mice having body masses such that the difference between the lightest and the heaviest does not exceed 5 g.

Preparation of test toxin Prepare the test toxin from a sterile filtrate of an approximately 5-day culture in liquid medium of *Cl. septicum*. Treat the filtrate with *ammonium sulfate R*, collect the precipitate, which contains the toxin, dry *in vacuo* over *diphosphorus pentoxide R*, powder and store dry.

Selection of test toxin Select a toxin for use as a test toxin by determining for mice the L+ dose and the LD_{50}, the observation period being 72 h. The test toxin has an L+ dose of 0.5 mg or less and contains not less than 25 LD_{50} in each L+ dose.

Determination of test dose of toxin (L+ dose) Prepare a solution of the reference preparation in a suitable liquid such that it contains 5 IU of antitoxin per millilitre.

Prepare a solution of the test toxin in a suitable liquid such that 1 mL contains a precisely known amount such as 20 mg.

Prepare mixtures of the solution of the reference preparation and the solution of the test toxin such that each contains 2.0 mL of the solution of the reference preparation, one of a graded series of volumes of the solution of the test toxin and

sufficient of a suitable liquid to bring the total volume to 5.0 mL. Allow the mixtures to stand at room temperature, protected from light, for 60 min. Using six mice for each mixture, inject a dose of 0.5 mL intravenously into each mouse. Observe the mice for 72 h.

The test dose of toxin is the quantity in 0.5 mL of the mixture made with the smallest amount of toxin capable of causing, despite partial neutralisation by the reference preparation, the death of all six mice injected with the mixture within the observation period.

Determination of potency of the antitoxin Prepare a solution of the reference preparation in a suitable liquid such that it contains 5 IU of antitoxin per millilitre.

Prepare a solution of the test toxin in a suitable liquid such that it contains five test doses per millilitre.

Prepare mixtures of the solution of the test toxin and the antitoxin to be examined such that each contains 2.0 mL of the solution of the test toxin, one of a graded series of volumes of the antitoxin to be examined and sufficient of a suitable liquid to bring the total volume to 5.0 mL. Also prepare mixtures of the solution of the test toxin and the solution of the reference preparation such that each contains 2.0 mL of the solution of the test toxin, one of a graded series of volumes of the solution of the reference preparation centred on that volume (2.0 mL) that contains 10 IU and sufficient of a suitable liquid to bring the total volume to 5.0 mL. Allow the mixtures to stand at room temperature, protected from light, for 60 min. Using six mice for each mixture, inject a dose of 0.5 mL intravenously into each mouse. Observe the mice for 72 h.

The mixture that contains the largest volume of antitoxin that fails to protect the mice from death contains 10 IU. This quantity is used to calculate the potency of the antitoxin in International Units per millilitre.

The test is not valid unless all the mice injected with mixtures containing 2.0 mL or less of the solution of the reference preparation die and all those injected with mixtures containing more survive.

⎯⎯⎯⎯⎯⎯⎯⎯⎯⎯⎯⎯⎯ *Ph Eur*

Mixed Gas-gangrene Antitoxin

(*Ph Eur monograph 0090*)

The label may state 'Gas/Ser'.

Ph Eur ⎯⎯⎯⎯⎯⎯⎯⎯⎯⎯⎯⎯⎯

DEFINITION

Mixed gas-gangrene antitoxin is prepared by mixing gas-gangrene antitoxin (novyi), gas-gangrene antitoxin (perfringens) and gas-gangrene antitoxin (septicum) in appropriate quantities.

IDENTIFICATION

It specifically neutralises the alpha toxins formed by *Clostridium novyi* (former nomenclature: *Clostridium oedematiens*), *Clostridium perfringens* and *Clostridium septicum*, rendering them harmless to susceptible animals.

ASSAY

Gas-gangrene antitoxin (novyi), not less than 1000 IU of antitoxin per millilitre; gas-gangrene antitoxin (perfringens), not less than 1000 IU of antitoxin per millilitre; gas-gangrene antitoxin (septicum) not less than 500 IU of antitoxin per millilitre.

Carry out the assay for each component, as prescribed in the monographs on *Gas-gangrene antitoxin (novyi) (0087)*, *Gas-gangrene antitoxin (perfringens) (0088)* and *Gas-gangrene antitoxin (septicum) (0089)*.

—————————————————————————— *Ph Eur*

Tetanus Antitoxin

(*Tetanus Antitoxin for Human Use,*
Ph Eur monograph 0091)
The label may state 'Tet/Ser'.

Ph Eur ——————————————————————

DEFINITION
Tetanus antitoxin for human use is a preparation containing antitoxic globulins that have the power of specifically neutralising the toxin formed by *Clostridium tetani*.

PRODUCTION
It is obtained by fractionation from the serum of horses, or other mammals, that have been immunised against tetanus toxin.

IDENTIFICATION
It specifically neutralises the toxin formed by *Cl. tetani*, rendering it harmless to susceptible animals.

POTENCY
Not less than 1000 IU of antitoxin per millilitre when intended for prophylactic use. Not less than 3000 IU of antitoxin per millilitre when intended for therapeutic use.

The potency of tetanus antitoxin is determined by comparing the dose necessary to protect guinea-pigs or mice against the paralytic effects of a fixed dose of tetanus toxin with the quantity of the standard preparation of tetanus antitoxin necessary to give the same protection. In countries where the paralysis method is not obligatory the lethal method may be used. For this method the number of animals and the procedure are identical with those described for the paralysis method but the end-point is the death of the animal rather than the onset of paralysis and the L+/10 dose is used instead of the Lp/10 dose. For this comparison a reference preparation of tetanus antitoxin, calibrated in International Units, and a suitable preparation of tetanus toxin, for use as a test toxin, are required. The potency of the test toxin is determined in relation to the reference preparation; the potency of the tetanus antitoxin to be examined is determined in relation to the potency of the test toxin by the same method.

The International Unit of antitoxin is the specific neutralising activity for tetanus toxin contained in a stated amount of the International Standard which consists of a quantity of dried immune horse serum. The equivalence in International Units of the International Standard is stated by the World Health Organisation.

Selection of animals   If mice are used, the body masses should be such that the difference between the lightest and the heaviest does not exceed 5 g.

Preparation of test toxin   Prepare the test toxin from a sterile filtrate of an approximately 9-day culture in liquid medium of *Cl. tetani*. To the filtrate add 1 to 2 volumes of glycerol and store slightly below 0 °C. Alternatively, treat the filtrate with *ammonium sulfate R*, collect the precipitate, which contains the toxin, dry *in vacuo* over *diphosphorus pentoxide R*, powder and store dry, either in sealed ampoules or *in vacuo* over *diphosphorus pentoxide R*.

Determination of test dose of toxin (Lp/10 dose)   Prepare a solution of the reference preparation in a suitable liquid such that it contains 0.5 IU of antitoxin per millilitre.

If the test toxin is stored dry, reconstitute it using a suitable liquid.

Prepare mixtures of the solution of the reference preparation and the test toxin such that each contains 2.0 mL of the solution of the reference preparation, one of a graded series of volumes of the test toxin and sufficient of a suitable liquid to bring the volume to 5.0 mL. Allow the mixtures to stand at room temperature, protected from light, for 60 min. Using six mice for each mixture, inject a dose of 0.5 mL subcutaneously into each mouse. Observe the mice for 96 h. Mice that become paralysed may be euthanised.

The test dose of toxin is the quantity in 0.5 mL of the mixture made with the smallest amount of toxin capable of causing, despite partial neutralisation by the reference preparation, paralysis in all six mice injected with the mixture within the observation period.

Determination of potency of the antitoxin   Prepare a solution of the reference preparation in a suitable liquid such that it contains 0.5 IU of antitoxin per millilitre.

Prepare a solution of the test toxin in a suitable liquid such that it contains five test doses per millilitre.

Prepare mixtures of the solution of the test toxin and the antitoxin to be examined such that each contains 2.0 mL of the solution of the test toxin, one of a graded series of volumes of the antitoxin to be examined and sufficient of a suitable liquid to bring the total volume to 5.0 mL. Also prepare mixtures of the solution of the test toxin and the solution of the reference preparation such that each contains 2.0 mL of the solution of the test toxin, one of a graded series of volumes of the solution of the reference preparation centred on that volume (2.0 mL) that contains 1 IU and sufficient of a suitable liquid to bring the total volume to 5.0 mL. Allow the mixtures to stand at room temperature, protected from light, for 60 min. Using six mice for each mixture, inject into each mouse subcutaneously a dose of 0.5 mL. Observe the mice for 96 h. Mice that become paralysed may be euthanised.

The mixture that contains the largest volume of antitoxin that fails to protect the mice from paralysis contains 1 IU. This quantity is used to calculate the potency of the antitoxin in International Units per millilitre.

The test is not valid unless all the mice injected with mixtures containing 2.0 mL or less of the solution of the reference preparation show paralysis and all those injected with mixtures containing more do not.

—————————————————————————— *Ph Eur*

VACCINES

(Vaccines for Human Use, Ph Eur monograph 0153)
Vaccines comply with the requirements of the European
Pharmacopoeia monograph for Vaccines for Human Use. These
requirements are reproduced below.

Ph Eur _____

DEFINITION

Vaccines for human use are preparations containing antigens capable of inducing a specific and active immunity in man against an infecting agent or the toxin or antigen elaborated by it. Immune responses include the induction of the innate and the adaptive (cellular, humoral) parts of the immune system. Vaccines for human use shall have been shown to have acceptable immunogenic activity and safety in man with the intended vaccination schedule.

Vaccines for human use may contain: whole micro-organisms (bacteria, viruses or parasites), inactivated by chemical or physical means that maintain adequate immunogenic properties; whole live micro-organisms that are naturally avirulent or that have been treated to attenuate their virulence whilst retaining adequate immunogenic properties; antigens extracted from the micro-organisms or secreted by the micro-organisms or produced by genetic engineering or chemical synthesis. The antigens may be used in their native state or may be detoxified or otherwise modified by chemical or physical means and may be aggregated, polymerised or conjugated to a carrier to increase their immunogenicity. Vaccines may contain an adjuvant. Where the antigen is adsorbed on a mineral adjuvant, the vaccine is referred to as 'adsorbed'.

Terminology used in monographs on vaccines for human use is defined in chapter 5.2.1.

Bacterial vaccines containing whole cells are suspensions of various degrees of opacity in colourless or almost colourless liquids, or may be freeze-dried. They may be adsorbed. The concentration of living or inactivated bacteria is expressed in terms of International Units of opacity or, where appropriate, is determined by direct cell count or, for live bacteria, by viable count.

Bacterial vaccines containing bacterial components are suspensions or freeze-dried products. They may be adsorbed. The antigen content is determined by a suitable validated assay.

Bacterial toxoids are prepared from toxins by diminishing their toxicity to an acceptable level or by completely eliminating it by physical or chemical procedures whilst retaining adequate immunogenic properties. The toxins are obtained from selected strains of micro-organisms. The method of production is such that the toxoid does not revert to toxin. The toxoids are purified. Purification is performed before and/or after detoxification. Toxoid vaccines may be adsorbed.

Viral vaccines are prepared from viruses grown in animals, in fertilised eggs, in suitable cell cultures or in suitable tissues, or by culture of genetically engineered cells. They are liquids that vary in opacity according to the type of preparation or may be freeze-dried. They may be adsorbed. Liquid preparations and freeze-dried preparations after reconstitution may be coloured if a pH indicator such as phenol red has been used in the culture medium.

Synthetic antigen vaccines are generally clear or colourless liquids. The concentration of the components is usually expressed in terms of specific antigen content.

Combined vaccines are multicomponent preparations formulated so that different antigens are administered simultaneously. The different antigenic components are intended to protect against different strains or types of the same organism and/or against different organisms.
A combined vaccine may be supplied by the manufacturer either as a single liquid or freeze-dried preparation or as several constituents with directions for admixture before use. Where there is no monograph to cover a particular combination, the vaccine complies with the monograph for each individual component, with any necessary modifications approved by the competent authority.

Adsorbed vaccines are suspensions and may form a sediment at the bottom of the container.

PRODUCTION
General provisions

The production method for a given product must have been shown to yield consistently batches comparable with the batch of proven clinical efficacy, immunogenicity and safety in man. Product specifications including in-process testing should be set. Specific requirements for production including in-process testing are included in individual monographs. Where justified and authorised, certain tests may be omitted where it can be demonstrated, for example by validation studies, that the production process consistently ensures compliance with the test.

Unless otherwise justified and authorised, vaccines are produced using a seed-lot system. The methods of preparation are designed to maintain adequate immunogenic properties, to render the preparation harmless and to prevent contamination with extraneous agents.

Where vaccines for human use are manufactured using materials of human or animal origin, the general requirements of chapter 5.1.7. *Viral safety* apply in conjunction with the more specific requirements relating to viral safety in this monograph, in chapters 5.2.2. *Chicken flocks free from specified pathogens for the production and quality control of vaccines*, 5.2.3. *Cell substrates for the production of vaccines for human use* and 2.6.16. *Tests for extraneous agents in viral vaccines for human use*, and in individual monographs.

Unless otherwise justified and authorised, in the production of a final lot of vaccine, the number of passages of a virus, or the number of subcultures of a bacterium, from the master seed lot shall not exceed that used for production of the vaccine shown to be satisfactory in clinical trials with respect to safety and efficacy or immunogenicity.

Vaccines are as far as possible free from ingredients known to cause toxic, allergic or other undesirable reactions in man. Suitable additives, including stabilisers and adjuvants may be incorporated. Penicillin and streptomycin are neither used at any stage of production nor added to the final product; however, master seed lots prepared with media containing penicillin or streptomycin may, where justified and authorised, be used for production.

Consistency of production is an important feature of vaccine production. Monographs on vaccines for human use give limits for various tests carried out during production and on the final lot. These limits may be in the form of maximum values, minimum values, or minimum and maximum tolerances around a given value. While compliance with these limits is required, it is not necessarily sufficient to ensure consistency of production for a given vaccine. For relevant tests, the manufacturer must therefore define for each product a suitable action or release limit or limits to be applied in view of the results found for batches tested clinically and those used to demonstrate consistency of production. These limits may subsequently be refined on a statistical basis in light of production data.

Substrates for propagation

Substrates for propagation comply with the relevant requirements of the Pharmacopoeia (*5.2.2, 5.2.3*) or in the absence of such requirements with those of the competent authority. Processing of cell banks and subsequent cell cultures is done under aseptic conditions in an area where no other cells are being handled. Serum and trypsin used in the preparation of cell suspensions shall be shown to be free from extraneous agents.

Seed lots/cell banks

The master seed lot or cell bank is identified by historical records that include information on its origin and subsequent manipulation. Suitable measures are taken to ensure that no extraneous agent or undesirable substance is present in a master or working seed lot or a cell bank.

Culture media

Culture media are as far as possible free from ingredients known to cause toxic, allergic or other undesirable reactions in man; if inclusion of such ingredients is necessary, it shall be demonstrated that the amount present in the final lot is reduced to such a level as to render the product safe. Approved animal (but not human) serum may be used in the growth medium for cell cultures but the medium used for maintaining cell growth during virus multiplication shall not contain serum, unless otherwise stated. Cell culture media may contain a pH indicator such as phenol red and approved antibiotics at the lowest effective concentration, although it is preferable to have a medium free from antibiotics during production.

Propagation and harvest

The seed cultures are propagated and harvested under defined conditions. The purity of the harvest is verified by suitable tests as defined in the monograph.

Control cells

For vaccines produced in cell cultures, control cells are maintained and tested as prescribed. In order to provide a valid control, these cells must be maintained in conditions that are essentially equivalent to those used for the production cell cultures, including use of the same batches of media and media changes.

Control eggs

For live vaccines produced in eggs, control eggs are incubated and tested as prescribed in the monograph.

Purification

Where applicable, validated purification procedures may be applied.

Inactivation

Inactivated vaccines are produced using a validated inactivation process whose effectiveness and consistency have been demonstrated. Where it is recognised that extraneous agents may be present in a harvest, for example in vaccines produced in eggs from healthy, non-SPF flocks, the inactivation process is also validated with respect to a panel of model extraneous agents representative of the potential extraneous agents. A test for effectiveness of the inactivation process is carried out as soon as possible after the inactivation process.

Test for sterility of intermediates prior to final bulk

Individual monographs on vaccines for human use may prescribe a test for sterility for intermediates.

In agreement with the competent authority, replacement of the sterility test by a bioburden test with a low bioburden limit based on batch data and process validation may be acceptable for intermediates preceding the final bulk, provided that a sterilising filtration is performed later in the production process.

It is a prerequisite that the intermediate is filtered through a bacteria-retentive filter prior to storage, that authorised pre-filtration bioburden limits have been established for this filtration, and that adequate measures are in place to avoid contamination and growth of micro-organisms during storage of the intermediate.

Final bulk

The final bulk is prepared by aseptically blending the ingredients of the vaccine. For non-liquid vaccines for administration by a non-parenteral route, the final bulk is prepared by blending the ingredients of the vaccine under suitable conditions.

Adjuvants   One or more adjuvants may be included in the formulation of a vaccine to potentiate and/or modulate the immune response to the antigen(s). Adjuvants may be included in the formulation of the final vaccine or presented separately. Suitable characterisation and quality control of the adjuvant(s), alone and in combination with the antigen(s), is essential for consistent production. Quality specifications are established for each adjuvant, alone and in combination with the antigen(s).

Adsorbents as adjuvants   Vaccines may be adsorbed on aluminium hydroxide, aluminium phosphate, calcium phosphate or other suitable adsorbents. The adsorbents are prepared in special conditions that confer the appropriate physical form and adsorptive properties.

Where an adsorbent is used as an adjuvant and is generated in *situ* during production of the vaccine, quality specifications are established for each of the ingredients and for the generated adsorbent in the vaccine. Quality specifications are intended to control, in particular:

— qualitative and quantitative chemical composition;
— physical form and associated adsorptive properties, where relevant, and particularly where the adjuvant will be present as an adsorbent;
— interaction between adjuvant and antigen;
— purity, including bacterial endotoxin content and microbiological quality;
— any other parameters identified as being critical for functionality.

The stability of each adjuvant, alone and in combination with the antigen(s), particularly for critical parameters, is established during development studies.

Antimicrobial preservatives   Antimicrobial preservatives are used to prevent spoilage or adverse effects caused by microbial contamination occurring during the use of a vaccine. Antimicrobial preservatives are not included in freeze-dried products. For single-dose liquid preparations, inclusion of antimicrobial preservatives is not normally acceptable. For multidose liquid preparations, the need for effective antimicrobial preservation is evaluated taking into account likely contamination during use and the maximum recommended period of use after broaching of the container. If an antimicrobial preservative is used, it shall be shown that it does not impair the safety or efficacy of the vaccine. Addition of antibiotics as antimicrobial preservatives is not normally acceptable.

During development studies, the effectiveness of the antimicrobial preservative throughout the period of validity shall be demonstrated to the satisfaction of the competent authority.

The efficacy of the antimicrobial preservative is evaluated as described in chapter *5.1.3*. If neither the A criteria nor the B criteria can be met, then in justified cases the following criteria are applied to vaccines for human use: bacteria, no increase at 24 h and 7 days, 3 log reduction at 14 days, no increase at 28 days; fungi, no increase at 14 days and 28 days.

Stability of intermediates

During production of vaccines, intermediates are obtained at various stages and are stored, sometimes for long periods. Such intermediates include:
— seed lots and cell banks;
— live or inactivated harvests;
— purified harvests that may consist of toxins or toxoids, polysaccharides, bacterial or viral suspensions;
— purified antigens;
— adsorbed antigens;
— conjugated polysaccharides;
— final bulk vaccine;
— vaccine in the final closed container stored at a temperature lower than that used for final-product stability studies and intended for release without re-assay.

Except where they are used within a short period of time, stability studies are carried out on the intermediates in the intended storage conditions to establish the expected extent of degradation. For final bulk vaccine, stability studies may be carried out on representative samples in conditions equivalent to those intended to be used for storage. For each intermediate (except for seed lots and cell banks), a period of validity applicable for the intended storage conditions is established, where appropriate in light of stability studies.

Final lot

The final lot is prepared by aseptically distributing the final bulk into sterile, tamper-proof containers, which, after freeze-drying where applicable, are closed so as to exclude contamination. For non-liquid vaccines for administration by a non-parenteral route, the final lot is prepared by distributing the final bulk under suitable conditions into sterile, tamper-proof containers. Where justified and authorised, certain tests prescribed for the final lot may be carried out on the final bulk, if it has been demonstrated that subsequent manufacturing operations do not affect compliance.

Appearance

Unless otherwise justified and authorised, each container (vial, syringe or ampoule) in each final lot is inspected visually or mechanically for acceptable appearance.

Degree of adsorption For an adsorbed vaccine, unless otherwise justified and authorised, a release specification for the degree of adsorption is established in light of results found for batches used in clinical trials. From the stability data generated for the vaccine it must be shown that at the end of the period of validity the degree of adsorption is not less than for batches used in clinical trials.

Thermal stability When the thermal stability test is prescribed in a monograph for a live attenuated vaccine, the test is carried out on the final lot to monitor the lot-to-lot consistency in heat-sensitivity of viral/bacterial particles in the product. Suitable conditions are indicated in the individual monograph. The test may be omitted as a routine test for a given product once the consistency of the production process has been demonstrated, in agreement with the competent authority, using relevant parameters, such as consistency in

yield, ratio of infectious viruses (viable bacteria) before and after freeze-drying, potency at release and real-time stability under the prescribed conditions as well as thermal stability. Where there is a significant change in the manufacturing procedure of the antigen(s) or formulation, the need for re-introduction of the test is considered.

Stability During development studies, maintenance of potency of the final lot throughout the period of validity shall be demonstrated; the loss of potency in the recommended storage conditions is assessed. Excessive loss even within the limits of acceptable potency may indicate that the vaccine is unacceptable.

Expiry date Unless otherwise stated, the expiry date is calculated from the beginning of the assay or from the beginning of the first assay for a combined vaccine.
For vaccines stored at a temperature lower than that used for stability studies and intended for release without re-assay, the expiry date is calculated from the date of removal from cold storage. If, for a given vaccine, an assay is not carried out, the expiry date for the final lot is calculated from the date of an approved stability-indicating test or, failing this, from the date of freeze-drying or the date of filling into the final containers. For a combined vaccine where components are presented in separate containers, the expiry date is that of the component which expires first.

The expiry date applies to vaccines stored in the prescribed conditions.

Animal tests

In accordance with the provisions of the European Convention for the Protection of Vertebrate Animals Used for Experimental and Other Scientific Purposes, tests must be carried out in such a way as to use the minimum number of animals and to cause the least pain, suffering, distress or lasting harm. The criteria for judging tests in monographs must be applied in light of this. For example, if it is indicated that an animal is considered to be positive, infected, etc. when typical clinical signs or death occur, then as soon as sufficient indication of a positive result is obtained the animal in question shall be either euthanised or given suitable treatment to prevent unnecessary suffering. In accordance with the General Notices, alternative test methods may be used to demonstrate compliance with the monograph and the use of such tests is particularly encouraged when this leads to replacement or reduction of animal use or reduction of suffering.

TESTS

Vaccines comply with the tests prescribed in individual monographs including, where applicable, the following:

pH *(2.2.3)*

Liquid vaccines, after reconstitution where applicable, comply with the limits for pH approved for the particular preparation.

Adjuvant

If the vaccine contains an adjuvant, the amount is determined and shown to be within acceptable limits with respect to the expected amount (see also the tests for aluminium and calcium below).

Aluminium *(2.5.13)*

Maximum 1.25 mg of aluminium (Al) per single human dose where an aluminium adsorbent has been used in the vaccine, unless otherwise stated.

Calcium (*2.5.14*)
Maximum 1.3 mg of calcium (Ca) per single human dose where a calcium adsorbent has been used in the vaccine, unless otherwise stated.

Free formaldehyde (*2.4.18*)
Maximum 0.2 g/L of free formaldehyde in the final product where formaldehyde has been used in the preparation of the vaccine, unless otherwise stated.

Phenol (*2.5.15*)
Maximum 2.5 g/L in the final product where phenol has been used in the preparation of the vaccine, unless otherwise stated.

Water (*2.5.12*)
Maximum 3.0 per cent *m/m* for freeze-dried vaccines, unless otherwise stated.

Extractable volume (*2.9.17*)
Unless otherwise justified and authorised, it complies with the requirement for extractable volume.

Bacterial endotoxins
Unless otherwise justified and authorised, a test for bacterial endotoxins is carried out on the final product. Where no limit is specified in the individual monograph, the content of bacterial endotoxins determined by a suitable method (*2.6.14*) is less than the limit approved for the particular product.

STORAGE
Store protected from light. Unless otherwise stated, the storage temperature is 5 ± 3 °C; liquid adsorbed vaccines must not be allowed to freeze.

LABELLING
The label states:
— the name of the preparation;
— a reference identifying the final lot;
— the recommended human dose and route of administration;
— the storage conditions;
— the expiry date;
— the name and amount of any antimicrobial preservative;
— the name of any antibiotic, adjuvant, flavour or stabiliser present in the vaccine;
— where applicable, that the vaccine is adsorbed;
— the name of any constituent that may cause adverse reactions and any contra-indications to the use of the vaccine;
— for freeze-dried vaccines:
  — the name or composition and the volume of the reconstituting liquid to be added;
  — the time within which the vaccine is to be used after reconstitution.

Ph Eur

Anthrax Vaccine for Human Use (Adsorbed, Prepared from Culture Filtrates)

(*Ph Eur monograph 2188*)
The label may state 'Anthrax'.

Ph Eur

DEFINITION
Anthrax vaccine for human use (adsorbed, prepared from culture filtrates) is a preparation of *Bacillus anthracis* antigens precipitated by aluminium potassium sulfate. The antigens are prepared from a sterile culture filtrate produced by a non-encapsulated strain, either avirulent or attenuated, of *B. anthracis*.

The main virulence components of *B. anthracis* are the polyglutamic aicd capsule and 2 binary anthrax toxins, namely lethal toxin and œdema toxin, formed from the respective combination of protective antigen (PA) with either lethal factor (LF) or œdema factor (EF).

LF is a zinc-dependent endopeptidase and EF is a potent calmodulin and calcium-dependent adenylate cyclase. Cell-free cultures of *B. anthracis* contain PA and because expression of the 3 toxin-component genes is co-ordinately regulated, LF and EF are also present. In addition, the vaccine is likely to contain many other *B. anthracis* antigens, including membrane proteins, secreted proteins, cytoplasmic proteins, peptidoglycans, nucleic acids and carbohydrates.

PRODUCTION
GENERAL PROVISIONS
Cultures are managed in a seed-lot system. The vaccine strain is toxigenic but lacks the plasmid with the necessary genes for synthesis of the capsule, an important virulence factor.

The production method must be shown to yield a consistent and active product with a safety and efficacy profile that is adequate or equivalent to previous lots. The vaccine must show a level of protection against a virulent strain of *B. anthracis*, in a suitable animal infection model, that is equal to or greater than that of a reference vaccine. The vaccine must not show a level of toxicity that exceeds that of a reference vaccine.

The production method and stability of the final lot and relevant intermediates are evaluated using one or more indicator tests. Such tests include potency and specific toxicity, and may be supported by tests confirming the presence of relevant antigens and associated proteins. Release and shelf-life specifications are established based upon the results of stability testing so as to ensure satisfactory product performance during the approved period of validity.

SEED LOTS
The attenuated non-encapsulated strain of *B. anthracis* used is identified by historical records that include information on its origin and subsequent manipulation and the tests used to characterise the strain. These include morphological, cultural, biochemical and genetic properties of the strain. Only a master seed lot or, where applicable, working seed lots, that comply with the following requirements may be used.

Identification
Each seed lot is identified as containing *B. anthracis*.

Phenotypic parameters
Each seed lot must have a known biochemical and enzymatic profile and have a known history of absence of antibiotic resistance.

Microbial purity

Each seed lot complies with the requirements for absence of contaminating organisms. Purity of bacterial cultures is verified by methods of suitable sensitivity.

Virulence test

The absence of bacterial capsule is demonstrated for each seed lot by McFadyean stain and the specific toxicity (oedema) test.

REFERENCE PREPARATION

The potency and toxicity of the vaccine bulk are verified using reference standards derived from representative vaccine batches. These batches are extensively characterised for their intended purpose and are stored in suitably sized aliquots under conditions ensuring their stability.

PROPAGATION AND HARVEST

The attenuated strain is grown using suitable liquid media. At the end of cultivation, the purity of the culture is tested. The culture medium is separated from the bacterial mass by filtration. The pH of the filtrate is determined after dilution with a 0.9 g/L solution of *sodium chloride R* and is shown to be within limits suitable for stability. A suitable test for absence of live B. anthracis, including spores, is carried out. Aluminium potassium sulfate or an alternative adjuvant may be added at this stage. An antimicrobial preservative may be added to the suspension to form the purified harvest.

Only a purified harvest that complies with the following requirements may be used in the preparation of the final lot.

Immunological identity

Confirm the presence of *B. anthracis* protective antigen by a suitable immunochemical method (*2.7.1*).

Antimicrobial preservative

Determine the amount of antimicrobial preservative by a suitable chemical method. The amount is not less than 85 per cent and not greater than 115 per cent of the intended content.

FINAL BULK VACCINE

The purified harvest is diluted aseptically with sterile saline solution to make the final bulk vaccine.

Only a final bulk vaccine that complies with the following requirement may be used in the preparation of the final lot.

Sterility (*2.6.1*)

Carry out the test for sterility, using 10 mL for each medium.

FINAL LOT

The final bulk vaccine is distributed aseptically into sterile, tamper-proof glass ampoules and heat-sealed to prevent contamination.

Only a final lot that is satisfactory with respect to each of the requirements given below under Identification, Tests and Assay may be released for use. Provided the potency assay, the specific toxicity (oedema) test and the test for antimicrobial preservative have been carried out with satisfactory results on the purified harvest, they may be omitted on the final lot.

IDENTIFICATION

The presence of *B. anthracis* protective antigen is confirmed by a suitable immunochemical method (*2.7.1*).

TESTS

Abnormal toxicity

Inject intraperitoneally up to 4 human doses of vaccine into each of at least 10 healthy mice, each weighing 17-22 g. Observe the mice daily for 7 days. The vaccine complies with the test if none of the animals shows signs of ill health.

Specific toxicity (oedema) test

Use not fewer than 2 rabbits per test. Prepare serial two-fold dilutions of vaccine with normal saline, corresponding to 4, 2, 1, 0.5 and 0.25 human doses. Inject intradermally 0.1 mL of each dilution of the test and of the reference vaccine into the shaved flanks of 2 rabbits. Each rabbit receives the 10 previously prepared injections (5 dilutions of the test vaccine and 5 dilutions of the reference vaccine). In one of the rabbits, the lower concentrations are injected at the anterior end and the higher concentrations at the posterior end. The reverse is used for the 2nd rabbit. The rabbits are monitored for 24 h for signs of oedema at the injection site. The vaccine complies with the test if the oedematous reaction is not greater than that observed with the reference vaccine.

Alternatively, specific *in vitro* assays for lethal factor and adenylate cyclase activity may be used, subject to validation.

Antimicrobial preservative

Determine the amount of antimicrobial preservative by a suitable chemical method. The content is not less than the minimum amount shown to be effective and is not greater than 115 per cent of the intended content.

Aluminium (*2.5.13*)

Maximum 1.25 mg per single human dose.

Sterility (*2.6.1*)

It complies with the test for sterility.

ASSAY

The potency of the anthrax vaccine is determined by comparing the dose required to protect guinea-pigs against intradermal challenge by a virulent strain of *B. anthracis* with the dose of a suitable reference preparation that gives the same protection. Use 9 groups of not fewer than 16 female guinea-pigs, each weighing 250-350 g. Prepare 4 dilutions of the vaccine and of the reference preparation containing 1.5, 0.5, 0.17 and 0.05 human doses in 0.5 mL. Allocate each dilution to a separate group. The remaining group receives 0.5 mL of saline and is used to verify the challenge dose. Inject subcutaneously into each guinea-pig 0.5 mL of the dilution allocated to its group on each of 2 occasions, 1 week apart. 7 days after the 2nd injection, inject intradermally into each guinea-pig 2000 spores of a virulent strain of *B. anthracis* (Vollum) in 0.1 mL. Observe the animals for 10 days and record the number of deaths per group. The test is not valid unless all the control animals die within 5 days of challenge. Using the proportions of animals that survive in each of the vaccinated groups, calculate the potency of the vaccine relative to the reference preparation using the usual statistical methods (*5.3*). The vaccine complies with the test if:

— the relative potency estimate exceeds 1.0, or;
— the 95 per cent confidence interval for the relative potency includes 1.0, and the lower 95 per cent confidence limit is not less than 50 per cent of the relative potency estimate.

LABELLING

The label states that the vaccine is not to be frozen.

_____ *Ph Eur*

Bacillus Calmette-Guérin Vaccine

BCG Vaccine

(*BCG Vaccine, Freeze-dried, Ph Eur monograph 0163*)

The label may state 'BCG'.

Ph Eur _____

DEFINITION

Freeze-dried BCG vaccine is a preparation of live bacteria derived from a culture of the bacillus of Calmette and Guérin (*Mycobacterium bovis* BCG) whose capacity to protect against tuberculosis has been established.

PRODUCTION

GENERAL PROVISIONS

BCG vaccine shall be produced by a staff consisting of healthy persons who do not work with other infectious agents; in particular they shall not work with virulent strains of *Mycobacterium tuberculosis*, nor shall they be exposed to a known risk of tuberculosis infection. Staff are examined periodically for tuberculosis. BCG vaccine is susceptible to sunlight: the procedures for the preparation of the vaccine shall be designed so that all cultures and vaccines are protected from direct sunlight and from ultraviolet light at all stages of manufacture, testing and storage.

Production of the vaccine is based on a seed-lot system. The production method shall have been shown to yield consistently BCG vaccines that induce adequate sensitivity to tuberculin in man, that have acceptable protective potency in animals and are safe. The vaccine is prepared from cultures which are derived from the master seed lot by as few subcultures as possible and in any case not more than 8 subcultures. During the course of these subcultures the preparation is not freeze-dried more than once.

If a bioluminescence test or other biochemical method is used instead of viable count, the method is validated against the viable count for each stage of the process at which it is used.

BACTERIAL SEED LOTS

The strain used to establish the master seed lot is chosen for and maintained to preserve its characteristics, its capacity to sensitise man to tuberculin and to protect animals against tuberculosis, and its relative absence of pathogenicity for man and laboratory animals. The strain used shall be identified by historical records that include information on its origin and subsequent manipulation.

A suitable batch of vaccine is prepared from the first working seed lot and is reserved for use as the comparison vaccine. When a new working seed lot is established, a suitable test for delayed hypersensitivity in guinea-pigs is carried out on a batch of vaccine prepared from the new working seed lot; the vaccine is shown to be not significantly different in activity from the comparison vaccine. Antimicrobial agent sensitivity testing is also carried out.

Only a working seed lot that complies with the following requirements may be used for propagation.

IDENTIFICATION

The bacteria in the working seed lot are identified as *Mycobacterium bovis* BCG using microbiological techniques, which may be supplemented by molecular biology techniques (for example, nucleic acid amplification and restriction-fragment-length polymorphism).

Bacterial and fungal contamination

Carry out the test for sterility (*2.6.1*), using 10 mL for each medium. The working seed lot complies with the test for sterility except for the presence of mycobacteria.

Virulent mycobacteria

Examine the working seed lot as prescribed under Tests, using 10 guinea-pigs.

PROPAGATION AND HARVEST

The bacteria are grown in a suitable medium for not more than 21 days by surface or submerged culture. The culture medium does not contain substances known to cause toxic or allergic reactions in humans or to cause the bacteria to become virulent for guinea-pigs. The culture is harvested and suspended in a sterile liquid medium that protects the viability of the vaccine as determined by a suitable method of viable count.

FINAL BULK VACCINE

The final bulk vaccine is prepared from a single harvest or by pooling a number of single harvests. A stabiliser may be added; if the stabiliser interferes with the determination of bacterial concentration in the final bulk vaccine, the determination is carried out before addition of the stabiliser.

Only final bulk vaccine that complies with the following requirements may be used in the preparation of the final lot.

Bacterial and fungal contamination

Carry out the test for sterility (*2.6.1*), using 10 mL for each medium. The final bulk vaccine complies with the test for sterility except for the presence of mycobacteria.

Count of viable units

Determine the number of viable units per millilitre by viable count on solid medium using a method suitable for the vaccine to be examined or by a suitable biochemical method. Carry out the test in parallel on a reference preparation of the same strain.

Bacterial concentration

Determine the total bacterial concentration by a suitable method, either directly by determining the mass of the micro-organisms, or indirectly by an opacity method that has been calibrated in relation to the mass of the organisms; if the bacterial concentration is determined before addition of a stabiliser, the concentration in the final bulk vaccine is established by calculation. The total bacterial concentration is within the limits approved for the particular product.

The ratio of the count of viable units to the total bacterial concentration is not less than that approved for the particular product.

FINAL LOT

The final bulk vaccine is distributed into sterile containers and freeze-dried to a moisture content favourable to the stability of the vaccine; the containers are closed either under vacuum or under an inert gas.

Except where the filled and closed containers are stored at a temperature of −20 °C or lower, the expiry date is not later than 4 years from the date of harvest.

Only a final lot that complies with the following requirement for count of viable units and with each of the requirements given below under Identification, Tests and Assay may be released for use. Provided the test for virulent mycobacteria has been carried out with satisfactory results on the final bulk vaccine, it may be omitted on the final lot. Provided the test for excessive dermal reactivity has been carried out with satisfactory results on the working seed lot and on 5 consecutive final lots produced from it, the test may be omitted on the final lot.

Count of viable units

Determine the number of viable units per millilitre of the reconstituted vaccine by viable count on solid medium using a method suitable for the vaccine to be examined or by a suitable biochemical method. The ratio of the count of viable units after freeze-drying to that before is not less than that approved for the particular product.

Thermal stability

Maintain containers of the final lot of freeze-dried vaccine in the dry state at 37 ± 1 °C for 4 weeks. Determine the number of viable units as described under Assay in parallel for the heated vaccine and for vaccine stored at the temperature recommended for storage. The number of viable units in the heated vaccine is not less than 20 per cent of that in the unheated vaccine.

IDENTIFICATION

BCG vaccine is identified by microscopic examination of the bacilli in stained smears demonstrating their acid-fast property and by the characteristic appearance of colonies grown on solid medium. Alternatively, molecular biology techniques (for example nucleic acid amplification) may be used.

TESTS

Virulent mycobacteria

Inject subcutaneously or intramuscularly into each of 6 guinea-pigs, each weighing 250-400 g and having received no treatment likely to interfere with the test, a quantity of vaccine equivalent to at least 50 human doses. Observe the animals for at least 42 days. At the end of this period, euthanise the guinea-pigs and examine by autopsy for signs of infection with tuberculosis, ignoring any minor reactions at the site of injection. Animals that die during the observation period are also examined for signs of tuberculosis.

The vaccine complies with the test if none of the guinea-pigs shows signs of tuberculosis and if not more than 1 animal dies during the observation period. If 2 animals die during this period and autopsy does not reveal signs of tuberculosis repeat the test on 6 other guinea-pigs. The vaccine complies with the test if not more than 1 animal dies during the 42 days following the injection and autopsy does not reveal any sign of tuberculosis.

Bacterial and fungal contamination

The reconstituted vaccine complies with the test for sterility (2.6.1) except for the presence of mycobacteria.

Excessive dermal reactivity

Use 6 healthy, white or pale-coloured guinea-pigs, each weighing not less than 250 g and having received no treatment likely to interfere with the test. Inject intradermally into each guinea-pig, according to a randomised plan, 0.1 mL of the reconstituted vaccine and of 2 tenfold serial dilutions of the vaccine and identical doses of the comparison vaccine. Observe the lesions formed at the site of the injection for 4 weeks. The vaccine complies with the test if the reaction it produces is not markedly different from that produced by the comparison vaccine.

Water

Not more than the limit approved for the particular product, determined by a suitable method.

ASSAY

Determine the number of viable units in the reconstituted vaccine by viable count on solid medium using a method suitable for the vaccine to be examined or by a suitable validated biochemical method. The number is within the range stated on the label. Determine the number of viable units in the comparison vaccine in parallel.

LABELLING

The label states:
— the minimum and maximum number of viable units per millilitre in the reconstituted vaccine,
— that the vaccine must be protected from direct sunlight.

_____ Ph Eur

BCG for Immunotherapy

(Ph Eur monograph 1929)

Ph Eur _____

DEFINITION

BCG for immunotherapy is a freeze-dried preparation of live bacteria derived from a culture of the bacillus of Calmette and Guérin (*Mycobacterium bovis* BCG) whose capacity for treatment has been established.

It complies with the monograph *Vaccines for human use (0153)*.

PRODUCTION

GENERAL PROVISIONS

BCG for immunotherapy shall be produced by a staff consisting of healthy persons who do not work with other infectious agents; in particular they shall not work with virulent strains of *Mycobacterium tuberculosis*, nor shall they be exposed to a known risk of tuberculosis infection. Staff are examined periodically for tuberculosis. BCG for immunotherapy is susceptible to sunlight: the procedures for production shall be so designed that all products are protected from direct sunlight and from ultraviolet light at all stages of manufacture, testing and storage.

Production is based on a seed-lot system. The production method shall have been shown to yield consistently BCG products that can be used for treatment of superficial bladder cancer and are safe. The product is prepared from cultures which are separated from the master seed lot by as few subcultures as possible and in any case not more than 8 subcultures. During the course of these subcultures the preparation is not freeze-dried more than once.

If a bioluminescence test or other biochemical method is used instead of viable count, the method is validated against the viable count for each stage of the process at which it is used.

SEED LOTS

The strain used to establish the master seed lot is chosen for and maintained to preserve its characteristics, its capacity to treat and prevent superficial bladder cancer, and its relative absence of pathogenicity for man and laboratory animals. The strain used shall be identified by historical records that include information on its origin and subsequent manipulation.

Before establishment of a working seed lot a batch is prepared and reserved for use as the comparison product. When a new working seed lot is established, a suitable test for delayed hypersensitivity in guinea-pigs is carried out on a batch of product prepared from the new working seed lot; the product is shown to be not significantly different in activity from the comparison product. Antimicrobial agent sensitivity testing is also carried out.

Only a working seed lot that complies with the following requirements may be used for propagation.

Identification

The bacteria in the working seed lot are identified as *Mycobacterium bovis BCG* using microbiological techniques, which may be supplemented by molecular biology techniques (for example, nucleic acid amplification and restriction-fragment-length polymorphism).

Bacterial and fungal contamination

Carry out the test for sterility (*2.6.1*), using 10 mL for each medium. The working seed lot complies with the test for sterility, except for the presence of mycobacteria.

Virulent mycobacteria

Examine the working seed lot as prescribed under Tests, using 10 guinea-pigs.

PROPAGATION AND HARVEST

The bacteria are grown in a suitable medium for not more than 21 days by surface or submerged culture. The culture medium does not contain substances known to cause toxic or allergic reactions in human beings or to cause the bacteria to become virulent for guinea-pigs. The culture is harvested and suspended in a sterile liquid medium that protects the viability of the culture as determined by a suitable method of viable count.

FINAL BULK

The final bulk is prepared from a single harvest or by pooling a number of single harvests. A stabiliser may be added; if the stabiliser interferes with the determination of bacterial concentration on the final bulk, the determination is carried out before addition of the stabiliser.

Only final bulk that complies with the following requirements may be used in the preparation of the final lot.

Bacterial and fungal contamination

Carry out the test for sterility (*2.6.1*), using 10 mL of final bulk for each medium. The final bulk complies with the test for sterility, except for the presence of mycobacteria.

Count of viable units

Determine the number of viable units per millilitre by viable count on solid medium using a method suitable for the product to be examined or by a suitable biochemical method. Carry out the test in parallel on a reference preparation of the same strain.

Bacterial concentration

Determine the total bacterial concentration by a suitable method, either directly by determining the mass of the micro-organisms, or indirectly by an opacity method that has been calibrated in relation to the mass of the micro-organisms; if the bacterial concentration is determined before addition of a stabiliser, the concentration in the final bulk is established by calculation. The total bacterial concentration is within the limits approved for the particular product.

The ratio of the count of viable units to the total bacterial concentration is not less than that approved for the particular product.

FINAL LOT

The final bulk is distributed into sterile containers and freeze-dried to a moisture content favourable to the stability of the product; the containers are closed either under vacuum or under an inert gas.

Except where the filled and closed containers are stored at a temperature of − 20 °C or lower, the expiry date is not later than 4 years from the date of harvest.

Only a final lot that complies with the following requirement for count of viable units and with each of the requirements given below under Identification, Tests and Assay may be released for use. Provided the test for virulent mycobacteria has been carried out with satisfactory results on the final bulk, it may be omitted on the final lot.

Count of viable units

Determine the number of viable units per millilitre of the reconstituted product by viable count on solid medium using a method suitable for the product to be examined, or by a suitable biochemical method. The ratio of the count of viable units after freeze-drying to that before is not less than that approved for the particular product.

IDENTIFICATION

BCG for immunotherapy is identified by microscopic examination of the bacilli in stained smears demonstrating their acid-fast property and by the characteristic appearance of colonies grown on solid medium. Alternatively, molecular biology techniques (for example, nucleic acid amplification) may be used.

TESTS

Virulent mycobacteria

Inject subcutaneously or intramuscularly into each of 6 guinea-pigs, each weighing 250-400 g and having received no treatment likely to interfere with the test, a quantity of the product to be examined equivalent to at least 1/25 of 1 human dose. Observe the animals for at least 42 days. At the end of this period, euthanise the guinea-pigs and examine by autopsy for signs of infection with tuberculosis, ignoring any minor reactions at the site of injection. Animals that die during the observation period are also examined for signs of tuberculosis. The product complies with the test if none of the guinea-pigs shows signs of tuberculosis and if not more than 1 animal dies during the observation period.
If 2 animals die during this period and autopsy does not reveal signs of tuberculosis, repeat the test on 6 other guinea-pigs. The product complies with the test if not more than 1 animal dies during the 42 days following the injection and autopsy does not reveal any sign of tuberculosis.

Bacterial and fungal contamination

The reconstituted product complies with the test for sterility (*2.6.1*) except for the presence of mycobacteria.

Water

Not more than the limit approved for the particular product, determined by a suitable method.

ASSAY

Determine the number of viable units in the reconstituted product by viable count on solid medium using a method suitable for the product to be examined or by a suitable validated biochemical method. The number is within the range stated on the label. Determine the number of viable units in the comparison control in parallel.

LABELLING

The label states:
— the minimum and the maximum number of viable units per dose in the reconstituted product;
— that the product must be protected from direct sunlight.

_____ *Ph Eur*

Cholera Vaccine

(*Ph Eur monograph 0154*)

The label may state 'Cholera'.

Ph Eur

DEFINITION

Cholera vaccine is a homogeneous suspension of a suitable strain or strains of *Vibrio cholerae* containing not less than 8 $\times$ 10^9 bacteria in each human dose. The human dose does not exceed 1.0 mL.

PRODUCTION

The vaccine is prepared using a seed-lot system. The vaccine consists of a mixture of equal parts of vaccines prepared from smooth strains of the 2 main serological types, Inaba and Ogawa. These may be of the classical biotype with or without the El-Tor biotype. A single strain or several strains of each type may be included. All strains must contain, in addition to their type O antigens, the heat-stable O antigen common to Inaba and Ogawa. If more than one strain each of Inaba and Ogawa are used, these may be selected so as to contain other O antigens in addition. The World Health Organisation recommends new strains which may be used if necessary, in accordance with the regulations in force in the signatory States of the Convention on the Elaboration of a European Pharmacopoeia. In order to comply with the requirements for vaccination certificates required for international travel, the vaccine must contain not less than 8 $\times$ 10^9 organisms of the classical biotype. Each strain is grown separately.

The bacteria are inactivated either by heating the suspensions (for example, at 56 °C for 1 h) or by treatment with formaldehyde or phenol or by a combination of the physical and chemical methods.

The production method is validated to demonstrate that the product, if tested, would comply with the test for abnormal toxicity for immunosera and vaccines for human use (*2.6.9*) modified as follows: inject 0.5 mL of the vaccine into each mouse and 1.0 mL into each guinea pig.

IDENTIFICATION

It is identified by specific agglutination tests.

TESTS

Phenol (*2.5.15*)

If phenol has been used in the preparation, the concentration is not more than 5 g/L.

Antibody production

Test the ability of the vaccine to induce antibodies (such as agglutinating, vibriocidal or haemagglutinating antibodies) in the guinea-pig, the rabbit or the mouse. Administer the vaccine to a group of at least 6 animals. At the end of the interval of time necessary for maximum antibody formation, determined in preliminary tests, collect sera from the animals and titrate them individually for the appropriate antibody using a suitable method. The vaccine to be examined passes the test if each serotype has elicited a significant antibody response.

Sterility (*2.6.1*)

It complies with the test for sterility.

LABELLING

The label states:
— the method used to inactivate the bacteria,
— the number of bacteria in each human dose.

Ph Eur

Cholera Vaccine, Freeze-dried

(*Ph Eur monograph 0155*)

The label may state 'Dried/Cholera'.

Ph Eur

DEFINITION

Freeze-dried cholera vaccine is a preparation of a suitable strain or strains of *Vibrio cholerae*. The vaccine is reconstituted as stated on the label to give a uniform suspension containing not less than 8 $\times$ 10^9 bacteria in each human dose. The human dose does not exceed 1.0 mL of the reconstituted vaccine.

PRODUCTION

The vaccine is prepared using a seed-lot system. The vaccine consists of a mixture of equal parts of vaccines prepared from smooth strains of the 2 main serological types, Inaba and Ogawa. These may be of the classical biotype with or without the El-Tor biotype. A single strain or several strains of each type may be included. All strains must contain, in addition to their type O antigens, the heat-stable O antigen common to Inaba and Ogawa. If more than one strain each of Inaba and Ogawa are used, these may be selected so as to contain other O antigens in addition. The World Health Organisation recommends new strains which may be used if necessary in accordance with the regulations in force in the signatory States of the Convention on the Elaboration of a European Pharmacopoeia. In order to comply with the requirements for vaccination certificates required for international travel, the vaccine must contain not less than 8 $\times$ 10^9 organisms of the classical biotype. Each strain is grown separately.

The bacteria are inactivated either by heating the suspensions (for example, at 56 °C for 1 h) or by treatment with formaldehyde or by a combination of the physical and chemical methods. Phenol is not used in the preparation. The vaccine is distributed into sterile containers and freeze-dried to a moisture content favourable to the stability of the vaccine. The containers are then closed so as to exclude contamination.

The production method is validated to demonstrate that the product, if tested, would comply with the test for abnormal toxicity for immunosera and vaccines for human use (*2.6.9*) modified as follows: inject 0.5 mL of the vaccine into each mouse and 1.0 mL into each guinea pig.

IDENTIFICATION

The vaccine reconstituted as stated on the label is identified by specific agglutination tests.

TESTS

Phenol (*2.5.15*)

If phenol has been used in the preparation, the concentration is not more than 5 g/L.

Antibody production

Test the ability of the vaccine to induce antibodies (such as agglutinating, vibriocidal or haemagglutinating antibodies) in the guinea-pig, the rabbit or the mouse. Administer the reconstituted vaccine to a group of at least 6 animals. At the end of the interval of time necessary for maximum antibody formation, determined in preliminary tests, collect sera from the animals and titrate them individually for the appropriate antibody using a suitable method. The vaccine to be examined passes the test if each serotype has elicited a significant antibody response.

Sterility (*2.6.1*)

The reconstituted vaccine complies with the test for sterility.

LABELLING

The label states:

— the method used to inactivate the bacteria,

— the number of bacteria in each human dose.

Ph Eur

Cholera Vaccine (Inactivated, Oral)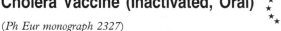

(*Ph Eur monograph 2327*)

The label may state Cholera(*oral*)

Ph Eur

DEFINITION

Cholera vaccine (inactivated, oral) is a homogeneous suspension of inactivated suitable strains of *Vibrio cholerae* serogroup O1, representing serotypes and biotypes of epidemic strains. The vaccine may contain the B subunit of cholera toxin (CTB). Just prior to ingestion, one dose of vaccine suspension is mixed with a suitable buffer as stated on the label.

PRODUCTION

GENERAL PROVISIONS

The production method must be validated to yield consistently vaccines comparable with the vaccine of proven clinical efficacy and safety in man.

The production process must be validated to show that no clinically significant quantities of active toxin are present in the product.

CHOICE OF VACCINE STRAIN

The vaccine consists of a mixture of epidemic *V. cholerae* strains inactivated by a suitable method such as heat or formalin inactivation. All strains express smooth lipopolysaccharide (LPS). The CTB is produced by recombinant DNA technology in a strain that lacks the gene for cholera toxin subunit A (*ctxA⁻*). Selected *V. cholerae* strains are low cholera-toxin producers.

The World Health Organisation (WHO) can recommend new vaccine strains or antigens that may be used if necessary, in accordance with the regulations in force in the signatory states of the Convention on the Elaboration of a European Pharmacopoeia.

SEED LOTS

The strains of *V. cholerae* used shall be identified by historical records that include information on the origin of the strains and their subsequent manipulation. Characterisation and maintenance of the recombinant strains and plasmids used for production of the recombinant B subunit of cholera toxin (rCTB) and the origin of the gene for cholera toxin subunit B (*ctxB*) are documented. The stability of the rCTB plasmid in the recombinant strain during storage and beyond the passage level used in production is confirmed.

Characterisation of the rCTB is undertaken using a variety of analytical techniques including determination of molecular size, charge and amino acid composition. Techniques suitable for such purposes include sodium dodecyl sulfate polyacrylamide gel electrophoresis (SDS-PAGE) and different liquid chromatographies. The identity of the product is confirmed by at least partial *N*-terminal and *C*-terminal amino acid sequencing.

Master seed lots are grown on agar plates, which may contain appropriate antibiotics. Colonies are used to produce working seed lots in liquid media that are free from antibiotics. Cultures derived from the working seed lot must have the same characteristics as the cultures of the strain from which the master seed lot was derived.

Only a seed lot that complies with the following requirements may be used in the preparation of the monovalent cell harvest.

Identification

Master seed lots are identified by colony morphology, and by biochemical characterisation, using suitable molecular assays or immunoassays. Working seed lots are identified by colony morphology and by molecular assays or immunoassays.

Purity

Purity of master seed lots and working seed lots is verified by methods of suitable sensitivity.

PROPAGATION AND HARVEST

Each strain is grown separately from the working seed lot.

Cultures are checked at different stages of fermentation (subcultures and main culture) for purity, identity, cell opacity, pH and biochemical characteristics. Unsatisfactory cultures must be discarded.

Production cultures are shown to be consistent in respect of growth rate, pH and yield of cells or cell products.

MONOVALENT CELL HARVEST

Only a monovalent harvest that complies with established specifications for the following tests may be used.

pH (*2.2.3*)

Within the range approved for the particular product.

Identification

Relevant antigenic characteristics are verified by suitable immunological or biochemical assays.

Purity

Samples of culture are examined by microscopy of Gram-stained smears, by inoculation of appropriate culture media or by another suitable procedure.

Opacity

The absorbance at 600 nm (*2.2.25*) is within the range approved for the particular product.

INACTIVATED MONOVALENT CELL BULK

To limit the possibility of contamination, inactivation is initiated as soon as possible after preparation. Bacteria are inactivated after washing, either by treatment with formaldehyde or by heating under conditions that ensure inactivation.

Only an inactivated monovalent cell bulk that complies with established specifications for the following tests may be used in the preparation of the final bulk.

pH (*2.2.3*)

Within the range approved for the particular product.

Identification

Verified by slide agglutination.

Inactivation

Complete inactivation is verified by a suitable culture method.

Sterility (*2.6.1*)

It complies with the test for sterility, carried out using 10 mL for each medium.

Opacity

The inactivation process may affect the accuracy of opacity measurements.

IMMUNOLOGICAL PRODUCTS

Purity

Samples of culture are examined by microscopy of Gram-stained smears, by inoculation of appropriate culture media or by another suitable procedure.

Smooth LPS content

Verified by a suitable immunoassay (*2.7.1*).

Residual cholera toxin

The absence of residual cholera toxin is verified by a suitable immunoassay (*2.7.1*) or biochemical assay.

Free formaldehyde (*2.4.18*)

Content to be determined where formaldehyde is used for inactivation.

PURIFIED RCTB

Production of the rCTB follows the guidelines for assuring the quality of pharmaceutical and biological products prepared by recombinant technology and is covered by the monograph *Products of recombinant DNA technology (0784)*. Prior to harvest, the cell culture is checked for purity and opacity. rCTB is harvested by suitable filtration, concentrated by diafiltration, purified by chromatography, filter-sterilised and stored under suitable conditions. The pH of the pooled eluate is adjusted prior to buffer exchange.

Only purified rCTB that complies with established specifications for the following tests may be used in the preparation of the final bulk.

pH (*2.2.3*)

Within the range approved for the particular product.

Purity

Verified by SDS-PAGE (*2.2.31*) and an appropriate liquid chromatography method (*2.2.29*).

Sterility (*2.6.1*)

It complies with the test for sterility, carried out using 10 mL for each medium.

rCTB

The amount of rCTB is determined by a suitable immunoassay (*2.7.1*).

FINAL BULK

The final bulk vaccine is prepared by aseptically mixing a suitable buffer with monovalent cell bulks. Where used, the rCTB bulk is added in appropriate amounts. Preservatives, if used, may be added at this stage.

Only a final bulk that complies with the following requirements may be used in the preparation of the final lot.

Sterility (*2.6.1*)

It complies with the test for sterility, carried out using 10 mL for each medium.

Antimicrobial preservative

Where applicable, determine the amount of antimicrobial preservative by a suitable chemical or physico-chemical method. The amount is not less than 85 per cent and not greater than 115 per cent of the intended amount.

FINAL LOT

The final bulk is mixed to homogeneity and filled aseptically into suitable containers.

Only a final lot that is within the limits approved for the particular product and is satisfactory with respect to each of the requirements given below under Identification, Tests and Assay may be released for use.

IDENTIFICATION

Serotypes are detected by a suitable immunoassay (*2.7.1*) or molecular assay. rCTB is detected by a suitable immunoassay

(*2.7.1*). The antigen-content assays may also serve as an identity test.

TESTS

pH (*2.2.3*)

Within the range approved for the particular product.

Sterility (*2.6.1*)

It complies with the test for sterility.

Free formaldehyde (*2.4.18*)

Maximum 0.2 g/L, where applicable.

Antimicrobial preservative

Where applicable, determine the amount of antimicrobial preservative by a suitable chemical or physico-chemical method. The amount is not less than 85 per cent and not greater than 115 per cent of the intended amount.

ASSAY

Antigen content

The amount of smooth LPS, and where applicable, the amount of rCTB, are within the limits approved for the particular product, determined by a suitable immunoassay (*2.7.1*).

LABELLING

The label states:
— the method of inactivation;
— the serogroup, serotypes and biotypes of vaccine strains;
— the number of bacteria per human dose;
— the amount of rCTB.

_____ Ph Eur

Adsorbed Diphtheria Vaccine

(Diphtheria Vaccine (Adsorbed),
Ph Eur monograph 0443)

Ph Eur _____

DEFINITION

Diphtheria vaccine (adsorbed) is a preparation of diphtheria formol toxoid with a mineral adsorbent. The formol toxoid is prepared from the toxin produced by the growth of *Corynebacterium diphtheriae*.

PRODUCTION

GENERAL PROVISIONS

Specific toxicity

The production method is validated to demonstrate that the product, if tested, would comply with the following test: inject subcutaneously 5 times the single human dose stated on the label into each of 5 healthy guinea-pigs, each weighing 250-350 g, that have not previously been treated with any material that will interfere with the test. If within 42 days of the injection any of the animals shows signs of or dies from diphtheria toxaemia, the vaccine does not comply with the test. If more than 1 animal dies from non-specific causes, repeat the test once; if more than 1 animal dies in the second test, the vaccine does not comply with the test.

BULK PURIFIED TOXOID

For the production of diphtheria toxin, from which toxoid is prepared, seed cultures are managed in a defined seed-lot system in which toxinogenicity is conserved and, where necessary, restored by deliberate reselection. A highly toxinogenic strain of *Corynebacterium diphtheriae* with known origin and history is grown in a suitable liquid medium. At the end of cultivation, the purity of each culture is tested and contaminated cultures are discarded. Toxin-containing culture medium is separated aseptically from the bacterial mass as soon as possible. The toxin content (Lf per millilitre) is checked (2.7.27) to monitor consistency of production. Single harvests may be pooled to prepare the bulk purified toxoid. The toxin is purified to remove components likely to cause adverse reactions in humans. The purified toxin is detoxified with formaldehyde by a method that avoids destruction of the immunogenic potency of the toxoid and reversion of the toxoid to toxin, particularly on exposure to heat. Alternatively, purification may be carried out after detoxification.

Only bulk purified toxoid that complies with the following requirements may be used in the preparation of the final bulk vaccine.

Sterility (2.6.1)
Carry out the test for sterility using 10 mL for each medium.

Absence of toxin and irreversibility of toxoid
Using the same buffer solution as for the final vaccine, without adsorbent, prepare a solution of bulk purified toxoid at 100 Lf/mL. Divide the solution into 2 equal parts. Maintain 1 part at 5 ± 3 °C and the other at 37 °C for 6 weeks. Carry out a test in Vero cells for active diphtheria toxin using 50 µL/well of both samples. The sample should not contain antimicrobial preservatives and detoxifying agents should be determined to be below the concentration toxic to Vero cells. Non-specific toxicity may be eliminated by dialysis.

Use freshly trypsinised Vero cells at a suitable concentration, for example 2.5×10^5 mL^{-1} and a reference diphtheria toxin diluted in 100 Lf/mL diphtheria toxoid. A suitable reference diphtheria toxin will contain either not less than 100 LD$_{50}$/mL or 67 to 133 lr/100 in 1 Lf and 25 000 to 50 000 minimal reacting doses for guinea-pig skin in 1 Lf (diphtheria toxin BRP is suitable for use as the reference toxin). Dilute the toxin in 100 Lf/mL diphtheria toxoid to a suitable concentration, for example 2×10^{-4} Lf/mL. Prepare serial twofold dilutions of the diluted diphtheria toxin and use undiluted test samples (50 µL/well). Distribute them in the wells of a sterile tissue culture plate containing a medium suitable for Vero cells. To ascertain that any cytotoxic effect noted is specific to diphtheria toxin, prepare in parallel dilutions where the toxin is neutralised by a suitable concentration of diphtheria antitoxin, for example 100 IU/mL. Include control wells without toxoid or toxin and with non-toxic toxoid at 100 Lf/mL on each plate to verify normal cell growth. Add cell suspension to each well, seal the plates and incubate at 37 °C for 5-6 days. Cytotoxic effect is judged to be present where there is complete metabolic inhibition of the Vero cells, indicated by the pH indicator of the medium. Confirm cytopathic effect by microscopic examination or suitable staining such as MTT dye. The test is invalid if 5×10^{-5} Lf/mL of reference diphtheria toxin in 100 Lf/mL toxoid has no cytotoxic effect on Vero cells or if the cytotoxic effect of this amount of toxin is not neutralised in the wells containing diphtheria antitoxin. The bulk purified toxoid complies with the test if no toxicity neutralisable by antitoxin is found in either sample.

Antigenic purity (2.7.27)
Not less than 1500 Lf per milligram of protein nitrogen.

FINAL BULK VACCINE
The final bulk vaccine is prepared by adsorption of a suitable quantity of bulk purified toxoid onto a mineral carrier such as hydrated aluminium phosphate or aluminium hydroxide; the resulting mixture is approximately isotonic with blood.

Suitable antimicrobial preservatives may be added. Certain antimicrobial preservatives, particularly those of the phenolic type, adversely affect the antigenic activity and must not be used.

Only a final bulk vaccine that complies with the following requirements may be used in the preparation of the final lot.

Antimicrobial preservative
Where applicable, determine the amount of antimicrobial preservative by a suitable chemical method. The amount is not less than 85 per cent and not greater than 115 per cent of the intended amount.

Sterility (2.6.1)
Carry out the test for sterility using 10 mL for each medium.

FINAL LOT
The final bulk vaccine is distributed aseptically into sterile, tamper-proof containers. The containers are closed so as to prevent contamination.

Only a final lot that is satisfactory with respect to each of the requirements given below under Identification, Tests and Assay may be released for use. Provided the test for antimicrobial preservative and the assay have been carried out with satisfactory results on the final bulk vaccine, they may be omitted on the final lot.

Provided the free formaldehyde content has been determined on the bulk purified antigens or on the final bulk and it has been shown that the content in the final lot will not exceed 0.2 g/L, the test for free formaldehyde may be omitted on the final lot.

IDENTIFICATION
Diphtheria toxoid is identified by a suitable immunochemical method (2.7.1). The following method, applicable to certain vaccines, is given as an example. Dissolve in the vaccine to be examined sufficient *sodium citrate R* to give a 100 g/L solution. Maintain at 37 °C for about 16 h and centrifuge until a clear supernatant liquid is obtained. The clear supernatant liquid reacts with a suitable diphtheria antitoxin, giving a precipitate.

TESTS
Aluminium (2.5.13)
Maximum 1.25 mg per single human dose, if aluminium hydroxide or hydrated aluminium phosphate is used as the absorbent.

Free formaldehyde (2.4.18)
Maximum 0.2 g/L.

Antimicrobial preservative
Where applicable, determine the amount of antimicrobial preservative by a suitable chemical method. The content is not less than the minimum amount shown to be effective and is not greater than 115 per cent of the quantity stated on the label.

Sterility (2.6.1)
The vaccine complies with the test for sterility.

ASSAY
Carry out one of the prescribed methods for the assay of diphtheria vaccine (adsorbed) (2.7.6).

The lower confidence limit ($P = 0.95$) of the estimated potency is not less than 30 IU per single human dose.

LABELLING
The label states:
— the minimum number of International Units per single human dose,

— where applicable, that the vaccine is intended for primary vaccination of children and is not necessarily suitable for reinforcing doses or for administration to adults,
— the name and the amount of the adsorbent,
— that the vaccine must be shaken before use,
— that the vaccine is not to be frozen.

Ph Eur

Diphtheria Vaccine (Adsorbed, Reduced Antigen Content)

Adsorbed Diphtheria Vaccine for Adults and Adolescents

(*Ph Eur monograph 0646*)

For a vaccine for use in the United Kingdom, the amount of toxoid used is adjusted so that the final vaccine contains not more than 2.0 flocculation equivalents (2.0 Lf) per dose.

Ph Eur _____

DEFINITION

Diphtheria vaccine (adsorbed, reduced antigen content) is a preparation of diphtheria formol toxoid with a mineral adsorbent. The formol toxoid is prepared from the toxin produced by the growth of *Corynebacterium diphtheriae*.
It shall have been demonstrated to the competent authority that the quantity of diphtheria toxoid used does not produce adverse reactions in subjects from the age groups for which the vaccine is intended.

PRODUCTION
GENERAL PROVISIONS

Specific toxicity

The production method is validated to demonstrate that the product, if tested, would comply with the following test: inject subcutaneously 5 times the single human dose stated on the label into each of 5 healthy guinea-pigs, each weighing 250-350 g, that have not previously been treated with any material that will interfere with the test. If within 42 days of the injection any of the animals shows signs of or dies from diphtheria toxaemia, the vaccine does not comply with the test. If more than one animal dies from non-specific causes, repeat the test once; if more than one animal dies in the second test, the vaccine does not comply with the test.

BULK PURIFIED TOXOID

The bulk purified toxoid is prepared as described in the monograph on *Diphtheria vaccine (adsorbed) (0443)* and complies with the requirements prescribed therein.

FINAL BULK VACCINE

The final bulk vaccine is prepared by adsorption of a suitable quantity of bulk purified toxoid onto a mineral carrier such as hydrated aluminium phosphate or aluminium hydroxide; the resulting mixture is approximately isotonic with blood. Suitable antimicrobial preservatives may be added. Certain antimicrobial preservatives, particularly those of the phenolic type, adversely affect the antigenic activity and must not be used.

Only a final bulk vaccine that complies with the following requirements may be used in the preparation of the final lot.

Antimicrobial preservative

Where applicable, determine the amount of antimicrobial preservative by a suitable chemical method. The amount is not less than 85 per cent and not greater than 115 per cent of the intended amount.

Sterility (*2.6.1*)

Carry out the test for sterility using 10 mL for each medium.

FINAL LOT

The final bulk vaccine is distributed aseptically into sterile, tamper-proof containers. The containers are closed so as to prevent contamination.

Only a final lot that is satisfactory with respect to each of the requirements given below under Identification, Tests and Assay may be released for use. Provided the test for antimicrobial preservative and the assay have been carried out with satisfactory results on the final bulk vaccine, they may be omitted on the final lot.

Provided the free formaldehyde content has been determined on the bulk purified toxoid or on the final bulk and it has been shown that the content in the final lot will not exceed 0.2 g/L, the test for free formaldehyde may be omitted on the final lot.

IDENTIFICATION

Diphtheria toxoid is identified by a suitable immunochemical method (*2.7.1*). The following method, applicable to certain vaccines, is given as an example. Dissolve in the vaccine to be examined sufficient *sodium citrate R* to give a 100 g/L solution. Maintain at 37 °C for about 16 h and centrifuge until a clear supernatant liquid is obtained. The clear supernatant liquid reacts with a suitable diphtheria antitoxin, giving a precipitate. If a satisfactory result is not obtained with a vaccine adsorbed on aluminium hydroxide, carry out the test as follows. Centrifuge 15 mL of the vaccine to be examined and suspend the residue in 5 mL of a freshly prepared mixture of 1 volume of a 56 g/L solution of *sodium edetate R* and 49 volumes of a 90 g/L solution of *disodium hydrogen phosphate R*. Maintain at 37 °C for not less than 6 h and centrifuge. The clear supernatant liquid reacts with a suitable diphtheria antitoxin, giving a precipitate.

TESTS

Aluminium (*2.5.13*)

Maximum 1.25 mg per single human dose, if aluminium hydroxide or hydrated aluminium phosphate is used as the adsorbent.

Free formaldehyde (*2.4.18*)

Maximum 0.2 g/L.

Antimicrobial preservative

Where applicable, determine the amount of antimicrobial preservative by a suitable chemical method. The content is not less than the minimum amount shown to be effective and is not greater than 115 per cent of the quantity stated on the label.

Sterility (*2.6.1*)

The vaccine complies with the test for sterility.

ASSAY

Carry out one of the prescribed methods for the assay of diphtheria vaccine (adsorbed) (*2.7.6*).

The lower confidence limit ($P = 0.95$) of the estimated potency is not less than 2 IU per single human dose.

LABELLING

The label states:
— the minimum number of International Units per single human dose;
— the name and the amount of the adsorbent;
— that the vaccine must be shaken before use;
— that the vaccine is not to be frozen.

Ph Eur

Adsorbed Diphtheria and Tetanus Vaccine

*(Diphtheria and Tetanus Vaccine (Adsorbed),
Ph Eur monograph 0444)*

The label may state 'DT'.

Ph Eur _____

DEFINITION

Diphtheria and tetanus vaccine (adsorbed) is a preparation of diphtheria formol toxoid and tetanus formol toxoid with a mineral adsorbent. The formol toxoids are prepared from the toxins produced by the growth of *Corynebacterium diphtheriae* and *Clostridium tetani*, respectively.

PRODUCTION

GENERAL PROVISIONS

Specific toxicity of the diphtheria and tetanus components

The production method is validated to demonstrate that the product, if tested, would comply with the following test: inject subcutaneously 5 times the single human dose stated on the label into each of 5 healthy guinea-pigs, each weighing 250-350 g, that have not previously been treated with any material that will interfere with the test. If within 42 days of the injection any of the animals shows signs of or dies from diphtheria toxaemia or tetanus, the vaccine does not comply with the test. If more than 1 animal dies from non-specific causes, repeat the test once; if more than 1 animal dies in the second test, the vaccine does not comply with the test.

BULK PURIFIED DIPHTHERIA AND TETANUS TOXOIDS

The bulk purified diphtheria and tetanus toxoids are prepared as described in the monographs on *Diphtheria vaccine (adsorbed) (0443)* and *Tetanus vaccine (adsorbed) (0452)* and comply with the requirements prescribed therein.

FINAL BULK VACCINE

The final bulk vaccine is prepared by adsorption of suitable quantities of bulk purified diphtheria toxoid and tetanus toxoid onto a mineral carrier such as hydrated aluminium phosphate or aluminium hydroxide; the resulting mixture is approximately isotonic with blood. Suitable antimicrobial preservatives may be added. Certain antimicrobial preservatives, particularly those of the phenolic type, adversely affect the antigenic activity and must not be used.

Only a final bulk vaccine that complies with the following requirements may be used in the preparation of the final lot.

Antimicrobial preservative

Where applicable, determine the amount of antimicrobial preservative by a suitable chemical method. The amount is not less than 85 per cent and not greater than 115 per cent of the intended amount.

Sterility (*2.6.1*)

Carry out the test for sterility using 10 mL for each medium.

FINAL LOT

The final bulk vaccine is distributed aseptically into sterile, tamper-proof containers. The containers are closed so as to prevent contamination.

Only a final lot that is satisfactory with respect to each of the requirements given below under Identification, Tests and Assay may be released for use. Provided the test for antimicrobial preservative and the assay have been carried out with satisfactory results on the final bulk vaccine, they may be omitted on the final lot.

Provided the free formaldehyde content has been determined on the bulk purified antigens or on the final bulk and it has been shown that the content in the final lot will not exceed 0.2 g/L, the test for free formaldehyde may be omitted on the final lot.

IDENTIFICATION

A. Diphtheria toxoid is identified by a suitable immunochemical method (*2.7.1*). The following method, applicable to certain vaccines, is given as an example. Dissolve in the vaccine to be examined sufficient *sodium citrate R* to give a 100 g/L solution. Maintain at 37 °C for about 16 h and centrifuge until a clear supernatant liquid is obtained. The clear supernatant liquid reacts with a suitable diphtheria antitoxin, giving a precipitate.

B. Tetanus toxoid is identified by a suitable immunochemical method (*2.7.1*). The following method, applicable to certain vaccines, is given as an example. The clear supernatant liquid obtained as described in identification test A reacts with a suitable tetanus antitoxin, giving a precipitate.

TESTS

Aluminium (*2.5.13*)

Maximum 1.25 mg per single human dose, if aluminium hydroxide or hydrated aluminium phosphate is used as the adsorbent.

Free formaldehyde (*2.4.18*)

Maximum 0.2 g/L.

Antimicrobial preservative

Where applicable, determine the amount of antimicrobial preservative by a suitable chemical method. The content is not less than the minimum amount shown to be effective and is not greater than 115 per cent of the quantity stated on the label.

Sterility (*2.6.1*)

The vaccine complies with the test for sterility.

ASSAY

Diphtheria component

Carry out one of the prescribed methods for the assay of diphtheria vaccine (adsorbed) (*2.7.6*).

The lower confidence limit ($P = 0.95$) of the estimated potency is not less than 30 IU per single human dose.

Tetanus component

Carry out one of the prescribed methods for the assay of tetanus vaccine (adsorbed) (*2.7.8*).

The lower confidence limit ($P = 0.95$) of the estimated potency is not less than 40 IU per single human dose.

LABELLING

The label states:
— the minimum number of International Units of each component per single human dose,
— where applicable, that the vaccine is intended for primary vaccination of children and is not necessarily suitable for reinforcing doses or for administration to adults,
— the name and the amount of the adsorbent,
— that the vaccine must be shaken before use,
— that the vaccine is not to be frozen.

_____ *Ph Eur*

IMMUNOLOGICAL PRODUCTS

Diphtheria and Tetanus Vaccine (Adsorbed, Reduced Antigen(s) Content)

Adsorbed Diphtheria and Tetanus Vaccine for Adults and Adolescents

(Ph Eur monograph 0647)

The label may state 'dT'.

For a vaccine for use in the United Kingdom, the amount of diphtheria toxoid used is adjusted so that the final vaccine contains not more than 2.0 flocculation equivalents (2.0 Lf) of diphtheria toxoid per dose.

Ph Eur _____

DEFINITION

Diphtheria and tetanus vaccine (adsorbed, reduced antigen(s) content) is a preparation of diphtheria formol toxoid and tetanus formol toxoid with a mineral adsorbent. The formol toxoids are prepared from the toxins produced by the growth of *Corynebacterium diphtheriae* and *Clostridium tetani*, respectively. It shall have been demonstrated to the competent authority that the quantity of diphtheria toxoid used does not produce adverse reactions in subjects from the age groups for which the vaccine is intended.

PRODUCTION

GENERAL PROVISIONS

Specific toxicity of the diphtheria and tetanus components

The production method is validated to demonstrate that the product, if tested, would comply with the following test: inject subcutaneously 5 times the single human dose stated on the label into each of 5 healthy guinea-pigs, each weighing 250-350 g, that have not previously been treated with any material that will interfere with the test. If within 42 days of the injection any of the animals shows signs of or dies from diphtheria toxaemia or tetanus, the vaccine does not comply with the test. If more than one animal dies from non-specific causes, repeat the test once; if more than one animal dies in the second test, the vaccine does not comply with the test.

BULK PURIFIED DIPHTHERIA TOXOID AND TETANUS TOXOIDS

The bulk purified diphtheria and tetanus toxoids are prepared as described in the monographs on *Diphtheria vaccine (adsorbed) (0443)* and *Tetanus vaccine (adsorbed) (0452)* and comply with the requirements prescribed therein.

FINAL BULK VACCINE

The vaccine is prepared by adsorption of suitable quantities of bulk purified diphtheria toxoid and tetanus toxoid onto a mineral carrier such as hydrated aluminium phosphate or aluminium hydroxide; the resulting mixture is approximately isotonic with blood. Suitable antimicrobial preservatives may be added. Certain antimicrobial preservatives, particularly those of the phenolic type, adversely affect the antigenic activity and must not be used.

Only a final bulk vaccine that complies with the following requirements may be used in the preparation of the final lot.

Antimicrobial preservative

Where applicable, determine the amount of antimicrobial preservative by a suitable chemical method. The amount is not less than 85 per cent and not greater than 115 per cent of the intended amount.

Sterility (2.6.1)

Carry out the test for sterility using 10 mL for each medium.

FINAL LOT

The final bulk vaccine is distributed aseptically into sterile, tamper-proof containers. The containers are closed so as to prevent contamination.

Only a final lot that is satisfactory with respect to each of the requirements given below under Identification, Tests and Assay may be released for use. Provided the test for antimicrobial preservative and the assay have been carried out with satisfactory results on the final bulk vaccine, they may be omitted on the final lot.

Provided the free formaldehyde content has been determined on the bulk purified toxoids or on the final bulk and it has been shown that the content in the final lot will not exceed 0.2 g/L, the test for free formaldehyde may be omitted on the final lot.

IDENTIFICATION

A. Diphtheria toxoid is identified by a suitable immunochemical method (2.7.1). The following method, applicable to certain vaccines, is given as an example. Dissolve in the vaccine to be examined sufficient *sodium citrate R* to give a 100 g/L solution. Maintain at 37 °C for about 16 h and centrifuge until a clear supernatant liquid is obtained. The clear supernatant liquid reacts with a suitable diphtheria antitoxin, giving a precipitate. If a satisfactory result is not obtained with a vaccine adsorbed on aluminium hydroxide, carry out the test as follows. Centrifuge 15 mL of the vaccine to be examined and suspend the residue in 5 mL of a freshly prepared mixture of 1 volume of a 56 g/L solution of *sodium edetate R* and 49 volumes of a 90 g/L solution of *disodium hydrogen phosphate R*. Maintain at 37 °C for not less than 6 h and centrifuge. The clear supernatant liquid reacts with a suitable diphtheria antitoxin, giving a precipitate.

B. Tetanus toxoid is identified by a suitable immunochemical method (2.7.1). The following method, applicable to certain vaccines, is given as an example. The clear supernatant liquid obtained during identification test A reacts with a suitable tetanus antitoxin, giving a precipitate.

TESTS

Aluminium (2.5.13)

Maximum 1.25 mg per single human dose, if aluminium hydroxide or hydrated aluminium phosphate is used as the adsorbent.

Free formaldehyde (2.4.18)

Maximum 0.2 g/L.

Antimicrobial preservative

Where applicable, determine the amount of antimicrobial preservative by a suitable chemical method. The content is not less than the minimum amount shown to be effective and is not greater than 115 per cent of the quantity stated on the label.

Sterility (2.6.1)

The vaccine complies with the test for sterility.

ASSAY

Diphtheria component

Carry out one of the prescribed methods for the assay of diphtheria vaccine (adsorbed) (2.7.6).

The lower confidence limit ($P = 0.95$) of the estimated potency is not less than 2 IU per single human dose.

Tetanus component

Carry out one of the prescribed methods for the assay of tetanus vaccine (adsorbed) (2.7.8).

The lower confidence limit ($P = 0.95$) of the estimated potency is not less than 20 IU per single human dose.

LABELLING
The label states:
— the minimum number of International Units of each component per single human dose;
— the name and the amount of the adsorbent;
— that the vaccine must be shaken before use;
— that the vaccine is not to be frozen.

_____ Ph Eur

Diphtheria, Tetanus and Hepatitis B (rDNA) Vaccine (Adsorbed)

(*Ph Eur monograph 2062*)
The label may state 'DT/HepB'.

Ph Eur _____

DEFINITION
Diphtheria, tetanus and hepatitis B (rDNA) vaccine (adsorbed) is a combined vaccine composed of: diphtheria formol toxoid; tetanus formol toxoid; hepatitis B surface antigen (HBsAg); a mineral adsorbent such as aluminium hydroxide or hydrated aluminium phosphate.

The formol toxoids are prepared from the toxins produced by the growth of *Corynebacterium diphtheriae* and *Clostridium tetani*, respectively.

HBsAg is a component protein of hepatitis B virus; the antigen is obtained by recombinant DNA technology.

PRODUCTION
GENERAL PROVISIONS
The production method shall have been shown to yield consistently vaccines comparable with the vaccine of proven clinical efficacy and safety in man.

The content of bacterial endotoxins (*2.6.14*) in the bulk purified diphtheria toxoid and tetanus toxoid is determined to monitor the purification procedure and to limit the amount in the final vaccine. For each component, the content of bacterial endotoxins is less than the limit approved for the particular vaccine and in any case the contents are such that the final vaccine contains less than 100 IU per single human dose.

Reference vaccine(s)   Provided valid assays can be performed, monocomponent reference vaccines may be used for the assays on the combined vaccine. If this is not possible because of interaction between the components of the combined vaccine or because of the difference in composition between monocomponent reference vaccine and the test vaccine, a batch of combined vaccine shown to be effective in clinical trials or a batch representative thereof is used as a reference vaccine. For the preparation of a representative batch, strict adherence to the production process used for the batch tested in clinical trials is necessary. The reference vaccine may be stabilised by a method that has been shown to have no effect on the assay procedure.

Specific toxicity of the diphtheria and tetanus components
The production method is validated to demonstrate that the product, if tested, would comply with the following test: inject subcutaneously 5 times the single human dose stated on the label into each of 5 healthy guinea-pigs, each weighing 250-350 g, that have not previously been treated with any material that will interfere with the test. If within 42 days of the injection any of the animals shows signs of or dies from diphtheria toxaemia or tetanus, the vaccine does not comply with the test. If more than 1 animal dies from non-specific causes, repeat the test once; if more than 1 animal dies in the second test, the vaccine does not comply with the test.

PRODUCTION OF THE COMPONENTS
The production of the components complies with the requirements of the monographs on *Diphtheria vaccine (adsorbed) (0443)*, *Tetanus vaccine (adsorbed) (0452)* and *Hepatitis B vaccine (rDNA) (1056)*.

FINAL BULK VACCINE
The final bulk vaccine is prepared by adsorption, separately or together, of suitable quantities of bulk purified diphtheria toxoid, tetanus toxoid and HBsAg onto a mineral carrier such as aluminium hydroxide or hydrated aluminium phosphate. Suitable antimicrobial preservatives may be added.

Only a final bulk vaccine that complies with the following requirements may be used in the preparation of the final lot.

Antimicrobial preservative
Where applicable, determine the amount of antimicrobial preservative by a suitable chemical method. The amount is not less than 85 per cent and not greater than 115 per cent of the intended content.

Sterility (*2.6.1*)
Carry out the test for sterility using 10 mL for each medium.

FINAL LOT
Only a final lot that is satisfactory with respect to the test for osmolality and with respect to each of the requirements given below under Identification, Tests and Assay may be released for use.

Provided the test for antimicrobial preservative and the assays for the diphtheria and tetanus components have been carried out with satisfactory results on the final bulk vaccine, they may be omitted on the final lot.

Provided the content of free formaldehyde has been determined on the bulk purified antigens or on the final bulk and it has been shown that the content in the final lot will not exceed 0.2 g/L, the test for free formaldehyde may be omitted on the final lot.

If an *in vivo* assay is used for the hepatitis B component, provided it has been carried out with satisfactory results on the final bulk vaccine, it may be omitted on the final lot.

Osmolality (*2.2.35*)
The osmolality of the vaccine is within the limits approved for the particular preparation.

IDENTIFICATION
A. Diphtheria toxoid is identified by a suitable immunochemical method (*2.7.1*). The following method, applicable to certain vaccines, is given as an example. Dissolve in the vaccine to be examined sufficient *sodium citrate R* to give a 100 g/L solution. Maintain at 37 °C for about 16 h and centrifuge until a clear supernatant liquid is obtained. The clear supernatant liquid reacts with a suitable diphtheria antitoxin, giving a precipitate.

B. Tetanus toxoid is identified by a suitable immunochemical method (*2.7.1*). The following method, applicable to certain vaccines, is given as an example. The clear supernatant liquid obtained during identification test A reacts with a suitable tetanus antitoxin, giving a precipitate.

C. The assay or, where applicable, the electrophoretic profile, serves also to identify the hepatitis B component of the vaccine.

TESTS

Aluminium (2.5.13)

Maximum 1.25 mg per single human dose, if aluminium hydroxide or hydrated aluminium phosphate is used as the adsorbent.

Free formaldehyde (2.4.18)

Maximum 0.2 g/L.

Antimicrobial preservative

Where applicable, determine the amount of antimicrobial preservative by a suitable chemical method. The content is not less than the minimum amount shown to be effective and is not greater than 115 per cent of the quantity stated on the label.

Sterility (2.6.1)

It complies with the test for sterility.

Pyrogens (2.6.8)

It complies with the test for pyrogens. Inject the equivalent of 1 human dose into each rabbit.

ASSAY

Diphtheria component

Carry out one of the prescribed methods for the assay of diphtheria vaccine (adsorbed) (2.7.6).

The lower confidence limit ($P = 0.95$) of the estimated potency is not less than 30 IU per single human dose.

Tetanus component

Carry out one of the prescribed methods for the assay of tetanus vaccine (adsorbed) (2.7.8).

The lower confidence limit ($P = 0.95$) of the estimated potency is not less than 40 IU per single human dose.

Hepatitis B component

It complies with the assay of hepatitis B vaccine (2.7.15).

LABELLING

The label states:

— the minimum number of International Units of diphtheria and tetanus toxoid per single human dose,
— the amount of HBsAg per single human dose,
— the type of cells used for production of the HBsAg component,
— where applicable, that the vaccine is intended for primary vaccination of children and is not necessarily suitable for reinforcing doses or for administration to adults,
— the name and the amount of the adsorbent,
— that the vaccine must be shaken before use,
— that the vaccine is not to be frozen.

_____ Ph Eur

Diphtheria, Tetanus and Pertussis (Whole Cell) Vaccine (Adsorbed)

Diphtheria, Tetanus and Pertussis Vaccine (Adsorbed)

(Ph Eur monograph 0445)

The label may state 'DTwP'.

Ph Eur _____

DEFINITION

Diphtheria, tetanus and pertussis (whole cell) vaccine (adsorbed) is a preparation of diphtheria formol toxoid and tetanus formol toxoid with a mineral adsorbent to which a suspension of inactivated *Bordetella pertussis* has been added. The formol toxoids are prepared from the toxins produced by the growth of *Corynebacterium diphtheriae* and *Clostridium tetani*, respectively.

PRODUCTION

GENERAL PROVISIONS

Specific toxicity of the diphtheria and tetanus components

The production method is validated to demonstrate that the product, if tested, would comply with the following test: inject subcutaneously 5 times the single human dose stated on the label into each of 5 healthy guinea-pigs, each weighing 250-350 g, that have not previously been treated with any material that will interfere with the test. If within 42 days of the injection any of the animals shows signs of or dies from diphtheria toxaemia or tetanus, the vaccine does not comply with the test. If more than 1 animal dies from non-specific causes, repeat the test once; if more than 1 animal dies in the second test, the vaccine does not comply with the test.

BULK PURIFIED DIPHTHERIA AND TETANUS TOXOIDS, BULK INACTIVATED B. PERTUSSIS SUSPENSION

The bulk purified diphtheria and tetanus toxoids and the inactivated *B. pertussis* suspension are prepared as described in the monographs *Diphtheria vaccine (adsorbed) (0443)*, *Tetanus vaccine (adsorbed) (0452)* and *Pertussis vaccine (whole cell, adsorbed) (0161)*, respectively, and comply with the requirements prescribed therein.

FINAL BULK VACCINE

The final bulk vaccine is prepared by adsorption of suitable quantities of bulk purified diphtheria toxoid and tetanus toxoid onto a mineral carrier such as hydrated aluminium phosphate or aluminium hydroxide and admixture of an appropriate quantity of a suspension of inactivated *B. pertussis*; the resulting mixture is approximately isotonic with blood. The *B. pertussis* concentration of the final bulk vaccine does not exceed that corresponding to an opacity of 20 IU per single human dose. If 2 or more strains of *B. pertussis* are used, the composition of consecutive lots of the final bulk vaccine shall be consistent with respect to the proportion of each strain as measured in opacity units. Suitable antimicrobial preservatives may be added to the bulk vaccine. Certain antimicrobial preservatives, particularly those of the phenolic type, adversely affect the antigenic activity and must not be used.

Only a final bulk vaccine that complies with the following requirements may be used in the preparation of the final lot.

Antimicrobial preservative

Where applicable, determine the amount of antimicrobial preservative by a suitable chemical method. The amount is not less than 85 per cent and not greater than 115 per cent of the intended amount.

Sterility (*2.6.1*)

Carry out the test for sterility using 10 mL for each medium.

FINAL LOT

The final bulk vaccine is distributed aseptically into sterile, tamper-proof containers. The containers are closed so as to prevent contamination.

Only a final lot that is satisfactory with respect to each of the requirements given below under Identification, Tests and Assay may be released for use. Provided the tests for specific toxicity of the pertussis component, antimicrobial preservative and the assay have been carried out with satisfactory results on the final bulk vaccine, they may be omitted on the final lot.

Provided the free formaldehyde content has been determined on the bulk purified antigens or on the final bulk and it has been shown that the content in the final lot will not exceed 0.2 g/L, the test for free formaldehyde may be omitted on the final lot.

IDENTIFICATION

A. Diphtheria toxoid is identified by a suitable immunochemical method (*2.7.1*). The following method, applicable to certain vaccines, is given as an example. Dissolve in the vaccine to be examined sufficient *sodium citrate R* to give a 100 g/L solution. Maintain at 37 °C for about 16 h and centrifuge until a clear supernatant liquid is obtained; reserve the precipitate for identification test C. The clear supernatant liquid reacts with a suitable diphtheria antitoxin, giving a precipitate.

B. Tetanus toxoid is identified by a suitable immunochemical method (*2.7.1*). The following method, applicable to certain vaccines, is given as an example. The clear supernatant liquid obtained during identification test A reacts with a suitable tetanus antitoxin, giving a precipitate.

C. Dissolve in the vaccine to be examined sufficient *sodium citrate R* to give a 100 g/L solution. Maintain at 37 °C for about 16 h and centrifuge to obtain a bacterial precipitate. Other suitable methods for separating the bacteria from the adsorbent may also be used. Identify pertussis vaccine by agglutination of the bacteria from the resuspended precipitate by antisera specific to *B. pertussis* or by the assay.

TESTS

Specific toxicity of the pertussis component

Use not fewer than 5 mice each weighing 14 - 16 g for the vaccine group and for the saline control. Use mice of the same sex or distribute males and females equally between the groups. Allow the animals access to food and water for at least 2 h before injection and during the test. Inject each mouse of the vaccine group intraperitoneally with 0.5 mL, containing a quantity of the vaccine equivalent to not less than half the single human dose. Inject each mouse of the control group with 0.5 mL of a 9 g/L sterile solution of *sodium chloride R*, preferably containing the same amount of antimicrobial preservative as that injected with the vaccine. Weigh the groups of mice immediately before the injection and 72 h and 7 days after the injection. The vaccine complies with the test if: (a) at the end of 72 h the total mass of the group of vaccinated mice is not less than that preceding the injection; (b) at the end of 7 days the average increase in mass per vaccinated mouse is not less than 60 per cent of that per control mouse; and (c) not more than 5 per cent of the vaccinated mice die during the test. The test may be repeated and the results of the tests combined.

Aluminium (*2.5.13*)

Maximum 1.25 mg per single human dose, if aluminium hydroxide or hydrated aluminium phosphate is used as the adsorbent.

Free formaldehyde (*2.4.18*)

Maximum 0.2 g/L.

Antimicrobial preservative

Where applicable, determine the amount of antimicrobial preservative by a suitable chemical method. The content is not less than the minimum amount shown to be effective and is not greater than 115 per cent of the quantity stated on the label.

Sterility (*2.6.1*)

The vaccine complies with the test for sterility.

ASSAY

Diphtheria component

Carry out one of the prescribed methods for the assay of diphtheria vaccine (adsorbed) (*2.7.6*).

The lower confidence limit ($P = 0.95$) of the estimated potency is not less than 30 IU per single human dose.

Tetanus component

Carry out one of the prescribed methods for the assay of tetanus vaccine (adsorbed) (*2.7.8*).

If the test is carried out in guinea-pigs, the lower confidence limit ($P = 0.95$) of the estimated potency is not less than 40 IU per single human dose; if the test is carried out in mice, the lower confidence limit ($P = 0.95$) of the estimated potency is not less than 60 IU per single human dose.

Pertussis component

Carry out the assay of pertussis vaccine (whole cell) (*2.7.7*).

The estimated potency is not less than 4.0 IU per single human dose and the lower confidence limit ($P = 0.95$) of the estimated potency is not less than 2.0 IU per single human dose.

LABELLING

The label states:
— the minimum number of International Units of each component per single human dose;
— where applicable, that the vaccine is intended for primary vaccination of children and is not necessarily suitable for reinforcing doses or for administration to adults;
— the name and the amount of the adsorbent;
— that the vaccine must be shaken before use;
— that the vaccine is not to be frozen.

Ph Eur

Adsorbed Diphtheria, Tetanus and Pertussis (Acellular Component) Vaccine

(Diphtheria, Tetanus and Pertussis (Acellular, Component) Vaccine (Adsorbed), Ph Eur monograph 1931)

The label may state 'DTaP'.

Ph Eur

DEFINITION

Diphtheria, tetanus and pertussis (acellular, component) vaccine (adsorbed) is a combined vaccine composed of: diphtheria formol toxoid; tetanus formol toxoid; individually purified antigenic components of *Bordetella pertussis*; a mineral adsorbent such as aluminium hydroxide or hydrated aluminium phosphate.

The formol toxoids are prepared from the toxins produced by the growth of *Corynebacterium diphtheriae* and *Clostridium tetani*, respectively.

The vaccine contains either pertussis toxoid or a pertussis-toxin-like protein free from toxic properties, produced by expression of a genetically modified form of the corresponding gene. Pertussis toxoid is prepared from pertussis toxin by a method that renders the latter harmless while maintaining adequate immunogenic properties and avoiding reversion to toxin. The vaccine may also contain filamentous haemagglutinin, pertactin (a 69 kDa outer-membrane protein) and other defined components of *B. pertussis* such as fimbrial-2 and fimbrial-3 antigens. The latter 2 antigens may be co-purified. The antigenic composition and characteristics are based on evidence of protection and freedom from unexpected reactions in the target group for which the vaccine is intended.

PRODUCTION

GENERAL PROVISIONS

The production method shall have been shown to yield consistently vaccines comparable with the vaccine of proven clinical efficacy and safety in man.

Specific toxicity of the diphtheria and tetanus components

The production method is validated to demonstrate that the product, if tested, would comply with the following test: inject subcutaneously 5 times the single human dose stated on the label into each of 5 healthy guinea-pigs, each weighing 250-350 g, that have not previously been treated with any material that will interfere with the test. If within 42 days of the injection any of the animals shows signs of or dies from diphtheria toxaemia or tetanus, the vaccine does not comply with the test. If more than 1 animal dies from non-specific causes, repeat the test once; if more than 1 animal dies in the second test, the vaccine does not comply with the test.

The content of bacterial endotoxins (2.6.14) in the bulk purified diphtheria toxoid, tetanus toxoid and pertussis components is determined to monitor the purification procedure and to limit the amount in the final vaccine. For each component, the content of bacterial endotoxins is less than the limit approved for the particular vaccine and, in any case, the contents are such that the final vaccine contains less than 100 IU per single human dose.

Reference vaccine(s) Provided valid assays can be performed, monocomponent reference vaccines may be used for the assays on the combined vaccine. If this is not possible because of interaction between the components of the combined vaccine or because of differences in composition between the monocomponent reference vaccine and the test vaccine, a batch of combined vaccine shown to be effective in clinical trials or a batch representative thereof is used as a reference vaccine. For the preparation of a representative batch, strict adherence to the production process used for the batch tested in clinical trials is necessary. The reference vaccine may be stabilised by a method that has been shown to have no effect on the assay procedure.

PRODUCTION OF THE COMPONENTS

The production of the components complies with the requirements of the monographs *Diphtheria vaccine (adsorbed) (0443)*, *Tetanus vaccine (adsorbed) (0452)* and *Pertussis vaccine (acellular, component, adsorbed) (1356)*.

FINAL BULK VACCINE

The final bulk vaccine is prepared by adsorption of suitable quantities of bulk purified diphtheria toxoid, tetanus toxoid and pertussis components separately or together onto a mineral carrier such as aluminium hydroxide or hydrated aluminium phosphate. Suitable antimicrobial preservatives may be added.

Only a final bulk vaccine that complies with the following requirements may be used in the preparation of the final lot.

Antimicrobial preservative

Where applicable, determine the amount of antimicrobial preservative by a suitable chemical method. The amount is not less than 85 per cent and not greater than 115 per cent of the intended content.

Sterility (2.6.1)

Carry out the test for sterility using 10 mL for each medium.

FINAL LOT

Only a final lot that is satisfactory with respect to the test for osmolality and with respect to each of the requirements given below under Identification, Tests and Assay may be released for use.

Provided the tests for residual pertussis toxin and irreversibility of pertussis toxoid, free formaldehyde and antimicrobial preservative and the assay have been carried out with satisfactory results on the final bulk vaccine, they may be omitted on the final lot.

Provided the free formaldehyde content has been determined on the bulk purified antigens or on the final bulk and it has been shown that the content in the final lot will not exceed 0.2 g/L, the test for free formaldehyde may be omitted on the final lot.

Osmolality (2.2.35)

The osmolality of the vaccine is within the limits approved for the particular preparation.

IDENTIFICATION

A. Diphtheria toxoid is identified by a suitable immunochemical method (2.7.1). The following method, applicable to certain vaccines, is given as an example. Dissolve in the vaccine to be examined sufficient *sodium citrate R* to give a 100 g/L solution. Maintain at 37 °C for about 16 h and centrifuge until a clear supernatant liquid is obtained. The clear supernatant liquid reacts with a suitable diphtheria antitoxin, giving a precipitate.

B. Tetanus toxoid is identified by a suitable immunochemical method (2.7.1). The following method, applicable to certain vaccines, is given as an example. The clear supernatant liquid obtained as described in identification test A reacts with a suitable tetanus antitoxin, giving a precipitate.

C. The pertussis components are identified by a suitable immunochemical method (2.7.1). The following method, applicable to certain vaccines, is given as an example. The clear supernatant liquid obtained as described in identification test A reacts with specific antisera to the pertussis components of the vaccine.

TESTS

Residual pertussis toxin and irreversibility of pertussis toxoid (2.6.33)

The final lot complies with the test.

Aluminium (2.5.13)

Maximum 1.25 mg per single human dose, if aluminium hydroxide or hydrated aluminium phosphate is used as the adsorbent.

Free formaldehyde (*2.4.18*)
Maximum 0.2 g/L.

Antimicrobial preservative
Where applicable, determine the amount of antimicrobial preservative by a suitable chemical method. The content is not less than the minimum amount shown to be effective and is not greater than 115 per cent of the quantity stated on the label.

Sterility (*2.6.1*)
The vaccine complies with the test for sterility.

ASSAY

Diphtheria component
Carry out one of the prescribed methods for the assay of diphtheria vaccine (adsorbed) (*2.7.6*).

The lower confidence limit ($P = 0.95$) of the estimated potency is not less than the minimum potency stated on the label.

Unless otherwise justified and authorised, the minimum potency stated on the label is 30 IU per single human dose.

Tetanus component
Carry out one of the prescribed methods for the assay of tetanus vaccine (adsorbed) (*2.7.8*).

The lower confidence limit ($P = 0.95$) of the estimated potency is not less than 40 IU per single human dose.

Pertussis component
Carry out one of the prescribed methods for the assay of pertussis vaccine (acellular) (*2.7.16*).

The capacity of the vaccine to induce antibodies for each included acellular pertussis antigen is not significantly ($P = 0.95$) less than that of the reference vaccine.

LABELLING

The label states:
— the minimum number of International Units of diphtheria and tetanus toxoid per single human dose;
— the names and amounts of the pertussis components per single human dose;
— where applicable, that the vaccine is intended for primary vaccination of children and is not necessarily suitable for reinforcing doses or for administration to adults;
— the name and the amount of the adsorbent;
— that the vaccine must be shaken before use;
— that the vaccine is not to be frozen;
— where applicable, that the vaccine contains a pertussis toxin-like protein produced by genetic modification.

Ph Eur

Adsorbed Diphtheria, Tetanus, Pertussis (Acellular Component) and Haemophilus Type b Conjugate Vaccine

(*Diphtheria, Tetanus, Pertussis (Acellular, Component) and Haemophilus Type b Conjugate Vaccine (Adsorbed), Ph Eur monograph 1932*)

The label may state 'DTaP/Hib'.

Ph Eur

DEFINITION

Diphtheria, tetanus, pertussis (acellular, component) and haemophilus type b conjugate vaccine (adsorbed) is a combined vaccine composed of: diphtheria formol toxoid; tetanus formol toxoid; individually purified antigenic components of *Bordetella pertussis*; polyribosylribitol phosphate (PRP) covalently bound to a carrier protein; a mineral absorbent such as aluminium hydroxide or hydrated aluminium phosphate. The product is presented either as a tetravalent liquid formulation in the same container, or as a trivalent liquid formulation with the haemophilus component in a separate container, the contents of which are mixed with the other components immediately before use.

The formol toxoids are prepared from the toxins produced by the growth of *Corynebacterium diphtheriae* and *Clostridium tetani* respectively.

The vaccine contains either pertussis toxoid or a pertussis-toxin-like protein free from toxic properties produced by expression of a genetically modified form of the corresponding gene. Pertussis toxoid is prepared from pertussis toxin by a method that renders the toxin harmless while maintaining adequate immunogenic properties and avoiding reversion to toxin. The acellular pertussis component may also contain filamentous haemagglutinin, pertactin (a 69 kDa outer-membrane protein) and other defined components of *B. pertussis* such as fimbrial-2 and fimbrial-3 antigens. The latter 2 antigens may be co-purified. The antigenic composition and characteristics are based on evidence of protection and freedom from unexpected reactions in the target group for which the vaccine is intended.

PRP is a linear copolymer composed of repeated units of 3-β-D-ribofuranosyl-(1→1)-ribitol-5-phosphate [($C_{10}H_{19}O_{12}P$)n], with a defined molecular size and derived from a suitable strain of *Haemophilus influenzae type b*.
The carrier protein, when conjugated to PRP, is capable of inducing a T-cell-dependent B-cell immune response to the polysaccharide.

PRODUCTION

GENERAL PROVISIONS

The production method shall have been shown to yield consistently vaccines comparable with the vaccine of proven clinical efficacy and safety in man.

Where the haemophilus component is presented in a separate container, as part of consistency studies the assays of the diphtheria, tetanus and pertussis components are carried out on a suitable number of batches of vaccine reconstituted as for use. For subsequent routine control, the assays of these components may be carried out without mixing with the haemophilus component.

Specific toxicity of the diphtheria and tetanus components
The production method is validated to demonstrate that the product, if tested, would comply with the following test: inject subcutaneously 5 times the single human dose stated on the label into each of 5 healthy guinea-pigs, each weighing 250-350 g, that have not previously been treated with any material that will interfere with the test. If within 42 days of the injection any of the animals shows signs of or dies from diphtheria toxaemia or tetanus, the vaccine does not comply with the test. If more than 1 animal dies from non-specific causes, repeat the test once; if more than 1 animal dies in the second test, the vaccine does not comply with the test.

The content of bacterial endotoxins (*2.6.14*) in bulk purified diphtheria toxoid, tetanus toxoid, pertussis components and bulk PRP conjugate is determined to monitor the purification procedure and to limit the amount in the final vaccine.
For each component, the content of bacterial endotoxins is

IMMUNOLOGICAL PRODUCTS

less than the limit approved for the particular vaccine; where the haemophilus component is presented in a separate container, the contents of the diphtheria, tetanus and pertussis antigens are in any case such that the final vial for these components contains less than 100 IU per single human dose.

The production method is validated to demonstrate that the product, if tested, would comply with the test for abnormal toxicity for immunosera and vaccines for human use (2.6.9).

During development studies and wherever revalidation is necessary, it shall be demonstrated by tests in animals that the vaccine induces a T-cell dependent B-cell immune response to PRP.

Where the haemophilus component is presented in a separate container, the production method is validated to demonstrate that the haemophilus component, if tested, would comply with the test for pyrogens (2.6.8), carried out as follows: inject per kilogram of the rabbit's mass a quantity of the vaccine equivalent to: 1 μg of PRP for a vaccine with diphtheria toxoid or CRM 197 diphtheria protein as carrier; 0.1 μg of PRP for a vaccine with tetanus toxoid as carrier; 0.025 μg of PRP for a vaccine with OMP (meningococcal group B outer membrane protein complex) as carrier.

Reference vaccine(s) Provided valid assays can be performed, monocomponent reference vaccines may be used for the assays on the combined vaccine. If this is not possible because of interaction between the components of the combined vaccine or because of differences in composition between the monocomponent reference vaccine and the test vaccine, a batch of combined vaccine shown to be effective in clinical trials or a batch representative thereof is used as a reference vaccine. For the preparation of a representative batch, strict adherence to the production process used for the batch tested in clinical trials is necessary. The reference vaccine may be stabilised by a method that has been shown to have no effect on the assay procedure.

PRODUCTION OF THE COMPONENTS

The production of the components complies with the requirements of the monographs *Diphtheria vaccine (adsorbed) (0443)*, *Tetanus vaccine (adsorbed) (0452)*, *Pertussis vaccine (acellular, component, adsorbed) (1356)* and *Haemophilus type b conjugate vaccine (1219)*.

FINAL BULK VACCINE

Different methods of preparation may be used: a final bulk vaccine may be prepared by adsorption, separately or together, of suitable quantities of bulk purified diphtheria toxoid, tetanus toxoid, acellular pertussis components and PRP conjugate onto a mineral carrier such as aluminium hydroxide or hydrated aluminium phosphate; or 2 final bulks may be prepared and filled separately, one containing the diphtheria, tetanus and pertussis components, the other the haemophilus component, which may be freeze-dried. Suitable antimicrobial preservatives may be added.

Only a final bulk vaccine that complies with the following requirements may be used in the preparation of the final lot.

Antimicrobial preservative

Where applicable, determine the amount of antimicrobial preservative by a suitable chemical method. The amount is not less than 85 per cent and not greater than 115 per cent of the intended content.

Sterility (2.6.1)

Carry out the test for sterility using 10 mL for each medium.

FINAL LOT

Only a final lot that is satisfactory with respect to the test for osmolality shown below and with respect to each of the requirements given below under Identification, Tests and Assay may be released for use.

Provided the test for residual pertussis toxin and irreversibility of pertussis toxoid, the test for antimicrobial preservative and the assay have been carried out with satisfactory results on the final bulk vaccine, they may be omitted on the final lot.

Provided the free formaldehyde content has been determined on the bulk purified antigens or the final bulk and it has been shown that the content in the final lot will not exceed 0.2 g/L, the test for free formaldehyde may be omitted on the final lot.

Osmolality (2.2.35)

The osmolality of the vaccine, reconstituted where applicable, is within the limits approved for the particular preparation.

pH (2.2.3)

The pH of the vaccine, reconstituted if necessary, is within the range approved for the particular product.

Free PRP

Unbound PRP is determined after removal of the conjugate, for example by anion-exchange, size-exclusion or hydrophobic chromatography, ultrafiltration or other validated methods. The amount of free PRP is not greater than that approved for the particular product.

IDENTIFICATION

Where the haemophilus component is presented in a separate container: identification tests A, B and C are carried out using the container containing the diphtheria, tetanus and pertussis components; identification test D is carried out on the container containing the haemophilus component.

A. Diphtheria toxoid is identified by a suitable immunochemical method (2.7.1). The following method, applicable to certain vaccines, is given as an example. Dissolve in the vaccine to be examined sufficient *sodium citrate R* to give a 100 g/L solution. Maintain at 37 °C for about 16 h and centrifuge until a clear supernatant liquid is obtained. The clear supernatant liquid reacts with a suitable diphtheria antitoxin, giving a precipitate.

B. Tetanus toxoid is identified by a suitable immunochemical method (2.7.1). The following method, applicable to certain vaccines, is given as an example. The clear supernatant liquid obtained as described in identification test A reacts with a suitable tetanus antitoxin, giving a precipitate.

C. The pertussis components are identified by a suitable immunochemical method (2.7.1). The following method, applicable to certain vaccines, is given as an example. The clear supernatant liquid obtained as described in identification test A reacts with specific antisera to the pertussis components of the vaccine.

D. The haemophilus component is identified by a suitable immunochemical method (2.7.1) for PRP.

TESTS

Where the product is presented with the haemophilus component in a separate container: the tests for residual pertussis toxin and irreversibility of pertussis toxoid, aluminium, free formaldehyde, antimicrobial preservative and sterility are carried out on the container with the diphtheria, tetanus and pertussis components; the tests for PRP content, water (where applicable), sterility and bacterial endotoxins are carried out on the container with the haemophilus component.

If the haemophilus component is freeze-dried, some tests may be carried out on the freeze-dried product rather than on the bulk conjugate where the freeze-drying process may affect the component to be tested.

Residual pertussis toxin and irreversibility of pertussis toxoid (2.6.33)

The final lot complies with the test.

PRP

Minimum 80 per cent of the amount of PRP stated on the label. PRP is determined either by assay of ribose (2.5.31) or phosphorus (2.5.18), by an immunochemical method (2.7.1) or by anion-exchange liquid chromatography (2.2.29) with pulsed-amperometric detection.

Aluminium (2.5.13)

Maximum 1.25 mg per single human dose, if aluminium hydroxide or hydrated aluminium phosphate is used as the adsorbent.

Free formaldehyde (2.4.18)

Maximum 0.2 g/L.

Antimicrobial preservative

Where applicable, determine the amount of antimicrobial preservative by a suitable chemical method. The content is not less than the minimum amount shown to be effective and is not greater than 115 per cent of the quantity stated on the label.

Water (2.5.12)

Maximum 3.0 per cent for the freeze-dried haemophilus component.

Sterility (2.6.1)

It complies with the test for sterility.

Bacterial endotoxins (2.6.14)

The content is within the limits approved by the competent authority for the haemophilus component of the particular product. If any components of the vaccine prevent the determination of endotoxin, a test for pyrogens is carried out as described under General provisions.

ASSAY

Diphtheria component

Carry out one of the prescribed methods for the assay of diphtheria vaccine (adsorbed) (2.7.6).

The lower confidence limit ($P = 0.95$) of the estimated potency is not less than the minimum potency stated on the label.

Unless otherwise justified and authorised, the minimum potency stated on the label is 30 IU per single human dose.

Tetanus component

Carry out one of the prescribed methods for the assay of tetanus vaccine (adsorbed) (2.7.8).

The lower confidence limit ($P = 0.95$) of the estimated potency is not less than 40 IU per single human dose.

Pertussis component

Carry out one of the prescribed methods for the assay of pertussis vaccine (acellular) (2.7.16).

The capacity of the vaccine to induce antibodies for each included acellular pertussis antigen is not significantly ($P = 0.95$) less than that of the reference vaccine.

LABELLING

The label states:
— the minimum number of International Units of diphtheria and tetanus toxoid per single human dose;
— the names and amounts of the pertussis components per single human dose;
— the number of micrograms of PRP per single human dose;
— the type and nominal amount of carrier protein per single human dose;
— where applicable, that the vaccine is intended for primary vaccination of children and is not necessarily suitable for reinforcing doses or for administration to adults;
— the name and the amount of the adsorbent;
— that the vaccine must be shaken before use;
— that the vaccine is not to be frozen;
— where applicable, that the vaccine contains a pertussis toxin-like protein produced by genetic modification.

—————————————— Ph Eur

Adsorbed Diphtheria, Tetanus, Pertussis (Acellular Component) and Hepatitis B (rDNA) Vaccine

(Diphtheria, Tetanus, Pertussis (Acellular, Component) and Hepatitis B (rDNA) Vaccine (Adsorbed), Ph Eur monograph 1933)

The label may state 'DTaP/HepB'.

Ph Eur —————————————————

DEFINITION

Diphtheria, tetanus, pertussis (acellular, component) and hepatitis B (rDNA) vaccine (adsorbed) is a combined vaccine composed of: diphtheria formol toxoid; tetanus formol toxoid; individually purified antigenic components of *Bordetella pertussis*; hepatitis B surface antigen; a mineral adsorbent such as aluminium hydroxide or hydrated aluminium phosphate.

The formol toxoids are prepared from the toxins produced by the growth of *Corynebacterium diphtheriae* and *Clostridium tetani*, respectively.

The vaccine contains either pertussis toxoid or a pertussis-toxin-like protein free from toxic properties, produced by expression of a genetically modified form of the corresponding gene. Pertussis toxoid is prepared from pertussis toxin by a method that renders the latter harmless while maintaining adequate immunogenic properties and avoiding reversion to toxin. The vaccine may also contain filamentous haemagglutinin, pertactin (a 69 kDa outer-membrane protein) and other defined components of *B. pertussis* such as fimbrial-2 and fimbrial-3 antigens. The latter 2 antigens may be co-purified. The antigenic composition and characteristics are based on evidence of protection and freedom from unexpected reactions in the target group for which the vaccine is intended.

Hepatitis B surface antigen is a component protein of hepatitis B virus; the antigen is obtained by recombinant DNA technology.

PRODUCTION

GENERAL PROVISIONS

The production method shall have been shown to yield consistently vaccines comparable with the vaccine of proven clinical efficacy and safety in man.

Specific toxicity of the diphtheria and tetanus components

The production method is validated to demonstrate that the product, if tested, would comply with the following test: inject subcutaneously 5 times the single human dose stated on the label into each of 5 healthy guinea-pigs, each weighing 250-350 g, that have not previously been treated with any material that will interfere with the test. If within 42 days of the injection any of the animals shows signs of or dies from diphtheria toxaemia or tetanus, the vaccine does not comply with the test. If more than 1 animal dies from non-specific causes, repeat the test once; if more than 1 animal dies in the second test, the vaccine does not comply with the test.

The content of bacterial endotoxins (2.6.14) in the bulk purified diphtheria toxoid, tetanus toxoid and pertussis components is determined to monitor the purification procedure and to limit the amount in the final vaccine. For each component, the content of bacterial endotoxins is less than the limit approved for the particular vaccine.

Reference vaccine(s) Provided valid assays can be performed, monocomponent reference vaccines may be used for the assays on the combined vaccine. If this is not possible because of interaction between the components of the combined vaccine or because of differences in composition between the monocomponent reference vaccine and the test vaccine, a batch of combined vaccine shown to be effective in clinical trials or a batch representative thereof is used as a reference vaccine. For the preparation of a representative batch, strict adherence to the production process used for the batch tested in clinical trials is necessary. The reference vaccine may be stabilised by a method that has been shown to have no effect on the assay procedure.

PRODUCTION OF THE COMPONENTS

The production of the components complies with the requirements of the monographs *Diphtheria vaccine (adsorbed) (0443), Tetanus vaccine (adsorbed) (0452), Pertussis vaccine (acellular, component, adsorbed) (1356)* and *Hepatitis B vaccine (rDNA) (1056)*.

FINAL BULK VACCINE

The final bulk vaccine is prepared by adsorption, separately or together, of suitable quantities of bulk purified diphtheria toxoid, tetanus toxoid, acellular pertussis components and hepatitis B surface antigen onto a mineral carrier such as aluminium hydroxide or hydrated aluminium phosphate. Suitable antimicrobial preservatives may be added.

Only a final bulk vaccine that complies with the following requirements may be used in the preparation of the final lot.

Antimicrobial preservative

Where applicable, determine the amount of antimicrobial preservative by a suitable chemical method. The amount is not less than 85 per cent and not greater than 115 per cent of the intended content.

Sterility (2.6.1)

Carry out the test for sterility using 10 mL for each medium.

FINAL LOT

Only a final lot that is satisfactory with respect to the test for osmolality and with respect to each of the requirements given below under Identification, Tests and Assay may be released for use.

Provided the test for residual pertussis toxin and irreversibility of pertussis toxoid, the test for antimicrobial preservative and the assays for the diphtheria, tetanus and pertussis components have been carried out with satisfactory results on the final bulk vaccine, they may be omitted on the final lot.

Provided the content of free formaldehyde has been determined on the bulk purified antigens or on the final bulk and it has been shown that the content in the final lot will not exceed 0.2 g/L, the test for free formaldehyde may be omitted on the final lot.

If an *in vivo* assay is used for the hepatitis B component, provided it has been carried out with satisfactory results on the final bulk vaccine, it may be omitted on the final lot.

Osmolality (2.2.35)

The osmolality of the vaccine is within the limits approved for the particular preparation.

IDENTIFICATION

A. Diphtheria toxoid is identified by a suitable immunochemical method (2.7.1). The following method, applicable to certain vaccines, is given as an example. Dissolve in the vaccine to be examined sufficient *sodium citrate R* to give a 100 g/L solution. Maintain at 37 °C for about 16 h and centrifuge until a clear supernatant liquid is obtained. The clear supernatant liquid reacts with a suitable diphtheria antitoxin, giving a precipitate.

B. Tetanus toxoid is identified by a suitable immunochemical method (2.7.1). The following method, applicable to certain vaccines, is given as an example. The clear supernatant liquid obtained as described in identification test A reacts with a suitable tetanus antitoxin, giving a precipitate.

C. The pertussis components are identified by a suitable immunochemical method (2.7.1). The following method, applicable to certain vaccines, is given as an example. The clear supernatant liquid obtained as described in identification test A reacts with specific antisera to the pertussis components of the vaccine.

D. The assay or, where applicable, the electrophoretic profile, serves also to identify the hepatitis B component of the vaccine.

TESTS

Residual pertussis toxin and irreversibility of pertussis toxoid (2.6.33)
The final lot complies with the test.

Aluminium (2.5.13)
Maximum 1.25 mg per single human dose, if aluminium hydroxide or hydrated aluminium phosphate is used as the adsorbent.

Free formaldehyde (2.4.18)
Maximum 0.2 g/L.

Antimicrobial preservative
Where applicable, determine the amount of antimicrobial preservative by a suitable chemical method. The content is not less than the minimum amount shown to be effective and is not greater than 115 per cent of the quantity stated on the label.

Sterility (2.6.1)
The vaccine complies with the test for sterility.

Pyrogens (2.6.8)
The vaccine complies with the test for pyrogens. Inject the equivalent of 1 human dose into each rabbit.

ASSAY

Diphtheria component
Carry out one of the prescribed methods for the assay of diphtheria vaccine (adsorbed) (2.7.6).

The lower confidence limit ($P = 0.95$) of the estimated potency is not less than the minimum potency stated on the label.

Unless otherwise justified and authorised, the minimum potency stated on the label is 30 IU per single human dose.

Tetanus component

Carry out one of the prescribed methods for the assay of tetanus vaccine (adsorbed) (*2.7.8*).

The lower confidence limit ($P = 0.95$) of the estimated potency is not less than 40 IU per single human dose.

Pertussis component

Carry out one of the prescribed methods for the assay of pertussis vaccine (acellular) (*2.7.16*).

The capacity of the vaccine to induce antibodies for each included acellular pertussis antigen is not significantly ($P = 0.95$) less than that of the reference vaccine.

Hepatitis B component

The vaccine complies with the assay of hepatitis B vaccine (*2.7.15*).

LABELLING

The label states:

— the minimum number of International Units of diphtheria and tetanus toxoid per single human dose;
— the names and amounts of the pertussis components per single human dose;
— the amount of HBsAg per single human dose;
— the type of cells used for production of the hepatitis B component;
— where applicable, that the vaccine is intended for primary vaccination of children and is not necessarily suitable for reinforcing doses or for administration to adults;
— the name and the amount of the adsorbent;
— that the vaccine must be shaken before use;
— that the vaccine is not to be frozen;
— where applicable, that the vaccine contains a pertussis toxin-like protein produced by genetic modification.

Ph Eur

Adsorbed Diphtheria, Tetanus, Pertussis (Acellular Component) and Inactivated Poliomyelitis Vaccine

(Diphtheria, Tetanus, Pertussis (Acellular, Component) and Poliomyelitis (Inactivated) Vaccine (Adsorbed), Ph Eur monograph 1934)

The label may state 'DTaP/IPV'.

Ph Eur

DEFINITION

Diphtheria, tetanus, pertussis (acellular, component) and poliomyelitis (inactivated) vaccine (adsorbed) is a combined vaccine containing: diphtheria formol toxoid; tetanus formol toxoid; individually purified antigenic components of *Bordetella pertussis*; suitable strains of human poliovirus types 1, 2 and 3 grown in suitable cell cultures and inactivated by a validated method; a mineral adsorbent such as aluminium hydroxide or hydrated aluminium phosphate.

The formol toxoids are prepared from the toxins produced by the growth of *Corynebacterium diphtheriae* and *Clostridium tetani* respectively.

The vaccine contains either pertussis toxoid or a pertussis-toxin-like protein free from toxic properties produced by expression of a genetically modified form of the corresponding gene. Pertussis toxoid is prepared from pertussis toxin by a method that renders the toxin harmless while maintaining adequate immunogenic properties and avoiding reversion to toxin. The vaccine may also contain filamentous haemagglutinin, pertactin (a 69 kDa outer-membrane protein) and other defined components of *B. pertussis* such as fimbrial-2 and fimbrial-3 antigens. The latter 2 antigens may be co-purified. The antigenic composition and characteristics are based on evidence of protection and freedom from unexpected reactions in the target group for which the vaccine is intended.

PRODUCTION

GENERAL PROVISIONS

The production method shall have been shown to yield consistently vaccines comparable with the vaccine of proven clinical efficacy and safety in man.

Specific toxicity of the diphtheria and tetanus components

The production method is validated to demonstrate that the product, if tested, would comply with the following test: inject subcutaneously 5 times the single human dose stated on the label into each of 5 healthy guinea-pigs, each weighing 250-350 g, that have not previously been treated with any material that will interfere with the test. If within 42 days of the injection any of the animals shows signs of or dies from diphtheria toxaemia or tetanus, the vaccine does not comply with the test. If more than 1 animal dies from non-specific causes, repeat the test once; if more than 1 animal dies in the second test, the vaccine does not comply with the test.

The content of bacterial endotoxins (*2.6.14*) in bulk purified diphtheria toxoid, tetanus toxoid, pertussis components and purified, inactivated monovalent poliovirus harvests is determined to monitor the purification procedure and to limit the amount in the final vaccine. For each component, the content of bacterial endotoxins is less than the limit approved for the particular vaccine and, in any case, the contents are such that the final vaccine contains less than 100 IU per single human dose.

Reference vaccine(s)   rovided valid assays can be performed, monocomponent reference vaccines may be used for the assays on the combined vaccine. If this is not possible because of interaction between the components of the combined vaccine or because of differences in composition between the monocomponent reference vaccine and the test vaccine, a batch of combined vaccine shown to be effective in clinical trials or a batch representative thereof is used as a reference vaccine. For the preparation of a representative batch, strict adherence to the production process used for the batch tested in clinical trials is necessary. The reference vaccine may be stabilised by a method that has been shown to have no effect on the assay procedure.

PRODUCTION OF THE COMPONENTS

The production of the components complies with the requirements of the monographs *Diphtheria vaccine (adsorbed) (0443)*, *Tetanus vaccine (adsorbed) (0452)*, *Pertussis vaccine (acellular, component, adsorbed) (1356)* and *Poliomyelitis vaccine (inactivated) (0214)*.

FINAL BULK VACCINE

The final bulk vaccine is prepared by adsorption onto a mineral carrier such as aluminium hydroxide or hydrated aluminium phosphate, separately or together, of suitable quantities of bulk purified diphtheria toxoid, tetanus toxoid, acellular pertussis components and admixture of suitable quantities of purified monovalent harvests of human poliovirus types 1, 2 and 3 or a suitable quantity of a trivalent pool of such purified monovalent harvests. Suitable antimicrobial preservatives may be added.

Only a final bulk vaccine that complies with the following requirements may be used in the preparation of the final lot.

Bovine serum albumin

Determined on the poliomyelitis components by a suitable immunochemical method (2.7.1) after virus harvest and before addition of the adsorbent in the preparation of the final bulk vaccine, the amount of bovine serum albumin is such that the content in the final vaccine will be not more than 50 ng per single human dose.

Antimicrobial preservative

Where applicable, determine the amount of antimicrobial preservative by a suitable chemical method. The amount is not less than 85 per cent and not greater than 115 per cent of the intended content.

Sterility (2.6.1)

Carry out the test for sterility using 10 mL for each medium.

FINAL LOT

Only a final lot that is satisfactory with respect to the test for osmolality and with respect to each of the requirements given below under Identification, Tests and Assay may be released for use.

Provided the test for residual pertussis toxin and irreversibility of pertussis toxoid, the test for antimicrobial preservative and the assays for the diphtheria, tetanus and pertussis components have been carried out with satisfactory results on the final bulk vaccine, they may be omitted on the final lot.

Provided the free formaldehyde content has been determined on the bulk purified antigens or on the final bulk and it has been shown that the content in the final lot will not exceed 0.2 g/L, the test for free formaldehyde may be omitted on the final lot.

Provided that the determination of D-antigen content has been carried out with satisfactory results during preparation of the final bulk before addition of the adsorbent, it may be omitted on the final lot.

Provided that the *in vivo* assay for the poliomyelitis component has been carried out with satisfactory results on the final bulk vaccine, it may be omitted on the final lot.

The *in vivo* assay for the poliomyelitis component may be omitted once it has been demonstrated for a given product and for each poliovirus type that the acceptance criteria for the D-antigen determination are such that it yields the same result as the *in vivo* assay in terms of acceptance or rejection of a batch. This demonstration must include testing of subpotent batches, produced experimentally if necessary, for example by heat treatment or other means of diminishing the immunogenic activity. Where there is a significant change in the manufacturing process of the antigens or their formulation, any impact on the *in vivo* and *in vitro* assays must be evaluated, and the need for revalidation considered.

Osmolality (2.2.35)

The osmolality of the vaccine is within the limits approved for the particular preparation.

IDENTIFICATION

A. Diphtheria toxoid is identified by a suitable immunochemical method (2.7.1). The following method, applicable to certain vaccines, is given as an example. Dissolve in the vaccine to be examined sufficient *sodium citrate R* to give a 100 g/L solution. Maintain at 37 °C for about 16 h and centrifuge until a clear supernatant liquid is obtained. The clear supernatant liquid reacts with a suitable diphtheria antitoxin, giving a precipitate.

B. Tetanus toxoid is identified by a suitable immunochemical method (2.7.1). The following method, applicable to certain vaccines, is given as an example. The clear supernatant liquid obtained as described in identification test A reacts with a suitable tetanus antitoxin, giving a precipitate.

C. The pertussis components are identified by a suitable immunochemical method (2.7.1). The following method, applicable to certain vaccines, is given as an example. The clear supernatant liquid obtained as described in identification test A reacts with specific antisera to the pertussis components of the vaccine.

D. The vaccine is shown to contain human poliovirus types 1, 2 and 3 by a suitable immunochemical method (2.7.1) such as the determination of D-antigen by enzyme-linked immunosorbent assay (ELISA).

TESTS

Residual pertussis toxin and irreversibility of pertussis toxoid (2.6.33)

The final lot complies with the test.

Aluminium (2.5.13)

Maximum 1.25 mg per single human dose if aluminium hydroxide or hydrated aluminium phosphate is used as the adsorbent.

Free formaldehyde (2.4.18)

Maximum 0.2 g/L.

Antimicrobial preservative

Where applicable, determine the amount of antimicrobial preservative by a suitable chemical method. The content is not less than the minimum amount shown to be effective and is not greater than 115 per cent of the quantity stated on the label.

Sterility (2.6.1)

It complies with the test for sterility.

ASSAY

Diphtheria component

Carry out one of the prescribed methods for the assay of diphtheria vaccine (adsorbed) (2.7.6).

The lower confidence limit ($P = 0.95$) of the estimated potency is not less than the minimum potency stated on the label.

Unless otherwise justified and authorised, the minimum potency stated on the label is 30 IU per single human dose.

Tetanus component

Carry out one of the prescribed methods for the assay of tetanus vaccine (adsorbed) (2.7.8).

The lower confidence limit ($P = 0.95$) of the estimated potency is not less than 40 IU per single human dose.

Pertussis component

Carry out one of the prescribed methods for the assay of pertussis vaccine (acellular) (2.7.16).

The capacity of the vaccine to induce antibodies for each included acellular pertussis antigen is not significantly ($P = 0.95$) less than that of the reference vaccine.

Poliomyelitis component

D-antigen content As a measure of consistency of production, determine the D-antigen content for human poliovirus types 1, 2 and 3 by a suitable immunochemical method (2.7.1) following desorption, using a reference preparation calibrated in European Pharmacopoeia Units of D-antigen. For each type, the content, expressed with reference to the amount of D-antigen stated on the label, is within the limits approved for the particular product.

Poliomyelitis vaccine (inactivated) BRP is calibrated in European Pharmacopoeia Units and intended for use in the assay of D-antigen. The European Pharmacopoeia Unit and the International Unit are equivalent.

In vivo test   The vaccine complies with the *in vivo* assay of poliomyelitis vaccine (inactivated) (*2.7.20*).

LABELLING

The label states:
— the minimum number of International Units of diphtheria and tetanus toxoid per single human dose;
— the names and amounts of the pertussis components per single human dose;
— the types of poliovirus contained in the vaccine;
— the nominal amount of poliovirus of each type (1, 2 and 3), expressed in European Pharmacopoeia Units of D-antigen, per single human dose;
— the type of cells used for production of the poliomyelitis component;
— where applicable, that the vaccine is intended for primary vaccination of children and is not necessarily suitable for reinforcing doses or for administration to adults;
— the name and the amount of the adsorbent;
— that the vaccine must be shaken before use;
— that the vaccine is not to be frozen;
— where applicable, that the vaccine contains a pertussis toxin-like protein produced by genetic modification.

Ph Eur

Diphtheria, Tetanus and Poliomyelitis (Inactivated) Vaccine (Adsorbed, Reduced Antigen(s) Content)

(*Ph Eur monograph 2328*)
The label may state 'Td/IPV'.

Ph Eur

DEFINITION

Diphtheria, tetanus and poliomyelitis (inactivated) vaccine (adsorbed, reduced antigen(s) content) is a combined vaccine containing: diphtheria formol toxoid; tetanus formol toxoid; suitable strains of human poliovirus types 1, 2 and 3 grown in suitable cell cultures and inactivated by a validated method; a mineral adsorbent such as aluminium hydroxide or hydrated aluminium phosphate.

The formol toxoids are prepared from the toxins produced by the growth of *Corynebacterium diphtheriae* and *Clostridium tetani* respectively.

The amount of diphtheria toxoid per single human dose is reduced compared to vaccines generally used for primary vaccination; the amount of tetanus toxoid may also be reduced.

PRODUCTION

GENERAL PROVISIONS

The production method shall have been shown to yield consistently vaccines comparable with the vaccine of proven clinical efficacy and safety in man.

Reference vaccine(s)   Provided valid assays can be performed, monocomponent reference vaccines may be used for the assays on the combined vaccine. If this is not possible because of interaction between the components of the

combined vaccine or because of the difference in composition between the monocomponent reference vaccine and the test vaccine, a batch of combined vaccine shown to be effective in clinical trials or a batch representative thereof is used as a reference vaccine. For the preparation of a representative batch, strict adherence to the production process used for the batch tested in clinical trials is necessary. The reference vaccine may be stabilised by a method that has been shown to have no effect on the assay procedure.

Specific toxicity of the diphtheria and tetanus components

The production method is validated to demonstrate that the product, if tested, would comply with the following test: inject subcutaneously 5 times the single human dose stated on the label into each of 5 healthy guinea-pigs, each weighing 250-350 g, that have not previously been treated with any material that will interfere with the test. If within 42 days of the injection any of the animals shows signs of or dies from diphtheria toxaemia or tetanus, the vaccine does not comply with the test. If more than one animal dies from non-specific causes, repeat the test once; if more than one animal dies in the second test, the vaccine does not comply with the test.

The content of bacterial endotoxins (*2.6.14*) in bulk purified diphtheria toxoid, tetanus toxoid and inactivated monovalent poliovirus harvests is determined to monitor the purification procedure and to limit the amount in the final vaccine. For each component, the content of bacterial endotoxins is less than the limit approved for the particular vaccine and, in any case, the contents are such that the final vaccine contains less than 100 IU per single human dose.

PRODUCTION OF THE COMPONENTS

The production of the components complies with the requirements of the monographs on *Diphtheria vaccine (adsorbed) (0443)*, *Tetanus vaccine (adsorbed) (0452)* and *Poliomyelitis vaccine (inactivated) (0214)*.

FINAL BULK VACCINE

The final bulk vaccine is prepared by adsorption onto a mineral carrier such as aluminium hydroxide or hydrated aluminium phosphate, separately or together, of suitable quantities of bulk purified diphtheria toxoid and tetanus toxoid, and an admixture of suitable quantities of purified monovalent harvests of human poliovirus types 1, 2 and 3 or a suitable quantity of a trivalent pool of such purified monovalent harvests. Suitable antimicrobial preservatives may be added.

Only a final bulk vaccine that complies with the following requirements may be used in the preparation of the final lot.

Bovine serum albumin

Determined on the poliomyelitis components by a suitable immunochemical method (*2.7.1*) after virus harvest and before addition of the adsorbent in the preparation of the final bulk vaccine, the amount of bovine serum albumin is such that the content in the final vaccine will be not more than 50 ng per single human dose.

Antimicrobial preservative

Where applicable, determine the amount of antimicrobial preservative by a suitable chemical method. The amount is not less than 85 per cent and not greater than 115 per cent of the intended content.

Sterility (*2.6.1*)

Carry out the test for sterility using 10 mL for each medium.

IMMUNOLOGICAL PRODUCTS

FINAL LOT

The final bulk vaccine is distributed aseptically into sterile, tamper-proof containers. The containers are closed so as to prevent contamination.

Only a final lot that is satisfactory with respect to the test for osmolality and with respect to each of the requirements given below under Identification, Tests and Assay may be released for use.

Provided the test for antimicrobial preservative and the assays for the diphtheria and tetanus components have been carried out with satisfactory results on the final bulk vaccine, they may be omitted on the final lot.

Provided the free formaldehyde content has been determined on the bulk purified antigens or on the final bulk and it has been shown that the content in the final lot will not exceed 0.2 g/L, the test for free formaldehyde may be omitted on the final lot.

Provided the determination of D-antigen content cannot be carried out on the final lot, it is carried out during preparation of the final bulk before addition of the adsorbent.

Provided the *in vivo* assay for the poliomyelitis component has been carried out with satisfactory results on the final bulk vaccine, it may be omitted on the final lot.

The *in vivo* assay for the poliomyelitis component may be omitted once it has been demonstrated for a given vaccine and for each poliovirus type that the acceptance criteria for the D-antigen determination are such that it yields the same result as the *in vivo* assay in terms of acceptance or rejection of a batch. This demonstration must include testing of subpotent batches, produced experimentally if necessary, for example by heat treatment or other means of diminishing the immunogenic activity. Where there is a significant change in the manufacturing process of the antigens or their formulation, any impact on the *in vivo* and *in vitro* assays must be evaluated, and the need for revalidation considered.

Osmolality (*2.2.35*)

The osmolality of the vaccine is within the limits approved for the particular preparation.

IDENTIFICATION

A. Diphtheria toxoid is identified by a suitable immunochemical method (*2.7.1*). The following method, applicable to certain vaccines, is given as an example. Dissolve in the vaccine to be examined sufficient *sodium citrate R* to give a 100 g/L solution. Maintain at 37 °C for about 16 h and centrifuge until a clear supernatant liquid is obtained. The clear supernatant liquid reacts with a suitable diphtheria antitoxin, giving a precipitate. If a satisfactory result is not obtained with a vaccine adsorbed on aluminium hydroxide, carry out the test as follows. Centrifuge 15 mL of the vaccine to be examined and suspend the residue in 5 mL of a freshly prepared mixture of 1 volume of a 56 g/L solution of *sodium edetate R* and 49 volumes of a 90 g/L solution of *disodium hydrogen phosphate R*. Maintain at 37 °C for not less than 6 h and centrifuge. The clear supernatant liquid reacts with a suitable diphtheria antitoxin, giving a precipitate.

B. Tetanus toxoid is identified by a suitable immunochemical method (*2.7.1*). The following method, applicable to certain vaccines, is given as an example. The clear supernatant liquid obtained as described in identification test A reacts with a suitable tetanus antitoxin, giving a precipitate.

C. The vaccine is shown to contain human poliovirus types 1, 2 and 3 by a suitable immunochemical method (*2.7.1*)

such as the determination of D-antigen by enzyme-linked immunosorbent assay (ELISA).

TESTS

Aluminium (*2.5.13*)

Maximum 1.25 mg per single human dose, if aluminium hydroxide or hydrated aluminium phosphate is used as the adsorbent.

Free formaldehyde (*2.4.18*)

Maximum 0.2 g/L.

Antimicrobial preservative

Where applicable, determine the amount of antimicrobial preservative by a suitable chemical method. The content is not less than the minimum amount shown to be effective and is not greater than 115 per cent of the quantity stated on the label.

Sterility (*2.6.1*)

It complies with the test for sterility.

ASSAY

Diphtheria component

Carry out one of the prescribed methods for the assay of diphtheria vaccine (adsorbed) (*2.7.6*).

The lower confidence limit ($P = 0.95$) of the estimated potency is not less than 2 IU per single human dose.

Tetanus component

Carry out one of the prescribed methods for the assay of tetanus vaccine (adsorbed) (*2.7.8*).

The lower confidence limit ($P = 0.95$) of the estimated potency is not less than 20 IU per single human dose.

Poliomyelitis component

D-antigen content   As a measure of consistency of production, determine the D-antigen content for human poliovirus types 1, 2 and 3 by a suitable immunochemical method (*2.7.1*) following desorption, using a reference preparation calibrated in European Pharmacopoeia Units of D-antigen. For each type, the content, expressed with reference to the amount of D-antigen stated on the label, is within the limits approved for the particular product.

Poliomyelitis vaccine (inactivated) BRP is calibrated in European Pharmacopoeia Units and intended for use in the assay of D-antigen. The European Pharmacopoeia Unit and the International Unit are equivalent.

In vivo test. The vaccine complies with the *in vivo* assay of poliomyelitis vaccine (inactivated) (*2.7.20*).

LABELLING

The label states:

— the minimum number of International Units of diphtheria and tetanus toxoid per single human dose;

— the types of poliovirus contained in the vaccine;

— the nominal amount of poliovirus of each type (1, 2 and 3), expressed in European Pharmacopoeia Units of D-antigen, per single human dose;

— the type of cells used for production of the poliomyelitis component;

— the name and the amount of the adsorbent;

— that the vaccine must be shaken before use;

— that the vaccine is not to be frozen.

Ph Eur

Diphtheria, Tetanus, Pertussis (Acellular, Component) and Poliomyelitis (Inactivated) Vaccine (Adsorbed, Reduced Antigen(s) Content)

(*Ph Eur monograph 2329*)

The label may state 'dTaP/IPV'.

Ph Eur _____

DEFINITION

Diphtheria, tetanus, pertussis (acellular, component) and poliomyelitis (inactivated) vaccine (adsorbed, reduced antigen(s) content) is a combined vaccine containing: diphtheria formol toxoid; tetanus formol toxoid; individually purified antigenic components of *Bordetella pertussis*; suitable strains of human poliovirus types 1, 2 and 3 grown in suitable cell cultures and inactivated by a validated method; a mineral adsorbent such as aluminium hydroxide or hydrated aluminium phosphate.

The formol toxoids are prepared from the toxins produced by the growth of *Corynebacterium diphtheriae* and *Clostridium tetani* respectively.

The amount of diphtheria toxoid per single human dose is reduced compared to vaccines generally used for primary vaccination; the amounts of tetanus toxoid and pertussis components may also be reduced.

The vaccine contains either pertussis toxoid or a pertussis-toxin-like protein free from toxic properties produced by expression of a genetically modified form of the corresponding gene. Pertussis toxoid is prepared from pertussis toxin by a method that renders the toxin harmless while maintaining adequate immunogenic properties and avoiding reversion to toxin. The vaccine may also contain filamentous haemagglutinin, pertactin (a 69 kDa outer-membrane protein) and other defined components of *B. pertussis* such as fimbrial-2 and fimbrial-3 antigens. The latter 2 antigens may be co-purified. The antigenic composition and characteristics are based on evidence of protection and freedom from unexpected reactions in the target group for which the vaccine is intended.

PRODUCTION

GENERAL PROVISIONS

The production method shall have been shown to yield consistently vaccines comparable with the vaccine of proven clinical efficacy and safety in man.

Reference vaccine(s) Provided valid assays can be performed, monocomponent reference vaccines may be used for the assays on the combined vaccine. If this is not possible because of interaction between the components of the combined vaccine or because of differences in composition between the monocomponent reference vaccine and the test vaccine, a batch of combined vaccine shown to be effective in clinical trials or a batch representative thereof is used as a reference vaccine. For the preparation of a representative batch, strict adherence to the production process used for the batch tested in clinical trials is necessary. The reference vaccine may be stabilised by a method that has been shown to have no effect on the assay procedure.

Specific toxicity of the diphtheria and tetanus components

The production method is validated to demonstrate that the product, if tested, would comply with the following test: inject subcutaneously 5 times the single human dose stated on the label into each of 5 healthy guinea-pigs, each weighing 250-350 g, that have not previously been treated with any material that will interfere with the test. If within 42 days of the injection any of the animals shows signs of or dies from diphtheria toxaemia or tetanus, the vaccine does not comply with the test. If more than 1 animal dies from non-specific causes, repeat the test once; if more than 1 animal dies in the second test, the vaccine does not comply with the test.

The content of bacterial endotoxins (*2.6.14*) in bulk purified diphtheria toxoid, tetanus toxoid, pertussis components and inactivated monovalent poliovirus harvests is determined to monitor the purification procedure and to limit the amount in the final vaccine. For each component, the content of bacterial endotoxins is less than the limit approved for the particular vaccine and, in any case, the contents are such that the final vaccine contains less than 100 IU per single human dose.

PRODUCTION OF THE COMPONENTS

The production of the components complies with the requirements of the monographs *Diphtheria vaccine (adsorbed) (0443)*, *Tetanus vaccine (adsorbed) (0452)*, *Pertussis vaccine (acellular, component, adsorbed) (1356)* and *Poliomyelitis vaccine (inactivated) (0214)*.

FINAL BULK VACCINE

The final bulk vaccine is prepared by adsorption onto a mineral carrier such as aluminium hydroxide or hydrated aluminium phosphate, separately or together, of suitable quantities of bulk purified diphtheria toxoid, tetanus toxoid and acellular pertussis components, and an admixture of suitable quantities of purified monovalent harvests of human poliovirus types 1, 2 and 3 or a suitable quantity of a trivalent pool of such purified monovalent harvests. Suitable antimicrobial preservatives may be added.

Only a final bulk vaccine that complies with the following requirements may be used in the preparation of the final lot.

Bovine serum albumin

Determined on the poliomyelitis components by a suitable immunochemical method (*2.7.1*) after virus harvest and before addition of the adsorbent in the preparation of the final bulk vaccine, the amount of bovine serum albumin is such that the content in the final vaccine will be not more than 50 ng per single human dose.

Antimicrobial preservative

Where applicable, determine the amount of antimicrobial preservative by a suitable chemical method. The amount is not less than 85 per cent and not greater than 115 per cent of the intended content.

Sterility (*2.6.1*)

Carry out the test for sterility using 10 mL for each medium.

FINAL LOT

The final bulk vaccine is distributed aseptically into sterile, tamper-proof containers. The containers are closed so as to prevent contamination.

Only a final lot that is satisfactory with respect to the test for osmolality and with respect to each of the requirements given below under Identification, Tests and Assay may be released for use.

Provided the test for residual pertussis toxin and irreversibility of pertussis toxoid, the test for antimicrobial preservative and the assays for the diphtheria, tetanus and pertussis components have been carried out with satisfactory results on the final bulk vaccine, they may be omitted on the final lot.

Provided the free formaldehyde content has been determined on the bulk purified antigens or on the final bulk and it has been shown that the content in the final lot will not exceed 0.2 g/L, the test for free formaldehyde may be omitted on the final lot.

Provided the determination of D-antigen content cannot be carried out on the final lot, it is carried out during preparation of the final bulk before addition of the adsorbent.

Provided the *in vivo* assay for the poliomyelitis component has been carried out with satisfactory results on the final bulk vaccine, it may be omitted on the final lot.

The *in vivo* assay for the poliomyelitis component may be omitted once it has been demonstrated for a given vaccine and for each poliovirus type that the acceptance criteria for the D-antigen determination are such that it yields the same result as the *in vivo* assay in terms of acceptance or rejection of a batch. This demonstration must include testing of subpotent batches, produced experimentally if necessary, for example by heat treatment or other means of diminishing the immunogenic activity. Where there is a significant change in the manufacturing process of the antigens or their formulation, any impact on the *in vivo* and *in vitro* assays must be evaluated, and the need for revalidation considered.

Osmolality (*2.2.35*)
The osmolality of the vaccine is within the limits approved for the particular preparation.

IDENTIFICATION

A. Diphtheria toxoid is identified by a suitable immunochemical method (*2.7.1*). The following method, applicable to certain vaccines, is given as an example. Dissolve in the vaccine to be examined sufficient *sodium citrate R* to give a 100 g/L solution. Maintain at 37 °C for about 16 h and centrifuge until a clear supernatant liquid is obtained.
The clear supernatant liquid reacts with a suitable diphtheria antitoxin, giving a precipitate. If a satisfactory result is not obtained with a vaccine adsorbed on aluminium hydroxide, carry out the test as follows. Centrifuge 15 mL of the vaccine to be examined and suspend the residue in 5 mL of a freshly prepared mixture of 1 volume of a 56 g/L solution of *sodium edetate R* and 49 volumes of a 90 g/L solution of *disodium hydrogen phosphate R*. Maintain at 37 °C for not less than 6 h and centrifuge. The clear supernatant liquid reacts with a suitable diphtheria antitoxin, giving a precipitate.

B. Tetanus toxoid is identified by a suitable immunochemical method (*2.7.1*). The following method, applicable to certain vaccines, is given as an example. The clear supernatant liquid obtained as described in identification test A reacts with a suitable tetanus antitoxin, giving a precipitate.

C. The pertussis components are identified by a suitable immunochemical method (*2.7.1*). The following method, applicable to certain vaccines, is given as an example. The clear supernatant liquid obtained as described in identification test A reacts with a specific antisera to the pertussis components of the vaccine.

D. The vaccine is shown to contain human poliovirus types 1, 2 and 3 by a suitable immunochemical method (*2.7.1*) such as the determination of D-antigen by enzyme-linked immunosorbent assay (ELISA).

TESTS

Residual pertussis toxin and irreversibility of pertussis toxoid (*2.6.33*)
The final lot complies with the test.

Aluminium (*2.5.13*)
Maximum 1.25 mg per single human dose, if aluminium hydroxide or hydrated aluminium phosphate is used as the adsorbent.

Free formaldehyde (*2.4.18*)
Maximum 0.2 g/L.

Antimicrobial preservative
Where applicable, determine the amount of antimicrobial preservative by a suitable chemical method. The content is not less than the minimum amount shown to be effective and is not greater than 115 per cent of the quantity stated on the label.

Sterility (*2.6.1*)
It complies with the test for sterility.

ASSAY

Diphtheria component
Carry out one of the prescribed methods for the assay of diphtheria vaccine (adsorbed) (*2.7.6*).

The lower confidence limit ($P = 0.95$) of the estimated potency is not less than 2 IU per single human dose.

Tetanus component
Carry out one of the prescribed methods for the assay of tetanus vaccine (adsorbed) (*2.7.8*).

The lower confidence limit ($P = 0.95$) of the estimated potency is not less than 20 IU per single human dose.

Pertussis component
Carry out one of the prescribed methods for the assay of pertussis vaccine (acellular) (*2.7.16*).

The capacity of the vaccine to induce antibodies for each included acellular pertussis antigen is not significantly ($P = 0.95$) less than that of the reference vaccine.

Poliomyelitis component
D-antigen content As a measure of consistency of production, determine the D-antigen content for human poliovirus types 1, 2 and 3 by a suitable immunochemical method (*2.7.1*) following desorption, using a reference preparation calibrated in European Pharmacopoeia Units of D-antigen. For each type, the content, expressed with reference to the amount of D-antigen stated on the label, is within the limits approved for the particular product. *Poliomyelitis vaccine (inactivated) BRP* is calibrated in European Pharmacopoeia Units and intended for use in the assay of D-antigen. The European Pharmacopoeia Unit and the International Unit are equivalent.

In vivo test The vaccine complies with the *in vivo* assay of poliomyelitis vaccine (inactivated) (*2.7.20*).

LABELLING
The label states:
— the minimum number of International Units of diphtheria and tetanus toxoid per single human dose;
— the names and amounts of the pertussis components per single human dose;
— where applicable, that the vaccine contains a pertussis toxin-like protein produced by genetic modification;
— the types of poliovirus contained in the vaccine;
— the nominal amount of poliovirus of each type (1, 2 and 3), expressed in European Pharmacopoeia Units of D-antigen, per single human dose;
— the type of cells used for production of the poliomyelitis component;
— the name and the amount of the adsorbent;
— that the vaccine must be shaken before use;
— that the vaccine is not to be frozen.

_____ *Ph Eur*

Diphtheria, Tetanus, Pertussis (Acellular, Component), Poliomyelitis (Inactivated) and Haemophilus Type b Conjugate Vaccine (Adsorbed)

(*Ph Eur monograph 2065*)

The label may state 'DTaP/IPV/Hib'.

Ph Eur _____

DEFINITION

Diphtheria, tetanus, pertussis (acellular, component), poliomyelitis (inactivated) and haemophilus type b conjugate vaccine (adsorbed) is a combined vaccine composed of: diphtheria formol toxoid; tetanus formol toxoid; individually purified antigenic components of *Bordetella pertussis*; suitable strains of human poliovirus types 1, 2 and 3 grown in suitable cell cultures and inactivated by a suitable method; polyribosylribitol phosphate (PRP) covalently bound to a carrier protein; a mineral adsorbent such as aluminium hydroxide or hydrated aluminium phosphate. The product is presented either as a pentavalent liquid formulation in the same container, or as a tetravalent liquid formulation with the freeze-dried haemophilus component in a separate container, the contents of which are mixed with the other components immediately before use.

The formol toxoids are prepared from the toxins produced by the growth of *Corynebacterium diphtheriae* and *Clostridium tetani* respectively.

The vaccine contains either pertussis toxoid or a pertussis-toxin-like protein free from toxic properties produced by expression of a genetically modified form of the corresponding gene. Pertussis toxoid is prepared from pertussis toxin by a method that renders the toxin harmless while maintaining adequate immunogenic properties and avoiding reversion to toxin. The acellular pertussis component may also contain filamentous haemagglutinin, pertactin (a 69 kDa outer-membrane protein) and other defined components of *B. pertussis* such as fimbrial-2 and fimbrial-3 antigens. The latter 2 antigens may be co-purified. The antigenic composition and characteristics are based on evidence of protection and freedom from unexpected reactions in the target group for which the vaccine is intended.

PRP is a linear copolymer composed of repeated units of 3-β-D-ribofuranosyl-(1→1)-ribitol-5-phosphate $[(C_{10}H_{19}O_{12}P)_n]$, with a defined molecular size and derived from a suitable strain of Haemophilus influenzae type b. The carrier protein, when conjugated to PRP, is capable of inducing a T-cell-dependent B-cell immune response to the polysaccharide.

PRODUCTION

GENERAL PROVISIONS

The production method shall have been shown to yield consistently vaccines comparable with the vaccine of proven clinical efficacy and safety in man.

Specific toxicity of the diphtheria and tetanus components

The production method is validated to demonstrate that the product, if tested, would comply with the following test: inject subcutaneously 5 times the single human dose stated on the label into each of 5 healthy guinea-pigs, each weighing 250-350 g, that have not previously been treated with any material that will interfere with the test. If within 42 days of the injection any of the animals shows signs of or dies from diphtheria toxaemia or tetanus, the vaccine does not comply with the test. If more than 1 animal dies from non-specific causes, repeat the test once; if more than 1 animal dies in the second test, the vaccine does not comply with the test.

Bacterial endotoxins (*2.6.14*)

The content of bacterial endotoxins in bulk purified diphtheria toxoid, tetanus toxoid, pertussis components, purified, inactivated monovalent poliovirus harvests and bulk PRP conjugate is determined to monitor the purification procedure and to limit the amount in the final vaccine. For each component, the content of bacterial endotoxins is less than the limit approved by the competent authority for the particular vaccine.

Development and consistency studies

During development studies and wherever revalidation is necessary, it shall be demonstrated by tests in animals that the vaccine induces a T-cell-dependent B-cell immune response to PRP.

Where the haemophilus component is presented in a separate container, and as part of consistency studies, the assays of the diphtheria, tetanus, pertussis and poliomyelitis components are carried out on a suitable number of batches of vaccine reconstituted as for use. For subsequent routine control, the assays of these components may be carried out without mixing with the haemophilus component.

Where the haemophilus component is presented in a separate container, the production method is validated to demonstrate that the haemophilus component, if tested, would comply with the test for pyrogens (*2.6.8*), carried out as follows: inject per kilogram of the rabbit's mass a quantity of the vaccine equivalent to: 1 μg of PRP for a vaccine with diphtheria toxoid or CRM 197 diphtheria protein as carrier; 0.1 μg of PRP for a vaccine with tetanus toxoid as carrier; 0.025 μg of PRP for a vaccine with OMP (meningococcal group B outer membrane protein complex) as carrier.

Reference vaccine(s)   Provided valid assays can be performed, monocomponent reference vaccines may be used for the assays on the combined vaccine. If this is not possible because of interaction between the components of the combined vaccine or because of differences in composition between the monocomponent reference vaccine and the test vaccine, a batch of combined vaccine shown to be effective in clinical trials or a batch representative thereof is used as a reference vaccine. For the preparation of a representative batch, strict adherence to the production process used for the batch tested in clinical trials is necessary. The reference vaccine may be stabilised by a method that has been shown to have no effect on the assay procedure.

PRODUCTION OF THE COMPONENTS

The production of the components complies with the requirements of the monographs *Diphtheria vaccine (adsorbed) (0443)*, *Tetanus vaccine (adsorbed) (0452)*, *Pertussis vaccine (acellular, component, adsorbed) (1356)*, *Poliomyelitis vaccine (inactivated) (0214)* and *Haemophilus type b conjugate vaccine (1219)*.

FINAL BULKS

The final tetravalent bulk of the diphtheria, tetanus, pertussis and poliomyelitis components is prepared by adsorption, separately or together, of suitable quantities of bulk purified diphtheria toxoid, bulk purified tetanus toxoid and bulk purified acellular pertussis components onto a mineral carrier such as aluminium hydroxide or hydrated aluminium phosphate, and admixture of suitable quantities of purified, monovalent harvests of human poliovirus types 1, 2 and 3 or a suitable quantity of a trivalent pool of such monovalent harvests. Suitable antimicrobial preservatives may be added.

Where the vaccine is presented with all 5 components in the same container, the final bulk is prepared by addition of a suitable quantity of the haemophilus bulk conjugate to the tetravalent bulk. Where the haemophilus component is presented in a separate container, the final bulk is prepared by dilution of the bulk conjugate with suitable diluents for freeze-drying. A stabiliser may be added.

Only final bulks that comply with the following requirements may be used in the preparation of the final lot.

Bovine serum albumin
Determined on the poliomyelitis components by a suitable immunochemical method (2.7.1) during preparation of the final bulk vaccine, before addition of the adsorbent, the amount of bovine serum albumin is such that the content in the final vaccine will be not more than 50 ng per single human dose.

Antimicrobial preservative
Where applicable, determine the amount of antimicrobial preservative by a suitable chemical method. The amount is not less than 85 per cent and not greater than 115 per cent of the intended content.

Sterility (2.6.1)
Carry out the test for sterility using 10 mL for each medium.

FINAL LOT
Where the haemophilus component is presented in a separate container, the final bulk of the haemophilus component is freeze-dried.

Only a final lot that is satisfactory with respect to the test for osmolality shown below and with respect to each of the requirements given below under Identification, Tests and Assay may be released for use.

Provided that the test for residual pertussis toxin and irreversibility of pertussis toxoid, the test for antimicrobial preservative and the assay have been carried out with satisfactory results on the final bulk vaccine, they may be omitted on the final lot.

Provided that the free formaldehyde content has been determined on the bulk purified antigens and the purified monovalent harvests or the trivalent pool of polioviruses or the final bulk and it has been shown that the content in the final lot will not exceed 0.2 g/L, the test for free formaldehyde may be omitted on the final lot.

If the *in vivo* assay for the poliomyelitis component is used, provided it has been carried out with satisfactory results on the final bulk vaccine, it may be omitted on the final lot.

The *in vivo* assay for the poliomyelitis component may be omitted once it has been demonstrated for a given product and for each poliovirus type that the acceptance criteria for the D-antigen determination are such that it yields the same result as the *in vivo* assay in terms of acceptance or rejection of a batch. This demonstration must include testing of subpotent batches, produced experimentally if necessary, for example by heat treatment or other means of diminishing the immunogenic activity. Where there is a significant change in the manufacturing process of the antigens or their formulation, any impact on the *in vivo* and *in vitro* assays must be evaluated, and the need for revalidation considered.

Osmolality (2.2.35)
The osmolality of the vaccine, reconstituted where applicable, is within the limits approved for the particular preparation.

Free PRP
Where the haemophilus component is presented in liquid formulation, the presence of other components may interfere in the assay and it may not be possible to separate the PRP from the adjuvant. The presence of free PRP may be determined on the bulk conjugate prior to the addition of other components or on the non-adsorbed fraction in the final combination.

Where the haemophilus component is presented in a separate container, a number of methods have been used to separate free PRP from the conjugate, including precipitation, gel filtration, size-exclusion, anion exchange and hydrophobic chromatography, ultrafiltration and ultracentrifugation. The free PRP can then be quantified by a range of techniques, including high-performance anion-exchange chromatography with pulsed amperometric detection (HPAEC-PAD) and immunoassays with anti-PRP antibodies. The amount of free PRP is not greater than that approved for the particular product.

IDENTIFICATION
Identification tests A, B, C and D are carried out using the vial containing the diphtheria, tetanus, pertussis and poliomyelitis components; identification test E is carried out either on the vial containing all 5 components, or on the vial containing the haemophilus component alone.

A. Diphtheria toxoid is identified by a suitable immunochemical method (2.7.1). The following method, applicable to certain vaccines, is given as an example. Dissolve in the vaccine to be examined sufficient *sodium citrate R* to give a 100 g/L solution. Maintain at 37 °C for about 16 h and centrifuge until a clear supernatant liquid is obtained. The clear supernatant liquid reacts with a suitable diphtheria antitoxin, giving a precipitate.

B. Tetanus toxoid is identified by a suitable immunochemical method (2.7.1). The following method, applicable to certain vaccines, is given as an example. The clear supernatant liquid obtained during identification test A reacts with a suitable tetanus antitoxin, giving a precipitate.

C. The pertussis components are identified by a suitable immunochemical method (2.7.1). The following method, applicable to certain vaccines, is given as an example. The clear supernatant liquid obtained during identification test A reacts with specific antisera to the pertussis components of the vaccine.

D. The vaccine is shown to contain human poliovirus types 1, 2 and 3 by a suitable immunochemical method (2.7.1), such as determination of D-antigen by enzyme-linked immunosorbent assay (ELISA).

E. The haemophilus component is identified by a suitable immunochemical method (2.7.1) for PRP.

TESTS
Where the haemophilus component is presented in a separate container, the tests for residual pertussis toxin and irreversibility of pertussis toxoid, aluminium, free formaldehyde, antimicrobial preservative and sterility are carried out on the container with the diphtheria, tetanus, pertussis and poliomyelitis components; the tests for PRP, water, sterility and bacterial endotoxins are carried out on the container with the haemophilus component alone.

Where the haemophilus component is presented in a separate container, some tests may be carried out on the freeze-dried product rather than on the bulk conjugate where the freeze-drying process may affect the component to be tested.

Residual pertussis toxin and irreversibility of pertussis toxoid (*2.6.33*)
The final lot complies with the test.

PRP
Not less than 80 per cent of the amount of PRP stated on the label. PRP is determined either by assay of ribose (*2.5.31*) or phosphorus (*2.5.18*), by an immunochemical method (*2.7.1*) or by anion-exchange liquid chromatography (*2.2.29*) with pulsed-amperometric detection.

Aluminium (*2.5.13*)
Maximum 1.25 mg per single human dose, if aluminium hydroxide or hydrated aluminium phosphate is used as the adsorbent.

Free formaldehyde (*2.4.18*)
Maximum 0.2 g/L.

Antimicrobial preservative
Where applicable, determine the amount of antimicrobial preservative by a suitable chemical method. The content is not less than the minimum amount shown to be effective and is not greater than 115 per cent of the quantity stated on the label.

Water (*2.5.12*)
Maximum 3.0 per cent for the freeze-dried haemophilus component.

Sterility (*2.6.1*)
It complies with the test for sterility.

Bacterial endotoxins (*2.6.14*)
The content is within the limits approved by the competent authority for the haemophilus component of the particular product. If any components of the vaccine prevent the determination of endotoxin, a test for pyrogens is carried out as described under General provisions.

ASSAY

Diphtheria component
Carry out one of the prescribed methods for the assay of diphtheria vaccine (adsorbed) (*2.7.6*).

Unless otherwise justified and authorised, the lower confidence limit (P = 0.95) of the estimated potency is not less than 30 IU per single human dose.

Tetanus component
Carry out one of the prescribed methods for the assay of tetanus vaccine (adsorbed) (*2.7.8*).

The lower confidence limit (*P* = 0.95) of the estimated potency is not less than 40 IU per single human dose.

Pertussis component
Carry out one of the prescribed methods for the assay of pertussis vaccine (acellular) (*2.7.16*).

The capacity of the vaccine to induce antibodies for each included acellular pertussis antigen is not significantly (*P* = 0.95) less than that of the reference vaccine.

Poliomyelitis component
D-antigen content   As a measure of consistency of production, determine the D-antigen content for human poliovirus types 1, 2 and 3 by a suitable immunochemical method (*2.7.1*) following desorption, using a reference preparation calibrated in European Pharmacopoeia Units of D-antigen. For each type, the content, expressed with reference to the amount of D-antigen stated on the label, is within the limits approved for the particular product. *Poliomyelitis vaccine (inactivated) BRP* is calibrated in European Pharmacopoeia Units and intended for use in the assay of D-antigen. The European Pharmacopoeia Unit and the International Unit are equivalent.

In vivo test   The vaccine complies with the *in vivo* assay of poliomyelitis vaccine (inactivated) (*2.7.20*).

LABELLING
The label states:
— the minimum number of International Units of diphtheria and tetanus toxoid per single human dose;
— the names and amounts of the pertussis components per single human dose;
— the nominal amount of poliovirus of each type (1, 2 and 3), expressed in European Pharmacopoeia Units of D-antigen, per single human dose;
— the type of cells used for production of the poliomyelitis component;
— the number of micrograms of PRP per single human dose;
— the type and nominal amount of carrier protein per single human dose;
— where applicable, that the vaccine is intended for primary vaccination of children and is not necessarily suitable for reinforcing doses or for administration to adults;
— the name and the amount of the adsorbent;
— that the vaccine must be shaken before use;
— that the vaccine is not to be frozen;
— where applicable, that the vaccine contains a pertussis-toxin-like protein produced by genetic modification.

————————————————— Ph Eur

Diphtheria, Tetanus, Pertussis (Acellular, Component), Hepatitis B (rDNA), Poliomyelitis (Inactivated) and Haemophilus Type b Conjugate Vaccine (Adsorbed)

(*Ph Eur monograph 2067*)
The label may state 'DTaP/HepB/IPV/Hib'.

Ph Eur ————————————————————————

DEFINITION
Diphtheria, tetanus, pertussis (acellular, component), hepatitis B (rDNA), poliomyelitis (inactivated) and haemophilus type b conjugate vaccine (adsorbed) is a combined vaccine composed of: diphtheria formol toxoid; tetanus formol toxoid; individually purified antigenic components of *Bordetella pertussis*; hepatitis B surface antigen (HBsAg); human poliovirus types 1, 2 and 3 grown in suitable cell cultures and inactivated by a suitable method; polyribosylribitol phosphate (PRP) covalently bound to a carrier protein. The antigens in the vaccine may be adsorbed on a mineral carrier such as aluminium hydroxide or hydrated aluminium phosphate. The product is presented either as a hexavalent liquid formulation in the same container, or as a pentavalent liquid formulation with the haemophilus component in a separate container, the contents of which are mixed with the other components immediately before or during use.

The formol toxoids are prepared from the toxins produced by the growth of *Corynebacterium diphtheriae* and *Clostridium tetani* respectively.

The vaccine contains either pertussis toxoid or a pertussis-toxin-like protein free from toxic properties produced by expression of a genetically modified form of the corresponding gene. Pertussis toxoid is prepared from pertussis toxin by a method that renders the toxin harmless while maintaining adequate immunogenic properties and avoiding reversion to toxin. The acellular pertussis component may also contain filamentous haemagglutinin, pertactin (a 69 kDa outer-membrane protein) and other defined components of *B. pertussis* such as fimbrial-2 and fimbrial-3 antigens. The latter 2 antigens may be co-purified. The antigenic composition and characteristics are based on evidence of protection and freedom from unexpected reactions in the target group for which the vaccine is intended.

Hepatitis B surface antigen is a component protein of hepatitis B virus; the antigen is obtained by recombinant DNA technology.

PRP is a linear copolymer composed of repeated units of 3-β-D-ribofuranosyl-(1→1)-ribitol-5-phosphate $[(C_{10}H_{19}O_{12}P)_n]$, with a defined molecular size and derived from a suitable strain of *Haemophilus influenzae* type b.

The carrier protein, when conjugated to PRP, is capable of inducing a T-cell-dependent B-cell immune response to the polysaccharide.

PRODUCTION

GENERAL PROVISIONS

The production method shall have been shown to yield consistently vaccines comparable with the vaccine of proven clinical efficacy and safety in man.

If the vaccine is presented with the haemophilus component in a separate container, as part of consistency studies the assays of the diphtheria, tetanus, pertussis, hepatitis B and poliomyelitis components are carried out on a suitable number of batches of vaccine reconstituted as for use. For subsequent routine control, the assays of these components may be carried out without mixing with the haemophilus component.

Specific toxicity of the diphtheria and tetanus components

The production method is validated to demonstrate that the product, if tested, would comply with the following test: inject subcutaneously 5 times the single human dose stated on the label into each of 5 healthy guinea-pigs, each weighing 250-350 g, that have not previously been treated with any material that will interfere with the test. If within 42 days of the injection any of the animals shows signs of or dies from diphtheria toxaemia or tetanus, the vaccine does not comply with the test. If more than 1 animal dies from non-specific causes, repeat the test once; if more than 1 animal dies in the second test, the vaccine does not comply with the test.

The content of bacterial endotoxins (*2.6.14*) in bulk purified diphtheria toxoid, tetanus toxoid and pertussis components, hepatitis B surface antigen, purified, inactivated monovalent poliovirus harvests and bulk PRP conjugate is determined to monitor the purification procedure and to limit the amount in the final vaccine. For each component, the content of bacterial endotoxins is not greater than the limit approved.

During development studies and wherever revalidation is necessary, a test for pyrogens in rabbits (*2.6.8*) is carried out by injection of a suitable dose of the final lot. The vaccine is shown to be acceptable with respect to absence of pyrogenic activity.

During development studies and wherever revalidation is necessary, it shall be demonstrated by tests in animals that the vaccine induces a T-cell-dependent B-cell immune response to PRP.

The stability of the final lot and relevant intermediates is evaluated using one or more indicator tests. For the haemophilus component, such tests may include determination of molecular size, determination of free PRP in the conjugate and kinetics of depolymerisation. Taking account of the results of the stability testing, release requirements are set for these indicator tests to ensure that the vaccine will be satisfactory at the end of the period of validity.

Reference vaccine(s)   Provided valid assays can be performed, monocomponent reference vaccines may be used for the assays on the combined vaccine. If this is not possible because of interaction between the components of the combined vaccine or because of differences in composition between the monocomponent reference vaccine and the test vaccine, a batch of combined vaccine shown to be effective in clinical trials or a batch representative thereof is used as a reference vaccine. For the preparation of a representative batch, strict adherence to the production process used for the batch tested in clinical trials is necessary. The reference vaccine may be stabilised by a method that has been shown to have no effect on the assay procedure.

PRODUCTION OF THE COMPONENTS

The production of the components complies with the requirements of the monographs *Diphtheria vaccine (adsorbed) (0443)*, *Tetanus vaccine (adsorbed) (0452)*, *Pertussis vaccine (acellular, component, adsorbed) (1356)*, *Hepatitis B vaccine (rDNA) (1056)*, *Poliomyelitis vaccine (inactivated) (0214)* and *Haemophilus type b conjugate vaccine (1219)*.

FINAL BULKS

Vaccine with all components in the same container   The final bulk is prepared by adsorption, separately or together, of suitable quantities of bulk purified diphtheria toxoid, tetanus toxoid, acellular pertussis components and hepatitis B surface antigen onto a mineral carrier such as aluminium hydroxide or hydrated aluminium phosphate and admixture of a suitable quantity of PRP conjugate and suitable quantities of purified and inactivated, monovalent harvests of human poliovirus types 1, 2 and 3 or a suitable quantity of a trivalent pool of such monovalent harvests. Suitable antimicrobial preservatives may be added.

Vaccine with the haemophilus component in a separate container   The final bulk of diphtheria, tetanus, pertussis, hepatitis B and poliovirus component is prepared by adsorption, separately or together, of suitable quantities of bulk purified diphtheria toxoid, tetanus toxoid, acellular pertussis components and hepatitis B surface antigen onto a mineral carrier such as aluminium hydroxide or hydrated aluminium phosphate and admixture of suitable quantities of purified and inactivated, monovalent harvests of human poliovirus types 1, 2 and 3 or a suitable pool of such monovalent harvests. This final bulk is filled separately. Suitable antimicrobial preservatives may be added. The final bulk of the haemophilus component is prepared by dilution of the bulk conjugate to the final concentration with a suitable diluent. A stabiliser may be added.

Only final bulks that comply with the following requirements may be used in the preparation of the final lot.

Bovine serum albumin

Determined on the poliomyelitis components by a suitable immunochemical method (*2.7.1*) after purification of the harvests and before preparation of the final bulk vaccine, before addition of the adsorbent, the amount of bovine serum albumin is such that the content in the final vaccine will be not more than 50 ng per single human dose.

Antimicrobial preservative

Where applicable, determine the amount of antimicrobial preservative by a suitable chemical method. The amount is not less than 85 per cent and not greater than 115 per cent of the intended content.

Sterility (2.6.1)

Carry out the test for sterility using 10 mL for each medium.

FINAL LOT

Where the haemophilus component is in a separate container, the final bulk of the haemophilus component is freeze-dried. Only a final lot that is satisfactory with respect to the test for osmolality shown below and with respect to each of the requirements given below under Identification, Tests and Assay may be released for use.

Provided that the test for osmolality, the test for residual pertussis toxin and irreversibility of pertussis toxoid, the test for antimicrobial preservative and the assays for the diphtheria, tetanus and pertussis components have been carried out with satisfactory results on the final bulk vaccine, they may be omitted on the final lot.

Provided the free formaldehyde content has been determined on the bulk purified antigens and the purified monovalent harvests or the trivalent pool of polioviruses or the final bulk and it has been shown that the content in the final lot will not exceed 0.2 g/L, the test for free formaldehyde may be omitted on the final lot.

Provided that the test for bovine serum albumin has been carried out with satisfactory results on the trivalent pool of inactivated monovalent harvests of polioviruses or on the final bulk vaccine, it may be omitted on the final lot.

If an *in vivo* assay is used for the hepatitis B component, provided it has been carried out with satisfactory results on the final bulk vaccine, it may be omitted on the final lot.

Provided the *in vivo* assay for the poliomyelitis component has been carried out with satisfactory results on the final bulk vaccine, it may be omitted on the final lot.

The *in vivo* assay for the poliomyelitis component may be omitted once it has been demonstrated for a given product and for each poliovirus type that the acceptance criteria for the D-antigen determination are such that it yields the same result as the *in vivo* assay in terms of acceptance or rejection of a batch. This demonstration must include testing of subpotent batches, produced experimentally if necessary, for example by heat treatment or other means of diminishing the immunogenic activity. Where there is a significant change in the manufacturing process of the antigens or their formulation, any impact on the *in vivo* and *in vitro* assays must be evaluated, and the need for revalidation considered.

Free PRP

For vaccines with all components in the same container, the free PRP content is determined on the non-absorbed fraction. Unbound PRP is determined on the haemophilus component after removal of the conjugate, for example by anion-exchange, size-exclusion or hydrophobic chromatography, ultrafiltration or other validated methods. The amount of free PRP is not greater than that approved for the particular product.

Bacterial endotoxins (2.6.14)

Less than the limit approved for the product concerned.

Osmolality (2.2.35)

The osmolality of the vaccine, reconstituted where applicable, is within the limits approved for the particular preparation.

IDENTIFICATION

If the vaccine is presented with the haemophilus component in a separate container: identification tests A, B, C, D and E are carried out using the container with the diphtheria, tetanus, pertussis, hepatitis B and poliomyelitis components; identification test F is carried out on the container with the haemophilus components.

A. Diphtheria toxoid is identified by a suitable immunochemical method (2.7.1). The following method is given as an example. Dissolve in the vaccine to be examined sufficient *sodium citrate R* to give a 100 g/L solution. Maintain at 37 °C for about 16 h and centrifuge until a clear supernatant liquid is obtained. The clear supernatant liquid reacts with a suitable diphtheria antitoxin, giving a precipitate.

B. Tetanus toxoid is identified by a suitable immunochemical method (2.7.1). The following method is given as an example. The clear supernatant liquid obtained during identification test A reacts with a suitable tetanus antitoxin, giving a precipitate.

C. The clear supernatant liquid obtained during identification test A reacts with specific antisera to the pertussis components of the vaccine when examined by suitable immunochemical methods (2.7.1).

D. The hepatitis B component is identified by a suitable immunochemical method (2.7.1), for example the *in vitro* assay, or by a suitable electrophoretic method (2.2.31).

E. The vaccine is shown to contain human poliovirus types 1, 2 and 3 by a suitable immunochemical method (2.7.1), such as determination of D-antigen by enzyme-linked immunosorbent assay (ELISA).

F. The PRP and its carrier protein are identified by a suitable immunochemical method (2.7.1).

TESTS

If the product is presented with the haemophilus component in a separate container, the tests for residual pertussis toxin and irreversibility of pertussis toxoid, free formaldehyde, aluminium, antimicrobial preservative and sterility are carried out on the container with the diphtheria, tetanus, pertussis, poliomyelitis and hepatitis B components; the tests for PRP, water, antimicrobial preservative (where applicable), aluminium (where applicable) and sterility are carried out on the container with the haemophilus component.

Some tests for the haemophilus component are carried out on the freeze-dried product rather than on the bulk conjugate where the freeze-drying process may affect the component to be tested.

Residual pertussis toxin and irreversibility of pertussis toxoid (2.6.33)

The final lot complies with the test.

PRP

Minimum 80 per cent of the amount of PRP stated on the label, for a vaccine with the haemophilus component in a separate container.

For a vaccine with all components in the same container: the PRP content determined on the non-absorbed fraction is not less than that approved for the product.

PRP is determined either by assay of ribose (2.5.31) or phosphorus (2.5.18), by an immunochemical method (2.7.1) or by anion-exchange liquid chromatography (2.2.29) with pulsed-amperometric detection.

IMMUNOLOGICAL PRODUCTS

Aluminium (*2.5.13*)

Maximum 1.25 mg per single human dose, if aluminium hydroxide or hydrated aluminium phosphate is used as the adsorbent.

Free formaldehyde (*2.4.18*)

Maximum 0.2 g/L of free formaldehyde per single human dose.

Antimicrobial preservative

Where applicable, determine the amount of antimicrobial preservative by a suitable chemical method. The content is not less than the minimum amount shown to be effective and is not greater than 115 per cent of the quantity stated on the label.

Water (*2.5.12*)

Maximum 3.0 per cent for the freeze-dried haemophilus component.

Sterility (*2.6.1*)

It complies with the test for sterility.

ASSAY

Diphtheria component

Carry out one of the prescribed methods for the assay of diphtheria vaccine (adsorbed) (*2.7.6*).

The lower confidence limit ($P = 0.95$) of the estimated potency is not less than the minimum potency stated on the label.

Unless otherwise justified and authorised, the minimum potency stated on the label is 30 IU per single human dose.

Tetanus component

Carry out one of the prescribed methods for the assay of tetanus vaccine (adsorbed) (*2.7.8*).

The lower confidence limit ($P = 0.95$) of the estimated potency is not less than 40 IU per single human dose.

Pertussis component

Carry out one of the prescribed methods for the assay of pertussis vaccine (acellular) (*2.7.16*).

The capacity of the vaccine to induce antibodies for each included acellular pertussis antigen is not significantly ($P = 0.95$) less than that of the reference vaccine.

Hepatitis B component

The vaccine complies with the assay of hepatitis B vaccine (*2.7.15*).

Poliomyelitis component

D-antigen content   As a measure of consistency of production, determine the D-antigen content for human poliovirus types 1, 2 and 3 by a suitable immunochemical method (*2.7.1*) following desorption, using a reference preparation calibrated in European Pharmacopoeia Units of D-antigen. For each type, the content, expressed with reference to the amount of D-antigen stated on the label, is within the limits approved for the particular product.

Poliomyelitis vaccine (inactivated) BRP is calibrated in European Pharmacopoeia Units and intended for use in the assay of D-antigen. The European Pharmacopoeia Unit and the International Unit are equivalent.

In vivo test   The vaccine complies with the *in vivo* assay of poliomyelitis vaccine (inactivated) (*2.7.20*).

LABELLING

The label states:

— the minimum number of International Units of diphtheria and tetanus toxoid per single human dose;

— the names and amounts of the pertussis components per single human dose;

— the amount of HBsAg per single human dose;

— the nominal amount of poliovirus of each type (1, 2 and 3), expressed in European Pharmacopoeia Units of D-antigen, per single human dose;

— the types of cells used for production of the poliomyelitis and the hepatitis B components;

— the number of micrograms of PRP per single human dose;

— the type and nominal amount of carrier protein per single human dose;

— where applicable, that the vaccine is intended for primary vaccination of children and is not necessarily suitable for reinforcing doses or for administration to adults;

— the name and the amount of the adsorbent;

— that the vaccine must be shaken before use;

— that the vaccine is not to be frozen;

— where applicable, that the vaccine contains a pertussis toxin-like protein produced by genetic modification.

————————— Ph Eur

Diphtheria, Tetanus, Pertussis (Whole Cell), Poliomyelitis (Inactivated) and Haemophilus Type b Conjugate Vaccine (Adsorbed)

Diphtheria, Tetanus, Pertussis, Poliomyelitis (Inactivated) and Haemophilus Type b Conjugate Vaccine (Adsorbed)

(Ph Eur monograph 2066)

The label may state 'DTwP/IPV/Hib'.

Ph Eur _____

DEFINITION

Diphtheria, tetanus, pertussis (whole cell), poliomyelitis (inactivated) and haemophilus type b conjugate vaccine (adsorbed) is a combined vaccine composed of: diphtheria formol toxoid; tetanus formol toxoid; an inactivated suspension of *Bordetella pertussis*; suitable strains of human poliovirus types 1, 2 and 3 grown in suitable cell cultures and inactivated by a suitable method; polyribosylribitol phosphate (PRP) covalently bound to a carrier protein; a mineral adsorbent such as aluminium hydroxide or hydrated aluminium phosphate. The product is presented with the haemophilus component in a separate container, the contents of which are mixed with the other components immediately before use.

The formol toxoids are prepared from the toxins produced by the growth of *Corynebacterium diphtheriae* and *Clostridium tetani* respectively.

PRP is a linear copolymer composed of repeated units of 3-β-D-ribofuranosyl-(1→1)-ribitol-5-phosphate $[(C_{10}H_{19}O_{12}P)_n]$, with a defined molecular size and derived from a suitable strain of *Haemophilus influenzae* type b.

The carrier protein, when conjugated to PRP, is capable of inducing a T-cell-dependent B-cell immune response to the polysaccharide.

PRODUCTION

GENERAL PROVISIONS

The production method shall have been shown to yield consistently vaccines comparable with the vaccine of proven clinical efficacy and safety in man.

During development studies and wherever revalidation is necessary, it shall be demonstrated by tests in animals that the vaccine induces a T-cell-dependent B-cell immune response to PRP.

As part of consistency studies the assays of the diphtheria, tetanus, pertussis and poliomyelitis components are carried out on a suitable number of batches of vaccine reconstituted as for use. For subsequent routine control, the assays of these components may be carried out without mixing with the haemophilus component.

For the haemophilus component, the production method is validated to demonstrate that the haemophilus component, if tested, would comply with the test for pyrogens (2.6.8), carried out as follows: inject per kilogram of the rabbit's mass a quantity of the vaccine equivalent to: 1 µg of PRP for a vaccine with diphtheria toxoid or CRM 197 diphtheria protein as carrier; 0.1 µg of PRP for a vaccine with tetanus toxoid as carrier; 0.025 µg of PRP for a vaccine with OMP (meningococcal group B outer membrane protein complex) as carrier.

Reference vaccine(s)   Provided valid assays can be performed, monocomponent reference vaccines may be used for the assays on the combined vaccine. If this is not possible because of interaction between the components of the combined vaccine or because of the difference in composition between monocomponent reference vaccine and the test vaccine, a batch of combined vaccine shown to be effective in clinical trials or a batch representative thereof is used as a reference vaccine. For the preparation of a representative batch, strict adherence to the production process used for the batch tested in clinical trials is necessary. The reference vaccine may be stabilised by a method that has been shown to have no effect on the assay procedure.

Specific toxicity of the diphtheria and tetanus components

The production method is validated to demonstrate that the product, if tested, would comply with the following test: inject subcutaneously 5 times the single human dose stated on the label into each of 5 healthy guinea-pigs, each weighing 250-350 g, that have not previously been treated with any material that will interfere with the test. If within 42 days of the injection any of the animals shows signs of or dies from diphtheria toxaemia or tetanus, the vaccine does not comply with the test. If more than 1 animal dies from non-specific causes, repeat the test once; if more than 1 animal dies in the second test, the vaccine does not comply with the test.

PRODUCTION OF THE COMPONENTS

The production of the components complies with the requirements of the monographs *Diphtheria vaccine (adsorbed) (0443), Tetanus vaccine (adsorbed) (0452), Pertussis vaccine (whole cell, adsorbed) (0161), Poliomyelitis vaccine (inactivated) (0214)* and *Haemophilus type b conjugate vaccine (1219)*.

FINAL BULKS

The final bulk of the diphtheria, tetanus, pertussis and poliomyelitis components is prepared by adsorption, separately or together, of suitable quantities of bulk purified diphtheria toxoid, and bulk purified tetanus toxoid onto a mineral carrier such as aluminium hydroxide or hydrated aluminium phosphate and admixture of suitable quantities of an inactivated suspension of *B. pertussis* and of purified, monovalent harvests of human poliovirus types 1, 2 and 3 or a suitable quantity of a trivalent pool of such monovalent harvests. Suitable antimicrobial preservatives may be added.

The final bulk of the haemophilus component is prepared by dilution of the bulk conjugate to the final concentration with a suitable diluent. A stabiliser may be added.

Only final bulks that comply with the following requirements may be used in the preparation of the final lot.

Bovine serum albumin

Determined on the poliomyelitis components by a suitable immunochemical method (2.7.1) during preparation of the final bulk vaccine, before addition of the adsorbent, the amount of bovine serum albumin is such that the content in the final vaccine will be not more than 50 ng per single human dose.

Antimicrobial preservative

Where applicable, determine the amount of antimicrobial preservative by a suitable chemical method. The amount is not less than 85 per cent and not greater than 115 per cent of the intended content.

Sterility (2.6.1)

Carry out the test for sterility using 10 mL for each medium.

FINAL LOT

The final bulk of the haemophilus component is freeze-dried.

Only a final lot that is satisfactory with respect to the test for osmolality shown below and with respect to each of the requirements given below under Identification, Tests and Assay may be released for use.

Provided the tests for specific toxicity of the pertussis component and antimicrobial preservative, and the assays for the diphtheria, tetanus and pertussis components have been carried out with satisfactory results on the final bulk vaccine, they may be omitted on the final lot.

Provided the free formaldehyde content has been determined on the bulk purified antigens, the inactivated *B. pertussis* suspension and the purified monovalent harvests or the trivalent pool of polioviruses or on the final bulk and it has been shown that the content in the final lot will not exceed 0.2 g/L, the test for free formaldehyde may be omitted on the final lot.

Provided the *in vivo* assay for the poliomyelitis component has been carried out with satisfactory results on the final bulk vaccine, it may be omitted on the final lot.

The *in vivo* assay for the poliomyelitis component may be omitted once it has been demonstrated for a given product and for each poliovirus type that the acceptance criteria for the D-antigen determination are such that it yields the same result as the *in vivo* assay in terms of acceptance or rejection of a batch. This demonstration must include testing of subpotent batches, produced experimentally if necessary, for example by heat treatment or other means of diminishing the immunogenic activity. Where there is a significant change in the manufacturing process of the antigens or their formulation, any impact on the *in vivo* and *in vitro* assays must be evaluated, and the need for revalidation considered.

Osmolality (2.2.35)

The osmolality of the vaccine, reconstituted where applicable, is within the limits approved for the particular preparation.

Free PRP

Unbound PRP is determined on the haemophilus component after removal of the conjugate, for example by anion-exchange, size-exclusion or hydrophobic chromatography, ultrafiltration or other validated methods. The amount of free PRP is not greater than that approved for the particular product.

IMMUNOLOGICAL PRODUCTS

IDENTIFICATION

Identification tests A, B, C and D are carried out using the vial containing the diphtheria, tetanus, pertussis and poliomyelitis components; identification test E is carried out on the vial containing the haemophilus component.

A. Diphtheria toxoid is identified by a suitable immunochemical method (*2.7.1*). The following method, applicable to certain vaccines, is given as an example. Dissolve in the vaccine to be examined sufficient *sodium citrate R* to give a 100 g/L solution. Maintain at 37 °C for about 16 h and centrifuge until a clear supernatant liquid is obtained. The clear supernatant liquid reacts with a suitable diphtheria antitoxin, giving a precipitate.

B. Tetanus toxoid is identified by a suitable immunochemical method (*2.7.1*). The following method, applicable to certain vaccines, is given as an example. The clear supernatant liquid obtained during identification test A reacts with a suitable tetanus antitoxin, giving a precipitate.

C. The centrifugation residue obtained in identification A may be used. Other suitable methods for separating the bacteria from the adsorbent may also be used. Identify pertussis vaccine by agglutination of the bacteria from the resuspended precipitate by antisera specific to *B. pertussis* or by the assay of the pertussis component prescribed under Assay.

D. The vaccine is shown to contain human poliovirus types 1, 2 and 3 by a suitable immunochemical method (*2.7.1*), such as determination of D-antigen by enzyme-linked immunosorbent assay (ELISA).

E. The haemophilus component is identified by a suitable immunochemical method (*2.7.1*) for PRP.

TESTS

The tests for specific toxicity of the pertussis component, aluminium, free formaldehyde, antimicrobial preservative and sterility are carried out on the container with diphtheria, tetanus, pertussis and poliomyelitis components; the tests for PRP, water, sterility and bacterial endotoxins are carried out on the container with the haemophilus component.

Some tests for the haemophilus component may be carried out on the freeze-dried product rather than on the bulk conjugate where the freeze-drying process may affect the component to be tested.

Specific toxicity of the pertussis component

Use not fewer than 5 healthy mice each weighing 14-16 g, for the vaccine group and for the saline control. Use mice of the same sex or distribute males and females equally between the groups. Allow the animals access to food and water for at least 2 h before injection and during the test. Inject each mouse of the vaccine group intraperitoneally with 0.5 mL, containing a quantity of the vaccine equivalent to not less than half the single human dose. Inject each mouse of the control group with 0.5 mL of a 9 g/L sterile solution of *sodium chloride R*, preferably containing the same amount of antimicrobial preservative as that injected with the vaccine. Weigh the groups of mice immediately before the injection and 72 h and 7 days after the injection. The vaccine complies with the test if: (a) at the end of 72 h the total mass of the group of vaccinated mice is not less than that preceding the injection; (b) at the end of 7 days the average increase in mass per vaccinated mouse is not less than 60 per cent of that per control mouse; and (c) not more than 5 per cent of the vaccinated mice die during the test. The test may be repeated and the results of the tests combined.

PRP

Minimum 80 per cent of the amount of PRP stated on the label. PRP is determined either by assay of ribose (*2.5.31*) or phosphorus (*2.5.18*), by an immunochemical method (*2.7.1*) or by anion-exchange liquid chromatography (*2.2.29*) with pulsed-amperometric detection.

Aluminium (*2.5.13*)

Maximum 1.25 mg per single human dose, if aluminium hydroxide or hydrated aluminium phosphate is used as the adsorbent.

Free formaldehyde (*2.4.18*)

Maximum 0.2 g/L.

Antimicrobial preservative

Where applicable, determine the amount of antimicrobial preservative by a suitable chemical method. The content is not less than the minimum amount shown to be effective and is not greater than 115 per cent of the quantity stated on the label.

Water (*2.5.12*)

Maximum 3.0 per cent for the haemophilus component.

Sterility (*2.6.1*)

It complies with the test for sterility.

Bacterial endotoxins (*2.6.14*)

The content is within the limits approved by the competent authority for the haemophilus component of the particular product. If any components of the vaccine prevent the determination of endotoxin, a test for pyrogens is carried out as described under General provisions.

ASSAY

Diphtheria component

Carry out one of the prescribed methods for the assay of diphtheria vaccine (adsorbed) (*2.7.6*).

The lower confidence limit ($P = 0.95$) of the estimated potency is not less than 30 IU per single human dose.

Tetanus component

Carry out one of the prescribed methods for the assay of tetanus vaccine (adsorbed) (*2.7.8*).

If the test is carried out in guinea-pigs, the lower confidence limit ($P = 0.95$) of the estimated potency is not less than 40 IU per single human dose; if the test is carried out in mice, the lower confidence limit ($P = 0.95$) of the estimated potency is not less than 60 IU per single human dose.

Pertussis component

Carry out the assay of pertussis vaccine (whole cell) (*2.7.7*).

The estimated potency is not less than 4.0 IU per single human dose and the lower confidence limit ($P = 0.95$) of the estimated potency is not less than 2.0 IU per single human dose.

Poliomyelitis component

D-antigen content As a measure of consistency of production, determine the D-antigen content for human poliovirus types 1, 2 and 3 by a suitable immunochemical method (*2.7.1*) following desorption using a reference preparation calibrated in European Pharmacopoeia Units of D-antigen. For each type, the content, expressed with reference to the amount of D-antigen stated on the label, is within the limits approved for the particular product. *Poliomyelitis vaccine (inactivated) BRP* is calibrated in European Pharmacopoeia Units and intended for use in the assay of D-antigen. The European Pharmacopoeia Unit and the International Unit are equivalent.

In vivo test The vaccine complies with the *in vivo* assay of poliomyelitis vaccine (inactivated) (*2.7.20*).

LABELLING

The label states:

— the minimum number of International Units of diphtheria and tetanus toxoid per single human dose;

— the minimum number of International Units of pertussis vaccine per single human dose;

— the nominal amount of poliovirus of each type (1, 2 and 3), expressed in European Pharmacopoeia Units of D-antigen, per single human dose;

— the type of cells used for production of the poliomyelitis component;

— the number of micrograms of PRP per single human dose;

— the type and nominal amount of carrier protein per single human dose;

— where applicable, that the vaccine is intended for primary vaccination of children and is not necessarily suitable for reinforcing doses or for administration to adults;

— the name and the amount of the adsorbent;

— that the vaccine must be shaken before use;

— that the vaccine is not to be frozen.

Ph Eur

Diphtheria, Tetanus, Pertussis (Whole Cell) and Poliomyelitis (Inactivated) Vaccine (Adsorbed)

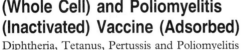

Diphtheria, Tetanus, Pertussis and Poliomyelitis (Inactivated) Vaccine (Adsorbed)

(Ph Eur monograph 2061)

The label may state 'DTwP/IPV'.

Ph Eur

DEFINITION

Diphtheria, tetanus, pertussis (whole cell) and poliomyelitis (inactivated) vaccine (adsorbed) is a combined vaccine containing: diphtheria formol toxoid; tetanus formol toxoid; an inactivated suspension of *Bordetella pertussis*; suitable strains of human poliovirus types 1, 2 and 3 grown in suitable cell cultures and inactivated by a validated method; a mineral adsorbent such as aluminium hydroxide or hydrated aluminium phosphate.

The formol toxoids are prepared from the toxins produced by the growth of *Corynebacterium diphtheriae* and *Clostridium tetani* respectively.

PRODUCTION

GENERAL PROVISIONS

The production method shall have been shown to yield consistently vaccines comparable with the vaccine of proven clinical efficacy and safety in man.

Reference vaccine(s) Provided valid assays can be performed, monocomponent reference vaccines may be used for the assays on the combined vaccine. If this is not possible because of interaction between the components of the combined vaccine or because of the difference in composition between monocomponent reference vaccine and the test vaccine, a batch of combined vaccine shown to be effective in clinical trials or a batch representative thereof is used as a reference vaccine. For the preparation of a representative batch, strict adherence to the production process used for the batch tested in clinical trials is necessary. The reference

vaccine may be stabilised by a method that has been shown to have no effect on the assay procedure.

Specific toxicity of the diphtheria and tetanus components

The production method is validated to demonstrate that the product, if tested, would comply with the following test: inject subcutaneously 5 times the single human dose stated on the label into each of 5 healthy guinea-pigs, each weighing 250-350 g, that have not previously been treated with any material that will interfere with the test. If within 42 days of the injection any of the animals shows signs of or dies from diphtheria toxaemia or tetanus, the vaccine does not comply with the test. If more than 1 animal dies from non-specific causes, repeat the test once; if more than 1 animal dies in the second test, the vaccine does not comply with the test.

PRODUCTION OF THE COMPONENTS

The production of the components complies with the requirements of the monographs *Diphtheria vaccine (adsorbed) (0443)*, *Tetanus vaccine (adsorbed) (0452)*, *Pertussis vaccine (whole cell, adsorbed) (0161)* and *Poliomyelitis vaccine (inactivated) (0214)*.

FINAL BULK VACCINE

The final bulk vaccine is prepared by adsorption onto a mineral carrier such as aluminium hydroxide or hydrated aluminium phosphate, separately or together, of suitable quantities of bulk purified diphtheria toxoid and bulk purified tetanus toxoid and admixture of suitable quantities of an inactivated suspension of *B. pertussis* and purified monovalent harvests of human poliovirus types 1, 2 and 3 or a suitable quantity of a trivalent pool of such purified monovalent harvests. Suitable antimicrobial preservatives may be added.

Only a final bulk vaccine that complies with the following requirements may be used in the preparation of the final lot.

Bovine serum albumin

Determined on the poliomyelitis components by a suitable immunochemical method *(2.7.1)* during preparation of the final bulk vaccine, before addition of the adsorbent, the amount of bovine serum albumin is such that the content in the final vaccine will be not more than 50 ng per single human dose.

Antimicrobial preservative

Where applicable, determine the amount of antimicrobial preservative by a suitable chemical method. The amount is not less than 85 per cent and not greater than 115 per cent of the intended content.

Sterility *(2.6.1)*

Carry out the test for sterility using 10 mL for each medium.

FINAL LOT

Only a final lot that is satisfactory with respect to the test for osmolality and with respect to each of the requirements given below under Identification, Tests and Assay may be released for use.

Provided that the tests for specific toxicity of the pertussis component and antimicrobial preservative, and the assays for the diphtheria, tetanus and pertussis components have been carried out with satisfactory results on the final bulk vaccine, they may be omitted on the final lot.

Provided that the free formaldehyde content has been determined on the bulk purified antigens, the inactivated *B. pertussis* suspension and the purified monovalent harvests or the trivalent pool of polioviruses or on the final bulk and it has been shown that the content in the final lot will not exceed 0.2 g/L, the test for free formaldehyde may be omitted on the final lot.

Provided that the *in vivo* assay for the poliomyelitis component has been carried out with satisfactory results on the final bulk vaccine, it may be omitted on the final lot.

The *in vivo* assay for the poliomyelitis component may be omitted once it has been demonstrated for a given product and for each poliovirus type that the acceptance criteria for the D-antigen determination are such that it yields the same result as the *in vivo* assay in terms of acceptance or rejection of a batch. This demonstration must include testing of subpotent batches, produced experimentally if necessary, for example by heat treatment or other means of diminishing the immunogenic activity. Where there is a significant change in the manufacturing process of the antigens or their formulation, any impact on the *in vivo* and *in vitro* assays must be evaluated, and the need for revalidation considered.

Osmolality (*2.2.35*)
The osmolality of the vaccine is within the limits approved for the particular preparation.

IDENTIFICATION

A. Diphtheria toxoid is identified by a suitable immunochemical method (*2.7.1*). The following method, applicable to certain vaccines, is given as an example. Dissolve in the vaccine to be examined sufficient *sodium citrate R* to give a 100 g/L solution. Maintain at 37 °C for about 16 h and centrifuge until a clear supernatant liquid is obtained. The clear supernatant liquid reacts with a suitable diphtheria antitoxin, giving a precipitate.

B. Tetanus toxoid is identified by a suitable immunochemical method (*2.7.1*). The following method, applicable to certain vaccines, is given as an example. The clear supernatant liquid obtained during identification test A reacts with a suitable tetanus antitoxin, giving a precipitate.

C. The centrifugation residue obtained in identification A may be used. Other suitable methods for separating the bacteria from the adsorbent may also be used.
Identify pertussis vaccine by agglutination of the bacteria from the resuspended precipitate by antisera specific to *B. pertussis* or by the assay of the pertussis component prescribed under Assay.

D. The vaccine is shown to contain human poliovirus types 1, 2 and 3 by a suitable immunochemical method (*2.7.1*) such as the determination of D-antigen by enzyme-linked immunosorbent assay (ELISA).

TESTS

Specific toxicity of the pertussis component
Use not fewer than 5 healthy mice each weighing 14-16 g for the vaccine group and for the saline control. Use mice of the same sex or distribute males and females equally between the groups. Allow the animals access to food and water for at least 2 h before injection and during the test. Inject each mouse of the vaccine group intraperitoneally with 0.5 mL, containing a quantity of the vaccine equivalent to not less than half the single human dose. Inject each mouse of the control group with 0.5 mL of a 9 g/L sterile solution of *sodium chloride R*, preferably containing the same amount of antimicrobial preservative as that injected with the vaccine. Weigh the groups of mice immediately before the injection and 72 h and 7 days after the injection. The vaccine complies with the test if: (a) at the end of 72 h the total mass of the group of vaccinated mice is not less than that preceding the injection; (b) at the end of 7 days the average increase in mass per vaccinated mouse is not less than 60 per cent of that per control mouse; and (c) not more than 5 per cent of the vaccinated mice die during the test.

The test may be repeated and the results of the tests combined.

Aluminium (*2.5.13*)
Maximum 1.25 mg per single human dose, if aluminium hydroxide or hydrated aluminium phosphate is used as the adsorbent.

Free formaldehyde (*2.4.18*)
Maximum 0.2 g/L.

Antimicrobial preservative
Where applicable, determine the amount of antimicrobial preservative by a suitable chemical method. The content is not less than the minimum amount shown to be effective and is not greater than 115 per cent of the quantity stated on the label.

Sterility (*2.6.1*)
It complies with the test for sterility.

ASSAY
Diphtheria component
Carry out one of the prescribed methods for the assay of diphtheria vaccine (adsorbed) (*2.7.6*).

The lower confidence limit ($P = 0.95$) of the estimated potency is not less than 30 IU per single human dose.

Tetanus component
Carry out one of the prescribed methods for the assay of tetanus vaccine (adsorbed) (*2.7.8*).

If the test is carried out in guinea pigs, the lower confidence limit ($P = 0.95$) of the estimated potency is not less than 40 IU per single human dose; if the test is carried out in mice, the lower confidence limit ($P = 0.95$) of the estimated potency is not less than 60 IU per single human dose.

Pertussis component
Carry out the assay of pertussis vaccine (whole cell) (*2.7.7*).

The estimated potency is not less than 4.0 IU per single human dose and the lower confidence limit ($P = 0.95$) of the estimated potency is not less than 2.0 IU per single human dose.

Poliomyelitis component
D-antigen content   As a measure of consistency of production, determine the D-antigen content for human poliovirus types 1, 2 and 3 by a suitable immunochemical method (*2.7.1*) following desorption, using a reference preparation calibrated in European Pharmacopoeia Units of D-antigen. For each type, the content, expressed with reference to the amount of D-antigen stated on the label, is within the limits approved for the particular product.
Poliomyelitis vaccine (inactivated) BRP is calibrated in European Pharmacopoeia Units and intended for use in the assay of D-antigen. The European Pharmacopoeia Unit and the International Unit are equivalent.

In vivo test   The vaccine complies with the in vivo assay of poliomyelitis vaccine (inactivated) (*2.7.20*).

LABELLING
The label states:
— the minimum number of International Units of diphtheria and tetanus toxoid per single human dose;
— the minimum number of International Units of pertussis vaccine per single human dose;
— the nominal amount of poliovirus of each type (1, 2 and 3), expressed in European Pharmacopoeia Units of D-antigen, per single human dose;
— the type of cells used for production of the poliomyelitis component;

— where applicable, that the vaccine is intended for primary vaccination of children and is not necessarily suitable for reinforcing doses or for administration to adults;
— the name and the amount of the adsorbent;
— that the vaccine must be shaken before use;
— that the vaccine is not to be frozen.

Ph Eur

Haemophilus Type b Conjugate Vaccine

(*Ph Eur monograph 1219*)
The label may state 'Hib'.

Ph Eur

DEFINITION
Haemophilus type b conjugate vaccine is a liquid or freeze-dried preparation of a polysaccharide, derived from a suitable strain of *Haemophilus influenzae* type b, covalently bound to a carrier protein. The polysaccharide, polyribosylribitol phosphate, referred to as PRP, is a linear copolymer composed of repeated units of 3-β-D-ribofuranosyl-(1→1)-ribitol-5-phosphate $[(C_{10}H_{19}O_{12}P)_n]$, with a defined molecular size. The carrier protein, when conjugated to PRP, is capable of inducing a T-cell-dependent B-cell immune response to the polysaccharide.

PRODUCTION
GENERAL PROVISIONS
The production method shall have been shown to yield consistently haemophilus type b conjugate vaccines of adequate safety and immunogenicity in man. The production of PRP and of the carrier protein are based on seed-lot systems.

The production method is validated to demonstrate that the product, if tested, would comply with the test for abnormal toxicity for immunosera and vaccines for human use (*2.6.9*) and also with the test for pyrogens (*2.6.8*), carried out as follows: inject per kilogram of the rabbit's mass a quantity of the vaccine equivalent to: 1 µg of PRP for a vaccine with diphtheria toxoid or CRM 197 diphtheria protein as carrier; 0.1 µg of PRP for a vaccine with tetanus toxoid as carrier; 0.025 µg of PRP for a vaccine with OMP (meningococcal group B outer membrane protein complex) as carrier.

During development studies and wherever revalidation of the manufacturing process is necessary, it shall be demonstrated by tests in animals that the vaccine consistently induces a T-cell-dependent B-cell immune response.

The stability of the final lot and relevant intermediates is evaluated using one or more indicator tests. Such tests may include determination of molecular size, determination of free PRP in the conjugate and the immunogenicity test in mice. Taking account of the results of the stability testing, release requirements are set for these indicator tests to ensure that the vaccine will be satisfactory at the end of the period of validity.

BACTERIAL SEED LOTS
The seed lots of *H. influenzae* type b are shown to be free from contamination by methods of suitable sensitivity. These may include inoculation into suitable media, examination of colony morphology, microscopic examination of Gram-stained smears and culture agglutination with suitable specific antisera.

No complex products of animal origin are included in the medium used for preservation of strain viability, either for freeze-drying or for frozen storage.

It is recommended that PRP produced by the seed lot be characterised using nuclear magnetic resonance spectrometry (*2.2.33*).

H. INFLUENZAE TYPE B POLYSACCHARIDE (PRP)
H. influenzae type b is grown in a liquid medium that does not contain high-molecular-mass polysaccharides; if any ingredient of the medium contains blood-group substances, the process shall be validated to demonstrate that after the purification step they are no longer detectable. The bacterial purity of the culture is verified by methods of suitable sensitivity. These may include inoculation into suitable media, examination of colony morphology, microscopic examination of Gram-stained smears and culture agglutination with suitable specific antisera. The culture may be inactivated. PRP is separated from the culture medium and purified by a suitable method. Volatile matter, including water, in the purified polysaccharide is determined by a suitable method; the result is used to calculate the results of certain tests with reference to the dried substance, as prescribed below.

Only PRP that complies with the following requirements may be used in the preparation of the conjugate.

Identification
PRP is identified by an immunochemical method (*2.7.1*) or other suitable method, for example ^{1}H nuclear magnetic resonance spectrometry (*2.2.33*).

Molecular-size distribution
The percentage of PRP eluted before a given K_0 value or within a range of K_0 values is determined by size-exclusion chromatography (*2.2.30*); an acceptable value is established for the particular product and each batch of PRP must be shown to comply with this limit. Limits for currently approved products, using the indicated stationary phases, are shown for information in Table 1219.-1. Where applicable, the molecular-size distribution is also determined after chemical modification of the polysaccharide.

Liquid chromatography (*2.2.29*) with multiple-angle laser light-scattering detection may also be used for determination of molecular-size distribution.

A validated determination of the degree of polymerisation or of the weight-average molecular weight and the dispersion of molecular masses may be used instead of the determination of molecular size distribution.

Ribose (*2.5.31*)
Within the limits approved by the competent authority for the particular product, calculated with reference to the dried substance.

Phosphorus (*2.5.18*)
Within the limits approved by the competent authority for the particular product, calculated with reference to the dried substance.

Protein (*2.5.16*)
Maximum 1.0 per cent, calculated with reference to the dried substance. Use sufficient PRP to allow detection of proteins at concentrations of 1 per cent or greater.

Nucleic acid (*2.5.17*)
Maximum 1.0 per cent, calculated with reference to the dried substance.

Bacterial endotoxins (*2.6.14*)
Less than 10 IU per microgram of PRP.

Table 1219.-1. – *Product characteristics and specifications for PRP and carrier protein in currently approved products*

Carrier			Haemophilus polysaccharide		Conjugation	
Type	Purity	Nominal amount per dose	Type of PRP	Nominal amount per dose	Coupling method	Procedure
Diphtheria toxoid	> 1500 Lf per milligram of nitrogen	18 µg	Size-reduced PRP K_0: 0.6-0.7, using cross-linked agarose for chromatography R	25 µg	cyanogen bromide activation of PRP	activated diphtheria toxoid (D-AH+), cyanogen bromide-activated PRP
Tetanus toxoid	> 1500 Lf per milligram of nitrogen	20 µg	PRP ≥ 50 % ≤ K_0: 0.30, using cross-linked agarose for chromatography R	10 µg	carbodiimide mediated	ADH-activated PRP (PRP-cov.-AH) + tetanus toxoid + EDAC
CRM 197 diphtheria protein	> 90 % of diphtheria protein	25 µg	Size-reduced PRP Dp = 15-35 or 10-35	10 µg	reductive amination (1-step method) or N-hydroxysuccinimide activation	direct coupling of PRP to CRM 197 (cyanoborohydride activated)
Meningococcal group B outer membrane protein (OMP)	outer membrane protein vesicles: ≤ 8 % of lipopolysaccharide	125 µg or 250 µg	Size-reduced PRP K_0 < 0.6, using cross-linked agarose for chromatography R or M_w > 50 × 10^3	7.5 µg or 15 µg	thioether bond	PRP activation by CDI PRP-IM + BuA2 + BrAc = PRP-BuA2-BrAc + thioactivated OMP

ADH = adipic acid dihydrazide	Dp = degree of polymerisation
BrAc = bromoacetyl chloride	EDAC = 1-ethyl-3-(3-dimethylaminopropyl)carbodiimide
BuA2 = butane-1,4-diamide	IM = imidazolium
CDI = carbonyldiimidazole	M_w = weight-average molecular weight

Residual reagents

Where applicable, tests are carried out to determine residues of reagents used during inactivation and purification. An acceptable value for each reagent is established for the particular product and each batch of PRP must be shown to comply with this limit. Where validation studies have demonstrated removal of a residual reagent, the test on PRP may be omitted.

CARRIER PROTEIN

The carrier protein is chosen so that when the PRP is conjugated it is able to induce a T-cell-dependent B-cell immune response. Currently approved carrier proteins and coupling methods are listed for information in Table 1219.-1. The carrier proteins are produced by culture of suitable micro-organisms; the bacterial purity of the culture is verified; the culture may be inactivated; the carrier protein is purified by a suitable method.

Only a carrier protein that complies with the following requirements may be used in the preparation of the conjugate.

Identification

The carrier protein is identified by a suitable immunochemical method (*2.7.1*).

Diphtheria toxoid

Diphtheria toxoid is produced as described in the monograph *Diphtheria vaccine (adsorbed) (0443)* and complies with the requirements prescribed therein for bulk purified toxoid except that the test for sterility (*2.6.1*) is not required.

Tetanus toxoid

Tetanus toxoid is produced as described in the monograph *Tetanus vaccine (adsorbed) (0452)* and complies with the requirements prescribed therein for bulk purified toxoid, except that the antigenic purity is not less than

1500 Lf per milligram of protein nitrogen and that the test for sterility (*2.6.1*) is not required.

Diphtheria protein CRM 197

Minimum 90 per cent, determined by a suitable method. Suitable tests are carried out, for validation or routinely, to demonstrate that the product is non-toxic.

OMP (meningococcal group B outer membrane protein complex)

OMP complies with the following requirements for lipopolysaccharide and pyrogens.

Lipopolysaccharide Maximum 8 per cent of lipopolysaccharide, determined by a suitable method.

Pyrogens (2.6.8) Inject into each rabbit 0.25 µg of OMP per kilogram of body mass.

BULK CONJUGATE

PRP is chemically modified to enable conjugation; it is usually partly depolymerised either before or during this procedure. Reactive functional groups or spacers may be introduced into the carrier protein or PRP prior to conjugation. As a measure of consistency, the extent of derivatisation is monitored. The conjugate is obtained by the covalent binding of PRP and carrier protein. Where applicable, unreacted but potentially reactogenic functional groups are made unreactive by means of capping agents; the conjugate is purified to remove reagents.

Only a bulk conjugate that complies with the following requirements may be used in the preparation of the final bulk vaccine. For each test and for each particular product, limits of acceptance are established and each batch of conjugate must be shown to comply with these limits. Limits applied to currently approved products for some of these tests are listed for information in Table 1219.-2. For a freeze-dried vaccine, some of the tests may be carried out on the final lot rather

Table 1219.-2. – *Bulk conjugate requirements for currently approved products*

Test	Protein carrier			
	Diphtheria toxoid	Tetanus toxoid	CRM 197	OMP
Free PRP	< 37 %	< 20 %	< 25 %	< 15 %
Free protein	< 4 %	< 1 %, where applicable	< 1 % or < 2 %, depending on the coupling method	not applicable
PRP to protein ratio	1.25 - 1.8	0.30 - 0.55	0.3 - 0.7	0.05 - 0.1
Molecular size (K_o):				
cross-linked agarose for chromatography R	95 % < 0.75	60 % < 0.2	50 % 0.3 - 0.6	85 % < 0.3
cross-linked agarose for chromatography R1	0.6 - 0.7	85 % < 0.5		

than on the bulk conjugate where the freeze-drying process may affect the component being tested.

PRP

The PRP content is determined by assay of phosphorus (*2.5.18*) or by assay of ribose (*2.5.31*) or by an immunochemical method (*2.7.1*).

Protein

The protein content is determined by a suitable chemical method (for example, *2.5.16*).

PRP to protein ratio

Determine the ratio by calculation.

Molecular-size distribution

Molecular-size distribution is determined by size-exclusion chromatography (*2.2.30*).

Free PRP

A number of methods have been used to separate free PRP from the conjugate, including precipitation, gel filtration, size-exclusion, anion exchange and hydrophobic chromatography, ultrafiltration and ultracentrifugation. The free PRP can then be quantified by a range of techniques, including high-performance anion-exchange chromatography with pulsed amperometric detection (HPAEC-PAD) and immunoassays with anti-PRP antibodies.

Free carrier protein

Determine the content by a suitable method, either directly or by deriving the content by calculation from the results of other tests. The amount is within the limits approved for the particular product.

Unreacted functional groups

No unreacted functional groups are detectable in the bulk conjugate unless process validation has shown that unreacted functional groups detectable at this stage are removed during the subsequent manufacturing process (for example, owing to short half-life).

Residual reagents

Removal of residual reagents such as cyanide, EDAC (ethyldimethylaminopropylcarbodiimide) and phenol is confirmed by suitable tests or by validation of the process.

Sterility (*2.6.1*)

Carry out the test using for each medium 10 mL or the equivalent of 100 doses, whichever is less.

FINAL BULK VACCINE

An adjuvant, an antimicrobial preservative and a stabiliser may be added to the bulk conjugate before dilution to the final concentration with a suitable diluent.

Only a final bulk vaccine that complies with the following requirements may be used in preparation of the final lot.

Antimicrobial preservative

Where applicable, determine the amount of antimicrobial preservative by a suitable chemical or physico-chemical method. The content is not less than 85 per cent and not greater than 115 per cent of the intended amount.

Sterility (*2.6.1*)

It complies with the test for sterility, carried out using 10 mL for each medium.

FINAL LOT

Only a final lot that is satisfactory with respect to each of the following requirements and the requirements given below under Identification and Tests may be released for use. Provided the test for antimicrobial preservative has been carried out on the final bulk vaccine, it may be omitted on the final lot.

pH (*2.2.3*)

The pH of the vaccine, reconstituted if necessary, is within the range approved for the particular product.

Free PRP

A number of methods have been used to separate free PRP from the conjugate, including precipitation, gel filtration, size-exclusion, anion exchange and hydrophobic chromatography, ultrafiltration and ultracentrifugation. The free PRP can then be quantified by a range of techniques, including HPAEC-PAD and immunoassays with anti-PRP antibodies. The amount of free PRP is not greater than that approved for the particular product.

IDENTIFICATION

The vaccine is identified by a suitable immunochemical method (*2.7.1*) for PRP.

TESTS

PRP

Minimum 80 per cent of the amount of PRP stated on the label. PRP is determined either by assay of ribose (*2.5.31*) or phosphorus (*2.5.18*), by an immunochemical method (*2.7.1*) or by anion-exchange liquid chromatography with pulsed amperometric detection (*2.2.29*).

Aluminium (*2.5.13*)

Maximum 1.25 mg per single human dose, if aluminium hydroxide or hydrated aluminium phosphate is used as the adsorbent.

Antimicrobial preservative

Where applicable, determine the amount of antimicrobial preservative by a suitable chemical or physico-chemical method. The content is not less than the minimum amount shown to be effective and not greater than 115 per cent of the quantity stated on the label.

Water (*2.5.12*)

Maximum 3.0 per cent for freeze-dried vaccines.

IMMUNOLOGICAL PRODUCTS

Sterility (*2.6.1*)
It complies with the test for sterility.

Bacterial endotoxins (*2.6.14*)
The content is within the limits approved by the competent authority for the particular product. If any components of the vaccine prevent the determination of endotoxin, a test for pyrogens is carried out as described under General provisions.

LABELLING

The label states:
— the number of micrograms of PRP per human dose;
— the type and nominal amount of carrier protein per single human dose.

Ph Eur

Haemophilus Type b and Meningococcal Group C Conjugate Vaccine

The label may state 'Hib/MenC'.

DEFINITION

Haemophilus Type b and Meningococcal Group C Conjugate Vaccine is a combined vaccine. It is prepared from purified polysaccharides derived from a suitable strain of *Neisseria meningitidis* group C and from a suitable strain of *Haemophilus influenzae*, type b covalently bound to a carrier protein.

The product is presented as a combined lyophilisate of the haemophilus type b and meningococcal group C components together with the solvent in a separate container. The final product is prepared by mixing the contents of the two containers immediately before use.

PRODUCTION

GENERAL PROVISIONS

The production method shall have been shown to yield consistently vaccines comparable with the vaccine of proven clinical efficacy and safety in man.

The production method is validated to demonstrate that the product, if tested, would comply with the *test for abnormal toxicity for immunosera and vaccines*, Appendix XIV E.
The stability of the final lot and relevant intermediates is evaluated using one or more indicator tests. Such tests may include determination of molecular size, determination of free saccharides in the conjugate or an immunogenicity test in animals. Taking account of the results of the stability testing, release requirements are set for these indicator tests to ensure that the vaccine will be satisfactory at the end of the period of validity.

During development studies and wherever revalidation of the manufacturing process is necessary, it shall be demonstrated by tests in animals that the vaccine consistently induces a T-cell-dependent B-cell immune responses to PRP and to meningococcal group C polysaccharides.

PRODUCTION OF THE COMPONENTS

The production of the vaccine components complies with the requirements of the monographs for Haemophilus Type b Conjugate Vaccine and Meningococcal Group C Conjugate Vaccine.

FINAL BULK VACCINE

A final bulk may be prepared by mixing suitable quantities of the haemophilus and meningococcal C bulk conjugates and dilution to the final concentration with a suitable diluent.

Different methods of preparation may be used. A suitable adjuvant, a suitable antimicrobial preservative and a stabiliser may be added to the components bulk conjugates.

Only a final bulk vaccine that complies with the following requirements may be used in the preparation of the final lot.

Antimicrobial preservative

Where applicable, determine the amount of antimicrobial preservative by a suitable chemical or physico-chemical method. The content is not less than the minimum amount shown to be effective and not greater than 115% of the intended amount.

Sterility

Carry out the *test for sterility*, Appendix XVI A, using 10 mL for each medium.

FINAL LOT

Only a final lot that is satisfactory with respect to each of the requirements given below under Identification and Tests may be released for use. Provided the test for antimicrobial preservative has been carried out on the final bulk vaccine, it may be omitted on the final lot.

Acidity or alkalinity

pH of the reconstituted vaccine is within the range approved by the competent authority for the particular product, Appendix V L.

Free PRP

Unbound PRP is determined after removal of the conjugate, for example by anion-exchange, size-exclusion or hydrophobic chromatography, ultrafiltration or other validated methods. The amount of free PRP is not greater than that approved by the competent authority for the particular product.

Free meningococcal C saccharide

Unbound saccharide is determined after removal of the conjugate, for example by anion-exchange liquid chromatography, size-exclusion or hydrophobic chromatography, ultrafiltration or other validated methods. The amount of free meningococcal C saccharide is not greater than that approved for the particular product.

The vaccine complies with the requirements stated under Vaccines and with the following requirements.

IDENTIFICATION

The haemophilus and menigococcal components are identified by a suitable immunochemical method, Appendix XIV B.

TESTS

PRP

Not less than 80% of the amount of PRP stated on the label. PRP is determined either by assay of ribose or phosphorus, Appendix XV G, by an immunochemical method, Appendix XIV B, or by anion-exchange liquid chromatography, Appendix III D, with pulsed-amperometric detection.

Meningococcal saccharide

Not less than 80% of the amount of meningococcal group C polysaccharide stated on the label. The saccharide content is determined by a suitable validated assay, for example sialic acid assay, Appendix XV G or anion-exchange liquid chromatography, Appendix III D, with pulsed-amperometric detection.

Antimicrobial preservative

Where applicable, determine the amount of antimicrobial preservative by a suitable chemical or physico-chemical method. The content is not less than the minimum amount shown to be effective and not greater than 115% of the quantity stated on the label.

Bacterial endotoxins
Carry out the *test for bacterial endotoxins*, Appendix XVI C. Less than 25 IU per single human dose.

Sterility
Complies with the *test for sterility*, Appendix XVI A.

LABELLING
The label states per human dose: (1) the number of micrograms of PRP; (2) the number of micrograms of meningococcal group C polysaccharide; (3) the type and nominal amount of carrier protein.

Inactivated Hepatitis A Vaccine

(Hepatitis A Vaccine (Inactivated, Adsorbed),
Ph Eur monograph 1107)
The label may state 'HepA'.

Ph Eur _____

DEFINITION
Hepatitis A vaccine (inactivated, adsorbed) is a suspension consisting of a suitable strain of hepatitis A virus grown in cell cultures, inactivated by a validated method and adsorbed on a mineral carrier.

PRODUCTION
GENERAL PROVISIONS
Production of the vaccine is based on a virus seed-lot system and a cell-bank system. The production method shall have been shown to consistently yield vaccines that comply with the requirements for immunogenicity, safety and stability.

The production method is validated to demonstrate that the product, if tested, would comply with the test for abnormal toxicity for immunosera and vaccines for human use (2.6.9).

Unless otherwise justified and authorised, the virus in the final vaccine shall not have undergone more passages from the master seed lot than were used to prepare the vaccine shown in clinical studies to be satisfactory with respect to safety and efficacy.

Reference preparation   A part of a batch shown to be at least as immunogenic in animals as a batch that, in clinical studies in young healthy adults, produced not less than 95 per cent seroconversion, corresponding to a level of neutralising antibody accepted to be protective, after a full-course primary immunisation is used as a reference preparation. An antibody level of 20 mIU/mL determined by enzyme-linked immunosorbent assay is recognised as being protective.

SUBSTRATE FOR VIRUS PROPAGATION
The virus is propagated in a human diploid cell line (5.2.3) or in a continuous cell line approved by the competent authority.

SEED LOTS
The strain of hepatitis A virus used to prepare the master seed lot shall be identified by historical records that include information on the origin of the strain and its subsequent manipulation.

Only a seed lot that complies with the following requirements may be used for virus propagation.

Identification
Each master and working seed lot is identified as hepatitis A virus using specific antibodies.

Virus concentration
The virus concentration of each master and working seed lot is determined to monitor consistency of production.

Extraneous agents
The working seed lot complies with the requirements for seed lots for virus vaccines (2.6.16). In addition, if primary monkey cells have been used for isolation of the strain, measures are taken to ensure that the strain is not contaminated with simian viruses such as simian immunodeficiency virus and filoviruses.

VIRUS PROPAGATION AND HARVEST
All processing of the cell bank and subsequent cell cultures is done under aseptic conditions in an area where no other cells are being handled. Animal serum (but not human serum) may be used in the cell culture media. Serum and trypsin used in the preparation of cell suspensions and media are shown to be free from extraneous agents. The cell culture media may contain a pH indicator, such as phenol red, and antibiotics at the lowest effective concentration. Not less than 500 mL of the cell cultures employed for vaccine production is set aside as uninfected cell cultures (control cells). Multiple harvests from the same production cell culture may be pooled and considered as a single harvest.

Only a single harvest that complies with the following requirements may be used in the preparation of the vaccine. When the determination of the ratio of virus concentration to antigen content has been carried out on a suitable number of single harvests to demonstrate production consistency, it may subsequently be omitted as a routine test.

Identification
The test for antigen content also serves to identify the single harvest.

Bacterial and fungal contamination
The single harvest complies with the test for sterility (2.6.1), carried out using 10 mL for each medium.

Mycoplasmas (2.6.7)
The single harvest complies with the test for mycoplasmas, carried out using 1 mL for each medium.

Control cells
The control cells of the production cell culture comply with a test for identification and the requirements for extraneous agents (2.6.16).

Antigen content
Determine the hepatitis A antigen content by a suitable immunochemical method (2.7.1) to monitor production consistency; the content is within the limits approved for the particular product.

Ratio of virus concentration to antigen content
The consistency of the ratio of the concentration of infectious virus, determined by a suitable cell culture method, to antigen content is established by validation on a suitable number of single harvests.

PURIFICATION AND PURIFIED HARVEST
The harvest, which may be a pool of several single harvests, is purified by validated methods. If continuous cell lines are used for production, the purification process shall have been shown to reduce consistently the level of host-cell DNA.

Only a purified harvest that complies with the following requirements may be used in the preparation of the inactivated harvest.

Virus concentration
The concentration of infectious virus in the purified harvest is determined by a suitable cell culture method to monitor

IMMUNOLOGICAL PRODUCTS

production consistency and as a starting point for monitoring the inactivation curve.

Antigen:total protein ratio

Determine the hepatitis A virus antigen content by a suitable immunochemical method (2.7.1). Determine the total protein by a validated method. The ratio of hepatitis A virus antigen content to total protein content is within the limits approved for the particular product.

Bovine serum albumin

Not more than 50 ng in the equivalent of a single human dose, determined by a suitable immunochemical method (2.7.1). Where appropriate in view of the manufacturing process, other suitable protein markers may be used to demonstrate effective purification.

Residual host-cell DNA

If a continuous cell line is used for virus propagation, the content of residual host-cell DNA, determined using a suitable method, is not greater than 100 pg in the equivalent of a single human dose.

Residual chemicals

If chemical substances are used during the purification process, tests for these substances are carried out on the purified harvest (or on the inactivated harvest), unless validation of the process has demonstrated total clearance. The concentration must not exceed the limits approved for the particular product.

INACTIVATION AND INACTIVATED HARVEST

Several purified harvests may be pooled before inactivation. In order to avoid interference with the inactivation process, virus aggregation must be prevented or aggregates must be removed immediately before and/or during the inactivation process. The virus suspension is inactivated by a validated method; the method shall have been shown to be consistently capable of inactivating hepatitis A virus without destroying the antigenic and immunogenic activity; for each inactivation procedure, an inactivation curve is plotted representing residual live virus concentration measured at not fewer than 3 points in time (for example, on days 0, 1 and 2 of the inactivation process). If formaldehyde is used for inactivation, the presence of excess free formaldehyde is verified at the end of the inactivation process.

Only an inactivated harvest that complies with the following requirements may be used in the preparation of the final bulk vaccine.

Inactivation

Carry out an amplification test for residual infectious hepatitis A virus by inoculating a quantity of the inactivated harvest equivalent to 5 per cent of the batch or, if the harvest contains the equivalent of 30 000 doses or more, not less than 1500 doses of vaccine into cell cultures of the same type as those used for production of the vaccine; incubate for a total of not less than 70 days making not fewer than one passage of cells within that period. At the end of the incubation period, carry out a test of suitable sensitivity for residual infectious virus. No evidence of hepatitis A virus multiplication is found in the samples taken at the end of the inactivation process. Use infectious virus inocula concurrently as positive controls to demonstrate cellular susceptibility and absence of interference.

Sterility (2.6.1)

The inactivated viral harvest complies with the test for sterility, carried out using 10 mL for each medium.

Bacterial endotoxins (2.6.14)

Less than 2 IU in the equivalent of a single human dose.

Antigen content

Determine the hepatitis A virus antigen content by a suitable immunochemical method (2.7.1).

Residual chemicals

See under Purification and purified harvest.

FINAL BULK VACCINE

The final bulk vaccine is prepared from one or more inactivated harvests. Approved adjuvants, stabilisers and antimicrobial preservatives may be added.

Only a final bulk vaccine that complies with the following requirements may be used in the preparation of the final lot.

Sterility (2.6.1)

The final bulk vaccine complies with the test for sterility, carried out using 10 mL for each medium.

Antimicrobial preservative

Where applicable, determine the amount of antimicrobial preservative by a suitable chemical or physico-chemical method. The amount is not less than 85 per cent and not greater than 115 per cent of the intended amount.

FINAL LOT

The final bulk vaccine is distributed aseptically into sterile containers. The containers are then closed so as to avoid contamination.

Only a final lot that complies with each of the requirements given below under Identification, Tests and Assay may be released for use. Provided that the tests for free formaldehyde (where applicable) and antimicrobial preservative content (where applicable) have been carried out on the final bulk vaccine with satisfactory results, these tests may be omitted on the final lot. If the assay is carried out using mice or other animals, then provided it has been carried out with satisfactory results on the final bulk vaccine, it may be omitted on the final lot.

IDENTIFICATION

The vaccine is shown to contain hepatitis A virus antigen by a suitable immunochemical method (2.7.1) using specific antibodies or by the in vivo assay (2.7.14).

TESTS

Aluminium (2.5.13)

Maximum 1.25 mg per single human dose, if aluminium hydroxide or hydrated aluminium phosphate is used as the adsorbent.

Free formaldehyde (2.4.18)

Maximum 0.2 g/L.

Antimicrobial preservative

Where applicable, determine the amount of antimicrobial preservative by a suitable chemical or physico-chemical method. The amount is not less than the minimum amount shown to be effective and is not greater than 115 per cent of that stated on the label.

Sterility (2.6.1)

The vaccine complies with the test for sterility.

ASSAY

The vaccine complies with the assay of hepatitis A vaccine (2.7.14).

LABELLING

The label states the biological origin of the cells used for the preparation of the vaccine.

Ph Eur

Hepatitis A Vaccine (Inactivated, Virosome)

(*Ph Eur monograph 1935*)

The label may state 'HepA'.

Ph Eur _____

DEFINITION

Hepatitis A vaccine (inactivated, virosome) is a suspension of a suitable strain of hepatitis A virus grown in cell cultures and inactivated by a validated method. Virosomes composed of influenza proteins of a strain approved for the particular product and phospholipids are used as adjuvants.

PRODUCTION

GENERAL PROVISIONS

The production method shall have been shown to yield consistently vaccines comparable with the vaccine of proven clinical efficacy and safety in man.

The production method is validated to demonstrate that the product, if tested, would comply with the test for abnormal toxicity for immunosera and vaccines for human use (*2.6.9*).

Reference preparation A reference preparation of inactivated hepatitis A antigen is calibrated against a batch of hepatitis A vaccine (inactivated, virosome) that, in clinical studies in young healthy adults, produced not less than 95 per cent seroconversion, corresponding to a level of neutralising antibody accepted to be protective, after a full-course primary immunisation. An antibody level not less than 20 mIU/mL determined by enzyme-linked immunosorbent assay is recognised as being protective.

PREPARATION OF HEPATITIS A ANTIGEN

Production of the hepatitis A antigen is based on a virus seed-lot system and a cell-bank system. The production method shall have been shown to consistently yield vaccines that comply with the requirements for immunogenicity, safety and stability.

Unless otherwise justified and authorised, the virus in the final vaccine shall not have undergone more passages from the master seed lot than were used to prepare the vaccine shown in clinical studies to be satisfactory with respect to safety and efficacy.

SUBSTRATE FOR PROPAGATION OF HEPATITIS A VIRUS

The virus is propagated in a human diploid cell line (*5.2.3*).

SEED LOTS OF HEPATITIS A VIRUS

The strain of hepatitis A virus used to prepare the master seed lot shall be identified by historical records that include information on the origin of the strain and its subsequent manipulation.

Only a seed lot that complies with the following requirements may be used for virus propagation.

Identification

Each master and working seed lot is identified as hepatitis A virus using specific antibodies.

Virus concentration

The virus concentration of each master and working seed lot is determined to monitor consistency of production.

Extraneous agents

The working seed lot complies with the requirements for seed lots for virus vaccines (*2.6.16*).

PROPAGATION AND HARVEST OF HEPATITIS A VIRUS

All processing of the cell bank and subsequent cell cultures is done under aseptic conditions in an area where no other cells are handled. Animal serum (but not human serum) may be used in the cell culture media. Serum and trypsin used in the preparation of cell suspensions and media are shown to be free from extraneous agents. The cell culture media may contain a pH indicator such as phenol red and antibiotics at the lowest effective concentration. Not less than 500 mL of the cell cultures employed for vaccine production is set aside as uninfected cell cultures (control cells). Multiple harvests from the same production cell culture may be pooled and considered as a single harvest.

Only a single harvest that complies with the following requirements may be used in the preparation of the vaccine. When the determination of the ratio of virus concentration to antigen content has been carried out on a suitable number of single harvests to demonstrate consistency, it may subsequently be omitted as a routine test.

Identification

The test for antigen content also serves to identify the single harvest.

Bacterial and fungal contamination

The single harvest complies with the test for sterility (*2.6.1*), carried out using 10 mL for each medium.

Mycoplasmas (*2.6.7*)

The single harvest complies with the test for mycoplasmas.

Control cells

The control cells of the production cell culture comply with a test for identity and the requirements for extraneous agents (*2.6.16*).

Antigen content

Determine the hepatitis A antigen content by a suitable immunochemical method (*2.7.1*) to monitor production consistency; the content is within the limits approved for the particular product.

Ratio of virus concentration to antigen content

The consistency of the ratio of the concentration of infectious virus, as determined by a suitable cell culture method, to antigen content is established by validation on a suitable number of single harvests.

PURIFICATION AND PURIFIED HARVEST OF HEPATITIS A VIRUS

The harvest, which may be a pool of several single harvests, is purified by validated methods. If continuous cell lines are used for production, the purification process shall have been shown to reduce consistently the level of host-cell DNA.

Only a purified harvest that complies with the following requirements may be used in the preparation of the inactivated harvest.

Virus concentration

The concentration of infective virus in the purified harvest is determined by a suitable cell culture method to monitor production consistency and as a starting point for monitoring the inactivation curve.

Ratio of antigen to total protein

Determine the hepatitis A virus antigen content by a suitable immunochemical method (*2.7.1*). Determine the total protein by a validated method. The ratio of hepatitis A virus antigen content to total protein content is within the limits approved for the particular product.

Bovine serum albumin

Maximum 50 ng per single human dose if foetal bovine serum is used, determined by a suitable immunochemical method (*2.7.1*). Where appropriate in view of the manufacturing process, other suitable protein markers may be used to demonstrate effective purification.

Residual chemicals

If chemical substances are used during the purification process, tests for these substances are carried out on the purified harvest (or on the inactivated harvest), unless validation of the process has demonstrated total clearance. The concentration must not exceed the limits approved for the particular product.

INACTIVATION AND INACTIVATED HARVEST OF HEPATITIS A VIRUS

Several purified harvests may be pooled before inactivation. In order to avoid interference with the inactivation process, virus aggregation must be prevented or aggregates must be removed immediately before and/or during the inactivation process. The virus suspension is inactivated by a validated method; the method shall have been shown to be consistently capable of inactivating hepatitis A virus without destroying the antigenic and immunogenic activity; for each inactivation procedure, an inactivation curve is plotted representing residual live virus concentration measured on at least 3 occasions (for example, on days 0, 1 and 2 of the inactivation process). If formaldehyde is used for inactivation, the presence of excess free formaldehyde is verified at the end of the inactivation process.

Only an inactivated harvest that complies with the following requirements may be used in the preparation of the final bulk vaccine.

Inactivation

Carry out an amplification test for residual infectious hepatitis A virus by inoculating a quantity of the inactivated harvest equivalent to 5 per cent of the batch or, if the harvest contains the equivalent of 30 000 doses or more, not less than 1500 doses of vaccine into cell cultures of the same type as those used for production of the vaccine; incubate for a total of not less than 70 days making not fewer than 1 passage of cells within that period. At the end of the incubation period, carry out a test of suitable sensitivity for residual infectious virus. No evidence of hepatitis A virus multiplication is found in the samples taken at the end of the inactivation process. Use infective virus inocula concurrently as positive controls to demonstrate cellular susceptibility and absence of interference.

Sterility (2.6.1)

The inactivated viral harvest complies with the test for sterility, carried out using 10 mL for each medium.

Bacterial endotoxins (2.6.14)

Less than 2 IU of endotoxin in the equivalent of a single human dose.

Antigen content

Determine the hepatitis A virus antigen content by a suitable immunochemical method (2.7.1).

Residual chemicals

See under Purification and purified harvest.

PREPARATION OF INACTIVATED INFLUENZA VIRUS

The production of influenza viruses is based on a seed-lot system. Working seed lots represent not more than 15 passages from the approved reassorted virus or the approved virus isolate. The final production represents 1 passage from the working seed lot. The strain of influenza virus to be used is approved by the competent authority.

SUBSTRATE FOR PROPAGATION OF INFLUENZA VIRUS

Influenza virus seed to be used in the production of vaccine is propagated in fertilised eggs from chicken flocks free from specified pathogens (5.2.2) or in suitable cell cultures (5.2.4), such as chick-embryo fibroblasts or chick kidney cells obtained from chicken flocks free from specified pathogens (5.2.2). For production, the virus is grown in the allantoic cavity of fertilised hens' eggs from healthy flocks.

SEED LOTS OF INFLUENZA VIRUS

The haemagglutinin and neuraminidase antigens of each seed lot are identified as originating from the correct strain of influenza virus by suitable methods.

Only a working virus seed lot that complies with the following requirements may be used in the preparation of the monovalent pooled harvest.

Bacterial and fungal contamination

Carry out the test for sterility (2.6.1), using 10 mL for each medium.

Mycoplasmas (2.6.7)

Carry out the test for mycoplasmas, using 10 mL.

PROPAGATION AND HARVEST OF INFLUENZA VIRUS

An antimicrobial agent may be added to the inoculum. After incubation at a controlled temperature, the allantoic fluids are harvested and combined to form the monovalent pooled harvest. An antimicrobial agent may be added at the time of harvest. At no stage in the production is penicillin or streptomycin used.

POOLED HARVEST OF INFLUENZA VIRUS

To limit the possibility of contamination, inactivation is initiated as soon as possible after preparation. The virus is inactivated by a method that has been demonstrated on 3 consecutive batches to be consistently effective for the manufacturer. The inactivation process shall have been shown to be capable of inactivating the influenza virus without destroying antigenicity of haemagglutinin.

The inactivation process shall also have been shown to be capable of inactivating avian leucosis viruses and mycoplasmas. If the monovalent pooled harvest is stored after inactivation, it is held at a temperature of 5 ± 3 °C. If formaldehyde solution is used, the concentration does not exceed 0.2 g/L of CH_2O at any time during inactivation; if betapropiolactone is used, the concentration does not exceed 0.1 per cent V/V at any time during inactivation.

Only a pooled harvest that complies with the following requirements may be used in the preparation of the virosomes.

Haemagglutinin antigen

Determine the content of haemagglutinin antigen by an immunodiffusion test (2.7.1), by comparison with a haemagglutinin antigen reference preparation or with an antigen preparation calibrated against it. Carry out the test at 20-25 °C.

Sterility (2.6.1)

Carry out the test for sterility, using 10 mL for each medium.

Viral inactivation

Inoculate 0.2 mL of the harvest into the allantoic cavity of each of 10 fertilised eggs and incubate at 33-37 °C for 3 days. The test is not valid unless at least 8 of the 10 embryos survive. Harvest 0.5 mL of the allantoic fluid from each surviving embryo and pool the fluids. Inoculate 0.2 mL of the pooled fluid into a further 10 fertilised eggs and incubate at 33-37 °C for 3 days. The test is not valid unless at least 8 of the 10 embryos survive. Harvest about 0.1 mL of the allantoic fluid from each surviving embryo and examine each individual harvest by a haemagglutination test. If haemagglutination is found for any of the fluids, carry out for that fluid a further passage in eggs and test for haemagglutination; no haemagglutination occurs.

IMMUNOLOGICAL PRODUCTS

Ovalbumin

Maximum 1 μg of ovalbumin in the equivalent of 1 human dose, determined by a suitable technique using a suitable reference preparation of ovalbumin.

Antimicrobial preservative

Where applicable, determine the amount of antimicrobial preservative by a suitable chemical method. The content is not less than 85 per cent and not greater than 115 per cent of the intended amount.

Residual chemicals

Tests are carried out on the monovalent pooled harvest for the chemicals used for inactivation, the limits being approved by the competent authority.

PREPARATION OF VIROSOMES

Inactivated influenza virions are solubilised using a suitable detergent and are purified by high-speed centrifugation in order to obtain supernatants containing mainly influenza antigens. After the addition of suitable phospholipids, virosomes are formed by removal of the detergent either by adsorption chromatography or another suitable technique.

Only virosomes that comply with the following requirements may be used in the preparation of the final bulk vaccine.

Haemagglutinin content

Determine the content of haemagglutinin antigen by an immunodiffusion test (*2.7.1*), by comparison with a haemagglutinin antigen reference preparation or with an antigen preparation calibrated against it.

Phospholipids

The content and identity of the phospholipids are determined by suitable immunochemical or physico-chemical methods.

Ratio of phospholipid to haemagglutinin

The ratio of phospholipid content to haemagglutinin content is within the limits approved for the particular product.

Residual chemicals

Tests are carried out for the chemicals used during the process. The concentration of each residual chemical is within the limits approved for the particular product.

FINAL BULK VACCINE

The bulk vaccine is prepared by adding virosomes to inactivated hepatitis A viruses to yield an approved hepatitis A antigen:haemagglutinin ratio. Several bulks may be pooled, and approved stabilisers and antimicrobial preservatives may be added.

Only a final bulk vaccine that complies with the following requirements may be used in the preparation of the final lot.

Protein content

The amount of protein is determined using a suitable technique, the limits being approved by the competent authority.

Phospholipids

The content and identity of the phospholipids are determined by suitable immunochemical or physico-chemical methods. The amount of phospholipids complies with the limits approved for the particular product.

Haemagglutinin content

Determine the content of haemagglutinin antigen by an immunodiffusion test (*2.7.1*). The amount of haemagglutinin must not exceed the limits approved for the particular product.

Hepatitis A antigen content

Determine the hepatitis A antigen content by a suitable immunochemical method. The amount of antigen must not exceed the limits approved for the particular product.

Ratio of hepatitis A antigen to haemagglutinin

The ratio of hepatitis A antigen content to haemagglutinin content is within the limits approved for the particular product.

Ovalbumin

Maximum 1 μg of ovalbumin per human dose, determined by a suitable technique using a suitable reference preparation of ovalbumin.

Virosome size

The size distribution of the virosome-hepatitis A virus mixture is within the limits approved for the particular product.

Sterility (*2.6.1*)

The final bulk vaccine complies with the test for sterility, carried out using 10 mL for each medium.

Antimicrobial preservative

Where applicable, determine the amount of antimicrobial preservative by a suitable chemical or physico-chemical method. The amount is not less than 85 per cent and not greater than 115 per cent of the intended amount.

Residual chemicals

If chemical substances are used during the formulation process, tests for these substances are carried out, the limits being approved by the competent authorithy.

FINAL LOT

The final bulk vaccine is distributed aseptically into sterile containers. The containers are then closed so as to avoid contamination.

Only a final lot that complies with each of the requirements given below under Identification, Tests and Assay may be released for use. Provided that the tests for free formaldehyde (where applicable) and antimicrobial preservative content (where applicable) have been carried out on the final bulk vaccine with satisfactory results, these tests may be omitted on the final lot. If the assay is carried out *in vivo*, provided it has been carried out with satisfactory results on the final bulk vaccine, it may be omitted on the final lot.

IDENTIFICATION

The vaccine is shown to contain hepatitis A virus antigen by a suitable immunochemical method (*2.7.1*) using specific antibodies.

TESTS

Free formaldehyde (*2.4.18*)

Maximum 0.2 g/L.

Antimicrobial preservative

Where applicable, determine the amount of antimicrobial preservative by a suitable chemical or physico-chemical method. The amount is not less than the minimum amount shown to be effective and is not greater than 115 per cent of that stated on the label.

Sterility (*2.6.1*)

The vaccine complies with the test for sterility.

Bacterial endotoxins (*2.6.14*)

Less than 2 IU of endotoxin per human dose.

ASSAY

Determine the antigen content of the vaccine using a suitable immunochemical method (*2.7.1*) by comparison with the reference preparation. The acceptance criteria are approved for a given reference preparation by the competent authority.

LABELLING

The label states:

IMMUNOLOGICAL PRODUCTS

— the biological origin of the cells used for the preparation of the vaccine,
— that the carrier contains influenza proteins prepared in eggs,
— that the vaccine is not to be frozen,
— that the vaccine is to be shaken before use.

Ph Eur

Hepatitis A (Inactivated, Adsorbed) and Typhoid Polysaccharide Vaccine

(Ph Eur monograph 2597)

The label may state 'HepA/Typhoid'

Ph Eur

DEFINITION

Hepatitis A (inactivated, adsorbed) and typhoid polysaccharide vaccine is a suspension consisting of a suitable strain of hepatitis A virus, grown in cell cultures and inactivated by a validated method, and of purified Vi capsular polysaccharide obtained from *Salmonella typhi* Ty 2 strain or some other suitable strain that has the capacity to produce Vi polysaccharide.

The hepatitis A antigen is adsorbed on a mineral carrier, such as aluminium hydroxide, and the Vi capsular polysaccharide consists of partly 3-*O*-acetylated repeated units of 2-acetylamino-2-deoxy-D-galactopyranuronic acid with α-(1→4) linkages.

The product is presented either as a liquid mixture containing the hepatitis A component and the typhoid Vi polysaccharide component or as 2 separate liquids, one containing the hepatitis A component and the other the typhoid Vi polysaccharide component, which are mixed together immediately before use.

PRODUCTION

GENERAL PROVISIONS

The 2 components are prepared as described in the monographs *Hepatitis A vaccine (inactivated, adsorbed) (1107)* and *Typhoid polysaccharide vaccine (1160)* and comply with the requirements prescribed therein.

The production method is validated to demonstrate that the product, if tested, would comply with the test for abnormal toxicity for immunosera and vaccines for human use *(2.6.9)*.

Reference preparation The hepatitis A reference preparation is part of a representative batch shown to be at least as immunogenic in animals as a batch that, in clinical studies in young healthy adults, produced not less than 95 per cent seroconversion, corresponding to a level of neutralising antibody accepted to be protective, after a full-course primary immunisation. An antibody level not less than 20 mIU/mL determined by enzyme-linked immunosorbent assay is recognised as being protective.

FINAL BULKS

The hepatitis A final bulk is prepared from 1 or more inactivated harvests of hepatitis A virus. Approved adjuvants, stabilisers and antimicrobial preservatives may be added.

The Vi polysaccharide final bulk is prepared from 1 or more batches of purified Vi polysaccharide which are dissolved in a suitable solvent, which may contain an antimicrobial preservative, so that the volume corresponding to 1 dose contains 25 µg of polysaccharide and the solution is isotonic with blood (250-350 mosmol/kg).

Where the vaccine is presented as a liquid mixture of both components, the final bulk is prepared by addition of a suitable quantity of the Vi capsular polysaccharide bulk to the hepatitis A bulk.

Only final bulks that comply with the following requirements may be used in the preparation of the final lot.

Antimicrobial preservative

Where applicable, determine the amount of antimicrobial preservative by a suitable chemical or physico-chemical method. The amount is not less than 85 per cent and not greater than 115 per cent of the intended amount.

Sterility *(2.6.1)*

Carry out the test for sterility using 10 mL for each medium.

FINAL LOT

The final bulks are distributed aseptically into sterile containers. The containers are then closed so as to avoid contamination.

Only a final lot that complies with each of the requirements given below under Identification, Tests and Assay may be released for use. Provided that the tests for free formaldehyde (where applicable), antimicrobial preservative (where applicable) and bacterial endotoxins have been carried out on the final bulks with satisfactory results, they may be omitted on the final lot. If the assay of the hepatitis A component is carried out *in vivo*, then provided it has been carried out with satisfactory results on the final bulk containing the hepatitis A component, it may be omitted on the final lot.

CHARACTERS

If the vaccine is presented as 2 separate liquids test A is carried out using the hepatitis A component and test B is carried out using the typhoid Vi polysaccharide component. Test C is carried out if the vaccine is presented as a liquid mixture of both components or immediately after mixing both components if the vaccine is presented as 2 separate liquids.

A. Whitish, cloudy suspension.

B. Clear, colourless liquid, free from visible particles.

C. Turbid liquid with a slow settling white deposit.

IDENTIFICATION

If the vaccine is presented as 2 separate liquids, identification test A is carried out using the hepatitis A component and identification test B is carried out using the typhoid Vi polysaccharide component. If the vaccine is presented as a liquid mixture, tests A and B are carried out.

A. Hepatitis A virus antigen is identified by a suitable immunochemical method *(2.7.1)* using specific antibodies or by the *in vivo* assay *(2.7.14)*.

B. Typhoid Vi polysaccharide is identified by a suitable immunochemical method *(2.7.1)* using specific antibodies.

TESTS

If the vaccine is presented as 2 separate liquids, the tests for pH, antimicrobial preservative and bacterial endotoxins are carried out on both components; the test for aluminium is carried out using the hepatitis A component and the test for O-acetyl groups is carried out using the typhoid Vi polysaccharide component; the tests for pH, free formaldehyde, osmolality and sterility are carried out immediately after mixing both components. If the vaccine is presented as a liquid mixture, the test for O-acetyl groups is carried out before the 2 components are mixed.

pH *(2.2.3)*
6.8 to 7.8 for the hepatitis A component and 6.5 to 7.5 for the typhoid Vi polysaccharide component; 6.6 to 7.6 for the vaccine presented as a liquid mixture or immediately after mixing both components if the vaccine is presented as 2 separate liquids.

Aluminium *(2.5.13)*
Maximum 1.25 mg per single human dose, if aluminium hydroxide is used as the adsorbent.

Free formaldehyde *(2.4.18)*
Maximum 0.2 g/L.

Antimicrobial preservative
Where applicable, determine the amount of antimicrobial preservative by a suitable chemical or physico-chemical method. The amount is not less than the minimum amount shown to be effective and is not greater than 115 per cent of the amount stated on the label.

Sterility *(2.6.1)*
The vaccine complies with the test for sterility.

Osmolality *(2.2.35)*
Where applicable, the osmolality of the vaccine is within the limits approved for the particular product.

Bacterial endotoxins *(2.6.14)*
The bacterial endotoxins content is less than 2 IU per human dose for the hepatitis A component and within the limit approved for the typhoid Vi polysaccharide component. If the vaccine is presented as a liquid mixture of hepatitis A component and typhoid Vi polysaccharide component the bacterial endotoxins content is within the limit approved for the specific product.

***O*-Acetyl groups** *(2.5.19)*
0.085 µmol (± 25 per cent) per dose (25 µg of polysaccharide).

ASSAY
Hepatitis A component
The vaccine complies with the assay of hepatitis A vaccine *(2.7.14)*.

Typhoid Vi polysaccharide component
Determine Vi polysaccharide by a suitable immunochemical method *(2.7.1)*, using a reference purified polysaccharide. The estimated amount of polysaccharide per dose is 80 per cent to 120 per cent of the content stated on the label. The confidence limits ($P = 0.95$) of the estimated amount of polysaccharide are not less than 80 per cent and not more than 120 per cent.

LABELLING
The label states:
— the amount of hepatitis A virus antigen per human dose;
— the number of micrograms of polysaccharide per human dose (25 µg);
— the total quantity of polysaccharide in the container;
— the type of cells used for production of the vaccine;
— the name and amount of the adsorbent used;
— that the vaccine must be shaken before use;
— that the vaccine must not be frozen.

———————————————————— Ph Eur

Hepatitis A (Inactivated) and Hepatitis B (rDNA) Vaccine

(Hepatitis A (Inactivated) and Hepatitis B (rDNA) Vaccine (Adsorbed), Ph Eur monograph 1526)
The label may state 'HepA/HepB'.

Ph Eur ————————————————————

DEFINITION
Hepatitis A (inactivated) and hepatitis B (rDNA) vaccine (adsorbed) is a suspension consisting of a suitable strain of hepatitis A virus, grown in cell cultures and inactivated by a validated method, and of hepatitis B surface antigen (HBsAg), a component protein of hepatitis B virus obtained by recombinant DNA technology; the antigens are adsorbed on a mineral carrier, such as aluminium hydroxide or hydrated aluminium phosphate.

PRODUCTION
GENERAL PROVISIONS
The two components are prepared as described in the monographs on *Hepatitis A vaccine (inactivated, adsorbed) (1107)* and *Hepatitis B vaccine (rDNA) (1056)* and comply with the requirements prescribed therein.

The production method is validated to demonstrate that the product, if tested, would comply with the test for abnormal toxicity for immunosera and vaccines for human use *(2.6.9)*.

Reference preparation The reference preparation is part of a representative batch shown to be at least as immunogenic in animals as a batch that, in clinical studies in young healthy adults, produced not less than 95 per cent seroconversion, corresponding to a level of neutralising antibody recognised to be protective, after a full-course primary immunisation. For hepatitis A, an antibody level not less than 20 mIU/mL determined by enzyme-linked immunosorbent assay is recognised as being protective. For hepatitis B, an antibody level not less than 10 mIU/mL against HBsAg is recognised as being protective.

FINAL BULK VACCINE
The final bulk vaccine is prepared from one or more inactivated harvests of hepatitis A virus and one or more batches of purified antigen.

Only a final bulk vaccine that complies with the following requirements may be used in the preparation of the final lot.

Antimicrobial preservative
Where applicable, determine the amount of antimicrobial preservative by a suitable chemical or physico-chemical method. The amount is not less than 85 per cent and not greater than 115 per cent of the intended amount.

Sterility *(2.6.1)*
The final bulk vaccine complies with the test for sterility, carried out using 10 mL for each medium.

FINAL LOT
Only a final lot that complies with each of the requirements given below under Identification, Tests and Assay may be released for use. Provided that the tests for free formaldehyde (where applicable) and antimicrobial preservative content (where applicable) have been carried out on the final bulk vaccine with satisfactory results, they may be omitted on the final lot. If the assay of the hepatitis A and/or the hepatitis B component is carried out *in vivo*, then provided it has been carried out with satisfactory results on the final bulk vaccine, it may be omitted on the final lot.

IDENTIFICATION

The vaccine is shown to contain hepatitis A virus antigen and hepatitis B surface antigen by suitable immunochemical methods (*2.7.1*), using specific antibodies or by the mouse immunogenicity tests described under Assay.

TESTS

Aluminium (*2.5.13*)

Maximum 1.25 mg per single human dose, if aluminium hydroxide or hydrated aluminium phosphate is used as the adsorbent.

Free formaldehyde (*2.4.18*)

Maximum 0.2 g/L.

Antimicrobial preservative

Where applicable, determine the amount of antimicrobial preservative by a suitable chemical or physico-chemical method. The amount is not less than the minimum amount shown to be effective and is not greater than 115 per cent of that stated on the label.

Sterility (*2.6.1*)

The vaccine complies with the test for sterility.

Bacterial endotoxins (*2.6.14*)

Less than 2 IU per human dose.

ASSAY

Hepatitis A component

The vaccine complies with the assay of hepatitis A vaccine (*2.7.14*).

Hepatitis B component

The vaccine complies with the assay of hepatitis B vaccine (rDNA) (*2.7.15*).

LABELLING

The label states:
— the amount of hepatitis A virus antigen and hepatitis B surface antigen per container,
— the type of cells used for production of the vaccine,
— the name and amount of the adsorbent used,
— that the vaccine must be shaken before use,
— that the vaccine must not be frozen.

Ph Eur

Hepatitis B Vaccine (rDNA)

(*Ph Eur monograph 1056*)

The label may state 'HepB'.

Ph Eur

DEFINITION

Hepatitis B vaccine (rDNA) is a preparation of hepatitis B surface antigen (HBsAg), a component protein of hepatitis B virus; the antigen may be adsorbed on a mineral carrier such as aluminium hydroxide or hydrated aluminium phosphate. The vaccine may also contain the adjuvant 3-*O*-desacyl-4'-monophosphoryl lipid A. The antigen is obtained by recombinant DNA technology.

PRODUCTION

GENERAL PROVISIONS

The vaccine shall have been shown to induce specific, protective antibodies in man. The production method shall have been shown to yield consistently vaccines that comply with the requirements for immunogenicity and safety.

The production method is validated to demonstrate that the product, if tested, would comply with the test for abnormal toxicity for immunosera and vaccines for human use (*2.6.9*).

Hepatitis B vaccine (rDNA) is produced by the expression of the viral gene coding for HBsAg in yeast (*Saccharomyces cerevisiae*) or mammalian cells (Chinese hamster ovary (CHO) cells or other suitable cell lines), purification of the resulting HBsAg and the rendering of this antigen into an immunogenic preparation. The suitability and safety of the cells are approved by the competent authority.

The vaccine may contain the product of the S gene (major protein), a combination of the S gene and pre-S2 gene products (middle protein) or a combination of the S gene, the pre-S2 gene and pre-S1 gene products (large protein).

Reference preparation Part of a representative batch shown to be at least as immunogenic in animals as a batch that, in clinical studies in young, healthy adults, produced not less than 95 per cent seroconversion, corresponding to a level of HBsAg neutralising antibody recognised to be protective, after a full-course primary immunisation. An antibody level not less than 10 mIU/mL is recognised as being protective.

CHARACTERISATION OF THE SUBSTANCE

Development studies are carried out to characterise the antigen. The complete protein, lipid and carbohydrate structure of the antigen is established. The morphological characteristics of the antigen particles are established by electron microscopy. The mean buoyant density of the antigen particles is determined by a physico-chemical method, such as gradient centrifugation. The antigenic epitopes are characterised. The protein fraction of the antigen is characterised in terms of the primary structure (for example, by determination of the amino-acid composition, by partial amino-acid sequence analysis and by peptide mapping).

CULTURE AND HARVEST

Identity, microbial purity, plasmid retention and consistency of yield are determined at suitable production stages. If mammalian cells are used, tests for extraneous agents and mycoplasmas are performed in accordance with general chapter *2.6.16. Tests for extraneous agents in viral vaccines for human use*, but using 200 mL of harvest in the test in cell culture for other extraneous agents.

PURIFIED ANTIGEN

Only a purified antigen that complies with the following requirements may be used in the preparation of the final bulk vaccine.

Total protein

The total protein is determined by a validated method. The content is within the limits approved for the specific product.

Antigen content and identification

The quantity and specificity of HBsAg is determined in comparison with the International Standard for HBsAg subtype *ad* or an in-house reference, by a suitable immunochemical method (*2.7.1*) such as radio-immunoassay (RIA), enzyme-linked immunosorbent assay (ELISA), immunoblot (preferably using a monoclonal antibody directed against a protective epitope) or single radial diffusion. The antigen/protein ratio is within the limits approved for the specific product.

The molecular weight of the major band revealed following sodium dodecyl sulfate polyacrylamide gel electrophoresis (SDS-PAGE) performed under reducing conditions corresponds to the value expected from the known nucleic acid and polypeptide sequences and possible glycosylation.

Antigenic purity
The purity of the antigen is determined by comparison with a reference preparation using liquid chromatography or other suitable methods such as SDS-PAGE with staining by acid blue 92 and silver. A suitable method is sensitive enough to detect a potential contaminant at a concentration of 1 per cent of total protein. Not less than 95 per cent of the total protein consists of hepatitis B surface antigen.

Composition
The content of proteins, lipids, nucleic acids and carbohydrates is determined.

Host-cell- and vector-derived DNA
If mammalian cells are used for production, not more than 10 pg of DNA in the quantity of purified antigen equivalent to a single human dose of vaccine.

Caesium
If a caesium salt is used during production, a test for residual caesium is carried out on the purified antigen. The content is within the limits approved for the specific product.

Sterility (2.6.1)
The purified antigen complies with the test, carried out using 10 mL for each medium.

Additional tests on the purified antigen may be required depending on the production method used: for example, a test for residual animal serum where mammalian cells are used for production or tests for residual chemicals used during extraction and purification.

ADSORBED 3-O-DESACYL-4′-MONOPHOSPHORYL LIPID A BULK
If 3-O-desacyl-4′-monophosphoryl lipid A is included in the vaccine it complies with the monograph *3-O-desacyl-4′-monophosphoryl lipid A (2537)*. Where 3-O-desacyl-4′-monophosphoryl lipid A liquid bulk is adsorbed prior to inclusion in the vaccine, the adsorbed 3-O-desacyl-4′-monophosphoryl lipid A bulk complies with the following requirements.

Degree of adsorption of 3-*O*-desacyl-4′-monophosphoryl lipid A
The content of non-adsorbed 3-O-desacyl-4′-monophosphoryl lipid A in the adsorbed 3-*O*-desacyl-4′-monophosphoryl lipid A bulk is determined by a suitable method, for example gas chromatographic quantification of the *3-O-desacyl-4′-monophosphoryl lipid A (2537)* fatty acids in the supernatant, evaporated to dryness, after centrifugation.

pH (2.2.3)
The pH is within the limits approved for the particular preparation.

Sterility (2.6.1)
It complies with the test, carried out using 10 mL for each medium.

FINAL BULK VACCINE
An antimicrobial preservative, a mineral carrier, such as aluminium hydroxide or hydrated aluminium phosphate, and the adjuvant 3-O-desacyl-4′-monophosphoryl lipid A may be included in the formulation of the final bulk.

Only a final bulk vaccine that complies with the following requirements may be used in the preparation of the final lot.

Antimicrobial preservative
Where applicable, determine the amount of antimicrobial preservative by a suitable chemical or physico-chemical method. The amount is not less than 85 per cent and not greater than 115 per cent of the intended amount.

Sterility (2.6.1)
The final bulk vaccine complies with the test, carried out using 10 mL for each medium.

FINAL LOT
Only a final lot that complies with each of the requirements given below under Identification, Tests and Assay may be released for use. Provided that the tests for free formaldehyde (where applicable) and antimicrobial preservative content (where applicable) have been carried out on the final bulk vaccine with satisfactory results, they may be omitted on the final lot. If the assay is carried out *in vivo*, then provided it has been carried out with satisfactory results on the final bulk vaccine, it may be omitted on the final lot.

Degree of adsorption
The degree of adsorption of the antigen and, where applicable, 3-O-desacyl-4′-monophosphoryl lipid A is assessed.

IDENTIFICATION
The assay or, where applicable, the electrophoretic profile, serves also to identify the vaccine. In addition, where applicable, the test for 3-O-desacyl-4′-monophosphoryl lipid A content also serves to identify the 3-O-desacyl-4′-monophosphoryl lipid A-containing vaccine.

TESTS
ALUMINIUM (2.5.13)
Maximum 1.25 mg per single human dose, if aluminium hydroxide or hydrated aluminium phosphate is used as the adsorbent.

3-*O*-Desacyl-4′-monophosphoryl lipid A
Minimum 80 per cent and maximum 120 per cent of the intended amount.

Where applicable, determine the content of 3-O-desacyl-4′-monophosphoryl lipid A by a suitable method, for example gas chromatography (2.2.28).

FREE FORMALDEHYDE (2.4.18)
Maximum 0.2 g/L.

ANTIMICROBIAL PRESERVATIVE
Where applicable, determine the content of antimicrobial preservative by a suitable chemical or physico-chemical method. The amount is not less than the minimum amount shown to be effective and is not greater than 115 per cent of that stated on the label.

Sterility (2.6.1)
The vaccine complies with the test.

PYROGENS (2.6.8)
The vaccine complies with the test for pyrogens. Inject the equivalent of one human dose into each rabbit or, if the vaccine contains 3-O-desacyl-4′-monophosphoryl lipid A, inject per kilogram of the rabbit's mass an amount of the vaccine containing 2.5 µg of 3-O-desacyl-4′-monophosphoryl lipid A.

ASSAY
The vaccine complies with the assay of hepatitis B vaccine (rDNA) (2.7.15).

LABELLING
The label states:
— the amount of HBsAg per container;
— the type of cells used for production of the vaccine;
— the name and amount of the adjuvant and/or adsorbent used;

IMMUNOLOGICAL PRODUCTS

— that the vaccine must be shaken before use;
— that the vaccine must not be frozen.

Ph Eur

Inactivated Influenza Vaccine (Whole Virion)

(Influenza Vaccine (Whole Virion, Inactivated),
Ph Eur monograph 0159)

The label may state 'Flu'.

When Inactivated Influenza Vaccine or Influenza Vaccine is prescribed or demanded and the form is not stated, Inactivated Influenza Vaccine (Whole Virion), Inactivated Influenza Vaccine (Split Virion) or Inactivated Influenza Vaccine (Surface Antigen) may be dispensed or supplied.

Ph Eur

DEFINITION

Influenza vaccine (whole virion, inactivated) is a sterile, aqueous suspension of a strain or strains of influenza virus, type A or B, or a mixture of strains of the 2 types grown individually in fertilised hens' eggs and inactivated in such a manner that their antigenic properties are retained.

The stated amount of haemagglutinin antigen for each strain present in the vaccine is 15 µg per dose, unless clinical evidence supports the use of a different amount.

The vaccine is a slightly opalescent liquid.

PRODUCTION

The production method is validated to demonstrate that the product, if tested, would comply with the test for abnormal toxicity for immunosera and vaccines for human use (2.6.9).

CHOICE OF VACCINE STRAIN

The World Health Organisation reviews the world epidemiological situation annually and if necessary recommends the strains that correspond to this epidemiological evidence.

Such strains are used in accordance with the regulations in force in the signatory States of the Convention on the Elaboration of a European Pharmacopoeia. It is now common practice to use reassorted strains giving high yields of the appropriate surface antigens. The origin and passage history of virus strains shall be approved by the competent authority.

SUBSTRATE FOR VIRUS PROPAGATION

Influenza virus seed to be used in the production of vaccine is propagated in fertilised eggs from chicken flocks free from specified pathogens (SPF) (5.2.2) or in suitable cell cultures (5.2.4), such as chick-embryo fibroblasts or chick kidney cells obtained from SPF chicken flocks (5.2.2). For production, the virus of each strain is grown in the allantoic cavity of fertilised hens' eggs from healthy flocks.

VIRUS SEED LOT

The production of vaccine is based on a seed-lot system. Working seed lots represent not more than 15 passages from the approved reassorted virus or the approved virus isolate. The final vaccine represents 1 passage from the working seed lot. The haemagglutinin and neuraminidase antigens of each seed lot are identified as originating from the correct strain of influenza virus by suitable methods.

Only a working virus seed lot that complies with the following requirements may be used in the preparation of the monovalent pooled harvest.

Bacterial and fungal contamination
Carry out the test for sterility (2.6.1), using 10 mL for each medium.

Mycoplasmas (2.6.7)
Carry out the test for mycoplasmas, using 10 mL.

VIRUS PROPAGATION AND HARVEST

An antimicrobial agent may be added to the inoculum. After incubation at a controlled temperature, the allantoic fluids are harvested and combined to form a monovalent pooled harvest. An antimicrobial agent may be added at the time of harvest. At no stage in the production is penicillin or streptomycin used.

MONOVALENT POOLED HARVEST

To limit the possibility of contamination, inactivation is initiated as soon as possible after preparation. The virus is inactivated by a method that has been demonstrated on 3 consecutive batches to be consistently effective for the manufacturer. The inactivation process shall have been shown to be capable of inactivating the influenza virus without destroying its antigenicity; the process should cause minimum alteration of the haemagglutinin and neuraminidase antigens. The inactivation process shall also have been shown to be capable of inactivating avian leucosis viruses and mycoplasmas. If the monovalent pooled harvest is stored after inactivation, it is held at 5 ± 3 °C.

If formaldehyde solution is used, the concentration does not exceed 0.2 g/L of CH_2O at any time during inactivation; if betapropiolactone is used, the concentration does not exceed 0.1 per cent *V/V* at any time during inactivation.

Before or after the inactivation process, the monovalent pooled harvest is concentrated and purified by high-speed centrifugation or other suitable method.

Only a monovalent pooled harvest that complies with the following requirements may be used in the preparation of the final bulk vaccine.

Haemagglutinin antigen
Determine the content of haemagglutinin antigen by an immunodiffusion test (2.7.1), by comparison with a haemagglutinin antigen reference preparation or with an antigen preparation calibrated against it [1]. Carry out the test at 20-25 °C.

Neuraminidase antigen
The presence and type of neuraminidase antigen are confirmed by suitable enzymatic or immunological methods on the first 3 monovalent pooled harvests from each working seed lot.

Sterility (2.6.1)
Carry out the test for sterility, using 10 mL for each medium.

Residual infectious virus
Carry out the test described below under Tests.

FINAL BULK VACCINE

Appropriate quantities of the monovalent pooled harvests are blended to make the final bulk vaccine.

Only a final bulk vaccine that complies with the following requirements may be used in the preparation of the final lot.

Antimicrobial preservative
Where applicable, determine the amount of antimicrobial preservative by a suitable chemical method. The content is

---

[1] *Reference haemagglutinin antigens are available from the National Institute for Biological Standards and Control, Blanche Lane, South Mimms, Potters Bar, Hertfordshire, EN6 3QG, Great Britain*

not less than 85 per cent and not greater than 115 per cent of the intended amount.

Sterility (*2.6.1*)
Carry out the test for sterility using 10 mL for each medium.

FINAL LOT
The final bulk vaccine is distributed aseptically into sterile, tamper-proof containers. The containers are closed so as to prevent contamination.

Only a final lot that is satisfactory with respect to each of the requirements given below under Tests and Assay may be released for use. Provided that the test for residual infectious virus has been performed with satisfactory results on each monovalent pooled harvest and that the tests for free formaldehyde, ovalbumin and total protein have been performed with satisfactory results on the final bulk vaccine, they may be omitted on the final lot.

IDENTIFICATION
The assay serves to confirm the antigenic specificity of the vaccine.

TESTS
Residual infectious virus. Inoculate 0.2 mL of the vaccine into the allantoic cavity of each of 10 fertilised eggs and incubate at 33-37 °C for 3 days. The test is not valid unless at least 8 of the 10 embryos survive. Harvest 0.5 mL of the allantoic fluid from each surviving embryo and pool the fluids. Inoculate 0.2 mL of the pooled fluid into a further 10 fertilised eggs and incubate at 33-37 °C for 3 days. The test is not valid unless at least 8 of the 10 embryos survive. Harvest about 0.1 mL of the allantoic fluid from each surviving embryo and examine each individual harvest for live virus by a haemagglutination test. If haemagglutination is found for any of the fluids, carry out for that fluid a further passage in eggs and test for haemagglutination; no haemagglutination occurs.

Antimicrobial preservative
Where applicable, determine the amount of antimicrobial preservative by a suitable chemical method. The content is not less than the minimum amount shown to be effective and is not greater than 115 per cent of the quantity stated on the label.

Free formaldehyde (*2.4.18*)
Maximum 0.2 g/L, where applicable.

Ovalbumin
Not more than the quantity stated on the label and in any case not more than 1 µg per human dose, determined by a suitable immunochemical method (*2.7.1*) using a suitable reference preparation of ovalbumin.

Total protein
Not more than 6 times the total haemagglutinin content of the vaccine as determined in the assay, but in any case, not more than 100 µg of protein per virus strain per human dose and not more than a total of 300 µg of protein per human dose.

Sterility (*2.6.1*)
It complies with the test for sterility.

Bacterial endotoxins (*2.6.14*)
Less than 100 IU per human dose.

ASSAY
Determine the content of haemagglutinin antigen by an immunodiffusion test (*2.7.1*), by comparison with a haemagglutinin antigen reference preparation or with an antigen preparation calibrated against it [1]. Carry out the test at 20-25 °C. The confidence limits ($P = 0.95$) are not less than 80 per cent and not more than 125 per cent of the estimated haemagglutinin antigen content. The lower confidence limit ($P = 0.95$) is not less than 80 per cent of the amount stated on the label for each strain.

LABELLING
The label states:
— that the vaccine has been prepared on eggs,
— the strain or strains of influenza virus used to prepare the vaccine,
— the method of inactivation,
— the haemagglutinin content in micrograms per virus strain per dose,
— the maximum amount of ovalbumin,
— the season during which the vaccine is intended to protect.

_____ *Ph Eur*

Influenza Vaccine (Whole Virion, Inactivated, Prepared in Cell Cultures)

(*Ph Eur monograph 2308*)
The label may state 'Flu' or 'Flu(adj)' as appropriate.

_____ *Ph Eur*

DEFINITION
Influenza vaccine (whole virion, inactivated, prepared in cell cultures) is a sterile, aqueous suspension of a strain or strains of influenza virus, type A or B, or a mixture of strains of the 2 types grown individually in cell cultures and inactivated in such a manner that their antigenic properties are retained. The stated amount of haemagglutinin antigen for each strain present in the vaccine is 15 µg per dose, unless clinical evidence supports the use of a different amount. The vaccine is a slightly opalescent or opalescent liquid. The vaccine may contain an adjuvant. This monograph applies to vaccines produced in diploid or continuous cell lines of mammalian origin.

PRODUCTION
GENERAL PROVISIONS
Production of the vaccine is based on a virus seed-lot system and a cell-bank system. The production method shall have been shown to yield consistently vaccines that comply with the requirements for immunogenicity, safety and stability.

The production method is validated to demonstrate that the product, if tested, would comply with the test for abnormal toxicity for immunosera and vaccines for human use (*2.6.9*).

The production method is validated to demonstrate suitable reduction of residual host-cell protein. With the agreement of the competent authority and for each specific product, routine testing for residual host-cell proteins may be omitted based on the results of validation studies for the product. Guidance on the principles of such validation studies is given, for example, in the monograph *Products of recombinant DNA technology (0784)*, in particular in the sections 'Validation of the production process - Extraction and

_____

[1] *Reference haemagglutinin antigens are available from the National Institute for Biological Standards and Control, Blanche Lane, South Mimms, Potters Bar, Hertfordshire, EN6 3QG, Great Britain*

purification' and 'Production consistency - Host-cell-derived proteins'.

CHOICE OF VACCINE STRAIN

The World Health Organisation reviews the world epidemiological situation annually and if necessary recommends new strains corresponding to this epidemiological evidence.

Such strains are used in accordance with the regulations in force in the signatory states of the Convention on the Elaboration of a European Pharmacopoeia. It is now common practice to use reassorted strains giving high yields of the appropriate surface antigens. The origin and passage history of virus strains shall be approved by the competent authority.

SUBSTRATE FOR VIRUS PROPAGATION

Influenza virus used in the preparation of seed lots is propagated in fertilised eggs from chicken flocks free from specified pathogens (SPF) (5.2.2) or in suitable cell cultures (5.2.3), such as chick-embryo fibroblasts, chick kidney cells obtained from SPF chicken flocks (5.2.2), or a diploid or continuous cell line. The final passage for establishment of the working seed lot is prepared in the cell line used for routine production. For this production, the virus of each strain is propagated in a diploid or continuous cell line (5.2.3).

VIRUS SEED LOT

The production of vaccine is based on a seed-lot system. Each of the strains of influenza virus used shall be identified by historical records that include information on the origin of the strain and its subsequent manipulation. Working seed lots represent not more than 15 passages from the approved reassorted virus or the approved virus isolate. The final vaccine represents 1 passage from the working seed lot.

Only a seed lot that complies with the following requirements may be used for virus propagation.

Identification

The haemagglutinin and neuraminidase antigens of each master and working seed lot are identified as originating from the correct strain of influenza virus by suitable methods.

Virus concentration

The virus concentration of each working seed lot is determined. Where applicable, the virus concentration of each master seed lot is determined.

Extraneous agents (2.6.16)

The working seed lots comply with the requirements for seed lots. It is recognised that due to a seasonal change in one or more of the influenza vaccine strains, timely testing of a virus seed for extraneous agents according to general chapter 2.6.16 may be problematic (e.g. duration of *in vivo* tests, timely availability of specific neutralising antisera).

In agreement with the competent authority, and in light of a risk assessment, rapid assays (e.g. multiplex PCR) may be applied as alternatives to general chapter 2.6.16 following validation.

Such risk assessment and validation includes more general considerations on potential contaminants of the virus isolates, the susceptibility of the cell substrate to such viruses and the capacity of the production process for viral removal or inactivation; validation includes also comparative data on testing of seeds according to general chapter 2.6.16 and the proposed rapid assays. Each applied PCR/NAT test (2.6.21) must be shown to be suitable for its intended use by appropriate analytical validation. The risk assessment is reviewed when new information becomes available on

potential viral contaminants, and the justification of the chosen PCR panel of extraneous agents tested for is provided to the competent authority within the annual update. This update also includes vaccine strain-specific aspects such as specific PCR inhibitory effects.

If an agent is detected in a virus seed and the mammalian cells used for production are shown to be susceptible to this agent, the virus seed is not used for vaccine production.

If an agent is detected in a virus seed and the mammalian cells are not susceptible to the agent, validation of the production process to demonstrate removal or inactivation of the agent is carried out. If removal or inactivation cannot be demonstrated, the inactivated monovalent harvest is tested to demonstrate absence of any contaminant identified in the virus seed.

PROPAGATION AND SINGLE HARVEST

All processing of the cell bank and subsequent cell cultures is done under aseptic conditions in an area where no other cells are being handled at the same time. Approved animal serum (but not human serum) may be used in the cell culture media. Serum and trypsin used in the preparation of cell suspensions or media are shown to be free from extraneous agents. The cell culture media may contain a pH indicator, such as phenol red, and antibiotics at the lowest effective concentration. A sufficient quantity of the cell cultures employed for vaccine production are set aside as uninfected cell cultures (control cells).

Only a single harvest that complies with the following requirements may be used in the preparation of the vaccine.

Identification

The test for antigen content also serves to identify the single harvest.

Bacterial and fungal contamination

Carry out the test for sterility (2.6.1), using 10 mL for each medium.

Mycoplasmas (2.6.7)

Carry out the test for mycoplasmas, using 10 mL for each medium.

Control cells

The control cells of the production cell culture comply with a test for identification and the requirements for extraneous agents (2.6.16).

Haemagglutinin antigen

Determine the haemagglutinin antigen content by a suitable immunochemical method (2.7.1).

INACTIVATED AND PURIFIED MONOVALENT HARVEST

The harvest, which may be a pool of several single harvests of the same strain, is inactivated and purified by validated methods. Before or after the inactivation process, the monovalent harvest is concentrated and purified by high-speed centrifugation or another suitable method. The influenza virus is inactivated by a method that has been demonstrated on 3 consecutive batches to be consistently effective for the manufacturer. The inactivation process shall have been shown to be capable of inactivating the influenza virus without destroying its antigenicity; the process is designed so as to cause minimum alteration of the haemagglutinin and neuraminidase antigens.

If continuous cell lines are used for production, the purification process shall have been validated to reduce consistently host-cell DNA to a suitable level.

Only an inactivated, purified monovalent harvest that complies with the following requirements may be used in the preparation of the final bulk vaccine.

Haemagglutinin antigen
Determine the haemagglutinin antigen content by a suitable immunochemical method (2.7.1).

Antigen/total protein ratio
Determine the haemagglutinin antigen content by a suitable immunodiffusion test. Determine the total protein by a validated method. The ratio of haemagglutinin antigen content to total protein content is within the limits approved for the particular product.

Neuraminidase antigen
The presence and type of neuraminidase antigen are confirmed by suitable enzymatic or immunological methods on the first 3 monovalent harvests from each working seed lot.

Sterility (2.6.1)
Carry out the test for sterility, using 10 mL for each medium.

Residual infectious virus
Carry out the test described below under Tests.

FINAL BULK VACCINE
Appropriate quantities of the inactivated, purified monovalent pooled harvests are blended to make the final bulk vaccine. An adjuvant may be added.

Only a final bulk vaccine that complies with the following requirements may be used in the preparation of the final lot.

Antimicrobial preservative
Where applicable, determine the amount of antimicrobial preservative by a suitable chemical method. The content is not less than 85 per cent and not greater than 115 per cent of the intended amount.

Sterility (2.6.1)
Carry out the test for sterility, using 10 mL for each medium.

Residual host-cell DNA
If a continuous cell line is used for virus propagation, the content of residual host-cell DNA, determined using a suitable method, is not greater than 10 ng in the equivalent of a single human dose.

FINAL LOT
The final bulk vaccine is distributed aseptically into sterile, tamper-proof containers. The containers are closed so as to prevent contamination.

Only a final lot that is satisfactory with respect to each of the requirements given below under Tests and Assay may be released for use. Provided that the test for residual infectious virus has been performed with satisfactory results on each inactivated and purified monovalent harvest and that the tests for free formaldehyde, bovine serum albumin and total protein have been performed with satisfactory results on the final bulk vaccine, they may be omitted on the final lot.

If the vaccine contains an adjuvant, suitable tests for identity and other relevant quality criteria are carried out on the final lot. These tests may include chemical and physical analysis, determination of particle size and determination of the number of particles per unit volume.

IDENTIFICATION
The assay serves to confirm the antigenic specificity of the vaccine.

TESTS
Residual infectious virus. Carry out an amplification test for residual infectious influenza virus by inoculating not less than 4 mL of the vaccine into cell cultures of the same type as used for production of the vaccine; incubate for not less than 7 days at 32 ± 2 °C. Inoculate not less than 10 mL of the cell culture harvested medium into a new semi-confluent cell culture and incubate as before. At the end of the incubation period, examine for live virus by a haemagglutination test. If haemagglutination is found for any of the fluids, carry out for that fluid a further passage on cell cultures and test for haemagglutination; no haemagglutination occurs.

Antimicrobial preservative
Where applicable, determine the amount of antimicrobial preservative by a suitable chemical method. The content is not less than the minimum amount shown to be effective and is not greater than 115 per cent of the quantity stated on the label.

Free formaldehyde (2.4.18)
Maximum 0.2 g/L, where applicable.

Bovine serum albumin
Maximum 50 ng per human dose, determined by a suitable immunochemical method (2.7.1).

Total protein
Not more than 6 times the total haemagglutinin content of the vaccine as determined in the assay, but in any case, not more than 100 μg of protein per virus strain per human dose.

Sterility (2.6.1)
It complies with the test for sterility.

Bacterial endotoxins (2.6.14)
Less than 25 IU per human dose.

ASSAY
Determine the content of haemagglutinin antigen by an immunodiffusion test (2.7.1), by comparison with a haemagglutinin antigen reference preparation[1] or with an antigen preparation calibrated against it. Carry out the test at 20-25 °C. The confidence limits ($P = 0.95$) are not less than 80 per cent and not more than 125 per cent of the estimated content. The lower confidence limit ($P = 0.95$) is not less than 80 per cent of the amount stated on the label for each strain.

LABELLING
The label states:
— the biological origin of the cells used for the preparation of the vaccine;
— the strain or strains of influenza virus used to prepare the vaccine;
— the method of inactivation;
— the haemagglutinin antigen content in micrograms per virus strain per dose;
— the season during which the vaccine is intended to protect;
— where applicable, the name and the quantity of adjuvant used.

_____ _Ph Eur_

[1] _Reference haemagglutinin antigens are available from the National Institute for Biological Standards and Control, Blanche Lane, South Mimms, Potters Bar, Hertfordshire, EN6 3QG, Great Britain_

Inactivated Influenza Vaccine (Split Virion)

(Influenza Vaccine (Split Virion, Inactivated), Ph Eur monograph 0158)

The label may state 'Flu'.

When Inactivated Influenza Vaccine or Influenza Vaccine is prescribed or demanded and the form is not stated, Inactivated Influenza Vaccine (Whole Virion), Inactivated Influenza Vaccine (Split Virion) or Inactivated Influenza Vaccine (Surface Antigen) may be dispensed or supplied.

Ph Eur _____

DEFINITION

Influenza vaccine (split virion, inactivated) is a sterile, aqueous suspension of a strain or strains of influenza virus, type A or B, or a mixture of strains of the 2 types grown individually in fertilised hens' eggs, inactivated and treated so that the integrity of the virus particles has been disrupted without diminishing the antigenic properties of the haemagglutinin and neuraminidase antigens. The stated amount of haemagglutinin antigen for each strain present in the vaccine is 15 μg per dose, unless clinical evidence supports the use of a different amount.

The vaccine is a slightly opalescent liquid.

PRODUCTION

The production method is validated to demonstrate that the product, if tested, would comply with the test for abnormal toxicity for immunosera and vaccines for human use *(2.6.9)*.

CHOICE OF VACCINE STRAIN

The World Health Organisation reviews the world epidemiological situation annually and if necessary recommends the strains that correspond to this epidemiological evidence.

Such strains are used in accordance with the regulations in force in the signatory States of the Convention on the Elaboration of a European Pharmacopoeia. It is now common practice to use reassorted strains giving high yields of the appropriate surface antigens. The origin and passage history of virus strains shall be approved by the competent authority.

SUBSTRATE FOR VIRUS PROPAGATION

Influenza virus seed to be used in the production of vaccine is propagated in fertilised eggs from chicken flocks free from specified pathogens (SPF) *(5.2.2)* or in suitable cell cultures *(5.2.4)*, such as chick-embryo fibroblasts or chick kidney cells obtained from SPF chicken flocks *(5.2.2)*. For production, the virus of each strain is grown in the allantoic cavity of fertilised hens' eggs from healthy flocks.

VIRUS SEED LOT

The production of vaccine is based on a seed-lot system. Working seed lots represent not more than 15 passages from the approved reassorted virus or the approved virus isolate. The final vaccine represents 1 passage from the working seed lot. The haemagglutinin and neuraminidase antigens of each seed lot are identified as originating from the correct strain of influenza virus by suitable methods.

Only a working virus seed lot that complies with the following requirements may be used in the preparation of the monovalent pooled harvest.

Bacterial and fungal contamination

Carry out the test for sterility *(2.6.1)*, using 10 mL for each medium.

Mycoplasmas *(2.6.7)*

Carry out the test for mycoplasmas, using 10 mL.

VIRUS PROPAGATION AND HARVEST

An antimicrobial agent may be added to the inoculum. After incubation at a controlled temperature, the allantoic fluids are harvested and combined to form a monovalent pooled harvest. An antimicrobial agent may be added at the time of harvest. At no stage in the production is penicillin or streptomycin used.

MONOVALENT POOLED HARVEST

To limit the possibility of contamination, inactivation is initiated as soon as possible after preparation. The virus is inactivated by a method that has been demonstrated on 3 consecutive batches to be consistently effective for the manufacturer. The inactivation process shall have been shown to be capable of inactivating the influenza virus without destroying its antigenicity; the process should cause minimum alteration of the haemagglutinin and neuraminidase antigens. The inactivation process shall also have been shown to be capable of inactivating avian leucosis viruses and mycoplasmas. If the monovalent pooled harvest is stored after inactivation, it is held at 5 ± 3 °C.

If formaldehyde solution is used, the concentration does not exceed 0.2 g/L of CH_2O at any time during inactivation; if betapropiolactone is used, the concentration does not exceed 0.1 per cent *V/V* at any time during inactivation.

Before or after the inactivation procedure, the monovalent pooled harvest is concentrated and purified by high-speed centrifugation or other suitable method and the virus particles are disrupted into component subunits by the use of approved procedures. For each new strain, a validation test is carried out to show that the monovalent bulk consists predominantly of disrupted virus particles.

Only a monovalent pooled harvest that complies with the following requirements may be used in the preparation of the final bulk vaccine.

Haemagglutinin antigen

Determine the content of haemagglutinin antigen by an immunodiffusion test *(2.7.1)*, by comparison with a haemagglutinin antigen reference preparation or with an antigen preparation calibrated against it[1] . Carry out the test at 20-25 °C.

For some vaccines, the physical form of the haemagglutinin particles prevents quantitative determination by immunodiffusion after inactivation of the virus. For these vaccines, a determination of haemagglutinin antigen is made on the monovalent pooled harvest before inactivation. The production process is validated to demonstrate suitable conservation of haemagglutinin antigen and a suitable tracer is used for formulation, for example, protein content.

Neuraminidase antigen

The presence and type of neuraminidase antigen are confirmed by suitable enzymatic or immunological methods on the first 3 monovalent pooled harvests from each working seed lot.

Sterility *(2.6.1)*

Carry out the test for sterility, using 10 mL for each medium.

Residual infectious virus

Carry out the test described below under Tests.

_____

[1] *Reference haemagglutinin antigens are available from the National Institute for Biological Standards and Control, Blanche Lane, South Mimms, Potters Bar, Hertfordshire, EN6 3QG, Great Britain*

Chemicals used for disruption

Tests are carried out on the monovalent pooled harvest for the chemicals used for disruption, the limits being approved by the competent authority.

FINAL BULK VACCINE

Appropriate quantities of the monovalent pooled harvests are blended to make the final bulk vaccine.

Only a final bulk vaccine that complies with the following requirements may be used in the preparation of the final lot.

Antimicrobial preservative

Where applicable, determine the amount of antimicrobial preservative by a suitable chemical method. The content is not less than 85 per cent and not greater than 115 per cent of the intended amount.

Sterility (2.6.1)

Carry out the test for sterility, using 10 mL for each medium.

FINAL LOT

The final bulk vaccine is distributed aseptically into sterile, tamper-proof containers. The containers are closed so as to prevent contamination.

Only a final lot that is satisfactory with respect to each of the requirements given below under Tests and Assay may be released for use. Provided that the test for residual infectious virus has been performed with satisfactory results on each monovalent pooled harvest and that the tests for free formaldehyde, ovalbumin and total protein have been performed with satisfactory results on the final bulk vaccine, they may be omitted on the final lot.

IDENTIFICATION

The assay serves to confirm the antigenic specificity of the vaccine.

TESTS

Residual infectious virus

Inoculate 0.2 mL of the vaccine into the allantoic cavity of each of 10 fertilised eggs and incubate at 33-37 °C for 3 days. The test is not valid unless at least 8 of the 10 embryos survive. Harvest 0.5 mL of the allantoic fluid from each surviving embryo and pool the fluids. Inoculate 0.2 mL of the pooled fluid into a further 10 fertilised eggs and incubate at 33-37 °C for 3 days. The test is not valid unless at least 8 of the 10 embryos survive. Harvest about 0.1 mL of the allantoic fluid from each surviving embryo and examine each individual harvest for live virus by a haemagglutination test. If haemagglutination is found for any of the fluids, carry out for that fluid a further passage in eggs and test for haemagglutination; no haemagglutination occurs.

Antimicrobial preservative

Where applicable, determine the amount of antimicrobial preservative by a suitable chemical method. The content is not less than the minimum amount shown to be effective and is not greater than 115 per cent of the quantity stated on the label.

Free formaldehyde (2.4.18)

Maximum 0.2 g/L, where applicable.

Ovalbumin

Not more than the quantity stated on the label and in any case not more than 1 µg per human dose, determined by a suitable immunochemical method (2.7.1) using a suitable reference preparation of ovalbumin.

Total protein

Not more than 6 times the total haemagglutinin content of the vaccine as determined in the assay, but in any case, not

more than 100 µg of protein per virus strain per human dose and not more than a total of 300 µg of protein per human dose.

Sterility (2.6.1)

It complies with the test for sterility.

Bacterial endotoxins (2.6.14)

Less than 100 IU per human dose.

ASSAY

Determine the content of haemagglutinin antigen by an immunodiffusion test (2.7.1), by comparison with a haemagglutinin antigen reference preparation or with an antigen preparation calibrated against it[1]. Carry out the test at 20-25 °C. The confidence limits ($P = 0.95$) are not less than 80 per cent and not more than 125 per cent of the estimated haemagglutinin antigen content. The lower confidence limit ($P = 0.95$) is not less than 80 per cent of the amount stated on the label for each strain.

For some vaccines, quantitative determination of haemagglutinin antigen with respect to available reference preparations is not possible. An immunological identification of the haemagglutinin antigen and a semi-quantitative determination are carried out instead by suitable methods.

LABELLING

The label states:
— that the vaccine has been prepared on eggs,
— the strain or strains of influenza virus used to prepare the vaccine,
— the method of inactivation,
— the haemagglutinin content in micrograms per virus strain per dose,
— the maximum amount of ovalbumin,
— the season during which the vaccine is intended to protect.

_____ _Ph Eur_

Inactivated Influenza Vaccine (Surface Antigen)

(Influenza Vaccine (Surface Antigen, Inactivated), Ph Eur monograph 0869)

The label may state 'Flu' or 'Flu(adj)' as appropriate.

When Inactivated Influenza Vaccine or Influenza Vaccine is prescribed or demanded and the form is not stated, Inactivated Influenza Vaccine (Whole Virion), Inactivated Influenza Vaccine (Split Virion) or Inactivated Influenza Vaccine (Surface Antigen) may be dispensed or supplied.

Ph Eur _____

DEFINITION

Influenza vaccine (surface antigen, inactivated) is a sterile suspension of a strain or strains of influenza virus, type A or B, or a mixture of strains of the 2 types grown individually in fertilised hens' eggs, inactivated and treated so that the preparation consists predominantly of haemagglutinin and neuraminidase antigens, without diminishing the antigenic properties of these antigens. The stated amount of haemagglutinin antigen for each strain present in the vaccine

_____
[1] _Reference haemagglutinin antigens are available from the National Institute for Biological Standards and Control, Blanche Lane, South Mimms, Potters Bar, Hertfordshire, EN6 3QG, Great Britain_

IMMUNOLOGICAL PRODUCTS

is 15 µg per dose, unless clinical evidence supports the use of a different amount. The vaccine may contain an adjuvant.

PRODUCTION

The production method is validated to demonstrate that the product, if tested, would comply with the test for abnormal toxicity for immunosera and vaccines for human use (2.6.9).

CHOICE OF VACCINE STRAIN

The World Health Organisation reviews the world epidemiological situation annually and if necessary recommends the strains that correspond to this epidemiological evidence.

Such strains are used in accordance with the regulations in force in the signatory states of the Convention on the Elaboration of a European Pharmacopoeia. It is now common practice to use reassorted strains giving high yields of the appropriate surface antigens. The origin and passage history of virus strains shall be approved by the competent authority.

SUBSTRATE FOR VIRUS PROPAGATION

Influenza virus seed to be used in the production of vaccine is propagated in fertilised eggs from chicken flocks free from specified pathogens (SPF) (5.2.2) or in suitable cell cultures (5.2.4), such as chick-embryo fibroblasts or chick kidney cells obtained from SPF chicken flocks (5.2.2). For production, the virus of each strain is grown in the allantoic cavity of fertilised hens' eggs from healthy flocks.

VIRUS SEED LOT

The production of vaccine is based on a seed-lot system. Working seed lots represent not more than 15 passages from the approved reassorted virus or the approved virus isolate. The final vaccine represents one passage from the working seed lot. The haemagglutinin and neuraminidase antigens of each seed lot are identified as originating from the correct strain of influenza virus by suitable methods.

Only a working virus seed lot that complies with the following requirements may be used in the preparation of the monovalent pooled harvest.

Bacterial and fungal contamination
Carry out the test for sterility (2.6.1), using 10 mL for each medium.

Mycoplasmas (2.6.7)
Carry out the test for mycoplasmas, using 10 mL.

VIRUS PROPAGATION AND HARVEST

An antimicrobial agent may be added to the inoculum. After incubation at a controlled temperature, the allantoic fluids are harvested and combined to form a monovalent pooled harvest. An antimicrobial agent may be added at the time of harvest. At no stage in the production is penicillin or streptomycin used.

MONOVALENT POOLED HARVEST

To limit the possibility of contamination, inactivation is initiated as soon as possible after preparation. The virus is inactivated by a method that has been demonstrated on 3 consecutive batches to be consistently effective for the manufacturer. The inactivation process shall have been shown to be capable of inactivating the influenza virus without destroying its antigenicity; the process should cause minimum alteration of the haemagglutinin and neuraminidase antigens. The inactivation process shall also have been shown to be capable of inactivating avian leucosis viruses and mycoplasmas. If the monovalent pooled harvest is stored after inactivation, it is held at 5 ± 3 °C.

If formaldehyde solution is used, the concentration does not exceed 0.2 g/L of CH_2O at any time during inactivation; if betapropiolactone is used, the concentration does not exceed 0.1 per cent V/V at any time during inactivation.

Before or after the inactivation process, the monovalent pooled harvest is concentrated and purified by high-speed centrifugation or other suitable method. Virus particles are disrupted into component subunits by approved procedures and further purified so that the monovalent bulk consists mainly of haemagglutinin and neuraminidase antigens.

Only a monovalent pooled harvest that complies with the following requirements may be used in the preparation of the final bulk vaccine.

Haemagglutinin antigen
Determine the content of haemagglutinin antigen by an immunodiffusion test (2.7.1), by comparison with a haemagglutinin antigen reference preparation or with an antigen preparation calibrated against it [1]. Carry out the test at 20-25 °C.

Neuraminidase antigen
The presence and type of neuraminidase antigen are confirmed by suitable enzymatic or immunological methods on the first 3 monovalent pooled harvests from each working seed lot.

Sterility (2.6.1)
Carry out the test for sterility, using 10 mL for each medium.

Residual infectious virus
Carry out the test described below under Tests.

Purity
The purity of the monovalent pooled harvest is examined by polyacrylamide gel electrophoresis or by other approved techniques. Mainly haemagglutinin and neuraminidase antigens shall be present.

Chemicals used for disruption and purification
Tests are carried out on the monovalent pooled harvest for the chemicals used for disruption and purification, the limits being approved by the competent authority.

FINAL BULK VACCINE

Appropriate quantities of the monovalent pooled harvests are blended to make the final bulk vaccine. An adjuvant may be added.

Only a final bulk vaccine that complies with the following requirements may be used in the preparation of the final lot.

Antimicrobial preservative
Where applicable, determine the amount of antimicrobial preservative by a suitable chemical method. The content is not less than 85 per cent and not greater than 115 per cent of the intended amount.

Sterility (2.6.1)
Carry out the test for sterility, using 10 mL for each medium.

FINAL LOT

The final bulk vaccine is distributed aseptically into sterile, tamper-proof containers. The containers are closed so as to prevent contamination.

Only a final lot that is satisfactory with respect to each of the requirements given below under Tests and Assay may be released for use. Provided that the test for residual infectious virus has been performed with satisfactory results on each

---

[1] *Reference haemagglutinin antigens are available from the National Institute for Biological Standards and Control, Blanche Lane, South Mimms, Potters Bar, Hertfordshire, EN6 3QG, Great Britain*

monovalent pooled harvest and that the tests for free formaldehyde, ovalbumin and total protein have been performed with satisfactory results on the final bulk vaccine, they may be omitted on the final lot.

If the ovalbumin and formaldehyde content cannot be determined on the final lot, owing to interference from the adjuvant, they are determined on the monovalent pooled harvest, the acceptance limits being set to ensure that the limits for the final product will not be exceeded.

If the vaccine contains an adjuvant, suitable tests for identity and other relevant quality criteria are carried out on the final lot. These tests may include chemical and physical analysis, determination of particle size and determination of the number of particles per unit volume.

IDENTIFICATION

The assay serves to confirm the antigenic specificity of the vaccine.

TESTS

Residual infectious virus

Inoculate 0.2 mL of the vaccine into the allantoic cavity of each of 10 fertilised eggs and incubate at 33-37 °C for 3 days. The test is not valid unless at least 8 of the 10 embryos survive. Harvest 0.5 mL of the allantoic fluid from each surviving embryo and pool the fluids. Inoculate 0.2 mL of the pooled fluid into a further 10 fertilised eggs and incubate at 33-37 °C for 3 days. The test is not valid unless at least 8 of the 10 embryos survive. Harvest about 0.1 mL of the allantoic fluid from each surviving embryo and examine each individual harvest for live virus by a haemagglutination test. If haemagglutination is found for any of the fluids, carry out for that fluid a further passage in eggs and test for haemagglutination; no haemagglutination occurs.

Antimicrobial preservative

Where applicable, determine the amount of antimicrobial preservative by a suitable chemical method. The content is not less than the minimum amount shown to be effective and is not greater than 115 per cent of the quantity stated on the label.

Free formaldehyde (2.4.18)

Maximum 0.2 g/L, where applicable.

Ovalbumin

Not more than the quantity stated on the label and in any case not more than 1 μg per human dose, determined by a suitable immunochemical method (2.7.1) using a suitable reference preparation of ovalbumin.

Total protein

Not more than 40 μg of protein other than haemagglutinin per virus strain per human dose and not more than a total of 120 μg of protein other than haemagglutinin per human dose.

Sterility

It complies with the test for sterility (2.6.1).

Bacterial endotoxins (2.6.14)

Less than 100 IU per human dose.

ASSAY

Determine the content of haemagglutinin antigen by an immunodiffusion test (2.7.1), by comparison with a haemagglutinin antigen reference preparation or with an antigen preparation calibrated against it [1]. Carry out the test

---

[1] *Reference haemagglutinin antigens are available from the National Institute for Biological Standards and Control, Blanche Lane, South Mimms, Potters Bar, Hertfordshire, EN6 3QG, Great Britain*

at 20-25 °C. The confidence limits ($P = 0.95$) are not less than 80 per cent and not more than 125 per cent of the estimated content. The lower confidence limit ($P = 0.95$) haemagglutinin antigen is not less than 80 per cent of the amount stated on the label for each strain.

LABELLING

The label states:
— that the vaccine has been prepared on eggs,
— the strain or strains of influenza virus used to prepare the vaccine,
— the method of inactivation,
— the haemagglutinin content in micrograms per virus strain per dose,
— the season during which the vaccine is intended to protect,
— the maximum amount of ovalbumin,
— where applicable, the name and the quantity of adjuvant used.

_____ Ph Eur

Influenza Vaccine (Surface Antigen, Inactivated, Prepared in Cell Cultures)

(*Ph Eur monograph 2149*)

The label may state 'Flu' or 'Flu(adj)' as appropriate.

Ph Eur _____

DEFINITION

Influenza vaccine (surface antigen, inactivated, prepared in cell cultures) is a sterile, aqueous suspension of a strain or strains of influenza virus, type A or B, or a mixture of strains of the 2 types grown individually in cell cultures, inactivated and treated so that the preparation consists predominantly of haemagglutinin and neuraminidase antigens, preserving adequate antigenic properties of these antigens. The stated amount of haemagglutinin antigen for each strain present in the vaccine is 15 μg per dose, unless clinical evidence supports the use of a different amount. The vaccine is a clear or slightly opalescent liquid. The vaccine may contain an adjuvant. This monograph applies to vaccines produced in diploid or continuous cell lines of mammalian origin.

PRODUCTION

GENERAL PROVISIONS

Production of the vaccine is based on a virus seed-lot system and a cell-bank system. The production method shall have been shown to yield consistently vaccines that comply with the requirements for immunogenicity, safety and stability.

The production method is validated to demonstrate that the product, if tested, would comply with the test for abnormal toxicity for immunosera and vaccines for human use (2.6.9).

The production method is validated to demonstrate suitable reduction of residual host-cell protein. With the agreement of the competent authority and for each specific product, routine testing for residual host-cell proteins may be omitted based on the results of validation studies for the product. Guidance on the principles of such validation studies is given, for example, in the monograph *Products of recombinant DNA technology (0784)*, in particular in the sections 'Validation of the production process - Extraction and purification' and 'Production consistency - Host-cell-derived proteins'.

CHOICE OF VACCINE STRAIN
The World Health Organisation reviews the world epidemiological situation annually and if necessary recommends new strains corresponding to this epidemiological evidence.

Such strains are used in accordance with the regulations in force in the signatory states of the Convention on the Elaboration of a European Pharmacopoeia. It is now common practice to use reassorted strains giving high yields of the appropriate surface antigens. The origin and passage history of virus strains shall be approved by the competent authority.

SUBSTRATE FOR VIRUS PROPAGATION
Influenza virus used in the preparation of seed lots is propagated in fertilised eggs from chicken flocks free from specified pathogens (SPF) (5.2.2) or in suitable cell cultures (5.2.3), such as chick-embryo fibroblasts, chick kidney cells obtained from SPF chicken flocks (5.2.2), or a diploid or continuous cell line. The final passage for establishment of the working seed lot is prepared in the cell line used for routine production. For this production, the virus of each strain is propagated in a diploid or continuous cell line (5.2.3).

VIRUS SEED LOT
The production of vaccine is based on a seed-lot system. Each of the strains of influenza virus used shall be identified by historical records that include information on the origin of the strain and its subsequent manipulation. Working seed lots represent not more than 15 passages from the approved reassorted virus or the approved virus isolate. The final vaccine represents 1 passage from the working seed lot.

Only a seed lot that complies with the following requirements may be used for virus propagation.

Identification
The haemagglutinin and neuraminidase antigens of each master and working seed lot are identified as originating from the correct strain of influenza virus by suitable methods.

Virus concentration
The virus concentration of each working seed lot is determined. Where applicable, the virus concentration of each master seed lot is determined.

Extraneous agents (2.6.16)
The working seed lots comply with the requirements for seed lots. It is recognised that due to a seasonal change in one or more of the influenza vaccine strains, timely testing of a virus seed for extraneous agents according to general chapter 2.6.16 may be problematic (e.g. duration of in vivo tests, timely availability of specific neutralising antisera).

In agreement with the competent authority, and in light of a risk assessment, rapid assays (e.g. multiplex PCR) may be applied as alternatives to general chapter 2.6.16 following validation.

Such risk assessment and validation includes more general considerations on potential contaminants of the virus isolates, the susceptibility of the cell substrate to such viruses and the capacity of the production process for viral removal or inactivation; validation includes also comparative data on testing of seeds according to general chapter 2.6.16 and the proposed rapid assays. Each applied PCR/NAT test (2.6.21) must be shown to be suitable for its intended use by appropriate analytical validation. The risk assessment is reviewed when new information becomes available on potential viral contaminants, and the justification of the chosen PCR panel of extraneous agents tested for is provided to the competent authority within the annual update. This update also includes vaccine strain-specific aspects such as specific PCR inhibitory effects.

If an agent is detected in a virus seed and the mammalian cells used for production are shown to be susceptible to this agent, the virus seed is not used for vaccine production.

If an agent is detected in a virus seed and the mammalian cells are not susceptible to the agent, validation of the production process to demonstrate removal or inactivation of the agent is carried out. If removal or inactivation cannot be demonstrated, the inactivated monovalent harvest is tested to demonstrate absence of any contaminant identified in the virus seed.

PROPAGATION AND SINGLE HARVEST
All processing of the cell bank and subsequent cell cultures is done under aseptic conditions in an area where no other cells are being handled at the same time. Approved animal serum (but not human serum) may be used in the cell culture media. Serum and trypsin used in the preparation of cell suspensions or media are shown to be free from extraneous agents. The cell culture media may contain a pH indicator, such as phenol red, and antibiotics at the lowest effective concentration. Not less than 500 mL of the cell cultures employed for vaccine production are set aside as uninfected cell cultures (control cells).

Only a single harvest that complies with the following requirements may be used in the preparation of the vaccine.

Identification
The test for antigen content also serves to identify the single harvest.

Bacterial and fungal contamination
Carry out the test for sterility (2.6.1), using 10 mL for each medium.

Mycoplasmas (2.6.7)
Carry out the test for mycoplasmas, using 10 mL for each medium.

Control cells
The control cells of the production cell culture comply with a test for identification and the requirements for extraneous agents (2.6.16).

Haemagglutinin antigen
Determine the haemagglutinin antigen content by a suitable immunochemical method (2.7.1).

INACTIVATED AND PURIFIED MONOVALENT HARVEST
The harvest, which may be a pool of several single harvests of the same strain, is inactivated and purified by validated methods. Before or after the inactivation process, the monovalent harvest is concentrated and purified by high-speed centrifugation or another suitable method.

The influenza virus is inactivated by a method that has been demonstrated on 3 consecutive batches to be consistently effective for the manufacturer. The inactivation process shall have been shown to be capable of inactivating the influenza virus without destroying its antigenicity; the process is designed so as to cause minimum alteration of the haemagglutinin and neuraminidase antigens.

Virus particles are disrupted into component subunits by approved procedures and further purified so that the monovalent bulk consists mainly of haemagglutinin and neuraminidase antigens.

If continuous cell lines are used for production, the purification process shall have been validated to reduce consistently host-cell DNA to a suitable level.

Only an inactivated, purified monovalent harvest that complies with the following requirements may be used in the preparation of the final bulk vaccine.

Haemagglutinin antigen
Determine the haemagglutinin antigen content by a suitable immunochemical method (*2.7.1*).

Antigen/total protein ratio
Determine the haemagglutinin antigen content by a suitable immunodiffusion test. Determine the total protein by a validated method. The ratio of haemagglutinin antigen content to total protein content is within the limits approved for the particular product.

Neuraminidase antigen
The presence and type of neuraminidase antigen are confirmed by suitable enzymatic or immunological methods on the first 3 monovalent harvests from each working seed lot.

Sterility (*2.6.1*)
Carry out the test for sterility, using 10 mL for each medium.

Residual infectious virus
Carry out the test described below under Tests.

Purity
The purity of the monovalent harvest is examined by polyacrylamide gel electrophoresis or by other approved techniques. Mainly haemagglutinin and neuraminidase antigens are present.

Chemicals used for disruption and purification
Tests are carried out on the monovalent harvest for the chemicals used for disruption and purification, unless validation of the process has demonstrated total clearance. The concentration must not exceed the limits approved by the competent authority for the particular product.

FINAL BULK VACCINE
Appropriate quantities of the inactivated, purified monovalent pooled harvests are blended to make the final bulk vaccine. An adjuvant may be added.

Only a final bulk vaccine that complies with the following requirements may be used in the preparation of the final lot.

Antimicrobial preservative
Where applicable, determine the amount of antimicrobial preservative by a suitable chemical method. The content is not less than 85 per cent and not greater than 115 per cent of the intended amount.

Sterility (*2.6.1*)
Carry out the test for sterility, using 10 mL for each medium.

Residual host-cell DNA
If a continuous cell line is used for virus propagation, the content of residual host-cell DNA, determined using a suitable method, is not greater than 10 ng in the equivalent of a single human dose.

FINAL LOT
The final bulk vaccine is distributed aseptically into sterile, tamper-proof containers. The containers are closed so as to prevent contamination.

Only a final lot that is satisfactory with respect to each of the requirements given below under Tests and Assay may be released for use. Provided that the test for residual infectious virus has been performed with satisfactory results on each inactivated and purified monovalent harvest and that the tests for free formaldehyde, bovine serum albumin and total

protein have been performed with satisfactory results on the final bulk vaccine, they may be omitted on the final lot.

If the vaccine contains an adjuvant, suitable tests for identity and other relevant quality criteria are carried out on the final lot. These tests may include chemical and physical analysis, determination of particle size and determination of the number of particles per unit volume.

IDENTIFICATION
The assay serves to confirm the antigenic specificity of the vaccine.

TESTS
Residual infectious virus
Carry out an amplification test for residual infectious influenza virus by inoculating not less than 0.2 mL of the vaccine into cell cultures of the same type as used for production of the vaccine; incubate for not less than 4 days at 37 °C. Inoculate not less than 0.2 mL of the cell culture harvested medium into a new semiconfluent cell culture and incubate as before. At the end of the incubation period, examine for live virus by a haemagglutination test.
If haemagglutination is found for any of the fluids, carry out for that fluid a further passage on cell cultures and test for haemagglutination; no haemagglutination occurs.

Antimicrobial preservative
Where applicable, determine the amount of antimicrobial preservative by a suitable chemical method. The content is not less than the minimum amount shown to be effective and is not greater than 115 per cent of the quantity stated on the label.

Free formaldehyde (*2.4.18*)
Maximum 0.2 g/L, where applicable.

Bovine serum albumin
Maximum 50 ng per human dose, determined by a suitable immunochemical method (*2.7.1*).

Total protein
Maximum 40 μg of protein other than haemagglutinin per virus strain per human dose.

Sterility (*2.6.1*)
It complies with the test for sterility.

Bacterial endotoxins (*2.6.14*)
Less than 25 IU per human dose.

ASSAY
Determine the content of haemagglutinin antigen by an immunodiffusion test (*2.7.1*), by comparison with a haemagglutinin antigen reference preparation [1] or with an antigen preparation calibrated against it. Carry out the test at 20-25 °C. The confidence limits ($P = 0.95$) are not less than 80 per cent and not more than 125 per cent of the estimated content. The lower confidence limit ($P = 0.95$) is not less than 80 per cent of the amount stated on the label for each strain.

LABELLING
The label states:
— the biological origin of the cells used for the preparation of the vaccine;
— the strain or strains of influenza virus used to prepare the vaccine;
— the method of inactivation;

IMMUNOLOGICAL PRODUCTS

[1] *Reference haemagglutinin antigens are available from the National Institute for Biological Standards and Control, Blanche Lane, South Mimms, Potters Bar, Hertfordshire, EN6 3QG, Great Britain*

- the haemagglutinin antigen content in micrograms per virus strain per dose;
- the season during which the vaccine is intended to protect;
- where applicable, the name and the quantity of adjuvant used.

———————————————— Ph Eur

Influenza Vaccine (Surface Antigen, Inactivated, Virosome)

(Ph Eur monograph 2053)

The label may state 'Flu'.

Ph Eur ————————————————

DEFINITION

Influenza vaccine (surface antigen, inactivated, virosome) is a sterile, aqueous suspension of a strain or strains of influenza virus, type A or B, or a mixture of strains of the 2 types grown individually in fertilised hens' eggs, inactivated and treated so that the preparation consists predominantly of haemagglutinin and neuraminidase antigens reconstituted to virosomes and without diminishing the antigenic properties of the antigens. The stated amount of haemagglutinin antigen for each strain present in the vaccine is 15 μg per dose, unless clinical evidence supports the use of a different amount.

The vaccine is a slightly opalescent liquid.

PRODUCTION

GENERAL PROVISIONS

The production method is validated to demonstrate that the product, if tested, would comply with the test for abnormal toxicity for immunosera and vaccines for human use (2.6.9).

CHOICE OF VACCINE STRAIN

The World Health Organisation reviews the world epidemiological situation annually and if necessary recommends the strains that correspond to this epidemiological evidence.

Such strains are used in accordance with the regulations in force in the signatory states of the Convention on the Elaboration of a European Pharmacopoeia. It is now common practice to use reassorted strains giving high yields of the appropriate surface antigens. The origin and passage history of virus strains shall be approved by the competent authority.

SUBSTRATE FOR VIRUS PROPAGATION

Influenza virus seed to be used in the production of vaccine is propagated in fertilised eggs from chicken flocks free from specified pathogens (SPF) (5.2.2) or in suitable cell cultures (5.2.4), such as chick-embryo fibroblasts or chick kidney cells obtained from SPF chicken flocks (5.2.2). For production, the virus of each strain is grown in the allantoic cavity of fertilised hens' eggs from healthy flocks.

VIRUS SEED LOT

The production of vaccine is based on a seed lot system. Working seed lots represent not more than 15 passages from the approved reassorted virus or the approved virus isolate. The final vaccine represents 1 passage from the working seed lot. The haemagglutinin and neuraminidase antigens of each seed lot are identified as originating from the correct strain of influenza virus by suitable methods.

Only a working virus seed lot that complies with the following requirements may be used in the preparation of the monovalent pooled harvest.

Bacterial and fungal contamination

Carry out the test for sterility (2.6.1), using 10 mL for each medium.

Mycoplasmas (2.6.7)

Carry out the test for mycoplasmas, using 10 mL.

VIRUS PROPAGATION AND HARVEST

An antimicrobial agent may be added to the inoculum. After incubation at a controlled temperature, the allantoic fluids are harvested and combined to form a monovalent pooled harvest. An antimicrobial agent may be added at the time of harvest.

MONOVALENT POOLED HARVEST

To limit the possibility of contamination, inactivation is initiated as soon as possible after preparation. The virus is inactivated by a method that has been demonstrated on 3 consecutive batches to be consistently effective for the manufacturer. The inactivation process shall have been shown to be capable of inactivating the influenza virus without destroying its antigenicity; the process is designed so as to cause minimum alteration of the haemagglutinin and neuraminidase antigens. The inactivation process shall also have been shown to be capable of inactivating avian leucosis viruses and mycoplasmas. If the monovalent pooled harvest is stored after inactivation, it is held at a temperature of 5 ± 3 °C. If formaldehyde solution is used, the concentration does not exceed 0.2 g/L of CH_2O at any time during inactivation; if betapropiolactone is used, the concentration does not exceed 0.1 per cent V/V at any time during inactivation.

Before or after the inactivation process, the monovalent pooled harvest is concentrated and purified by high-speed centrifugation or another suitable method.

Only a monovalent pooled harvest that complies with the following requirements may be used for the preparation of virosomes.

Provided the tests for haemagglutinin antigen, neuraminidase antigen and residual infectious virus have been carried out with satisfactory results on the monovalent virosomal preparation, they may be omitted on the monovalent pooled harvest when the manufacturing process is continuous between the monovalent pooled harvest and the monovalent virosomal preparation.

Haemagglutinin antigen

Determine the content of haemagglutinin antigen by an immunodiffusion test (2.7.1), by comparison with a haemagglutinin antigen reference preparation [1] or with an antigen preparation calibrated against it. Carry out the test at 20-25 °C.

Neuraminidase antigen

The presence and type of neuraminidase antigen are confirmed by suitable enzymatic or immunological methods on the first 3 monovalent pooled harvests from each working seed lot.

Residual infectious virus

Carry out the test described under Tests.

————————————————

[1] *Reference haemagglutinin antigens are available from the National Institute for Biological Standards and Control, Blanche Lane, South Mimms, Potters Bar, Hertfordshire, EN6 3QG, Great Britain*

PREPARATION OF MONOVALENT VIROSOMES
Virus particles are disrupted into component subunits by approved procedures and further purified so that the monovalent bulk consists mainly of haemagglutinin and neuraminidase antigens. Additional phospholipids may be added and virosomes may be formed by removal of the detergent either by adsorption chromatography or another suitable technique. Several monovalent virosomal preparations may be pooled.

Only a monovalent virosomal preparation that complies with the following requirements may be used in the preparation of the final bulk vaccine.

Haemagglutinin antigen
Determine the content of haemagglutinin antigen by an immunodiffusion test (2.7.1), by comparison with a haemagglutinin antigen reference preparation [1] or with an antigen preparation calibrated against it. Carry out the test at 20-25 °C.

Neuraminidase antigen
The presence and type of neuraminidase antigen are confirmed by suitable enzymatic or immunological methods on the first 3 virosomal preparations from each working seed lot.

Residual infectious virus
Carry out the test described under Tests. Provided this test has been carried out with satisfactory results on the monovalent pooled harvest, it may be omitted on the preparation of monovalent virosomes.

Sterility (2.6.1)
Carry out the test for sterility, using 10 mL for each medium.

Purity
The purity of the monovalent virosomal preparation is examined by polyacrylamide gel electrophoresis (2.2.31) or by other approved techniques. Mainly haemagglutinin and neuraminidase antigens are present.

Chemicals used for disruption and purification
Tests for the chemicals used for disruption and purification are carried out on the monovalent virosomal preparation, the limits being approved by the competent authority.

Phospholipids
The content and identity of the phospholipids are determined by suitable immunochemical or physico-chemical methods.

Ratio of haemagglutinin to phospholipid
The ratio of haemagglutinin content to phospholipid content is within the limits approved for the particular product.

Virosome size
The average virosome diameter, determined by a suitable method such as photon-correlation spectroscopy, is not less than 100 nm and not greater than 300 nm.
The polydispersity index is not greater than 0.4.

FINAL BULK VACCINE
Appropriate quantities of the monovalent virosomal preparations are blended to make the final bulk vaccine.

Only a final bulk vaccine that complies with the following requirements may be used in the preparation of the final lot.

Antimicrobial preservative
Where applicable, determine the amount of antimicrobial

[1] *Reference haemagglutinin antigens are available from the National Institute for Biological Standards and Control, Blanche Lane, South Mimms, Potters Bar, Hertfordshire, EN6 3QG, Great Britain*

preservative by a suitable chemical or physico-chemical method. The content is not less than 85 per cent and not greater than 115 per cent of the intended amount.

Sterility (2.6.1)
Carry out the test for sterility, using 10 mL for each medium.

FINAL LOT
The final bulk vaccine is distributed aseptically into sterile, tamper-proof containers. The containers are closed so as to prevent contamination.

Only a final lot that is satisfactory with respect to each of the requirements given under Tests and Assay may be released for use. Provided that the test for residual infectious virus has been performed with satisfactory results on each monovalent pooled harvest or, where appropriate, on the monovalent virosomal preparations, and that the tests for phospholipids, ratio of haemagglutinin to phospholipid, free formaldehyde, ovalbumin and total protein have been performed with satisfactory results on the final bulk vaccine, they may be omitted on the final lot.

IDENTIFICATION
The assay serves to confirm the antigenic specificity of the vaccine.

TESTS
Residual infectious virus
Inoculate 0.2 mL of the vaccine into the allantoic cavity of each of 10 fertilised eggs and incubate at 33-37 °C for 3 days. The test is not valid unless at least 8 of the 10 embryos survive. Harvest 0.5 mL of the allantoic fluid from each surviving embryo and pool the fluids. Inoculate 0.2 mL of the pooled fluid into a further 10 fertilised eggs and incubate at 33-37 °C for 3 days. The test is not valid unless at least 8 of the 10 embryos survive. Harvest about 0.1 mL of the allantoic fluid from each surviving embryo and examine each individual harvest for live virus by a haemagglutination test. If haemagglutination is found for any of the fluids, carry out for that fluid a further passage in eggs and test for haemagglutination; no haemagglutination occurs.

pH (2.2.3)
6.5 to 7.8

Phospholipids
The content and identity of the phospholipids is determined by a suitable immunochemical or physico-chemical method.

Ratio of haemagglutinin to phospholipid
The ratio of haemagglutinin content to phospholipid content is within the limits approved for the particular product.

Antimicrobial preservative
Where applicable, determine the amount of antimicrobial preservative by a suitable chemical or physico-chemical method. The content is not less than the minimum amount shown to be effective and is not greater than 115 per cent of the quantity stated on the label.

Free formaldehyde (2.4.18)
Maximum 0.2 g/L, where applicable.

Ovalbumin
Not more than the quantity stated on the label and in any case not more than 1 µg per human dose, determined by a suitable immunochemical method (2.7.1) using a suitable reference preparation of ovalbumin.

Total protein
Not more than 40 µg of protein other than haemagglutinin per virus strain per human dose, and not more than a total of 120 µg of protein other than hemagglutinin per human dose.

IMMUNOLOGICAL PRODUCTS

Sterility (2.6.1)

It complies with the test for sterility.

Virosome size

The average virosome diameter, determined by a suitable method such as photon-correlation spectroscopy, is not less than 100 nm and not greater than 300 nm.

The polydispersity index is not greater than 0.4.

Bacterial endotoxins (2.6.14)

Less than 100 IU per human dose.

ASSAY

Determine the content of haemagglutinin antigen by an immunodiffusion test (2.7.1), by comparison with a haemagglutinin antigen reference preparation [1] or with an antigen preparation calibrated against it. Carry out the test at 20-25 °C. The confidence limits (P = 0.95) are not less than 80 per cent and not more than 125 per cent of the estimated haemagglutinin antigen content. The lower confidence limit (P = 0.95) is not less than 80 per cent of the amount stated on the label for each strain.

LABELLING

The label states:

— that the vaccine has been prepared on eggs;
— the strain or strains of influenza virus used to prepare the vaccine;
— the method of inactivation;
— the haemagglutinin content, in micrograms per virus strain per dose;
— the maximum amount of ovalbumin;
— the season during which the vaccine is intended to protect.

Ph Eur

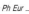

Measles Vaccine, Live

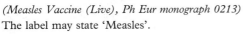

(Measles Vaccine (Live), Ph Eur monograph 0213)

The label may state 'Measles'.

Ph Eur

DEFINITION

Measles vaccine (live) is a freeze-dried preparation of a suitable attenuated strain of measles virus. The vaccine is reconstituted immediately before use, as stated on the label, to give a clear liquid that may be coloured owing to the presence of a pH indicator.

PRODUCTION

The production of vaccine is based on a virus seed-lot system and, if the virus is propagated in human diploid cells, a cell-bank system. The production method shall have been shown to yield consistently live measles vaccines of adequate immunogenicity and safety in man. Unless otherwise justified and authorised, the virus in the final vaccine shall have undergone no more passages from the master seed lot than were used to prepare the vaccine shown in clinical studies to be satisfactory with respect to safety and efficacy; even with authorised exceptions, the number of passages beyond the level used for clinical studies shall not exceed 5.

The potential neurovirulence of the vaccine strain is

considered during preclinical development, based on available epidemiological data on neurovirulence and neurotropism, primarily for the wild-type virus. In light of this, a risk analysis is carried out. Where necessary and if available, a test is carried out on the vaccine strain using an animal model that differentiates wild-type and attenuated virus; tests on strains of intermediate attenuation may also be needed.

The production method is validated to demonstrate that the product, if tested, would comply with the test for abnormal toxicity for immunosera and vaccines for human use (2.6.9).

SUBSTRATE FOR VIRUS PROPAGATION

The virus is propagated in human diploid cells (5.2.3) or in cultures of chick-embryo cells derived from a chicken flock free from specified pathogens (5.2.2).

SEED LOT

The strain of measles virus used shall be identified by historical records that include information on the origin of the strain and its subsequent manipulation. Virus seed lots are prepared in large quantities and stored at temperatures below − 20 °C if freeze-dried, or below − 60 °C if not freeze-dried.

Only a seed lot that complies with the following requirements may be used for virus propagation.

Identification

The master and working seed lots are identified as measles virus by serum neutralisation in cell culture, using specific antibodies.

Virus concentration

The virus concentration of the master and working seed lots is determined to monitor consistency of production.

Extraneous agents (2.6.16)

The working seed lot complies with the requirements for seed lots.

PROPAGATION AND HARVEST

All processing of the cell bank and subsequent cell cultures is done under aseptic conditions in an area where no other cells are handled during production. Suitable animal (but not human) serum may be used in the growth medium, but the final medium for maintaining cells during virus multiplication does not contain animal serum. Serum and trypsin used in the preparation of cell suspensions and culture media are shown to be free from extraneous agents. The cell culture medium may contain a pH indicator such as phenol red and suitable antibiotics at the lowest effective concentration. It is preferable to have a substrate free from antibiotics during production. Not less than 500 mL of the production cell cultures is set aside as uninfected cell cultures (control cells). The viral suspensions are harvested at a time appropriate to the strain of virus being used.

Only a single harvest that complies with the following requirements may be used in the preparation of the final bulk vaccine.

Identification

The single harvest contains virus that is identified as measles virus by serum neutralisation in cell culture, using specific antibodies.

Virus concentration

The virus concentration in the single harvest is determined as prescribed under Assay to monitor consistency of production and to determine the dilution to be used for the final bulk vaccine.

---

[1] *Reference haemagglutinin antigens are available from the National Institute for Biological Standards and Control, Blanche Lane, South Mimms, Potters Bar, Hertfordshire, EN6 3QG, Great Britain*

Extraneous agents (2.6.16)

The single harvest complies with the tests for extraneous agents.

Control cells

If human diploid cells are used for production, the control cells comply with a test for identification. They comply with the tests for extraneous agents (2.6.16).

FINAL BULK VACCINE

Virus harvests that comply with the above tests are pooled and clarified to remove cells. A suitable stabiliser may be added and the pooled harvests diluted as appropriate.

Only a final bulk vaccine that complies with the following requirement may be used in the preparation of the final lot.

Bacterial and fungal contamination

The final bulk vaccine complies with the test for sterility (2.6.1), carried out using 10 mL for each medium.

FINAL LOT

A minimum virus concentration for release of the product is established such as to ensure, in light of stability data, that the minimum concentration stated on the label will be present at the end of the period of validity.

Only a final lot that complies with the requirements for minimum virus concentration for release, with the following requirement for thermal stability and with each of the requirements given below under Identification and Tests may be released for use. Provided that the test for bovine serum albumin has been carried out with satisfactory results on the final bulk vaccine, it may be omitted on the final lot.

Thermal stability

Maintain at least 3 vials of the final lot of freeze-dried vaccine in the dry state at 37 ± 1 °C for 7 days. Determine the virus concentration as described under Assay in parallel for the heated vaccine and for vaccine stored at the temperature recommended for storage. The virus concentration of the heated vaccine is not more than 1.0 log lower than that of the unheated vaccine.

IDENTIFICATION

When the vaccine reconstituted as stated on the label is mixed with specific measles antibodies, it is no longer able to infect susceptible cell cultures.

TESTS

Bacterial and fungal contamination

The reconstituted vaccine complies with the test for sterility (2.6.1).

Bovine serum albumin

Not more than 50 ng per single human dose, determined by a suitable immunochemical method (2.7.1).

Water (2.5.12)

Not more than 3.0 per cent, determined by the semi-micro determination of water.

ASSAY

Titrate the vaccine for infective virus, using at least 3 separate vials of vaccine and inoculating a suitable number of wells for each dilution step. Titrate 1 vial of an appropriate virus reference preparation in triplicate to validate each assay. The virus concentration of the reference preparation is monitored using a control chart and a titre is established on a historical basis by each laboratory. The relation with the appropriate European Pharmacopoeia Biological Reference Preparation is established and monitored at regular intervals if a manufacturer's reference preparation is used. Calculate the individual virus concentration for each vial of vaccine and for each replicate

of the reference preparation as well as the corresponding combined virus concentrations, using the usual statistical methods (for example, 5.3). The combined estimate of the virus concentration for the 3 vials of vaccine is not less than that stated on the label; the minimum virus concentration stated on the label is not less than 3.0 log CCID$_{50}$ per single human dose.

The assay is not valid if:
— the confidence interval ($P = 0.95$) of the estimated virus concentration of the reference preparation for the 3 replicates combined is greater than $\pm$ 0.3 log CCID$_{50}$;
— the virus concentration of the reference preparation differs by more than 0.5 log CCID$_{50}$ from the established value.

The assay is repeated if the confidence interval ($P = 0.95$) of the combined virus concentration of the vaccine is greater than $\pm$ 0.3 log CCID$_{50}$; data obtained from valid assays only are combined by the usual statistical methods (for example, 5.3) to calculate the virus concentration of the sample.

The confidence interval ($P = 0.95$) of the combined virus concentration is not greater than $\pm$ 0.3 log CCID$_{50}$.

Measles vaccine (live) BRP is suitable for use as a reference preparation.

Where justified and authorised, different assay designs may be used; this may imply the application of different validity and acceptance criteria. However, the vaccine must comply if tested as described above.

LABELLING

The label states:
— the strain of virus used for the preparation of the vaccine;
— the type and origin of the cells used for the preparation of the vaccine;
— the minimum virus concentration;
— that contact between the vaccine and disinfectants is to be avoided.

Ph Eur

Measles, Mumps and Rubella Vaccine, Live

(Measles, Mumps and Rubella Vaccine (Live), Ph Eur monograph 1057)

The label may state 'MMR'.

Ph Eur

DEFINITION

Measles, mumps and rubella vaccine (live) is a freeze-dried preparation of suitable attenuated strains of measles virus, mumps virus and rubella virus.

The vaccine is reconstituted immediately before use, as stated on the label, to give a clear liquid that may be coloured owing to the presence of a pH indicator.

PRODUCTION

The 3 components are prepared as described in the monographs *Measles vaccine (live) (0213)*, *Mumps vaccine (live) (0538)* and *Rubella vaccine (live) (0162)* and comply with the requirements prescribed therein.

The production method is validated to demonstrate that the product, if tested, would comply with the test for abnormal toxicity for immunosera and vaccines for human use (2.6.9).

FINAL BULK VACCINE

Virus harvests for each component are pooled and clarified to remove cells. A suitable stabiliser may be added and the pooled harvests diluted as appropriate. Suitable quantities of the pooled harvest for each component are mixed.

Only a final bulk vaccine that complies with the following requirement may be used in the preparation of the final lot.

Bacterial and fungal contamination

Carry out the test for sterility (2.6.1), using 10 mL for each medium.

FINAL LOT

For each component, a minimum virus concentration for release of the product is established such as to ensure, in light of stability data, that the minimum concentration stated on the label will be present at the end of the period of validity.

Only a final lot that complies with the requirements for minimum virus concentration of each component for release, with the following requirement for thermal stability and with each of the requirements given below under Identification and Tests may be released for use. Provided that the tests for bovine serum albumin and, where applicable, for ovalbumin have been carried out with satisfactory results on the final bulk vaccine, they may be omitted on the final lot.

Thermal stability

Maintain at least 3 vials of the final lot of freeze-dried vaccine in the dry state at 37 ± 1 °C for 7 days. Determine the virus concentration as described under Assay in parallel for the heated vaccine and for vaccine stored at the temperature recommended for storage. For each component, the virus concentration of the heated vaccine is not more than 1.0 log lower than that of the unheated vaccine.

IDENTIFICATION

When the vaccine reconstituted as stated on the label is mixed with antibodies specific for measles virus, mumps virus and rubella virus, it is no longer able to infect cell cultures susceptible to these viruses. When the vaccine reconstituted as stated on the label is mixed with quantities of specific antibodies sufficient to neutralise any 2 viral components, the 3rd viral component infects susceptible cell cultures.

TESTS

Bacterial and fungal contamination

The reconstituted vaccine complies with the test for sterility (2.6.1).

Bovine serum albumin

Not more than 50 ng per single human dose, determined by a suitable immunochemical method (2.7.1).

Ovalbumin

If the mumps component is produced in chick embryos, the vaccine contains not more than 1 µg of ovalbumin per single human dose, determined by a suitable immunochemical method (2.7.1).

Water (2.5.12)

Not more than 3.0 per cent, determined by the semi-micro determination of water.

ASSAY

The cell lines and/or neutralising antisera are chosen to ensure that each component is assayed without interference from the other 2 components.

Titrate the vaccine for infective measles, mumps and rubella virus, using at least 3 separate vials of vaccine and inoculating a suitable number of wells for each dilution step. Titrate 1 vial of the appropriate virus reference preparation in triplicate to validate each assay. The virus concentration of the reference preparation is monitored using a control chart and a titre is established on a historical basis by each

laboratory. The relation with the appropriate European Pharmacopoeia Biological Reference Preparation is established and monitored at regular intervals if a manufacturer's reference preparation is used. Calculate the individual virus concentration for each vial of vaccine and for each replicate of the reference preparation as well as the corresponding combined virus concentrations, using the usual statistical methods (for example, 5.3).

The combined estimates of the measles, mumps and rubella virus concentrations for the 3 vials of vaccine are not less than that stated on the label; the minimum measles virus concentration stated on the label is not less than 3.0 log $CCID_{50}$ per single human dose; the minimum mumps virus concentration stated on the label is not less than 3.7 log $CCID_{50}$ per single human dose; the minimum rubella virus concentration stated on the label is not less than 3.0 log $CCID_{50}$ per single human dose.

The assay is not valid if:
— the confidence interval ($P = 0.95$) of the estimated virus concentration of the reference preparation for the 3 replicates combined is greater than $\pm$ 0.3 log $CCID_{50}$;
— the virus concentration of the reference preparation differs by more than 0.5 log $CCID_{50}$ from the established value.

The assay is repeated if the confidence interval ($P = 0.95$) of the combined virus concentration of the vaccine is greater than $\pm$ 0.3 log $CCID_{50}$; data obtained from valid assays only are combined by the usual statistical methods (for example, 5.3) to calculate the virus concentration of the sample. The confidence interval ($P = 0.95$) of the combined virus concentration is not greater than $\pm$ 0.3 log $CCID_{50}$.

Measles vaccine (live) BRP is suitable for use as a reference preparation.

Mumps vaccine (live) BRP is suitable for use as a reference preparation.

Rubella vaccine (live) BRP is suitable for use as a reference preparation.

Where justified and authorised, different assay designs may be used; this may imply the application of different validity and acceptance criteria. However, the vaccine must comply if tested as described above.

LABELLING

The label states:
— the strains of virus used in the preparation of the vaccine;
— where applicable, that chick embryos have been used for the preparation of the vaccine;
— the type and origin of the cells used for the preparation of the vaccine;
— the minimum virus concentration for each component of the vaccine;
— that contact between the vaccine and disinfectants is to be avoided.

_____ *Ph Eur*

Measles, Mumps, Rubella and Varicella Vaccine (Live)

(*Ph Eur monograph 2442*)

The label may state 'MMRVar'.

Ph Eur _____

DEFINITION

Measles, mumps, rubella and varicella vaccine (live) is a freeze-dried preparation of suitable attenuated strains of measles virus, mumps virus, rubella virus and human herpesvirus 3. The vaccine is reconstituted immediately before use, as stated on the label, to give a clear liquid that may be coloured owing to the presence of a pH indicator.

PRODUCTION

The 4 components are prepared as described in the monographs *Measles vaccine (live) (0213)*, *Mumps vaccine (live) (0538)*, *Rubella vaccine (live) (0162)* and *Varicella vaccine (live) (0648)* and comply with the requirements prescribed therein.

The production method is validated to demonstrate that the product, if tested, would comply with the test for abnormal toxicity for immunosera and vaccines for human use (*2.6.9*).

FINAL BULK VACCINE

Virus harvests for each component are pooled and clarified to remove cells. A suitable stabiliser may be added and for each component the pooled harvests diluted as appropriate. Suitable quantities of the pooled harvest for each component are mixed.

Only a final bulk vaccine that complies with the following requirement may be used in the preparation of the final lot.

Bacterial and fungal contamination

Carry out the test for sterility (*2.6.1*), using 10 mL for each medium.

FINAL LOT

For each component, a minimum virus concentration for release of the product is established such as to ensure, in light of stability data, that the minimum concentration stated on the label will be present at the end of the period of validity. The final bulk vaccine is distributed aseptically into sterile, tamper-proof containers and freeze-dried to a moisture content shown to be favourable to the stability of the vaccine. The containers are then closed so as to prevent contamination and the introduction of moisture.

Only a final lot that complies with the requirements for minimum virus concentration of each component for release, with the following requirements for thermal stability, bovine serum albumin and water, and with each of the requirements given under Identification and Tests may be released for use. Provided that the test for bovine serum albumin has been carried out with satisfactory results on the final bulk vaccine, it may be omitted on the final lot.

Thermal stability

For the measles, mumps and rubella components maintain at least 3 containers of the final lot of freeze-dried vaccine in the dry state at 37 ± 1 °C for 7 days. Determine the virus concentration as described under Assay in parallel for the heated vaccine and for vaccine stored at the temperature recommended for storage. For each component, the virus concentration of the heated vaccine is not more than 1.0 log lower than that of the unheated vaccine.

Bovine serum albumin

Not more than the amount approved by the competent authority, determined by a suitable immunochemical method (*2.7.1*).

Water (*2.5.12*)

Not more than the amount shown to ensure stability of the vaccines as approved by the competent authority, determined by the semi-micro determination of water.

IDENTIFICATION

When the vaccine reconstituted as stated on the label is mixed with antibodies specific for measles virus, mumps virus, rubella virus and human herpesvirus 3, it is no longer able to infect cell cultures susceptible to these viruses. When the vaccine reconstituted as stated on the label is mixed with quantities of specific antibodies sufficient to neutralise any 3 viral components, the 4th viral component infects susceptible cell cultures.

TESTS

Bacterial and fungal contamination

The reconstituted vaccine complies with the test for sterility (*2.6.1*).

ASSAY

The cell lines and/or neutralising antisera are chosen to ensure that each component is assayed without interference from the other 3 components.

Titrate the vaccine for infective measles virus, mumps virus, rubella virus and human herpesvirus 3 using at least 3 separate containers of vaccine and inoculating a suitable number of wells for each dilution step. Titrate 1 container of the appropriate virus reference preparation in triplicate to validate each assay. The virus concentration of the reference preparation is monitored using a control chart and a titre is established on a historical basis by each laboratory. Unless otherwise justified and authorised, for the measles, mumps, rubella and human herpesvirus 3 viruses the relation with the appropriate European Pharmacopoeia Biological Reference Preparation is established and monitored at regular intervals if a manufacturer's reference preparation is used. Calculate the individual virus concentration for each container of vaccine and for each replicate of the reference preparation as well as the corresponding combined virus concentrations, using the usual statistical methods (for example, *5.3*).

The combined estimates of the measles virus, mumps virus, rubella virus and human herpesvirus 3 concentrations for the 3 containers of vaccine are not less than that stated on the label; the minimum measles virus concentration stated on the label is not less than 3.0 log $CCID_{50}$ per single human dose; the minimum mumps virus concentration stated on the label is not less than 3.7 log $CCID_{50}$ per single human dose; the minimum rubella virus concentration stated on the label is not less than 3.0 log $CCID_{50}$ per single human dose.

The assay is not valid if:
— the confidence interval ($P = 0.95$) of the estimated virus concentration of the reference preparation for the 3 replicates combined is greater than $\pm$ 0.3 log $CCID_{50}$ (measles virus, mumps virus and rubella virus) or $\pm$ 0.3 log PFU (human herpesvirus 3);
— the virus concentration of the reference preparation differs by more than 0.5 log $CCID_{50}$ (measles virus, mumps virus and rubella virus) or 0.5 log PFU (human herpesvirus 3) from the established value.

The assay is repeated if the confidence interval ($P = 0.95$) of the combined virus concentration of the vaccine is greater than $\pm$ 0.3 log $CCID_{50}$ (measles virus, mumps virus and

IMMUNOLOGICAL PRODUCTS

rubella virus) or $\pm$ 0.3 log PFU (human herpesvirus 3); data obtained from valid assays only are combined by using the usual statistical methods (for example, 5.3) to calculate the virus concentration of the sample. The confidence interval ($P = 0.95$) of the combined virus concentration is not greater than $\pm$ 0.3 log CCID$_{50}$ (measles virus, mumps virus and rubella virus) or $\pm$ 0.3 log PFU (human herpesvirus 3).

Measles vaccine (live) BRP is suitable for use as a reference preparation.

Mumps vaccine (live) BRP is suitable for use as a reference preparation.

Rubella vaccine (live) BRP is suitable for use as a reference preparation.

Varicella vaccine (live) BRP is suitable for use as a reference preparation.

Where justified and authorised, different assay designs may be used; this may imply the application of different validity and acceptance criteria. However, the vaccine must comply if tested as described above.

LABELLING
The label states:
— the strains of virus used in the preparation of the vaccine;
— the type and origin of the cells used for the preparation of the vaccine;
— the minimum virus concentration for each component of the vaccine;
— that contact between the vaccine and disinfectants is to be avoided.

———————————————————— Ph Eur

Meningococcal Group C Conjugate Vaccine

(Ph Eur monograph 2112)
The label may state 'MenC(*conj*)'.

Ph Eur —————————————————————————

DEFINITION
Meningococcal group C conjugate vaccine is a liquid or freeze-dried preparation of purified capsular polysaccharide derived from a suitable strain of *Neisseria meningitidis* group C covalently linked to a carrier protein. Meningococcal group C polysaccharide consists of partly *O*-acetylated or *O*-deacetylated repeating units of sialic acids, linked with $2\alpha{\rightarrow}9$ glycosidic bonds. The carrier protein, when conjugated to group C polysaccharide, is capable of inducing a T-cell-dependent B-cell immune response to the polysaccharide. The vaccine may contain an adjuvant.

PRODUCTION
GENERAL PROVISIONS
The production method shall consistently have been shown to yield meningococcal group C conjugate vaccines of satisfactory immunogenicity and safety in man.
The production of meningococcal group C polysaccharide and of the carrier protein are based on seed-lot systems.
During development studies and wherever revalidation is necessary, a test for pyrogens in rabbits (*2.6.8*) is carried out by injection of a suitable dose of the final lot. The vaccine is shown to be acceptable with respect to absence of pyrogenic activity. The production method is validated to demonstrate that the vaccine, if tested, would comply with the test for

abnormal toxicity for immunosera and vaccines for human use (*2.6.9*).

During development studies and wherever revalidation of the manufacturing process is necessary, it shall be demonstrated by tests in animals that the vaccine consistently induces a T-cell-dependent B-cell immune response.

The stability of the final lot and relevant intermediates is evaluated using 1 or more indicator tests. Such tests may include determination of molecular size, determination of free saccharide in the conjugate or an immunogenicity test in animals.

BACTERIAL SEED LOTS
The bacterial strains used for master seed lots shall be identified by historical records that include information on their origin and the tests used to characterise the strain. Cultures from the working seed lot shall have the same characteristics as the strain that was used to prepare the master seed lot.

Purity of bacterial cultures is verified by methods of suitable sensitivity. These may include inoculation into suitable media, examination of colony morphology, microscopic examination of Gram-stained smears and culture agglutination with suitable specific antisera.

MENINGOCOCCAL GROUP C POLYSACCHARIDE
N. meningitidis is grown in a liquid medium that does not contain high-molecular-mass polysaccharides and is free from ingredients that will form a precipitate upon addition of cetyltrimethylammonium bromide (CTAB). The culture may be inactivated by heat and filtered before the polysaccharide is precipitated by addition of CTAB. The precipitate is further purified using suitable methods to remove nucleic acids, proteins and lipopolysaccharides and the final purification step consists of ethanol precipitation.

An *O*-deacetylation step may also be included. Volatile matter, including water, in the purified polysaccharide is determined by a suitable method such as thermogravimetry (*2.2.34*). The value is used to calculate the results of other tests with reference to the dried substance, as prescribed below.

Only meningococcal group C polysaccharide that complies with the following requirements may be used in the preparation of the conjugate.

Protein (*2.5.16*)
Maximum 1.0 per cent, calculated with reference to the dried substance.

Nucleic acid (*2.5.17*)
Maximum 1.0 per cent, calculated with reference to the dried substance.

O-acetyl groups
Examine by a suitable method (for example *2.5.19*).
An acceptable value is established for the particular product and each batch of meningococcal group C polysaccharide must be shown to comply with this limit.

Sialic acid (*2.5.23*)
Minimum 0.800 g of sialic acid per gram of meningococcal group C polysaccharide using *N-acetylneuraminic acid R* to prepare the reference solution.

Residual reagents
Where applicable, tests are carried out to determine residues of reagents used during inactivation and purification.
An acceptable value for each reagent is established for the particular product and each batch of meningococcal group C polysaccharide must be shown to comply with this limit.
Where validation studies have demonstrated removal of a

residual reagent, the test on purified meningococcal group C polysaccharide may be omitted.

Molecular-size distribution

Examine by size-exclusion chromatography (2.2.30). An acceptable value is established for the particular product and each batch of meningococcal group C polysaccharide must be shown to comply with this limit. Where applicable, the molecular-size distribution is also determined after chemical modification of the meningococcal group C polysaccharide.

Identification and serological specificity

The identity and serological specificity are determined by a suitable immunochemical method (2.7.1) or other suitable method, for example ^{1}H nuclear magnetic resonance spectrometry (2.2.33).

Bacterial endotoxins (2.6.14)

Less than 100 IU per microgram of meningococcal group C polysaccharide.

CARRIER PROTEIN

The carrier protein is chosen so that when meningococcal group C polysaccharide is conjugated it is able to induce a T-cell-dependent immune response. Tetanus toxoid and the non-toxic mutant of diphtheria toxin-like protein, CRM 197, are suitable. The carrier protein is produced by culture of a suitable microorganism, the bacterial purity of which is verified.

Only a carrier protein that complies with the following requirements may be used in preparation of the conjugate.

Identification

The carrier protein is identified by a suitable immunochemical method (2.7.1).

CRM 197

Where CRM 197 is used as the carrier protein, it is not less than 90 per cent pure, determined by a suitable method. Suitable tests are carried out, for validation or routinely, to demonstrate that the product is non-toxic.

Tetanus toxoid

Where tetanus toxoid is used as the carrier, it is produced as described in the monograph *Tetanus vaccine (adsorbed) (0452)* and complies with the requirements prescribed therein for bulk purified toxoid, except that the antigenic purity (2.7.27) is not less than 1500 Lf per milligram of protein nitrogen and that the test for sterility (2.6.1) is not required.

BULK CONJUGATE

Meningococcal group C polysaccharide is chemically modified to enable conjugation; it is usually partly depolymerised either before or during this procedure. The conjugate is obtained by the covalent bonding of activated meningococcal group C oligosaccharide and carrier protein. The conjugate purification procedures are designed to remove residual reagents used for conjugation. The removal of residual reagents and reaction by-products is confirmed by suitable tests or by validation of the purification process.

Only a bulk conjugate that complies with the following requirements may be used in the preparation of the final bulk vaccine. For each test and for each particular product, limits of acceptance are established and each batch of conjugate must be shown to comply with these limits.

Molecular-size distribution

Examine by size-exclusion chromatography (2.2.30). An acceptable value is established for the particular product and each batch of bulk conjugate must be shown to comply with this limit.

Saccharide

The saccharide content is determined by a suitable validated assay (for example 2.5.23). Anion-exchange liquid chromatography with pulsed amperometric detection (2.2.29) may also be used for determination of saccharide content. An acceptable value is established for the particular product and each batch of bulk conjugate must be shown to comply with this limit.

Protein

The protein content is determined by a suitable chemical method (for example 2.5.16). An acceptable value is established for the particular product and each batch of bulk conjugate must be shown to comply with this limit.

Saccharide-to-protein ratio

Determine the ratio by calculation.

Free saccharide

Unbound saccharide is determined after removal of the conjugate, for example by anion-exchange liquid chromatography, size-exclusion or hydrophobic chromatography, ultrafiltration or other validated methods. An acceptable value is established for the particular product and each batch of bulk conjugate must be shown to comply with this limit.

Free carrier protein

Determine the content, either directly by a suitable method or by deriving the content by calculation from the results of other tests. An acceptable value is established for the particular product and each batch of bulk conjugate must be shown to comply with this limit.

Residual reagents

Removal of residual reagents such as cyanide is confirmed by suitable tests or by validation of the process.

Sterility (2.6.1)

It complies with the test for sterility, carried out using 10 mL for each medium or the equivalent of 100 doses, whichever is less.

FINAL BULK VACCINE

An adjuvant and a stabiliser may be added to the bulk conjugate before dilution to the final concentration with a suitable diluent.

Only a final bulk vaccine that complies with the following requirement and is within the limits approved for the particular product may be used in preparation of the final lot.

Sterility (2.6.1)

It complies with the test for sterility, carried out using 10 mL for each medium.

FINAL LOT

Only a final lot that is within the limits approved for the particular product and is satisfactory with respect to each of the requirement given below under Identification, Tests, and Assay may be released for use.

IDENTIFICATION

The vaccine is identified by a suitable immunochemical method (2.7.1).

TESTS

pH (2.2.3)

The pH of the vaccine, reconstituted if necessary, is within $\pm$ 0.5 pH units of the limit approved for the particular product.

Aluminium (2.5.13)

Maximum 1.25 mg per single human dose, if aluminium hydroxide or hydrated aluminium phosphate is used as the adsorbent.

Water (2.5.12)

Maximum 3.0 per cent for freeze-dried vaccines.

Free saccharide

Unbound saccharide is determined after removal of the conjugate, for example by anion-exchange liquid chromatography, size-exclusion or hydrophobic chromatography, ultrafiltration or other validated methods. An acceptable value consistent with adequate immunogenicity, as shown in clinical trials, is established for the particular product and each final lot must be shown to comply with this limit.

Sterility (2.6.1)

It complies with the test for sterility.

Bacterial endotoxins (2.6.14)

Less than 25 IU per single human dose.

ASSAY

Saccharide

Minimum 80 per cent of the amount of meningococcal group C polysaccharide stated on the label. The saccharide content is determined by a suitable validated assay, for example sialic acid assay (2.5.23) or anion-exchange liquid chromatography with pulsed amperometric detection (2.2.29).

LABELLING

The label states:
— the number of micrograms of meningococcal group C polysaccharide per human dose;
— the type and number of micrograms of carrier protein per human dose.

Ph Eur

Meningococcal Polysaccharide Vaccine

(*Ph Eur monograph 0250*)

The label may state 'Men' plus relevant antigen. For example, 'MenAC'.

Ph Eur

DEFINITION

Meningococcal polysaccharide vaccine is a freeze-dried preparation of one or more purified capsular polysaccharides obtained from one or more suitable strains of *Neisseria meningitidis* group A, group C, group Y and group W135 that are capable of consistently producing polysaccharides.

N. meningitidis group A polysaccharide consists of partly *O*-acetylated repeating units of *N*-acetylmannosamine, linked with 1α→6 phosphodiester bonds.

N. meningitidis group C polysaccharide consists of partly *O*-acetylated repeating units of sialic acid, linked with 2α→9 glycosidic bonds.

N. meningitidis group Y polysaccharide consists of partly *O*-acetylated alternating units of sialic acid and D-glucose, linked with 2α→6 and 1α→4 glycosidic bonds.

N. meningitidis group W135 polysaccharide consists of partly *O*-acetylated alternating units of sialic acid and D-galactose, linked with 2α→6 and 1α→4 glycosidic bonds.

The polysaccharide component or components stated on the label together with calcium ions and residual moisture account for over 90 per cent of the mass of the preparation.

PRODUCTION

Production of the meningococcal polysaccharides is based on a seed-lot system. The production method shall have been shown to yield consistently meningococcal polysaccharide vaccines of satisfactory immunogenicity and safety in man.

The production method is validated to demonstrate that the product, if tested, would comply with the test for abnormal toxicity for immunosera and vaccines for human use (2.6.9).

SEED LOTS

The strains of *N. meningitidis* used for the master seed lots shall be identified by historical records that include information on their origin and by their biochemical and serological characteristics.

Cultures from each working seed lot shall have the same characteristics as the strain that was used to prepare the master seed lot. The strains have the following characteristics:
— colonies obtained from a culture are rounded, uniform in shape and smooth with a mucous, opalescent, greyish appearance,
— Gram staining reveals characteristic Gram-negative diplococci in "coffee-bean" arrangement,
— the oxidase test is positive,
— the culture utilises glucose and maltose,
— suspensions of the culture agglutinate with suitable specific antisera.

Purity of bacterial strains used for the seed lots is verified by methods of suitable sensitivity. These may include inoculation into suitable media, examination of colony morphology, microscopic examination of Gram-stained smears and culture agglutination with suitable specific antisera.

PROPAGATION AND HARVEST

The working seed lots are cultured on solid media that do not contain blood-group substances or ingredients of mammalian origin. The inoculum may undergo 1 or more subcultures in liquid medium before being used for inoculating the final medium. The liquid media used and the final medium are semisynthetic and free from substances precipitated by cetrimonium bromide (hexadecyltrimethylammonium bromide) and do not contain blood-group substances or high-molecular-mass polysaccharides.

The bacterial purity of the culture is verified by methods of suitable sensitivity. These may include inoculation into suitable media, examination of colony morphology, microscopic examination of Gram-stained smears and culture agglutination with suitable specific antisera.

The cultures are centrifuged and the polysaccharides precipitated from the supernatant by addition of cetrimonium bromide. The precipitate obtained is harvested and may be stored at − 20 °C awaiting further purification.

PURIFIED POLYSACCHARIDES

The polysaccharides are purified, after dissociation of the complex of polysaccharide and cetrimonium bromide, using suitable procedures to remove successively nucleic acids, proteins and lipopolysaccharides.

The final purification step consists of ethanol precipitation of the polysaccharides which are then dried and stored at − 20 °C. The loss on drying is determined by thermogravimetry (2.2.34) and the value is used to calculate the results of the other chemical tests with reference to the dried substance.

Only purified polysaccharides that comply with the following requirements may be used in the preparation of the final bulk vaccine.

Protein (2.5.16)
Not more than 10 mg of protein per gram of purified polysaccharide, calculated with reference to the dried substance.

Nucleic acids (2.5.17)
Not more than 10 mg of nucleic acids per gram of purified polysaccharide, calculated with reference to the dried substance.

O-Acetyl groups (2.5.19)
Not less than 2 mmol of O-acetyl groups per gram of purified polysaccharide for group A, not less than 1.5 mmol per gram of polysaccharide for group C, not less than 0.3 mmol per gram of polysaccharide for groups Y and W135, all calculated with reference to the dried substance.

Phosphorus (2.5.18)
Not less than 80 mg of phosphorus per gram of group A purified polysaccharide, calculated with reference to the dried substance.

Sialic acid (2.5.23)
Not less than 800 mg of sialic acid per gram of group C polysaccharide and not less than 560 mg of sialic acid per gram of purified polysaccharide for groups Y and W135, all calculated with reference to the dried substance. Use the following reference solutions.

Group C polysaccharide: a 150 mg/L solution of N-acetylneuraminic acid R.

Group Y polysaccharide: a solution containing 95 mg/L of N-acetylneuraminic acid R and 55 mg/L of glucose R.

Group W135 polysaccharide: a solution containing 95 mg/L of N-acetylneuraminic acid R and 55 mg/L of galactose R.

Calcium
If a calcium salt is used during purification, a determination of calcium is carried out on the purified polysaccharide; the content is within the limits approved for the particular product.

Distribution of molecular size
Examine by size-exclusion chromatography (2.2.30) using agarose for chromatography R or cross-linked agarose for chromatography R. Use a column about 0.9 m long and 16 mm in internal diameter equilibrated with a solvent having an ionic strength of 0.2 mol/kg and a pH of 7.0-7.5. Apply to the column about 2.5 mg of polysaccharide in a volume of about 1.5 mL and elute at about 20 mL/h. Collect fractions of about 2.5 mL and determine the content of polysaccharide by a suitable method. At least 65 per cent of group A polysaccharide, 75 per cent of group C polysaccharide, 80 per cent of group Y polysaccharide and 80 per cent of group W135 polysaccharide is eluted before a distribution coefficient (K_0) of 0.50 is reached. In addition, the percentages eluted before this distribution coefficient are within the limits approved for the particular product.

Identification and serological specificity
The identity and serological specificity are determined by a suitable immunochemical method (2.7.1). Identity and purity of each polysaccharide shall be confirmed; it shall be shown that there is not more than 1 per cent m/m of group-heterologous N. meningitidis polysaccharide.

Pyrogens (2.6.8)
The polysaccharide complies with the test for pyrogens. Inject into each rabbit per kilogram of body mass 1 mL of a solution containing 0.025 µg of purified polysaccharide per millilitre.

FINAL BULK VACCINE
One or more purified polysaccharides of 1 or more N. meningitidis groups are dissolved in a suitable solvent that may contain a stabiliser. When dissolution is complete, the solution is filtered through a bacteria-retentive filter.

Only a final bulk vaccine that complies with the following requirement may be used in the preparation of the final lot.

Sterility (2.6.1)
The final bulk vaccine complies with the test for sterility, carried out using 10 mL for each medium.

FINAL LOT
The final bulk vaccine is distributed aseptically into sterile containers. The containers are then closed so as to avoid contamination.

Only a final lot that is satisfactory with respect to each of the requirements prescribed below under Identification, Tests and Assay may be released for use.

CHARACTERS
A white or cream-coloured powder or pellet, freely soluble in water.

IDENTIFICATION
Carry out an identification test for each polysaccharide present in the vaccine by a suitable immunochemical method (2.7.1).

TESTS
Distribution of molecular size
Examine by size-exclusion chromatography (2.2.30). Use a column about 0.9 m long and 16 mm in internal diameter equilibrated with a solvent having an ionic strength of 0.2 mol/kg and a pH of 7.0-7.5. Apply to the column about 2.5 mg of each polysaccharide in a volume of about 1.5 mL and elute at about 20 mL/h. Collect fractions of about 2.5 mL and determine the content of polysaccharide by a suitable method.

For a divalent vaccine (group A + group C), use cross-linked agarose for chromatography R. The vaccine complies with the test if:
— 65 per cent of group A polysaccharide is eluted before $K_0 = 0.50$,
— 75 per cent of group C polysaccharide is eluted before $K_0 = 0.50$.

For a tetravalent vaccine (group A + group C + group Y + group W135), use cross-linked agarose for chromatography R1 and apply a suitable immunochemical method (2.7.1) to establish the elution pattern of the different polysaccharides. The vaccine complies with the test if K_0 for the principal peak is:
— not greater than 0.70 for group A and group C polysaccharide,
— not greater than 0.57 for group Y polysaccharide,
— not greater than 0.68 for group W135 polysaccharide.

Water (2.5.12)
Not more than 3.0 per cent, determined by the semi-micro determination of water.

Sterility (2.6.1)
It complies with the test for sterility.

Pyrogens (*2.6.8*)

It complies with the test for pyrogens. Inject per kilogram of the rabbit's mass 1 mL of a solution containing:

— 0.025 µg of polysaccharide for a monovalent vaccine,
— 0.050 µg of polysaccharide for a divalent vaccine,
— 0.10 µg of polysaccharide for a tetravalent vaccine.

ASSAY

Carry out an assay of each polysaccharide present in the vaccine.

For a divalent vaccine (group A + group C), use measurement of phosphorus (*2.5.18*) to determine the content of polysaccharide A and measurement of sialic acid (*2.5.23*) to determine the content of polysaccharide C. To determine sialic acid, use as reference solution a 150 mg/L solution of *N-acetylneuraminic acid R*.

For a tetravalent vaccine (group A + group C + group Y + group W135) a suitable immunochemical method (*2.7.1*) is used with a reference preparation of purified polysaccharide for each group.

The vaccine contains not less than 70 per cent and not more than 130 per cent of the quantity of each polysaccharide stated on the label.

LABELLING

The label states:

— the group or groups of polysaccharides (A, C, Y or W135) present in the vaccine,
— the number of micrograms of polysaccharide per human dose.

Ph Eur

Mumps Vaccine, Live

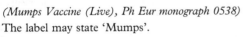

(*Mumps Vaccine (Live)*, *Ph Eur monograph 0538*)
The label may state 'Mumps'.

Ph Eur

DEFINITION

Mumps vaccine (live) is a freeze-dried preparation of a suitable attenuated strain of mumps virus. The vaccine is reconstituted immediately before use, as stated on the label, to give a clear liquid that may be coloured owing to the presence of a pH indicator.

PRODUCTION

The production of vaccine is based on a virus seed-lot system and, if the virus is propagated in human diploid cells, a cell-bank system. The production method shall have been shown to yield consistently live mumps vaccines of adequate immunogenicity and safety in man. Unless otherwise justified and authorised, the virus in the final vaccine shall have undergone no more passages from the master seed lot than were used to prepare the vaccine shown in clinical studies to be satisfactory with respect to safety and efficacy.

The potential neurovirulence of the vaccine strain is considered during preclinical development, based on available epidemiological data on neurovirulence and neurotropism, primarily for the wild-type virus. In light of this, a risk analysis is carried out. Where necessary and if available, a test is carried out on the vaccine strain using an animal model that differentiates wild-type and attenuated virus; tests on strains of intermediate attenuation may also be needed.

The production method is validated to demonstrate that the product, if tested, would comply with the test for abnormal toxicity for immunosera and vaccines for human use (*2.6.9*).

SUBSTRATE FOR VIRUS PROPAGATION

The virus is propagated in human diploid cells (*5.2.3*) or in chick-embryo cells or in the amniotic cavity of chick embryos derived from a chicken flock free from specified pathogens (*5.2.2*).

SEED LOT

The strain of mumps virus used shall be identified by historical records that include information on the origin of the strain and its subsequent manipulation. Virus seed lots are prepared in large quantities and stored at temperatures below − 20 °C if freeze-dried, or below − 60 °C if not freeze-dried.

Only a seed lot that complies with the following requirements may be used for virus propagation.

Identification

The master and working seed lots are identified as mumps virus by serum neutralisation in cell culture, using specific antibodies.

Virus concentration

The virus concentration of the master and working seed lots is determined to ensure consistency of production.

Extraneous agents (*2.6.16*)

The working seed lot complies with the requirements for seed lots.

PROPAGATION AND HARVEST

All processing of the cell bank and subsequent cell cultures is done under aseptic conditions in an area where no other cells are handled during the production. Suitable animal (but not human) serum may be used in the culture media. Serum and trypsin used in the preparation of cell suspensions and culture media are shown to be free from extraneous agents. The cell culture medium may contain a pH indicator such as phenol red and suitable antibiotics at the lowest effective concentration. It is preferable to have a substrate free from antibiotics during production. Not less than 500 mL of the production cell cultures is set aside as uninfected cell cultures (control cells). If the virus is propagated in chick embryos, 2 per cent but not less than 20 eggs are set aside as uninfected control eggs. The viral suspensions are harvested at a time appropriate to the strain of virus being used.

Only a single harvest that complies with the following requirements may be used in the preparation of the final bulk vaccine.

Identification

The single harvest contains virus that is identified as mumps virus by serum neutralisation in cell culture, using specific antibodies.

Virus concentration

The virus concentration in the single harvest is determined as prescribed under Assay to monitor consistency of production and to determine the dilution to be used for the final bulk vaccine.

Extraneous agents (*2.6.16*)

The single harvest complies with the tests for extraneous agents.

Control cells or eggs

If human diploid cells are used for production, the control cells comply with a test for identification; the control cells and the control eggs comply with the tests for extraneous agents (*2.6.16*).

FINAL BULK VACCINE

Single harvests that comply with the above tests are pooled and clarified to remove cells. A suitable stabiliser may be added and the pooled harvests diluted as appropriate.

Only a final bulk vaccine that complies with the following requirement may be used in the preparation of the final lot.

Bacterial and fungal contamination

The final bulk vaccine complies with the test for sterility (2.6.1), carried out using 10 mL for each medium.

FINAL LOT

A minimum virus concentration for release of the product is established such as to ensure, in light of stability data, that the minimum concentration stated on the label will be present at the end of the period of validity.

Only a final lot that complies with the requirements for minimum virus concentration for release, with the following requirement for thermal stability and with each of the requirements given below under Identification and Tests may be released for use. Provided that the tests for bovine serum albumin and, where applicable, for ovalbumin have been carried out with satisfactory results on the final bulk vaccine, they may be omitted on the final lot.

Thermal stability

Maintain at least 3 vials of the final lot of freeze-dried vaccine in the dry state at 37 ± 1 °C for 7 days. Determine the virus concentration as described under Assay in parallel for the heated vaccine and for vaccine stored at the temperature recommended for storage. The virus concentration of the heated vaccine is not more than 1.0 log lower than that of the unheated vaccine.

IDENTIFICATION

When the vaccine reconstituted as stated on the label is mixed with specific mumps antibodies, it is no longer able to infect susceptible cell cultures.

TESTS

Bacterial and fungal contamination

The reconstituted vaccine complies with the test for sterility (2.6.1).

Bovine serum albumin

Not more than 50 ng per single human dose, determined by a suitable immunochemical method (2.7.1).

Ovalbumin

If the vaccine is produced in chick embryos, it contains not more than 1 µg of ovalbumin per single human dose, determined by a suitable immunochemical method (2.7.1).

Water (2.5.12)

Not more than 3.0 per cent, determined by the semi-micro determination of water.

ASSAY

Titrate the vaccine for infective virus, using at least 3 separate vials of vaccine and inoculating a suitable number of wells for each dilution step. Titrate 1 vial of an appropriate virus reference preparation in triplicate to validate each assay. The virus concentration of the reference preparation is monitored using a control chart and a titre is established on a historical basis by each laboratory.
The relation with the appropriate European Pharmacopoeia Biological Reference Preparation is established and monitored at regular intervals if a manufacturer's reference preparation is used. Calculate the individual virus concentration for each vial of vaccine and for each replicate of the reference preparation as well as the corresponding combined virus concentrations, using the usual statistical

methods (for example, 5.3). The combined estimate of the virus concentration for the 3 vials of vaccine is not less than that stated on the label; the minimum virus concentration stated on the label is not less than 3.7 log $CCID_{50}$ per single human dose.

The assay is not valid if:
— the confidence interval ($P = 0.95$) of the estimated virus concentration of the reference preparation for the 3 replicates combined is greater than $\pm$ 0.3 log $CCID_{50}$;
— the virus concentration of the reference preparation differs by more than 0.5 log $CCID_{50}$ from the established value.

The assay is repeated if the confidence interval ($P = 0.95$) of the combined virus concentration of the vaccine is greater than $\pm$ 0.3 log $CCID_{50}$; data obtained from valid assays only are combined by the usual statistical methods (for example, 5.3) to calculate the virus concentration of the sample.
The confidence interval ($P = 0.95$) of the combined virus concentration is not greater than $\pm$ 0.3 log $CCID_{50}$.

Mumps vaccine (live) BRP is suitable for use as a reference preparation.

Where justified and authorised, different assay designs may be used; this may imply the application of different validity and acceptance criteria. However, the vaccine must comply if tested as described above.

LABELLING

The label states:
— the strain of virus used for the preparation of the vaccine;
— that the vaccine has been prepared in chick embryos or the type and origin of cells used for the preparation of the vaccine;
— the minimum virus concentration;
— that contact between the vaccine and disinfectants is to be avoided.

_____ *Ph Eur*

Human Papillomavirus Vaccine (rDNA)

(*Ph Eur monograph 2441*)
The label may state 'HPV'.

Ph Eur _____

DEFINITION

Human papillomavirus vaccine (rDNA) is a preparation of purified virus-like particles (VLPs) composed of the major capsid protein (L1) of one or more human papillomavirus (HPV) genotypes; the antigens may be adsorbed on a mineral carrier such as aluminium hydroxide or hydrated aluminium phosphate. The vaccine may also contain the adjuvant 3-*O*-desacyl-4′-monophosphoryl lipid A.
The antigens are obtained by recombinant DNA technology.

PRODUCTION

GENERAL PROVISIONS

The vaccine shall have been shown to induce specific neutralising antibodies in man. The production method shall have been shown to yield consistently vaccines comparable in quality with the vaccine of proven clinical efficacy and safety in man.

The production method is validated to demonstrate that the product, if tested, would comply with the test for abnormal toxicity for immunosera and vaccines for human use (2.6.9).

The vaccine is produced by the expression of the viral genes coding for the capsid proteins in yeast or in an insect cell/baculovirus expression vector system, purification of the resulting VLPs and the rendering of these particles into an immunogenic preparation. The suitability and safety of the expression systems are approved by the competent authority. Production of the vaccine is based on a seed lot/cell bank system. Unless otherwise justified and authorised, the virus and cells used for vaccine production shall not have undergone more passages from the master seed lot/cell bank than was used to prepare the vaccine shown in clinical studies to be satisfactory with respect to safety and efficacy.

Reference preparation   A batch of vaccine shown to be effective in clinical trials or a batch representative thereof is used as a reference vaccine. The reference vaccine is preferably stabilised and the stabilisation method shall have been shown to have no significant effect on the assay validity.

CHARACTERISATION

Characterisation of the VLPs is performed on lots produced during vaccine development, including the process validation batches. Characterisation includes protein composition, for example using techniques such as sodium dodecyl sulfate polyacrylamide gel electrophoresis (SDS-PAGE) and Western blotting or mass spectrometry, peptide mapping and/or terminal amino acid sequence analysis. Morphological characteristics of the VLPs and degree of aggregation are determined to confirm the presence of the conformational epitopes that are essential for efficacy. VLP characterisation may be done by atomic force microscopy and transmission electron microscopy, dynamic light scattering, epitope mapping and reactivity with neutralising monoclonal antibodies. In addition, the protein, lipid, nucleic acid and carbohydrate content are measured where applicable. The level of residual host-cell protein derived from insect cells meets acceptable safety criteria as set by the competent authority.

CELL BANKS AND SEED LOTS

Production in recombinant yeast cells   Only cell banks that have been satisfactorily characterised for identity, microbial purity, growth characteristics and stability shall be used for production. Gene homogeneity is studied for the master and working cell banks. A full description of the biological characteristics of the host cell and expression vectors is given. The physiological measures used to promote and control the expression of the cloned gene in the host cell are described in detail. This includes genetic markers of the host cell, the construction, genetics and structure of the expression vector, and the origin and identification of the gene that is being cloned. The nucleotide sequence of the gene insert and of adjacent segments of the vector and restriction-enzyme mapping of the vector containing the gene insert are provided. Data that demonstrates the stability of the expression system during storage of the recombinant working cell bank up to or beyond the passage level used for production is provided.

Production in an insect cell/baculovirus expression vector system
— *Insect cell substrate.* Only cell banks that have been satisfactorily characterised for identity, purity, growth characteristics, stability, extraneous agents and tumorigenicity shall be used for production. Such characterisation is performed at suitable stages of production in accordance with general chapters *5.2.3. Cell substrates for the production of vaccines for human use* and *2.6.16. Tests for extraneous agents in viral vaccines for human use.* Special attention is given to insect-borne

viruses, in particular insect-borne potential human pathogens (e.g. arboviruses). Adventitious infectious agents of insect cells may be without cytopathic effect. Tests therefore include nucleic acid amplification techniques, and other tests such as electron microscopy and co-cultivation.
— *Recombinant baculovirus.* The use of the recombinant baculovirus vector is based on a seed-lot system with a defined number of passages between the original virus and the master and the working seed-lots, as approved by the competent authorities. The recombinant baculovirus expression vector contains the coding sequence of the HPV L1 antigen. Segments of the expression construct are analysed using nucleic acid amplification techniques in conjunction with other tests performed on the purified recombinant protein for assuring the quality and consistency of the expressed HPV L1 antigens. The recombinant baculovirus used in the production of HPV vaccines is identified by historical records, which include information on the origin and identity of the gene being cloned as well as the construction, genetics and structure of the baculovirus expression vector(s). The genetic stability of the expression construct is demonstrated from the baculovirus master seed up to at least the highest level used in production and preferably beyond this level.

Recombinant baculovirus seed lots are prepared in large quantities and stored at temperatures favourable for stability.

Only a seed lot that complies with the following requirements may be used for virus propagation.

Identification
The master and working seed lots are identified by the HPV type of the inserted gene of origin, by an appropriate method such as nucleic acid amplification techniques (NAT) (*2.6.21*).

Virus concentration
The virus concentration of the master and working seed lots is determined to monitor consistency of production.

Extraneous agents (*2.6.16*)
The working seed lot complies with the requirements for seed lots and control cells. Special attention is given to *Spiroplasma* spp. and insect-borne viruses, in particular insect-borne potential human pathogens (e.g. arboviruses).

PROPAGATION AND HARVEST
All processing of the cell banks and baculovirus seed lots and subsequent cell cultures is done under aseptic conditions in an area where no other cells are being handled.

Where justified and authorised for production in an insect cell/baculovirus expression vector system, a stored virus intermediate culture that complies with the 5 following tests may be used for virus propagation.

Identification
Each stored virus intermediate culture is identified by HPV type, by an immunological assay using specific antibodies or by a molecular identity test such as NAT (*2.6.21*).

Bacterial and fungal contamination
Each stored virus intermediate culture complies with the test for sterility (*2.6.1*), carried out using 10 mL for each medium.

Virus concentration
The virus concentration of each stored baculovirus intermediate culture is determined by a suitable method such as plaque assay or NAT (*2.6.21*) in order to monitor consistency of production.

Extraneous agents (*2.6.16*)

Each stored virus intermediate culture complies with the tests for extraneous agents.

Control cells

The control cells of the production cell culture from which each stored virus intermediate is derived comply with a test for identity and with the requirements for extraneous agents (*2.6.16*).

Production in recombinant yeast cells   Identity, microbial purity, plasmid retention and consistency of yield are determined at suitable production stages.

Production in an insect cell/baculovirus expression vector system   Insect cell cultures are inoculated with recombinant baculovirus at a defined multiplicity of infection as approved by the competent authority. Several single harvests may be pooled before testing. No antibiotics are added at the time of harvesting or at any later stage of manufacturing.

SINGLE HARVESTS

Only a single harvest or a pool of single harvests that complies with the following requirements may be used in the preparation of the purified monovalent antigen.

Identification

Each single harvest is identified as the appropriate HPV type by immunological assay or by a molecular biology-based assay, for example hybridisation or polymerase chain reaction (PCR).

Bacterial and fungal contamination

In case of production in an insect cell/baculovirus expression vector system the single harvest complies with the test for sterility (*2.6.1*). In case of production in yeast cells the single harvest is tested for culture purity by inoculation of suitable medium to ensure no growth other than the host organism.

Extraneous agents (*2.6.16*)

In case of production in an insect cell/baculovirus expression vector system the single harvest complies with the tests for extraneous agents. Special attention is given to insect-borne viruses as mentioned under Cell banks and seed lots.

Control cells

In case of production in an insect cell/baculovirus expression vector system the control cells comply with a test for identification and with the requirements for extraneous agents (*2.6.16*). Special attention is given to insect-borne viruses as mentioned under Cell banks and seed lots.

PURIFIED MONOVALENT ANTIGEN

Harvests are purified using validated methods. When an insect cell/baculovirus expression vector system substrate is used, the production process is validated for its capacity to eliminate (by removal and/or inactivation) adventitious viruses and recombinant baculoviruses.

Only a purified monovalent antigen that complies with the following requirements may be used in the preparation of the final bulk. In agreement with the competent authority one or more of the tests mentioned below may be omitted if performed on the adsorbed monovalent antigen.

Total protein

The total protein is determined by a validated method. The content is within the limits approved for the particular product.

Antigen content and identification

The quantity and specificity of each antigen type is determined by a suitable immunochemical method (*2.7.1*) such as radio-immunoassay (RIA), enzyme-linked immunosorbent assay (ELISA), immunoblot (preferably using a monoclonal antibody directed against a protective epitope) or single radial diffusion. The antigen/protein ratio may be determined and is within the limits approved for the particular product.

Antigenic purity

The purity of each purified monovalent antigen is determined by a suitable method, such as SDS-PAGE with quantification by densitometric analysis, the limit of detection being 1 per cent of impurities or better with respect to total protein. A reference preparation is used to validate each test. The protein purity is calculated as the ratio of the L1 protein-related bands relative to the total protein bands, expressed as a percentage. For the genotypes included in the vaccine, the value calculated for purity is within the limits approved for the particular product.

Percent intact L1 monomer

The antigenic purity assay serves also to assess the integrity of the L1 monomer. The percent intact L1 monomer is the ratio of the intact L1 monomer to the total protein, expressed as a percentage.

VLP size and structure

The size and structure of the VLPs is established and monitored by a suitable method such as dynamic light scattering. The size is within the limits approved for the particular product.

Composition

The protein, lipid, nucleic acid and carbohydrate contents are determined, where applicable.

Host-cell and vector-derived DNA

Maximum 10 ng of DNA in a quantity of purified antigen equivalent to a single human dose of vaccine, determined in each monovalent purified antigen by sensitive methods.

Residual host-cell proteins

Tests for residual host-cell proteins are carried out. The content is within the limits approved for the particular product.

Chemicals used for disruption and purification

Tests for the chemicals used for purification or other stages of production are carried out. The content is within the limits approved for the particular products.

Sterility (*2.6.1*)

Each purified monovalent antigen complies with the test, carried out using 10 mL for each medium.

ADSORBED MONOVALENT ANTIGEN

The purified monovalent antigens may be adsorbed onto a mineral vehicle such as an aluminium salt.

Only an adsorbed monovalent antigen that complies with the following requirements may be used in the preparation of the final bulk.

Sterility (*2.6.1*)

Each adsorbed monovalent antigen complies with the test, carried out using 10 mL for each medium.

Bacterial endotoxins (*2.6.14*)

Each adsorbed monovalent antigen is tested for bacterial endotoxins. The content is within the limits approved for the particular product.

Antigen content and identification

Each antigen type is identified by a suitable immunochemical method (*2.7.1*) such as radio-immunoassay (RIA), enzyme-linked immunosorbent assay (ELISA), immunoblot (preferably using a monoclonal antibody directed against a protective epitope) or single radial diffusion.
The antigen/protein ratio is determined.

IMMUNOLOGICAL PRODUCTS

Mineral vehicle concentration

Where applicable, each adsorbed monovalent antigen is tested for the content of mineral vehicle. The content is within the limits approved for the particular product.

ADSORBED 3-O-DESACYL-4′-MONOPHOSPHORYL LIPID A BULK

If 3-O-desacyl-4′-monophosphoryl lipid A is included in the vaccine it complies with the monograph *3-O-desacyl-4′-monophosphoryl lipid A (2537)*. Where 3-O-desacyl-4′-monophosphoryl lipid A is adsorbed prior to inclusion in the vaccine, the adsorbed 3-O-desacyl-4′-monophosphoryl lipid A bulk complies with the following requirements.

Degree of adsorption of 3-O-desacyl-4′-monophosphoryl lipid A

The content of non-adsorbed 3-O-desacyl-4′-monophosphoryl lipid A in the adsorbed 3-O-desacyl-4′-monophosphoryl lipid A bulk is determined by a suitable method, for example gas chromatographic quantification of the *3-O-desacyl-4′-monophosphoryl lipid A (2537)* fatty acids in the supernatant, evaporated to dryness, after centrifugation.

pH (2.2.3)

The pH is within the limits approved for the particular preparation.

Sterility (2.6.1)

It complies with the test, carried out using 10 mL for each medium.

FINAL BULK VACCINE

The final bulk vaccine is prepared directly from each purified monovalent antigen HPV type or adsorbed purified monovalent antigen HPV type. An antimicrobial preservative, a mineral vehicle such as an aluminium salt and the adjuvant 3-O-desacyl-4′-monophosphoryl lipid A may be included in the formulation of the final bulk.

Only a final bulk that complies with the following requirements may be used in the preparation of the final lot.

Antimicrobial preservative

Where applicable, determine the amount of antimicrobial preservative by a suitable chemical or physico-chemical method. The amount is not less than 85 per cent and not greater than 115 per cent of the intended content.

Sterility (2.6.1)

The final bulk vaccine complies with the test, carried out using 10 mL for each medium.

FINAL LOT

Only a final lot that complies with each of the requirements given below under Identification, Tests and Assay may be released for use. Provided that the test for antimicrobial preservative content (where applicable) has been carried out with satisfactory results on the final bulk vaccine, it may be omitted on the final lot. If an *in vivo* assay is carried out, then provided it has been carried out with satisfactory results on the final bulk vaccine, it may be omitted on the final lot.

Adjuvants

If the vaccine contains an adjuvant, the amount is determined and shown to be within acceptable limits with respect to the expected amount. A suitable method for 3-O-desacyl-4′-monophosphoryl lipid A is, for example, gas chromatography.

Degree of adsorption

The degree of adsorption of each antigen and, where applicable, 3-O-desacyl-4′-monophosphoryl lipid A is assessed.

IDENTIFICATION

The vaccine is shown to contain the different types of HPV antigen by a suitable immunochemical method (2.7.1). The *in vitro* assay may serve to identify the vaccine. In addition, where applicable, the test for 3-O-desacyl-4′-monophosphoryl lipid A content also serves to identify the 3-O-desacyl-4′-monophosphoryl lipid A-containing vaccine.

TESTS

Aluminium (2.5.13)

Maximum 1.25 mg per single human dose, if aluminium hydroxide or hydrated aluminium phosphate is used as the adsorbent.

3-O-Desacyl-4′-monophosphoryl lipid A

Minimum 80 per cent and maximum 120 per cent of the intended amount.

Where applicable, determine the content of 3-O-desacyl-4′-monophosphoryl lipid A by a suitable method, for example gas chromatography (2.2.28).

Antimicrobial preservative

Where applicable, determine the content of antimicrobial preservative by a suitable chemical or physico-chemical method. The amount is not less than the minimum amount shown to be effective and is not greater than 115 per cent of that stated on the label.

Sterility (2.6.1)

The vaccine complies with the test.

Bacterial endotoxins (2.6.14)

Maximum 5 IU per single human dose. If the adjuvant prevents the determination of endotoxin, a suitable in-process test is carried out.

ASSAY

The assay is performed by an *in vivo* test or an in vitro test having acceptance criteria established by correlation studies against an *in vivo* test.

In vivo test

A suitable *in vivo* assay method consists of the injection of not fewer than 3 dilutions of the vaccine to be examined and of a reference vaccine preparation, using for each dilution a group of a suitable number of female mice of a suitable strain. The vaccine is diluted in a solution of *sodium chloride R* containing the aluminium adjuvant used for the vaccine production. The mice are 6-8 weeks old at the time of injection, and each mouse is given a 0.5 mL injection. A preimmunisation serum sample is taken prior to inoculation, and a final serum sample is taken at a defined time between days 21 and 28. Assay the individual sera for specific neutralising antibodies against each HPV type by a suitable immunochemical method (2.7.1).

The test is not valid unless:
— for both the vaccine to be examined and the reference vaccine, the ED_{50} lies between the smallest and the largest doses given to the animals;
— the statistical analysis shows no significant deviation from linearity or parallelism;
— the confidence limits ($P = 0.95$) are within the limits approved for the particular product.

In vitro test

Carry out an immunochemical determination (2.7.1) of each antigen genotype content. Enzyme-linked immunosorbent assay (ELISA) and radio-immunoassay (RIA) using monoclonal antibodies specific for protection-inducing epitopes of the L1 protein have been shown to be suitable. Suitable numbers of dilutions of the vaccine to be examined and a manufacturer's reference preparation are used and a suitable model is used to analyse the data. For each type, the antigen content is within the limits approved for the particular product.

LABELLING
The label states:
— the amount of L1 proteins and the genotype of HPV contained in the vaccine;
— the cell substrate used for production of the vaccine;
— the name and amount of the adjuvant and/or adsorbent used;
— that the vaccine must not be frozen.

Ph Eur

Pertussis Vaccine (Whole Cell, Adsorbed)

(*Ph Eur monograph 0161*)
The label may state 'wP'.

Ph Eur

DEFINITION
Pertussis vaccine (whole cell, adsorbed) is a sterile suspension of inactivated whole cells of one or more strains of *Bordetella pertussis*, treated to minimise toxicity and retain potency. The vaccine contains a mineral adsorbent such as hydrated aluminium phosphate or aluminium hydroxide.

PRODUCTION
GENERAL PROVISIONS
The production process shall have been shown to yield consistently vaccines comparable with the vaccine of proven clinical efficacy and safety in man.

Levels of pertussis toxin, active heat-labile toxin (dermonecrotic toxin) or tracheal cytotoxin must be comparable to the levels present in the vaccine of proven clinical efficacy and safety in man and be approved by the competent authority.

CHOICE OF VACCINE STRAIN
The vaccine consists of a mixture of one or more strains of B. pertussis. Strains of *B. pertussis* used in preparing vaccines are well characterised and chosen in such a way that the final vaccine contains predominantly phase I cells that display fimbriae 2 and 3, as determined by an agglutination test or other suitable immunochemical method (*2.7.1*).

SEED LOTS
The production of pertussis vaccine is based on a seed-lot system.

The strains of *B. pertussis* used are identified by a full historical record, including information on the origin of the strain and its subsequent manipulation, characteristics on isolation, and particularly on all tests carried out periodically to verify the strain's characters.

The media chosen for growing *B. pertussis* are carefully selected and enable the micro-organism to retain phase I characteristics.

When animal blood or animal blood products are used, they are removed by washing the harvested bacteria.

Human blood or human blood products are not used in any culture media for propagating bacteria, either for seed or for vaccine.

PROPAGATION AND HARVEST
Each strain is grown separately from the working seed lot.

Cultures are checked at different stages of fermentation (subcultures and main culture) for purity, identity, cell opacity and pH. Unsatisfactory cultures must be discarded.

Production cultures are shown to be consistent in respect of growth rate, pH and yield of cells or cell products.

The bacteria are harvested and may be washed to remove substances derived from the medium and suspended in a 9 g/L solution of sodium chloride or other suitable isotonic solution.

MONOVALENT CELL HARVEST
Consistency of production is monitored in respect of growth rate, pH, yield and demonstration of characteristics of phase I organisms in the culture, such as presence of fimbriae 2 and 3 and haemolytic activity. Single harvests are not used for the final bulk vaccine unless they have been shown to contain *B. pertussis* cells with the same characteristics with regard to growth and agglutinogens as the parent strain, and to be free from contaminating bacteria and fungi.

Only a monovalent harvest that complies with the following requirements may be used in further production.

Purity
Samples of single harvests taken before inactivation are examined by microscopy of Gram-stained smears or by inoculation into appropriate culture media or by another suitable procedure.

Opacity
The opacity of each single harvest is measured not later than 2 weeks after harvest and before the bacterial suspension has been subjected to any process capable of altering its opacity, by comparison with the International Reference Preparation of Opacity, and used as the basis of calculation for subsequent stages in vaccine preparation. The equivalence in International Units of the International Reference Preparation is stated by the World Health Organization.

A spectrophotometric method validated against the opacity reference preparation may be used and absorbance may, for example, be measured at 600 nm (*2.2.25*).

INACTIVATION AND DETOXIFICATION OF B. PERTUSSIS SUSPENSION
Inactivation is initiated as soon as possible after taking samples of single harvests for purity control and opacity measurement. The bacteria are killed and detoxified in controlled conditions by means of a suitable chemical agent or by heating or by a combination of these methods. The suspension is maintained at 5 ± 3 °C for a suitable period to diminish its toxicity.

Only an inactivated monovalent cell bulk that complies with established specifications for the following tests may be used in the preparation of the final bulk.

Residual live *B. pertussis*
Inactivation of the whole cells of *B. pertussis* is verified by a suitable culture medium.

Pertussis toxin
Presence of pertussis toxin is measured by a CHO cell culture assay using a semi-quantitative technique and range determined for the particular product.

pH (*2.2.3*)
Within the range approved for the particular product.

Identification
Verified by agglutination assay or suitable immunodiffusion assay.

Sterility (2.6.1)

It complies with the test for sterility, carried out using 10 mL for each medium.

Opacity

The opacity of each single harvest is measured in the final phase, at the end of the main fermentation process, by comparison with the International Reference Preparation of Opacity. The equivalence in International Units of the International Reference Preparation is stated by the World Health Organization. The absorbance, for example measured at 600 nm (2.2.25), is within the range approved for the particular product.

FINAL BULK

The final bulk vaccine is prepared by aseptically mixing suitable quantities of the inactivated single harvests.

If 2 or more strains of *B. pertussis* are used, the composition of consecutive lots of the final bulk vaccine shall be consistent with respect to the proportion of each strain as measured in opacity units. The bacterial concentration of the final bulk vaccine does not exceed that corresponding to an opacity of 20 IU per single human dose. The opacity measured on the single harvests is used to calculate the bacterial concentration in the final bulk. A mineral adsorbent such as hydrated aluminium phosphate or aluminium hydroxide is added to the cell suspension. Suitable antimicrobial preservatives may be added. Phenol is not used as a preservative.

Only a final bulk that complies with the following requirements may be used in the preparation of the final lot.

Fimbriae

Each bulk is examined, before adsorbent is added, for the presence of fimbriae 2 and 3 to ensure that appropriate expression has occurred during bacterial growth.

Sterility (2.6.1)

It complies with the test for sterility, carried out using 10 mL for each medium.

Antimicrobial preservative

Where applicable, determine the amount of antimicrobial preservative by a suitable chemical or physico-chemical method. The amount is not less than 85 per cent and not greater than 115 per cent of the intended amount.

FINAL LOT

The final bulk is mixed to homogeneity and filled aseptically into suitable containers.

Only a final lot that is within the limits approved for the particular product and is satisfactory with respect to each of the requirements given below under Identification, Tests and Assay may be released for use. Provided the tests for specific toxicity, free formaldehyde and antimicrobial preservative and the determination of potency have been carried out with satisfactory results on the final bulk vaccine, they may be omitted on the final lot.

IDENTIFICATION

Dissolve in the vaccine to be examined sufficient *sodium citrate R* to give a 100 g/L solution. Maintain at 37 °C for about 16 h and centrifuge to obtain a bacterial precipitate. Identity of pertussis vaccine is based on an immunological reaction, for example agglutination of the resuspended bacteria with a specific anti-pertussis serum or another suitable immunochemical method (2.7.1).

TESTS

Specific toxicity

Use not fewer than 5 healthy mice each weighing 14-16 g for the vaccine group and for the saline control. Use mice of the same sex or distribute males and females equally between the groups. Inject each mouse of the vaccine group intraperitoneally with 0.5 mL, containing a quantity of the vaccine equivalent to not less than half the single human dose. Inject each mouse of the control group with 0.5 mL of a 9 g/L sterile solution of *sodium chloride R*, preferably containing, where applicable, the same amount of antimicrobial preservative as that injected with the vaccine. Weigh the groups of mice immediately before the injection and 72 h and 7 days after the injection. The vaccine complies with the test if: (a) at the end of 72 h the average weight of the group of vaccinated mice is not less than that preceding the injection; (b) at the end of 7 days the average increase in mass per vaccinated mouse is not less than 60 per cent of that per control mouse; and (c) not more than 5 per cent of the vaccinated mice die during the test. If the test is carried out using 5 mice and 1 vaccinated mouse dies, the test may be repeated using 15 mice and the results of both tests combined.

Aluminium (2.5.13)

Maximum 1.25 mg per single human dose, if aluminium hydroxide or hydrated aluminium phosphate is used as the adsorbent.

Free formaldehyde (2.4.18)

Maximum 0.2 g/L, where applicable.

Antimicrobial preservative

Where applicable, determine the amount of antimicrobial preservative by a suitable chemical method. The content is not less than the minimum amount shown to be effective and is not greater than 115 per cent of the quantity stated on the label.

Sterility (2.6.1)

It complies with the test for sterility.

ASSAY

Carry out the assay of pertussis vaccine (whole cell) (2.7.7).

The estimated potency is not less than 4.0 IU per single human dose and the lower confidence limit ($P = 0.95$) of the estimated potency is not less than 2.0 IU per single human dose.

LABELLING

The label states:

— the minimum number of International Units per single human dose;

— the method used for inactivation;

— the name and the amount of the adsorbent;

— that the vaccine must be shaken before use;

— that the vaccine is not to be frozen.

Ph Eur

Adsorbed Pertussis Vaccine (Acellular Component)

(Pertussis Vaccine (Acellular, Component, Adsorbed),
Ph Eur monograph 1356)
The label may state 'aP'.

Ph Eur

DEFINITION

Pertussis vaccine (acellular, component, adsorbed) is a preparation of individually prepared and purified antigenic components of *Bordetella pertussis* adsorbed on a mineral carrier such as aluminium hydroxide or hydrated aluminium phosphate.

The vaccine contains either pertussis toxoid or a pertussis-toxin-like protein free from toxic properties, produced by expression of a genetically modified form of the corresponding gene. Pertussis toxoid is prepared from pertussis toxin by a method that renders the latter harmless while maintaining adequate immunogenic properties and avoiding reversion to toxin. The vaccine may also contain filamentous haemagglutinin, pertactin (a 69 kDa outer-membrane protein) and other defined components of *B. pertussis* such as fimbrial-2 and fimbrial-3 antigens. The latter 2 antigens may be co-purified. The antigenic composition and characteristics are based on evidence of protection and freedom from unexpected reactions in the target group for which the vaccine is intended.

PRODUCTION

GENERAL PROVISIONS

The production method shall have been shown to yield consistently vaccines comparable with the vaccine of proven clinical efficacy and safety in man.

Where a genetically modified form of *B. pertussis* is used, production consistency and genetic stability shall be established in conformity with the requirements of the monograph *Products of recombinant DNA technology (0784)*.

Reference vaccine A batch of vaccine shown to be effective in clinical trials or a batch representative thereof is used as a reference vaccine. For the preparation of a representative batch, strict adherence to the production process used for the batch tested in clinical trials is necessary. The reference vaccine is preferably stabilised by a method that has been shown to have no significant effect on the assay procedure when the stabilised and non-stabilised batches are compared.

CHARACTERISATION OF COMPONENTS

During development of the vaccine, the production process shall be validated to demonstrate that it yields consistently individual components that comply with the following requirements; after demonstration of consistency, the tests need not be applied routinely to each batch.

Adenylate cyclise

Not more than 500 ng in the equivalent of 1 dose of the final vaccine, determined by immunoblot analysis or another suitable method.

Tracheal cytotoxin

Not more than 2 pmol in the equivalent of 1 dose of the final vaccine, determined by a suitable method such as a biological assay or liquid chromatography (*2.2.29*).

Absence of residual dermonecrotic toxin

Inject intradermally into each of 3 unweaned mice, in a volume of 0.1 mL, the amount of component or antigenic fraction equivalent to 1 dose of the final vaccine. Observe for 48 h. No dermonecrotic reaction is demonstrable.

Specific properties

The components of the vaccine are analysed by one or more of the methods shown below in order to determine their identity and specific properties (activity per unit amount of protein) in comparison with reference preparations.

Pertussis toxin Chinese hamster ovary (CHO) cell-clustering effect and haemagglutination as *in vitro* methods; lymphocytosis-promoting activity, histamine-sensitising activity and insulin secretory activity as *in vivo* methods. The toxin shows ADP-ribosyl transferase activity using transducin as the acceptor.

Filamentous haemagglutinin Haemagglutination and inhibition by a specific antibody.

Pertactin, fimbrial-2 and fimbrial-3 antigens Reactivity with specific antibodies.

Pertussis toxoid The toxoid induces in animals production of antibodies capable of inhibiting all the properties of pertussis toxin.

PURIFIED COMPONENTS

Production of each component is based on a seed-lot system. The seed cultures from which toxin is prepared are managed to conserve or, where necessary, restore toxinogenicity by deliberate selection.

None of the media used at any stage contains blood or blood products of human origin. Media used for the preparation of seed lots and inocula may contain blood or blood products of animal origin.

Pertussis toxin and, where applicable, filamentous haemagglutinin and pertactin are purified and, after appropriate characterisation, detoxified using suitable chemical reagents, by a method that avoids reversion of the toxoid to toxin, particularly on storage or exposure to heat. Other components such as fimbrial-2 and fimbrial-3 antigens are purified either separately or together, characterised and shown to be free from toxic substances. The purification procedure is validated to demonstrate appropriate clearance of substances used during culture or purification.

The content of bacterial endotoxins (*2.6.14*) is determined to monitor the purification procedure and to limit the amount in the final vaccine. The limits applied for the individual components are such that the final vaccine contains less than 100 IU per single human dose.

Before detoxification, the purity of the components is determined by a suitable method such as polyacrylamide gel electrophoresis (PAGE) or liquid chromatography. SDS-PAGE or immunoblot analysis with specific monoclonal or polyclonal antibodies may be used to characterise subunits. Requirements are established for each individual product.

Only purified components that comply with the following requirements may be used in the preparation of the final bulk vaccine.

Sterility (*2.6.1*)

Carry out the test for sterility using for each medium a quantity of purified component equivalent to not less than 100 doses.

Residual pertussis toxin (*2.6.33*)

It complies with the test.

A validated test based on the clustering effect of the toxin for Chinese hamster ovary (CHO) cells may be used instead of the test in mice.

IMMUNOLOGICAL PRODUCTS

Residual detoxifying agents and other reagents

The content of residual detoxifying agents and other reagents is determined and shown to be below approved limits unless validation of the process has demonstrated acceptable clearance.

Antigen content

Determine the antigen content by a suitable immunochemical method (2.7.1) and protein nitrogen by sulfuric acid digestion (2.5.9) or another suitable method. The ratio of antigen content to protein nitrogen is within the limits established for the product.

FINAL BULK VACCINE

The vaccine is prepared by adsorption of suitable quantities of purified components, separately or together, onto aluminium hydroxide or hydrated aluminium phosphate. A suitable antimicrobial preservative may be added.

Only a final bulk vaccine that complies with the following requirements may be used in the preparation of the final lot.

Antimicrobial preservative

Where applicable, determine the amount of antimicrobial preservative by a suitable chemical or physico-chemical method. The amount is not less than 85 per cent and not greater than 115 per cent of the intended content.

Sterility (2.6.1)

Carry out the test for sterility using 10 mL for each medium.

FINAL LOT

Only a final lot that is satisfactory with respect to each of the requirements given below under Identification, Tests and Assay may be released for use. Provided that the tests for residual pertussis toxin and irreversibility of pertussis toxoid, antimicrobial preservative, free formaldehyde and the assay have been carried out with satisfactory results on the final bulk vaccine, these tests may be omitted on the final lot.

IDENTIFICATION

Subject the vaccine to a suitable desorption procedure such as the following: dissolve in the vaccine to be examined sufficient *sodium citrate R* to give a 10 g/L solution; maintain at 37 °C for about 16 h and centrifuge until a clear supernatant liquid is obtained. Examined by a suitable immunochemical method (2.7.1), the clear supernatant liquid reacts with specific antisera to the components stated on the label.

TESTS

Residual pertussis toxin and irreversibility of pertussis toxoid (2.6.33)

The final lot complies with the test.

Aluminium (2.5.13)

Maximum 1.25 mg per single human dose, if aluminium hydroxide or hydrated aluminium phosphate is used as the adsorbent.

Free formaldehyde (2.4.18)

Maximum 0.2 g/L.

Antimicrobial preservative

Where applicable, determine the amount of antimicrobial preservative by a suitable chemical or physico-chemical method. The amount is not less than the minimum amount shown to be effective and is not greater than 115 per cent of the quantity stated on the label.

Sterility (2.6.1)

It complies with the test for sterility.

ASSAY

Carry out one of the prescribed methods for the assay of pertussis vaccine (acellular) (2.7.16).

The capacity of the vaccine to induce antibodies for each included acellular pertussis antigen is not significantly (*P* = 0.95) less than that of the reference vaccine.

LABELLING

The label states:

— the names and amounts of the components present in the vaccine;
— where applicable, that the vaccine contains a pertussis toxin-like protein produced by genetic modification;
— the name and amount of the adsorbent;
— that the vaccine must be shaken before use;
— that the vaccine is not to be frozen.

———————————————— Ph Eur

Adsorbed Pertussis Vaccine (Acellular, Co-purified)

(Pertussis Vaccine (Acellular, Co-purified, Adsorbed), Ph Eur monograph 1595)

The label may state 'aP'.

Ph Eur ————————————————

DEFINITION

Pertussis vaccine (acellular, co-purified, adsorbed) is a preparation of antigenic components of *Bordetella pertussis* adsorbed on a mineral carrier such as aluminium hydroxide or hydrated aluminium phosphate.

The vaccine contains an antigenic fraction purified without separation of the individual components. The antigenic fraction is treated by a method that transforms pertussis toxin to toxoid, rendering it harmless while maintaining adequate immunogenic properties of all the components and avoiding reversion to toxin. The antigenic fraction is composed of pertussis toxoid, filamentous haemagglutinin, pertactin (a 69 kDa outer-membrane protein) and other defined components of *B. pertussis* such as fimbrial-2 and fimbrial-3 antigens. It may contain residual pertussis toxin up to a maximum level approved by the competent authority. The antigenic composition and characteristics are based on evidence of protection and freedom from unexpected reactions in the target group for which the vaccine is intended.

PRODUCTION

GENERAL PROVISIONS

The production method shall have been shown to yield consistently vaccines comparable with the vaccine of proven clinical efficacy and safety in man.

Reference vaccine A batch of vaccine shown to be effective in clinical trials or a batch representative thereof is used as a reference vaccine. For the preparation of a representative batch, strict adherence to the production process used for the batch tested in clinical trials is necessary. The reference vaccine is preferably stabilised, by a method that has been shown to have no significant effect on the assay procedure when the stabilised and non-stabilised batches are compared.

CHARACTERISATION OF COMPONENTS

During development of the vaccine, the production process shall be validated to demonstrate that it yields consistently an antigenic fraction that complies with the following requirements; after demonstration of consistency, the tests need not be applied routinely to each batch.

Adenylate cyclise

Not more than 500 ng in the equivalent of 1 dose of the final vaccine, determined by immunoblot analysis or another suitable method.

Tracheal cytotoxin

Not more than 2 pmol in the equivalent of 1 dose of the final vaccine, determined by a suitable method such as a biological assay or liquid chromatography (2.2.29).

Absence of residual dermonecrotic toxin

Inject intradermally into each of 3 unweaned mice, in a volume of 0.1 mL, the amount of antigenic fraction equivalent to 1 dose of the final vaccine. Observe for 48 h. No dermonecrotic reaction is demonstrable.

Specific properties

The antigenic fraction is analysed by one or more of the methods shown below in order to determine the identity and specific properties (activity per unit amount of protein) of its components in comparison with reference preparations.

Pertussis toxin   Chinese hamster ovary (CHO) cell-clustering effect and haemagglutination as *in vitro* methods; lymphocytosis-promoting activity, histamine-sensitising activity and insulin secretory activity as *in vivo* methods. The toxin shows ADP-ribosyl transferase activity using transducin as the acceptor.

Filamentous haemagglutinin   Haemagglutination and inhibition by a specific antibody.

Pertactin, fimbrial-2 and fimbrial-3 antigens   Reactivity with specific antibodies.

Pertussis toxoid   The toxoid induces in animals the production of antibodies capable of inhibiting all the properties of pertussis toxin.

PURIFIED ANTIGENIC FRACTION

Production of the antigenic fraction is based on a seed-lot system. The seed cultures are managed to conserve or, where necessary, restore toxinogenicity by deliberate selection.

None of the media used at any stage contains blood or blood products of human origin. Media used for the preparation of seed batches and inocula may contain blood or blood products of animal origin.

The antigenic fraction is purified and, after appropriate characterisation, detoxified using suitable reagents by a method that ensures minimal reversion of toxoid to toxin, particularly on storage or exposure to heat. The purification procedure is validated to demonstrate appropriate clearance of substances used during culture or purification.

The content of bacterial endotoxins (2.6.14) is determined to monitor the purification procedure and to limit the amount in the final vaccine. The limits applied are such that the final vaccine contains not more than 100 IU per single human dose.

Before detoxification, the purity of the antigenic fraction is determined by a suitable method such as polyacrylamide gel electrophoresis (PAGE) or liquid chromatography. SDS-PAGE or immunoblot analysis with specific monoclonal or polyclonal antibodies may be used to characterise subunits. Requirements are established for each individual product.

Only a purified antigenic fraction that complies with the following requirements may be used in the preparation of the final bulk vaccine.

Sterility

Carry out the test for sterility (2.6.1) using for each medium a quantity of purified antigenic fraction equivalent to not less than 100 doses of the final vaccine.

Residual pertussis toxin (2.6.33)

The purified antigenic fraction complies with the test.

A validated test based on the clustering effect of the toxin for Chinese hamster ovary (CHO) cells may be used instead of the test in mice.

Residual detoxifying agents and other reagents

The content of residual detoxifying agents and other reagents is determined and shown to be below approved limits unless validation of the process has demonstrated acceptable clearance.

Antigen content

Determine the complete quantitative antigen composition of the antigenic fraction by suitable immunochemical methods (2.7.1) and protein nitrogen by sulfuric acid digestion (2.5.9) or another suitable method. The ratio of total antigen content to protein nitrogen is within the limits established for the product.

FINAL BULK VACCINE

The vaccine is prepared by adsorption of a suitable quantity of the antigenic fraction onto aluminium hydroxide or hydrated aluminium phosphate. A suitable antimicrobial preservative may be added.

Only a final bulk vaccine that complies with the following requirements may be used in the preparation of the final lot.

Antimicrobial preservative

Where applicable, determine the amount of antimicrobial preservative by a suitable chemical or physico-chemical method. The amount is not less than 85 per cent and not greater than 115 per cent of the intended content.

Sterility

The final bulk vaccine complies with the test for sterility (2.6.1), carried out using 10 mL for each medium.

FINAL LOT

Only a final lot that is satisfactory with respect to each of the requirements given below under Identification, Tests and Assay may be released for use.

Provided that the tests for residual pertussis toxin and irreversibility of pertussis toxoid, antimicrobial preservative, free formaldehyde and the assay have been carried out with satisfactory results on the final bulk vaccine, these tests may be omitted on the final lot.

IDENTIFICATION

Subject the vaccine to a suitable desorption procedure such as the following: dissolve in the vaccine to be examined sufficient *sodium citrate R* to give a 10 g/L solution; maintain at 37 °C for about 16 h and centrifuge until a clear supernatant liquid is obtained. Examined by a suitable immunochemical method (2.7.1), the clear supernatant liquid reacts with specific antisera to the components in the vaccine.

TESTS

Residual pertussis toxin and irreversibility of pertussis toxoid (2.6.33)

The final lot complies with the test.

Antimicrobial preservative

Where applicable, determine the amount of antimicrobial preservative by a suitable chemical or physico-chemical method. The amount is not less than the minimum amount shown to be effective and is not greater than 115 per cent of the quantity stated on the label.

Aluminium (*2.5.13*)

Maximum 1.25 mg per single human dose, if aluminium hydroxide or hydrated aluminium phosphate is used as the adsorbent.

Free formaldehyde (*2.4.18*)

Maximum 0.2 g/L.

Sterility

It complies with the test for sterility (*2.6.1*).

ASSAY

Carry out one of the prescribed methods for the assay of pertussis vaccine (acellular) (*2.7.16*).

The capacity of the vaccine to induce antibodies for each included acellular pertussis antigen is not significantly (*P* = 0.95) less than that of the reference vaccine.

LABELLING

The label states:

— the names and amounts of the antigenic components present in the vaccine,

— the maximum amount of residual pertussis toxin present in the vaccine,

— the maximum degree of reversion of toxoid to toxin during the period of validity,

— the name and amount of the adsorbent,

— that the vaccine must be shaken before use,

— that the vaccine is not to be frozen.

—————————————————————————— Ph Eur

Pneumococcal Polysaccharide Vaccine

(*Ph Eur monograph 0966*)

The label may state 'Pneumo'.

Ph Eur _____

DEFINITION

Pneumococcal polysaccharide vaccine consists of a mixture of equal parts of purified capsular polysaccharide antigens prepared from suitable pathogenic strains of *Streptococcus pneumoniae* whose capsules have been shown to be made up of polysaccharides that are capable of inducing satisfactory levels of specific antibodies in man. It contains the 23 immunochemically different capsular polysaccharides listed in Table 0966-1.

The vaccine is a clear, colourless liquid.

PRODUCTION

Production of the vaccine is based on a seed-lot system for each type. The production method shall have been shown to yield consistently pneumococcal polysaccharide vaccines of adequate safety and immunogenicity in man.

The production method is validated to demonstrate that the product, if tested, would comply with the test for abnormal toxicity for immunosera and vaccines for human use (*2.6.9*) modified as follows for the test in guinea-pigs: inject 10 human doses into each guinea-pig and observe for 12 days.

MONOVALENT BULK POLYSACCHARIDES

The bacteria are grown in a suitable liquid medium that does not contain blood-group substances or high-molecular-mass polysaccharides. The bacterial purity of the culture is verified and the culture is inactivated with phenol. Impurities are removed by such techniques as fractional precipitation, enzymatic digestion and ultrafiltration. The polysaccharide is obtained by fractional precipitation, washed, and dried in a vacuum to a residual moisture content shown to be favourable to the stability of the polysaccharide. The residual moisture content is determined by drying under reduced pressure over diphosphorus pentoxide or by thermogravimetric analysis and the value obtained is used to calculate the results of the tests shown below with reference to the dried substance. The monovalent bulk polysaccharide is stored at a suitable temperature in conditions that avoid the uptake of moisture.

Only a monovalent bulk polysaccharide that complies with the following requirements may be used in the preparation of the final bulk vaccine. Percentage contents of components, determined by the methods prescribed below, are shown in Table 0966-1.

Protein (*2.5.16*).

Nucleic acids (*2.5.17*).

Total nitrogen (*2.5.9*).

Phosphorus (*2.5.18*).

Molecular size

Determine by size-exclusion chromatography (*2.2.30*) using *cross-linked agarose for chromatography R* or *cross-linked agarose for chromatography R1*.

Uronic acids (*2.5.22*).

Hexosamines (*2.5.20*).

Methylpentoses (*2.5.21*).

***O*-Acetyl groups** (*2.5.19*).

Identification (*2.7.1*)

Confirm the identity of the monovalent bulk polysaccharide by double immunodiffusion or electroimmunodiffusion (except for polysaccharides 7F, 14 and 33F), using specific antisera.

Specificity

No reaction occurs when the antigens are tested against all the antisera specific for the other polysaccharides of the vaccine, including factor sera for distinguishing types within groups. The polysaccharides are tested at a concentration of 50 µg/mL using a method capable of detecting 0.5 µg/mL.

FINAL BULK VACCINE

The final bulk vaccine is obtained by aseptically mixing the different polysaccharide powders. The uniform mixture is aseptically dissolved in a suitable isotonic solution so that one human dose of 0.50 mL contains 25 µg of each polysaccharide. An antimicrobial preservative may be added. The solution is sterilised by filtration through a bacteria-retentive filter.

Only a final bulk vaccine that complies with the following requirements may be used in the preparation of the final lot.

Antimicrobial preservative

Where applicable, determine the amount of antimicrobial preservative by a suitable chemical method. The content is not less than 85 per cent and not greater than 115 per cent of the intended amount.

Sterility (*2.6.1*)

The final bulk vaccine complies with the test for sterility, using 10 mL for each medium.

FINAL LOT

The final bulk vaccine is distributed aseptically into sterile, tamper-proof containers.

Only a final lot that is satisfactory with respect to each of the requirements given below under identification, tests and assay

Table 0966.-1 – *Percentage contents of components of monovalent bulk polysaccharides*

Molecular type*	Protein	Nucleic acids	Total nitrogen	Phosphorus	Molecular size (K_0) **	***	Uronic acids	Hexos-amines	Methyl-pentoses	O-acetyl Groups
1	≤ 2	≤ 2	3.5-6	0-1.5	≤ 0.15		≥ 45			≥ 1.8
2	≤ 2	≤ 2	0-1	0-1.0	≤ 0.15		≥ 15		≥ 38	
3	≤ 5	≤ 2	0-1	0-1.0	≤ 0.15		≥ 40			
4	≤ 3	≤ 2	4-6	0-1.5	≤ 0.15			≥ 40		
5	≤ 7.5	≤ 2	2.5-6.0	≤ 2		≤ 0.60	≥ 12	≥ 20		
6B	≤ 2	≤ 2	0-2	2.5-5.0		≤ 0.50			≥ 15	
7F	≤ 5	≤ 2	1.5-4.0	0-1.0	≤ 0.20				≥13	
8	≤ 2	≤ 2	0-1	0-1.0	≤ 0.15		≥ 25			
9N	≤ 2	≤ 1	2.2-4	0-1.0	≤ 0.20		≥ 20	≥ 28		
9V	≤ 2	≤ 2	0.5-3	0-1.0		≤ 0.45	≥ 15	≥ 13		
10A	≤ 7	≤ 2	0.5-3.5	1.5-3.5		≤ 0.65		≥ 12		
11A	≤ 3	≤ 2	0-2.5	2.0-5.0		≤ 0.40				≥ 9
12F	≤ 3	≤ 2	3-5	0-1.0	≤ 0.25			≥ 25		
14	≤ 5	≤ 2	1.5-4	0-1.0	≤ 0.30			≥ 20		
15B	≤ 3	≤ 2	1-3	2.0-4.5		≤0.55		≥ 15		
17A or 17F	≤ 2	≤ 2	0-1.5	0-3.5		≤ 0.45			≥ 20	
18C	≤ 3	≤ 2	0-1	2.4-4.9	≤ 0.15				≥ 14	
19A	≤ 2	≤ 2	0.6-3.5	3.0-7.0	≤ 0.45			≥ 12	≥ 20	
19F	≤ 3	≤ 2	1.4-3.5	3.0-5.5	≤ 0.20			≥ 12.5	≥ 20	
20	≤ 2	≤ 2	0.5-2.5	1.5-4.0		≤ 0.60		≥ 12		
22F	≤ 2	≤ 2	0-2	0-1.0		≤ 0.55	≥ 15		≥ 25	
23F	≤ 2	≤ 2	0-1	3.0-4.5	≤ 0.15				≥ 37	
33F	≤ 2.5	≤ 2	0-2	0-1.0		≤ 0.50				

* The different types are indicated using the Danish nomenclature.

** *Cross-linked agarose for chromatography R.*

*** *Cross-linked agarose for chromatography R1.*

may be released for use. Provided that the tests for phenol and for antimicrobial preservative have been carried out with satisfactory results on the final bulk vaccine, they may be omitted on the final lot. When consistency of production has been established on a suitable number of consecutive batches, the assay may be replaced by a qualitative test that identifies each polysaccharide, provided that an assay has been performed on each monovalent bulk polysaccharide used in the preparation of the final lot.

IDENTIFICATION

The assay serves also to identify the vaccine.

TESTS

pH (*2.2.3*)

The pH of the vaccine is 4.5 to 7.4.

Antimicrobial preservative

Where applicable, determine the amount of antimicrobial preservative by a suitable chemical method. The content is not less than the minimum amount shown to be effective and is not greater than 115 per cent of the quantity stated on the label.

Phenol (*2.5.15*)

Not more than 2.5 g/L.

Sterility (*2.6.1*)

It complies with the test for sterility.

Pyrogens (*2.6.8*)

It complies with the test for pyrogens. Inject per kilogram of the rabbit's mass 1 mL of a dilution of the vaccine containing 2.5 μg/mL of each polysaccharide.

ASSAY

Determine the content of each polysaccharide by a suitable immunochemical method (*2.7.1*), using antisera specific for each polysaccharide contained in the vaccine, including factor sera for types within groups, and purified polysaccharides of each type as standards.

The vaccine contains not less than 70 per cent and not more than 130 per cent of the quantity stated on the label for each polysaccharide. The confidence limits ($P = 0.95$) are not less than 80 per cent and not more than 120 per cent of the estimated content.

LABELLING

The label states:

— the number of micrograms of each polysaccharide per human dose,

— the total amount of polysaccharide in the container.

Ph Eur

Pneumococcal Polysaccharide Conjugate Vaccine (Adsorbed)

(*Ph Eur monograph 2150*)

The label may state 'Pneumo(conj)'.

Ph Eur

DEFINITION

Pneumococcal polysaccharide conjugate vaccine (adsorbed) is a sterile suspension of purified capsular polysaccharides obtained from *Streptococcus pneumoniae* serotypes individually conjugated to a carrier protein. The carrier protein used may vary for the various polysaccharide conjugates contained in a multivalent vaccine. The vaccine may be adsorbed on a suitable adjuvant or adsorbant.

Each serotype, produced from suitable pathogenic strains of *S. pneumoniae*, is grown in an appropriate medium.

The individual polysaccharides are purified through suitable purification methods (for example centrifugation, precipitation, ultrafiltration and column chromatography).

Each polysaccharide has a defined composition and a defined molecular size range.

The choice of polysaccharide depends on the frequency of the serotypes responsible for acute pathologies and their geographical distribution. The vaccine contains immunochemically different capsular polysaccharides.

PRODUCTION

GENERAL PROVISIONS

The production method shall have been shown to yield consistently *S. pneumoniae* conjugate vaccines of adequate safety and immunogenicity in man. The production of polysaccharides and of the carrier(s) is based on a seed-lot system.

During development studies and wherever revalidation is necessary, a test for pyrogens in rabbits (*2.6.8*) is carried out. The vaccine is shown to be acceptable with respect to absence of pyrogenic activity.

The production method is validated to demonstrate that the product, if tested, would comply with the test for abnormal toxicity for immunosera and vaccines for human use (*2.6.9*).

During development studies and whenever revalidation of the manufacturing process is necessary, it shall be demonstrated by tests in animals that the vaccine consistently induces a T-cell-dependent B-cell immune response.

The stability of the conjugated bulk and/or final lot and pneumococcal saccharide is evaluated using suitable indicator tests. Such tests may include determination of molecular size, quantification of saccharide content and free polysaccharide content in the conjugate.

BACTERIAL SEED LOTS

The bacterial strains used for master seed lots shall be identified by historical records that include information on their origin and the tests used to characterise the strain.

Cultures obtained from the working seed lot shall have the same characteristics as the strain that was used to prepare the master seed lot.

Purity of bacterial cultures is verified by methods of suitable sensitivity. These may include inoculation into suitable media, examination of colony morphology, microscopic examination of Gram-stained smears and culture agglutination with suitable specific antisera.

PNEUMOCOCCAL POLYSACCHARIDES

Each strain of *S. pneumoniae* serotypes is individually grown in a liquid medium that does not contain high-molecular-mass polysaccharides; if any ingredient of the medium contains blood-group substances, the process is validated to demonstrate that after the purification step they are no longer detectable. The bacterial purity of the culture is verified by suitable methods. The culture is then inactivated. Each polysaccharide is separated from the liquid culture and purified by suitable methods. Volatile matter, including water, in the purified polysaccharide is determined by a suitable method such as thermogravimetry (*2.2.34*), semi-micro determination of water (*2.5.12*) or, where applicable, determination of solvent and/or alcohol content by spectrometry. The values are used to calculate the results of other chemical tests with reference to the dried substance, as prescribed below.

Only polysaccharides that comply with the following requirements may be used in the preparation of the conjugate.

Identification

Each polysaccharide is identified by an immunochemical method (*2.7.1*) or other suitable methods, for example ^{1}H nuclear magnetic resonance spectrometry (*2.2.33*).

Protein (*2.5.16*)

Depending on the serotype used, not more than the limit approved for the product, calculated with reference to the dried substance.

Nucleic acid (*2.5.17*)

Depending on the serotype used, not more than the limit approved for the product, calculated with reference to the dried substance.

Molecular size

The molecular size is evaluated by liquid chromatography (*2.2.29*) with multiple-angle laser light scattering detection (MALLS) or other suitable methods, such as size-exclusion chromatography (*2.2.30*) using *cross-linked agarose for chromatography R* or *cross-linked agarose for chromatography R1*. The values are within the limits approved for each serotype. A validated determination of the degree of polymerisation or of the weight-average molecular weight and the dispersion of molecular masses may be used instead of the determination of molecular-size distribution.

Bacterial endotoxins (*2.6.14*)

Less than 0.5 IU of endotoxin per microgram of polysaccharide.

Residual reagents

Where applicable, suitable tests are carried out to determine residues of reagents used during inactivation and purification. An acceptable value for each reagent is established for the particular product and each batch of polysaccharide must be shown to comply with this limit. Where validation studies have demonstrated removal of residual reagents, the test on polysaccharides may be omitted.

Water

Where applicable, the values are within the limits approved for each serotype, determined by a suitable method.

Depending on the chemical composition of a pneumococcal polysaccharide serotype, not all of the following tests may be applicable. The values are within the limits approved.

Suitable limits for some pneumococcal polysaccharide

serotypes are given in the monograph *Pneumococcal polysaccharide vaccine (0966)*.

Total nitrogen (*2.5.9*).

Phosphorus (*2.5.18*).

Uronic acids (*2.5.22*).

Hexosamines (*2.5.20*).

Methylpentoses (*2.5.21*).

O-Acetyl groups (*2.5.19*).

MODIFIED PNEUMOCOCCAL POLYSACCHARIDES
Before conjugation, the polysaccharide can be depolymerised by chemical or mechanical means followed by a concentration step to obtain polysaccharides of a desired molecular size range. Polysaccharides or depolymerised polysaccharides are modified by an activation process.

Only modified polysaccharides that comply with the following requirements may be used in the preparation of the conjugate.

Molecular size
In the case of a size-reduced modified pneumococcal polysaccharide, the molecular size is evaluated by liquid chromatography (*2.2.29*) with MALLS detection or other suitable methods, such as size-exclusion chromatography (*2.2.30*) using *cross-linked agarose for chromatography R* or *cross-linked agarose for chromatography R1*. The values are within the limits approved for each serotype.

Degree of oxidation
Where applicable, the degree of oxidation is represented by the ratio of moles of saccharide repeat unit per mole of aldehyde and determined by a suitable method. The values are within the limits approved for each serotype.

CARRIER PROTEIN
The carrier protein is produced by culture of suitable (including inducible recombinant) micro-organisms; the bacterial purity of the culture is verified. The culture is inactivated. The carrier protein is purified by a suitable method. Suitable tests are carried out, for validation or routinely, to demonstrate that, where applicable, the product is free from specific toxins.

Where diphtheria toxoid is used, it is produced as described in the monograph *Diphtheria vaccine (adsorbed) (0443)* and complies with the requirements prescribed therein for bulk purified toxoid, except that the test for sterility (*2.6.1*) is not required.

Where CRM 197 is used as the carrier protein, it is not less than 90 per cent pure, determined by a suitable method.

Where tetanus toxoid is used as the carrier protein, it is produced as described in the monograph *Tetanus vaccine (adsorbed) (0452)* and complies with the requirements prescribed therein for purified bulk toxoid, except that the antigenic purity (*2.7.27*) is not less than 1500 Lf per milligram of protein nitrogen and that the test for sterility (*2.6.1*) is not required.

Where protein D is used, a specific strain of *Escherichia coli* is modified by a plasmid carrying the protein D coding sequence in order to express this outer-surface protein of *Haemophilus influenzae*. The modified strain is grown in a suitable liquid medium to express protein D. At the end of cultivation, protein D is purified and sterilised by suitable methods. The product contains not less than 95 per cent of protein D.

Only a carrier protein that complies with the following requirements may be used in the preparation of the conjugate.

Identification
The carrier protein is identified by a suitable immunochemical method (*2.7.1*).

Bacterial endotoxins (*2.6.14*)
Less than 1 IU per microgram of protein.

Carrier protein
Not less than 90 per cent of the total protein content, determined by a suitable method.

MONOVALENT BULK CONJUGATE
The conjugate is obtained by the covalent binding of activated polysaccharides to the carrier protein.

The conjugate purification procedures are designed to remove residual reagents used for conjugation. The removal of residual reagents is confirmed by suitable tests or by validation of the purification process.

Only a bulk conjugate that complies with the following requirements may be used in the preparation of the final bulk vaccine. For each test, limits of acceptance are established and each batch of conjugate must be shown to comply with these limits.

Saccharide
The polysaccharide content is determined by a suitable physical or chemical method or by an immunochemical method (*2.7.1*). The value complies with the requirement approved for each serotype.

Protein
The protein content is determined by a suitable physical or chemical method (for example, *2.5.16*). The value complies with the requirement approved for each serotype.

Saccharide-to-protein ratio
Determine the saccharide-to-protein ratio by calculation. The value complies with the requirement approved for each serotype.

Free saccharide
Unbound polysaccharide is determined after removal of the conjugate, for example by anion-exchange, size-exclusion or hydrophobic chromatography, ultrafiltration, or other validated methods. A value consistent with adequate immunogenicity as shown in clinical trials is established for each serotype and each lot must be shown to comply with this limit.

Free carrier protein
Determine the content by a suitable method, either directly or by deriving the content by calculation from the results of other tests. The value complies with the requirement approved for each serotype.

Molecular size
The molecular size is evaluated by liquid chromatography (*2.2.29*) with MALLS detection or other suitable methods. The values are within the limits approved for each serotype.

Residual reagents
Where applicable, suitable tests are carried out to determine residues of reagents used during inactivation and purification. An acceptable value for each reagent is established for the particular product and each batch of conjugate must be shown to comply with this limit. Where validation studies have demonstrated removal of residual reagents, the test on conjugate polysaccharides may be omitted.

Sterility (*2.6.1*)
It complies with the test for sterility, carried out using 10 mL for each medium or the equivalent of 100 doses for each medium, whichever is less.

Bacterial endotoxins (*2.6.14*)

Less than 0.75 IU of endotoxin per microgram of polysaccharide.

ADSORBED MONOVALENT BULK CONJUGATE

An aluminium-containing adjuvant may be added to each of the monovalent bulk conjugates prior to formulation of the final bulk. Once the conjugates are adsorbed on a sterile adjuvant, sterility is assured by aseptic processing.

Only an adsorbed monovalent bulk conjugate that complies with the following requirements may be used in the preparation of the final bulk vaccine.

Identification

Each adsorbed polysaccharide conjugate is identified by an immunochemical method (*2.7.1*) or other suitable methods.

Sterility (*2.6.1*)

It complies with the test for sterility, carried out using 10 mL or the equivalent of 100 doses for each medium, whichever is less.

Saccharide

The polysaccharide content is determined by a suitable physical or chemical method or by an immunochemical method (*2.7.1*). The value complies with the requirement approved for each serotype.

Free saccharide

Centrifuge the adsorbed monovalent bulk conjugate. In the supernatant the unbound polysaccharide is determined after removal of the conjugate, for example by anion-exchange, size-exclusion or hydrophobic liquid chromatography, ultrafiltration, or other validated methods. An acceptable value consistent with adequate immunogenicity as shown in clinical trials is established for each serotype and each lot must be shown to comply with this limit.

Degree of adsorption

The degree of adsorption of each polysaccharide conjugate is assessed.

FINAL BULK VACCINE

A final bulk vaccine may be formulated from the individually adsorbed monovalent bulk conjugates, or from the mixture of the monovalent bulk conjugates that is adsorbed on an aluminium-containing adjuvant.

Where a final bulk vaccine is formulated as a release intermediate, it complies with the following requirements and is within the limits approved for the particular product.

Only a final bulk vaccine that complies with the following requirements may be used in the preparation of the final lot.

Sterility (*2.6.1*)

It complies with the test for sterility, carried out using 10 mL or the equivalent of 100 doses for each medium, whichever is less.

FINAL LOT

Only a final lot that is within the limits approved for the particular product and is satisfactory with respect to each of the requirements given below under Identification, Tests and Assay may be released for use.

IDENTIFICATION

Each polysaccharide present in the vaccine is identified by a suitable immunochemical method (*2.7.1*).

TESTS

Aluminium (*2.5.13*)

Maximum 1.25 mg per single human dose.

Sterility (*2.6.1*)

It complies with the test for sterility.

Bacterial endotoxins (*2.6.14*)

Less than 12.5 IU per single human dose, unless otherwise justified and authorised.

ASSAY

Saccharide content

The polysaccharide content for each serotype is determined by a suitable immunochemical method (for example, nephelometry assay or enzyme-linked immunosorbent assay (ELISA)). The vaccine contains not less than 70 per cent and not more than 130 per cent of the quantity stated on the label for each polysaccharide. The confidence limits ($P = 0.95$) are not less than 80 per cent and not more than 120 per cent of the estimated content.

LABELLING

The label states:

— the pneumococcal serotype and carrier protein present in each single human dose;

— the number of micrograms of each polysaccharide per single human dose;

— the number of micrograms of carrier protein per single human dose;

— if applicable, the name and amount of adsorbent;

— if applicable, that the vaccine must be shaken before use;

— if applicable, that the vaccine must not be frozen.

——————————— Ph Eur

Inactivated Poliomyelitis Vaccine

*(Poliomyelitis Vaccine (Inactivated),
Ph Eur monograph 0214)*

The label may state 'IPV'.

Ph Eur —————————————————

DEFINITION

Poliomyelitis vaccine (inactivated) is a liquid preparation of suitable strains of human poliovirus types 1, 2 and 3 grown in suitable cell cultures and inactivated by a validated method. It is a clear liquid that may be coloured owing to the presence of a pH indicator.

PRODUCTION

The production method shall have been shown to yield consistently vaccines of acceptable safety and immunogenicity in man.

Production of the vaccine is based on a virus seed-lot system. Cell lines are used according to a cell-bank system.

If primary, secondary or tertiary monkey kidney cells are used, production complies with the requirements indicated below.

Unless otherwise justified and authorised, the virus in the final vaccine shall not have undergone more passages from the master seed lot than was used to prepare the vaccine shown in clinical studies to be satisfactory with respect to safety and efficacy.

The production method is validated to demonstrate that the product, if tested, would comply with the test for abnormal toxicity for immunosera and vaccines for human use (*2.6.9*).

SUBSTRATE FOR VIRUS PROPAGATION

The virus is propagated in a human diploid cell line (*5.2.3*), in a continuous cell line (*5.2.3*) or in primary, secondary or tertiary monkey kidney cells.

Primary, secondary or tertiary monkey kidney cells

The following special requirements for the substrate for virus propagation apply to primary, secondary or tertiary monkey kidney cells.

Monkeys used in the preparation of kidney cell cultures for production and control of the vaccine The animals used are of a species approved by the competent authority, in good health and, unless otherwise justified and authorised, have not been previously employed for experimental purposes. Kidney cells used for vaccine production and control are derived from monitored, closed colonies of monkeys bred in captivity, not from animals caught in the wild; a previously approved seed lot prepared using virus passaged in cells from wild monkeys may, subject to approval by the competent authority, be used for vaccine production if historical data on safety justify this.

Monitored, closed colonies of monkeys The monkeys are kept in groups in cages. Freedom from extraneous agents is achieved by the use of animals maintained in closed colonies that are subject to continuous and systematic veterinary and laboratory monitoring for the presence of infectious agents. The supplier of animals is certified by the competent authority. Each monkey is tested serologically at regular intervals during a quarantine period of not less than 6 weeks imposed before entering the colony, and then during its stay in the colony.

The monkeys used are shown to be tuberculin-negative and free from antibodies to simian virus 40 (SV40) and simian immunodeficiency virus. The blood sample used in testing for SV40 antibodies must be taken as close as possible to the time of removal of the kidneys. If *Macaca* sp. monkeys are used for production, the monkeys are also shown to be free from antibodies to herpesvirus B (cercopithecine herpesvirus 1) infection. Human herpesvirus 1 has been used as an indicator for freedom from herpesvirus B antibodies on account of the danger of handling herpesvirus B (cercopithecine herpesvirus 1).

Monkeys from which kidneys are to be removed are thoroughly examined, particularly for evidence of tuberculosis and herpesvirus B (cercopithecine herpesvirus 1) infection. If a monkey shows any pathological lesion relevant to the use of its kidneys in the preparation of a seed lot or vaccine, it is not to be used nor are any of the remaining monkeys of the group concerned unless it is evident that their use will not impair the safety of the product.

All the operations described in this section are conducted outside the area where the vaccine is produced.

Monkey cell cultures for vaccine production Kidneys that show no pathological signs are used for preparing cell cultures. Each group of cell cultures derived from a single monkey forms a separate production cell culture giving rise to a separate single harvest.

The primary monkey kidney cell suspension complies with the test for mycobacteria (2.6.2); disrupt the cells before carrying out the test.

If secondary or tertiary cells are used, it shall be demonstrated by suitable validation tests that cell cultures beyond the passage level used for production are free from tumorigenicity.

SEED LOTS

Each of the 3 strains of poliovirus used shall be identified by historical records that include information on the origin of the strain and its subsequent manipulation.

Only a working seed lot that complies with the following requirements may be used for virus propagation.

Identification

Each working seed lot is identified as human poliovirus types 1, 2 or 3 by virus neutralisation in cell cultures using specific antibodies.

Virus concentration

The virus concentration of each working seed lot is determined to define the quantity of virus to be used for inoculation of production cell cultures.

Extraneous agents

The working seed lot complies with the requirements for seed lots for virus vaccines (2.6.16). In addition, if primary, secondary or tertiary monkey kidney cells have been used for isolation of the strain, measures are taken to ensure that the strain is not contaminated with simian viruses such as simian immunodeficiency virus, simian virus 40, filoviruses and herpesvirus B (cercopithecine herpesvirus 1). A working seed lot produced in primary, secondary or tertiary monkey kidney cells complies with the requirements given below under Virus propagation and harvest for single harvests produced in such cells.

PROPAGATION AND HARVEST

All processing of the cell bank and cell cultures is done under aseptic conditions in an area where no other cells or viruses are being handled. Approved animal serum (but not human serum) may be used in the cell culture media. Serum and trypsin used in the preparation of cell suspensions and media are shown to be free from extraneous agents. The cell culture media may contain a pH indicator such as phenol red and approved antibiotics at the lowest effective concentration. Not less than 500 mL of the cell cultures employed for vaccine production is set aside as uninfected cell cultures (control cells); where continuous cell lines in a fermenter are used for production, 200×10^6 cells are set aside to prepare control cells; where primary, secondary or tertiary monkey kidney cells are used for production, a cell sample equivalent to at least 500 mL of the cell suspension, at the concentration employed for vaccine production, is taken to prepare control cells.

Only a single harvest that complies with the following requirements may be used in the preparation of the vaccine. The tests for identification and bacterial and fungal contamination may be carried out instead on the purified, pooled monovalent harvest. After demonstration of consistency of production at the stage of the single harvest, the test for virus concentration may be carried out instead on the purified, pooled monovalent harvest.

Control cells

The control cells of the production cell culture comply with a test for identification (if a cell-bank system is used for production) and with the requirements for extraneous agents (2.6.16; *where primary, secondary or tertiary monkey kidney cells are used, the tests in cell cultures are carried out as shown below under Test in rabbit kidney cell cultures and Test in cercopithecus kidney cell cultures*).

Test in rabbit kidney cell cultures Test a sample of at least 10 mL of the pooled supernatant fluid from the control cultures for the absence of herpesvirus B (cercopithecine herpesvirus 1) and other viruses by inoculation onto rabbit kidney cell cultures. The dilution of supernatant in the nutrient medium is not greater than 1/4 and the area of the cell layer is at least 3 cm^2 per millilitre of inoculum. Set aside one or more containers of each batch of cells with the same medium as non-inoculated control cells. Incubate the cultures at 37 °C and observe for at least 2 weeks. The test is not valid if more than 20 per cent of the control cell cultures are discarded for non-specific, accidental reasons.

Test in cercopithecus kidney cell cultures   Test a sample of at least 10 mL of the pooled supernatant fluid from the control cultures for the absence of SV40 virus and other extraneous agents by inoculation onto cell cultures prepared from the kidneys of cercopithecus monkeys, or other cells shown to be at least as sensitive for SV40, by the method described under Test in rabbit kidney cell cultures. The test is not valid if more than 20 per cent of the control cell cultures are discarded for non-specific, accidental reasons.

Identification
The single harvest is identified as containing human poliovirus types 1, 2 or 3 by virus neutralisation in cell cultures using specific antibodies.

Virus concentration
The virus concentration of each single harvest is determined by titration of infectious virus in cell cultures.

Bacterial and fungal contamination
The single harvest complies with the test for sterility (*2.6.1*), carried out using 10 mL for each medium.

Mycoplasmas (*2.6.7*)
The single harvest complies with the test for mycoplasmas, carried out using 10 mL.

Test in rabbit kidney cell cultures
Where primary, secondary or tertiary monkey kidney cells are used for production, test a sample of at least 10 mL of the single harvest for the absence of herpesvirus B (cercopithecine herpesvirus 1) and other viruses by inoculation onto rabbit kidney cell cultures as described above for the control cells.

Test in cercopithecus kidney cell cultures
Where primary, secondary or tertiary monkey kidney cells are used for production, test a sample of at least 10 mL of the single harvest for the absence of SV40 virus and other extraneous agents. Neutralise the sample by a high-titre antiserum against the specific type of poliovirus. Test the sample in primary cercopithecus kidney cell cultures or cells that have been demonstrated to be at least as susceptible for SV40. Incubate the cultures at 37 °C and observe for 14 days. At the end of this period, make at least one subculture of fluid in the same cell culture system and observe both primary cultures and subcultures for an additional 14 days.

PURIFICATION AND PURIFIED MONOVALENT HARVEST
Several single harvests of the same type may be pooled and may be concentrated. The monovalent harvest or pooled monovalent harvest is purified by validated methods.

If continuous cell lines are used for production, the purification process shall have been shown to reduce consistently the content of substrate-cell DNA to not more than 100 pg per single human dose.

Only a purified monovalent harvest that complies with the following requirements may be used for the preparation of the inactivated monovalent harvest.

Identification
The virus is identified by virus neutralisation in cell cultures using specific antibodies or by determination of D-antigen.

Virus concentration
The virus concentration is determined by titration of infectious virus.

Specific activity
The ratio of the virus concentration or the D-antigen content, determined by a suitable immunochemical method (*2.7.1*), to the total protein content (specific activity) of the purified monovalent harvest is within the limits approved for the particular product.

INACTIVATION AND INACTIVATED MONOVALENT HARVEST
Several purified monovalent harvests of the same type may be mixed before inactivation. To avoid failures in inactivation caused by the presence of virus aggregates, filtration is carried out before and during inactivation; inactivation is started within a suitable period, preferably not more than 24 h and in any case not more than 72 h, of the prior filtration. The virus suspension is inactivated by a validated method that has been shown to inactivate poliovirus without destruction of immunogenicity; during validation studies, an inactivation curve with at least 4 points (for example, time 0 h, 24 h, 48 h and 96 h) is established showing the decrease in concentration of live virus with time. If formaldehyde is used for inactivation, the presence of an excess of formaldehyde at the end of the inactivation period is verified. The inactivation kinetics tests mentioned below are carried out on each batch to ensure consistency of the inactivation process.

Only an inactivated monovalent harvest that complies with the following requirements may be used in the preparation of a trivalent pool of inactivated monovalent harvests or a final bulk vaccine.

Test for effective inactivation
After neutralisation of the formaldehyde with sodium bisulfite (where applicable), verify the absence of residual live poliovirus by inoculation on suitable cell cultures of 2 samples of each inactivated monovalent harvest, corresponding to at least 1500 human doses. Cells used for the test must be of optimal sensitivity regarding residual infectious poliovirus, for example kidney cells from certain monkey species (*Macaca*, *Cercopithecus* or *Papio*), or Hep-2 cells. If other cells are used, they must have been shown to possess at least the same sensitivity as those specified above. Take one sample not later than 3/4 of the way through the inactivation period and the other at the end. Inoculate the samples in cell cultures such that the dilution of vaccine in the nutrient medium is not greater than 1/4 and the area of the cell layer is at least 3 cm^2 per millilitre of inoculum. Set aside one or more containers with the same medium as non-inoculated control cells. Observe the cell cultures for at least 3 weeks. Make not fewer than 2 passages from each container, one at the end of the observation period and the other 1 week before; for the passages, use cell culture supernatant and inoculate as for the initial sample. Observe the subcultures for at least 2 weeks. No sign of poliovirus multiplication is present in the cell cultures. At the end of the observation period, test the susceptibility of the cell culture used by inoculation of live poliovirus of the same type as that present in the inactivated monovalent harvest.

Inactivation kinetics
Kinetics of inactivation are established and approved by the competent authority. Adequate data on inactivation kinetics are obtained and consistency of the inactivation process is monitored.

Sterility (*2.6.1*)
The inactivated monovalent harvest complies with the test for sterility, carried out using 10 mL for each medium.

D-antigen content

The content of D-antigen determined by a suitable immunochemical method (2.7.1) is within the limits approved for the particular preparation.

FINAL BULK VACCINE

The final bulk vaccine is prepared directly from the inactivated monovalent harvests of human poliovirus types 1, 2 and 3 or from a trivalent pool of inactivated monovalent harvests. A suitable stabiliser and a suitable antimicrobial preservative may be added.

Only a final bulk vaccine that complies with the following requirements may be used in the preparation of the final lot.

Sterility (2.6.1)

The final bulk vaccine complies with the test for sterility, carried out using 10 mL for each medium.

Antimicrobial preservative

Where applicable, determine the amount of antimicrobial preservative by a suitable chemical or physicochemical method. The amount is not less than 85 per cent and not greater than 115 per cent of the intended amount.

FINAL LOT

Only a final lot that complies with each of the requirements given below under Identification, Tests and Assay may be released for use. Provided that the tests for free formaldehyde and antimicrobial preservative and the *in vivo* assay have been performed with satisfactory results on the final bulk vaccine, they may be omitted on the final lot.

The *in vivo* assay may be omitted once it has been demonstrated for a given product and for each poliovirus type that the acceptance criteria for the D-antigen determination are such that it yields the same result as the *in vivo* assay in terms of acceptance or rejection of a batch. This demonstration must include testing of subpotent batches, produced experimentally if necessary, for example by heat treatment or other means of diminishing the immunogenic activity. Where there is a significant change in the manufacturing process of the antigens or their formulation, any impact on the *in vivo* and *in vitro* assays must be evaluated, and the need for revalidation considered.

Provided that the protein content has been determined on the purified monovalent harvests or on the inactivated monovalent harvests and that it has been shown that the content in the final lot will not exceed 10 µg per single human dose, the test for protein content may be omitted on the final lot.

Provided that the test for bovine serum albumin has been performed with satisfactory results on the trivalent pool of inactivated monovalent harvests or on the final bulk vaccine, it may be omitted on the final lot.

IDENTIFICATION

The vaccine is shown to contain human poliovirus types 1, 2 and 3 by a suitable immunochemical method (2.7.1) such as the determination of D-antigen by enzyme-linked immunosorbent assay (ELISA).

TESTS

Free formaldehyde (2.4.18)

Maximum 0.2 g/L.

Antimicrobial preservative

Where applicable, determine the amount of antimicrobial preservative by a suitable chemical or physicochemical method. The amount is not less than the minimum amount shown to be effective and is not greater than 115 per cent of that stated on the label.

Protein content (2.5.33, Method 2)

Maximum 10 µg per single human dose.

Bovine serum albumin

Maximum 50 ng per single human dose, determined by a suitable immunochemical method (2.7.1).

Sterility (2.6.1)

It complies with the test.

Bacterial endotoxins (2.6.14)

Less than 5 IU per single human dose.

ASSAY

D-antigen content

As a measure of consistency of production, determine the D-antigen content for human poliovirus types 1, 2 and 3 by a suitable immunochemical method (2.7.1) using a reference preparation calibrated in European Pharmacopoeia Units of D-antigen. For each type, the content, expressed with reference to the amount of D-antigen stated on the label, is within the limits approved for the particular product. *Poliomyelitis vaccine (inactivated) BRP* is calibrated in European Pharmacopoeia Units and intended for use in the assay of D-antigen. The European Pharmacopoeia Unit and the International Unit are equivalent.

***In vivo* test**

The vaccine complies with the *in vivo* assay of poliomyelitis vaccine (inactivated) (2.7.20).

LABELLING

The label states:
— the types of poliovirus contained in the vaccine;
— the nominal amount of virus of each type (1, 2 and 3), expressed in European Pharmacopoeia Units of D-antigen, per single human dose;
— the cell substrate used to prepare the vaccine.

_____ *Ph Eur*

Poliomyelitis Vaccine, Live (Oral)

*(Poliomyelitis Vaccine (Oral),
Ph Eur monograph 0215)*

The label may state 'OPV'.

Ph Eur _____

DEFINITION

Oral poliomyelitis vaccine is a preparation of approved strains of live attenuated poliovirus type 1, 2 or 3 grown in *in vitro* cultures of approved cells, containing any one type or any combination of the 3 types of Sabin strains, presented in a form suitable for oral administration.

The vaccine is a clear liquid that may be coloured owing to the presence of a pH indicator.

PRODUCTION

The vaccine strains and the production method shall have been shown to yield consistently vaccines that are both immunogenic and safe in man.

The production of vaccine is based on a virus seed-lot system. Cell lines are used according to a cell-bank system. If primary monkey kidney cell cultures are used, production complies with the requirements indicated below. Unless otherwise justified and authorised, the virus in the final vaccine shall not have undergone more than 2 passages from the master seed lot.

REFERENCE STANDARDS
Poliomyelitis vaccine (oral) BRP is suitable for use as a virus reference preparation for the assay.

The International Standards for poliovirus type 2 (Sabin) for MAPREC (Mutant Analysis by PCR and Restriction Enzyme Cleavage) assays and poliovirus, type 3 (Sabin) synthetic DNA for MAPREC assays are suitable for use in the tests for genetic markers and the molecular tests for consistency of production.

Reference preparations of each poliovirus type at the Sabin Original + 2 passage level, namely WHO (SO + 2)/I for type 1 virus, WHO (SO + 2)/II for type 2 virus and WHO (SO + 2)/III for type 3 virus are available for comparison of the *in vivo* neurovirulence with that of homotypic vaccines. Requests for the WHO reference preparations for *in vivo* neurovirulence tests are to be directed to WHO, Biologicals, Geneva, Switzerland.

A suitable reference preparation is to be included in each test.

SUBSTRATE FOR VIRUS PROPAGATION
The virus is propagated in human diploid cells (*5.2.3*), in continuous cell lines (*5.2.3*) or in primary monkey kidney cell cultures (including serially passaged cells from primary monkey kidney cells).

Primary monkey kidney cell cultures
The following special requirements for the substrate for virus propagation apply to primary monkey kidney cell cultures.

Monkeys used for preparation of primary monkey kidney cell cultures and for testing of virus   If the vaccine is prepared in primary monkey kidney cell cultures, animals of a species approved by the competent authority, in good health, kept in closed or intensively monitored colonies and not previously employed for experimental purposes shall be used.

The monkeys shall be kept in well-constructed and adequately ventilated animal rooms in cages spaced as far apart as possible. Adequate precautions shall be taken to prevent cross-infection between cages. Not more than 2 monkeys shall be housed per cage and cage-mates shall not be interchanged. The monkeys shall be kept in the country of manufacture of the vaccine in quarantine groups for a period of not less than 6 weeks before use. A quarantine group is a colony of selected, healthy monkeys kept in one room, with separate feeding and cleaning facilities, and having no contact with other monkeys during the quarantine period. If at any time during the quarantine period the overall death rate of a shipment consisting of one or more groups reaches 5 per cent (excluding deaths from accidents or where the cause was specifically determined not to be an infectious disease), monkeys from that entire shipment shall continue in quarantine from that time for a minimum of 6 weeks. The groups shall be kept continuously in isolation, as in quarantine, even after completion of the quarantine period, until the monkeys are used. After the last monkey of a group has been taken, the room that housed the group shall be thoroughly cleaned and decontaminated before being used for a fresh group. If kidneys from near-term monkeys are used, the mother is quarantined for the term of pregnancy.

Monkeys from which kidneys are to be removed shall be anaesthetised and thoroughly examined, particularly for evidence of tuberculosis and cercopithecid herpesvirus 1 (B virus) infection.

If a monkey shows any pathological lesion relevant to the use of its kidneys in the preparation of a seed lot or vaccine, it shall not be used, nor shall any of the remaining monkeys of the quarantine group concerned be used unless it is evident that their use will not impair the safety of the product.

All the operations described in this section shall be conducted outside the areas where the vaccine is produced.

The monkeys used shall be shown to be free from antibodies to simian virus 40 (SV40), simian immunodeficiency virus and spumaviruses. The blood sample used in testing for SV40 antibodies must be taken as close as possible to the time of removal of the kidneys. If *Macaca* spp. are used for production, the monkeys shall also be shown to be free from antibodies to cercopithecid herpesvirus 1 (B virus). Human herpesvirus has been used as an indicator for freedom from B virus antibodies on account of the danger of handling cercopithecid herpesvirus 1 (B virus). Monkeys used for the production of new seed lots are shown to be free from antibodies to simian cytomegalovirus (sCMV).

Primary monkey kidney cell cultures for vaccine production   Kidneys that show no pathological signs are used for preparing cell cultures. If the monkeys are from a colony maintained for vaccine production, serially passaged monkey kidney cell cultures from primary monkey kidney cells may be used for virus propagation, otherwise the monkey kidney cells are not propagated in series. Virus for the preparation of vaccine is grown by aseptic methods in such cultures. If animal serum is used in the propagation of the cells, the maintenance medium after virus inoculation shall contain no added serum.

Each group of cell cultures derived from a single monkey or from foetuses from no more than 10 near-term monkeys is prepared and tested as an individual group.

VIRUS SEED LOTS
The strains of poliovirus used shall be identified by historical records that include information on the origin and subsequent manipulation of the strains.

Working seed lots are prepared by a single passage from a master seed lot and at an approved passage level from the original Sabin virus. Virus seed lots are prepared in large quantities and stored at a temperature below $-60\ ^\circ C$.

Only a virus seed lot that complies with the following requirements may be used for virus propagation.

Identification
Each working seed lot is identified as polio virus of the given type, using specific antibodies.

Virus concentration
Determined by the method described below, the virus concentration is the basis for the quantity of virus used in the neurovirulence test.

Extraneous agents (*2.6.16*)
If the working seed lot is produced in human diploid cells or in a continuous cell line, it complies with the requirements for seed lots for virus vaccines. If the working seed lot is produced in primary monkey kidney cell cultures, it complies with the requirements given below under Virus Propagation and Harvest and Monovalent Pooled Harvest and with the tests in adult mice, suckling mice and guinea-pigs given in chapter *2.6.16*.

In addition to the requirements in chapter *2.6.16*, for vaccines produced in cell lines and when the seed lot was produced in primary monkey kidney cell cultures, a validated test for sCMV is performed.

Working seed lots shall be free from detectable DNA sequences from simian virus 40 (SV40).

Neurovirulence

Each master and working seed lot complies with the test for neurovirulence of poliomyelitis vaccine (oral) in monkeys (*2.6.19*). In addition, at least the first 4 consecutive batches of monovalent pooled harvest prepared from these seed lots shall be shown to comply with the test for neurovirulence of poliomyelitis vaccine (oral) in monkeys (*2.6.19*) before the seed lot is deemed suitable for use. Furthermore, the seed lot shall cease to be used in vaccine production if the frequency of failure of the monovalent pooled harvests produced from it is greater than predicted statistically. This statistical prediction is calculated after each test on the basis of all the monovalent pooled harvests tested; it is equal to the probability of false rejection on the occasion of a first test (i.e. 1 per cent), the probability of false rejection on retest being negligible. If the test is carried out only by the manufacturer, the test slides are provided to the control authority for assessment.

Genetic markers

Each working seed lot is tested for its replicating properties at temperatures ranging from 36 °C to 40 °C as described under Monovalent pooled harvest. A profile (i.e. percentage of mutant) of the seed virus using the MAPREC assay is prepared. Type 3 virus seed lots comply with the MAPREC assay as described under Monovalent pooled harvest.

VIRUS PROPAGATION AND HARVEST

All processing of the cell banks and subsequent cell cultures is done under aseptic conditions in an area where no other cells are handled during the production. Suitable animal (but not human) serum may be used in the culture media, but the final medium for maintaining cell growth during virus multiplication does not contain animal serum. Serum and trypsin used in the preparation of cell suspensions and media are shown to be free from live extraneous agents. The cell-culture medium may contain a pH indicator such as phenol red and suitable antibiotics at the lowest effective concentration. It is preferable to have a substrate free from antibiotics during production. On the day of inoculation with the virus working seed lot, not less than 5 per cent or 1000 mL, whichever is the less, of the cell cultures employed for vaccine production are set aside as uninfected cell cultures (control cells). Special requirements, given below, apply to control cells when the vaccine is produced in primary monkey kidney cell cultures. The virus suspension is harvested not later than 4 days after virus inoculation. After inoculation of the production cell culture with the virus working seed lot, inoculated cells are maintained at a fixed temperature, shown to be suitable, within the range 33-35 °C; the temperature is maintained constant to ± 0.5 °C; control cell cultures are maintained at 33-35 °C for the relevant incubation periods.

Only a single virus harvest that complies with the following requirements may be used in the preparation of the monovalent pooled harvest.

Virus concentration

The virus concentration of virus harvests is determined as prescribed under Assay to monitor consistency of production and to determine the dilution to be used for the final bulk vaccine.

Molecular tests for consistency of production

The MAPREC assay is performed on each virus harvest. The acceptance/rejection criteria for consistency of production are determined for each manufacturer and for each working seed by agreement with the competent authority. These criteria are periodically reviewed and updated to the satisfaction of the competent authority. An investigation of consistency occurs if a virus harvest gives results that are inconsistent with previous production history.

Control cells

The control cells of the production cell culture from which the virus harvest is derived comply with a test for identity and with the requirements for extraneous agents (*2.6.16*) or, where primary monkey kidney cell cultures are used, as shown below.

Primary monkey kidney cell cultures

The following special requirements apply to virus propagation and harvest in primary monkey kidney cell cultures.

Cell cultures   On the day of inoculation with the virus working seed lot, each cell culture is examined for degeneration caused by an infective agent. If, in this examination, evidence is found of the presence in a cell culture of any extraneous agent, the entire group of cultures concerned shall be rejected.

On the day of inoculation with the virus working seed lot, a sample of at least 30 mL of the pooled fluid removed from the cell cultures of the kidneys of each single monkey or from foetuses from not more than 10 near-term monkeys is divided into 2 equal portions. 1 portion of the pooled fluid is tested in monkey kidney cell cultures prepared from the same species, but not the same animal, as that used for vaccine production. The other portion of the pooled fluid is, where necessary, tested in monkey kidney cell cultures from another species so that tests on the pooled fluids are done in cell cultures from at least 1 species known to be sensitive to SV40. The pooled fluid is inoculated into bottles of these cell cultures in such a way that the dilution of the pooled fluid in the nutrient medium does not exceed 1 in 4. The area of the cell sheet is at least 3 cm²/ml of pooled fluid. At least 1 bottle of each type of cell culture remains uninoculated to serve as a control. If the monkey species used for vaccine production is known to be sensitive to SV40, a test in a 2nd species is not required. Animal serum may be used in the propagation of the cells, provided that it does not contain SV40 antibody, but the maintenance medium after inoculation of test material contains no added serum except as described below.

The cultures are incubated at a temperature of 35-37 °C and are observed for a total period of at least 4 weeks. During this observation period and after not less than 2 weeks' incubation, at least 1 subculture of fluid is made from each of these cultures in the same cell culture system. The subcultures are also observed for at least 2 weeks.

Serum may be added to the original culture at the time of subculturing, provided that the serum does not contain SV40 antibody.

Fluorescent-antibody techniques may be useful for detecting SV40 virus and other viruses in the cells.

A further sample of at least 10 mL of the pooled fluid is tested for cercopithecid herpesvirus 1 (B virus) and other viruses in rabbit kidney cell cultures. Serum used in the nutrient medium of these cultures shall have been shown to be free from inhibitors of B virus. Human herpesvirus has been used as an indicator for freedom from B virus inhibitors on account of the danger of handling cercopithecid herpesvirus 1 (B virus). The sample is inoculated into bottles of these cell cultures in such a way that the dilution of the pooled fluid in the nutrient medium does not exceed 1 in 4. The area of the cell sheet is at least 3 cm²/ml of pooled fluid. At least 1 bottle of the cell cultures remains uninoculated to serve as a control.

IMMUNOLOGICAL PRODUCTS

The cultures are incubated at a temperature of 35-37 °C and observed for at least 2 weeks.

A further sample of 10 mL of the pooled fluid removed from the cell cultures on the day of inoculation with the seed lot virus is tested for the presence of extraneous agents by inoculation into human cell cultures sensitive to measles virus.

The tests are not valid if more than 20 per cent of the culture vessels have been discarded for non-specific accidental reasons by the end of the respective test periods.

If, in these tests, evidence is found of the presence of an extraneous agent, the single harvest from the whole group of cell cultures concerned is rejected.

If the presence of cercopithecid herpesvirus 1 (B virus) is demonstrated, the manufacture of oral poliomyelitis vaccine shall be discontinued and the competent authority shall be informed. Manufacturing shall not be resumed until a thorough investigation has been completed and precautions have been taken against any reappearance of the infection, and then only with the approval of the competent authority.

If these tests are not done immediately, the samples of pooled cell-culture fluid shall be kept at a temperature of −60 °C or below, with the exception of the sample for the test for B virus, which may be held at 4 °C, provided that the test is done not more than 7 days after it has been taken.

Control cell cultures   On the day of inoculation with the virus working seed lot, 25 per cent (but not more than 2.5 litres) of the cell suspension obtained from the kidneys of each single monkey or from not more than 10 near-term monkeys is taken to prepare uninoculated control cell cultures. These control cell cultures are incubated in the same conditions as the inoculated cultures for at least 2 weeks and are examined during this period for evidence of cytopathic changes.

The tests are not valid if more than 20 per cent of the control cell cultures have been discarded for non-specific, accidental reasons. At the end of the observation period, the control cell cultures are examined for degeneration caused by an infectious agent. If this examination or any of the tests required in this section shows evidence of the presence in a control culture of any extraneous agent, the poliovirus grown in the corresponding inoculated cultures from the same group shall be rejected.

Tests for haemadsorbing viruses   At the time of harvest or within 4 days of inoculation of the production cultures with the virus working seed lot, a sample of 4 per cent of the control cell cultures is taken and tested for haemadsorbing viruses. At the end of the observation period, the remaining control cell cultures are similarly tested. The tests are carried out as described in chapter *2.6.16*.

Tests for other extraneous agents   At the time of harvest, or within 7 days of the day of inoculation of the production cultures with the working seed lot, a sample of at least 20 mL of the pooled fluid from each group of control cultures is taken and tested in 2 kinds of monkey kidney cell culture, as described above.

At the end of the observation period for the original control cell cultures, similar samples of the pooled fluid are taken and the tests referred to in this section in the 2 kinds of monkey kidney cell culture and in the rabbit cell cultures are repeated, as described above under Cell cultures.

If the presence of cercopithecid herpesvirus 1 (B virus) is demonstrated, the production cell cultures shall not be used and the measures concerning vaccine production described above must be undertaken.

The fluids collected from the control cell cultures at the time of virus harvest and at the end of the observation period may be pooled before testing for extraneous agents. A sample of 2 per cent of the pooled fluid is tested in each of the cell culture systems specified.

Single harvests

Tests for neutralised single harvests in primary monkey kidney cell cultures   A sample of at least 10 mL of each single harvest is neutralised by a type-specific poliomyelitis antiserum prepared in animals other than monkeys. In preparing antisera for this purpose, the immunising antigens used shall be prepared in non-simian cells.

Half of the neutralised suspension (corresponding to at least 5 mL of single harvest) is tested in monkey kidney cell cultures prepared from the same species, but not the same animal, as that used for vaccine production. The other half of the neutralised suspension is tested, if necessary, in monkey kidney cell cultures from another species so that the tests on the neutralised suspension are done in cell cultures from at least 1 species known to be sensitive to SV40.

The neutralised suspensions are inoculated into bottles of these cell cultures in such a way that the dilution of the suspension in the nutrient medium does not exceed 1 in 4. The area of the cell sheet is at least 3 cm^2/ml of neutralised suspension. At least 1 bottle of each type of cell culture remains uninoculated to serve as a control and is maintained by nutrient medium containing the same concentration of the specific antiserum used for neutralisation.

Animal serum may be used in the propagation of the cells, provided that it does not contain SV40 antibody, but the maintenance medium, after the inoculation of the test material, contains no added serum other than the poliovirus neutralising antiserum, except as described below.

The cultures are incubated at a temperature of 35-37 °C and observed for a total period of at least 4 weeks. During this observation period and after not less than 2 weeks' incubation, at least 1 subculture of fluid is made from each of these cultures in the same cell-culture system.

The subcultures are also observed for at least 2 weeks.

Serum may be added to the original cultures at the time of subculturing, provided that the serum does not contain SV40 antibody.

Additional tests are made for extraneous agents on a further sample of the neutralised single harvests by inoculation of 10 mL into human cell cultures sensitive to measles virus. This test is also validated for the detection of sCMV.

Fluorescent-antibody techniques may be useful for detecting SV40 virus and other viruses in the cells.

The tests are not valid if more than 20 per cent of the culture vessels have been discarded for non-specific accidental reasons by the end of the respective test periods.

If any cytopathic changes occur in any of the cultures, the causes of these changes are investigated. If the cytopathic changes are shown to be due to unneutralised poliovirus, the test is repeated. If there is evidence of the presence of SV40 or other extraneous agents attributable to the single harvest, that single harvest is rejected.

MONOVALENT POOLED HARVEST

Monovalent pooled harvests are prepared by pooling a number of satisfactory single harvests of the same virus type. Monovalent pooled harvests from continuous cell lines may be purified. Each monovalent pooled harvest is filtered through a bacteria-retentive filter.

Only a monovalent pooled harvest that complies with the following requirements may be used in the preparation of the final bulk vaccine.

Identification

Each monovalent pooled harvest is identified as poliovirus of the given type, using specific antibodies.

Virus concentration

The virus concentration is determined by the method described below and serves as the basis for calculating the dilutions for preparation of the final bulk, for the quantity of virus used in the neurovirulence test and to establish and monitor production consistency.

Genetic markers

For Sabin poliovirus type 3, a validated MAPREC assay is performed. In this analysis the amount of the mutation at position 472 of the genome (472-C) is estimated and expressed as a ratio relative to the International Standard for MAPREC analysis of poliovirus type 3 (Sabin). A poliovirus type 3 monovalent pooled harvest found to have significantly more 472-C than the International Standard for MAPREC analysis of poliovirus type 3 (Sabin) fails in the MAPREC assay.

The MAPREC analysis of poliovirus type 3 (Sabin) is carried out using a standard operating procedure approved by the competent authority. A suitable procedure (*Mutant analysis by PCR and restriction enzyme cleavage (MAPREC) for oral poliovirus (Sabin) vaccine*) is available from WHO, Quality and Safety of Biologicals (QSB), Geneva. A laboratory must demonstrate to the competent authority that it is competent to perform the assay. The manufacturer and the competent authority shall agree on the procedure and the criteria for deciding whether a monovalent pooled harvest contains significantly more 472-C than the International Standard.

Acceptance/rejection criteria for assessment of consistency of production are determined for each manufacturer and for each working seed lot by agreement with the competent authority. These criteria are updated as each new bulk is prepared and analysed. An investigation of consistency occurs if a monovalent pooled harvest gives results that are inconsistent with previous production history.

As the MAPREC assay for type 3 poliovirus (Sabin) is highly predictive of *in vivo* neurovirulence, if a filtered monovalent pooled harvest of type 3 poliovirus (Sabin) fails the MAPREC assay then this triggers an investigation of the consistency of the manufacturing process. This investigation also includes a consideration of the suitability of the working seed lot.

Monovalent pooled harvests passing the MAPREC assay are subsequently tested for *in vivo* neurovirulence.

For poliovirus type 3, results from the MAPREC assay and the monkey neurovirulence test (*2.6.19*) are used concomitantly to assess the impact of changes in the production process or when a new manufacturer starts production.

Pending validation of MAPREC assays for poliovirus types 1 and 2, for these viruses filtered bulk suspension is tested for the property of reproducing at temperatures of 36 °C and 40 °C. A ratio of the replication capacities of the virus in the monovalent pooled harvest is obtained over a temperature range between 36 °C and 40 °C in comparison with the seed lot or a reference preparation for the marker tests and with appropriate rct/40− and rct/40+ strains of poliovirus of the same type. The incubation temperatures used in this test are controlled to within ± 0.1 °C. The monovalent pooled harvest passes the test if, for both the virus in the harvest and the appropriate reference material, the titre determined at 36 °C is at least 5.0 log greater than that determined at 40 °C. If growth at 40 °C is so low that a valid comparison cannot be established, a temperature in the region of 39.0-39.5 °C is used, at which temperature the reduction in titre of the reference material must be in the range 3.0-5.0 log of its value at 36 °C; the acceptable minimum reduction is determined for each virus strain at a given temperature. If the titres obtained for 1 or more of the reference viruses are not concordant with the expected values, the test must be repeated.

Neurovirulence (*2.6.19*)

Each monovalent pooled harvest complies with the test for neurovirulence of poliomyelitis vaccine (oral). If the monkey neurovirulence test is carried out only by the manufacturer, the test slides are provided to the competent authority for assessment. The TgPVR21 transgenic mouse model provides a suitable alternative to the monkey neurovirulence test for neurovirulence testing of types 1, 2 or 3 vaccines once a laboratory qualifies as being competent to perform the test and the experience gained is to the satisfaction of the competent authority. The test is carried out using a standard operating procedure approved by the competent authority. A suitable procedure (*Neurovirulence test of type 1, 2 or 3 live poliomyelitis vaccines (oral) in transgenic mice susceptible to poliovirus*) is available from WHO, Quality and Safety of Biologicals, Geneva.

Primary monkey kidney cell cultures

The following special requirements apply to monovalent pooled harvests derived from primary monkey kidney cell cultures.

Retroviruses   The monovalent pooled harvest is examined using a reverse transcriptase assay. No indication of the presence of retroviruses is found.

Test in rabbits   A sample of the monovalent pooled harvest is tested for cercopithecid herpesvirus 1 (B virus) and other viruses by injection of not less than 100 mL into not fewer than 10 healthy rabbits each weighing 1.5-2.5 kg. Each rabbit receives not less than 10 mL and not more than 20 mL, of which 1 mL is given intradermally at multiple sites since the maximum volume to be given intradermally at each site is 0.1 mL, and the remainder subcutaneously. The rabbits are observed for at least 3 weeks for death or signs of illness.

All rabbits that die after the first 24 h of the test and those showing signs of illness are examined by autopsy, and the brain and organs removed for detailed examination to establish the cause of death.

The test is not valid if more than 20 per cent of the inoculated rabbits show signs of intercurrent infection during the observation period. The monovalent pooled harvest passes the test if none of the rabbits shows evidence of infection with B virus or with other extraneous agents or lesions of any kind attributable to the bulk suspension.

If the presence of B virus is demonstrated, the measures concerning vaccine production described above under Cell cultures are taken.

Test in guinea-pigs   If the primary monkey kidney cell cultures are not derived from monkeys kept in a closed colony, the monovalent pooled harvest shall be shown to comply with the following test. Administer to each of not fewer than 5 guinea-pigs, each weighing 350-450 g, 0.1 mL of the monovalent pooled harvest by intracerebral injection (0.05 mL in each cerebral hemisphere) and 0.5 mL by intraperitoneal injection. Measure the rectal temperature of each animal on each working day for 6 weeks. At the end of the observation period carry out autopsy on each animal.

In addition, administer to not fewer than 5 guinea-pigs 0.5 mL by intraperitoneal injection and observe as described above for 2-3 weeks. At the end of the observation period, carry out a passage from these animals to not fewer than 5 guinea-pigs using blood and a suspension of liver or spleen tissue. Measure the rectal temperature of the latter guinea-pigs for 2-3 weeks. Examine by autopsy all animals that, after the first day of the test, die or are euthanised because they show disease, or show on 3 consecutive days a body temperature higher than 40.1 °C; carry out histological examination to detect infection with filoviruses; in addition, inject a suspension of liver or spleen tissue or of blood intraperitoneally into not fewer than 3 guinea-pigs. If any signs of infection with filoviruses are noted, confirmatory serological tests are carried out on the blood of the affected animals. The monovalent pooled harvest complies with the test if not fewer than 80 per cent of the guinea-pigs survive to the end of the observation period and remain in good health, and no animal shows signs of infection with filoviruses.

FINAL BULK VACCINE
The final bulk vaccine is prepared from one or more satisfactory monovalent pooled harvests and may contain more than one virus type. Suitable flavouring substances and stabilisers may be added.

Only a final bulk vaccine that complies with the following requirement may be used in the preparation of the final lot.

Bacterial and fungal contamination
Carry out the test for sterility (2.6.1), using 10 mL for each medium.

FINAL LOT
Only a final lot that complies with the following requirement for thermal stability and is satisfactory with respect to each of the requirements given below under Identification, Tests and Assay may be released for use.

Thermal stability
Maintain not fewer than 3 containers of the final lot at 37 ± 1 °C for 48 h. Determine the total virus concentration as described under Assay in parallel for the heated vaccine and for vaccine maintained at the temperature recommended for storage. The total virus concentration of the heated vaccine is not more than 0.5 log lower than that of the unheated vaccine.

IDENTIFICATION
The vaccine is shown to contain poliovirus of each type stated on the label, using specific antibodies.

TESTS
Bacterial and fungal contamination
The vaccine complies with the test for sterility (2.6.1).

ASSAY
Titrate the vaccine for infectious virus, using not fewer than 3 separate containers of vaccine, following the method described below. Titrate 1 container of an appropriate virus reference preparation in triplicate to validate each assay. The virus concentration of the reference preparation is monitored using a control chart and a titre is established on a historical basis by each laboratory. If the vaccine contains more than one poliovirus type, titrate each type separately, using an appropriate type-specific antiserum (or preferably a monoclonal antibody) to neutralise each of the other types present.

Calculate the individual virus concentration for each container of vaccine and for each replicate of the reference preparation as well as the corresponding combined virus concentrations, using the usual statistical methods (for example, 5.3).

For a trivalent vaccine, the combined estimated virus titres per single human dose must be:
— not less than 6.0 log infectious virus units ($CCID_{50}$) for type 1;
— not less than 5.0 log infectious virus units ($CCID_{50}$) for type 2; and
— not less than 5.5 log infectious virus units ($CCID_{50}$) for type 3.

For a monovalent or divalent vaccine, the minimum virus titres are decided by the competent authority.

Method Inoculate a suitable number of wells in a microtitre plate with a suitable volume of each of the selected dilutions of virus followed by a suitable volume of a cell suspension of the Hep-2 (Cincinnati) line. Examine the cultures between days 7 and 9.

The assay is not valid if:
— the confidence interval ($P = 0.95$) of the estimated virus concentration of the reference preparation for the 3 replicates combined is greater than ± 0.3 log $CCID_{50}$;
— the virus concentration of the reference preparation differs by more than 0.5 log $CCID_{50}$ from the established value. The relation with the appropriate European Pharmacopoeia Biological Reference Preparation is established and monitored at regular intervals when a manufacturer's reference preparation is used.

The assay is repeated if the confidence interval ($P = 0.95$) of the combined virus concentration of the vaccine is greater than ± 0.3 log $CCID_{50}$; data obtained from valid assays only are combined by the usual statistical methods (for example, 5.3) to calculate the virus concentration of the sample. The confidence interval ($P = 0.95$) of the combined virus concentration is not greater than ± 0.3 log $CCID_{50}$.

Poliomyelitis vaccine (oral) BRP is suitable for use as a reference preparation.

Where justified and authorised, different assay designs may be used; this may imply the application of different validity and acceptance criteria. However, the vaccine must comply if tested as described above.

LABELLING
The label states:
— the types of poliovirus contained in the vaccine;
— the minimum amount of virus of each type contained in a single human dose;
— the cell substrate used for the preparation of the vaccine.

_____ *Ph Eur*

Rabies Vaccine

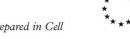

(Rabies Vaccine for Human Use Prepared in Cell Cultures, Ph Eur monograph 0216)
The label may state 'Rab'.

Ph Eur _____

DEFINITION
Rabies vaccine for human use prepared in cell cultures is a freeze-dried preparation of a suitable strain of fixed rabies virus grown in cell cultures and inactivated by a validated method.

The vaccine is reconstituted immediately before use as stated on the label to give a clear liquid that may be coloured owing to the presence of a pH indicator.

PRODUCTION
GENERAL PROVISIONS
The production of the vaccine is based on a virus seed-lot system and, if a cell line is used for virus propagation, a cell-bank system. The production method shall have been shown to yield consistently vaccines that comply with the requirements for immunogenicity, safety and stability. Unless otherwise justified and authorised, the virus in the final vaccine must not have undergone more passages from the master seed lot than were used to prepare the vaccine shown in clinical studies to be satisfactory with respect to safety and efficacy; even with authorised exceptions, the number of passages beyond the level used for clinical studies must not exceed 5.

The production method is validated to demonstrate that the product, if tested, would comply with the test for abnormal toxicity for immunosera and vaccines for human use (2.6.9).

SUBSTRATE FOR VIRUS PROPAGATION
The virus is propagated in a human diploid cell line (5.2.3), in a continuous cell line approved by the competent authority, or in cultures of chick-embryo cells derived from a flock free from specified pathogens (5.2.2).

SEED LOTS
The strain of rabies virus used shall be identified by historical records that include information on the origin of the strain and its subsequent manipulation.

Working seed lots are prepared by not more than 5 passages from the master seed lot.

Only a working seed lot that complies with the following tests may be used for virus propagation.

Identification
Each working seed lot is identified as rabies virus using specific antibodies.

Virus concentration
The virus concentration of each working seed lot is determined by a cell culture method using immunofluorescence, to ensure consistency of production.

Extraneous agents (2.6.16)
The working seed lot complies with the requirements for virus seed lots. If the virus has been passaged in mouse brain, specific tests for murine viruses are carried out.

VIRUS PROPAGATION AND HARVEST
All processing of the cell bank and subsequent cell cultures is done under aseptic conditions in an area where no other cells are handled. Approved animal (but not human) serum may be used in the media, but the final medium for maintaining cell growth during virus multiplication does not contain animal serum; the media may contain human albumin. Serum and trypsin used in the preparation of cell suspensions and media are shown to be free from extraneous agents. The cell culture media may contain a pH indicator such as phenol red and approved antibiotics at the lowest effective concentration. Not less than 500 mL of the cell cultures employed for vaccine production are set aside as uninfected cell cultures (control cells). The virus suspension is harvested on one or more occasions during incubation. Multiple harvests from the same production cell culture may be pooled and considered as a single harvest.

Only a single harvest that complies with the following requirements may be used in the preparation of the inactivated viral harvest.

Identification
The single harvest contains virus that is identified as rabies virus using specific antibodies.

Virus concentration
Titrate for infective virus in cell cultures; the titre is used to monitor consistency of production.

Control cells
The control cells of the production cell culture from which the single harvest is derived comply with a test for identification and with the requirements for extraneous agents (2.6.16).

PURIFICATION AND INACTIVATION
The virus harvest may be concentrated and/or purified by suitable methods; the virus harvest is inactivated by a validated method at a fixed, well-defined stage of the process, which may be before, during or after any concentration or purification. The method shall have been shown to be capable of inactivating rabies virus without destruction of the immunogenic activity. If betapropiolactone is used, the concentration shall at no time exceed 1:3500.

Only an inactivated viral suspension that complies with the following requirements may be used in the preparation of the final bulk vaccine.

Residual infectious virus
Carry out an amplification test for residual infectious rabies virus immediately after inactivation or using a sample frozen immediately after inactivation and stored at − 70 °C. Inoculate a quantity of inactivated viral suspension equivalent to not less than 25 human doses of vaccine into cell cultures of the same type as those used for production of the vaccine. A passage may be made after 7 days. Maintain the cultures for a total of 21 days and then examine the cell cultures for rabies virus using an immunofluorescence test.

The inactivated virus harvest complies with the test if no rabies virus is detected.

Residual host-cell DNA
If a continuous cell line is used for virus propagation, the content of residual host-cell DNA, determined using a suitable method as described in *Products of recombinant DNA technology (0784)*, is not greater than 10 ng per single human dose.

FINAL BULK VACCINE
The final bulk vaccine is prepared from one or more inactivated viral suspensions. An approved stabiliser may be added to maintain the activity of the product during and after freeze-drying.

Only a final bulk vaccine that complies with the following requirements may be used in the preparation of the final lot.

Glycoprotein content
Determine the glycoprotein content by a suitable immunochemical method (2.7.1), for example, single-radial immunodiffusion, enzyme-linked immunosorbent assay or an antibody-binding test. The content is within the limits approved for the particular product.

Sterility (2.6.1)
The final bulk vaccine complies with the test for sterility, carried out using 10 mL for each medium.

FINAL LOT
The final bulk vaccine is distributed aseptically into sterile containers and freeze-dried to a moisture content shown to be favourable to the stability of the vaccine. The containers are then closed so as to avoid contamination and the introduction of moisture.

Only a final lot that complies with each of the requirements given below under Identification, Tests and Assay may be released for use. Provided that the test for residual infectious

IMMUNOLOGICAL PRODUCTS

virus has been carried out with satisfactory results on the inactivated viral suspension and the test for bovine serum albumin has been carried out with satisfactory results on the final bulk vaccine, these tests may be omitted on the final lot.

IDENTIFICATION

The vaccine is shown to contain rabies virus antigen by a suitable immunochemical method (2.7.1) using specific antibodies, preferably monoclonal; alternatively, the assay serves also to identify the vaccine.

TESTS

Residual infectious virus

Inoculate a quantity equivalent to not less than 25 human doses of vaccine into cell cultures of the same type as those used for production of the vaccine. A passage may be made after 7 days. Maintain the cultures for a total of 21 days and then examine the cell cultures for rabies virus using an immunofluorescence test. The vaccine complies with the test if no rabies virus is detected.

Bovine serum albumin

Maximum 50 ng per single human dose, determined by a suitable immunochemical method (2.7.1).

Sterility (2.6.1)

It complies with the test.

Bacterial endotoxins (2.6.14)

Less than 25 IU per single human dose.

Pyrogens (2.6.8)

It complies with the test. Unless otherwise justified and authorised, inject into each rabbit a single human dose of the vaccine diluted to 10 times its volume.

Water (2.5.12)

Maximum 3.0 per cent.

ASSAY

The potency of rabies vaccine is determined by comparing the dose necessary to protect mice against the effects of a lethal dose of rabies virus, administered intracerebrally, with the quantity of a reference preparation of rabies vaccine necessary to provide the same protection. For this comparison a reference preparation of rabies vaccine, calibrated in International Units, and a suitable preparation of rabies virus for use as the challenge preparation are necessary.

The International Unit is the activity contained in a stated quantity of the International Standard. The equivalence in International Units of the International Standard is stated by the World Health Organisation.

The test described below uses a parallel-line model with at least 3 points for the vaccine to be examined and the reference preparation. Once the analyst has experience with the method for a given vaccine, it is possible to carry out a simplified test using a single dilution of the vaccine to be examined. Such a test enables the analyst to determine that the vaccine has a potency significantly higher than the required minimum, but does not give full information on the validity of each individual potency determination. The use of a single dilution allows a considerable reduction in the number of animals required for the test and must be considered by each laboratory in accordance with the provisions of the European Convention for the Protection of Vertebrate Animals used for Experimental and other Scientific Purposes.

Selection and distribution of the test animals   Use healthy female mice, about 4 weeks old, each weighing 11-15 g, and from the same stock. Distribute the mice into 6 groups of a size suitable to meet the requirements for validity of the test and, for titration of the challenge suspension, 4 groups of 5.

Preparation of the challenge suspension   Inoculate mice intracerebrally with the Challenge Virus Standard (CVS) strain of rabies virus and when the mice show signs of rabies, but before they die, euthanise them, then remove the brains and prepare a homogenate of the brain tissue in a suitable diluent. Separate gross particulate matter by centrifugation and use the supernatant liquid as the challenge suspension. Distribute the suspension in small volumes in ampoules, seal and store at a temperature below $- 60$ °C. Thaw one ampoule of the suspension and make serial dilutions in a suitable diluent. Allocate each dilution to a group of 5 mice and inject intracerebrally into each mouse 0.03 mL of the dilution allocated to its group. Observe the mice for 14 days. Calculate the LD_{50} of the undiluted suspension using the number in each group that, between the 5th and 14th days, die or develop signs of rabies.

Determination of potency of the vaccine   Prepare 3 fivefold serial dilutions of the vaccine to be examined and 3 fivefold serial dilutions of the reference preparation. Prepare the dilutions such that the most concentrated suspensions may be expected to protect more than 50 per cent of the animals to which they are administered and the least concentrated suspensions may be expected to protect less than 50 per cent of the animals to which they are administered. Allocate the 6 dilutions, 1 to each of the 6 groups of mice, and inject by the intraperitoneal route into each mouse 0.5 mL of the dilution allocated to its group. After 7 days, prepare 3 identical dilutions of the vaccine to be examined and of the reference preparation and repeat the injections. 7 days after the second injection, prepare a suspension of the challenge virus such that, on the basis of the preliminary titration, 0.03 mL contains about 50 LD_{50}. Inject intracerebrally into each vaccinated mouse 0.03 mL of this suspension. Prepare 3 suitable serial dilutions of the challenge suspension. Allocate the challenge suspension and the 3 dilutions, 1 to each of the 4 groups of 5 control mice, and inject intracerebrally into each mouse 0.03 mL of the suspension or dilution allocated to its group. Observe the animals in each group for 14 days and record the number in each group that die or show signs of rabies in the period 5-14 days after challenge.

The test is not valid unless:

— for both the vaccine to be examined and the reference preparation the 50 per cent protective dose lies between the largest and smallest doses given to the mice;

— the titration of the challenge suspension shows that 0.03 mL of the suspension contained not less than 10 LD_{50};

— the statistical analysis shows a significant slope and no significant deviations from linearity or parallelism of the dose-response curves;

— the confidence limits ($P = 0.95$) are not less than 25 per cent and not more than 400 per cent of the estimated potency.

The vaccine complies with the test if the estimated potency is not less than 2.5 IU per human dose.

Application of alternative end-points   Once a laboratory has established the above assay for routine use, the lethal end-point is replaced by an observation of clinical signs and application of an end-point earlier than death to reduce animal suffering. The following is given as an example.

The progress of rabies infection in mice following intracerebral injection can be represented by 5 stages defined by typical clinical signs:

Stage 1: ruffled fur, hunched back;

Stage 2: slow movements, loss of alertness (circular movements may also occur);

Stage 3: shaky movements, trembling, convulsions;

Stage 4: signs of paresis or paralysis;

Stage 5: moribund state.

Mice are observed at least twice daily from day 4 after challenge. Clinical signs are recorded using a chart such as that shown in Table 0216.-1. Experience has shown that using stage 3 as an end-point yields assay results equivalent to those found when a lethal end-point is used. This must be verified by each laboratory by scoring a suitable number of assays using both the clinical signs and the lethal end-point.

Table 0216.-1. – *Example of a chart used to record clinical signs in the rabies vaccine potency test*

Clinical signs	Days after challenge							
	4	5	6	7	8	9	10	11
Ruffled fur Hunched back								
Slow movements Loss of alertness Circular movements								
Shaky movements Trembling Convulsions								
Paresis Paralysis								
Moribund state								

LABELLING

The label states the biological origin of the cells used for the preparation of the vaccine.

Ph Eur

Rotavirus Vaccine (Live, Oral)

(*Ph Eur monograph 2417*)

The label may state 'Rotavirus (live, oral)'.

Ph Eur

DEFINITION

Rotavirus vaccine (live, oral) is a preparation of one or more suitable virus serotypes, grown in an approved cell substrate and presented in a form suitable for oral administration.

The vaccine is a clear liquid or it may be a freeze-dried preparation to be reconstituted immediately before use, as stated on the label, to give a slightly turbid liquid.

The vaccine ready for administration may be coloured owing to the presence of a pH indicator.

PRODUCTION

GENERAL PROVISIONS

The vaccine strains and the production method shall have been shown to yield consistently vaccines comparable with the vaccine of proven clinical efficacy and safety in man. The vaccine is formulated so as to avoid inactivation by gastric fluids. Where the vaccine is freeze-dried, the antacid capacity of the solvent and its stability are established.

The production of vaccine is based on a virus seed-lot system and a cell-bank system. Unless otherwise justified and authorised, the virus in the final vaccine shall have undergone no more passages from the master seed lot than were used to prepare the vaccine shown in clinical studies to be satisfactory with respect to safety and efficacy.

If purification steps are present, the reduction of selected process-related impurities and residuals such as residual host-cell proteins, residual cellular DNA, endotoxins, bovine serum, trypsin, and antibiotics is monitored to establish consistency of the purification process.

REFERENCE PREPARATION

A suitable reference preparation that is representative of batches of vaccine shown to be effective in clinical trials is established for use in tests to determine virus concentration. The differences in the composition and characteristics of rotavirus vaccines mean that there will be a specific reference preparation for each one.

SUBSTRATE FOR VIRUS PROPAGATION

The virus is propagated in a suitable cell line (*5.2.3*).

VIRUS SEED LOTS

The strain(s) of rotavirus used shall be identified by historical records that include information on the origin of each strain and its subsequent manipulation including the method of attenuation, whether the strains have been biologically cloned prior to generation of the master seed lot, genetic sequence information, the phenotypic and genotypic stability of the master and working seed lots when passaged up to the single harvest level, and the passage level at which attenuation for humans was demonstrated by clinical trials. Virus seed lots are stored at temperatures below -20 °C if freeze-dried, or below -60 °C if not freeze-dried.

Only a seed lot that complies with the following requirements may be used for virus propagation.

Identification

The master and working seed lots are shown to be of the required rotavirus type by an immunological assay using specific antibodies or by a molecular identity test such as polyacrylamide gel electrophoresis of RNA, RNA/RNA hybridisation, or restriction-enzyme mapping of genetic sequences of polymerase chain reaction (PCR)-amplified VP7 gene segments.

Virus concentration

The virus concentration of the master and working seed lots is determined to monitor consistency of production. Direct cell-culture based methods and nucleic acid amplification techniques (NAT) (*2.6.21*) such as PCR quantification of virus replication in cell culture may be used.

Extraneous agents (*2.6.16*)

Each working seed lot complies with the requirements for virus seed lots.

VIRUS PROPAGATION, SINGLE HARVEST, MONOVALENT POOLED HARVEST

All processing of the cell bank and subsequent cell cultures is done under aseptic conditions in an area where no other cells are being handled. Suitable animal (but not human) serum may be used in the culture media, but the final medium for maintaining cell growth during virus multiplication does not contain animal serum. Serum and trypsin used in the preparation of cell suspensions and culture media are shown to be free from extraneous agents. The cell culture medium may contain a pH indicator such as phenol red and suitable antibiotics at the lowest effective concentration. It is preferable to have a substrate free from antibiotics during production.

STORED VIRUS INTERMEDIATE CULTURE

Where a stored virus intermediate culture, prepared from the working seed lot, is used for inoculation, on the day of inoculation not less than 5 per cent or 500 mL of the cell cultures employed, whichever is greater, are set aside as uninfected cell cultures (control cells). Stored virus intermediate cultures are harvested at a time appropriate to the strain of virus and stored at temperatures below – 60°C.

Only a stored virus intermediate culture that complies with the following requirements may be used for virus propagation.

Identification

Each stored virus intermediate culture is identified by rotavirus type by an immunological assay using specific antibodies or by a molecular identity test such as NAT (2.6.21).

Bacterial and fungal contamination

Each stored virus intermediate culture complies with the test for sterility (2.6.1), carried out using 10 mL for each medium.

Virus concentration

The virus concentration of each stored virus intermediate culture is determined as prescribed under Assay to monitor consistency of production. Both direct cell-culture based methods and NAT (2.6.21) such as PCR quantification of virus replication in cell culture may be used.

Extraneous agents (2.6.16)

Each stored virus intermediate culture complies with the tests for extraneous agents.

Control cells

The control cells of the production cell culture from which each stored virus intermediate culture is derived comply with a test for identity and with the requirements for extraneous agents (2.6.16).

VIRUS PROPAGATION AND SINGLE HARVEST

On the day of inoculation with the virus working seed lot or stored virus intermediate culture, cell cultures employed for vaccine production are set aside as uninfected cell cultures (control cells). If bioreactor technology is used, the size and handling of the cell sample to be examined is approved by the competent authority. The virus suspensions are harvested at a time appropriate to the strain of virus being used.

Only a single virus harvest that complies with the following requirements may be used for further processing.

Bacterial and fungal contamination

Each single virus harvest complies with the test for sterility (2.6.1), carried out using 10 mL for each medium.

Control cells

The control cells of the production cell culture from which each single harvest is derived comply with a test for identity and with the requirements for extraneous agents (2.6.16).

MONOVALENT POOLED HARVEST

Monovalent pooled harvests are prepared by pooling a number of single harvests of the same virus type. If no monovalent pooled harvest is prepared, the tests below are carried out on each single harvest.

Only a single harvest or a monovalent pooled harvest that complies with the following requirements may be used in the preparation of the purified monovalent harvest.

Identification

Each single harvest or monovalent pooled harvest is identified by rotavirus type by an immunological assay using specific antibodies or by a molecular identity test such as NAT (2.6.21).

Bacterial and fungal contamination

Each single harvest or monovalent pooled harvest complies with the test for sterility (2.6.1), carried out using 10 mL for each medium.

Virus concentration

The virus concentration of each single harvest or monovalent pooled harvest is determined as prescribed under Assay to monitor consistency of production. Both direct cell-culture based methods and NAT (2.6.21) such as PCR quantification of virus replication in cell culture may be used.

Extraneous agents (2.6.16)

Each single harvest or monovalent pooled harvest complies with the tests for extraneous agents.

PURIFIED MONOVALENT HARVEST

The purified monovalent harvest is prepared from a single harvest or a pooled monovalent harvest. The single harvest or pooled monovalent harvest is clarified to remove cell debris and may be further purified.

Only a purified monovalent harvest that complies with the following requirements may be used in the preparation of the final bulk vaccine.

Bacterial and fungal contamination

The purified monovalent harvest complies with the test for sterility (2.6.1), carried out using 10 mL for each medium.

Virus concentration

The virus concentration of the purified monovalent harvest is determined as prescribed under Assay to monitor consistency of production. Both direct cell-culture based methods and NAT (2.6.21) such as PCR quantification of virus replication in cell culture may be used.

Residual cellular DNA

Maximum 100 μg of cellular DNA per human dose for viruses grown in continuous cells lines.

FINAL BULK VACCINE

The final bulk vaccine is prepared from one or more satisfactory purified monovalent harvests and may contain more than one virus type. Suitable stabilisers may be added.

Only a final bulk vaccine that complies with the following requirement may be used in the preparation of the final lot.

Bacterial and fungal contamination

The final bulk vaccine complies with the test for sterility (2.6.1), carried out using 10 mL for each medium.

FINAL LOT

The final bulk vaccine is distributed aseptically into sterile containers and may be freeze-dried to a moisture content shown to be favourable to the stability of the vaccine. The containers are then closed so as to avoid contamination and the introduction of moisture.

An approved minimum virus concentration for release of the product is established for each virus type to ensure, in light of stability data, that the minimum concentration stated on the label will be present at the end of the period of validity.

For freeze-dried vaccines, tests for identity, pH, volume, sterility and content of key components are carried out on the solvent.

Only a final lot that complies with the following requirement for thermal stability and is satisfactory with respect to each of the requirements given below under Identification, Tests and Assay may be released for use.

Thermal stability

Maintain not fewer than 3 containers of the final lot at an elevated temperature for a defined time period, using conditions found suitable for the particular product as approved by the competent authority. Determine the virus concentration as described under Assay in parallel for the heated vaccine and for vaccine maintained at the temperature recommended for storage. The virus concentration of the containers that have been heated does not decrease by more than an approved amount during the period of exposure. For a multivalent vaccine, if there is no significant difference in the virus loss between serotypes, the loss may be determined from total virus concentration.

IDENTIFICATION

The vaccine is shown to contain rotavirus of each type stated on the label by an immunological assay using specific antibodies or by a molecular identity test. If PCR is used for the assay, this may serve as the identity test.

TESTS

Bacterial and fungal contamination

The vaccine complies with the test for sterility (2.6.1).

Water (2.5.12)

Maximum 3.0 per cent for each final lot of freeze-dried vaccine.

ASSAY

The assay of rotavirus vaccine is carried out by inoculation of suitable cell cultures with dilutions of the vaccine and evaluation of the rotavirus concentration, either by visualisation of infected areas of a cell monolayer or by comparison of the capacity of the vaccine to produce viral RNA following infection of cells with the corresponding capacity of an approved reference preparation.

For the assay based on visualisation of infected areas of a cell monolayer, titrate the vaccine for infective virus using at least 3 separate containers. Titrate the contents of 1 container of an appropriate virus reference preparation in triplicate to validate each assay. If the vaccine contains more than 1 rotavirus type, titrate each type separately using a method of suitable specificity. The virus concentration of the reference preparation is monitored using a control chart and a titre is established on a historical basis by each laboratory.

Calculate the individual virus concentration for each container of vaccine and for each replicate of the reference preparation as well as the corresponding combined virus concentrations, using the usual statistical methods (for example, 5.3).

The assay is not valid if:

— the confidence interval ($P = 0.95$) of the estimated virus concentration of the reference preparation for the 3 replicates combined is greater than $\pm$ 0.3 log $CCID_{50}$ (or an equivalent value expressed with a unit suitable for the method used for the assay);

— the virus concentration of the reference preparation differs by more than 0.5 log $CCID_{50}$ (or an equivalent value expressed with a unit suitable for the method used for the assay) from the established value.

The assay is repeated if the confidence interval ($P = 0.95$) of the combined virus concentration of the vaccine is greater than $\pm$ 0.3 log $CCID_{50}$ (or an equivalent value expressed with a unit suitable for the method used for the assay); data generated from valid assays only are combined by the usual statistical methods (for example, 5.3) to calculate the virus

concentration of the sample. The confidence interval ($P = 0.95$) of the combined virus concentration is not greater than $\pm$ 0.3 log $CCID_{50}$ (or an equivalent value expressed with a unit suitable for the method used for the assay).

Where justified and authorised, different assay designs may be used; this may imply the application of different validity and acceptance criteria. However, the vaccine must comply if tested as described above.

For the assay based on comparison of the capacity of the vaccine to produce viral RNA following infection of cells with the corresponding capacity of an approved reference preparation, a suitable number of cell cultures in a microtitre plate are infected in parallel with serial dilutions of the vaccine and the reference preparation. After incubation to allow virus replication, viral RNA in the individual wells is released from the cells and quantified by NAT (2.6.21), such as real-time quantitative reverse-transcriptase polymerase chain reaction (RT-PCR) technology.

Not fewer than 3 separate containers of the vaccine are assayed against a container of the reference preparation titrated in triplicate.

Calculate the individual virus concentration for each container of vaccine against the reference preparation as well as the corresponding combined virus concentrations, using the usual statistical methods (for example, 5.3).

The combined estimate of the virus concentration for the 3 containers of vaccine is not less than that stated on the label.

The assay is not valid unless:

— the negative external NAT control is unambiguously negative;

— the positive external NAT control is unambiguously positive;

— the negative matrix control (uninfected cells) is unambiguously negative;

— the positive matrix control (cells spiked with viral RNA) is unambiguously positive;

— the statistical analysis shows a significant slope and no significant deviations from linearity or parallelism of the dose-response curves.

The assay is repeated if the confidence interval ($P = 0.95$) of the combined virus concentration of the vaccine is greater than $\pm$ 0.3 log infectious units; data generated from valid assays only are combined by the usual statistical methods (for example, 5.3) to calculate the virus concentration of the sample. The confidence interval ($P = 0.95$) of the combined virus concentration is not greater than $\pm$ 0.3 log infectious units.

LABELLING

The label states:

— the type or types of rotavirus contained in the vaccine;

— the minimum amount of each type of virus contained in 1 single human dose;

— the cell substrate used for the preparation of the vaccine.

Ph Eur

IMMUNOLOGICAL PRODUCTS

Rubella Vaccine, Live

(Ph Eur monograph 0162)

The label may state 'Rubella'.

Ph Eur _____

DEFINITION

Rubella vaccine (live) is a freeze-dried preparation of a suitable attenuated strain of rubella virus. The vaccine is reconstituted immediately before use, as stated on the label, to give a clear liquid that may be coloured owing to the presence of a pH indicator.

PRODUCTION

The production of vaccine is based on a virus seed-lot system and a cell-bank system. The production method shall have been shown to yield consistently live rubella vaccines of adequate immunogenicity and safety in man. Unless otherwise justified and authorised, the virus in the final vaccine shall have undergone no more passages from the master seed lot than were used to prepare the vaccine shown in clinical studies to be satisfactory with respect to safety and efficacy.

The potential neurovirulence of the vaccine strain is considered during preclinical development, based on available epidemiological data on neurovirulence and neurotropism, primarily for the wild-type virus. In light of this, a risk analysis is carried out. Where necessary and if available, a test is carried out on the vaccine strain using an animal model that differentiates wild-type and attenuated virus; tests on strains of intermediate attenuation may also be needed.

The production method is validated to demonstrate that the product, if tested, would comply with the test for abnormal toxicity for immunosera and vaccines for human use (*2.6.9*).

SUBSTRATE FOR VIRUS PROPAGATION

The virus is propagated in human diploid cells (*5.2.3*).

SEED LOT

The strain of rubella virus used shall be identified by historical records that include information on the origin of the strain and its subsequent manipulation. Virus seed lots are prepared in large quantities and stored at temperatures below − 20 °C if freeze-dried, or below − 60 °C if not freeze-dried.

Only a seed lot that complies with the following requirements may be used for virus propagation.

Identification

The master and working seed lots are identified as rubella virus by serum neutralisation in cell culture, using specific antibodies.

Virus concentration

The virus concentration of the master and working seed lots is determined to ensure consistency of production.

Extraneous agents (*2.6.16*)

The working seed lot complies with the requirements for seed lots.

PROPAGATION AND HARVEST

All processing of the cell bank and subsequent cell cultures is done under aseptic conditions in an area where no other cells are handled during the production. Suitable animal (but not human) serum may be used in the growth medium, but the final medium for maintaining cell growth during virus multiplication does not contain animal serum. Serum and trypsin used in the preparation of cell suspensions and culture media are shown to be free from extraneous agents. The cell culture medium may contain a pH indicator such as phenol red and suitable antibiotics at the lowest effective concentration. It is preferable to have a substrate free from antibiotics during production. Not less than 500 mL of the production cell cultures is set aside as uninfected cell cultures (control cells). The temperature of incubation is controlled during the growth of the virus. The virus suspension is harvested, on one or more occasions, within 28 days of inoculation. Multiple harvests from the same production cell culture may be pooled and considered as a single harvest.

Only a single harvest that complies with the following requirements may be used in the preparation of the final bulk vaccine.

Identification

The single harvest contains virus that is identified as rubella virus by serum neutralisation in cell culture, using specific antibodies.

Virus concentration

The virus concentration in the single harvest is determined as prescribed under Assay to monitor consistency of production and to determine the dilution to be used for the final bulk vaccine.

Extraneous agents (*2.6.16*)

The single harvest complies with the tests for extraneous agents.

Control cells

The control cells comply with a test for identification and with the tests for extraneous agents (*2.6.16*).

FINAL BULK VACCINE

Single harvests that comply with the above tests are pooled and clarified to remove cells. A suitable stabiliser may be added and the pooled harvests diluted as appropriate.

Only a final bulk vaccine that complies with the following requirement may be used in the preparation of the final lot.

Bacterial and fungal contamination

The final bulk vaccine complies with the test for sterility (*2.6.1*), carried out using 10 mL for each medium.

FINAL LOT

A minimum virus concentration for release of the product is established such as to ensure, in light of stability data, that the minimum concentration stated on the label will be present at the end of the period of validity.

Only a final lot that complies with the requirements for minimum virus concentration for release, with the following requirement for thermal stability and with each of the requirements given below under Identification and Tests may be released for use. Provided that the test for bovine serum albumin has been carried out with satisfactory results on the final bulk vaccine, it may be omitted on the final lot.

Thermal stability

Maintain at least 3 vials of the final lot of freeze-dried vaccine in the dry state at 37 ± 1 °C for 7 days. Determine the virus concentration as described under Assay in parallel for the heated vaccine and for vaccine stored at the temperature recommended for storage. The virus concentration of the heated vaccine is not more than 1.0 log lower than that of the unheated vaccine.

IDENTIFICATION

When the vaccine reconstituted as stated on the label is mixed with specific rubella antibodies, it is no longer able to infect susceptible cell cultures.

TESTS

Bacterial and fungal contamination

The reconstituted vaccine complies with the test for sterility (2.6.1).

Bovine serum albumin

Not more than 50 ng per single human dose, determined by a suitable immunochemical method (2.7.1).

Water (2.5.12)

Not more than 3.0 per cent, determined by the semi-micro determination of water.

ASSAY

Titrate the vaccine for infective virus, using at least 3 separate vials of vaccine and inoculating a suitable number of wells for each dilution step. Titrate 1 vial of an appropriate virus reference preparation in triplicate to validate each assay. The virus concentration of the reference preparation is monitored using a control chart and a titre is established on a historical basis by each laboratory.

The relation with the appropriate European Pharmacopoeia Biological Reference Preparation is established and monitored at regular intervals if a manufacturer's reference preparation is used. Calculate the individual virus concentration for each vial of vaccine and for each replicate of the reference preparation as well as the corresponding combined virus concentrations, using the usual statistical methods (for example, 5.3). The combined estimate of the virus concentration for the 3 vials of vaccine is not less than that stated on the label; the minimum virus concentration stated on the label is not less than 3.0 log $CCID_{50}$ per single human dose.

The assay is not valid if:
— the confidence interval (P = 0.95) of the estimated virus concentration of the reference preparation for the 3 replicates combined is greater than ± 0.3 log $CCID_{50}$;
— the virus concentration of the reference preparation differs by more than 0.5 log $CCID_{50}$ from the established value.

The assay is repeated if the confidence interval (P = 0.95) of the combined virus concentration of the vaccine is greater than ± 0.3 log $CCID_{50}$; data obtained from valid assays only are combined by the usual statistical methods (for example, 5.3) to calculate the virus concentration of the sample.

The confidence interval (P = 0.95) of the combined virus concentration is not greater than ± 0.3 log $CCID_{50}$.

Rubella vaccine (live) BRP is suitable for use as a reference preparation.

Where justified and authorised, different assay designs may be used; this may imply the application of different validity and acceptance criteria. However, the vaccine must comply if tested as described above.

LABELLING

The label states:
— the strain of virus used for the preparation of the vaccine;
— the type and origin of the cells used for the preparation of the vaccine;
— the minimum virus concentration;
— that contact between the vaccine and disinfectants is to be avoided.

———————————— Ph Eur

Shingles (Herpes Zoster) Vaccine (Live)

(*Ph Eur monograph 2418*)

The label may state 'Shingles (live)'.

Ph Eur ———————————————————————

DEFINITION

Shingles (herpes zoster) vaccine (live) is a freeze-dried preparation of a suitable attenuated strain of human herpesvirus 3. The vaccine is reconstituted immediately before use, as stated on the label, to give a clear or slightly opalescent liquid, almost white suspension or pale yellow liquid that may be coloured owing to the presence of a pH indicator. It is intended for administration to adults.

PRODUCTION

The production of vaccine is based on a virus seed-lot system and a cell-bank system. The production method shall have been shown to yield consistently live shingles vaccines of adequate immunogenicity and safety in man. The virus in the final vaccine shall not have been passaged in cell cultures beyond a defined number of passages approved by the competent authority from the original isolated virus.

The potential neurovirulence of the vaccine strain is considered during preclinical development, based on available epidemiological data on neurovirulence and neurotropism, primarily for the wild-type virus. In light of this, a risk analysis is carried out. Where necessary and if available, a test is carried out on the vaccine strain using an animal model that differentiates wild-type and attenuated virus; tests on strains of intermediate attenuation may also be needed.

The production method is validated to demonstrate that the product, if tested, would comply with the test for abnormal toxicity for immunosera and vaccines for human use (2.6.9).

SUBSTRATE FOR VIRUS PROPAGATION

The virus is propagated in human diploid cells (5.2.3).

VIRUS SEED LOT

The strain of human herpesvirus 3 shall be identified as being suitable by historical records that include information on the origin of the strain and its subsequent manipulation. The virus shall at no time have been passaged in continuous cell lines. Seed lots are prepared in the same kind of cells as those used for the production of the final vaccine. Virus seed lots are prepared in large quantities and stored at temperatures below − 20 °C if freeze-dried, or below − 60 °C if not freeze-dried.

Only a virus seed lot that complies with the following requirements may be used for virus propagation.

Identification

The master and working seed lots are identified as human herpesvirus 3 by serum neutralisation in cell culture, using specific antibodies.

Virus concentration

The virus concentration of the master and working seed lots is determined as prescribed under Assay to monitor consistency of production.

Extraneous agents (2.6.16)

The working seed lot complies with the requirements for seed lots for live virus vaccines; a sample of 50 mL is taken for the test in cell cultures.

VIRUS PROPAGATION AND HARVEST

All processing of the cell bank and subsequent cell cultures is done under aseptic conditions in an area where no other cells or virus are being handled. Approved animal (but not human) serum may be used in the culture media. Serum and trypsin used in the preparation of cell suspensions and media are shown to be free from extraneous agents. The cell culture medium may contain a pH indicator such as phenol red and approved antibiotics at the lowest effective concentration. It is preferable to have a substrate free from antibiotics during production. 5 per cent, but not less than 50 mL, of the cell cultures employed for vaccine production is set aside as uninfected cell cultures (control cells). The infected cells constituting a single harvest are washed, released from the support surface and pooled. The cell suspension is disrupted by sonication.

Only a virus harvest that complies with the following requirements may be used in the preparation of the final bulk vaccine.

Identification
The virus harvest contains virus that is identified as human herpesvirus 3 by serum neutralisation in cell culture, using specific antibodies.

Virus concentration
The concentration of infective virus in virus harvests is determined as prescribed under Assay to monitor consistency of production and to determine the dilution to be used for the final bulk vaccine.

Extraneous agents (2.6.16)
Use 50 mL for the test in cell cultures.

Control cells
The control cells of the production cell culture from which the single harvest is derived comply with a test for identity and with the requirements for extraneous agents (2.6.16).

FINAL BULK VACCINE
Virus harvests that comply with the above tests are pooled and clarified to remove cells. A suitable stabiliser may be added and the pooled harvests diluted as appropriate.

Only a final bulk vaccine that complies with the following requirements may be used in the preparation of the final lot.

Bacterial and fungal contamination
Carry out the test for sterility (2.6.1) using 10 mL for each medium.

FINAL LOT
The final bulk vaccine is distributed aseptically into sterile, tamper-proof containers and freeze-dried to a moisture content shown to be favourable to the stability of the vaccine. The containers are then closed so as to prevent contamination and the introduction of moisture.

Only a final lot that is satisfactory with respect to the test for water and each of the requirements given below under Identification, Tests and Assay may be released for use. Provided that the test for bovine serum albumin has been carried out with satisfactory results on the final bulk vaccine, it may be omitted on the final lot.

Water (2.5.12)
Not more than the amount shown to ensure stability of the vaccine as approved by the competent authority, determined by the semi-micro determination of water.

IDENTIFICATION
When the vaccine reconstituted as stated on the label is mixed with specific human herpesvirus 3 antibodies, it is no longer able to infect susceptible cell cultures.

TESTS
Bacterial and fungal contamination
The reconstituted vaccine complies with the test for sterility (2.6.1).

Bovine serum albumin
Maximum 0.65 µg per human dose, determined by a suitable immunochemical method (2.7.1).

ASSAY
Titrate the vaccine for infective virus, using at least 3 separate vials of vaccine. Titrate 1 vial of an appropriate virus reference preparation in triplicate to validate each assay. The virus concentration of the reference preparation is monitored using a control chart and a titre is established on a historical basis by each laboratory. Calculate the individual virus concentration for each vial of vaccine and for each replicate of the reference preparation as well as the corresponding combined virus concentrations, using the usual statistical methods (for example, 5.3). The combined estimate of the virus concentration for the 3 vials of vaccine is not less than that stated on the label.

The assay is not valid if:
— the confidence interval ($P = 0.95$) of the estimated virus concentration of the reference preparation for the 3 replicates combined is greater than $\pm$ 0.3 log PFU;
— the virus concentration of the reference preparation differs by more than 0.5 log PFU from the established value.

The assay is repeated if the confidence interval ($P = 0.95$) of the combined virus concentration of the vaccine is greater than $\pm$ 0.3 log PFU; data obtained from valid assays only are combined by the usual statistical methods (for example, 5.3) to calculate the virus concentration of the sample. The confidence interval ($P = 0.95$) of the combined virus concentration is not greater than $\pm$ 0.3 log PFU.

Where justified and authorised, different assay designs may be used; this may imply the application of different validity and acceptance criteria. However, the vaccine must comply if tested as described above.

LABELLING
The label states:
— the strain of virus used for the preparation of the vaccine;
— the type and origin of the cells used for the preparation of the vaccine;
— the minimum virus concentration;
— that contact between the vaccine and disinfectants is to be avoided;
— that the vaccine is not to be administered to pregnant women.

Ph Eur

Smallpox Vaccine (Live)

(*Ph Eur monograph 0164*)
The label may state 'SMV(live)'.

Ph Eur

DEFINITION
Smallpox vaccine (live) is a liquid or freeze-dried preparation of live vaccinia virus grown *in ovo* in the membranes of the chick embryo, in cell cultures or in the skin of living animals.

This monograph applies to vaccines produced using strains of confirmed efficacy in man, in particular those used during eradication of smallpox, for example the Lister strain (sometimes referred to as the Lister/Elstree strain) and the New York City Board of Health (NYCBOH) strain. It does not apply to non-replicative strains such as Modified Virus Ankara (MVA).

PRODUCTION

GENERAL PROVISIONS

The production method shall have been shown to yield consistently smallpox vaccines of adequate safety and immunogenicity in man. The strain used shall have been shown to produce typical vaccinia skin lesions in man. Production is based on a seed-lot system.

The production method is validated to demonstrate that the product, if tested, would comply with the test for abnormal toxicity of immunosera and vaccines for human use (2.6.9).

The International Reference Preparation for smallpox vaccine is suitable for use as a reference preparation in virus titration.

SUBSTRATE FOR VIRUS PROPAGATION

Animals used for production of skin-derived vaccines

If the vaccine is prepared in animals skins, the animals used are of a species approved by the competent authority, are in good health, are kept in closed or intensively monitored colonies, and have not previously been employed for experimental purposes. Only animals susceptible to infection by dermal inoculations with vaccinia virus may be used for vaccine production.

The animals are kept in well-constructed and adequately ventilated animals rooms with cages spaced as far apart as possible. Adequate precautions are taken to prevent cross-infection between cages. Not more than 1 large animal is housed per stall. Not more than 2 small animals are housed per cage and cage-mates must not be interchanged. The animals must be kept in the country of production of the vaccine in quarantine groups for a period of not less than 6 weeks before use.

If at any time during the quarantine period the overall death rate of the group reaches 5 per cent, no animals from that entire group may be used for vaccine production.

The groups are kept continuously in isolation, as in quarantine, even after completion of the quarantine period, until the animals are used. After the last animal of a group has been taken, the room that housed the group is thoroughly cleaned and decontaminated before receiving a new group.

Animals that are to be inoculated are anaesthetised and thoroughly examined. If an animal shows any pathological lesion, it is not used in the preparation of a seed lot or a vaccine, nor are any of the remaining animals of the quarantine group concerned unless it is evident that their use will not impair the safety of the product.

The prophylactic and diagnostic measures adopted to exclude the presence of infectious disease are approved by the competent authority. According to the species of animals used and the diseases to which that animal is liable in the country where the vaccine is being produced, these measures may vary. Consideration must also be given to the danger of spreading diseases to other countries to which the vaccine may be shipped. Special attention must always be given to foot-and-mouth disease, brucellosis, Q fever, tuberculosis and dermatomycosis, and it may also be necessary to consider diseases such as contagious pustular dermatitis (orf), anthrax, rinderpest, haemorrhagic septicaemia, Rift valley fever and others.

Embryonated eggs

Embryonated eggs used for production are obtained from a flock free from specified pathogens (SPF) (5.2.2).

Human diploid cells, continuous cell lines

Human diploid cells and continuous cell lines comply with the requirements for cell substrates (5.2.3).

Primary chick embryo cells

Primary chick embryo cells are derived from an SPF flock (5.2.2).

Primary rabbit kidney cells

Only healthy rabbits derived from a closed colony approved by the competent authority are used as a source.

The animals, preferably 2-4 weeks old, are tested to ensure freedom from specified pathogens or their antibodies.

Where new animals are introduced into the colony, they are maintained in quarantine for a minimum of 2 months and shown to be free from specified pathogens. Animals to be used to provide kidneys shall not have been previously employed for experimental purposes, especially those involving infectious agents. The colony is monitored for zoonotic viruses and markers of contamination at regular intervals.

At the time the colony is established, all animals are tested to determine freedom from antibodies to possible viral contaminants for which there is evidence of capacity for infecting humans or evidence of capacity to replicate *in vitro* in cells of human origin. A test for retroviruses using a sensitive polymerase chain reaction (PCR)-based reverse transcriptase assay is also included. Nucleic acid amplification tests (2.6.21) for retroviruses may also be used.

After the colony is established, it is monitored by testing a representative group of at least 5 per cent of the animals, which are then bled at suitable (for example monthly) intervals. In addition, the colony is screened for pathogenic micro-organisms, including mycobacteria, fungi and mycoplasmas. The screening programme is designed to ensure that all animals are tested within a given period of time.

Any animal that dies is examined to determine the cause of death. If the presence of a causative infectious agent is demonstrated in the colony, the production of smallpox vaccine is discontinued.

At the time of kidney harvest, the animals are examined for the presence of abnormalities and, if any are noted, the animals are not used for vaccine production.

Each set of control cultures derived from a single group of animals used to produce a single virus harvest must remain identifiable as such until all testing, especially for extraneous agents, is completed.

VIRUS SEED LOT

The vaccinia virus isolate used for the master seed lot is identified by historical records that include information on its origin and the tests used in its characterisation.

Virus from the working seed lot must have the same characteristics as the strain that was used to prepare the master seed lot. The number of passages required to produce single harvests from the original isolate is limited and approved by the competent authority. Vaccine is produced from the working seed with a minimum number of intervening passages.

Since cell culture production and clonal selection (for example, plaque purification) may lead to altered characteristics of the virus, the master seed virus must be characterised as fully as possible, for example by comparing the safety profile and biological characteristics of the strain with that of the parental isolate. The characterisation shall include the following:

— antigenic analyses using specific antisera and/or monoclonal antibodies;

— biological studies such as infectivity titre, chorioallantoic membrane (CAM) assay, *in vitro* yield and *in vivo* growth characteristics in a suitable animal model;
— genetic analyses such as restriction mapping/southern blotting, PCR analyses and limited sequencing studies;
— phenotypic and genetic stability upon passage in the substrate;
— neurovirulence testing and immunogenicity studies.

The characterisation tests are also carried out on each working seed lot and on 3 batches of vaccine from the first working seed lot to verify genetic stability of the vaccine strain.

Only a virus seed that complies with the following requirements may be used for virus propagation.

Identification
Each working seed lot is identified as vaccinia virus using specific antibodies and molecular tests. Suitable tests are conducted to exclude the presence of variola virus and other orthopoxviruses.

Virus concentration
Determine by the CAM assay or by a suitable validated *in vitro* assay (plaque assay or $CCID_{50}$ assay). The virus concentration is the basis for the quantity of virus used in the neurovirulence test.

Extraneous agents (*2.6.16*)
If the working seed lot is produced in embryonated eggs, human diploid cells, or in a continuous cell line, it complies with the requirements for seed lots for virus vaccines. Seed lots produced in embryonated eggs and seed lots produced in primary cell cultures comply with the additional requirements described below.

Where the tests prescribed cannot be carried out because complete neutralisation of the seed virus is not possible, the seed lot may be diluted to a concentration equivalent to that of the dilution used as inoculum for production of vaccine prior to testing for extraneous viruses. Supplementary specific testing for extraneous viruses using validated nucleic acid amplification techniques (*2.6.21*) or immunochemical methods (*2.7.1*) may be envisaged. Where the indicator cell culture method for mycoplasma detection (*2.6.7*) cannot be carried out, nucleic acid amplification testing is performed instead.

Seed lots to be used for embryonated egg or cell culture production are in addition to be tested for carry-over of potential extraneous agents from the original seed. Given that the complete passage history of the original seed is unlikely to be known and that more than one species may have been used, this additional testing must at least cover important extraneous agents of concern.

The bioburden of master and working seed lots prepared in animal skins is limited by meticulous controls of facilities, personnel, and animals used for production, and by specific tests on the seeds. However, it may be difficult to ensure that seed lots produced in animal skins are totally free from extraneous agents, and consideration must be given to production procedures which remove or reduce them. Such lots must comply with the requirements indicated below. The absence of specific human pathogens is confirmed by additional testing procedures, for example, bacterial and fungal cultures, virus culture, nucleic acid amplification testings (*2.6.21*) for viral agents.

Neurovirulence
The neurovirulence of master and working seed lots is assessed using a suitable animal model, for example in monkeys or mice. The parental isolate is used as comparator. Where the original isolate is not available for this purpose, equivalent materials may be used.

VIRUS PROPAGATION AND HARVEST
Vaccine produced in living animals
Before inoculation the animals are cleaned and thereafter kept in scrupulously clean stalls until the vaccinia material is harvested. For 5 days before inoculation and during incubation the animals remain under veterinary supervision and must remain free from any sign of disease; daily rectal temperatures are recorded. If any abnormal rise in temperature occurs or any clinical sign of disease is observed, the production of vaccine from the group of animals concerned must be suspended until the cause has been resolved.

The inoculation of seed virus is carried out on such parts of the animal that are not liable to be soiled by urine and faeces. The surface used for inoculation is shaved and cleaned so as to achieve conditions that are as close as possible to surgical asepsis. If any antiseptic substance deleterious to the virus is used in the cleaning process it is removed by thorough rinsing with sterile water prior to inoculation. During inoculation the exposed surface of the animal not used for inoculation is covered with a sterile covering. By historical experience the ventral surface of female animals is appropriate for inoculation and inoculation of male animals is more appropriate on the flank.

Before the collection of the vaccinia material, any antibiotic is removed and the inoculated area is cleaned. The uninoculated surfaces are covered with a sterile covering. Before harvesting the animals are euthanised and exsanguinated to avoid heavy mixtures of the vaccinia material with blood. The vaccinia material from each animal is collected separately with aseptic precautions. All animals used in the production of vaccine are examined by autopsy. If evidence of any generalised or systemic disease other than vaccinia is found, the vaccinia material from that animal is discarded. If the disease is considered to be a communicable one, the harvest from the entire group of animals exposed must be discarded unless otherwise justified and authorised.

Vaccine produced in eggs
All processing of embryonated eggs is done under aseptic conditions in an area where no other infectious agents or cells are handled at the same time. After inoculation and incubation at a controlled temperature only living and suitable chick embryos are harvested. The age of the embryos at the time of virus harvest is reckoned from the initial introduction of the egg into the incubator and shall be not more than 12 days. After homogenisation and clarification by centrifugation, the extract of embryonic pulp is tested as described below and kept at −70 °C or below until further processing. Virus harvests that comply with the prescribed tests may be pooled. No human protein is added to the virus suspension at any stage during production. If stabilisers are added, they shall have been shown to have no antigenic or sensitising properties for man.

Only a single harvest that complies with the following requirements may be used in the preparation of the final bulk vaccine.

Control eggs
Control eggs comply with the tests for extraneous agents (*2.6.16*). A sample of 2 per cent of uninoculated embryonated eggs (not less than 20 and not more than 50) from the batch used for vaccine production shall be incubated under the same conditions as the inoculated eggs.

At the time of virus harvest the uninoculated eggs are processed in the same manner as the inoculated eggs.

Sterility (*2.6.1*)
It complies with the test for sterility, carried out using 10 mL for each medium.

Vaccine produced in cell cultures (primary chick embryo cells, primary rabbit kidney cells, human diploid cells or continuous cell lines)
All processing of the cell bank and subsequent cell cultures is done under aseptic conditions in an area where no other cells are handled at the same time during production. Suitable animal (but not human) serum may be used in the culture media, but the final medium for maintaining cell growth during virus multiplication does not contain animal serum. Serum and trypsin used in the preparation of cell suspensions and media are shown to be free from extraneous agents. The cell culture medium may contain a pH indicator such as phenol red and suitable antibiotics at the lowest effective concentration. It is preferable to have a substrate free from antibiotics during production. On the day of inoculation with the virus working seed lot, not less than 5 per cent or 1000 mL, whichever is the least, of the cell cultures employed for vaccine production are set aside as uninfected cell cultures (control cells); special requirements, given below, apply to control cells when the vaccine is produced in primary rabbit kidney cell cultures.

After inoculation of the production cell culture with the working seed lot, inoculated cells are maintained at a suitable fixed temperature, and the virus suspension is harvested after a suitable incubation period.

Only a single harvest that complies with the following requirements may be used in the preparation of the monovalent pooled harvest.

Control cells
The control cells of the production cell culture from which the virus harvest is derived comply with a test for identity and with the requirements for extraneous agents (*2.6.16*) or, where primary rabbit kidney cells cultures are used, with specific tests as mentioned hereafter. The test is invalid if more than 20 per cent of the control cell cultures have been discarded at the end of the observation period.

Extraneous agents (*2.6.16*)
The single harvest complies with the tests for extraneous agents. Complete neutralisation of vaccinia virus may be difficult to achieve at high virus concentration. In this case specific tests such as nucleic acid amplification (*2.6.21*) and immunochemical tests (*2.7.1*) can replace non-specific testing in cell culture or eggs. To save biological reagents such as vaccinia neutralising antisera, testing for extraneous agents may be performed on the final bulk instead of on the single harvests.

Vaccine prepared in primary chick embryo cells   A sample of fluids pooled from the control cultures is tested for adenoviruses and for avian retroviruses such as avian leukosis virus. In addition, a volume of each neutralised virus pool equivalent to 100 human doses of vaccine or 10 mL, whichever is the greater, is tested in a group of fertilised eggs by the allantoic route of inoculation, and a similar sample is tested in a separate group of eggs by the yolk-sac route of inoculation. In both cases 0.5 mL of inoculum is used per egg. The virus pool passes the test if, after 3-7 days, there is no evidence of the presence of any extraneous agent.

Vaccine prepared in primary rabbit kidney cell cultures   The following special requirements apply to virus propagation,

harvest and testing. On the day of inoculation with virus working seed, a sample of at least 30 mL of the pooled fluid is removed from the cell cultures of the kidneys of each group of animals used to prepare the primary cell suspension. The pooled fluid is inoculated in primary kidney cell cultures in such a way that the dilution of the pooled fluid does not exceed 1 in 4. The cultures are incubated at a temperature of 34-36 °C and observed for a period of at least 4 weeks. During this observation period and after not less than 2 weeks of incubation, at least 1 subculture of fluid is made from each of these cultures and observed also for a period of 2 weeks. The test is invalid if more than 20 per cent of the cultures are discarded. If evidence is found of the presence of an extraneous agent, no cell cultures from the entire group may be used for vaccine production.

— *Control cell cultures.* Cultures prepared on the day of inoculation with the working virus seed lot from 25 per cent of the cell suspensions obtained from the kidneys of each group of animals are maintained as controls. These control cell cultures are incubated under the same conditions as the inoculated cultures for at least 2 weeks. The test is invalid if more than 20 per cent of the control cell cultures are discarded for non-specific reasons.

— *Test for haemadsorbing viruses.* At the time of harvest or not more than 4 days after the day of inoculation of the production cultures with the virus working seed, a sample of 4 per cent of the control cell cultures is tested for haemadsorbing viruses by addition of guinea-pig red blood cells.

— *Test for other extraneous agents.* At the time of harvest or not more than 7 days after the day of inoculation of the production cultures with the virus working seed, a sample of at least 20 mL of the pooled fluid from each group of control cultures is tested for other extraneous agents.

— *Tests of neutralised single harvest in primary rabbit kidney cell cultures.* Each neutralised single harvest is additionally tested in primary kidney cell cultures prepared from a different group of animals to that used for production.

POOLED HARVEST
Only a pooled harvest that complies with the following requirements and is within the limits approved for the product may be used in the preparation of the final lot.

Identity
The vaccinia virus in the pooled harvest is identified by serological methods, which may be supplemented by molecular methods. Molecular tests such as restriction fragment length polymorphism or partial sequencing, especially of terminal DNA sequences which show the greatest variation between vaccinia strains, may be useful.

Virus concentration
The vaccinia virus concentration of the pooled harvest is determined by chick egg CAM assay or in cell cultures. A reference preparation is assayed in the same system in parallel for validation of the pooled harvest titration. The virus concentration serves as the basis for the quantity of virus used in the neurovirulence test in mice.

Consistency of virus characteristics
Vaccinia virus in the pooled harvest or the final bulk is examined by tests that are able to determine that the phenotypic and genetic characteristics of the vaccinia virus have not undergone changes during the multiplication in the production system. The master seed or an equivalent preparation is used as a comparator in these tests and the

IMMUNOLOGICAL PRODUCTS

comparator and the tests to be used are approved by the competent authority.

Neurovirulence

The neurovirulence of the pooled harvest is assessed versus a comparator original seed (or equivalent) by intracerebral inoculation into suckling mice. Other tests may be useful to discriminate between acceptable and unacceptable batches.

Residual DNA

For viruses grown in continuous cells the pooled harvest is tested for residual DNA. The production process demonstrates a level of cellular DNA of less than 10 ng per human dose.

Bacterial and fungal contamination

For vaccines other than those prepared on animal skins, the final bulk complies with the test for sterility (2.6.1) using 10 mL for each medium.

Mycoplasma (2.6.7)

For vaccines other than those prepared on animal skins, the final bulk complies with the test for mycoplasma, carried out using 10 mL.

FINAL BULK VACCINE

A minimum virus concentration for release of the product is established such as to ensure, in the light of stability data, that the minimum concentration stated on the label will be present at the end of the period of validity.

Vaccine produced in living animals

The pooled harvest is centrifuged. If the vaccine is intended for issue in the liquid form, treatment to reduce the presence of extraneous agents may consist of the addition of glycerol or another suitable diluent, with or without an antimicrobial substance, and temporary storage at a suitable temperature. If the vaccine is intended for issue in the dried form, the treatment may consist of the addition of a suitable antimicrobial substance. The following special requirements apply to the bulk vaccine for vaccines produced in living animals.

Only a final bulk vaccine that complies with the following requirements may be used in the preparation of the final lot.

Total bacterial count

For vaccines produced on animal skins only, maximum 50 per millilitre, determined by plate count using a suitable volume of the final bulk vaccine.

Escherichia coli

At least 1 mL samples of a 1:100 dilution of the final bulk vaccine is cultured on plates of a medium suitable for differentiating E. coli from other bacteria. The plates are incubated at 35-37 °C for 48 h. If E. coli is detected the final bulk is discarded or, subject to approval by the competent authority, processed further.

Haemolytic streptococci, coagulase-positive staphylococci or any other pathogenic micro-organisms which are known to be harmful to man by vaccination

At least 1 mL samples of a 1:100 dilution of the final bulk vaccine are cultured on blood agar. The plates are incubated at 35-37 °C for 48 h. If micro-organisms are detected, the final bulk vaccine is discarded.

Bacillus anthracis

Any colony seen on any of the plates that morphologically resembles B. anthracis is examined. If the organisms contained in the colony are non-motile, further tests for the cultural character of B. anthracis are carried out, including pathogenicity tests in suitable animals. If B. anthracis is found to be present, the final bulk vaccine and any other associated

bulks are discarded. Additional validated molecular testing may be performed.

Clostridium tetani and other pathogenic spore-forming anaerobes

A total volume of not less than 10 mL of the final bulk vaccine is distributed in equal amounts into 10 tubes, each containing not less than 10 mL of suitable medium for the growth of anaerobic micro-organisms. The tubes are kept at 65 °C for 1 h in order to reduce the content of non-spore-forming organisms, after which they are anaerobically incubated at 35-37 °C for at least 1 week. From every tube or plate showing growth, subcultures are made on plates of a suitable medium. Tubes and plates are incubated anaerobically at the same temperature. All anaerobic colonies are examined and identified and if C. tetani or other pathogenic spore-forming anaerobes are present, the final bulk is discarded.

Vaccine produced in eggs

The pooled harvest is clarified and may be further purified.

Vaccine produced in cell cultures (primary chick embryos fibroblasts, human diploid cells or continuous cell lines)

The pooled harvest is clarified to remove cells and may be further purified.

FINAL LOT

Only a final lot that complies with the requirements for minimum virus concentration for release, with the following requirement for thermal stability and with each of the requirements given below under Identification, Tests and Assay may be released for use. Provided that the tests for antimicrobial preservative, protein content, bovine serum albumin and ovalbumin have been carried out with satisfactory results on the final bulk vaccine, they may be omitted on the final lot.

Thermal stability

For liquid products, maintain not fewer than 3 containers of the final lot at an elevated temperature for a defined time period, using conditions found suitable for the particular product as approved by the competent authority. Determine the virus concentration as described under Assay in parallel for the heated vaccine and for vaccine stored at the temperature recommended for storage. The virus concentration of the containers that have been heated does not decrease by more than an approved amount during the period of exposure. The conditions of the test and the requirements are approved by the competent authority.

For freeze-dried products, maintain at least 3 containers of the final lot in the dry state at 37 ± 1 °C for 28 days. Determine the virus concentration as described under Assay in parallel for the heated vaccine and for vaccine stored at the temperature recommended for storage. The virus concentration of the heated vaccine is not more than 1.0 log lower than that of the unheated vaccine.

IDENTIFICATION

The vaccinia virus is identified by an appropriate method.

TESTS

Antimicrobial preservative

Where applicable determine the amount of antimicrobial preservative by a suitable chemical method. The content is not less than the minimum amount shown to be effective and is not greater than 115 per cent of the quantity stated on the label.

Phenol (2.5.15)

Maximum 0.5 per cent, if phenol is used.

Protein content

The protein content of each filling lot, if not done on the final bulk, is determined and is within the limits approved by the competent authority.

Bovine serum albumin

Maximum 50 ng per single human dose, determined by a suitable immunochemical method (2.7.1), where bovine serum albumin is used during cell culture.

Ovalbumin

For vaccines produced in embryonated eggs, the ovalbumin content is within the limits approved by the competent authority.

Residual moisture

The residual moisture content of each final lot of freeze-dried vaccines is within the limits approved by the competent authority.

Bacterial count

For skin-derived vaccines, examine the vaccine by suitable microscopic and culture methods for micro-organisms pathogenic for man and, in particular, haemolytic streptococci, staphylococci, pathogenic spore-bearing organisms, especially *B. anthracis*, and *E. coli*. The vaccine is free from such contaminants. The total number of non-pathogenic bacteria does not exceed 50 per millilitre.

Sterility (2.6.1)

Except for skin-derived vaccines, the vaccine complies with the test for sterility.

Bacterial endotoxins (2.6.14)

The vaccine complies with the specification approved by the competent authority.

ASSAY

Reconstitue the vaccine if necessary and titrate for infectious virus using at least 3 separate containers of vaccine. Titrate 1 container of an appropriate virus reference preparation in triplicate to validate each assay. The virus concentration of the reference preparation is monitored using a control chart and a titre is established on a historical basis by each laboratory. Calculate the individual virus concentration for each container of vaccine and for each replicate of the reference preparation as well as the corresponding combined virus concentrations, using the usual statistical methods (for example, 5.3). The combined virus concentration for the 3 containers of vaccine is not less than 8.0 log pock-forming units per millilitre or the validated equivalent in plaque-forming units or 50 per cent cell culture infective doses, unless a lower titre is justified by clinical studies.

The assay is not valid if:
— the confidence interval ($P = 0.95$) of the estimated virus concentration of the reference preparation for the 3 replicates combined is greater than ± 0.5 log infectious units;
— the virus concentration of the reference preparation differs by more than 0.5 log infectious units from the established value.

The assay is repeated if the confidence interval ($P = 0.95$) of the combined virus concentration of the vaccine is greater than ± 0.5 log infectious units; data obtained from valid assays only are combined by the usual statistical methods (for example, 5.3) to calculate the virus concentration of the sample. The confidence interval ($P = 0.95$) of the combined virus concentration is not greater than ± 0.5 log infectious units.

Where justified and authorised, different assay designs may be used; this may imply the application of different validity and acceptance criteria. However, the vaccine must comply if tested as described above.

LABELLING

The label states:
— the designation of the vaccinia virus strain;
— the minimum amount of virus per millilitre;
— the substrate used for the preparation of the vaccine;
— the nature and amount of stabiliser, preservative or additive present in the vaccine and/or in the diluent.

———————————————————— Ph Eur

Adsorbed Tetanus Vaccine

(Tetanus Vaccine (Adsorbed),
Ph Eur monograph 0452)

The label may state 'Tet'.

When Tetanus Vaccine is prescribed or demanded and the form is not stated, Adsorbed Tetanus Vaccine may be dispensed or supplied.

Ph Eur ————————————————————

DEFINITION

Tetanus vaccine (adsorbed) is a preparation of tetanus formol toxoid with a mineral adsorbent. The formol toxoid is prepared from the toxin produced by the growth of *Clostridium tetani*.

PRODUCTION

GENERAL PROVISIONS

Specific toxicity

The production method is validated to demonstrate that the product, if tested, would comply with the following test: inject subcutaneously 5 times the single human dose stated on the label into each of 5 healthy guinea-pigs, each weighing 250-350 g, that have not previously been treated with any material that will interfere with the test. If within 21 days of the injection any of the animals shows signs of or dies from tetanus, the vaccine does not comply with the test. If more than 1 animal dies from non-specific causes, repeat the test once; if more than 1 animal dies in the second test, the vaccine does not comply with the test.

BULK PURIFIED TOXOID

For the production of tetanus toxin, from which toxoid is prepared, seed cultures are managed in a defined seed-lot system in which toxinogenicity is conserved and, where necessary, restored by deliberate reselection. A highly toxinogenic strain of *Clostridium tetani* with known origin and history is grown in a suitable liquid medium. At the end of cultivation, the purity of each culture is tested and contaminated cultures are discarded. Toxin-containing culture medium is collected aseptically. The toxin content (Lf per millilitre) is checked (2.7.27) to monitor consistency of production. Single harvests may be pooled to prepare the bulk purified toxoid. The toxin is purified to remove components likely to cause adverse reactions in humans. The purified toxin is detoxified with formaldehyde by a method that avoids destruction of the immunogenic potency of the toxoid and reversion of toxoid to toxin, particularly on exposure to heat. Alternatively, purification may be carried out after detoxification.

Only bulk purified toxoid that complies with the following requirements may be used in the preparation of the final bulk vaccine.

Sterility (*2.6.1*)

Carry out the test for sterility using 10 mL for each medium.

Absence of toxin and irreversibility of toxoid

Using the same buffer solution as for the final vaccine, without adsorbent, prepare a solution of bulk purified toxoid at the same concentration as in the final vaccine. Divide the dilution into 2 equal parts. Keep one of them at 5 ± 3 °C and the other at 37 °C for 6 weeks. Test both dilutions as described below. Use 15 guinea-pigs, each weighing 250-350 g and that have not previously been treated with any material that will interfere with the test. Inject subcutaneously into each of 5 guinea-pigs 5 mL of the dilution incubated at 5 ± 3 °C. Inject subcutaneously into each of 5 other guinea-pigs 5 mL of the dilution incubated at 37 °C. Inject subcutaneously into each of 5 guinea-pigs at least 500 Lf of the non-incubated bulk purified toxoid in a volume of 1 mL. The bulk purified toxoid complies with the test if during the 21 days following the injection no animal shows signs of or dies from tetanus. If more than 1 animal dies from non-specific causes, repeat the test; if more than 1 animal dies in the second test, the toxoid does not comply with the test.

Antigenic purity (*2.7.27*)

Not less than 1000 Lf per milligram of protein nitrogen.

FINAL BULK VACCINE

The final bulk vaccine is prepared by adsorption of a suitable quantity of bulk purified toxoid onto a mineral carrier such as hydrated aluminium phosphate or aluminium hydroxide; the resulting mixture is approximately isotonic with blood. Suitable antimicrobial preservatives may be added. Certain antimicrobial preservatives, particularly those of the phenolic type, adversely affect the antigenic activity and must not be used.

Only final bulk vaccine that complies with the following requirements may be used in the preparation of the final lot.

Antimicrobial preservative

Where applicable, determine the amount of antimicrobial preservative by a suitable chemical method. The amount is not less than 85 per cent and not greater than 115 per cent of the intended amount.

Sterility (*2.6.1*)

Carry out the test for sterility using 10 mL for each medium.

FINAL LOT

The final bulk vaccine is distributed aseptically into sterile, tamper-proof containers. The containers are closed so as to prevent contamination.

Only a final lot that is satisfactory with respect to each of the requirements given below under Identification, Tests and Assay may be released for use. Provided the test for antimicrobial preservative and the assay have been carried out with satisfactory results on the final bulk vaccine, they may be omitted on the final lot.

Provided the free formaldehyde content has been determined on the bulk purified toxoid or on the final bulk and it has been shown that the content in the final lot will not exceed 0.2 g/L, the test for free formaldehyde may be omitted on the final lot.

IDENTIFICATION

Tetanus toxoid is identified by a suitable immunochemical method (*2.7.1*). The following method, applicable to certain vaccines, is given as an example. Dissolve in the vaccine to be examined sufficient *sodium citrate R* to give a 100 g/L solution. Maintain at 37 °C for about 16 h and centrifuge until a clear supernatant liquid is obtained. The clear supernatant liquid reacts with a suitable tetanus antitoxin, giving a precipitate.

TESTS

Aluminium (*2.5.13*)

Maximum 1.25 mg per single human dose, if aluminium hydroxide or hydrated aluminium phosphate is used as the adsorbent.

Free formaldehyde (*2.4.18*)

Maximum 0.2 g/L.

Antimicrobial preservative

Where applicable, determine the amount of antimicrobial preservative by a suitable chemical method. The content is not less than the minimum amount shown to be effective and is not greater than 115 per cent of the quantity stated on the label.

Sterility (*2.6.1*)

The vaccine complies with the test for sterility.

ASSAY

Carry out one of the prescribed methods for the assay of tetanus vaccine (adsorbed) (*2.7.8*).

The lower confidence limit ($P = 0.95$) of the estimated potency is not less than 40 IU per single human dose.

LABELLING

The label states:

— the minimum number of International Units per single human dose,

— the name and the amount of the adsorbent,

— that the vaccine must be shaken before use,

— that the vaccine is not to be frozen.

Ph Eur

Tick-borne Encephalitis Vaccine, Inactivated

(*Tick-borne Encephalitis Vaccine (Inactivated),*
Ph Eur monograph 1375)

The label may state 'Tic/enceph'.

Ph Eur

DEFINITION

Tick-borne encephalitis vaccine (inactivated) is a liquid preparation of a suitable strain of tick-borne encephalitis virus grown in cultures of chick-embryo cells or other suitable cell cultures and inactivated by a suitable, validated method.

PRODUCTION

GENERAL PROVISIONS

Production of the vaccine is based on a virus seed-lot system. The production method shall have been shown to yield consistently vaccines comparable with the vaccine of proven clinical efficacy and safety in man. Unless otherwise justified and authorised, the virus in the final vaccine shall not have undergone more passages from the master seed lot than the virus in the vaccine used in clinical trials.

The production method is validated to demonstrate that the product, if tested, would comply with the test for abnormal toxicity for immunosera and vaccines for human use (*2.6.9*).

SUBSTRATE FOR VIRUS PROPAGATION

The virus is propagated in chick embryo cells prepared from eggs derived from a chicken flock free from specified pathogens (5.2.2) or in other suitable cell cultures (5.2.3).

SEED LOTS

The strain of virus used is identified by historical records that include information on the origin of the strain and its subsequent manipulation. Virus seed lots are stored at or below − 60 °C.

Only a seed lot that complies with the following requirements may be used for virus propagation.

Identification

Each seed lot is identified as containing the vaccine strain of tick-borne encephalitis virus by a suitable immunochemical method (2.7.1), preferably using monoclonal antibodies.

Virus concentration

The virus concentration of each seed lot is determined by titration in suitable cell cultures to monitor consistency of production.

Extraneous agents (2.6.16)

Each seed lot complies with the requirements for extraneous agents in viral vaccines for human use. For neutralisation of the vaccine virus, the use of monoclonal antibodies is preferable.

VIRUS PROPAGATION AND HARVEST

If the virus has been passaged in mouse brain during preparation of the master seed lot, not fewer than 2 passages of the master seed virus in cell culture are made before inoculation of the production cell culture.

All processing of the cell cultures is performed under aseptic conditions in an area where no other cells are being handled. Serum and trypsin used in the preparation of cell suspensions and media used must be shown to be free from extraneous agents. The cell culture media may contain a pH indicator such as phenol red and approved antibiotics at the lowest effective concentration. At least 500 mL of the cell cultures employed for vaccine production is set aside as uninfected cell cultures (control cells).

Only a single harvest that complies with the following requirements may be used in the preparation of the inactivated harvest.

Identification

The single harvest is shown to contain tick-borne encephalitis virus by a suitable immunochemical method (2.7.1), preferably using monoclonal antibodies, or by virus neutralisation in cell cultures.

Bacterial and fungal contamination

The single harvest complies with the test for sterility (2.6.1), carried out using 10 mL for each medium.

Mycoplasmas (2.6.7)

The single harvest complies with the test for mycoplasmas carried out using 1 mL for each medium.

Control cells

The control cells comply with the tests for extraneous agents (2.6.16). If the vaccine is produced using a cell-bank system, the control cells comply with a test for identification.

Virus concentration

Determine the virus concentration by titration in suitable cell cultures to monitor consistency of production.

INACTIVATION

To avoid interference, viral aggregates are removed, where necessary, by filtration immediately before the inactivation process. The virus suspension is inactivated by a validated method; the method shall have been shown to be consistently capable of inactivating tick-borne encephalitis virus without destroying the antigenic and immunogenic activity; as part of the validation studies, an inactivation curve is plotted representing residual live virus concentration measured on not fewer than 3 occasions. If formaldehyde is used for inactivation, the presence of an excess of free formaldehyde is verified at the end of the inactivation process.

Only an inactivated harvest that complies with the following requirements may be used in the preparation of the final bulk vaccine.

Residual infective virus

Inoculate a quantity of the inactivated harvest equivalent to not less than 10 human doses of vaccine in the final lot into primary chicken fibroblast cell cultures, or other cells shown to be at least as sensitive to tick-borne encephalitis virus, with not less than 3 cm2 of cell sheet per millilitre of inoculum. Incubate at 37 ± 1 °C for 14 days. No cytopathic effect is detected at the end of the incubation period. Collect the culture fluid and examine for the presence of infective tick-borne encephalitis virus by the following test in mice or by a validated in vitro method: inoculate 0.03 mL intracerebrally into each of not fewer than 10 mice about 4 weeks old. Observe the mice for 14 days. They show no evidence of tick-borne encephalitis virus infection.

PURIFICATION

Several inactivated single harvests may be pooled before concentration and purification by suitable methods, preferably by continuous-flow, sucrose density-gradient centrifugation.

Several purified inactivated harvests may be pooled.

Only a purified, inactivated harvest that complies with the following requirements may be used in the preparation of the final bulk vaccine.

Sterility (2.6.1)

The purified, inactivated harvest complies with the test for sterility carried out using 10 mL for each medium.

Specific activity

Determine the antigen content of the purified, inactivated harvest by a suitable immunochemical method (2.7.1). Determine the total protein content by a suitable method. The specific activity, calculated as the antigen content per unit mass of protein, is within the limits approved for the specific product.

FINAL BULK VACCINE

The final bulk vaccine is prepared from one or more purified, inactivated harvests.

Only a final bulk vaccine that complies with the following requirement may be used in the preparation of the final lot.

Sterility (2.6.1)

The final bulk vaccine complies with the test for sterility, carried out using 10 mL for each medium.

FINAL LOT

Only a final lot that is satisfactory with respect to each of the requirements given below under Identification, Tests and Assay may be released for use. Provided that the tests for free formaldehyde, bovine serum albumin (where applicable) and pyrogens and the assay have been carried out with satisfactory results on the final bulk vaccine, they may be omitted on the final lot.

IDENTIFICATION

The vaccine is shown to contain tick-borne encephalitis virus antigen by a suitable immunochemical method (2.7.1) using specific antibodies. The assay also serves to identify the vaccine.

TESTS
Aluminium (2.5.13)
Maximum 1.25 mg per single human dose, if aluminium hydroxide or hydrated aluminium phosphate is used as the adsorbent.

Free formaldehyde (2.4.18)
Maximum 0.1 g/L.

Bovine serum albumin
Maximum 50 ng per single human dose, determined by a suitable immunochemical method (2.7.1), if bovine serum albumin has been used during production.

Sterility (2.6.1)
The vaccine complies with the test for sterility.

Pyrogens (2.6.8)
The vaccine complies with the test for pyrogens. Inject into each rabbit, per kilogram of body mass, 1 dose of vaccine.

ASSAY
The potency is determined by comparing the dose necessary to protect a given proportion of mice against the effects of a lethal dose of tick-borne encephalitis virus, administered intraperitoneally, with the quantity of a reference preparation of tick-borne encephalitis vaccine necessary to provide the same protection. For this comparison an approved reference preparation and a suitable preparation of tick-borne encephalitis virus from an approved strain for use as the challenge preparation are necessary.

The following is cited as an example of a method that has been found suitable for a given vaccine.

Selection and distribution of test animals Use healthy mice weighing 11-17 g and derived from the same stock. Distribute the mice into not fewer than 6 groups of a suitable size to meet the requirements for validity of the test; for titration of the challenge suspension, use not fewer than 4 groups of 10 mice. Use mice of the same sex or distribute males and females equally between groups.

Determination of potency of the vaccine Prepare not fewer than 3 suitable dilutions of the vaccine to be examined and of the reference preparation; in order to comply with validity criteria 4 or 5 dilutions will usually be necessary. Prepare dilutions such that the most concentrated suspension is expected to protect more than 50 per cent of the animals and the least concentrated suspension less than 50 per cent. Allocate each dilution to a different group of mice and inject subcutaneously into each mouse 0.2 mL of the dilution allocated to its group. 7 days later make a second injection using the same dilution scale. 14 days after the second injection prepare a suspension of the challenge virus containing not less than 100 LD_{50} in 0.2 mL. Inject 0.2 mL of this virus suspension intraperitoneally into each vaccinated mouse. To verify the challenge dose, prepare a series of not fewer than 3 dilutions of the challenge virus suspension at not greater than one-hundredfold intervals. Allocate the challenge suspension and all of the dilutions, one to each of the groups of 10 mice, and inject intraperitoneally into each mouse 0.2 mL of the challenge suspension or the dilution allocated to its group. Observe the animals for 21 days after the challenge and record the number of mice that die in the period between 7 and 21 days after the challenge. Humane endpoints may be used to avoid unnecessary suffering of animals after the virulent challenge.

Calculations Calculate the results for an assay with quantal responses by the usual statistical methods (for example, 5.3).

Validity criteria The test is not valid unless:
— the concentration of the challenge virus is not less than 100 LD_{50},
— for both the vaccine to be examined and the reference preparation the 50 per cent protective dose (PD_{50}) lies between the largest and smallest doses given to the mice,
— the statistical analysis shows a significant slope and no significant deviation from linearity and parallelism of the dose-response lines,
— the confidence limits ($P = 0.95$) are not less than 33 per cent and not more than 300 per cent of the estimated potency.

Potency requirement Include all valid tests to estimate the mean potency and the confidence limits ($P = 0.95$) for the mean potency; compute weighted means with the inverse of the squared standard error as weights. The vaccine complies with the test if the estimated potency is not less than that approved by the competent authority, based on data from clinical efficacy trials.

LABELLING
The label states:
— the strain of virus used in preparation,
— the type of cells used for production of the vaccine.

Ph Eur

Typhoid Polysaccharide Vaccine

(*Ph Eur monograph 1160*)
The label may state 'Typhoid'.

Ph Eur

DEFINITION
Typhoid polysaccharide vaccine is a preparation of purified Vi capsular polysaccharide obtained from *Salmonella typhi* Ty 2 strain or some other suitable strain that has the capacity to produce Vi polysaccharide.

Capsular Vi polysaccharide consists of partly 3-*O*-acetylated repeated units of 2-acetylamino-2-deoxy-D-galactopyranuronic acid with α-(1→4) linkages.

PRODUCTION
The production of Vi polysaccharide is based on a seed-lot system. The method of production shall have been shown to yield consistently typhoid polysaccharide vaccines of adequate immunogenicity and safety in man.

The production method is validated to demonstrate that the product, if tested, would comply with the test for abnormal toxicity for immunosera and vaccines for human use (2.6.9).

BACTERIAL SEED LOTS
The strain of *S. typhi* used for the master seed lot shall be identified by historical records that include information on its origin and by its biochemical and serological characteristics. Cultures from the working seed lot shall have the same characteristics as the strain that was used to prepare the master seed lot.

Only a strain that has the following characteristics may be used in the preparation of the vaccine: (a) stained smears from a culture are typical of enterobacteria; (b) the culture utilises glucose without production of gas; (c) colonies on agar are oxidase-negative; (d) a suspension of the culture agglutinates specifically with a suitable Vi antiserum or colonies form haloes on an agar plate containing a suitable Vi antiserum.

Purity of bacterial strain used for the seed lot is verified by methods of suitable sensitivity. These may include inoculation into suitable media, examination of colony morphology, microscopic examination of Gram-stained smears and culture agglutination with suitable specific antisera.

CULTURE AND HARVEST

The working seed lot is cultured on a solid medium, which may contain blood-group substances, or a liquid medium; the inoculum obtained is transferred to a liquid medium which is used to inoculate the final medium. The liquid medium used and the final medium are semi-synthetic, free from substances that are precipitated by cetrimonium bromide and do not contain blood-group substances or high-molecular-mass polysaccharides, unless it has been demonstrated that they are removed by the purification process.

The bacterial purity of the culture is verified by methods of suitable sensitivity. These may include inoculation into suitable media, examination of colony morphology, microscopic examination of Gram-stained smears and culture agglutination with suitable specific antisera.

The culture is then inactivated at the beginning of the stationary phase by the addition of formaldehyde. Bacterial cells are eliminated by centrifugation; the polysaccharide is precipitated from the culture medium by addition of hexadecyltrimethylammonium bromide (cetrimonium bromide). The precipitate is harvested and may be stored at − 20 °C before purification.

PURIFIED VI POLYSACCHARIDE

The polysaccharide is purified, after dissociation of the polysaccharide/cetrimonium bromide complex, using suitable procedures to eliminate successively nucleic acids, proteins and lipopolysaccharides. The polysaccharide is precipitated as the calcium salt in the presence of ethanol and dried at 2-8 °C; the powder obtained constitutes the purified Vi polysaccharide. The loss on drying is determined by thermogravimetry (*2.2.34*) and is used to calculate the results of the chemical tests shown below with reference to the dried substance.

Only a purified Vi polysaccharide that complies with the following requirements may be used in the preparation of the final bulk.

Protein (*2.5.16*)

Maximum 10 mg per gram of polysaccharide, calculated with reference to the dried substance.

Nucleic acids (*2.5.17*)

Maximum 20 mg per gram of polysaccharide, calculated with reference to the dried substance.

O-Acetyl groups (*2.5.19*)

Minimum 2 mmol per gram of polysaccharide, calculated with reference to the dried substance.

Molecular size

Examine by size-exclusion chromatography (*2.2.30*) using *cross-linked agarose for chromatography R*. Use a column 0.9 m long and 16 mm in internal diameter equilibrated with a solvent having an ionic strength of 0.2 mol/kg and a pH of 7.0-7.5. Apply about 5 mg of polysaccharide in a volume of 1 mL to the column and elute at about 20 mL/h. Collect fractions of about 2.5 mL. Determine the point corresponding to $K_0 = 0.25$ and make 2 pools consisting of fractions eluted before and after this point. Determine O-acetyl groups on the 2 pools (*2.5.19*). Not less than

50 per cent of the polysaccharide is found in the pool containing fractions eluted before $K_0 = 0.25$.

Identification

Carry out an identification test using a suitable immunochemical method (*2.7.1*).

Bacterial endotoxins

The content of bacterial endotoxins determined by a suitable method (*2.6.14*) is within the limits approved for the specific product.

FINAL BULK VACCINE

One or more batches of purified Vi polysaccharide are dissolved in a suitable solvent, which may contain an antimicrobial preservative, so that the volume corresponding to 1 dose contains 25 μg of polysaccharide and the solution is isotonic with blood (250 mosmol/kg to 350 mosmol/kg).

Only a final bulk vaccine that complies with the following tests may be used in the preparation of the final lot.

Sterility (*2.6.1*)

The final bulk vaccine complies with the test for sterility, carried out using 10 mL for each medium.

Antimicrobial preservative

Where applicable, determine the amount of antimicrobial preservative by a suitable physicochemical method.

The amount is not less than 85 per cent and not greater than 115 per cent of the intended amount.

FINAL LOT

The final bulk vaccine is distributed aseptically into sterile tamper-proof containers that are then closed so as to prevent contamination.

Only a final lot that is satisfactory with respect to each of the requirements prescribed below under Identification, Tests and Assay and with the requirement for bacterial endotoxins may be released for use. Provided the tests for free formaldehyde and antimicrobial preservative have been carried out on the final bulk vaccine, they may be omitted on the final lot.

Bacterial endotoxins

The content of bacterial endotoxins determined by a suitable method (*2.6.14*) is within the limit approved for the specific product.

CHARACTERS

Clear colourless liquid, free from visible particles.

IDENTIFICATION

Carry out an identification test using a suitable immunochemical method (*2.7.1*).

TESTS

pH (*2.2.3*)
6.5 to 7.5.

O-Acetyl groups

0.085 (± 25 per cent) μmol per dose (25 μg of polysaccharide).

Test solution   Place 3 mL of the vaccine in each of 3 tubes (2 reaction solutions and 1 correction solution).

Reference solutions   Dissolve 0.150 g of *acetylcholine chloride R* in 10 mL of *water R* (stock solution containing 15 g/L of acetylcholine chloride). Immediately before use, dilute 0.5 mL of the stock solution to 50 mL with *water R* (working dilution containing 150 μg/mL of acetylcholine chloride). In 10 tubes, place in duplicate (reaction and correction solutions) 0.1 mL, 0.2 mL, 0.5 mL, 1.0 mL and 1.5 mL of the working dilution.

Prepare a blank using 3 mL of *water R*.

Make up the volume in each tube to 3 mL with *water R*. Add 0.5 mL of a mixture of 1 volume of *water R* and 2 volumes of *dilute hydrochloric acid R* to each of the correction tubes and to the blank. Add 1.0 mL of *alkaline hydroxylamine solution R* to each tube. Allow the reaction to proceed for exactly 2 min and add 0.5 mL of a mixture of 1 volume of *water R* and 2 volumes of *dilute hydrochloric acid R* to each of the reaction tubes. Add 0.5 mL of a 200 g/L solution of *ferric chloride R* in *0.2 M hydrochloric acid* to each tube, stopper the tubes and shake vigorously to remove bubbles.

Measure the absorbance (*2.2.25*) of each solution at 540 nm using the blank as the compensation liquid. For each reaction solution, subtract the absorbance of the corresponding correction solution. Draw a calibration curve from the corrected absorbances for the 5 reference solutions and the corresponding content of acetylcholine chloride and read from the curve the content of acetylcholine chloride in the test solution for each volume tested. Calculate the mean of the 2 values.

1 mole of acetylcholine chloride (181.7 g) is equivalent to 1 mole of *O*-acetyl (43.05 g).

Free formaldehyde (*2.4.18*)
Maximum 0.2 g/L.

Antimicrobial preservative
Where applicable, determine the amount of antimicrobial preservative by a suitable physicochemical method.
The content is not less than the minimum amount shown to be effective and not more than 115 per cent of the content stated on the label. If phenol has been used in the preparation, the content is not more than 2.5 g/L (*2.5.15*).

Sterility (*2.6.1*)
The vaccine complies with the test for sterility.

ASSAY
Determine Vi polysaccharide by a suitable immunochemical method (*2.7.1*), using a reference purified polysaccharide. The estimated amount of polysaccharide per dose is 80 per cent to 120 per cent of the content stated on the label. The confidence limits ($P = 0.95$) of the estimated amount of polysaccharide are not less than 80 per cent and not more than 120 per cent.

LABELLING
The label states:
— the number of micrograms of polysaccharide per human dose (25 µg),
— the total quantity of polysaccharide in the container.

Ph Eur

Typhoid Vaccine

(*Ph Eur monograph 0156*)
The label may state 'Typhoid'.

Ph Eur

DEFINITION
Typhoid vaccine is a sterile suspension of inactivated *Salmonella typhi* containing not less than 5×10^8 and not more than 1×10^9 bacteria (*S. typhi*) per human dose. The human dose does not exceed 1.0 mL.

PRODUCTION
The vaccine is prepared using a seed-lot system from a suitable strain, such as Ty 2 [1], of *S. typhi*. The final vaccine represents not more than 3 subcultures from the strain on which were made the laboratory and clinical tests that showed it to be suitable. The bacteria are inactivated by acetone, by formaldehyde, by phenol or by heating or by a combination of the last 2 methods.

The production method is validated to demonstrate that the product, if tested, would comply with the test for abnormal toxicity for immunosera and vaccines for human use (*2.6.9*) modified as follows: inject 0.5 mL of the vaccine into each mouse and 1.0 mL into each guinea pig.

IDENTIFICATION
It is identified by specific agglutination.

TESTS
Phenol (*2.5.15*)
If phenol has been used in the preparation, the concentration is not more than 5 g/L.

Antigenic power
When injected into susceptible laboratory animals, it elicits anti-O, anti-H and, to a lesser extent, anti-Vi agglutinins.

Sterility (*2.6.1*)
It complies with the test for sterility.

LABELLING
The label states:
— the method used to inactivate the bacteria,
— the number of bacteria per human dose.

Ph Eur

Typhoid Vaccine, Freeze-dried

(*Ph Eur monograph 0157*)
The label may state 'Typhoid'.

Ph Eur

DEFINITION
Freeze-dried typhoid vaccine is a freeze-dried preparation of inactivated *Salmonella typhi*. The vaccine is reconstituted as stated on the label to give a uniform suspension containing not less than 5×10^8 and not more than 1×10^9 bacteria (*S. typhi*) per human dose. The human dose does not exceed 1.0 mL of the reconstituted vaccine.

PRODUCTION
The vaccine is prepared using a seed-lot system from a suitable strain, such as Ty 2 [1], of *S. typhi*. The final vaccine represents not more than 3 subcultures from the strain on which were made the laboratory and clinical tests that showed it to be suitable. The bacteria are inactivated either by acetone or by formaldehyde or by heat. Phenol is not used in the preparation. The vaccine is distributed into sterile containers and freeze-dried to a moisture content favourable to the stability of the vaccine. The containers are then closed so as to exclude contamination.

The production method is validated to demonstrate that the product, if tested, would comply with the test for abnormal toxicity for immunosera and vaccines for human use (*2.6.9*) modified as follows: inject 0.5 mL of the vaccine into each

---

[1] *This strain is issued by the World Health Organisation Collaborating Centre for Reference and Research on Bacterial Vaccines, Human Serum and Vaccine Institute, Szallas Utea 5, H-1107, Budapest, Hungary.*

mouse and 1.0 mL into each guinea pig.

IDENTIFICATION

The vaccine reconstituted as stated on the label is identified by specific agglutination.

TESTS

Phenol (*2.5.15*)

If phenol has been used in the preparation, the concentration is not more than 5 g/L.

Antigenic power

When injected into susceptible laboratory animals, the reconstituted vaccine elicits anti-O, anti-H and, to a lesser extent, anti-Vi agglutinins.

Sterility (*2.6.1*)

The reconstituted vaccine complies with the test for sterility.

LABELLING

The label states:
— the method used to inactivate the bacteria,
— the number of bacteria per human dose,
— that the vaccine should be used within 8 h of reconstitution.

Ph Eur

Typhoid (Strain Ty 21a) Vaccine, Live (Oral)

(Typhoid Vaccine (Live, Oral, Strain Ty 21a), Ph Eur monograph 1055)

The label may state 'Typhoid (live, oral)'.

Ph Eur

DEFINITION

Typhoid vaccine (live, oral, strain Ty 21a) is a freeze-dried preparation of live *Salmonella typhi* strain Ty 21a grown in a suitable medium. When presented in capsules, the vaccine complies with the monograph on *Capsules (0016)*.

PRODUCTION

CHOICE OF VACCINE STRAIN

The main characteristic of the strain is the defect of the enzyme uridine diphosphate-galactose-4-epimerase. The activities of galactopermease, galactokinase and galactose-1-phosphate uridyl-transferase are reduced by 50 per cent to 90 per cent. Whatever the growth conditions, the strain does not contain Vi antigen. The strain agglutinates to anti-O:9 antiserum only if grown in medium containing galactose. It contains the flagellar H:d antigen and does not produce hydrogen sulfide on Kligler iron agar. The strain is nonvirulent for mice. Cells of strain Ty 21a lyse if grown in the presence of 1 per cent of galactose.

BACTERIAL SEED LOTS

The vaccine is prepared using a seed-lot system. The working seed lots represent not more than one subculture from the master seed lot. The final vaccine represents not more than four subcultures from the original vaccine on which were made the laboratory and clinical tests showing the strain to be suitable.

Only a master seed lot that complies with the following requirements may be used in the preparation of working seed lots.

Galactose metabolism

In a spectrophotometric assay, no activity of the enzyme uridine diphosphate-galactose-4-epimerase is found in the cytoplasm of strain Ty 21a compared to strain Ty 2.

Biosynthesis of lipopolysaccharide

Lipopolysaccharides are extracted by the hot-phenol method and examined by size-exclusion chromatography. Strain Ty 21a grown in medium free of galactose shows only the rough (R) type of lipopolysaccharide.

Serological characteristics

Strain Ty 21a grown in a synthetic medium without galactose does not agglutinate to specific anti-O:9 antiserum. Whatever the growth conditions, strain Ty 21a does not agglutinate to Vi antiserum. Strain Ty 21a agglutinates to H:d flagellar antiserum.

Biochemical markers

Strain Ty 21a does not produce hydrogen sulfide on Kligler iron agar. This property serves to distinguish Ty 21a from other galactose-epimerase-negative *S. typhi* strains.

Cell growth

Strain Ty 21a cells lyse when grown in the presence of 1 per cent of galactose.

BACTERIAL PROPAGATION AND HARVEST

The bacteria from the working seed lot are multiplied in a preculture, subcultured once and are then grown in a suitable medium containing 0.001 per cent of galactose at 30 °C for 13 h to 15 h. The bacteria are harvested. The harvest must be free from contaminating micro-organisms.

Only a single harvest that complies with the following requirements may be used for the preparation of the freeze-dried harvest.

pH

The pH of the culture is 6.8 to 7.5.

Optical density

The optical density of the culture, measured at 546 nm, is 6.5 to 11.0. Before carrying out the measurement, dilute the culture so that a reading in the range 0.1 to 0.5 is obtained and correct the reading to take account of the dilution.

Identification

Culture bacteria on an agar medium containing 1 per cent of galactose and bromothymol blue. Light blue, concave colonies, transparent due to lysis of cells, are formed. No yellow colonies (galactose-fermenting) are found.

FREEZE-DRIED HARVEST

The harvest is mixed with a suitable stabiliser and freeze-dried by a process that ensures the survival of at least 10 per cent of the bacteria and to a water content shown to be favourable to the stability of the vaccine. No antimicrobial preservative is added to the vaccine.

Only a freeze-dried harvest that complies with the following tests may be used for the preparation of the final bulk.

Identification

Culture bacteria are examined on an agar medium containing 1 per cent of galactose and bromothymol blue. Light blue, concave colonies, transparent due to lysis of cells, are formed. No yellow colonies (galactose-fermenting) are found.

Number of live bacteria

Not fewer than 1×10^{11} live *S. typhi* strain Ty 21a per gram.

Water (*2.5.12*)

1.5 per cent to 4.0 per cent, determined by the semi-micro determination of water.

FINAL BULK VACCINE

The final bulk vaccine is prepared by mixing under suitable conditions one or more freeze-dried harvests with suitable excipients.

Only a final bulk that complies with the following requirement may be used in the preparation of the final lot.

Number of live bacteria

Not fewer than 40×10^9 live *S. typhi* strain Ty 21a per gram.

FINAL LOT

The final bulk vaccine is distributed under suitable conditions into capsules with a gastro-resistant shell or into suitable containers.

Only a final lot that is satisfactory with respect to each of the requirements given below under Identification, Tests and Number of live bacteria may be released for use, except that in the determination of the number of live bacteria each dosage unit must contain not fewer than 4×10^9 live bacteria.

IDENTIFICATION

Culture bacteria from the vaccine to be examined on an agar medium containing 1 per cent of galactose and bromothymol blue. Light blue, concave colonies, transparent due to lysis of cells, are formed. No yellow colonies (galactose-fermenting) are found.

TESTS

Contaminating micro-organisms (*2.6.12, 2.6.13*)
Carry out the test using suitable selective media. Determine the total viable count using the plate-count method. The number of contaminating micro-organisms per dosage unit is not greater than 10^2 bacteria and 20 fungi. No pathogenic bacterium, particularly *Escherichia coli, Staphylococcus aureus, Pseudomonas aeruginosa,* and no salmonella other than strain Ty 21a are found.

Water (*2.5.12*)
1.5 per cent to 4.0 per cent, determined on the contents of the capsule or of the container by the semi-micro determination of water.

NUMBER OF LIVE BACTERIA

Carry out the test using not fewer than five dosage units. Homogenise the contents of the dosage units in a 9 g/L solution of *sodium chloride R* at 4 °C using a mixer in a cold room with sufficient glass beads to emerge from the liquid. Immediately after homogenisation prepare a suitable dilution of the suspension using cooled diluent and inoculate brain heart infusion agar; incubate at 36 ± 1 °C for 20 h to 36 h. The vaccine contains not fewer than 2×10^9 live *S. typhi* Ty 21a bacteria per dosage unit.

LABELLING

The label states:
— the minimum number of live bacteria per dosage unit,
— that the vaccine is for oral use only.

Ph Eur

Varicella Vaccine (Live)

(*Ph Eur monograph 0648*)
The label may state 'Var(live)'.

Ph Eur

DEFINITION

Varicella vaccine (live) is a freeze-dried preparation of a suitable attenuated strain of human herpesvirus 3. The vaccine is reconstituted immediately before use, as stated on the label, to give a clear liquid that may be coloured owing to the presence of a pH indicator.

PRODUCTION

The production of vaccine is based on a virus seed-lot system and a cell-bank system. The production method shall have been shown to yield consistently live varicella vaccines of adequate immunogenicity and safety in man. The virus in the final vaccine shall not have been passaged in cell cultures beyond a defined number of passages approved by the competent authority from the original isolated virus.

The potential neurovirulence of the vaccine strain is considered during preclinical development, based on available epidemiological data on neurovirulence and neurotropism, primarily for the wild-type virus. In light of this, a risk analysis is carried out. Where necessary and if available, a test is carried out on the vaccine strain using an animal model that differentiates wild-type and attenuated virus; tests on strains of intermediate attenuation may also be needed.

The production method is validated to demonstrate that the product, if tested, would comply with the test for abnormal toxicity for immunosera and vaccines for human use (*2.6.9*).

SUBSTRATE FOR VIRUS PROPAGATION

The virus is propagated in human diploid cells (*5.2.3*).

VIRUS SEED LOT

The strain of human herpesvirus 3 used shall be identified as being suitable by historical records that include information on the origin of the strain and its subsequent manipulation. The virus shall at no time have been passaged in continuous cell lines. Seed lots are prepared in the same kind of cells as those used for the production of the final vaccine. Virus seed lots are prepared in large quantities and stored at temperatures below -20 °C if freeze-dried, or below -60 °C if not freeze-dried.

Only a virus seed lot that complies with the following requirements may be used for virus propagation.

Identification
The master and working seed lots are identified as human herpesvirus 3 by serum neutralisation in cell culture, using specific antibodies.

Virus concentration
The virus concentration of the master and working seed lots is determined as prescribed under Assay to monitor consistency of production.

Extraneous agents (*2.6.16*)
The working seed lot complies with the requirements for seed lots for live virus vaccines; a sample of 50 mL is taken for the test in cell cultures.

VIRUS PROPAGATION AND HARVEST

All processing of the cell bank and subsequent cell cultures is done under aseptic conditions in an area where no other cells or viruses are being handled. Approved animal (but not human) serum may be used in the culture media. Serum and trypsin used in the preparation of cell suspensions and media are shown to be free from extraneous agents. The cell culture medium may contain a pH indicator such as phenol red and approved antibiotics at the lowest effective concentration. It is preferable to have a substrate free from antibiotics during production. 5 per cent, but not less than 50 mL, of the cell cultures employed for vaccine production is set aside as uninfected cell cultures (control cells). The infected cells constituting a single harvest are washed, released from the support surface and pooled. The cell suspension is disrupted by sonication.

Only a virus harvest that complies with the following requirements may be used in the preparation of the final bulk vaccine.

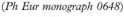

Identification

The virus harvest contains virus that is identified as human herpesvirus 3 by serum neutralisation in cell culture, using specific antibodies.

Virus concentration

The concentration of infective virus in virus harvests is determined as prescribed under Assay to monitor consistency of production and to determine the dilution to be used for the final bulk vaccine.

Extraneous agents (2.6.16)

Use 50 mL for the test in cell cultures.

Control cells

The control cells of the production cell culture from which the single harvest is derived comply with a test for identity and with the requirements for extraneous agents (2.6.16).

FINAL BULK VACCINE

Virus harvests that comply with the above tests are pooled and clarified to remove cells. A suitable stabiliser may be added and the pooled harvests diluted as appropriate.

Only a final bulk vaccine that complies with the following requirements may be used in the preparation of the final lot.

Bacterial and fungal contamination

Carry out the test for sterility (2.6.1) using 10 mL for each medium.

FINAL LOT

The final bulk vaccine is distributed aseptically into sterile, tamper-proof containers and freeze-dried to a moisture content shown to be favourable to the stability of the vaccine. The containers are then closed so as to prevent contamination and the introduction of moisture.

Only a final lot that is satisfactory with respect to the test for water and each of the requirements given below under Identification, Tests and Assay may be released for use. Provided that the test for bovine serum albumin has been carried out with satisfactory results on the final bulk vaccine, it may be omitted on the final lot.

Water (2.5.12)

Not more than the amount shown to ensure stability of the vaccines as approved by the competent authority, determined by the semi-micro determination of water.

IDENTIFICATION

When the vaccine reconstituted as stated on the label is mixed with specific human herpesvirus 3 antibodies, it is no longer able to infect susceptible cell cultures.

TESTS

Bacterial and fungal contamination

The reconstituted vaccine complies with the test for sterility (2.6.1).

Bovine serum albumin

Maximum 0.5 μg per human dose, determined by a suitable immunochemical method (2.7.1).

ASSAY

Titrate the vaccine for infective virus, using at least 3 separate vials of vaccine. Titrate 1 vial of an appropriate virus reference preparation in triplicate to validate each assay. The virus concentration of the reference preparation is monitored using a control chart and a titre is established on a historical basis by each laboratory. The relation with the appropriate European Pharmacopoeia Biological Reference Preparation is established and monitored at regular intervals if a manufacturer's reference preparation is used. Calculate the individual virus concentration for each vial of vaccine and

for each replicate of the reference preparation as well as the corresponding combined virus concentrations, using the usual statistical methods (for example, 5.3). The combined estimate of the virus concentration for the 3 vials of vaccine is not less than that stated on the label.

The assay is not valid if:
— the confidence interval ($P = 0.95$) of the estimated virus concentration of the reference preparation for the 3 replicates combined is greater than $\pm$ 0.3 log PFU;
— the virus concentration of the reference preparation differs by more than 0.5 log PFU from the established value.

The assay is repeated if the confidence interval ($P = 0.95$) of the combined virus concentration of the vaccine is greater than $\pm$ 0.3 log PFU; data obtained from valid assays only are combined by the usual statistical methods (for example, 5.3) to calculate the virus concentration of the sample. The confidence interval ($P = 0.95$) of the combined virus concentration is not greater than $\pm$ 0.3 log PFU.

Varicella vaccine (live) BRP is suitable for use as a reference preparation.

Where justified and authorised, different assay designs may be used; this may imply the application of different validity and acceptance criteria. However, the vaccine must comply if tested as described above.

LABELLING

The label states:
— the strain of virus used for the preparation of the vaccine;
— the type and origin of the cells used for the preparation of the vaccine;
— the minimum virus concentration;
— that contact between the vaccine and disinfectants is to be avoided.

Ph Eur

Yellow Fever Vaccine, Live

(Yellow Fever Vaccine (Live),
Ph Eur monograph 0537)

The label may state 'Yel(live).'

Ph Eur

DEFINITION

Yellow fever vaccine (live) is a freeze-dried preparation of yellow fever virus derived from the 17D strain and grown in fertilised hen eggs. The vaccine is reconstituted immediately before use, as stated on the label, to give a clear liquid.

PRODUCTION

The production of vaccine is based on a virus seed-lot system. The production method shall have been shown to yield consistently yellow fever vaccine (live) of acceptable immunogenicity and safety for man.

The production method is validated to demonstrate that the product, if tested, would comply with the test for abnormal toxicity for immunosera and vaccines for human use (2.6.9) modified as follows for the test in guinea-pigs: inject 10 human doses into each guinea-pig at 2 different injection sites and observe for 21 days.

Reference preparation In the test for neurotropism, a suitable batch of vaccine known to have satisfactory properties in man is used as the reference preparation.

A reference preparation calibrated in International Units per ampoule is used to verify the titre of the virus inoculum in the tests for viraemia (viscerotropism) and immunogenicity, and to titrate the vaccine batch in the potency assay.

The International Unit is the activity contained in a stated quantity of the International Standard. The equivalence in International Units of the International Standard is stated by the World Health Organization.

SUBSTRATE FOR VIRUS PROPAGATION
Virus for the preparation of master and working seed lots and of all vaccine batches is grown in the tissues of chick embryos from a flock free from specified pathogens (SPF) (5.2.2).

SEED LOTS
The 17D strain shall be identified by historical records that include information on the origin of the strain and its subsequent manipulation. Virus seed lots are prepared in large quantities and stored at a temperature below −60 °C. Master and working seed lots shall not contain any human protein, added serum or antibiotics.

Unless otherwise justified and authorised, the virus in the final vaccine shall be between passage levels 204 and 239 from the original isolate of strain 17D. A working seed lot shall be only 1 passage from a master seed lot. A working seed lot shall be used without intervening passage as the inoculum for infecting the tissues used in the production of a vaccine lot, so that no vaccine virus is more than 1 passage from a seed lot that has passed all the safety tests.

Only a virus seed lot that complies with the following requirements may be used for virus propagation.

Identification
The master and working seed lots are identified as containing yellow fever virus by serum neutralisation in cell culture using specific antibodies, or by molecular methods (e.g. nucleic acid amplification techniques (NAT), sequencing).

Extraneous agents (2.6.16)
Each master seed lot complies with the following tests:
— bacterial and fungal sterility (as described in chapter 2.6.16 under Virus seed lot and virus harvests);
— mycoplasmas (as described in chapter 2.6.16 under Virus seed lot and virus harvests);
— mycobacteria (as described in chapter 2.6.16 under Virus seed lot and virus harvests).

Avian leucosis viruses (2.6.24)
Each master seed lot complies with the test for avian leucosis viruses.

Extraneous agents (2.6.16)
Each working seed lot complies with the following tests:
— test in adult mice (intraperitoneal inoculation only) (as described in chapter 2.6.16 under Virus seed lot);
— test in guinea-pigs (as described in chapter 2.6.16 under Virus seed lot);
— bacterial and fungal sterility (as described in chapter 2.6.16 under Virus seed lot and virus harvests);
— mycoplasmas (as described in chapter 2.6.16 under Virus seed lot and virus harvests);
— mycobacteria (as described in chapter 2.6.16 under Virus seed lot and virus harvests);
— test in cell culture for other extraneous agents: a neutralised sample of 5 mL of working seed lot, representing at least 500 000 (5.7 $\log_{10}$) IU, is tested for the presence of extraneous agents by inoculation into continuous simian kidney and human cell cultures as well as into primary chick-embryo-fibroblast cells; the cells are incubated at 36 ± 1 °C and observed for a period of 14 days; the working seed lot passes the test if there is no

evidence of the presence of any extraneous agents; the test is not valid unless at least 80 per cent of the cell cultures remain viable;
— avian viruses: a neutralised sample of 1 mL of working seed lot, representing at least 100 000 (5.0 $\log_{10}$) IU, is tested for the presence of avian viruses by inoculation by the allantoic route into a group of at least 20 fertilised, 9- to 11-day-old, SPF eggs (5.2.2), and by inoculation into the yolk sac of a group of at least 20 fertilised, 5- to 7-day-old, SPF eggs (5.2.2); incubate for 7 days; the working seed lot complies if the allantoic and yolk sac fluids show no signs of haemagglutinating agents and if the embryos and chorio-allantoic membranes examined to detect any macroscopic pathology are typical; the test is not valid unless at least 80 per cent of the inoculated eggs survive during the 7-day observation period.

Avian leucosis viruses (2.6.24)
Each working seed lot complies with the test for avian leucosis viruses.

Tests in monkeys
Each master and working seed lot complies with the following tests in monkeys for viraemia (viscerotropism), immunogenicity and neurotropism.

The monkeys shall be *Macaca* sp. susceptible to yellow fever virus and shall have been shown to be non-immune to yellow fever at the time of injecting the seed virus. They shall be healthy and shall not have received previously intracerebral or intraspinal inoculation. Furthermore, they shall not have been inoculated by other routes with neurotropic viruses or with antigens related to yellow fever virus. Not fewer than 10 monkeys are used for each test.

Use a test dose of 0.25 mL containing the equivalent of not less than 5000 (3.7 $\log_{10}$) IU and not more than 50 000 (4.7 $\log_{10}$) IU, determined by an *in vitro* titration for infectious virus in cell culture. Inject the test dose into 1 frontal lobe of each monkey under anaesthesia and observe the monkeys for not less than 30 days.

Viraemia (Viscerotropism) Viscerotropism is indicated by the amount of virus present in serum. Take blood from each of the test monkeys on the 2nd, 4th and 6th days after inoculation and prepare serum from each sample. Prepare 1:10, 1:100 and 1:1000 dilutions from each serum and inoculate each dilution into a group of at least 4 cell culture vessels used for the determination of the virus concentration. The seed lot complies with the test if none of the sera contains more than the equivalent of 500 (2.7 $\log_{10}$) IU in 0.03 mL and at most 1 serum contains more than the equivalent of 100 (2.0 $\log_{10}$) IU in 0.03 mL.

Immunogenicity Take blood from each monkey 30 days after the injection of the test dose and prepare serum from each sample. The seed lot complies with the test if at least 90 per cent of the test monkeys are shown to be immune, as determined by examining their sera in the test for neutralisation of yellow fever virus described below.

It has been shown that a low dilution of serum (for example, 1:10) may contain non-specific inhibitors that influence this test; such serum shall be treated to remove inhibitors. Mix dilutions of at least 1:10, 1:40 and 1:160 of serum from each monkey with an equal volume of 17D vaccine virus at a dilution that will yield an optimum number of plaques with the titration method used. Incubate the serum-virus mixtures in a water-bath at 37 °C for 1 h and then cool in iced water; add 0.2 mL of each serum-virus mixture to each of 4 cell-culture plates and proceed as for the determination of virus concentration. Inoculate similarly 10 plates with the same amount of virus, plus an equal volume of a 1:10 dilution of monkey serum known to contain no neutralising antibodies to yellow fever virus. At the end of the observation period, compare the mean number of plaques in the plates receiving virus plus non-immune serum with the mean number of plaques in the plates receiving virus plus dilutions of each monkey serum. Not more than 10 per cent of the test monkeys have serum that fails to reduce the number of plaques by 50 per cent at the 1:10 dilution.

Neurotropism   Neurotropism is assessed from clinical evidence of encephalitis, from incidence of clinical manifestations and by evaluation of histological lesions, in comparison with 10 monkeys injected with the reference preparation. The seed lot is not acceptable if either the onset and duration of the febrile reaction or the clinical signs of encephalitis and pathological findings are such as to indicate a change in the properties of the virus.

Clinical evaluation

The monkeys are examined daily for 30 days by personnel familiar with clinical signs of encephalitis in primates (if necessary, the monkeys are removed from their cage and examined for signs of motor weakness or spasticity).

The seed lot is not acceptable if in the monkeys injected with it the incidence of severe signs of encephalitis, such as paralysis or inability to stand when stimulated, or mortality is greater than for the reference vaccine. These and other signs of encephalitis, such as paresis, incoordination, lethargy, tremors or spasticity are assigned numerical values for the severity of symptoms by a grading method. Each day each monkey in the test is given a score based on the following scale:

— grade 1: rough coat, not eating;
— grade 2: high-pitched voice, inactive, slow moving;
— grade 3: shaky movements, tremors, incoordination, limb weakness;
— grade 4: inability to stand, limb paralysis or death (a dead monkey receives a daily score of 4 from the day of death until day 30).

A clinical score for a particular monkey is the average of its daily scores; the clinical score for the group is the arithmetic mean of the individual monkey scores. The seed lot is not acceptable if the mean of the clinical severity scores for the group of monkeys inoculated with it is significantly greater ($P = 0.95$) than the mean for the group of monkeys injected with the reference preparation. In addition, special consideration is given to any animal showing unusually severe signs when deciding on the acceptability of the seed lot.

Histological evaluation

5 levels of the brain are examined including:

— block I: the corpus striatum at the level of the optic chiasma;
— block II: the thalamus at the level of the mamillary bodies;
— block III: the mesencephalon at the level of the superior colliculi;
— block IV: the pons and cerebellum at the level of the superior olives;
— block V: the medulla oblongata and cerebellum at the level of the mid-inferior olivary nuclei.

Cervical and lumbar enlargements of the spinal cord are each divided equally into 6 blocks; 15 µm sections are cut from the tissue blocks embedded in paraffin wax and stained with gallocyanin. Numerical scores are given to each hemisection of the cord and to structures in each hemisection of the brain as listed below. Lesions are scored as follows:

— grade 1 - minimal: 1 to 3 small focal inflammatory infiltrates; degeneration or loss of a few neurons;
— grade 2 - moderate: 4 or more focal inflammatory infiltrates; degeneration or loss of neurons affecting not more than one third of cells;
— grade 3 - severe: moderate focal or diffuse inflammatory infiltration; degeneration or loss of 33-90 per cent of the neurons;
— grade 4 - overwhelming: variable but often severe inflammatory reaction; degeneration or loss of more than 90 per cent of neurons.

It has been found that inoculation of yellow fever vaccine into the monkey brain causes histological lesions in different anatomical formations of the central nervous system with varying frequency and severity (I. S. Levenbook *et al.*, *Journal of Biological Standardization*, 1987, 15, 305-313). Based on these 2 indicators, the anatomical structures can be divided into target, spared and discriminator areas. Target areas are those that show more severe specific lesions in a majority of monkeys irrespective of the degree of neurovirulence of the seed lot. Spared areas are those that show only minimal specific lesions and in a minority of monkeys. Discriminator areas are those where there is a significant increase in the frequency of more severe specific lesions with seed lots having a higher degree of neurovirulence. Discriminator and target areas for *Macaca cynomolgus* and *Macaca rhesus* monkeys are shown in the table below.

Type of monkey	Discriminator areas	Target areas
Macaca cynomolgus	Globus pallidus	Substantia nigra
	Putamen	
	Anterior/median thalamic nucleus	
	Lateral thalamic nucleus	
Macaca rhesus	Caudate nucleus	Substantia nigra
	Globus pallidus	Cervical enlargement
	Putamen	Lumbar enlargement
	Anterior/median thalamic nucleus	
	Lateral thalamic nucleus	
	Cervical enlargement	
	Lumbar enlargement	

Scores for discriminator and target areas are used for the final evaluation of the seed lot. The individual monkey score is calculated from the sum of individual target area scores in each hemisection divided by the number of areas examined. A separate score is calculated similarly for the discriminator areas.

Mean scores for the test group are calculated in 2 ways: (1) by dividing the sum of the individual monkey discriminator scores by the number of monkeys; and (2) by dividing the sum of the individual monkey target and discriminator scores by the number of monkeys. These 2 mean scores are taken into account when deciding on the acceptability of the seed lot. The seed lot is not acceptable if either of the mean lesion scores is significantly greater ($P = 0.95$) than for the reference preparation.

PROPAGATION AND HARVEST

All processing of the fertilised eggs is done under aseptic conditions in an area where no other infectious agents or cells are handled at the same time. At least 2 per cent but

IMMUNOLOGICAL PRODUCTS

not fewer than 20 and not more than 80 eggs are maintained as uninfected control eggs. After inoculation and incubation at a controlled temperature, only living and typical chick embryos are harvested. At the time of harvest, the control eggs are treated in the same way as the inoculated eggs to obtain a control embryonic pulp. The age of the embryo at the time of virus harvest is reckoned from the initial introduction of the egg into the incubator and shall be not more than 12 days. After homogenisation and clarification by centrifugation, the extract of embryonic pulp is tested as described below and kept at -70 °C or colder until further processing. Virus harvests may be pooled. No human protein is added to the virus suspension at any stage during production. If stabilisers are added, they shall have been shown to have no antigenic or sensitising properties for man.

Only a single harvest or, where applicable, a pool of single harvests that complies with the following requirements may be used in the preparation of the final bulk vaccine.

Identification
The single harvest or pool of single harvests contains virus that is identified as yellow fever virus by serum neutralisation in cell culture using specific antibodies, or by molecular methods (e.g. NAT, sequencing).

Bacterial and fungal contamination
The single harvest complies with the test for sterility (2.6.1), carried out using 10 mL for each medium.

Mycoplasmas (2.6.7)
The single harvest or pool of single harvests complies with the test for mycoplasmas, carried out using 10 mL.

Mycobacteria (2.6.2)
A 5 mL sample of the single harvest or pool of single harvests is tested for the presence of *Mycobacterium* spp. by culture methods known to be sensitive for the detection of these organisms.

Embryonic pulp of control eggs
The extract of the control eggs shows no evidence of the presence of any extraneous agents in the tests described below.

Test in cell culture for other extraneous agents   Inoculate a 5 mL sample of embryonic pulp of the control eggs into continuous simian kidney and human cell cultures as well as into primary chick-embryo-fibroblast cells. The cells are incubated at 36 ± 1 °C and observed for a period of 14 days. The embryonic pulp of the control eggs passes the test if there is no evidence of the presence of any extraneous agents. The test is not valid unless at least 80 per cent of the cell cultures remain viable.

Avian viruses   Using 0.1 mL per egg, inoculate the embryonic pulp of control eggs: by the allantoic route into a group of 10 fertilised, 9- to 11-day-old, SPF eggs (5.2.2); and into the yolk sac of a group of 10 fertilised, 5- to 7-day-old, SPF eggs (5.2.2). Incubate for 7 days. The embryonic pulp lot of the control eggs complies if the allantoic and yolk sac fluids show no signs of haemagglutinating agents and if the embryos and chorio-allantoic membranes examined to detect any macroscopic pathology are typical. The test is not valid unless at least 80 per cent of the inoculated eggs survive during the 7 day observation period.

Virus concentration
In order to calculate the dilution for formulation of the final bulk, each single harvest is titrated as described under Assay.

FINAL BULK VACCINE
Single harvests or pools of single harvests that comply with the tests prescribed above are pooled and clarified again.

A test for protein nitrogen content is carried out. A suitable stabiliser may be added and the pooled harvests diluted as appropriate.

Only a final bulk vaccine that complies with the following requirements may be used in the preparation of the final lot.

Bacterial and fungal contamination
The final bulk vaccine complies with the test for sterility (2.6.1), carried out using 10 mL for each medium.

Protein nitrogen content
Maximum 0.25 mg per human dose before the addition of any stabiliser.

FINAL LOT
The final bulk vaccine is distributed aseptically into sterile, tamper-proof containers and freeze-dried to a moisture content shown to be favourable to the stability of the vaccine. The containers are then closed so as to prevent contamination and the introduction of moisture.

Only a final lot that is satisfactory with respect to thermal stability and each of the requirements given below under Identification, Tests and Assay may be released for use. Provided that the test for ovalbumin has been performed with satisfactory results on the final bulk vaccine, it may be omitted on the final lot.

Thermal stability
Maintain at least 3 containers of the final lot of freeze-dried vaccine in the dry state at 37 ± 1 °C for 14 days. Determine the virus concentration as described under Assay in parallel for the heated vaccine and for vaccine stored at the temperature recommended for storage. The virus concentration of the heated vaccine is not more than 1.0 $\log_{10}$ lower than that of the unheated vaccine.

IDENTIFICATION
When the vaccine reconstituted as stated on the label is mixed with specific yellow fever virus antibodies, there is a significant reduction in its ability to infect susceptible cell cultures. Alternatively, the vaccine reconstituted as stated on the label contains virus that is identified as yellow fever virus by molecular methods (e.g. NAT, sequencing).

TESTS
Ovalbumin
Maximum 5 µg of ovalbumin per human dose, determined by a suitable immunochemical method (2.7.1).

Water (2.5.12)
Maximum 3.0 per cent.

Bacterial and fungal contamination
The reconstituted vaccine complies with the test for sterility (2.6.1).

Bacterial endotoxins (2.6.14)
Less than 5 IU per single human dose.

ASSAY
Titrate for infective virus in cell cultures using at least 3 separate containers of vaccine. Titrate 1 container of an appropriate virus reference preparation in triplicate to validate each assay. The virus concentration of the reference preparation is monitored using a control chart and a titre is established on a historical basis by each laboratory. Calculate the individual virus concentration for each container of vaccine and for each replicate of the reference preparation as well as the corresponding combined virus concentrations using the usual statistical methods (for example, 5.3).

The combined virus concentration for the 3 containers of vaccine is compared to the results of the reference preparation titrated in parallel, to obtain results in

International Units. The combined virus concentration of the vaccine is not less than 3.0 $\log_{10}$ IU per human dose and not more than the upper limit approved for the particular product by the competent authority.

The assay is not valid if:

— the confidence interval ($P = 0.95$) of the estimated virus concentration of the reference preparation for the 3 replicates combined is greater than $\pm$ 0.3 $\log_{10}$ IU;

— the virus concentration of the reference preparation differs by more than 0.5 $\log_{10}$ IU from the established value.

The assay is repeated if the confidence interval ($P = 0.95$) of the combined virus concentration of the vaccine is greater than $\pm$ 0.3 $\log_{10}$ IU; data obtained from valid assays only are combined by the usual statistical methods (for example, 5.3) to calculate the virus concentration of the sample. The confidence interval ($P = 0.95$) of the combined virus concentration is not greater than $\pm$ 0.3 $\log_{10}$ IU.

Where justified and authorised, different assay designs may be used; this may imply the application of different validity and acceptance criteria. However, the vaccine must comply if tested as described above.

LABELLING

The label states:

— the strain of virus used in preparation of the vaccine;

— that the vaccine has been prepared in chick embryos;

— the minimum virus concentration;

— that contact between the vaccine and disinfectants is to be avoided.

_____ *Ph Eur*

DIAGNOSTIC PREPARATIONS

Old Tuberculin

(Tuberculin for Human Use, Old,
Ph Eur monograph 0152)

Ph Eur _____

DEFINITION

Old tuberculin for human use consists of a filtrate, concentrated by heating, containing the soluble products of the culture and lysis of one or more strains of *Mycobacterium bovis* and/or *Mycobacterium tuberculosis* that is capable of demonstrating a delayed hypersensitivity in an animal sensitised to micro-organisms of the same species.

Old tuberculin for human use in concentrated form is a transparent, viscous, yellow or brown liquid.

PRODUCTION

GENERAL PROVISIONS

The production of old tuberculin is based on a seed-lot system. The production method shall have been shown to yield consistently old tuberculin of adequate potency and safety in man. A batch of old tuberculin, calibrated in International Units by the method described under Assay and for which adequate clinical information is available as to its activity in man, is set aside to serve as a reference preparation.

The International Unit is the activity of a stated quantity of the International Standard. The equivalence in International Units of the International Standard is stated by the World Health Organisation.

SEED LOTS

The strains of mycobacteria used shall be identified by historical records that include information on their origin and subsequent manipulation.

The working seed lots used to inoculate the media for the production of a concentrated harvest shall not have undergone more than 4 subcultures from the master seed lot.

Only seed lots that comply with the following requirements may be used for propagation.

Identification

The species of mycobacterium of the master and working seed lots is identified.

Bacterial and fungal contamination

Carry out the test for sterility (*2.6.1*), using 10 mL for each medium. The working seed lot complies with the test for sterility except for the presence of mycobacteria.

PROPAGATION AND HARVEST

The bacteria are grown in a liquid medium which may be a glycerolated broth or a synthetic medium. Growth must be typical for the strain. The culture is inactivated by a suitable method, such as treatment in an autoclave (121 °C for not less than 30 min) or in flowing steam at a temperature not less than 100 °C for at least 1 h. The culture liquid, from which the micro-organisms may or may not have been separated by filtration, is concentrated by evaporation, usually to one-tenth of its initial volume. The preparation is free from live mycobacteria. The concentrated harvest is shown to comply with the test for mycobacteria (*2.6.2*) before addition of any antimicrobial preservative or other substance that might interfere with the test. Phenol (5 g/L)

or another suitable antimicrobial preservative that does not give rise to false positive reactions may be added.

Only a concentrated harvest that complies with the following requirements may be used in the preparation of the final bulk tuberculin.

pH (*2.2.3*)

The pH of the concentrated harvest is 6.5 to 8.

Glycerol

Where applicable, determine the glycerol content of the concentrated harvest. The amount is within the limits approved for the particular product.

Antimicrobial preservative

Where applicable, determine the amount of antimicrobial preservative by a suitable chemical or physico-chemical method. The content is not less than 85 per cent and not more than 115 per cent of the intended amount. If phenol has been used in the preparation, the concentration is not more than 5 g/L (*2.5.15*).

Sensitisation

Carry out the test described under Tests.

Sterility (*2.6.1*)

The concentrated harvest complies with the test for sterility, carried out using 10 mL for each medium.

Potency

Determine the potency as described under Assay.

FINAL BULK TUBERCULIN

The concentrated harvest is diluted aseptically.

Only a final bulk tuberculin that complies with the following requirement may be used in the preparation of the final lot.

Sterility (*2.6.1*)

The final bulk tuberculin complies with the test for sterility, carried out using 10 mL for each medium.

FINAL LOT

The final bulk tuberculin is distributed aseptically into sterile containers which are then closed so as to prevent contamination.

Only a final lot that is satisfactory with respect to each of the requirements given below under Identification, Tests and Assay may be released for use.

The following tests may be omitted on the final lot if they have been carried out at the stages indicated:
— live mycobacteria: concentrated harvest,
— sensitisation: concentrated harvest,
— toxicity: concentrated harvest or final bulk tuberculin,
— antimicrobial preservative: final bulk tuberculin.

IDENTIFICATION

Inject increasing doses of the preparation to be examined intradermally into healthy, white or pale-coloured guinea-pigs, specifically sensitised (for example, as described under Assay). A reaction varying from erythema to necrosis is produced at the site of the injection. Similar injections administered to non-sensitised guinea-pigs do not stimulate a reaction. The assay may also serve as identification.

TESTS

Old tuberculin for human use in concentrated form
(≥ 100 000 IU/mL) complies with each of the tests prescribed
below; the diluted product complies with the tests for antimicrobial
preservative and sterility.

Toxicity

Inject a quantity equivalent to 50 000 IU subcutaneously into each of two healthy guinea-pigs weighing 250 g to 350 g and which have not been subjected to any treatment likely to interfere with the test. Observe the animals for 7 days. No adverse effect is produced.

Sensitisation

Use 3 guinea-pigs that have not been subjected to any treatment likely to interfere with the test. On 3 occasions at intervals of 5 days, inject intradermally into each guinea-pig about 500 IU of the preparation to be examined in a volume of 0.1 mL. 2 to 3 weeks after the third injection, administer the same dose intradermally to the same animals and to a control group of 3 guinea-pigs of the same mass that have not previously received injections of tuberculin. After 24 h to 72 h, the reactions in the 2 groups of animals are not substantially different.

Antimicrobial preservative

Where applicable, determine the amount of antimicrobial preservative by a suitable chemical or physico-chemical method. The content is not less than the minimum amount shown to be effective and not more than 115 per cent of the amount stated on the label. If phenol has been used in the preparation, the concentration is not more than 5 g/L (*2.5.15*).

Live mycobacteria (*2.6.2*)

It complies with the test for mycobacteria.

Sterility (*2.6.1*)

It complies with the test for sterility.

ASSAY

The potency of old tuberculin is determined by comparing the reactions produced by the intradermal injection of increasing doses of the preparation to be examined into sensitised guinea-pigs with the reactions produced by known concentrations of the reference preparation.

Prepare a suspension containing a suitable amount (0.1 mg to 0.4 mg/mL) of heat-inactivated, dried mycobacteria in mineral oil with or without emulsifier; use mycobacteria of a strain of the same species as that used in the preparation to be examined. Sensitise not fewer than 6 pale-coloured guinea-pigs weighing not less than 300 g by injecting intramuscularly or intradermally a total of about 0.5 mL of the suspension, divided between several sites if necessary. Carry out the test after the period of time required for optimal sensitisation which is usually 4 to 8 weeks after sensitisation. Depilate the flanks of the animals so that it is possible to make at least three injections on each side and not more than a total of 12 injection points per animal. Use at least three different doses of the reference preparation and at least 3 different doses of the preparation to be examined. For both preparations, use doses such that the highest dose is about 10 times the lowest dose. Choose the doses such that when they are injected the lesions produced have a diameter of not less than 8 mm and not more than 25 mm. In any given test, the order of the dilutions injected at each point is chosen at random in a Latin square design. Inject each dose intradermally in a constant volume of 0.1 mL or 0.2 mL. Measure the diameters of the lesions 24 h to 48 h later and calculate the results of the test by the usual statistical methods, assuming that the diameters of the lesions are directly proportional to the logarithm of the concentration of the preparation.

The estimated potency is not less than 80 per cent and not more than 125 per cent of the stated potency.

The confidence limits (P = 0.95) are not less than 64 per cent and not more than 156 per cent of the stated potency.

STORAGE

Store protected from light.

LABELLING

The label states:
— the number of International Units per millilitre,
— the species of mycobacterium used to prepare the product,
— the name and quantity of any antimicrobial preservative or any other excipient,
— the expiry date,
— where applicable, that old tuberculin is not to be injected in its concentrated form but diluted so as to administer not more than 100 IU per dose.

———————————————————————— Ph Eur

Tuberculin Purified Protein Derivative

Tuberculin P.P.D.

(*Tuberculine Purified Protein Derivative for Human Use, Ph Eur monograph 0151*)

Ph Eur ————————————————————————

DEFINITION

Tuberculin purified protein derivative (tuberculin PPD) for human use is a preparation obtained by precipitation from the heated products of the culture and lysis of *Mycobacterium bovis* and/or *Mycobacterium tuberculosis* and capable of demonstrating a delayed hypersensitivity in an animal sensitised to micro-organisms of the same species.

Tuberculin PPD is a colourless or pale-yellow liquid; the diluted preparation may be a freeze-dried powder which upon dissolution gives a colourless or pale-yellow liquid.

PRODUCTION

GENERAL PROVISIONS

The production of tuberculin PPD is based on a seed-lot system. The production method shall have been shown to yield consistently tuberculin PPD of adequate potency and safety in man. A batch of tuberculin PPD, calibrated in International Units by method A described under Assay and for which adequate clinical information is available as to its activity in man, is set aside to serve as a reference preparation.

The International Unit is the activity of a stated quantity of the International Standard. The equivalence in International Units of the International Standard is stated by the World Health Organisation.

SEED LOTS

The strains of mycobacteria used shall be identified by historical records that include information on their origin and subsequent manipulation.

The working seed lots used to inoculate the media for production of a concentrated harvest shall not have undergone more than 4 subcultures from the master seed lot.

Only seed lots that comply with the following requirements may be used for propagation.

Identification

The species of mycobacterium of the master and working seed lots is identified.

Bacterial and fungal contamination

Carry out the test for sterility (2.6.1), using 10 mL for each medium. The working seed lot complies with the test for sterility except for the presence of mycobacteria.

PROPAGATION AND HARVEST

The bacteria are grown in a liquid synthetic medium. Growth must be typical for the strain. The culture is inactivated by a suitable method such as treatment in an autoclave (121 °C for not less than 30 min) or in flowing steam at a temperature not less than 100 °C for at least 1 h and filtered. The active fraction of the filtrate, consisting mainly of protein, is isolated by precipitation, washed and re-dissolved. The preparation is free from mycobacteria. The concentrated harvest is shown to comply with the test for mycobacteria (2.6.2) before addition of any antimicrobial preservative or other substance that might interfere with the test. Phenol (5 g/L) or another suitable antimicrobial preservative that does not give rise to false positive reactions may be added; a suitable stabiliser intended to prevent adsorption on glass or plastic surfaces may be added. The concentrated harvest may be freeze-dried. Phenol is not added to preparations that are to be freeze-dried.

Only a concentrated harvest that complies with the following requirements may be used in the preparation of the final bulk tuberculin PPD.

Antimicrobial preservative

Where applicable, determine the amount of antimicrobial preservative by a suitable chemical or physico-chemical method. The content is not less than 85 per cent and not more than 115 per cent of the intended amount. If phenol has been used in the preparation, the concentration is not more than 5 g/L (2.5.15).

Sensitisation

Carry out the test described under Tests.

Sterility (2.6.1)

The concentrated harvest, reconstituted if necessary, complies with the test for sterility, carried out using 10 mL for each medium.

Potency

Determine the potency as described under Assay.

FINAL BULK TUBERCULIN PPD

The concentrated harvest is diluted aseptically, after reconstitution if necessary.

Only a final bulk tuberculin PPD that complies with the following requirement may be used in the preparation of the final lot.

Sterility (2.6.1)

The final bulk tuberculin PPD complies with the test for sterility, carried out using 10 mL for each medium.

FINAL LOT

The final bulk tuberculin PPD is distributed aseptically into sterile containers which are then closed so as to prevent contamination. It may be freeze-dried.

Only a final lot that is satisfactory with respect to each of the requirements given below under Identification, Tests and Assay may be released for use.

The following tests may be omitted on the final lot if they have been carried out at the stages indicated:

— live mycobacteria: concentrated harvest
— sensitisation: concentrated harvest
— toxicity: concentrated harvest or final bulk tuberculin PPD
— antimicrobial preservative: final bulk tuberculin PPD.

IDENTIFICATION

Inject increasing doses of the preparation to be examined intradermally into healthy, white or pale-coloured guinea-pigs, specifically sensitised (for example as described under Assay). A reaction varying from erythema to necrosis is produced at the site of the injection. Similar injections administered to non-sensitised guinea-pigs do not stimulate a reaction. The assay may also serve as identification.

TESTS

Tuberculin purified protein derivative for human use in concentrated form (≥ 100 000 IU/mL) complies with each of the tests prescribed below; the diluted product complies with the tests for pH, antimicrobial preservative and sterility.

pH (2.2.3)

The pH of the preparation, reconstituted if necessary as stated on the label, is 6.5 to 7.5.

Toxicity

Inject subcutaneously 50 000 IU of the preparation to be examined into each of two healthy guinea-pigs weighing 250 g to 350 g and which have not been subjected to any treatment likely to interfere with the test. Observe the animals for 7 days. No adverse effect is produced.

Sensitisation

Use 3 guinea-pigs that have not been subjected to any treatment likely to interfere with the test. On 3 occasions at intervals of 5 days, inject intradermally into each guinea-pig about 500 IU of the preparation to be examined in a volume of 0.1 mL. 2 to 3 weeks after the third injection, administer the same dose intradermally to the same animals and to a control group of three guinea-pigs of the same mass that have not previously received injections of tuberculin. After 24 h to 72 h, the reactions in the 2 groups of animals are not substantially different.

Antimicrobial preservative

Where applicable, determine the amount of antimicrobial preservative by a suitable chemical or physico-chemical method. The content is not less than the minimum amount shown to be effective and not more than 115 per cent of the amount stated on the label. If phenol has been used in the preparation, the concentration is not more than 5 g/L (2.5.15).

Live mycobacteria (2.6.2)

It complies with the test for mycobacteria.

Sterility (2.6.1)

It complies with the test for sterility.

ASSAY

Use method A or, where the preparation contains 1 IU to 2 IU, use method B.

METHOD A

The potency of tuberculin PPD is determined by comparing the reactions produced by the intradermal injection of increasing doses of the preparation to be examined into sensitised guinea-pigs with the reactions produced by known concentrations of the reference preparation.

Prepare a suspension containing a suitable amount (0.1 mg/mL to 0.4 mg/mL) of heat-inactivated, dried mycobacteria in mineral oil with or without emulsifier; use mycobacteria of a strain of the same species as that used in the preparation to be examined. Sensitise not fewer than six pale-coloured guinea-pigs weighing not less than 300 g by injecting intramuscularly or intradermally a total of about 0.5 mL of the suspension, divided between several sites if necessary. Carry out the test after the period of time required for optimal sensitisation which is usually 4 to 8 weeks after sensitisation. Depilate the flanks of the animals so that it is possible to make at least 3 injections on each side but not more than a total of 12 injection points per animal. Prepare dilutions of the preparation to be examined and of the reference preparation using isotonic phosphate-buffered saline (pH 6.5 to 7.5) containing 50 mg/L of *polysorbate 80 R*. If the preparation to be examined is freeze-dried and does not contain a stabiliser, reconstitute it using the liquid described above. Use at least 3 different doses of the reference preparation and at least 3 different doses of the preparation to be examined. For both preparations, use doses such that the highest dose is about 10 times the lowest dose. Choose the doses such that when they are injected the lesions produced have a diameter of not less than 8 mm and not more than 25 mm. In any given test, the order of the dilutions injected at each point is chosen at random in a Latin square design. Inject each dose intradermally in a constant volume of 0.1 mL or 0.2 mL. Measure the diameters of the lesions 24 h to 48 h later and calculate the results of the test by the usual statistical methods, assuming that the diameters of the lesions are directly proportional to the logarithm of the concentration of the preparation.

The estimated potency is not less than 80 per cent and not more than 125 per cent of the stated potency.

The confidence limits (P = 0.95) are not less than 64 per cent and not more than 156 per cent of the stated potency.

METHOD B

The potency of tuberculin PPD is determined by comparing the reactions produced by the intradermal injection of the preparation to be examined into sensitised guinea-pigs with the reactions produced by known concentrations of the reference preparation.

Prepare a suspension in mineral oil with or without emulsifier and containing a suitable amount (0.1 mg/mL to 0.4 mg/mL) of heat-inactivated, dried mycobacteria; use mycobacteria of a strain of the same species as that used in the preparation to be examined. Sensitise not fewer than 6 pale-coloured guinea-pigs weighing not less than 300 g by injecting intramuscularly or intradermally a total of about 0.5 mL of the suspension, divided between several sites if necessary. Carry out the test after the period of time required for optimal sensitisation which is usually 4 to 8 weeks after sensitisation. Depilate the flanks of the animals so that it is possible to make at least 3 injections on each side but not more than a total of 12 injection points per animal. Prepare dilutions of the reference preparation using isotonic phosphate-buffered saline (pH 6.5 to 7.5) containing 50 mg/L of *polysorbate 80 R*. Use at least 3 different doses of the reference preparation such that the highest dose is about 10 times the lowest dose and the median dose is the same as that of the preparation to be examined. In any given test, the order of the dilutions injected at each point is chosen at random in a Latin square design. Inject the preparation to be examined and each dilution of the reference preparation intradermally in a constant volume of 0.1 mL or 0.2 mL. Measure the diameters of the lesions 24 h to 48 h later and calculate the results of the test by the usual statistical methods, assuming that the areas of the lesions are directly proportional to the logarithm of the concentration of the preparation to be examined. (This dose relationship applies to this assay and not necessarily to other test systems.)

The estimated potency is not less than 80 per cent and not more than 125 per cent of the stated potency.

The confidence limits (P = 0.95) are not less than 64 per cent and not more than 156 per cent of the stated potency.

STORAGE

Store protected from light.

LABELLING

The label states:
— the number of International Units per container,
— the species of mycobacteria used to prepare the product,
— the name and quantity of any antimicrobial preservative or any other excipient,
— the expiry date,
— for freeze-dried products, a statement that the product is to be reconstituted using the liquid provided by the manufacturer,
— where applicable, that tuberculin PPD is not to be injected in its concentrated form but diluted so as to administer not more than 100 IU per dose.

If the package does not contain a leaflet warning that the inhalation of concentrated tuberculin PPD may produce toxic effects, this warning must be shown on the label on the container together with a statement that the powder must be handled with care.

_____ *Ph Eur*

Monographs

Radiopharmaceutical Preparations

Radiopharmaceutical Preparations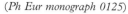

(Ph Eur monograph 0125)

Radiopharmaceutical Preparations comply with the requirements of the European Pharmacopoeia. These requirements are reproduced below.

Ph Eur

DEFINITIONS

Radiopharmaceutical preparations or radiopharmaceuticals are medicinal products which, when ready for use, contain 1 or more radionuclides (radioactive isotopes) included for a medicinal purpose.

For the purpose of this general monograph radiopharmaceutical preparations also cover:

— radionuclide generators: any system incorporating a fixed parent radionuclide from that is produced a daughter radionuclide that is to be obtained by elution or by any other method and used in a radiopharmaceutical preparation;

— kits for radiopharmaceutical preparation: any preparation to be reconstituted or combined with radionuclides in the final radiopharmaceutical preparation, usually prior to its administration;

— radionuclide precursors: any radionuclide produced for radiolabelling of another substance prior to administration;

— chemical precursors: non-radioactive substances for combination with a radionuclide.

Radionuclide precursors may be supplied as solutions for radiolabelling.

A nuclide is a species of atom characterised by the number of protons and neutrons in its nucleus (and hence by its atomic number Z, and mass number A) and also by its nuclear energy state. Isotopes of an element are nuclides with the same atomic number but different mass numbers. Nuclides containing an unstable arrangement of protons and neutrons will transform spontaneously to either a stable or another unstable combination of protons and neutrons with a constant statistical probability. Such nuclides are said to be radioactive and are called radionuclides. The initial unstable nuclide is referred to as the parent radionuclide and the resulting nuclide as the daughter nuclide.

Decay or transformation of radionuclides may involve the emission of charged particles, electron capture (EC) or isomeric transition (IT). The charged particles emitted from nuclei may be alpha particles (nuclei of 4He) or beta particles (negatively charged, generally called electrons, or positively charged, generally called positrons). Alpha decay usually concerns heavy nuclei (Z > 82). Radionuclides with a deficit of protons usually decay by emitting electrons. Radionuclides with a deficit of neutrons usually decay by electron capture or by emitting positrons. In the latter case, radionuclides are called positron emitters. Positrons are annihilated after interaction with electrons in the surrounding matter. The annihilation results in the emission of 2 gamma photons, each with energy of 0.511 MeV, generally emitted at 180° to each other (annihilation radiation). All decay modes may be accompanied by an emission of gamma rays. The emission of gamma rays may be partly or completely replaced by the ejection of electrons, known as internal conversion electrons. This phenomenon, like the process of electron capture, causes a secondary emission of X-rays (due to a reorganisation of the electrons in the atom). This secondary emission may itself be partly replaced by the ejection of electrons, known as Auger electrons.

Radioactivity

Generally the term 'radioactivity' is used both to describe the phenomenon of radioactive decay and to express the physical quantity of this phenomenon.

The radioactivity of a preparation is the number of nuclear disintegrations or transformations per unit time.

In the International System (SI), radioactivity is expressed in becquerel (Bq), which is 1 nuclear transformation per second. Absolute radioactivity measurements require a specialised laboratory but identification of radioactivity and quantitative measurement of radioactivity can be carried out relatively by comparing the measured samples with standardised preparations provided by laboratories recognised by the competent authority or by using a calibrated instrument.

Radioactive decay

Any radionuclide decays at an exponential rate with its characteristic decay constant.

The curve of exponential decay (decay curve) is described by the following expression:

$$A_t = A_0 e^{-\lambda t}$$

A_t = the radioactivity at time t;
A_0 = the radioactivity at time t = 0;
λ = the decay constant, characteristic of each radionuclide;
e = the base of Napierian logarithms.

The half-life ($T_{1/2}$) is the time in which a given radioactivity (amount) of a radionuclide decays to half its initial value.

It is related to the decay constant (λ) by the following equation:

$$T_{1/2} = \frac{ln\,2}{\lambda}$$

The equation of exponential decay can thus be expressed also in the following way, useful for the fast estimation of the radioactivity left after elapsing time *t*:

$$A_t = A_0 \left(\frac{1}{2}\right)^{\frac{t}{T_{1/2}}}$$

The penetrating power of each radiation varies considerably according to its nature and its energy. Alpha particles are completely absorbed in a thickness of a few micrometres to some tens of micrometres of matter. Beta particles are completely absorbed in a thickness of several millimetres to several centimetres of matter. Gamma rays are not completely absorbed but only attenuated and a tenfold reduction may require, for example, several centimetres of lead. The denser the absorbent, the shorter the range of alpha and beta particles and the greater the attenuation of gamma rays.

Each radionuclide is characterised by an invariable half-life, expressed in units of time and by the nature and energy of its radiation or radiations. The energy is expressed in electronvolts (eV), kilo-electronvolts (keV) or mega-electronvolts (MeV).

Radionuclidic purity

The ratio, expressed as a percentage, of the radioactivity of the radionuclide concerned to the total radioactivity of the radiopharmaceutical preparation. The relevant potential radionuclidic impurities are listed with their limits in the individual monographs.

Radiochemical purity

The ratio, expressed as a percentage, of the radioactivity of the radionuclide concerned which is present in the radiopharmaceutical preparation in the stated chemical form, to the total radioactivity of that radionuclide present in the radiopharmaceutical preparation. The relevant potential radiochemical impurities are listed with their limits in the individual monographs.

Chemical purity

In monographs on radiopharmaceutical preparations, chemical purity is controlled by specifying limits for chemical impurities.

Isotopic carrier

A stable isotope of the element concerned either present in or added to the radioactive preparation in the same chemical form as that in which the radionuclide is present.

Carrier-free preparation

A preparation free from stable isotopes of the same element as the radionuclide concerned present in the preparation in the stated chemical form or at the position of the radionuclide in the molecule concerned.

No-carrier-added preparation

A preparation to which no stable isotopes of the same element as the radionuclide concerned are intentionally added in the stated chemical form or at the position of the radionuclide in the molecule concerned.

Specific radioactivity

The radioactivity of a radionuclide per unit mass of the element or of the chemical form concerned, e.g. becquerel per gram or becquerel per mole.

Radioactivity concentration

The radioactivity of a radionuclide per unit volume or unit mass of the preparation. For radiopharmaceutical solutions, it is expressed as radioactivity per unit volume of the preparation.

Total radioactivity

The radioactivity of the radionuclide, expressed per unit (vial, capsule, ampoule, generator, etc).

Chemical precursors for synthesis of radioactive substances

If the active substance of a radiopharmaceutical preparation is not isolated, the chemical precursor for its synthesis is considered as a substance for pharmaceutical use.

It is recommended to test each batch of chemical precursor material in production runs before its use for the manufacture of radiopharmaceutical preparations to ensure that, under specified production conditions, the substance yields the radiopharmaceutical preparation in the desired quantity and of the quality specified.

Period of validity

The time during which specifications described in the monograph must be fulfilled.

PRODUCTION

A radiopharmaceutical preparation contains its radionuclide:
— as an element in atomic or molecular form, e.g. ^{133}Xe, [^{15}O]O$_2$;
— as an ion, e.g. [^{131}I]iodide, [^{99m}Tc]pertechnetate;
— included in, adsorbed on or attached to molecules by chelation, e.g. [^{111}In]indium oxine, or by covalent bonding, e.g. 2-[^{18}F]fluoro-2-deoxy-D-glucose.

Radionuclides can be produced in the following ways:

— in reactions of neutrons (target irradiation in nuclear reactors);
— in reactions of charged particles (target irradiation using accelerators, in particular cyclotrons);
— by its separation from radionuclide generators.

The probability of nuclear reaction occurrence depends on the nature and energy of the incident particles (protons, neutrons, deuterons etc.) and on the nature of the nucleus that is irradiated by them. The rate of production (yield) of a given radionuclide resulting from the irradiation depends in addition on the isotopic composition of the target material and its chemical purity, and in the case of neutrons on their flux, and in the case of charged particles on beam current.

In addition to the desired nuclear reaction, simultaneous transformations usually occur. Probability of their occurrence is given by the same factors as mentioned in the previous paragraph. Such simultaneous transformations may give rise to radionuclidic impurities.

The nuclear reaction (transformation) can be written in the form: target nucleus (incident particle, emitted particle) produced nucleus.

Examples:

$$^{58}Fe(n,\gamma)^{59}Fe$$

$$^{18}O(p,n)^{18}F$$

NEUTRON IRRADIATION

Irradiation of stable radionuclides in nuclear reactors usually results in proton-deficient nuclei, i.e. electron emitters that are formed in (n,γ) reactions (so-called radiative capture). The product is isotopic with the target nucleus and it may thus contain a considerable amount of carrier.

A number of nuclides with high atomic number are fissionable by neutrons. Nuclear fission, denoted as (n, f) reaction, results in a large number of radionuclides of various masses and half-lives. The most frequently used fission is that of ^{235}U. Iodine-131, molybdenum-99 and xenon-133 can be produced by irradiation of ^{235}U in nuclear reactors and by their separation from more than 200 radionuclides formed in that process.

CHARGED PARTICLE IRRADIATION

Irradiation of stable radionuclides with charged particles usually results in neutron-deficient nuclei that decay either by electron capture or by positron emission. They are formed in particular in (p, xn) reactions (where x is the number of emitted neutrons). The product is not isotopic with the target nucleus and its specific radioactivity might be close to that of a carrier-free preparation.

RADIONUCLIDE GENERATORS

Radionuclide generator systems use a parent radionuclide which decays to a daughter radionuclide with a shorter half-life.

By separating the daughter radionuclide from the parent radionuclide by a chemical or physical process, it is possible to use the daughter radionuclide at a considerable distance from the production site of the generator despite its short half-life.

TARGET MATERIALS

The isotopic composition and purity of the target material together with other factors such as the nature and energy of incident particles will determine the relative percentages of the principal radionuclide and radionuclidic impurities produced by irradiation. The use of isotopically enriched target material in which the abundance of the required target nuclide has been artificially increased, can improve the production yield and the purity of the desired radionuclide.

The chemical form, the purity and the physical state of the target material and the chemical additives, as well as the irradiation conditions and the direct physical and chemical environment, determine the chemical state and chemical purity of the radionuclides that are produced. In the production of radionuclides, and particularly of radionuclides with a short half-life, it may not be possible to determine any of these quality criteria before further processing and manufacture of radiopharmaceutical preparations. Therefore the quality of each batch of target material is assessed before its use in routine radionuclide production and manufacture of radiopharmaceutical preparations.

The target material is contained in a holder in gaseous, liquid or solid state, in order to be irradiated by a beam of particles. For neutron irradiation, the target material is commonly contained in quartz ampoules or high-purity aluminium or titanium containers. It is necessary to ascertain that no interaction can occur between the container and its contents under the irradiation conditions.

For charged particle irradiation, the holder for target material is constructed of an appropriate metal, possibly with inlet and outlet ports, a surrounding cooling system and usually a thin metal foil target window.

To evaluate all effects on the efficiency of the production of the radionuclide in terms of quality and quantity, the production procedure must clearly describe and take into consideration: the target material, the construction of the holder for target material, method of irradiation and separation of the desired radionuclide.

CHARACTERS

The *Table of physical characteristics of radionuclides (5.7)* summarises the most commonly accepted physical characteristics of radionuclides used in preparations that are the subject of monographs in the European Pharmacopoeia. In addition, the Table states the physical characteristics of the main potential radionuclidic impurities of the radionuclides mentioned in the monographs.

The term 'transition probability' means the probability of the transformation of a nucleus in a given energy state, via the transition concerned. Instead of 'probability' the term 'abundance' is also used.

The term 'emission probability' means the probability that an atom of a radionuclide gives rise to the emission of the particles or radiation concerned.

Irrespective of which meaning is intended, probability is usually stated as a percentage.

IDENTIFICATION

A radionuclide is generally identified by its half-life or by the nature and energy of its radiation or radiations or by both, as prescribed in the monograph.

Approximate half-life

The half-life as determined over a relatively short time period to allow release for use of radiopharmaceutical preparations.

The calculated approximate half-life is within the range of the values stated in the individual monograph.

Determination of the nature and energy of the radiation

The nature and energy of the radiation emitted are determined using spectrometry. The nature and energy of the radiation of positron emitters is usually not determined; their

identification is performed by determination of their half-life and gamma-ray spectrum.

TESTS

It is sometimes difficult to carry out some of the following tests before releasing the batch for use when the half-life of the radionuclide in the preparation is short. The individual monograph indicates the tests that need not be completed before release for use. These tests then constitute a control of the quality of production.

Non-radioactive substances and related substances

This section prescribes the determination of non-radioactive substances and related substances that can be present.

Residual solvents

Residual solvents are limited according to general chapter *5.4. Residual solvents,* using the methods given in general chapter *2.4.24. Identification and control of residual solvents* or another suitable method.

RADIONUCLIDIC PURITY

Radionuclidic impurities may arise during the production and decay of a radionuclide. Potential radionuclidic impurities may be mentioned in the monographs and their characteristics are described in general chapter 5.7. *Table of physical characteristics of radionuclides mentioned in the European Pharmacopoeia.*

In most cases, to establish the radionuclidic purity of a radiopharmaceutical preparation, the identity of every radionuclide present and its radioactivity must be known. Generally, the most useful method for examination of the radionuclidic purity of gamma- and X-ray emitting radionuclides is gamma-ray spectrometry. The use of sodium iodide detectors may cause a problem: the peaks due to gamma-ray emitting impurities may be concealed in the spectrum of the principal radionuclide or left unresolved from peaks of other radionuclidic impurities in the preparation. Alpha- and beta-particle emitting impurities that do not emit gamma- or X-rays cannot be detected in this way. For alpha- and beta-emitters other methods must be employed.

The individual monographs prescribe the radionuclidic purity required and may set limits for specific radionuclidic impurities (for example, molybdenum-99 in technetium-99^{m}). While these requirements are necessary, they are not in themselves sufficient to ensure that the radionuclidic purity of a preparation is sufficient for its clinical use.

The manufacturer must examine the product in detail and especially must examine preparations of radionuclides with a short half-life for impurities with a long half-life after a suitable period of decay. In this way, information on the suitability of the manufacturing processes and the adequacy of the testing procedures is obtained. In cases where 2 or more positron-emitting radionuclides need to be identified and/or differentiated, for example the presence of ^{18}F-impurities in ^{13}N-preparations, half-life determinations need to be carried out in addition to gamma-ray spectrometry.

Due to differences in the half-lives of the different radionuclides present in a radiopharmaceutical preparation, the radionuclidic purity changes with time.

RADIOCHEMICAL PURITY

Radiochemical impurities may originate from:
— radionuclide production;
— subsequent chemical procedures;
— incomplete preparative separation;
— chemical changes during storage.

The determination of radiochemical purity requires separation of the different chemical substances containing the radionuclide and determination of the percentage of radioactivity of the radionuclide concerned associated with the stated chemical form. The radiochemical purity section of an individual monograph may include limits for specified radiochemical impurities, including isomers.

In principle, any method of analytical separation may be used in the determination of radiochemical purity. For example, the monographs for radiopharmaceutical preparations may include paper chromatography (2.2.26), thin-layer chromatography (2.2.27), electrophoresis (2.2.31), size-exclusion chromatography (2.2.30), gas chromatography (2.2.28) and liquid chromatography (2.2.29). The technical description of these analytical methods is set out in the monographs. Moreover, certain precautions special to radiopharmaceuticals must also be considered, such as radiation protection, measurement geometry, detector linearity, use of carriers, dilution of the preparation.

Specific radioactivity

Specific radioactivity is usually calculated taking into account the radioactivity concentration and the concentration of the chemical substance being studied, after verification that the radioactivity is attributable only to the radionuclide (radionuclidic purity) and the chemical species (radiochemical purity) concerned.

Specific radioactivity changes with time. The statement of the specific radioactivity therefore includes reference to a date and, if necessary, time.

Physiological distribution

Tests involving animals should be avoided wherever possible. Where the tests for identity and for radiochemical purity are not adequate to completely define and control the radiochemical species in a radiopharmaceutical preparation, a physiological distribution test may be required.

The distribution pattern of radioactivity observed in specified organs, tissues or other body compartments of an appropriate animal species can be a reliable indication of the suitability for the intended purpose.

Alternatively, a physiological distribution test can serve to establish the biological equivalence of the preparation under test with similar preparations known to be clinically effective.

The individual monograph prescribes the details concerning the conduct of the test and the physiological distribution requirements that must be met.

In general, the test is performed as follows.

Each of 3 animals is injected intravenously with the preparation. In some cases, dilution immediately before injection may be necessary.

Immediately after injection each animal is placed in a separate cage for collection of excreta and prevention of contamination of the body surface of the animal. At the specified time after injection, the animals are euthanised by an appropriate method and dissected. Selected organs and tissues are assayed for their radioactivity. The physiological distribution is then calculated and expressed in terms of the percentage of the administered radioactivity that is found in each of the selected organs or tissues, taking into account corrections for radioactive decay. For some radiopharmaceutical preparations it is necessary to determine the ratio of the radioactivity in weighed samples of selected tissues (radioactivity/mass).

A preparation meets the requirements of the test if the distribution of radioactivity in at least 2 of the 3 animals complies with all the specified criteria.

Disregard the results from any animal showing evidence of extravasation of the injection (observed at the time of injection or revealed by subsequent assay of tissue radioactivity). In that case the test may be repeated.

Sterility

Radiopharmaceutical preparations for parenteral administration comply with the test for sterility. They must be prepared using precautions designed to exclude microbial contamination and to ensure sterility. The test for sterility is carried out as described in the general method (2.6.1). Special difficulties arise with radiopharmaceutical preparations because of the short half-life of some radionuclides, the small size of batches and the radiation hazards. In the case that the monograph states that the preparation can be released for use before completion of the test for sterility, the sterility test must be started as soon as practically possible in relation to the radiation. If not started immediately, samples are stored under conditions that are shown to be appropriate in order to prevent false negative results. Parametric release (5.1.1) of the product manufactured by a fully validated process is the method of choice in such cases. When aseptic manufacturing is used, the test for sterility has to be performed as a control of the quality of production.

When the size of a batch of the radiopharmaceutical preparation is limited to 1 or a few samples, sampling the batch for sterility testing according to the recommendations of the general method (2.6.1) may not be applicable.

When the half-life of the radionuclide is less than 5 min, the administration of the radiopharmaceutical preparation to the patient is generally on-line with a validated production system.

For safety reasons (high level of radioactivity) it is not possible to use the quantity of radiopharmaceutical preparations as required in the test for sterility (2.6.1). The method of membrane filtration is preferred to limit irradiation of personnel.

Notwithstanding the requirements concerning the use of antimicrobial preservatives in the monograph *Parenteral preparations (0520)*, their addition to radiopharmaceutical preparations in multidose containers is not obligatory, unless prescribed in the monograph.

Bacterial endotoxins - pyrogens

Radiopharmaceuticals for parenteral administration comply with the test for bacterial endotoxins (2.6.14) or with the test for pyrogens (2.6.8).

Eluates of radionuclide generators, solutions for radiolabelling and kits for radiopharmaceutical preparations also comply with the test for bacterial endotoxins if they are intended for the preparation of radiopharmaceuticals for parenteral administration without further purification.

Radionuclide precursors and chemical precursors comply with the test for bacterial endotoxins if intended for use in the manufacture of parenteral preparations without a further appropriate procedure for the removal of bacterial endotoxins.

The test for bacterial endotoxins is carried out as described in the general method (2.6.14), taking the necessary precautions to limit irradiation of the personnel carrying out the test. The limit for bacterial endotoxins is indicated in the individual monograph or calculated according to general chapter 5.1.10. *Guidelines for using the test for bacterial endotoxins*.

When the nature of the radiopharmaceutical preparation or the precursor results in an interference in the test for bacterial endotoxins by inhibition or activation and it is not possible to eliminate the interfering factor(s), the test for pyrogens (*2.6.8*) may be specifically prescribed.

STORAGE

Store preparations containing radioactive substances in an airtight container that is sufficiently shielded to protect personnel from irradiation by primary or secondary emissions and that complies with national and international regulations concerning the storage of radioactive substances. During storage, containers may darken due to irradiation. Such darkening does not necessarily involve deterioration of the preparations.

LABELLING

The labelling of radiopharmaceutical preparations complies with the relevant national and European legislation.

For preparations prepared at the site of use, the labelling can be modified.

The radioactivity of a preparation is stated at a given date. If the half-life is less than 70 days the time is also indicated, with reference to a time zone. The radioactivity at other times may be calculated from the decay equation or from tables.

In addition to the above, the label on the container, the package, a leaflet accompanying the package or a certificate of analysis accompanying the radiopharmaceutical preparation states:

— the route of administration;
— if applicable, the maximum recommended dose in millilitres;
— the name and concentration of any added antimicrobial preservative;
— where applicable, any special storage conditions.

For chemical precursors, the accompanying information recommends testing the substance in 1 or more production runs before its use for the manufacture of radiopharmaceutical preparations to ensure that, under specified production conditions, the substance yields the radiopharmaceutical preparation in the desired quantity and of the quality specified.

MEASUREMENT OF RADIOACTIVITY

The radioactivity of a preparation is stated at a given date and, if necessary, time.

The absolute measurement of the radioactivity of a given sample may be carried out if the decay scheme of the radionuclide is known, but in practice many corrections are required to obtain accurate results. For this reason it is common to carry out the measurement with the aid of a primary standard source. Primary standards may not be available for short-lived radionuclides e.g. positron emitters. Measuring instruments are calibrated using suitable standards for the particular radionuclides. Standards are available from the laboratories recognised by the competent authority. Ionisation chambers and Geiger-Müller counters may be used to measure beta and beta/gamma emitters; scintillation or semiconductor counters or ionisation chambers may be used for measuring gamma emitters; low-energy beta emitters require a liquid-scintillation counter. For the detection and measurement of alpha emitters, specialised equipment and techniques are required. For an accurate comparison of radioactive sources, it is essential for samples and standards to be measured under similar conditions.

Low-energy beta emitters may be measured by liquid-scintillation counting. The sample is dissolved in a solution containing one or more often two organic fluorescent substances (primary and secondary scintillators), which convert part of the energy of disintegration into photons of light, which are detected by a photomultiplier and converted into electrical impulses. When using a liquid-scintillation counter, comparative measurements are corrected for light-quenching effects. Direct measurements are made, wherever possible, under similar conditions, (e.g. volumes and type of solutions) for the source to be examined and the standard source.

All measurements of radioactivity must be corrected by subtracting the background due to radioactivity in the environment and to spurious signals generated in the equipment itself.

With some equipment, when measurements are made at high levels of radioactivity, it may be necessary to correct for loss by coincidence due to the finite resolving time of the detector and its associated electronic equipment. For a counting system with a fixed dead time τ following each count, the correction is:

$$N = \frac{N_{obs}}{1 - N_{obs}\tau}$$

N = the true count rate per second;
N_{obs} = the observed count rate per second;
τ = the dead time, in seconds.

With some equipment this correction is made automatically. Corrections for loss by coincidence must be made before the correction for background radiation.

If the time of an individual measurement, t_m is not negligible short compared with the half-life, $T_{1/2}$, the decay during this measurement time must be taken into account. After having corrected the instrument reading (count rate, ionisation current, etc.) for background and, if necessary, for losses due to electronic effects, the decay correction during measurement time is:

$$R_{corr} = \frac{R\dfrac{t_m \ln 2}{T_{1/2}}}{1 - \exp\left(-\dfrac{t_m \ln 2}{T_{1/2}}\right)}$$

R_{corr} = instrument reading corrected to the beginning of the individual measurement;
R = instrument reading before decay correction, but already corrected for background, etc.

The results of determinations of radioactivity show variations which derive mainly from the random nature of nuclear transformation. A sufficient number of counts must be registered in order to compensate for variations in the number of transformations per unit of time. The standard deviation is the square root of the counts, so at least 10 000 counts are necessary to obtain a relative standard deviation of not more than 1 per cent (confidence interval: 1 sigma).

All statements of radioactive content are accompanied by a statement of the date and, if necessary, the time at which the measurement was made. This statement of the radioactive content must be made with reference to a time zone (GMT, CET). The radioactivity at other times may be calculated from the exponential decay equation or from tables.

The radioactivity of a solution is expressed per unit volume to give the radioactive concentration.

Table of Physical Characteristics of Radionuclides Mentioned in the European Pharmacopoeia

The following table is given to complete the general monograph *Radiopharmaceutical preparations (0125)*.

The values are obtained from the database of the National Nuclear Data Center (NNDC) at Brookhaven National Laboratory, Upton. N.Y., USA, directly accessible via Internet at the address: 'http://www.nndc.bnl.gov/nndc/nudat/radform.html'.

In case another source of information is preferred (more recent values), this source is explicitly mentioned.

Other data sources:

* DAMRI (Département des Applications et de la Métrologie des Rayonnements Ionisants, CEA Gif-sur-Yvette, France),

** PTB (Physikalisch-Technische Bundesanstalt, Braunschweig, Germany),

*** NPL (National Physical Laboratory, Teddington, Middlesex, UK).

The uncertainty of the half-lives are given in parentheses. In principle the digits in parentheses are the standard uncertainty of the corresponding last digits of the indicated numerical value ('Guide to the Expression of Uncertainty in Measurement', International Organisation for Standardisation (ISO), 1993, ISBN 92-67-10188-9).

The following abbreviations are used:

e_A = Auger electrons,
ce = conversion electrons,
β^- = electrons,
β^+ = positrons,
γ = gamma rays,
X = X-rays.

Radionuclide	Half-life	Electronic emission			Photon emission		
		Type	Energy (MeV)	Emission probability (per 100 disintegrations)	Type	Energy (MeV)	Emission probability (per 100 disintegrations)
Tritium (^{3}H)	*12.33 (6) years	*β^-	*0.006 (I) (max: 0.019)	*100			
Carbon-11 (^{11}C)	20.385 (20) min	β^+	0.386 (I) (max: 0.960)	99.8	γ	0.511	199.5 (II)
Nitrogen-13 (^{13}N)	9.965 (4) min	β^+	0.492 (I) (max: 1.198)	99.8	γ	0.511	199.6 (II)
Oxygen-15 (^{15}O)	122.24 (16) s	β^+	0.735 (I) (max: 1.732)	99.9	γ	0.511	199.8 (II)
Fluorine-18 (^{18}F)	109.77 (5) min	β^+	0.250 (I) (max: 0.633)	96.7	γ	0.511	193.5 (II)
Phosphorus-32 (^{32}P)	14.26 (4) days	β^-	0.695 (I) (max: 1.71)	100			
Phosphorus-33 (^{33}P)	25.34 (12) days	β^-	0.076 (I) (max: 0.249)	100			
Sulphur-35 (^{35}S)	87.51 (12) days	β^-	0.049 (I) (max: 0.167)	100			
Chromium-51 (^{51}Cr)	27.7025 (24) days	e_A	0.004	67	X	0.005	22.3
					γ	0.320	9.9

(I) Mean energy of the β spectrum.
(II) Maximum emission probability corresponding to a total annihilation in the source per 100 disintegrations.

Radionuclide	Half-life	Electronic emission			Photon emission		
		Type	Energy (MeV)	Emission probability (per 100 disintegrations)	Type	Energy (MeV)	Emission probability (per 100 disintegrations)
Cobalt-56 (^{56}Co)	77.27 (3) days	e_A	0.006	47	X	0.006-0.007	25
		β^+	0.179 [I]	0.9	γ	0.511	38.0 [II]
			0.631 [I]	18.1		0.847	100.0
						1.038	14.1
						1.175	2.2
						1.238	66.1
						1.360	4.3
						1.771	15.5
						2.015	3.0
						2.035	7.8
						2.598	17.0
						3.202	3.1
						3.253	7.6
Cobalt-57 (^{57}Co)	271.79 (9) days	e_A+ce	0.006-0.007	177.4	X	0.006-0.007	57
		ce	0.014	7.4	γ	0.014	9.2
			0.115	1.8		0.122	85.6
			0.129	1.3		0.136	10.7
						0.692	0.15
Cobalt-58 (^{58}Co)	70.86 (7) days	e_A	0.006	49.4	X	0.006-0.007	26.3
		β^+	0.201 [I]	14.9	γ	0.511	29.9 [II]
						0.811	99.4
						0.864	0.7
						1.675	0.5
Cobalt-60 (^{60}Co)	5.2714 (5) years	β^-	0.096 [I] (max: 0.318)	99.9	γ	1.173	100.0
						1.333	100.0

(I) Mean energy of the β spectrum.
(II) Maximum emission probability corresponding to a total annihilation in the source per 100 disintegrations.

RADIOPHARMACEUTICAL PREPARATIONS

Radionuclide	Half-life	Electronic emission			Photon emission		
		Type	Energy (MeV)	Emission probability (per 100 disintegrations)	Type	Energy (MeV)	Emission probability (per 100 disintegrations)
Gallium-66 (^{66}Ga)	9.49 (7) hours	e_A	0.008	21	X	0.009-0.010	19.1
		β^+	0.157 (I)	1	γ	0.511	112 (II)
			0.331 (I)	0.7		0.834	5.9
			0.397 (I)	3.8		1.039	37
			0.782 (I)	0.3		1.333	1.2
			1.90 (I)	50		1.919	2.1
						2.190	5.6
						2.423	1.9
						2.752	23.4
						3.229	1.5
						3.381	1.5
						3.792	1.1
						4.086	1.3
						4.295	4.1
						4.807	1.8
Gallium-67 (^{67}Ga)	3.2612 (6) days	e_A	0.008	62	X	0.008-0.010	57
		ce	0.082-0.084	30.4	γ	0.091-0.093	42.4
			0.090-0.092	3.6		0.185	21.2
			0.175	0.3		0.209	2.4
						0.300	16.8
						0.394	4.7
						0.888	0.15
Germanium-68 (^{68}Ge) in equilibrium with Gallium-68 (^{68}Ga)	270.82 (27) days	e_A	0.008	42.4	X	0.009-0.010	44.1
	(^{68}Ga: 67.629 (24) min)	β^+	0.353 (I)	1.2	γ	0.511	178.3
			0.836 (I)	88.0		1.077	3.0
Gallium-68 (^{68}Ga)	67.629 (24) min	e_A	0.008	5.1	X	0.009-0.010	4.7
		β^+	0.353 (I)	1.2	γ	0.511	178.3
			0.836 (I)	88.0		1.077	3.0
Krypton-81m (^{81}mKr)	13.10 (3) s	ce	0.176	26.4	X	0.012-0.014	17.0
			0.189	4.6			
					γ	0.190	67.6

(I) Mean energy of the β spectrum.
(II) Maximum emission probability corresponding to a total annihilation in the source per 100 disintegrations.

Radionuclide	Half-life	Electronic emission			Photon emission		
		Type	Energy (MeV)	Emission probability (per 100 disintegrations)	Type	Energy (MeV)	Emission probability (per 100 disintegrations)
Rubidium-81 (^{81}Rb) in equilibrium with Krypton-81m (^{81m}Kr)	4.576 (5) hours	e_A	0.011	31.3	X	0.013-0.014	57.2
		ce	0.176	25.0	γ	0.190	64
			0.188	4.3		0.446	23.2
						0.457	3.0
		$β^+$	0.253 [I]	1.8		0.510	5.3
			0.447 [I]	25.0		0.511	54.2
	(^{81m}Kr: 13.10 (3) s)					0.538	2.2
Strontium-89 (^{89}Sr) in equilibrium with Yttrium-89m (^{89m}Y)	50.53 (7) days	$β^-$	0.583 [I] (max: 1.492)	99.99	γ	0.909	0.01
	(^{89m}Y: 16.06 (4) s)						
Strontium-90 (^{90}Sr) in equilibrium with Yttrium-90 (^{90}Y)	28.74 (4) years	$β^-$	0.196 [I] (max: 0.546)	100			
	(^{90}Y: 64.10 (8) hours)						
Yttrium-90 (^{90}Y)	64.10 (8) hours	$β^-$	0.934 [I] (max: 2.280)	100			
Molybdene-99 (^{99}Mo) in equilibrium with Technetium-99m (^{99m}Tc)	65.94 (1) hours	$β^-$	0.133 [I]	16.4	X	0.018-0.021	3.6
			0.290 [I]	1.1			
			0.443 [I]	82.4	γ	0.041	1.1
						0.141	4.5
						0.181	6
						0.366	1.2
	(^{99m}Tc: 6.01 (1) hours)					0.740	12.1
						0.778	4.3
Technetium-99m (^{99m}Tc)	6.01 (1) hours	ce	0.002	74	X	0.018-0.021	7.3
		e_A	0.015	2.1	γ	0.141	89.1
		ce	0.120	9.4			
			0.137-0.140	1.3			
Technetium-99 (^{99}Tc)	2.11×10^5 years	$β^-$	0.085 [I] (max: 0.294)	100			

(I) Mean energy of the β spectrum.
(II) Maximum emission probability corresponding to a total annihilation in the source per 100 disintegrations.

RADIOPHARMACEUTICAL PREPARATIONS

Radionuclide	Half-life	Electronic emission			Photon emission		
		Type	Energy (MeV)	Emission probability (per 100 disintegrations)	Type	Energy (MeV)	Emission probability (per 100 disintegrations)
Ruthenium-103 (^{103}Ru) in equilibrium with Rhodium-103m (^{103m}Rh)	39.26 (2) days	e_A+ce	0.017	12	X	0.020-0.023	9.0
		ce	0.030-0.039	88.3	γ	0.497	91
						0.610	5.8
	(^{103m}Rh: 56.114 (20) min)	β⁻	0.031 (I)	6.6			
			0.064 (I)	92.2			
Indium-110 (^{110}In)	4.9 (1) hours	e_A	0.019	13.4	X	0.023-0.026	70.5
					γ	0.642	25.9
						0.658	98.3
						0.885	92.9
						0.938	68.4
						0.997	10.5
Indium-110m (^{110m}In)	69.1 (5) min	e_A	0.019	5.3	X	0.023-0.026	27.8
		β⁺	1.015 (I)	61	γ	0.511	123.4 (II)
						0.658	97.8
						2.129	2.1
Indium-111 (^{111}In)	2.8047 (5) days	e_A	0.019	15.6	X	0.003	6.9
						0.023-0.026	82.3
		ce	0.145	7.8			
			0.167-0.171	1.3	γ	0.171	90.2
			0.219	4.9		0.245	94.0
			0.241-0.245	1.0			
Indium-114m (^{114m}In) in equilibrium with Indium-114 (^{114}In)	49.51 (1) days	ce	0.162	40	X	0.023-0.027	36.3
			0.186-0.190	40			
					γ	0.190	15.6
		˙β⁻	0.777 (I) (max: 1.985)	95		0.558	3.2
	(^{114}In: 71.9 (1) s)					0.725	3.2
Tellurium-121m (^{121m}Te) in equilibrium with Tellure-121 (^{121}Te)	154.0 (7) days	e_A	0.003	88.0	X	0.026-0.031	50.5
			0.022-0.023	7.4			
					γ	0.212	81.4
		ce	0.050	33.2		1.102	2.5
	(^{121}Te: 19.16 (5) days)		0.077	40.0			
			0.180	6.1			

(I) Mean energy of the β spectrum.

(II) Maximum emission probability corresponding to a total annihilation in the source per 100 disintegrations.

Radionuclide	Half-life	Electronic emission			Photon emission		
		Type	Energy (MeV)	Emission probability (per 100 disintegrations)	Type	Energy (MeV)	Emission probability (per 100 disintegrations)
Tellurium-121 (^{121}Te)	¨19.16 (5) days	e_A	0.022	11.6	X	0.026-0.030	75.6
					γ	0.470	1.4
						0.508	17.7
						0.573	80.3
Iodine-123 (^{123}I)	13.27 (8) hours	e_A	0.023	12.3	X	0.004	9.3
						0.027-0.031	86.6
		ce	0.127	13.6			
			0.154	1.8	γ	0.159	83.3
			0.158	0.4		0.346	0.1
						0.440	0.4
						0.505	0.3
						0.529	1.4
						0.538	0.4
Iodine-125 (^{125}I)	59.402 (14) days	e_A+ce	0.004	80	X	0.004	15.5
			0.023-0.035	33		0.027	114
						0.031	26
					γ	0.035	6.7
Iodine-126 (^{126}I)	13.11 (5) days	e_A	0.023	6	X	0.027-0.031	42.2
		ce	0.354	0.5	γ	0.388	34
			0.634	0.1		0.491	2.9
						0.511	2.3 [II]
		$β^-$	0.109 [I]	3.6		0.666	33
			0.290 [I]	32.1		0.754	4.2
			0.459 [I]	8.0		0.880	0.8
						1.420	0.3
		$β^+$	0.530 [I]	1			

(I) Mean energy of the β spectrum.
(II) Maximum emission probability corresponding to a total annihilation in the source per 100 disintegrations.

Radionuclide	Half-life	Electronic emission			Photon emission		
		Type	Energy (MeV)	Emission probability (per 100 disintegrations)	Type	Energy (MeV)	Emission probability (per 100 disintegrations)
Iodine-131 (^{131}I)	8.02070 (11) days	ce	0.46	3.5	X	0.029-0.030	3.9
			0.330	1.6			
					γ	0.080	2.6
		β⁻	0.069 (I)	2.1		0.284	6.1
			0.097 (I)	7.3		0.365	81.7
			0.192 (I)	89.9		0.637	7.2
						0.723	1.8
Xenon-131m (^{131m}Xe)	11.84 (7) days	e$_A$	0.025	6.8	X	0.004	8.3
						0.030	44.0
		ce	0.129	61		0.034	10.2
			0.159	28.5			
			0.163	8.3	γ	0.164	2.0
Iodine-133 (^{133}I) (decays to radioactive Xenon-133)	20.8 (1) hours	β⁻	0.140 (I)	3.8	γ	0.530	87
			0.162 (I)	3.2		0.875	4.5
			0.299 (I)	4.2		1.298	2.4
			0.441 (I)	83			
Xenon-133 (^{133}Xe)	5.243 (1) days	e$_A$	0.026	5.8	X	0.004	6.3
						0.031	40.3
		ce	0.045	55.1		0.035	9.4
			0.075-0.080	9.9			
					γ	0.080	38.3
		β⁻	0.101 (I)	99.0			
Xenon-133m (^{133m}Xe) (decays to radioactive Xenon-133)	2.19 (1) days	e$_A$	0.025	7	X	0.004	7.8
						0.030	45.9
		ce	0.199	64.0		0.034	10.6
			0.228	20.7			
			0.232	4.6	γ	0.233	10.0

(I) Mean energy of the β spectrum.
(II) Maximum emission probability corresponding to a total annihilation in the source per 100 disintegrations.

Radionuclide	Half-life	Electronic emission			Photon emission		
		Type	Energy (MeV)	Emission probability (per 100 disintegrations)	Type	Energy (MeV)	Emission probability (per 100 disintegrations)
Iodine-135 (^{135}I) (decays to radioactive Xenon-135)	6.57 (2) hours	β^-	0.140 (I)	7.4	γ	˙0.527	13.8
			0.237 (I)	8		0.547	7.2
			0.307 (I)	8.8		0.837	6.7
			0.352 (I)	21.9		1.039	8.0
			0.399 (I)	8		1.132	22.7
			0.444 (I)	7.5		1.260	28.9
			0.529 (I)	23.8		1.458	8.7
						1.678	9.6
						1.791	7.8
Xenon-135 (^{135}Xe)	9.14 (2) hours	ce	0.214	5.5	X	0.031-0.035	5.0
		β^-	0.171	3.1	γ	0.250	90.2
			0.308	96.0		0.608	2.9
Caesium-137 (^{137}Cs) in equilibrium with Barium-137m (^{137m}Ba)	30.04 (3) years	e_A	0.026	0.8	X	0.005	1
						0.032-0.036	7
		ce	0.624	8.0			
			0.656	1.4	γ	0.662	85.1
	(^{137m}Ba: 2.552 (1) min)	β^-	0.174 (I)	94.4			
			0.416 (I)	5.6			
Thallium-200 (^{200}Tl)	26.1 (1) hours	ce	0.285	3.4	X	0.010	32.0
			0.353	1.4		0.069-0.071	63.3
						0.08	17.5
		β^+	0.495 (I)	0.3			
					γ	0.368	87.2
						0.579	13.8
						0.828	10.8
						1.206	29.9
						1.226	3.4
						1.274	3.3
						1.363	3.4
						1.515	4.0

(I) Mean energy of the β spectrum.
(II) Maximum emission probability corresponding to a total annihilation in the source per 100 disintegrations.

Radionuclide	Half-life	Electronic emission			Photon emission		
		Type	Energy (MeV)	Emission probability (per 100 disintegrations)	Type	Energy (MeV)	Emission probability (per 100 disintegrations)
Lead-201 (²⁰¹Pb) (decays to radioactive Thallium-201)	9.33 (3) hours	e_A	0.055	3	X	0.070-0.073	69
						0.083	19
		ce	0.246	8.5			
			0.276	2	γ	0.331	79
			0.316	2.3		0.361	9.9
						0.406	2.0
						0.585	3.6
						0.692	4.3
						0.767	3.2
						0.826	2.4
						0.908	5.7
						0.946	7.9
						1.099	1.8
						1.277	1.6
Thallium-201 (²⁰¹Tl)	72.912 (17) hours	ce	0.016-0.017	17.7	X	0.010	46.0
			0.027-0.029	4.1		0.069-0.071	73.7
			0.052	7.2		0.080	20.4
			0.084	15.4			
			0.153	2.6	γ	0.135	2.6
						0,167	10.0
Thallium-202 (²⁰²Tl)	12.23 (2) days	e_A	0.054	2.8	X	0.010	31.0
						0.069-0.071	61.6
		ce	0.357	2.4		0.080	17.1
					γ	0.440	91.4
Lead-203 (²⁰³Pb)	51.873 (9) hours	e_A	0.055	3.0	X	0.010	37.0
						0.071-0.073	69.6
		ce	0.194	13.3		0.083	19.4
					γ	0.279	80.8
						0.401	3.4

(I) Mean energy of the β spectrum.
(II) Maximum emission probability corresponding to a total annihilation in the source per 100 disintegrations.

Iobenguane Sulfate for Radiopharmaceutical Preparations

Iobenguane Sulphate for Radiopharmaceutical Preparations

(Ph Eur monograph 2351)

$C_{16}H_{20}I_2N_6,H_2SO_4$ 648   *87862-25-7*

Ph Eur _____

DEFINITION
Bis[(3-iodobenzyl)guanidine] sulfate.

Content
98.0 per cent to 102.0 per cent (dried substance).

CHARACTERS
Appearance
White or almost white crystals.

IDENTIFICATION
A. Infrared absorption spectrophotometry *(2.2.24)*.

Comparison   Ph. Eur. reference spectrum of iobenguane sulfate.

B. Dissolve about 10 mg in 1 mL of *water R* with gentle heating. The solution gives reaction (a) of sulfates *(2.3.1)*.

TESTS
Impurity A
Liquid chromatography *(2.2.29)*. *Prepare the solutions and the mobile phase immediately before use.*

Test solution   Dissolve 10.0 mg of the substance to be examined in 1 mL of the mobile phase and dilute to 5.0 mL with the mobile phase.

Reference solution (a)   Dissolve 10.0 mg of *iobenguane sulfate CRS* in 1 mL of the mobile phase and dilute to 5.0 mL with the mobile phase.

Reference solution (b)   Dissolve 23.1 mg of *3-iodobenzylammonium chloride R* (salt of impurity A) in 1 mL of the mobile phase and dilute to 10.0 mL with the mobile phase.

Reference solution (c)   Mix 1 mL of reference solution (a) and 1 mL of reference solution (b).

Reference solution (d)   Dilute 0.1 mL of reference solution (b) to 10.0 mL with the mobile phase.

Column:
— *size: l* = 0.25 m, Ø = 4.0 mm;
— *stationary phase: silica gel for chromatography R* (5 µm);
— *temperature*: maintain at a constant temperature between 20 °C and 30 °C.

Mobile phase   Mix 40 mL of an 80 g/L solution of *ammonium nitrate R*, 80 mL of *dilute ammonia R2* and 1080 mL of *methanol R*.

Flow rate   1 mL/min.

Detection   Spectrophotometer at 254 nm.

Injection   20 µL of the test solution and reference solutions (c) and (d).

Run time   15 min.

Relative retention   With reference to iobenguane (retention time = about 7 min): impurity A = about 0.2.

System suitability   Reference solution (c):

— *resolution*: minimum 4.0 between the peaks due to impurity A and iobenguane.

Limit:
— *impurity A*: not more than the area of the corresponding peak in the chromatogram obtained with reference solution (d) (1.0 per cent).

Loss on drying *(2.2.32)*
Maximum 3.0 per cent, determined on 0.100 g by drying in an oven at 105 °C.

Bacterial endotoxins *(2.6.14)*
Less than 10 IU/mg, if intended for use without a further appropriate procedure for the removal of bacterial endotoxins.

ASSAY
Liquid chromatography *(2.2.29)* as described in the test for related substances with the following modification.

Injection
Test solution and reference solution (a).

Calculate the percentage content of $C_{16}H_{22}I_2N_6O_4S$ from the declared content of *iobenguane sulfate CRS*.

STORAGE
Protected from light, at a temperature below 25 °C.

LABELLING
The label recommends testing the substance in a production test before its use for the manufacture of radiopharmaceutical preparations. This ensures that, under specified production conditions, the substance yields the radiopharmaceutical preparation in the desired quantity and quality specified.

IMPURITIES
Specified impurities   A.

A. 1-(3-iodophenyl)methanamine.

_____ *Ph Eur*

Medronic Acid for Radiopharmaceutical Preparations

(Ph Eur monograph 2350)

$CH_6O_6P_2$ 176   *1984-15-2*

Action and use
Bisphosphonate; used for bone scanning.

Ph Eur _____

DEFINITION
Methylenediphosphonic acid.

Content
99.0 per cent to 101.0 per cent (dried substance).

CHARACTERS

Appearance

White or almost white, amorphous or crystalline, hygroscopic powder.

Solubility

Very soluble in water, very slightly soluble in anhydrous ethanol, practically insoluble in methylene chloride.

IDENTIFICATION

First identification A.

Second identification B.

A. ¹H Nuclear magnetic resonance spectrometry (2.2.33).

Preparation 100 g/L solution in *deuterium oxide R*.

Comparison 100 g/L solution of *medronic acid CRS* in *deuterium oxide R*.

B. Infrared absorption spectrophotometry (2.2.24).

Comparison *medronic acid CRS*.

TESTS

Impurities A and B

¹H Nuclear magnetic resonance spectrometry (2.2.33).

Test solution To 1.0 g of the substance to be examined add 10 mL of *deuterated chloroform R*. Stir for 1 hour. Pass the resulting solution through a sintered-glass filter to remove the precipitate containing medronic acid. Evaporate the filtrate to about 0.5 mL.

Reference solution (a) Mix 10 µL of *medronic acid impurity A CRS* with 1.0 mL of *deuterated chloroform R*.

Reference solution (b) Mix 10 µL of *medronic acid impurity B CRS* with 1.0 mL of *deuterated chloroform R*.

Reference solution (c) After recording the NMR spectrum of the test solution, add 10 µL of *medronic acid impurity A CRS* and 10 µL of *medronic acid impurity B CRS* to the test solution.

Apparatus NMR spectrometer operating at minimum 250 MHz.

Record the ¹H NMR spectra of the test solution and the reference solutions, if necessary using *tetramethylsilane R* as a chemical shift internal reference compound.

Position of the signals Deuterated chloroform = about 7.3 ppm;
impurity A = about 4.4 ppm and 1.3 ppm;
impurity B = about 4.7 ppm, 2.4 ppm and 1.3 ppm.

System suitability:
— the positions of the signals due to impurities A and B in the spectrum obtained with reference solution (c) do not differ significantly from those in the spectra obtained with reference solutions (a) and (b).

Limits:
— *integration*: integrate the multiplet at 4.4 ppm due to impurity A and the multiplet at 2.4 ppm due to impurity B in the spectra obtained with the test solution and reference solution (c) to obtain the areas of the peaks used in the comparison of impurity contents;
— *impurities A, B*: for each impurity, not more than 0.5 times the area of the corresponding peak in the spectrum obtained with reference solution (c) (1 per cent).

Phosphates (2.4.11)

Maximum 1.0 per cent.

Dissolve 0.100 g in 10 mL of *water R* and dilute to 100.0 mL with the same solvent. Dilute 1.0 mL of this solution to 100.0 mL with *water R*.

Loss on drying (2.2.32)

Maximum 0.5 per cent, determined on 0.500 g by drying in an oven at 105 °C.

Bacterial endotoxins (2.6.14)

Less than 2.0 IU/mg.

ASSAY

Dissolve 75 mg in *water R* and dilute to 50 mL with the same solvent. Titrate with *0.1 M sodium hydroxide*, using 0.1 mL of *bromocresol green solution R* as indicator.

1 mL of *0.1 M sodium hydroxide* is equivalent to 8.80 mg of $CH_6O_6P_2$.

STORAGE

In an airtight container, protected from light.

LABELLING

The label recommends testing the substance in a production test before its use for the manufacture of radiopharmaceutical preparations. This ensures that, under specified production conditions, the substance yields the radiopharmaceutical preparation in the desired quantity and quality specified.

IMPURITIES

Specified impurities A, B.

A. tris(1-methylethoxy)phosphane,

B. tetrakis(1-methylethyl) methylenediphosphonate.

Pentetate Sodium Calcium for Radiopharmaceutical Preparations

(*Ph Eur monograph 2353*)

$C_{14}H_{18}CaN_3Na_3O_{10},xH_2O$ 497.4

(anhydrous substance)

Ph Eur _____

DEFINITION

Trisodium [1,1′,1″,1‴-
[[(carboxylatomethyl)imino]bis(ethylenenitrilo)]tetraacetato]
calciate(3-).

It is a starting material for the preparation of technetium
(^{99m}Tc) pentetate injection.

Content

98.0 per cent to 102.0 per cent (anhydrous substance).

CHARACTERS

Appearance

White or almost white, hygroscopic powder or crystals.

Solubility

Freely soluble in water, practically insoluble in ethanol
(96 per cent).

IDENTIFICATION

A. Infrared absorption spectrophotometry (*2.2.24*).

Comparison   pentetate sodium calcium CRS.

B. Ignite. The residue gives reaction (b) of calcium (*2.3.1*).

C. The substance to be examined gives reaction (a) of
sodium (*2.3.1*).

TESTS

Solution S

Dissolve 5.0 g in *carbon dioxide-free water R* and dilute to
25.0 mL with the same solvent.

Appearance of solution

Solution S is clear (*2.2.1*) and colourless (*2.2.2, Method II*).

pH (*2.2.3*)

8.0 to 9.5 for solution S.

Impurity A

Liquid chromatography (*2.2.29*). *Carry out the test protected
from light.*

Solvent mixture   Dissolve 10 g of *ferric sulfate pentahydrate R*
in 20 mL of *0.5 M sulfuric acid* and add 780 mL of *water R*.
Adjust to pH 2.0 with *1 M sodium hydroxide* and dilute to
1000 mL with *water R*.

Test solution   Dissolve 0.100 g of the substance to be
examined in the solvent mixture and dilute to 25.0 mL with
the solvent mixture.

Reference solution (a)   Dissolve 0.100 g of *sodium calcium
edetate R* in the solvent mixture and dilute to 25.0 mL with
the solvent mixture.

Reference solution (b)   Dissolve 40.0 mg of *nitrilotriacetic
acid R* (impurity A) in the solvent mixture and dilute to
100.0 mL with the solvent mixture. To 10.0 mL of the
solution add 1 mL of reference solution (a) and dilute to
100.0 mL with the solvent mixture. Dilute 1.0 mL of this
solution to 10.0 mL with the solvent mixture.

Column:
— *size: l* = 0.10 m, $\emptyset$ = 4.6 mm;
— *stationary phase*: spherical *graphitised carbon for
   chromatography R1* (5 μm) with a specific surface area of
   120 m^2/g and a pore size of 25 nm.

Mobile phase   Dissolve 50 mg of *ferric sulfate pentahydrate R*
in 50 mL of *0.5 M sulfuric acid* and add 750 mL of *water R*;
adjust to pH 1.5 with *0.5 M sulfuric acid* or *1 M sodium
hydroxide*, add 20 mL of *ethylene glycol R* and dilute to
1000 mL with *water R*.

Flow rate   1 mL/min.

Detection   Spectrophotometer at 273 nm.

Injection   20 μL of the test solution and reference solution
(b); filter the solutions and inject immediately.

Run time   4 times the retention time of the iron complex of
impurity A.

Retention time   iron complex of impurity A = about 5 min;
iron complex of edetic acid = about 10 min; the iron
complex of pentetic acid elutes with the void volume.

System suitability   Reference solution (b):
— *resolution*: minimum 7 between the peaks due to the iron
   complex of impurity A and the iron complex of edetic
   acid;
— *signal-to-noise ratio*: minimum 50 for the peak due to the
   iron complex of impurity A.

Limit:
— *impurity A*: not more than the area of the corresponding
   peak in the chromatogram obtained with reference
   solution (b) (0.1 per cent).

Impurity B

Maximum 1.0 per cent.

Dissolve 5.0 g of the substance to be examined in 250 mL of
water R. Add 10 mL of *ammonium chloride buffer solution
pH 10.0 R* and 50 mg of *mordant black 11 triturate R*.
Not more than 1.3 mL of *0.1 M magnesium chloride* is
required to change the colour of the indicator to violet.

Chlorides

Maximum 0.1 per cent.

Dissolve 0.7 g in *water R* and dilute to 20 mL with the same
solvent. Add 30 mL of *dilute nitric acid R*, allow to stand for
30 min and filter. Dilute 10 mL of the filtrate to 50 mL with
water R. Use this solution as the test solution. Prepare the
reference solution using 0.40 mL of *0.01 M hydrochloric acid*,
add 6 mL of *dilute nitric acid R* and dilute to 50 mL with
water R. Filter both solutions if necessary. Add 1 mL of *silver
nitrate solution R2* to the test solution and the reference
solution. Mix and allow to stand for 5 min protected from
light. Any opalescence in the test solution is not more intense
than that in the reference solution.

Iron (*2.4.9*)

Maximum 20 ppm.

Dilute 2.5 mL of solution S to 10 mL with *water R*.
Add 0.25 g of *calcium chloride R* to the test solution and the
standard before the addition of the *thioglycollic acid R*.

Heavy metals (*2.4.8*)

Maximum 20 ppm.

1.0 g complies with test F. For the digestion replace *sulfuric acid R* by *nitric acid R*. Prepare the reference solution using 2 mL of *lead standard solution (10 ppm Pb) R*.

Water (*2.5.12*)
Maximum 15.0 per cent, determined on 0.100 g.

Bacterial endotoxins (*2.6.14*)
Less than 0.1 IU/mg, if intended for use in the manufacture of parenteral preparations without a further appropriate procedure for the removal of bacterial endotoxins.

ASSAY
Dissolve 0.100 g in *water R* and dilute to 50.0 mL with the same solvent. To 25.0 mL of this solution add 80 mL of *water R* and adjust to pH 2.3 with *dilute nitric acid R*. Titrate with *0.01 M bismuth nitrate* using 0.1 mL of a 1 g/L solution of *xylenol orange R* as indicator. The colour of the solution changes from yellow to red.

1 mL of *0.01 M bismuth nitrate* is equivalent to 4.974 mg of $C_{14}H_{18}CaN_3Na_3O_{10}$.

STORAGE
In an airtight container, protected from light.

LABELLING
The label recommends testing the substance in a production test before its use for the manufacture of radiopharmaceutical preparations. This ensures that, under specified production conditions, the substance yields the radiopharmaceutical preparation in the desired quantity and of the quality specified.

IMPURITIES
Specified impurities   A, B.

A. nitrilotriacetic acid,

B. [[(carboxymethyl)imino]bis(ethylenenitrilo)]tetraacetic acid (pentetic acid).

Ph Eur

Sodium Iodohippurate Dihydrate for Radiopharmaceutical Preparations

(*Ph Eur monograph 2352*)

$C_9H_7INNaO_3,2H_2O$ 363.1   *5990-94-3*

Ph Eur

DEFINITION
Sodium (2-iodobenzamido)acetate dihydrate.

Content
99.0 per cent to 101.0 per cent (anhydrous substance).

CHARACTERS
Appearance
White or almost white, crystalline powder.

Solubility
Soluble in water and in ethanol (96 per cent), practically insoluble in methylene chloride.

IDENTIFICATION
A. Infrared absorption spectrophotometry (*2.2.24*).
Comparison   sodium iodohippurate CRS.

B. It gives reaction (b) of sodium (*2.3.1*).

TESTS
Related substances
Liquid chromatography (*2.2.29*).

Test solution   Dissolve 0.100 g of the substance to be examined in the mobile phase and dilute to 10.0 mL with the mobile phase.

Reference solution (a)   Dilute 1.0 mL of the test solution to 100.0 mL with the mobile phase. Dilute 1.0 mL of this solution to 10.0 mL with the mobile phase.

Reference solution (b)   Dissolve 10 mg of *2-iodobenzoic acid R* (impurity A) in *methanol R* and dilute to 100.0 mL with the same solvent.

Reference solution (c)   Dissolve 10 mg of *benzoic acid R* in the mobile phase, add 1 mL of the test solution and dilute to 100 mL with the mobile phase.

Column:
— *size*: l = 0.25 m, $\emptyset$ = 4.6 mm;
— *stationary phase*: *end-capped polar-embedded octadecylsilyl amorphous organosilica polymer R* (5 µm).

Mobile phase   acetic acid R, methanol R, water R (1:50:50 *V/V/V*).

Flow rate   1 mL/min.

Detection   Spectrophotometer at 230 nm.

Injection   20 µL.

Run time   7 times the retention time of 2-iodohippuric acid.

Identification of impurities   Use the chromatogram obtained with reference solution (b) to identify the peak due to impurity A.

Relative retention   With reference to 2-iodohippuric acid (retention time = about 4.5 min): benzoic acid = about 1.6; impurity A = about 2.1.

System suitability   Reference solution (c):

— *resolution*: minimum 5.0 between the peaks due to 2-iodohippuric acid and benzoic acid.

Limits:

— *impurity A*: not more than 5 times the area of the principal peak in the chromatogram obtained with reference solution (a) (0.5 per cent);

— *unspecified impurities*: for each impurity, not more than the area of the principal peak in the chromatogram obtained with reference solution (a) (0.10 per cent);

— *total*: not more than 5 times the area of the principal peak in the chromatogram obtained with reference solution (a) (0.5 per cent);

— *disregard limit*: 0.5 times the area of the principal peak in the chromatogram obtained with reference solution (a) (0.05 per cent).

Water (*2.5.12*)
8.0 per cent to 12.0 per cent, determined on 0.100 g.

Bacterial endotoxins (*2.6.14*)
Less than 2 IU/mg, if intended for use in the manufacture of parenteral preparations without a further appropriate procedure for the removal of bacterial endotoxins.

ASSAY
Dissolve 0.250 g in 20 mL of *glacial acetic acid R*. Titrate with *0.1 M perchloric acid*, determining the end-point potentiometrically (*2.2.20*).

1 mL of *0.1 M perchloric acid* is equivalent to 32.71 mg of $C_9H_7INNaO_3$.

STORAGE
Protected from light.

LABELLING
The label recommends testing the substance in a production test before its use for the manufacture of radiopharmaceutical preparations. This ensures that, under specified production conditions, the substance yields the radiopharmaceutical preparation in the desired quantity and of the quality specified.

IMPURITIES
Specified impurities *A*.

A. 2-iodobenzoic acid.

_____ *Ph Eur*

Tetra-*O*-Acetyl-Mannose Triflate for Radiopharmaceutical Preparations

(*Ph Eur monograph 2294*)

$C_{15}H_{19}F_3O_{12}S$ 480.4   92051-23-5

Ph Eur _____

DEFINITION
1,3,4,6-Tetra-*O*-acetyl-2-*O*-trifluoromethanesulfonyl-β-D-mannopyranose.

Content
97.0 per cent to 102.0 per cent (dried substance).

CHARACTERS
Appearance
White or almost white, crystalline, hygroscopic powder.

Solubility
Practically insoluble in water, very soluble in acetonitrile, freely soluble in methylene chloride, slightly soluble in ethanol (96 per cent).

IDENTIFICATION
Infrared absorption spectrophotometry (*2.2.24*).

Comparison   tetra-*O*-acetyl-mannose triflate CRS.

TESTS
Specific optical rotation (*2.2.7*)
−12.0 to −16.0 (dried substance), measured at 20 °C.
Dissolve 0.250 g in *acetonitrile R* and dilute to 10.0 mL with the same solvent.

Impurity B
^{19}F Nuclear magnetic resonance spectrometry (*2.2.33*).
Prepare the solutions immediately before use.

Test solution   Dissolve 20.0 mg of the substance to be examined in *deuterated acetonitrile R* and dilute to 1.0 mL with the same solvent.

Reference solution (a).   Dissolve 20.0 mg of *tetra-O-acetyl-mannose triflate CRS* in *deuterated acetonitrile R* and dilute to 1.0 mL with the same solvent.

Reference solution (b)   Dissolve 4.0 mg of *lithium trifluoromethanesulfonate R* (lithium salt of impurity B) in *deuterated acetonitrile R* and dilute to 1.0 mL with the same solvent.

Reference solution (c)   Mix 1.0 mL of reference solution (a) and 10 μL of reference solution (b).

Limit   The peak area identified in the spectrum obtained with the test solution at about −78 ppm is smaller than the peak area identified in the spectrum obtained with reference solution (c) at the same chemical shift (0.2 per cent).

Related substances
Liquid chromatography (*2.2.29*). *Prepare the solutions immediately before use.*

Test solution (a)   Dissolve 0.200 g of the substance to be examined in *acetonitrile R* and dilute to 2.0 mL with the same solvent.

Test solution (b)   Dissolve 10.0 mg of the substance to be examined in *acetonitrile R* and dilute to 5.0 mL with the same solvent.

Reference solution (a)   Dissolve 10.0 mg of *tetra-O-acetyl-mannose triflate CRS* in *acetonitrile R* and dilute to 5.0 mL with the same solvent.

Reference solution (b)   Dilute 1.0 mL of test solution (a) to 10.0 mL with *acetonitrile R*. Dilute 1.0 mL of this solution to 100.0 mL with *acetonitrile R*.

Reference solution (c)   Dissolve 10 mg of *1,3,4,6-tetra-O-acetyl-β-D-mannopyranose R* (impurity A) in 5 mL of *acetonitrile R*. Mix 1 mL of this solution and 1 mL of reference solution (a).

Column:
— *size: l* = 0.25 m, Ø = 4.0 mm;
— *stationary phase: octadecylsilyl silica gel for chromatography R* (5 μm);
— *temperature:* 25 °C.

Mobile phase:
— *mobile phase A: water R*;
— *mobile phase B: acetonitrile R1*;

Time (min)	Mobile phase A (per cent V/V)	Mobile phase B (per cent V/V)
0 - 1	80	20
1 - 20	80 → 55	20 → 45
20 - 35	55	45
35 - 45	55 → 0	45 → 100
45 - 50	0	100

Flow rate   1 mL/min.

Detection   Spectrophotometer at 220 nm.

Injection   20 μL of test solution (a) and reference solutions (b) and (c).

Relative retention   With reference to tetra-O-acetyl-mannose triflate (retention time = about 29 min): impurity A = about 0.2.

System suitability   Reference solution (c):
— *resolution*: minimum 5.0 between the peaks due to impurity A and tetra-O-acetyl-mannose triflate.

Limits:
— *impurity A*: not more than twice the area of the principal peak in the chromatogram obtained with reference solution (b) (0.2 per cent);
— *any other impurity*: for each impurity, not more than the area of the principal peak in the chromatogram obtained with reference solution (b) (0.10 per cent);
— *total*: not more than 5 times the area of the principal peak in the chromatogram obtained with reference solution (b) (0.5 per cent);
— *disregard limit*: 0.5 times the area of the principal peak in the chromatogram obtained with reference solution (b) (0.05 per cent).

Loss on drying
Maximum 0.6 per cent, determined on 25 mg by thermogravimetry (*2.2.34*). Heat to 80 °C at a rate of 2.5 °C/min.

ASSAY
Liquid chromatography (*2.2.29*) as described in the test for related substances with the following modification.

Injection   Test solution (b) and reference solution (a).
Calculate the percentage content of $C_{15}H_{19}F_3O_{12}S$ from the declared content of *tetra-O-acetyl-mannose triflate CRS*.

STORAGE
In an airtight container, protected from light, at a temperature of 2 °C to 8 °C.

LABELLING
The label recommends testing the substance in a production run before its use for the manufacture of radiopharmaceutical preparations. This ensures that, under specified production conditions, the substance yields the radiopharmaceutical preparation in the desired quantity and of the quality specified.

IMPURITIES
Specified impurities   A, B.

A. 1,3,4,6-tetra-O-acetyl-β-D-mannopyranose,

B. trifluoromethanesulfonic acid.

———————————— *Ph Eur*

Iodinated (^{125}I) Albumin Injection

(Human Albumin Injection Iodinated (^{125}I),
Ph Eur monograph 1922)

Ph Eur ————————————

DEFINITION
Sterile, endotoxin-free solution of human albumin labelled with iodine-125. It may contain a suitable buffer and an antimicrobial preservative. The human albumin used complies with the requirements of the monograph on *Human albumin solution (0255)*.

Content
90 per cent to 110 per cent of the declared iodine-125 radioactivity at the date stated on the label.
Purity:
— minimum of 99.0 per cent of the total radioactivity corresponds to iodine-125,
— minimum of 80 per cent of the total radioactivity is associated with the albumin fractions II to V,
— maximum of 5 per cent of the total radioactivity corresponds to unbound iodide.

Content of albumin
95 per cent to 105 per cent of the declared albumin content stated on the label.

CHARACTERS
Appearance
Clear, colourless to yellowish solution.

Half-life and nature of radiation of iodine-125

See general chapter *5.7. Table of physical characteristics of radionuclides.*

IDENTIFICATION

A. Gamma-ray and X-ray spectrometry.

Comparison Standardised iodine-125 solution, or by using a calibrated instrument. Standardised iodine-125 solutions and/or standardisation services are available from the competent authority.

Results The spectrum obtained with the preparation to be examined does not differ significantly from that obtained with a standardised iodine-125 solution, apart from any differences attributable to the presence of iodine-126. The most prominent photon has an energy of 0.027 MeV, corresponding to the characteristic X-ray of tellurium, gamma photons of an energy of 0.035 MeV are also present. Iodine-126 has a half-life of 13.11 days and its most prominent gamma photons have energies of 0.388 MeV and 0.666 MeV.

B. Examine by a suitable immunoelectrophoresis technique *(2.7.1)*. Using antiserum to normal human serum, compare normal human serum and the preparation to be examined, both diluted if necessary. The main component of the preparation to be examined corresponds to the main component of the normal human serum. The diluted solution may show the presence of small quantities of other plasma proteins.

TESTS

pH *(2.2.3)*

5.0 to 9.0.

Albumin

Reference solution Dilute *human albumin solution R* with a 9 g/L solution of *sodium chloride R* to a concentration of 5 mg of albumin per millilitre.

To 1.0 mL of the preparation to be examined and to 1.0 mL of the reference solution add 4.0 mL of *biuret reagent R* and mix. After exactly 30 min, measure the absorbance *(2.2.25)* of each solution at 540 nm, using as the compensation liquid a 9 g/L solution of *sodium chloride R* treated in the same manner. From the absorbances measured, calculate the content of albumin in the injection to be examined in milligrams per millilitre.

Sterility

It complies with the test for sterility prescribed in the monograph on *Radiopharmaceutical preparations (0125)*.

Bacterial endotoxins *(2.6.14)*

Less than 175/V IU/mL, V being the maximum recommended dose in millilitres.

RADIONUCLIDIC PURITY

Iodine-125

Minimum 99.0 per cent of the total radioactivity.

Gamma-ray and X-ray spectroscopy.

Comparison Standardised solution of iodine-125.

Determine the relative amounts of iodine-125 and iodine-126 present.

RADIOCHEMICAL PURITY

Iodine-125 in albumin fractions II to V, iodine-125 corresponding to unbound iodide

Size-exclusion chromatography *(2.2.30)*.

Test solution Mix 0.25 mL of the preparation to be examined with 0.25 mL of the mobile phase.
Use immediately after mixing.

Reference solution *Human albumin solution R* or another appropriate human albumin standard diluted with the mobile phase to a suitable albumin concentration.

Column:
— *size: l* = 0.6 m, Ø = 7.5 mm,
— *stationary phase: silica gel for size-exclusion chromatography R,*
— *temperature:* 25 °C.

Mobile phase Dissolve 11.24 g of *potassium dihydrogen phosphate R,* 42.0 g of disodium *hydrogen phosphate R,* 11.70 g of *sodium chloride R* in 2000 mL of *water R.*

Flow rate 0.6 mL/min.

Detection Spectrophotometer at 280 nm and radioactivity detector set for iodine-125 connected in series.

Injection Loop injector.

Run time 85 min.

Retention times:

Peak No.	Fraction	Description of the compound	Retention time (min)
1	I	High molecular mass compound	18 - 20
2	II	Poly III albumin	23 - 24
3	III	Poly II albumin	25 - 26
4	IV	Poly I albumin	28
5	V	Human serum albumin	29 - 31
6	VI	Iodide	43 - 45

The main peak in the chromatogram obtained with the reference solution corresponds to fraction V.

Limits:
— *radioactivity in fractions II to V:* minimum 80 per cent of the total radioactivity applied to the column,
— *iodine-125 in fraction VI:* maximum 5 per cent of the total radioactivity.

RADIOACTIVITY

Measure the radioactivity using suitable equipment by comparison with a standardised iodine-125 solution or by measurement with a calibrated instrument.

LABELLING

The label states:
— the amount of albumin,
— the maximum volume to be injected.

_____ Ph Eur

Ammonia (^{13}N) Injection

(Ph Eur monograph 1492)

Ph Eur _____

DEFINITION

Sterile solution of [^{13}N]ammonia for diagnostic use.

Nitrogen-13

90 per cent to 110 per cent of the declared nitrogen-13 radioactivity at the date and time stated on the label.

CHARACTERS

Appearance

Clear, colourless solution.

Half-life and nature of radiation of nitrogen-13

See general chapter 5.7. *Table of physical characteristics of radionuclides*.

IDENTIFICATION

A. Gamma-ray spectrometry.

Results   The only gamma photons have an energy of 0.511 MeV and, depending on the measurement geometry, a sum peak of 1.022 MeV may be observed.

B Test A for radionuclidic purity (see Tests).

C. Examine the chromatograms obtained in the test for radiochemical purity (see Tests).

Result   The principal peak in the radiochromatogram obtained with the test solution has approximately the same retention time as the principal peak in the radiochromatogram obtained with the reference solution.

TESTS

pH *(2.2.3)*

5.5 to 8.5.

Sterility

It complies with the test for sterility prescribed in the monograph *Radiopharmaceutical preparations (0125)*. The preparation may be released for use before completion of the test.

Bacterial endotoxins *(2.6.14)*

Less than $175/V$ IU/mL, V being the maximum recommended dose in millilitres. The preparation may be released for use before completion of the test.

Aluminium

Maximum 2 ppm. The preparation may be released for use before completion of the test.

Test solution   In a test-tube about 12 mm in internal diameter, mix 1 mL of *acetate buffer solution pH 4.6 R* and 2 mL of a 1 in 20 dilution of the preparation to be examined in *water R*. Add 0.05 mL of a 10 g/L *solution of chromazurol S R*.

Reference solution   Prepare at the same time and in the same manner as the test solution using 2 mL of a 1 in 20 dilution of *aluminium standard solution (2 ppm Al) R*.

After 3 min, the colour of the test solution is not more intense than that of the reference solution.

RADIONUCLIDIC PURITY

The preparation may be released for use before completion of tests A and B.

A. *Half-life*. The half-life is between 9 min and 11 min.

B. *Gamma emitting impurities*: maximum 1.0 per cent of the total radioactivity.

Gamma-ray spectrometry   Retain a sample of the preparation to be examined for 2 h. Examine the gamma-ray spectrum of the decayed material for the presence of radionuclidic impurities, which should, where possible, be identified and quantified.

RADIOCHEMICAL PURITY

[^{13}N]Ammonia

Liquid chromatography *(2.2.29)*.

The preparation may be released for use before completion of the test.

Test solution   The preparation to be examined.

Reference solution   Dilute 1.0 mL of *dilute ammonia R2* to 10.0 mL with *water R*.

Column:
— *size*: $l = 0.04$ m, $\varnothing = 4.0$ mm;
— *stationary phase*: *cation exchange resin R* (10 µm);
— *temperature*: constant at 20-30 °C.

Mobile phase   *0.002 M nitric acid*.

Flow rate   2 mL/min.

Detection   Suitable radioactivity detector and conductivity detector.

System suitability   The chromatogram obtained with the test solution and the radioactivity detector shows a principal peak with approximately the same retention time as the peak in the chromatogram obtained with the reference solution and the conductivity detector.

Limit:
— *[^{13}N]ammonia*: minimum 99 per cent of the total radioactivity due to nitrogen-13.

RADIOACTIVITY

Determine the radioactivity using a calibrated instrument.

IMPURITIES

A. [^{13}N]O$_2^-$,

B. [^{13}N]O$_3^-$,

C. [^{18}F$^-$],

D. H$_2$[^{15}O].

Ph Eur

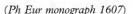

Carbon Monoxide (^{15}O)

(Ph Eur monograph 1607)

Ph Eur

DEFINITION

Mixture of carbon [^{15}O]monoxide in the gaseous phase and a suitable vehicle such as *Medicinal air (1238)*, for diagnostic use.

Purity:
— minimum 99 per cent of the total radioactivity corresponds to oxygen-15,
— minimum 97 per cent of the total radioactivity corresponds to oxygen-15 in the form of carbon monoxide (CO).

PRODUCTION

RADIONUCLIDE PRODUCTION

Oxygen-15 is a radioactive isotope of oxygen which may be produced by various nuclear reactions such as proton irradiation of nitrogen-15 or deuteron irradiation of nitrogen-14.

RADIOCHEMICAL SYNTHESIS

In order to recover oxygen-15 as molecular oxygen from the nitrogen target gas, carrier oxygen is added at concentrations generally ranging from 0.2 per cent V/V to 1.0 per cent V/V. After irradiation, the target gas is usually reacted with activated charcoal at a temperature of about 950 °C. The activated charcoal is preconditioned before use by flushing an inert gas at the production flow rate at a temperature of about 950 °C for not less than 1 h. The carbon [^{15}O]monoxide obtained is purified by passage through a carbon dioxide scavenger, such as soda lime, before mixing with the vehicle.

CHARACTERS

Appearance

Colourless gas.

Half-life and nature of radiation of oxygen-15

See general chapter *5.7. Table of physical characteristics of radionuclides*.

IDENTIFICATION

A. Gamma spectrometry.

Results   The only gamma photons have an energy of 0.511 MeV and, depending on the measurement geometry, a sum peak of 1.022 MeV may be observed.

B. Radionuclidic purity (see Tests).

C. Examine the chromatograms obtained in the test for radiochemical purity.

Results   The principal peaks in the chromatogram obtained with the test gas using the radioactivity detector are similar in retention times to the principal peaks corresponding to carbon monoxide in the chromatogram obtained with reference gas (a) using the thermal conductivity detector.

TESTS

The following tests are performed on carbon [¹⁵O]monoxide as described under radiochemical synthesis before mixing with the vehicle.

Carbon monoxide

Gas chromatography (*2.2.28*) as described in the test for radiochemical purity.

The concentration of carbon monoxide in the test sample is determined before administration and is used to calculate the amount of carbon monoxide to be administered to the patient.

Injection   Test sample, reference gas (b).

Examine the chromatogram obtained with the thermal conductivity detector and calculate the content of carbon monoxide.

RADIONUCLIDIC PURITY

Oxygen-15

Minimum 99 per cent of the total radioactivity.

A. Gamma spectrometry.

Comparison   Standardised fluorine-18 solution, or by using an instrument calibrated with the aid of such a solution. Standardised fluorine-18 solutions and/or standardisation services are available from the competent authority.

Results   The spectrum obtained with the solution to be examined does not differ significantly from that obtained with a standardised fluorine-18 solution.

B. Half-life: 1.9 min to 2.2 min.

The preparation may be released for use before completion of the test.

RADIOCHEMICAL PURITY

Carbon [¹⁵O]monoxide

Gas chromatography (*2.2.28*): use the normalisation procedure.

Test sample   Carbon [¹⁵O]monoxide as described under radiochemical synthesis.

Reference gas (a)   *Nitrogen gas mixture R.*

Reference gas (b)   *Nitrogen R, containing 2.0 per cent V/V of carbon monoxide R1.*

Column:
— *size: l = 1.8 m, Ø1 = 6.3 mm and Ø2 = 3.2 mm,*
— *stationary phase: GC concentrical column R,*

Carrier gas   *helium for chromatography R.*

Flow rate   65 mL/min.

Temperature:
— *column*: 40 °C,
— *injection port*: 40 °C,
— *thermal conductivity detector*: 70 °C.

Detection   Thermal conductivity detector and radioactivity detector connected in series.

Injection   Loop injector.

Run time   10 min.

Retention times   Oxygen, nitrogen and carbon monoxide eluting from the inner column = about 0.4 min; carbon dioxide eluting from the inner column = about 0.8 min; oxygen eluting from the outer column = about 2.1 min; nitrogen eluting from the outer column = about 3.1 min; carbon monoxide eluting from the outer column = about 6.2 min.

System suitability   Reference gas (a):
— 5 clearly separated principal peaks are observed in the chromatogram obtained using the thermal conductivity detector,
— *resolution*: minimum of 1.5 between the peaks due to carbon dioxide eluting from the inner column and oxygen eluting from the outer column, in the chromatogram obtained using the thermal conductivity detector.

Limits   Examine the chromatogram obtained with the radioactivity detector and calculate the percentage content of oxygen-15 substances from the peak areas.
— *carbon [¹⁵O]monoxide*: minimum 97 per cent of the total radioactivity.
— *disregard* the first peak corresponding to components co-eluting from the inner column.

RADIOACTIVITY

The radioactive concentration is determined before administration.

Measure the radioactivity using suitable equipment by comparison with a standardised fluorine-18 solution or by measurement in an instrument calibrated with the aid of such a solution.

_____ *Ph Eur*

Chromium (⁵¹Cr) Edetate Injection

(Ph Eur monograph 0266)

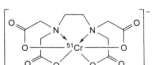

Ph Eur _____

DEFINITION

Sterile solution containing chromium-51 in the form of a complex of chromium(III) with (ethylenedinitrilo)tetraacetic acid, the latter being present in excess. It may be made isotonic by the addition of sodium chloride and may contain a suitable antimicrobial preservative such as benzyl alcohol.

Chromium-51

90 per cent to 110 per cent of the declared chromium-51 radioactivity at the date and time stated on the label.

Chromium

Maximum 1 mg/mL.

CHARACTERS

Appearance

Clear, violet solution.

Half-life and nature of radiation of chromium-51

See general chapter 5.7. *Table of physical characteristics of radionuclides.*

IDENTIFICATION

A. Radionuclidic purity (see Tests).

B. Examine the chromatograms obtained in the test for radiochemical purity (see Tests).

Result The principal peak in the radiochromatogram obtained with the test solution is similar in retardation factor to the principal peak in the chromatogram obtained with the reference solution.

TESTS

pH (2.2.3)

3.5 to 6.5.

Chromium

Maximum 1 mg/mL.

Ultraviolet and visible absorption spectrophotometry (2.2.25).

Test solution The preparation to be examined.

Reference solution Dissolve 0.96 g of *chromic potassium sulfate R* and 2.87 g of *sodium edetate R* in 50 mL of *water R*, boil for 10 min, cool, adjust to pH 3.5-6.5 with *dilute sodium hydroxide solution R* and dilute to 100.0 mL with *water R*.

Measure the absorbance of the test solution and the reference solution at the absorption maximum at 560 nm.

Result The absorbance of the test solution is not greater than that of the reference solution.

Sterility

It complies with the test for sterility prescribed in the monograph *Radiopharmaceutical preparations (0125)*.
The preparation may be released for use before completion of the test.

RADIONUCLIDIC PURITY

Chromium-51

Minimum 99.9 per cent of the total radioactivity.

A. Gamma-ray spectrometry.

Results The only gamma photons have an energy of 0.320 MeV.

B. Gamma-ray spectrometry.

Determine the relative amount of radionuclidic impurities.

Results The total radioactivity due to radionuclidic impurities is not more than 0.1 per cent.

RADIOCHEMICAL PURITY

[^{51}Cr]Chromium edetate

Descending paper chromatography (2.2.26).

Test solution The preparation to be examined.

Reference solution Use the reference solution from the test for chromium.

Chromate carrier solution Dissolve 0.1 g of *potassium chromate R* in 1 mL of *concentrated ammonia R1* and dilute to 100 mL with *water R*.

Paper paper for chromatography R.

Mobile phase concentrated ammonia R1, ethanol (96 per cent) R, water R (1:2:5 V/V/V).

Application Apply a band of a 50 g/L solution of *lead acetate R* to the paper at about 4 cm from the origin and dry in hot air. Apply 10 µL of the chromate carrier solution at the origin, followed by 10 µL of the test solution on the same spot. On a separate sheet, repeat the above procedure, applying 10 µL of the reference solution instead of the test solution.

Development Immediately, over a path of 14 cm.

Drying In air.

Detection Suitable detector to determine the distribution of radioactivity.

Retardation factors Impurity A = 0; impurity B = 0.2 to 0.4; [^{51}Cr]chromium edetate = 0.8 to 0.9.

System suitability The band of lead acetate turns yellow due to reaction with the chromate carrier solution.
The retardation factor of the radioactive spot due to [^{51}Cr]chromium edetate in the radiochromatogram obtained with the test solution is similar to that of the violet spot in the chromatogram obtained with the reference solution.

Limit:
— *[^{51}Cr]chromium edetate*: minimum 97.0 per cent of the total radioactivity due to chromium-51.

RADIOACTIVITY

Determine the radioactivity using a calibrated instrument.

IMPURITIES

A. [^{51}Cr]chromium(III) ion,

B. [^{51}Cr]chromate ion.

Ph Eur

Cyanocobalamin (^{57}Co) Capsules

(Ph Eur monograph 0710)

Ph Eur

DEFINITION

Capsules containing [^{57}Co]-α-(5,6-dimethylbenzimidazol-1-yl)cobamide cyanide; they may contain suitable excipients.

The capsules comply with the requirements for hard capsules prescribed in the monograph *Capsules (0016)*, unless otherwise justified and authorised.

Cobalt-57

90 per cent to 110 per cent of the declared cobalt-57 radioactivity at the date stated on the label.

CHARACTERS

Appearance

Hard, gelatin capsules.

Half-life and nature of radiation of cobalt-57

See general chapter 5.7. *Table of physical characteristics of radionuclides.*

IDENTIFICATION

A. Gamma-ray spectrometry.

Result The most prominent gamma photon of cobalt-57 has an energy of 0.122 MeV.

B. Examine the chromatograms obtained in the test for radiochemical purity (see Tests).

Result The principal peak in the radiochromatogram obtained with the test solution is similar in retention time to the principal peak in the chromatogram obtained with the reference solution.

TESTS

Disintegration

The capsules comply with the test for disintegration of tablets and capsules (2.9.1), except that 1 capsule is used in the test instead of 6.

Uniformity of content

Determine, by measurement in a suitable counting assembly and under identical geometrical conditions, the radioactivity of each of not fewer than 10 capsules. Calculate the average radioactivity per capsule. The radioactivity of no capsule differs by more than 10 per cent from the average.

The relative standard deviation is less than 3.5 per cent.

RADIONUCLIDIC PURITY

Cobalt-57

Minimum 99.9 per cent of the total radioactivity.

Gamma-ray spectrometry.

Determine the relative amounts of cobalt-57, cobalt-56 and cobalt-58 present.

RADIOCHEMICAL PURITY

[^{57}Co]Cyanocobalamin

Liquid chromatography (2.2.29).

Test solution   Dissolve the contents of a capsule in 1.0 mL of *water R* and allow to stand for 10 min. Centrifuge at 2000 r/min for 10 min. Use the supernatant.

Reference solution   Dissolve 10 mg of *cyanocobalamin CRS* in the mobile phase and dilute to 100 mL with the mobile phase. Dilute 2 mL of this solution to 100 mL with the mobile phase. *Use within 1 h of preparation.*

Column:
— *size: l* = 0.25 m, Ø = 4.0 mm;
— *stationary phase*: octylsilyl silica gel for chromatography R (5 μm).

Mobile phase   26.5 volumes of *methanol R* and 73.5 volumes of a 10 g/L solution of *disodium hydrogen phosphate R* adjusted to pH 3.5 using *phosphoric acid R*. *Use within 2 days of preparation.*

Flow rate   1.0 mL/min.

Detection   Radioactivity detector adjusted for cobalt-57 and spectrophotometer at 361 nm.

Injection   100 μL.

Run time   3 times the retention time of cyanocobalamin for the test solution; 30 min for the reference solution.

Limit:
— *[^{57}Co]cyanocobalamin*: minimum 90 per cent of the total radioactivity due to cobalt-57.

RADIOACTIVITY

Determine the radioactivity using a calibrated instrument.

STORAGE

In an airtight container, protected from light, at a temperature of 2 °C to 8 °C.

IMPURITIES

A. cobalt-56,

B. cobalt-58.

_____ *Ph Eur*

Cyanocobalamin (^{57}Co) Solution

(*Ph Eur monograph 0269*)

Ph Eur _____

DEFINITION

Solution of [^{57}Co]-α-(5,6-dimethylbenzimidazol-1-yl)cobamide cyanide and may contain a stabiliser and an antimicrobial preservative.

Cobalt-57

90 per cent to 110 per cent of the declared cobalt-57 radioactivity at the date stated on the label.

CHARACTERS

Appearance

Clear, colourless or slightly pink solution.

Half-life and nature of radiation of cobalt-57

See general chapter 5.7. *Table of physical characteristics of radionuclides.*

IDENTIFICATION

A. Gamma-ray spectrometry.

Result   The most prominent gamma photon of cobalt-57 has an energy of 0.122 MeV.

B. Examine the chromatograms obtained in the test for radiochemical purity (see Tests).

Result   The principal peak in the radiochromatogram obtained with the test solution is similar in retention time to the principal peak in the chromatogram obtained with the reference solution.

TESTS

pH (2.2.3)

4.0 to 6.0.

RADIONUCLIDIC PURITY

Cobalt-57

Minimum 99.9 per cent of the total radioactivity.

Gamma-ray spectrometry.

Determine the relative amounts of cobalt-57, cobalt-56 and cobalt-58 present.

RADIOCHEMICAL PURITY

[^{57}Co]Cyanocobalamin

Liquid chromatography (2.2.29).

Test solution   The preparation to be examined.

Reference solution   Dissolve 10 mg of *cyanocobalamin CRS* in the mobile phase and dilute to 100 mL with the mobile phase. Dilute 2 mL of this solution to 100 mL with the mobile phase. *Use within 1 h after preparation.*

Column:
— *size: l* = 0.25 m, Ø = 4.0 mm;
— *stationary phase*: octylsilyl silica gel for chromatography R (5 μm).

Mobile phase   26.5 volumes of *methanol R* and 73.5 volumes of a 10 g/L solution of *disodium hydrogen phosphate R* adjusted to pH 3.5 using *phosphoric acid R* (use within 2 days after preparation).

Flow rate   1.0 mL/min.

Detection   Radioactivity detector adjusted for cobalt-57 and spectrophotometer at 361 nm.

Injection   100 μL.

Run time   3 times the retention time of cyanocobalamin for the test solution; 30 min for the reference solution.

Limit:
— *[^{57}Co]cyanocobalamin:* minimum 90 per cent of the radioactivity due to cobalt-57.

RADIOACTIVITY

Determine the radioactivity using a calibrated instrument.

STORAGE

Protected from light, at a temperature of 2 °C to 8 °C.

IMPURITIES

A. cobalt-56,

B. cobalt-58.

———————————————————————————————— *Ph Eur*

Cyanocobalamin (^{58}Co) Capsules

(Ph Eur monograph 1505)

Ph Eur ——————————————————————————————————

DEFINITION

Capsules containing [^{58}Co]-α-(5,6-dimethylbenzimidazol-1-yl)cobamide cyanide; they may contain suitable excipients.

The capsules comply with the requirements for hard capsules in the monograph *Capsules (0016)*, unless otherwise justified and authorised.

Cobalt-58

Average between 90 per cent and 110 per cent of the declared cobalt-58 radioactivity at the date stated on the label.

CHARACTERS

Appearance

Hard gelatin capsules.

Half-life and nature of radiation of cobalt-58

See general chapter 5.7. *Table of physical characteristics of radionuclides.*

IDENTIFICATION

A. Gamma-ray spectrometry.

Results The most prominent gamma photons of cobalt-58 have energies of 0.511 MeV (annihilation radiation) and 0.811 MeV.

B. Examine the chromatograms obtained in the test for radiochemical purity (see Tests).

Result The principal peak in the radiochromatogram obtained with the test solution is similar in retention time to the principal peak in the chromatogram obtained with the reference solution.

TESTS

Disintegration

The capsules comply with the test for disintegration of tablets and capsules (*2.9.1*) except that 1 capsule is used in the test instead of 6.

Uniformity of content

Determine by measurement in a suitable counting assembly and under identical geometrical conditions the radioactivity of each of not less than 10 capsules. Calculate the average radioactivity per capsule. The radioactivity of no capsule differs by more than 10 per cent from the average. The relative standard deviation is less than 3.5 per cent.

RADIONUCLIDIC PURITY

Cobalt-58

Minimum 98 per cent of the total radioactivity.

Gamma-ray spectrometry.

Determine the relative amounts of cobalt-58, cobalt-57 and cobalt-60 present.

Result:
— *cobalt-60:* maximum 1 per cent of the total radioactivity.

RADIOCHEMICAL PURITY

[^{58}Co]Cyanocobalamin

Liquid chromatography (*2.2.29*).

Test solution Dissolve the contents of a capsule in 1.0 mL of *water R* and allow to stand for 10 min. Centrifuge at 2000 r/min for 10 min. Use the supernatant.

Reference solution Dissolve 10 mg of *cyanocobalamin CRS* in the mobile phase and dilute to 100 mL with the mobile phase. Dilute 2 mL of this solution to 100 mL with the mobile phase. *Use within 1 h after preparation.*

Column:
— size: *l* = 0.25 m, Ø = 4.0 mm;
— stationary phase: *octylsilyl silica gel for chromatography R* (5 μm).

Mobile phase 26.5 volumes of *methanol R* and 73.5 volumes of a 10 g/L solution of *disodium hydrogen phosphate R*, adjusted to pH 3.5 with *phosphoric acid R* (use within 2 days).

Flow rate 1.0 mL/min.

Detection Radioactivity detector adjusted for cobalt-58 and spectrophotometer at 361 nm.

Injection 100 μL.

Run time 3 times the retention time of cyanocobalamin for the test solution; 30 min for the reference solution.

Limit:
— *[^{58}Co]cyanocobalamin:* minimum 84 per cent of the total radioactivity due to cobalt-58.

RADIOACTIVITY

Determine the radioactivity using a calibrated instrument.

STORAGE

In an airtight container, protected from light, at a temperature of 2 °C to 8 °C.

IMPURITIES

A. cobalt-57,

B. cobalt-60.

———————————————————————————————— *Ph Eur*

Cyanocobalamin (^{58}Co) Solution

(Ph Eur monograph 0270)

Ph Eur ——————————————————————————————————

DEFINITION

Solution of [^{58}Co]-α-(5,6-dimethylbenzimidazol-1-yl)cobamide cyanide and may contain a stabiliser and an antimicrobial preservative.

Cobalt-58

90 per cent to 110 per cent of the declared cobalt-58 radioactivity at the date stated on the label.

CHARACTERS

Appearance

Clear, colourless or slightly pink solution.

Half-life and nature of radiation of cobalt-58

See general chapter 5.7. *Table of physical characteristics of radionuclides.*

IDENTIFICATION
A. Gamma-ray spectrometry.

Results The most prominent gamma photons of cobalt-58 have energies of 0.511 MeV (annihilation radiation) and 0.811 MeV.

B. Examine the chromatograms obtained in the test for radiochemical purity (see Tests).

Result The principal peak in the radiochromatogram obtained with the test solution is similar in retention time to the principal peak in the chromatogram obtained with the reference solution.

TESTS
pH (*2.2.3*)
4.0 to 6.0.

RADIONUCLIDIC PURITY

Cobalt-58
Minimum 98 per cent of the total radioactivity.

Gamma-ray spectrometry.

Determine the relative amounts of cobalt-58, cobalt-57 and cobalt-60 present.

Result:
— cobalt-60: maximum 1 per cent of the total radioactivity.

RADIOCHEMICAL PURITY

[⁵⁸Co]Cyanocobalamin
Liquid chromatography (*2.2.29*).

Test solution The preparation to be examined.

Reference solution Dissolve 10 mg of *cyanocobalamin CRS* in the mobile phase and dilute to 100 mL with the mobile phase. Dilute 2 mL of this solution to 100 mL with the mobile phase. *Use within 1 h after preparation.*

Column:
— *size: l = 0.25 m, Ø = 4.0 mm;*
— *stationary phase: octylsilyl silica gel for chromatography R* (5 μm).

Mobile phase 26.5 volumes of *methanol R* and 73.5 volumes of a 10 g/L solution of *disodium hydrogen phosphate R* adjusted to pH 3.5 using *phosphoric acid R* (use within 2 days).

Flow rate 1.0 mL/min.

Detection Radioactivity detector adjusted for cobalt-58 and spectrophotometer at 361 nm.

Injection 100 μL.

Run time 3 times the retention time of cyanocobalamin for the test solution; 30 min for the reference solution.

Limit:
— *[⁵⁸Co]cyanocobalamin*: minimum 90 per cent of the radioactivity due to cobalt-58.

RADIOACTIVITY
Determine the radioactivity using a calibrated instrument.

STORAGE
Protected from light, at a temperature of 2 °C to 8 °C.

IMPURITIES
A. cobalt-57,
B. cobalt-60.

_____ *Ph Eur*

Fludeoxyglucose (¹⁸F) Injection

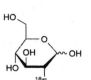

(*Ph Eur monograph 1325*)

Ph Eur _____

DEFINITION
Sterile solution containing 2-[¹⁸F]fluoro-2-deoxy-D-glucopyranose (2-[¹⁸F]fluoro-2-deoxy-D-glucose) prepared by nucleophilic substitution. It may also contain 2-[¹⁸F]fluoro-2-deoxy-D-mannose.

Fluorine-18
90 per cent to 110 per cent of the declared fluorine-18 radioactivity at the date and time stated on the label.

2-Fluoro-2-deoxy-d-glucose
Maximum 0.5 mg per maximum recommended dose, in millilitres.

CHARACTERS
Appearance
Clear, colourless or slightly yellow solution.

Half-life and nature of radiation of fluorine-18
See general chapter 5.7. *Table of physical characteristics of radionuclides.*

IDENTIFICATION
A. Test A for radionuclidic purity (see Tests).

B. Determine the approximate half-life by no fewer than 3 measurements of the activity of a sample in the same geometrical conditions within a suitable period of time (for example, 30 min).

Result 105 to 115 min.

C. Examine the chromatograms obtained in test A for radiochemical purity (see Tests).

Result The principal peak in the radiochromatogram obtained with the test solution is similar in retention time to the principal peak in the chromatogram obtained with reference solution (a).

TESTS
Particular tests for chemical impurities may be omitted if the substances mentioned are not used or cannot be formed in the production process.

pH (*2.2.3*)
4.5 to 8.5.

2-Fluoro-2-deoxy-d-glucose and impurity A
Liquid chromatography (*2.2.29*).

Test solution The preparation to be examined.

Reference solution (a) Dissolve 1.0 mg of *2-fluoro-2-deoxy-D-glucose R* in *water R* and dilute to 2.0 mL with the same solvent. Dilute 1.0 mL of the solution to *V* with *water R*, *V* being the maximum recommended dose in millilitres.

Reference solution (b) Dissolve 1.0 mg of *2-chloro-2-deoxy-D-glucose R* (impurity A) in *water R* and dilute to 2.0 mL with the same solvent. Dilute 1.0 mL of the solution to *V* with *water R*, *V* being the maximum recommended dose in millilitres.

Reference solution (c) Dissolve 1.0 mg of *2-fluoro-2-deoxy-D-mannose R* in *water R* and dilute to 2.0 mL with the same solvent. Mix 0.5 mL of this solution with 0.5 mL of reference solution (a).

Column:
— *size:* $l = 0.25$ m, Ø $= 4.0$ mm;
— *stationary phase:* strongly basic anion exchange resin for chromatography *R* (10 μm);
— *temperature:* constant, between 20-25 °C.

Mobile phase 4 g/L solution of *sodium hydroxide R* in *carbon dioxide-free water R*.

Flow rate 1 mL/min.

Detection Detector suitable for carbohydrates in the required concentration range, such as pulse amperometric detector and radioactivity detector connected in series.

Injection 20 μL.

Run time Twice the retention time of 2-fluoro-2-deoxy-D-glucose.

Relative retention With reference to 2-fluoro-2-deoxy-D-glucose (retention time = about 12 min): 2-fluoro-2-deoxy-D-mannose = about 0.9; impurity A = about 1.1.

System suitability Reference solution (c), using the carbohydrate detector:
— *resolution:* minimum 1.5 between the peaks due to 2-fluoro-2-deoxy-D-mannose and 2-fluoro-2-deoxy-D-glucose;
— *signal-to-noise ratio:* minimum 10 for the peak due to 2-fluoro-2-deoxy-D-glucose.

Limits In the chromatogram obtained with the carbohydrate detector:
— *2-fluoro-2-deoxy-D-glucose:* not more than the area of the corresponding peak in the chromatogram obtained with reference solution (a) (0.5 mg/V);
— *impurity A:* not more than the area of the corresponding peak in the chromatogram obtained with reference solution (b) (0.5 mg/V).

Impurity B
Spot test.

Test solution The preparation to be examined.

Reference solution (a) *water R.*

Reference solution (b) Dissolve 11.0 mg of *aminopolyether R* (impurity B) in *water R* and dilute to 5.0 mL with the same solvent. Dilute 1 mL of the solution to V with *water R*, V being the maximum recommended dose in millilitres.

Plate TLC silica gel plate for aminopolyether test *R.*

Application 2.5 μL; in addition, apply 2.5 μL of the test solution and then 2.5 μL of reference solution (b) at the same place.

Detection Visually compare the spots 1 min after application.

System suitability:
— the spot due to the successive application of the test solution and reference solution (b) is similar in appearance to the spot due to reference solution (b), which is characterised by a number of concentric circles; the darker innermost circle (of intensity proportional to the concentration of impurity B) may be surrounded by a bluish-black ring, outside of which is a lighter circle surrounded by a peripheral dark edge;
— the spot due to reference solution (a) has a more diffuse inner circle, which is brownish-pink and without a distinct margin between it and the surrounding lighter zone;

— the spot due to reference solution (b) is clearly different from the spot due to reference solution (a).

Limit:
— the central portion of the spot due to the test solution is less intense than that of the spot due to reference solution (b) (2.2 mg/V).

Impurity C
Liquid chromatography (2.2.29).

Test solution The preparation to be examined.

Reference solution (a) Dilute 2.1 mL of a 25.95 g/L solution of *tetrabutylammonium hydroxide R* (impurity C) to 20.0 mL with *water R*. Dilute 1.0 mL of this solution to V with *water R*, V being the maximum recommended dose in millilitres.

Reference solution (b) Dilute 1 mL of a 25.95 g/L solution of *tetrabutylammonium hydroxide R* to 10 mL with *water R*. Dilute 1 mL of this solution to 25 mL with *water R*.

Column:
— *size:* $l = 0.10$ m, Ø $= 4.6$ mm;
— *stationary phase:* octadecylsilyl silica gel for chromatography *R* (3 μm);
— *temperature:* constant, between 20-25 °C.

Mobile phase 25 volumes of a 0.95 g/L solution of *toluenesulfonic acid R* and 75 volumes of *acetonitrile R.*

Flow rate 0.6 mL/min.

Detection Spectrophotometer at 254 nm.

Injection 20 μL.

Run time Twice the retention time of tetrabutylammonium ions.

Retention time tetrabutylammonium hydroxide = about 3.3 min.

System suitability Reference solution (b):
— *signal-to-noise ratio:* minimum 10 for the principal peak;
— *symmetry factor:* maximum 1.8 for the principal peak.

Limit:
— *impurity C:* not more than the area of the corresponding peak in the chromatogram obtained with reference solution (a) (2.75 mg/V).

Impurity D
Maximum 0.02 mg/V.

Ultraviolet and visible absorption spectrophotometry (2.2.25).

Test solution The preparation to be examined.

Reference solution Dissolve 20.0 mg of *4-(4-methylpiperidin-1-yl)pyridine R* (impurity D) in *water R* and dilute to 100.0 mL with the same solvent. Dilute 0.1 mL of the solution to V with *water R*, V being the maximum recommended dose in millilitres.

Measure the absorbance of the test solution and the reference solution at the absorption maximum of 263 nm.

Result The absorbance of the test solution is not greater than that of the reference solution.

Residual solvents
Limited according to the principles defined in general chapter 5.4. The preparation may be released for use before completion of the test.

Sterility
It complies with the test for sterility prescribed in the monograph *Radiopharmaceutical preparations (0125).*
The preparation may be released for use before completion of the test.

Bacterial endotoxins (*2.6.14*)

Less than 175/*V* IU/mL, *V* being the maximum recommended dose in millilitres. The preparation may be released for use before completion of the test.

RADIONUCLIDIC PURITY

The preparation may be released for use before completion of test B.

A. Gamma-ray spectrometry.

Results   The only gamma photons have an energy of 0.511 MeV and, depending on the measurement geometry, a sum peak of 1.022 MeV may be observed.

B. Gamma-ray spectrometry.

Determine the amount of fluorine-18 and radionuclidic impurities with a half-life longer than 2 h. For the detection and quantification of impurities, retain the preparation to be examined for at least 24 h to allow the fluorine-18 to decay to a level that permits the detection of impurities.

Results   The total radioactivity due to radionuclidic impurities is not more than 0.1 per cent.

RADIOCHEMICAL PURITY

A. Liquid chromatography (*2.2.29*) as described in the test for 2-fluoro-2-deoxy-D-glucose and impurity A. If necessary, dilute the test solution with *water R* to obtain a radioactivity concentration suitable for the radioactivity detector.

Injection   Test solution and reference solutions (a) and (c).

Relative retention   With reference to 2-[^{18}F]fluoro-2-deoxy-D-glucose (retention time = about 12 min): 2-[^{18}F]fluoro-2-deoxy-D-mannose = about 0.9. Partially or fully acetylated derivatives of both compounds hydrolyse under the chromatographic conditions and therefore elute as 2-[^{18}F]fluoro-2-deoxy-D-glucose and 2-[^{18}F]fluoro-2-deoxy-D-mannose.

Locate the peaks due to 2-[^{18}F]fluoro-2-deoxy-D-glucose and 2-[^{18}F]fluoro-2-deoxy-D-mannose using the chromatograms obtained with the carbohydrate detector and reference solutions (a) and (c).

Limits:

— *[^{18}F]fluorine in the form of 2-[^{18}F]fluoro-2-deoxy-D-glucose and 2-[^{18}F]fluoro-2-deoxy-D-mannose*: minimum 95 per cent of the total radioactivity due to fluorine-18;

— *2-[^{18}F]fluoro-2-deoxy-D-mannose*: maximum 10 per cent of the total radioactivity due to 2-[^{18}F]fluoro-2-deoxy-D-glucose and 2-[^{18}F]fluoro-2-deoxy-D-mannose.

B. Thin-layer chromatography (*2.2.27*).

Test solution   The preparation to be examined.

Reference solution   Dissolve, with gentle heating, 30 mg of *1,2,3,4-tetra-O-acetyl-β-D-glucopyranose R* and 20 mg of *glucose R* in 1 mL of *water R*.

Plate   TLC silica gel plate R.

Mobile phase   water R, acetonitrile R (5:95 *V/V*).

Application   About 2 μL.

Development   Over a path of 8 cm.

Drying   In air for 15 min.

Detection   Suitable detector to determine the distribution of radioactivity; immerse the plate in a 75 g/L solution of *sulfuric acid R* in *methanol R* and dry with a heat gun or at 150 °C until the appearance of dark spots in the chromatogram obtained with the reference solution.

Retardation factors   [^{18}F]fluoride = about 0; 2-[^{18}F]fluoro-2-deoxy-D-glucose and 2-[^{18}F]fluoro-2-deoxy-D-mannose = about 0.45; partially or fully acetylated

derivatives of 2-[^{18}F]fluoro-2-deoxy-D-glucose and 2-[^{18}F]fluoro-2-deoxy-D-mannose = about 0.8 to 0.95.

System suitability   Reference solution:

— the chromatogram shows 2 clearly separated spots.

Limits:

— *[^{18}F]fluorine in the form of 2-[^{18}F]fluoro-2-deoxy-D-glucose and 2-[^{18}F]fluoro-2-deoxy-D-mannose*: minimum 95 per cent of the total radioactivity due to fluorine-18;

— *[^{18}F]fluorine in the form of fluoride and partially or fully acetylated derivatives of 2-[^{18}F]fluoro-2-deoxy-D-glucose and 2-[^{18}F]fluoro-2-deoxy-D-mannose*: maximum 5 per cent of the total radioactivity due to fluorine-18.

RADIOACTIVITY

Determine the radioactivity using a calibrated instrument.

LABELLING

The label states the maximum recommended dose, in millilitres.

IMPURITIES

Specified impurities   *A, B, C, D, E.*

A. 2-chloro-2-deoxy-D-glucopyranose (2-chloro-2-deoxy-D-glucose),

B. 4,7,13,16,21,24-hexaoxa-1,10-diazabicyclo[8.8.8]hexacosane (aminopolyether),

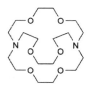

C. *N,N,N*-tributylbutan-1-aminium (tetrabutylammonium),

D. 4-(4-methylpiperidin-1-yl)pyridine,

E. [^{18}F]fluoride.

Ph Eur

Flumazenil (*N*-[¹¹C]methyl) Injection

(*Ph Eur monograph 1917*)

Ph Eur _____

DEFINITION

Sterile solution of ethyl 8-fluoro-5-[¹¹C]methyl-6-oxo-5,6-dihydro-4*H*-imidazo[1,5-*a*][1,4]benzodiazepine-3-carboxylate which may contain a stabiliser such as ascorbic acid.

Content

90 per cent to 110 per cent of the declared carbon-11 radioactivity at the date and time stated on the label.

Content of flumazenil

Maximum 50 µg in the maximum recommended dose in millilitres.

PRODUCTION

RADIONUCLIDE PRODUCTION

Carbon-11 is a radioactive isotope of carbon which is most commonly produced by proton irradiation of nitrogen. Depending on the addition of either trace amounts of oxygen or small amounts of hydrogen, the radioactivity is obtained as [¹¹C]carbon dioxide or [¹¹C]methane, respectively.

RADIOCHEMICAL SYNTHESIS

[5-Methyl-¹¹C]flumazenil may be prepared by *N*-alkylation of ethyl 8-fluoro-6-oxo-5,6-dihydro-4*H*-imidazo[1,5-*a*][1,4]benzodiazepine-3-carboxylate (demethylflumazenil) with iodo[¹¹C]methane or [¹¹C]methyl trifluoromethanesulfonate.

Synthesis of iodo[¹¹C]methane

Iodo[¹¹C]methane may be produced from [¹¹C]carbon dioxide or from [¹¹C]methane. The most frequently used method is reduction of [¹¹C]carbon dioxide with lithium aluminium hydride. The [¹¹C]methanolate formed is reacted with hydriodic acid. Alternatively [¹¹C]methane, either obtained directly in the target or by on-line processes from [¹¹C]carbon dioxide, is reacted with iodine.

Synthesis of [¹¹C]methyl trifluoromethanesulfonate

[¹¹C]methyl trifluoromethanesulfonate may be prepared from iodo[¹¹C]methane using a solid support such as graphitised carbon, impregnated with silver trifluoromethanesulfonate.

Synthesis of [5-methyl-¹¹C]flumazenil

The most widely used method to obtain [5-methyl-¹¹C]flumazenil is the *N*-alkylation of demethylflumazenil with iodo[¹¹C]methane in alkaline conditions in a solvent such as dimethylformamide or acetone. The resulting [5-methyl-¹¹C]flumazenil can be purified by semi-preparative liquid chromatography. For example, a column packed with octadecylsilyl silica gel for chromatography eluted with a mixture of ethanol and water is suitable.

PRECURSOR FOR SYNTHESIS

Demethylflumazenil

Melting point (*2.2.14*): 286 °C to 289 °C.

Infrared absorption spectrophotometry (*2.2.24*).

Comparison Ph. Eur. reference spectrum of demethylflumazenil.

CHARACTERS

Appearance

Clear, colourless solution.

Half-life and nature of radiation of carbon-11

See general chapter *5.7*. *Table of physical characteristics of radionuclides.*

IDENTIFICATION

A. Gamma-ray spectrometry.

Results The only gamma photons have an energy of 0.511 MeV and, depending on the measurement geometry, a sum peak of 1.022 MeV may be observed.

B. It complies with test B for radionuclidic purity (see Tests).

C. Examine the chromatograms obtained in the test for radiochemical purity.

Results The principal peak in the radiochromatogram obtained with the test solution is similar in retention time to the principal peak in the chromatogram obtained with reference solution (a).

TESTS

pH (*2.2.3*)

6.0 to 8.0.

Sterility

It complies with the test for sterility prescribed in the monograph on *Radiopharmaceutical preparations (0125)*. The injection may be released for use before completion of the test.

Bacterial endotoxins (*2.6.14*)

Less than $175/V$ IU/mL, V being the maximum recommended dose in millilitres. The injection may be released for use before completion of the test.

Flumazenil and impurity A

Liquid chromatography (*2.2.29*).

Test solution The preparation to be examined.

Reference solution (a) Dissolve 2.5 mg of *flumazenil R* in 5 mL of *methanol R*.

Reference solution (b) Dissolve 2.5 mg of *demethylflumazenil R* in 50 mL of *methanol R*.

Reference solution (c) To 0.1 mL of reference solution (a) add 0.1 mL of reference solution (b) and dilute to V with a 0.9 g/L solution of *sodium chloride R*, V being the maximum recommended dose in millilitres.

Reference solution (d) Dilute 0.1 mL of reference solution (a) to 50 mL with *methanol R*. Dilute 1.0 mL of this solution to V with a 0.9 g/L solution of *sodium chloride R*, V being the maximum recommended dose in millilitres.

Column:
— *size: l* = 0.15 m, Ø = 3.9 mm,
— *stationary phase:* spherical *octadecylsilyl silica gel for chromatography R* (5 µm) with a specific surface area of 440 m²/g, a pore size of 100 nm and a carbon loading of 19 per cent,
— *temperature:* maintain at a constant temperature between 20-30 °C.

Mobile phase methanol R, water R (45:55 *V/V*).

Flow rate 1 mL/min.

Detection Spectrophotometer at 260 nm and radioactivity detector connected in series.

Injection 100 µL.

Run time 10 min.

Relative retention   With reference to flumazenil:
impurity A = about 0.74.

System suitability   Reference solution (c):
— *resolution*: minimum 2.5 between the peaks due to
   flumazenil and impurity A.

Limits   Examine the chromatogram obtained with the
spectrophotometer:
— *flumazenil*: not more than the area of the corresponding
   peak in the chromatogram obtained with reference
   solution (c) (50 μg/*V*),
— *impurity A*: not more than the area of the corresponding
   peak in the chromatogram obtained with reference
   solution (c) (5 μg/*V*),
— *any other impurity*: not more than the area of the principal
   peak in the chromatogram obtained with reference
   solution (d) (1 μg/*V*).

Residual solvents
Are limited according to the principles defined in the general
chapter (*5.4*), using the general method (*2.4.24*).
The preparation may be released for use before completion
of the test.

RADIONUCLIDIC PURITY

Carbon-11
Minimum 99 per cent of the total radioactivity.
The preparation may be released for use before completion
of the test.

A. Gamma-ray spectrometry.

Results   The spectrum obtained with the solution to be
examined does not differ significantly from that obtained
with a standardised fluorine-18 solution.

B. Half-life: 19.9 min to 20.9 min.

RADIOCHEMICAL PURITY
Liquid chromatography (*2.2.29*) as described in the test for
flumazenil and impurity A, with the following modifications.

Injection   Test solution and reference solution (a);
if necessary, dilute the test solution to a radioactivity
concentration suitable for the detector.

Limit   Examine the chromatogram obtained with the
radioactivity detector:
— *[5-methyl-^{11}C]flumazenil*: minimum 95 per cent of the
   total radioactivity.

RADIOACTIVITY
Determine the radioactivity using a calibrated instrument.

LABELLING
The label states the maximum recommended dose in
millilitres.

IMPURITIES

A. R = H: ethyl 8-fluoro-6-oxo-5,6-dihydro-4*H*-imidazo[1,5-
a][1,4]benzodiazepine-3-carboxylate (demethylflumazenil),

B. R = CH$_2$-CO-CH$_3$: ethyl 8-fluoro-6-oxo-9-(2-oxopropyl)-
5,6-dihydro-4*H*-imidazo[1,5-*a*][1,4]benzodiazepine-3-
carboxylate (acetone addition compound of
demethylflumazenil).

——————————————— *Ph Eur*

Fluoride (^{18}F) Solution for Radiolabelling

(*Ph Eur monograph 2390*)

Ph Eur _____

DEFINITION
Alkaline solution containing fluorine-18 in the form of
[^{18}F]fluoride.

Content
90 per cent to 110 per cent of the declared fluorine-18
radioactivity at the date and time stated on the label.

CHARACTERS
Appearance
Clear, colourless solution.

Half-life and nature of radiation of fluorine-18
See general chapter *5.7. Table of physical characteristics of
radionuclides.*

IDENTIFICATION
A. Gamma-ray spectrometry.

Result   The principal photons have an energy of 0.511 MeV
and, depending on the measurement geometry, a sum peak
of 1.022 MeV may be observed.

B. Determine the approximate half-life by no fewer than 3
measurements of the activity of a sample in the same
geometrical conditions within a suitable period of time (for
example, 30 min).

Result   105 min to 115 min.

C. Examine the chromatograms obtained in the test for
radiochemical purity (see Tests).

Results   The principal peak in the radiochromatogram
obtained with the test solution is similar in retention time to
the principal peak in the chromatogram obtained with the
reference solution; in the chromatogram obtained with the
reference solution, the signal due to fluoride is negative.

TESTS
pH
8.0 to 14.0, using a *pH indicator strip R*.

Bacterial endotoxins (*2.6.14*)
Less than 20 IU/mL, if intended for use in the manufacture
of parenteral preparations without a further appropriate
procedure for the removal of bacterial endotoxins.
The preparation may be released for use before completion
of the test.

RADIONUCLIDIC PURITY
The preparation may be released for use before completion
of test B.

Fluorine-18
Minimum 99.9 per cent of the total radioactivity.

A. Gamma-ray spectrometry. Preliminary test.

Limit   Peaks in the gamma spectrum corresponding to
photons with an energy different from 0.511 MeV or
1.022 MeV represent not more than 0.1 per cent of the total
radioactivity.

B. Gamma-ray spectrometry.

Determine the amount of fluorine-18 and radionuclidic
impurities with a half-life longer than 2 h. For the detection
and quantification of impurities, retain the preparation to be
examined for at least 24 h to allow the fluorine-18 to decay
to a level that permits the detection of impurities.

Result   The total radioactivity due to radionuclidic impurities
is not more than 0.1 per cent.

RADIOCHEMICAL PURITY

[^{18}F]fluoride

Liquid chromatography (2.2.29).

Test solution Dilute the preparation to be examined with *water R* to obtain a radioactivity concentration suitable for the radioactivity detector.

Reference solution Dissolve 10 mg of *potassium fluoride R* in *water R* and dilute to 10 mL with the same solvent.

Column:
— *size: l = 0.25 m, Ø = 4.0 mm;*
— *stationary phase: strongly basic anion-exchange resin for chromatography R* (10 μm).

Mobile phase 4 g/L solution of *sodium hydroxide R* in *carbon dioxide-free water R*, protected from atmospheric carbon dioxide.

Flow rate 1 mL/min.

Detection Spectrophotometer at 220 nm and a radioactivity detector connected in series.

Injection 20 μL.

Run time 12 min.

System suitability Reference solution:
— *signal-to-noise ratio:* minimum 10 for the principal peak;
— *retention time of fluoride:* minimum 3 times the hold-up time.

Examine the chromatogram obtained with the test solution using the radioactivity detector and locate the peak due to fluoride by comparison with the chromatogram obtained with the reference solution using the spectrophotometer.

Limit:
— *[^{18}F]fluoride:* minimum 98.5 per cent of the total radioactivity due to fluorine-18.

RADIOACTIVITY

Determine the radioactivity using a calibrated instrument.

LABELLING

The label states:
— that the solution is not for direct administration to humans;
— where applicable, that the substance is suitable for use in the manufacture of parenteral preparations.

Ph Eur

Fluorodopa (^{18}F) Injection

(Fluorodopa (^{18}F) (Prepared By Electrophilic Substitution) Injection, Ph Eur monograph 1918)

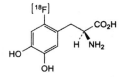

Ph Eur

DEFINITION

Sterile solution of (2*S*)-2-amino-3-(2-([^{18}F]fluoro)-4,5-dihydroxyphenyl)propanoic acid (6-[^{18}F]fluorolevodopa). It may contain stabilisers such as ascorbic acid and edetic acid.

This monograph applies to an injection containing 6-[^{18}F]fluorolevodopa produced by electrophilic substitution.

Content:
— *fluorine-18:* 90 per cent to 110 per cent of the declared fluorine-18 radioactivity at the date and time stated on the label;
— *dopa:* maximum 1 mg per maximum recommended dose in millilitres;
— *6-fluorolevodopa:* maximum 15 mg per maximum recommended dose in millilitres.

PRODUCTION

RADIONUCLIDE PRODUCTION

Fluorine-18 is a radioactive isotope of fluorine that may be produced by various nuclear reactions induced by proton irradiation of oxygen-18, deuteron irradiation of neon-20, or helium-3 or helium-4 irradiation of oxygen-16.

In order to obtain fluorine-18 in a chemical form suitable for electrophilic substitution reactions, such as fluorine gas or gaseous acetylhypofluorite, a small amount of non-radioactive fluorine gas (0.3-0.8 per cent of the target gas volume) must be added as a carrier at some step in the production process.

RADIOCHEMICAL SYNTHESIS

6-[^{18}F]Fluorolevodopa may be prepared by various radiochemical synthetic pathways, which lead to different products in terms of yield, specific radioactivity, by-products and possible impurities. Electrophilic pathways for production of 6-[^{18}F]fluorolevodopa may proceed by fluorodemetallation of a stannylated derivative of levodopa, with molecular [^{18}F]fluorine or [^{18}F]acetylhypofluorite, followed by hydrolysis of protecting groups and final purification by semipreparative liquid chromatography. Pathways using demercuration or dethallation must not be used.

CHARACTERS

Appearance

Clear, colourless solution.

Half-life and nature of radiation of fluorine-18

See general chapter 5.7. *Table of physical characteristics of radionuclides.*

IDENTIFICATION

A. Test A for radionuclidic purity (see Tests).

B. Determine the approximate half-life by at least 3 measurements of the activity of a sample in the same geometrical conditions over a suitable period of time, for example 30 min.

Results 105 min to 115 min.

C. Examine the chromatograms obtained in the test for radiochemical purity (see Tests).

Results The principal peak in the radiochromatogram obtained with the test solution is similar in retention time to the peak due to 6-fluorolevodopa in the chromatogram obtained with reference solution (a).

D. Examine the chromatograms obtained in the test for impurities C and D (see Tests).

Results The principal peak in the radiochromatogram obtained with the test solution is similar in retardation factor to the peak due to 6-fluorolevodopa in the chromatogram obtained with reference solution (b).

TESTS

pH (2.2.3)
4.0 to 5.5.

Sterility

It complies with the test for sterility prescribed in the monograph *Radiopharmaceutical preparations (0125)*. The injection may be released for use before completion of the test.

Bacterial endotoxins (*2.6.14*)

Less than $175/V$ IU/mL, V being the maximum recommended dose in millilitres. The injection may be released for use before completion of the test.

6-Fluorolevodopa, dopa, impurity A and impurity B

Liquid chromatography (*2.2.29*). *Prepare the reference solutions immediately before use.*

Test solution   The preparation to be examined.

Reference solution (a)   Dissolve 18.0 mg of *6-fluorolevodopa hydrochloride R* in 5.0 mL of the mobile phase and dilute to V with the mobile phase, V being the maximum recommended dose in millilitres.

Reference solution (b)   Dissolve 1.0 mg of *levodopa R* in 5 mL of the mobile phase and dilute to V with the mobile phase, V being the maximum recommended dose in millilitres.

Reference solution (c)   Dissolve 1.0 mg of *trimethyltin chloride R* (impurity A) in 2.0 mL of the mobile phase. Dilute 1.0 mL of this solution to V with the mobile phase, V being the maximum recommended dose in millilitres.

Reference solution (d)   Mix equal volumes of reference solutions (b) and (c).

Reference solution (e)   Dissolve 2.0 mg of *6-hydroxydopa R* (impurity B) in 20.0 mL of the mobile phase. Dilute 0.25 mL of this solution to V with the mobile phase, V being the maximum recommended dose in millilitres.

Column:
— *size:* $l = 0.25$ m, $\emptyset = 4.0$ mm;
— *stationary phase:* spherical *end-capped octadecylsilyl silica gel for chromatography R*;
— *temperature:* maintain at a constant temperature between 20 °C and 30 °C.

Mobile phase   6.9 g/L solution of *sodium dihydrogen phosphate R* adjusted to pH 2.4 with a 4.8 g/L solution of *phosphoric acid R*.

Flow rate   1 mL/min.

Detection   Spectrophotometer at 200 nm and radioactivity detector connected in series.

Injection   20 µL.

Run time   15 min.

Relative retention   With reference to 6-fluorolevodopa (retention time = about 6 min):
impurity A and impurity B = about 0.7; dopa = about 0.8.

System suitability   Reference solution (d):
— *resolution:* minimum 1.5 between the peaks due to dopa and impurity A.

Limits   Examine the chromatograms obtained with the spectrophotometer:
— *6-fluorolevodopa:* not more than the area of the corresponding peak in the chromatogram obtained with reference solution (a) (15 mg/V);
— *dopa:* not more than the area of the peak due to levodopa in the chromatogram obtained with reference solution (b) (1.0 mg/V);
— *sum of impurities A and B:* not more than the area of the principal peak in the chromatogram obtained with reference solution (e) (corresponding to a limit of 0.5 mg/V of impurity A or a limit of 0.025 mg/V of

impurity B, or to lower limits of each if both impurities are present).

Residual solvents

Limited according to the principles defined in general chapter *5.4*. The preparation may be released for use before completion of the test.

RADIONUCLIDIC PURITY

Fluorine-18

Minimum 99.9 per cent of the total radioactivity.

The preparation may be released for use before completion of test B.

A. Gamma-ray spectrometry

Results   The only gamma photons have an energy of 0.511 MeV and, depending on the measurement geometry, a sum peak of 1.022 MeV may be observed.

B. Gamma-ray spectrometry

Determine the amount of fluorine-18 and radionuclidic impurities with a half-life longer than 2 h. For the detection and quantification of impurities, retain the preparation to be examined for a sufficient time to allow the fluorine-18 to decay to a level that permits the detection of impurities.

Results   The spectrum obtained with the preparation to be examined does not differ significantly from a background spectrum.

RADIOCHEMICAL PURITY

Liquid chromatography (*2.2.29*) as described in the test for 6-fluorolevodopa, dopa, impurity A and impurity B.

Examine the chromatogram recorded using the radioactivity detector and locate the peak due to 6-[^{18}F]fluorolevodopa by comparison with the chromatogram obtained with reference solution (a) and the spectrophotometer.

Limit:
— *6-[^{18}F]fluorolevodopa:* minimum 95 per cent of the total radioactivity due to fluorine-18.

Impurities C and D

Thin-layer chromatography (*2.2.27*).

Test solution   The preparation to be examined.

Reference solution (a)   Dissolve 2 mg of DL-*6-fluorodopa hydrochloride R* in *water R* and dilute to 10 mL with the same solvent.

Reference solution (b)   Dissolve 2 mg of *6-fluorolevodopa hydrochloride R* in *water R* and dilute to 10 mL with the same solvent.

Plate   *octadecylsilyl TLC silica gel plate for chiral separations R*.

Mobile phase   *methanol R*, *water R* (50:50 *V/V*).

Application   2 µL.

Development   Over a path of 10 cm.

Drying   In air for 5 min.

Detection   Spray with a 2 g/L solution of *ninhydrin R* in *anhydrous ethanol R* and heat at 60 °C for 10 min; determine the distribution of radioactivity using a suitable detector.

Retardation factors   Impurity D = about 0; 6-[^{18}F]fluorolevodopa = about 0.3; impurity C = about 0.5.

System suitability   Reference solution (a):
— the chromatogram shows 2 clearly separated spots.

Limits:
— *impurity C:* maximum 2 per cent of the total radioactivity due to fluorine-18;
— *impurity D:* maximum 4 per cent of the total radioactivity due to fluorine-18.

RADIOACTIVITY

Measure the radioactivity using a calibrated instrument.

LABELLING

The label states the maximum recommended dose in millilitres.

IMPURITIES

A. Cl-Sn(CH₃)₃: chlorotrimethylstannane (trimethyltin chloride),

B. (2RS)-2-amino-3-(2,4,5-trihydroxyphenyl)propanoic acid (6-hydroxydopa),

C. (2R)-2-amino-3-(2-[¹⁸F]fluoro-4,5-dihydroxyphenyl)propanoic acid (6-[¹⁸F]fluorodextrodopa),

D. [¹⁸F]fluoride.

Ph Eur

Gallium (⁶⁷Ga) Citrate Injection

(Ph Eur monograph 0555)

Ph Eur _____

DEFINITION

Sterile solution of gallium-67 in the form of gallium citrate. It may be made isotonic by the addition of sodium chloride and sodium citrate and may contain a suitable antimicrobial preservative such as benzyl alcohol.

Gallium-67

90 per cent to 110 per cent of the declared gallium-67 radioactivity at the date and time stated on the label.

CHARACTERS

Appearance

Clear, colourless solution.

Half-life and nature of radiation of gallium-67

See general chapter 5.7. *Table of physical characteristics of radionuclides.*

IDENTIFICATION

A. Gamma-ray spectrometry.

Results The most prominent gamma photons have energies of 0.093 MeV, 0.185 MeV and 0.300 MeV.

B. To 0.2 mL of the preparation to be examined add 0.2 mL of a solution containing 1 g/L of *ferric chloride R* and 0.1 per cent V/V of *hydrochloric acid R* and mix. Compare the colour with that of a solution containing 7 g/L of *sodium chloride R* and 9 g/L of *benzyl alcohol R* treated in the same manner. A yellow colour develops in the test solution only.

TESTS

pH *(2.2.3)*

5.0 to 8.0.

Zinc

Maximum 5 ppm.

Test solution To 0.1 mL of the preparation to be examined add 0.9 mL of *water R*, 1 mL of a 250 g/L solution of *sodium thiosulfate R*, 5 mL of *acetate buffer solution pH 4.7 R* and 5.0 mL of a dithizone solution prepared as follows: dissolve 10 mg of *dithizone R* in 100 mL of *methyl ethyl ketone R* allow to stand for 5 min, filter and immediately before use dilute the solution to 10 times its volume with *methyl ethyl ketone R*. Shake vigorously for 2 min and allow the organic layer to separate.

Reference solution 0.1 mL of *zinc standard solution (5 ppm Zn) R* treated in the same manner as the test solution.

Measure the absorbance *(2.2.25)* of the organic layers at 530 nm, using the organic layer of a blank solution as the compensation liquid.

Results The absorbance of the organic layer obtained with the test solution is not greater than that of the organic layer obtained with the reference solution.

Sterility

It complies with the test for sterility prescribed in the monograph *Radiopharmaceutical preparations (0125)*.

The preparation may be released for use before completion of the test.

RADIONUCLIDIC PURITY

Gallium-67

Minimum 99.8 per cent of the total radioactivity.

Gamma-ray spectrometry.

Determine the relative amounts of gallium-66 and other radionuclidic impurities present.

RADIOACTIVITY

Determine the radioactivity using a calibrated instrument.

IMPURITIES

A. gallium-66.

Ph Eur

Gallium (⁶⁸Ga) Chloride Solution for Radiolabelling

(Ph Eur monograph 2464)

⁶⁸GaCl₃   174.3

Ph Eur _____

DEFINITION

Solution containing gallium-68 in the form of gallium chloride in dilute hydrochloric acid. The preparation may contain acetone.

Content:

— *gallium-68*: 90 per cent to 110 per cent of the declared gallium-68 radioactivity at the date and time stated on the label.

CHARACTERS

Appearance

Clear, colourless solution.

Half-life and nature of radiation of gallium-68
See general chapter *5.7. Table of physical characteristics of radionuclides.*

IDENTIFICATION
A. Gamma-ray spectrometry.

Result   The principal gamma photons have energies of 0.511 MeV and 1.077 MeV and, depending on the measurement geometry, a sum peak of 1.022 MeV may be observed.

B. Determine the approximate half-life by no fewer than 3 measurements of the activity of a sample in the same geometrical conditions within a suitable period of time (for example, 15 min).

Result   62 min to 74 min.

C. pH (see Tests).

D. To a volume of 20-100 μL of the solution to be examined add 1 mL of a 1.03 g/L solution of *hydrochloric acid R*. Apply this solution to the top of a column containing *strong cation-exchange resin R*, push 5 mL of air through the column and collect the eluate. Determine the radioactivity of the eluate (A1). Elute the column with 1 mL of a 1.03 g/L solution of *hydrochloric acid R*. Determine the radioactivity of the eluate (A2). Elute the column with 1 mL of a mixture of 2 volumes of *hydrochloric acid R* and 98 volumes of *acetone R* and push 5 mL of air through the column. Determine the radioactivity of the eluate (A3) and the residual activity on the column (A4).

Calculate the percentage of radioactivity in the A3 eluate using the following expression:

$$A3 \times 100 / (A1 + A2 + A3 + A4)$$

Result   The percentage of radioactivity in the A3 eluate is not less than 90 per cent.

E. To 100 μL of *silver nitrate solution R2* add 50 μL of the solution to be examined. A white precipitate is formed.

TESTS
pH
Maximum 2, using a *pH indicator strip R*.

Iron
Maximum 10 μg/GBq.

Atomic absorption spectrometry (*2.2.23, Method I*).

Modifier solution   14 g/L solution of *magnesium nitrate R*.

Test solution   Dilute the solution to be examined with a 1 per cent V/V solution of *nitric acid R* to obtain a radioactivity concentration of 2.5 MBq/mL.

Reference solutions   Prepare the reference solutions using *iron standard solution (20 ppm Fe) R*, diluting with a 1 per cent V/V solution of *nitric acid R*.

Source   Iron hollow-cathode lamp.

Wavelength   248.3 nm.

Atomisation device   Graphite furnace.

An example of the injection and instrument parameters for the graphic furnace atomic absorption analysis is shown below.

Internal and external protective gas   *argon R*.

Injection   20 μL of the test solution and the reference solutions, and 1 μL of the modifier solution.

Injection temperature   20°C

Furnace programme

Step	Final temperature (°C)	Ramp time (s)	Hold time (s)	Internal protective gas flow rate (mL/min)
Drying	110	1	30	250
Drying	130	15	30	250
Pyrolysis	1400	10	20	250
Atomisation	2100	0	5	0
Cleaning	2450	1	3	250

The solution may be released for use before completion of the test.

Zinc
Maximum 10 μg/GBq.

Atomic absorption spectrometry (*2.2.23, Method I*).

Test solution   Dilute the solution to be examined with a 1 per cent V/V solution of *nitric acid R* to obtain a radioactivity concentration of 50 MBq/mL.

Reference solutions   Prepare the reference solutions using *zinc standard solution (10 ppm Zn) R*, diluting with a 1 per cent V/V solution of *nitric acid R*.

Source   zinc hollow-cathode lamp.

Wavelength   213.9 nm.

Atomisation device   Air-acetylene flame.

The solution may be released for use before completion of the test.

Bacterial endotoxins (*2.6.14*)
Less than 175 IU/V, V being the maximum volume to be used for the preparation of a single patient dose, if intended for use in the manufacture of parenteral preparations without a further appropriate procedure for the removal of bacterial endotoxins. The solution may be released for use before completion of the test.

RADIONUCLIDIC PURITY
The solution may be released for use before completion of test B.

Gallium-68
Minimum 99.9 per cent of the total radioactivity.

A. Gamma-ray spectrometry.

Limit   Peaks in the gamma-ray spectrum corresponding to photons with an energy different from 0.511 MeV, 1.077 MeV, 1.022 MeV and 1.883 MeV represent not more than 0.1 per cent of the total radioactivity.

B. Germanium-68 and gamma-ray-emitting impurities. Gamma-ray spectrometry.

Determine the amount of gallium-68, germanium-68 and radionuclidic impurities with a half-life longer than 5 h. For the detection and quantification of germanium-68 and gamma-ray-emitting impurities, retain the solution to be examined for at least 48 h to allow the gallium-68 to decay to a level that permits the detection of impurities.

Result   The total radioactivity due to germanium-68 and gamma-ray-emitting impurities is not more than 0.001 per cent.

RADIOCHEMICAL PURITY
[⁶⁸Ga]Gallium(III) ion
Thin-layer chromatography (*2.2.27*).

Test solution   Adjust the solution to be examined to obtain a concentration of *hydrochloric acid R* of 10.3 g/L.

Reference solution (a) To 0.2 mL of the test solution add 0.3 mL of a 4 g/L solution of *sodium hydroxide R*. Use within 30 min of preparation.

Reference solution (b) To 1 mL of the test solution add 1 mL of a 10 g/L solution of *pentetic acid R* in a 4 g/L solution of *sodium hydroxide R*. Use within 30 min of preparation.

Plate TLC silica gel plate R; use a glass-fibre plate.

Mobile phase 77 g/L solution of *ammonium acetate R*, methanol R (50:50 V/V).

Application About 5 μL.

Development Immediately, over a path of at least 10 cm.

Drying In air.

Detection Suitable detector to determine the distribution of radioactivity.

Retardation factor [68Ga]Gallium(III) ion = 0-0.2.

System suitability The retardation factor of the principal peak in the chromatogram obtained with reference solution (a) is not more than 0.1; the retardation factor of the principal peak in the chromatogram obtained with reference solution (b) is not less than 0.7.

Limit:
— *[68Ga]gallium(III) ion*: minimum 95 per cent of the total radioactivity due to gallium-68.

RADIOACTIVITY

Determine the radioactivity using a calibrated instrument.

LABELLING

The label states:
— that the solution is not intended for direct administration to humans;
— the maximum volume that can be used for the preparation of a single patient dose;
— the concentration of hydrochloric acid;
— the concentration of acetone, if present;
— that the solution is intended for use in the preparation of gallium-68-labelled radiopharmaceuticals;
— a procedure to reduce the level of germanium-68 below 0.001 per cent of the total radioactivity.

IMPURITIES

A. germanium-68.

Ph Eur

Gallium (^{68}Ga) Edotreotide Injection

(*Ph Eur monograph 2482*)

$C_{65}H_{89}{}^{68}GaN_{14}O_{18}S_2$ 1487

Ph Eur

DEFINITION

Sterile solution of a complex of gallium-68 with edotreotide (*N*-[[4,7,10-tris(carboxymethyl)-1,4,7,10-

tetraazacyclododecan-1-yl]acetyl]-D-phenylalanyl-L-cysteinyl-L-tyrosyl-D-tryptophyl-L-lysyl-L-threonyl-*N*-[(1*R*,2*R*)-2-hydroxy-1-(hydroxymethyl)propyl]-L-cysteinamide cyclic (2→7)-disulfide) (gallium-68 DOTATOC).

Content:
— *gallium-68*: 90 per cent to 110 per cent of the declared gallium-68 radioactivity at the date and time stated on the label;
— *edotreotide*: maximum 50 μg per maximum recommended dose in millilitres.

CHARACTERS
Appearance
Clear, colourless solution.

Half-life and nature of radiation of gallium-68
See general chapter 5.7. *Table of physical characteristics of radionuclides.*

IDENTIFICATION
A. Gamma-ray spectrometry.

Result The principal gamma photons have energies of 0.511 MeV and 1.077 MeV and, depending on the measurement geometry, a sum peak of 1.022 MeV may be observed.

B. Determine the approximate half-life by no fewer than 3 measurements of the activity of a sample in the same geometrical conditions within a suitable period of time (for example, 15 min).

Result 62 min to 74 min.

C. Examine the chromatograms obtained in the test for other radiochemical impurities (see Tests).

Result The principal peak in the radiochromatogram obtained with the test solution has a relative retention of 1.3 with reference to the principal peak in the chromatogram obtained with reference solution (a) using the spectrophotometer.

TESTS
pH
4.0 to 8.0, using a *pH indicator strip R*.

Edotreotide, gallium edotreotide and other related substances
Liquid chromatography (*2.2.29*).

Test solution The preparation to be examined.

Reference solution (a) Prepare a 50 μg/*V* solution of *edotreotide R* in a 10.3 g/L solution of *hydrochloric acid R*, *V* being the maximum recommended dose in millilitres.

Reference solution (b) Prepare a 50 μg/*V* solution of *octreotide acetate R* in a 10.3 g/L solution of *hydrochloric acid R*, *V* being the maximum recommended dose in millilitres.

Reference solution (c) Mix 0.1 mL of reference solution (a) and 0.1 mL of reference solution (b).

Column:
— *size*: l = 0.15 m, Ø = 3.0 mm;
— *stationary phase*: base-deactivated octadecylsilyl silica gel for chromatography R (3 μm).

Mobile phase:
— *mobile phase A*: trifluoroacetic acid R, water R (0.1:99.9 V/V);
— *mobile phase B*: trifluoroacetic acid R, acetonitrile R (0.1:99.9 V/V);

Time (min)	Mobile phase A (per cent V/V)	Mobile phase B (per cent V/V)
0 - 8	76	24
8 - 9	76 → 40	24 → 60
9 - 14	40	60

Flow rate   0.6 mL/min.

Detection   Spectrophotometer at 220 nm and radioactivity detector connected in series.

Injection   20 µL.

Relative retention   With reference to edotreotide (retention time = about 3.3 min): gallium edotreotide = about 1.3; octreotide = about 2.6.

System suitability   Reference solution (c) using the spectrophotometer:
— *resolution*: minimum 5.0 between the peaks due to edotreotide and octreotide.

Limits   In the chromatogram obtained with the spectrophotometer:
— *edotreotide and metal complexes of edotreotide* (sum of the areas of the peaks with a relative retention with reference to edotreotide between 0.8 and 1.4): not more than the area of the principal peak in the chromatogram obtained with reference solution (a) (50 µg/V);
— *unspecified impurities*: for each impurity, not more than the area of the principal peak in the chromatogram obtained with reference solution (a) (50 µg/V); disregard any peak with a relative retention with reference to edotreotide of 0.5 or less.

Impurity D

Thin-layer chromatography (*2.2.27*).

Test solution   The preparation to be examined.

Reference solution   Dissolve 10 mg of *HEPES R* (impurity D) in *water R* and dilute to V with the same solvent, V being the maximum recommended dose in millilitres. Dilute 1.0 mL of the solution to 50.0 mL with *water R*.

Plate   *TLC silica gel F$_{254}$ plate R*; use an aluminium plate.

Mobile phase   *water R, acetonitrile R* (25:75 *V/V*).

Application   (V/2000) mL, V being the maximum recommended dose in millilitres; apply portions of 1 µL and dry with a current of warm air after each application.

Development   Over 2/3 of the plate.

Detection   Expose to iodine vapour for 4 min.

Retardation factor   Impurity D = about 0.3.

System suitability   Reference solution:
— the chromatogram shows a clearly visible spot.

Limit:
— *impurity D*: any spot due to impurity D is not more intense than the corresponding spot in the chromatogram obtained with the reference solution (200 µg/V).

Ethanol

Gas chromatography (*2.2.28*).

Internal standard solution   Dilute 1 mL of *propanol R* to 1000 mL with *water R*.

Test solution   Dilute 0.10 mL of the preparation to be examined to 10.0 mL with the internal standard solution.

Reference solution   Dilute 1.0 mL of *anhydrous ethanol R* to 100.0 mL with the internal standard solution. Dilute 1.0 mL of this solution to 10.0 mL with the internal standard solution.

Column:
— *material*: fused silica;
— *size*: l = 30 m, Ø = 0.53 mm;
— *stationary phase*: *macrogol 20 000 R* (film thickness 1.0 µm).

Carrier gas   *helium for chromatography R*.

Flow rate   10 mL/min.

Split ratio   1:10.

Temperature:
— *column*: 35 °C;
— *injection port*: 140 °C;
— *detector*: 220 °C.

Detection   Flame ionisation.

Injection   1.0 µL.

System suitability   Reference solution:
— *retention time*: ethanol = 2 min to 4 min;
— *resolution*: minimum 5.0 between the peaks due to ethanol and propanol.

Limit:
— *ethanol*: maximum 10 per cent *V/V* and maximum 2.5 g per administration, taking the density (*2.2.5*) to be 0.790 g/mL.

Sterility

It complies with the test for sterility prescribed in the monograph *Radiopharmaceutical preparations (0125)*.

The preparation may be released for use before completion of the test.

Bacterial endotoxins (*2.6.14*)

Less than 175/V IU/mL, V being the maximum recommended dose in millilitres. The preparation may be released for use before completion of the test.

RADIONUCLIDIC PURITY

The preparation may be released for use before completion of test B.

Gallium-68

Minimum 99.9 per cent of the total radioactivity.

A. Gamma-ray spectrometry.

Limit   Peaks in the gamma-ray spectrum corresponding to photons with an energy different from 0.511 MeV, 1.077 MeV, 1.022 MeV and 1.883 MeV represent not more than 0.1 per cent of the total radioactivity.

B. Germanium-68 and gamma-ray-emitting impurities. Gamma-ray spectrometry.

Determine the amount of gallium-68, germanium-68 and radionuclidic impurities with a half-life longer than 5 h. For the detection and quantification of germanium-68 and gamma-ray-emitting impurities, retain the preparation to be examined for at least 48 h to allow the gallium-68 to decay to a level that permits the detection of impurities.

Result   The total radioactivity due to germanium-68 and gamma-ray-emitting impurities is not more than 0.001 per cent.

RADIOCHEMICAL PURITY

— *[^{68}Ga]gallium edotreotide*: minimum 91 per cent of the total radioactivity due to gallium-68.

Impurity A

Thin-layer chromatography (*2.2.27*).

Test solution   The preparation to be examined.

Reference solution (a)   Dilute *gallium (^{68}Ga) chloride solution R* with *water R* to obtain a final concentration of 10 g/L of *hydrochloric acid R*. To 1 mL of this solution add 1.5 mL of a 4 g/L solution of *sodium hydroxide R*. Use within 30 min of preparation.

Reference solution (b)   Dilute *gallium (^{68}Ga) chloride solution R* with *water R* to obtain a final concentration of 10 g/L of *hydrochloric acid R*. To 1 mL of this solution add 1 mL of a solution containing 10 g/L of *pentetic acid R* and 4 g/L of *sodium hydroxide R*. Use within 30 min after preparation.

Plate   *TLC silica gel plate R*; use a glass-fibre plate.

Mobile phase   77 g/L solution of *ammonium acetate R* in *water R, methanol R* (50:50 *V/V*).

Application   5 µL.

Development   Immediately, over 2/3 of the plate.

Drying   In air.

Detection   Suitable detector to determine the distribution of radioactivity.

Retardation factors   Impurity A = 0.0-0.1; [⁶⁸Ga]gallium edotreotide = 0.8-1.0.

System suitability   The retardation factor of the principal signal in the chromatogram obtained with reference solution (a) is not more than 0.1; the retardation factor of the principal signal in the chromatogram obtained with reference solution (b) is more than 0.7.

Limit:
— *impurity A*: not more than 3 per cent of the total radioactivity due to gallium-68.

Other radiochemical impurities

Liquid chromatography (*2.2.29*) as described in the test for edotreotide, gallium edotreotide and other related substances. If necessary, dilute the test solution with *water R* to a radioactivity concentration suitable for the radioactivity detector.

Examine the chromatogram recorded using the radioactivity detector and locate the peak due to [⁶⁸Ga]gallium edotreotide by comparison with the chromatogram obtained with reference solution (a) and the spectrophotometer.

Relative retention   With reference to [⁶⁸Ga]gallium edotreotide (retention time = about 4.2 min): impurity B = about 0.3.

Limit:
— *impurity B*: not more than 2 per cent of the total radioactivity due to gallium-68.

Calculate the percentage of radioactivity due to [⁶⁸Ga]gallium edotreotide using the following expression:

$$(100 - A) \times T$$

A = percentage of radioactivity due to impurity A determined in the test for impurity A under radiochemical purity;

T = proportion of the area of the peak due to [⁶⁸Ga]gallium edotreotide relative to the total areas of the peaks in the chromatogram obtained with the test solution.

RADIOACTIVITY

Determine the radioactivity using a calibrated instrument.

LABELLING

The label states the percentage content of ethanol in the preparation.

IMPURITIES

Specified impurities   A, B, C, D.

A. [⁶⁸Ga]gallium in colloidal form,

B. [⁶⁸Ga]gallium(III) ion,

C. germanium-68,

D. 2-[4-(2-hydroxyethyl)piperazin-1-yl]ethanesulfonic acid (HEPES).

Indium (¹¹¹In) Chloride Solution

(*Ph Eur monograph 1227*)

Ph Eur

DEFINITION

Sterile solution of indium-111 as the chloride in aqueous hydrochloric acid containing no additives.

Indium-111

90 per cent to 110 per cent of the declared indium-111 radioactivity at the date and time stated on the label.

SPECIFIC RADIOACTIVITY

Minimum 1.85 GBq of indium-111 per microgram of indium.

PRODUCTION

No carrier indium is added.

CHARACTERS

Appearance

Clear, colourless solution.

Half-life and nature of radiation of indium-111

See general chapter *5.7. Table of physical characteristics of radionuclides*.

IDENTIFICATION

A. Gamma-ray and X-ray spectrometry. *Carry out the test after allowing sufficient time for short-lived impurities such as indium-110m to decay.*

Results   The most prominent gamma photons of indium-111 have energies of 0.171 MeV and 0.245 MeV.

B. To 100 µL of *silver nitrate solution R2* add 50 µL of the preparation to be examined. A white precipitate is formed.

C. pH (see Tests).

D. Examine the chromatogram obtained in the test for radiochemical purity (see Tests).

Result   The retardation factor of the principal peak in the radiochromatogram obtained with the test solution is 0.5 to 0.8.

TESTS

pH (*2.2.3*)

1.0 to 2.0.

Cadmium

Maximum 0.40 µg/mL.

Atomic absorption spectrometry (*2.2.23, Method I*).

Test solution   Dilute 0.05 mL of the preparation to be examined to a suitable volume with a suitable concentration of *hydrochloric acid R*.

Reference solutions   Prepare the reference solutions using *cadmium standard solution (0.1 per cent Cd) R*, diluting with the same concentration of *hydrochloric acid R* as in the test solution.

Source   Cadmium hollow-cathode lamp.

Wavelength   228.8 nm.

Atomisation device   Electrothermal.

Copper

Maximum 0.15 µg/mL.

Atomic absorption spectrometry (*2.2.23, Method I*).

Test solution   Dilute 0.1 mL of the preparation to be examined to a suitable volume with a suitable concentration of *hydrochloric acid R*.

Ph Eur

Reference solutions   Prepare the reference solutions using *copper standard solution (0.1 per cent) R* diluting with the same concentration of *hydrochloric acid R* as in the test solution.

Source   Copper hollow-cathode lamp.

Wavelength   324.8 nm.

Atomisation device   Electrothermal.

Iron

Maximum 0.60 µg/mL.

Atomic absorption spectrometry (*2.2.23, Method I*).

Test solution   Dilute 0.1 mL of the preparation to be examined to a suitable volume with a suitable concentration of *hydrochloric acid R*.

Reference solutions   Prepare the reference solutions using *iron standard solution (0.1 per cent Fe) R* diluting with the same concentration of *hydrochloric acid R* as in the test solution.

Source   Iron hollow-cathode lamp

Wavelength   248.3 nm.

Atomisation device   Electrothermal.

Sterility

It complies with the test for sterility prescribed in the monograph *Radiopharmaceutical preparations (0125)*.
The preparation may be released for use before completion of the test.

RADIONUCLIDIC PURITY

Indium-111

Gamma-ray and X-ray spectrometry.

Comparison   Standardised indium-111 solution.

Result   The spectrum obtained with the preparation to be examined does not differ significantly from that obtained with a standardised indium-111 solution apart from any differences due to the presence of indium-114m.

Impurity A

Maximum 0.25 per cent of the total radioactivity.

Gamma-ray spectrometry. *Carry out the test after allowing sufficient time for short-lived impurities such as indium-110m to decay.*

Take a volume equivalent to 30 MBq and record the gamma-ray spectrum using a suitable detector with a shield of lead, 6 mm thick, placed between the sample and the detector.

Results   The response in the region corresponding to the 0.558 MeV photon and the 0.725 MeV photon of indium-114m does not exceed that obtained using 75 kBq of a standardised indium-114m solution measured under the same conditions, when all measurements are calculated with reference to the date and time of administration.

RADIOCHEMICAL PURITY

[111In]Indium(III) ion

Thin-layer chromatography (*2.2.27*)

Test solution   The preparation to be examined.

Plate   TLC silica gel plate R. Use silica gel as the coating substance on a glass-fibre sheet.

Mobile phase   9.0 g/L solution of *sodium chloride R* adjusted to pH 2.3 ± 0.05 with *dilute hydrochloric acid R*.

Application   5 µL.

Development   Immediately over a path of 15 cm.

Drying   In a current of cold air.

Detection   Suitable detector to determine the distribution of radioactivity.

Retardation factor: [^{111}In]indium(III) ion = 0.5 to 0.8.

Limit:
— [^{111}In]indium(III) ion : minimum 95 per cent of the radioactivity due to indium-111.

RADIOACTIVITY

Determine the radioactivity using a calibrated instrument.

IMPURITIES

A. indium-114m.

_____ Ph Eur

Indium (^{111}In) Oxine Solution

(Ph Eur monograph 1109)

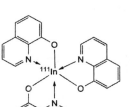

$C_{27}H_{18}[^{111}In]N_3O_3$ 547.2

Ph Eur _____

DEFINITION

Sterile solution of indium-111 in the form of a complex with 8-hydroxyquinoline. It may contain suitable surface active agents and may be made isotonic by the addition of sodium chloride and a suitable buffer.

Indium-111

90 per cent to 110 per cent of the declared indium-111 radioactivity at the date and time stated on the label.

Specific radioactivity

Minimum 1.85 GBq of indium-111 per microgram of indium.

PRODUCTION

No carrier indium is added.

CHARACTERS

Appearance

Clear, colourless solution.

Half-life and nature of radiation of indium-111

See general chapter *5.7. Table of physical characteristics of radionuclides.*

IDENTIFICATION

A. Gamma-ray and X-ray spectrometry. *Carry out the test after allowing sufficient time for short-lived impurities such as indium-110m to decay.*

Results   The most prominent gamma photons of indium-111 have energies of 0.171 MeV and 0.245 MeV.

B. Place 5-10 mg of *magnesium oxide R* in a glass container about 20 mm in internal diameter. Add 20 µL of the preparation to be examined. Examine in ultraviolet light at 365 nm. Bright yellow fluorescence is produced.

C. The distribution of radioactivity between the organic and aqueous phases in the test for radiochemical purity (see Tests) contributes to the identification of the preparation.

TESTS

pH (2.2.3)

6.0 to 7.5.

Sterility

It complies with the test for sterility prescribed in the monograph *Radiopharmaceutical preparations (0125)*. The preparation may be released for use before completion of the test.

RADIONUCLIDIC PURITY

Indium-111

Gamma-ray and X-ray spectrometry.

Comparison   Standardised indium-111 solution.

Result   The spectrum obtained with the preparation to be examined does not differ significantly from that obtained with a standardised indium-111 solution, apart from any differences due to the presence of indium-114m.

Impurity A

Maximum 0.25 per cent of the total radioactivity.

Gamma-ray spectrometry. *Carry out the test after allowing sufficient time for short-lived impurities such as indium-110m to decay.*

Take a volume equivalent to 30 MBq and record the gamma-ray spectrum using a suitable detector with a shield of lead, 6 mm thick, placed between the sample and the detector.

Results   The response in the region corresponding to the 0.558 MeV photon and the 0.725 MeV photon of indium-114m does not exceed that obtained using 75 kBq of a standardised indium-114m solution measured under the same conditions, when all measurements are calculated with reference to the date and time of administration.

RADIOCHEMICAL PURITY

[^{111}In]Indium oxine

To a silanised separating funnel containing 3 mL of a 9 g/L solution of *sodium chloride R* add 100 µL of the preparation to be examined and mix. Add 6 mL of *octanol R* and shake vigorously. Allow the phases to separate and then run the lower layer into a suitable vial for counting. Allow the upper layer to drain completely into a similar vial. Add 1 mL of *octanol R* to the separating funnel, shake vigorously and drain into the vial containing the organic fraction. Add 5 mL of *dilute hydrochloric acid R* to the separating funnel, shake vigorously and drain these rinsings into a 3rd vial. Seal each vial and, using a suitable instrument, measure the radioactivity in each. Calculate the radiochemical purity by expressing the radioactivity of the [^{111}In]indium oxine, found in the organic phase, as a percentage of the total radioactivity due to indium-111 measured in the 3 solutions.

Result   Minimum 90 per cent of the radioactivity due to indium-111.

RADIOACTIVITY

Determine the radioactivity using a calibrated instrument.

LABELLING

The label states that the solution is not for direct administration to humans.

IMPURITIES

A. indium-114m.

——————————— Ph Eur

Indium (^{111}In) Pentetate Injection

(Ph Eur monograph 0670)

Ph Eur ———————————

DEFINITION

Sterile solution containing indium-111 in the form of indium diethylenetriaminepenta-acetate. It may contain calcium and may be made isotonic by the addition of sodium chloride and a suitable buffer.

Indium-111

90 per cent to 110 per cent of the declared indium-111 radioactivity at the date and time stated on the label.

CHARACTERS

Appearance

Clear, colourless solution.

Half-life and nature of radiation of Indium-111

See general chapter 5.7. *Table of physical characteristics of radionuclides.*

IDENTIFICATION

A. Gamma-ray and X-ray spectrometry.

Results   The most prominent gamma photons of indium-111 have energies of 0.171 MeV and 0.245 MeV.

B. Examine the chromatogram obtained in the test for radiochemical purity (see Tests). The distribution of radioactivity contributes to the identification of the preparation.

TESTS

pH (2.2.3)

7.0 to 8.0.

Cadmium

Maximum 5 µg/mL.

Atomic absorption spectrometry (*2.2.23, Method II*).

Test solution   Mix 0.1 mL of the preparation to be examined with 0.9 mL of a mixture of 1 volume of *hydrochloric acid R* and 99 volumes of *water R*.

Reference solutions   Prepare the reference solutions using *cadmium standard solution (0.1 per cent Cd) R* and diluting with a mixture of 1 volume of *hydrochloric acid R* and 99 volumes of *water R*.

Source   Cadmium hollow-cathode lamp.

Wavelength   228.8 nm.

Atomisation device   Air-acetylene flame.

Uncomplexed diethylenetriaminepenta-acetic acid

Maximum 0.4 mg/mL.

In a micro test-tube, mix 100 µL of the preparation to be examined with 100 µL of a freshly prepared 1 g/L solution of *hydroxynaphthol blue, sodium salt R* in a 42 g/L solution of *sodium hydroxide R*. Add 50 µL of a 0.15 g/L solution of *calcium chloride R*. The solution remains pinkish-violet or changes from blue to pinkish-violet.

Sterility

It complies with the test for sterility prescribed in the monograph *Radiopharmaceutical preparations (0125)*. The preparation may be released for use before completion of the test.

Bacterial endotoxins (2.6.14)

Less than 14/V IU/mL, V being the maximum recommended dose in millilitres.

RADIONUCLIDIC PURITY

Indium-111

Gamma-ray and X-ray spectrometry.

Comparison   Standardised indium-111 solution.

Result   The spectrum obtained with the preparation to be examined does not differ significantly from that obtained with a standardised indium-111 solution apart from any differences due to the presence of indium-114m.

Impurity A

Maximum 0.2 per cent of the total radioactivity at the date and time of administration.

Gamma-ray spectrometry.

Retain a sample of the preparation to be examined for a sufficient time to allow the indium-111 radioactivity to decay to a sufficiently low level to permit the detection of radionuclidic impurities. Record the gamma-ray spectrum of the decayed material in a suitable instrument calibrated with the aid of a standardised indium-114m solution.

Result   Indium-114m has a half-life of 49.5 days and its most prominent gamma photon has an energy of 0.190 MeV.

RADIOCHEMICAL PURITY

[¹¹¹In]Indium pentetate

Thin-layer chromatography (*2.2.27*).

Test solution   The preparation to be examined.

Plate   TLC silica gel plate R; use silica gel as the coating substance on a glass-fibre sheet heated at 110 °C for 10 min.

Mobile phase   9 g/L solution of *sodium chloride R*.

Application   5-10 µL.

Development   Over a path of 10-15 cm in about 10 min.

Drying   In air.

Detection   Suitable detector to determine the distribution of radioactivity.

Identification of spots   [¹¹¹In]indium pentetate migrates near to the solvent front.

Limit:
— *[¹¹¹In]indium pentetate* : minimum 95 per cent of the radioactivity due to indium-111.

RADIOACTIVITY

Determine the radioactivity using a calibrated instrument.

IMPURITIES

A. indium-114m.

_____ *Ph Eur*

Iobenguane (¹²³I) Injection

(*Ph Eur monograph 1113*)

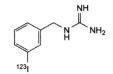

$C_8H_{10}[^{123}I]N_3$

Ph Eur _____

DEFINITION

Sterile, bacterial endotoxin-free solution of 1-(3-[¹²³I]iodobenzyl)guanidine or its salts. It may contain a suitable buffer, a suitable labelling catalyst such as ionic copper, a suitable labelling stabiliser such as ascorbic acid and antimicrobial preservatives.

Iodine-123

90 per cent to 110 per cent of the declared iodine-123 radioactivity at the date and time stated on the label.

Specific radioactivity

Minimum 10 GBq of iodine-123 per gram of iobenguane base.

CHARACTERS

Appearance

Clear, colourless or slightly yellow solution.

Half-life and nature of radiation of iodine-123

See general chapter 5.7. *Table of physical characteristics of radionuclides.*

IDENTIFICATION

A. Gamma-ray and X-ray spectrometry.

Result   The energy of the most prominent gamma photon of iodine-123 is 0.159 MeV.

B. Examine the chromatogram obtained in the test for radiochemical purity (see Tests). The distribution of the radioactivity contributes to the identification of the preparation.

TESTS

pH (*2.2.3*)

3.5 to 8.0.

Specific radioactivity

The specific radioactivity is calculated from the results obtained in the test for radiochemical purity. Determine the content of iobenguane sulfate from the areas of the peaks corresponding to iobenguane in the chromatograms obtained with the test solution and reference solution (b). Calculate the concentration as iobenguane base by multiplying the result obtained in the test by 0.85.

Sterility

It complies with the test for sterility prescribed in the monograph *Radiopharmaceutical preparations (0125)*.
The preparation may be released for use before completion of the test.

Bacterial endotoxins (*2.6.14*)

Less than $175/V$ IU/mL, V being the maximum recommended dose in millilitres.

RADIONUCLIDIC PURITY

The preparation may be released for use before completion of the test.

Radionuclides other than iodine-123

Maximum 0.35 per cent of the total radioactivity.

Gamma-ray and X-ray spectrometry.

Record the gamma-ray spectrum and the X-ray spectrum using a suitable instrument.

Determine the relative amounts of iodine-125, tellurium-121 and other radionuclidic impurities present. For their determination, retain the preparation to be examined for a sufficient time to allow iodine-123 to decay to a level which permits the detection of radionuclidic impurities.
No radionuclides with a half-life longer than that of iodine-125 are detected.

RADIOCHEMICAL PURITY

[¹²³I]Iobenguane

Liquid chromatography (*2.2.29*).

Test solution   The preparation to be examined.

Reference solution (a) Dissolve 0.100 g of *sodium iodide R* in the mobile phase and dilute to 100 mL with the mobile phase.

Reference solution (b) Dissolve 10.0 mg of *iobenguane sulfate CRS* in 25 mL of the mobile phase and dilute to 50.0 mL with the mobile phase.

Column:
— *size:* l = 0.25 m, Ø = 4.0 mm;
— *stationary phase: silica gel for chromatography R* (5 μm).

Mobile phase 80 g/L solution of *ammonium nitrate R, dilute ammonia R2, methanol R* (1:2:27 *V/V/V*).

Flow rate 1.0 mL/min.

Detection Suitable detector to determine the distribution of radioactivity and spectrophotometer at 254 nm, provided with a flow-cell.

Injection 10 μL.

Limits:
— *[^{123}I]iobenguane*: minimum 95 per cent of the radioactivity due to iodine-123;
— *impurity A*: maximum 4 per cent of the radioactivity due to iodine-123;
— *other impurities*: maximum 1 per cent of the radioactivity due to iodine-123.

RADIOACTIVITY
Determine the radioactivity using a calibrated instrument.

STORAGE
Protected from light.

LABELLING
The label states the specific radioactivity expressed in GBq of iodine-123 per gram of iobenguane base.

IMPURITIES
A. [^{123}I]iodide,

B. iodine-125,

C. tellurium-121.

Ph Eur

Iobenguane (^{131}I) Injection for Diagnostic Use

(*Ph Eur monograph 1111*)

$C_8H_{10}[^{131}I]N_3$

Ph Eur

DEFINITION
Sterile, bacterial endotoxin-free solution of 1-(3-[^{131}I]iodobenzyl)guanidine or its salts. It may contain a suitable buffer, a suitable labelling catalyst such as ionic copper, a suitable labelling stabiliser such as ascorbic acid, and antimicrobial preservatives.

Iodine-131
90 per cent to 110 per cent of the declared iodine-131 radioactivity at the date and time stated on the label.

Specific radioactivity
Minimum 20 GBq of iodine-131 per gram of iobenguane base.

CHARACTERS
Appearance
Clear, colourless or slightly yellow solution.

Half-life and nature of radiation of iodine-131
See general chapter *5.7. Table of physical characteristics of radionuclides.*

IDENTIFICATION
A. Gamma-ray spectrometry.

Result The most prominent gamma photon of iodine-131 has an energy of 0.365 MeV.

B. Examine the chromatogram obtained in the test for radiochemical purity (see Tests). The distribution of the radioactivity contributes to the identification of the preparation.

TESTS
pH (*2.2.3*)
3.5 to 8.0.

Specific radioactivity
The specific radioactivity is calculated from the results obtained in the test for radiochemical purity. Determine the content of iobenguane sulfate from the areas of the peaks corresponding to iobenguane in the chromatograms obtained with the test solution and reference solution (b). Calculate the concentration as iobenguane base by multiplying the result obtained in the test by 0.85.

Sterility
It complies with the test for sterility prescribed in the monograph *Radiopharmaceutical preparations (0125)*.
The preparation may be released for use before completion of the test.

Bacterial endotoxins (*2.6.14*)
Less than 175/*V* IU/mL, *V* being the maximum recommended dose in millilitres.

RADIONUCLIDIC PURITY

Iodine-131
Minimum 99.9 per cent of the total radioactivity.

Gamma-ray spectrometry.

Determine the relative amounts of iodine-131, iodine-133, iodine-135 and other radionuclidic impurities present.

RADIOCHEMICAL PURITY

[^{131}I]Iobenguane
Liquid chromatography (*2.2.29*).

Test solution The preparation to be examined.

Reference solution (a) Dissolve 0.100 g of *sodium iodide R* in the mobile phase and dilute to 100 mL with the mobile phase.

Reference solution (b) Dissolve 10.0 mg of *iobenguane sulfate CRS* in 25 mL of the mobile phase and dilute to 50.0 mL with the mobile phase.

Column:
— *size:* l = 0.25 m, Ø = 4.0 mm;
— *stationary phase: silica gel for chromatography R* (5 μm).

Mobile phase 80 g/L solution of *ammonium nitrate R, dilute ammonia R2, methanol R* (1:2:27 *V/V/V*).

Flow rate 1.0 mL/min.

Detection Suitable detector to determine the distribution of radioactivity and spectrophotometer at 254 nm, provided with a flow-cell.

Injection   10 µL.

Limits:

— *[¹³¹I]iobenguane*: minimum 94 per cent of the radioactivity due to iodine-131;

— *impurity A*: maximum 5 per cent of the radioactivity due to iodine-131;

— *other impurities*: maximum 1 per cent of the radioactivity due to iodine-131.

RADIOACTIVITY

Determine the radioactivity using a calibrated instrument.

STORAGE

Protected from light.

LABELLING

The label states the specific radioactivity expressed in GBq of iodine-131 per gram of iobenguane base.

IMPURITIES

A. [¹³¹I]iodide,

B. iodine-133,

C. iodine-135.

Ph Eur

Iobenguane (¹³¹I) Injection for Therapeutic Use

(Ph Eur monograph 1112)

$C_8H_{10}[^{131}I]N_3$

Ph Eur

DEFINITION

Sterile, bacterial endotoxin-free solution of 1-(3-[¹³¹I]iodobenzyl)guanidine or its salts. It may contain a suitable buffer, a suitable labelling catalyst such as ionic copper, a suitable labelling stabiliser such as ascorbic acid, and antimicrobial preservatives.

Iodine-131

90 per cent to 110 per cent of the declared iodine-131 radioactivity at the date and time stated on the label.

Specific radioactivity

Minimum 400 GBq of iodine-131 per gram of iobenguane base.

CHARACTERS

Appearance

Clear, colourless or slightly yellow solution.

Half-life and nature of radiation of iodine-131

See general chapter 5.7. *Table of physical characteristics of radionuclides.*

IDENTIFICATION

A. Gamma-ray spectrometry.

Result   The most prominent gamma photon of iodine-131 has an energy of 0.365 MeV.

B. Examine the chromatogram obtained in the test for radio-chemical purity (see Tests). The distribution of the radioactivity contributes to the identification of the preparation.

TESTS

pH *(2.2.3)*

3.5 to 8.0.

Specific radioactivity

The specific radioactivity is calculated from the results obtained in the test for radiochemical purity. Determine the content of iobenguane sulfate from the areas of the peaks corresponding to iobenguane in the chromatograms obtained with the test solution and reference solution (b). Calculate the concentration as iobenguane base by multiplying the result obtained in the test by 0.85.

Sterility

It complies with the test for sterility prescribed in the monograph *Radiopharmaceutical preparations (0125)*.

The preparation may be released for use before completion of the test.

Bacterial endotoxins *(2.6.14)*

Less than $175/V$ IU/mL, V being the maximum recommended dose in millilitres.

RADIONUCLIDIC PURITY

Iodine-131

Minimum 99.9 per cent of the total radioactivity.

Gamma-ray spectrometry.

Determine the relative amounts of iodine-131, iodine-133, iodine-135 and other radionuclidic impurities present.

RADIOCHEMICAL PURITY

[¹³¹I]Iobenguane

Liquid chromatography *(2.2.29)*.

Test solution   The preparation to be examined.

Reference solution (a)   Dissolve 0.100 g of *sodium iodide R* in the mobile phase and dilute to 100 mL with the mobile phase.

Reference solution (b)   Dissolve 10.0 mg of *iobenguane sulfate CRS* in 25 mL of the mobile phase and dilute to 50.0 mL with the mobile phase.

Column:

— *size: l* = 0.25 m, Ø = 4.0 mm;

— *stationary phase: silica gel for chromatography R* (5 µm).

Mobile phase   80 g/L solution of *ammonium nitrate R, dilute ammonia R2, methanol R* (1:2:27 *V/V/V*).

Flow rate   1.0 mL/min.

Detection   Suitable detector to determine the distribution of radioactivity and spectrophotometer at 254 nm, provided with a flow-cell.

Injection   10 µL.

Limits:

— *[¹³¹I]iobenguane*: minimum 92 per cent of the radioactivity due to iodine-131;

— *impurity A*: maximum 7 per cent of the radioactivity due to iodine-131;

— *other impurities*: maximum 1 per cent of the radioactivity due to iodine-131.

RADIOACTIVITY

Determine the radioactivity using a calibrated instrument.

STORAGE

Protected from light.

LABELLING

The label states the specific radioactivity expressed in GBq of iodine-131 per gram of iobenguane base.

IMPURITIES

A. [^{131}I]iodide,

B. iodine-133,

C. iodine-135.

_____ *Ph Eur*

Iodomethylnorcholesterol (^{131}I) Injection

Iodinated (^{131}I) Norcholesterol Injection

(Ph Eur monograph 0939)

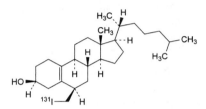

Ph Eur _____

DEFINITION

Sterile solution of 6β-[^{131}I]iodomethyl-19-norcholest-5(10)-en-3β-ol. It may contain a suitable emulsifier such as polysorbate 80 and a suitable antimicrobial preservative such as benzyl alcohol.

Iodine-131

90 per cent to 110 per cent of the declared iodine-131 radioactivity at the date and time stated on the label.

Specific radioactivity

3.7 GBq to 37 GBq per gram of 6β-iodomethylnorcholesterol.

CHARACTERS

Appearance

Clear or slightly turbid, colourless or pale yellow solution.

Half-life and nature of radiation of iodine-131: see general chapter *5.7. Table of physical characteristics of radionuclides.*

IDENTIFICATION

A. Gamma-ray spectrometry.

Result The most prominent photon of iodine-131 has an energy of 0.365 MeV.

B. Examine the chromatogram obtained in the test for radiochemical purity 6β-[^{131}I]iodomethyl-19-norcholest-5(10)-en-3β-ol (see Tests).

Result The retardation factor of the principal peak in the radiochromatogram obtained with the test solution is about 0.5.

TESTS

pH *(2.2.3)*

3.5 to 8.5.

Sterility

It complies with the test for sterility prescribed in the monograph *Radiopharmaceutical preparations (0125).*

The preparation may be released for use before completion of the test.

Bacterial endotoxins *(2.6.14)*

Less than 175/*V* IU/mL, *V* being the maximum recommended dose in millilitres.

RADIONUCLIDIC PURITY

Iodine-131

Minimum 99.9 per cent of the total radioactivity.

Gamma-ray spectrometry.

Determine the relative amounts of iodine-131, iodine-133, iodine-135 and other radionuclidic impurities present.

Radiochemical purity

6β-[^{131}I]Iodomethyl-19-norcholest-5(10)-en-3β-ol

Thin-layer chromatography *(2.2.27).*

Test solution The preparation to be examined.

Carrier solution Dissolve 10 mg of *potassium iodide R*, 20 mg of *potassium iodate R* and 0.1 g of *sodium hydrogen carbonate R* in *distilled water R* and dilute to 10 mL with the same solvent.

Plate TLC silica gel GF$_{254}$ plate R.

Mobile phase chloroform R.

Application Up to 5 μL of the test solution and 10 μL of the carrier solution on the same spot.

Development Over a path of 15 cm in about 60 min.

Drying In air.

Detection Ultraviolet light at 254 nm and suitable detector to determine the distribution of radioactivity.

Retardation factor 6β-[^{131}I]iodomethyl-19-norcholest-5(10)-en-3β-ol = about 0.5.

Identification of spots Impurity C remains near the point of application.

Limit:

— 6β-[^{131}I]iodomethyl-19-norcholest-5(10)-en-3β-ol: minimum 85 per cent of the total radioactivity due to iodine-131.

Impurity C

Thin-layer chromatography *(2.2.27).*

Test solution The preparation to be examined.

Carrier solution Dissolve 10 mg of *potassium iodide R*, 20 mg of *potassium iodate R* and 0.1 g of *sodium hydrogen carbonate R* in *distilled water R* and dilute to 10 mL with the same solvent.

Plate TLC silica gel GF$_{254}$ plate R.

Mobile phase chloroform R, anhydrous ethanol R (50:50 *V/V*).

Application 10 μL of the carrier solution and then up to 5 μL of the test solution on the same spot.

Development Over a path of 15 cm in about 90 min.

Drying In air.

Detection Ultraviolet light at 254 nm for 5 min and suitable detector to determine the distribution of radioactivity.

Retardation factor Impurity C (yellow spot) = about 0.5.

Identifications of spots The principal peak of radioactivity is near to the solvent front; other iodocholesterols migrate near the solvent front.

Limit:

— *impurity C*: maximum 5 per cent of the total radioactivity.

RADIOACTIVITY

Determine the radioactivity using a calibrated instrument.

STORAGE

Protected from light, at − 18 °C or below.

IMPURITIES

A. iodine-133,

B. iodine-135,

C. [^{131}I]iodide.

———————————————————— *Ph Eur*

Krypton (^{81m}Kr) Inhalation Gas

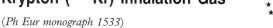

(*Ph Eur monograph 1533*)

Ph Eur ————————————————————

DEFINITION

Gaseous mixture of krypton-81m and a suitable vehicle such as air.

PRODUCTION

Krypton-81m is formed by decay of its parent radionuclide rubidium-81. Rubidium-81 has a half-life of 4.58 h.

The krypton-81m formed is separated from the rubidium-81 with a flow of a suitable gas in a rubidium/krypton generator. Rubidium-81 is produced by proton irradiation of krypton isotopes or by helium-3 or helium-4 irradiation of bromine. After separation of rubidium-81 from the target, it is retained by a suitable support.

Krypton-81m is eluted at a suitable flow rate with a vehicle such as air. The level of moisture required in the eluent depends on the type of generator used. The transport tube for administration has a defined length and inner diameter. The radioactivity concentration is determined before administration.

CHARACTERS

Appearance

Clear, colourless gas.

Half-life and nature of radiation of krypton-81m

See general chapter 5.7. *Table of physical characteristics of radionuclides.*

IDENTIFICATION

A. Gamma-ray and X-ray spectrometry.

Result   The gamma photon of krypton-81m has an energy of 0.190 MeV.

B. The half-life of krypton-81m is 11.8 s to 14.4 s.

TESTS

RADIONUCLIDIC PURITY

Radionuclides other than krypton-81m

Maximum 0.1 per cent of the radioactivity passed through the absorber, calculated with reference to the date and time of administration.

Gamma-ray and X-ray spectrometry   Elute the generator as prescribed. Pass a sufficient amount (2 L to 10 L) of eluate at a suitable flow rate through a suitable absorber such as water. Determine the amount of radioactivity eluted. Allow the krypton-81m to decay for 5 min and record the gamma and X-ray spectrum of the residual radioactivity on the absorber using a suitable instrument. Examine the gamma-ray and X-ray spectrum of the absorber for the presence of radioactive impurities, which must be identified and quantified.

RADIOACTIVITY

Determine the radioactive concentration of the preparation using suitable equipment such as an ionisation chamber or a gamma ray spectrometer. The radioactivity is measured

under defined operating conditions, such as gas flow rate and measurement geometry, that are identical to those used for the calibration of the instrument.

STORAGE

The storage conditions apply to the generator.

LABELLING

The labelling conditions apply to the generator.

———————————————————— *Ph Eur*

L-Methionine ([^{11}C]Methyl) Injection

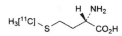

(*Ph Eur monograph 1617*)

Ph Eur ————————————————————

DEFINITION

Sterile solution of (2*S*)-2-amino-4-([^{11}C]methylsulfanyl)butanoic acid for diagnostic use.

Content

90 per cent to 110 per cent of the declared carbon-11 radioactivity at the date and time stated on the label.

Purity:

— minimum of 99 per cent of the total radioactivity corresponds to carbon-11,

— minimum of 95 per cent of the total radioactivity corresponds to carbon-11 in the form of L-[*methyl*-^{11}C]methionine and D-[*methyl*-^{11}C]methionine,

— maximum of 10 per cent of the total radioactivity corresponds to carbon-11 in the form of D-[*methyl*-^{11}C]methionine.

Content of methionine

Maximum of 2 mg per maximum recommended dose in millilitres.

PRODUCTION

RADIONUCLIDE PRODUCTION

Carbon-11 is a radioactive isotope of carbon which is most commonly produced by proton irradiation of nitrogen. Depending on the addition of either trace amounts of oxygen or small amounts of hydrogen, the radioactivity is obtained as [^{11}C]carbon dioxide or [^{11}C]methane.

RADIOCHEMICAL SYNTHESIS

L-[*Methyl*-^{11}C]methionine can be prepared by various chemical synthetic pathways. All methods rely on the alkylation of the sulfide anion of L-homocysteine with [^{11}C]methyl iodide or [^{11}C]methyl triflate. Variations in the procedures used to generate the sulfide anion of L-homocysteine and methods to obtain [^{11}C]methyl iodide lead to negligible differences with respect to quality in terms of specific radioactivity, enantiomeric purity and possible chemical and radiochemical impurities.

Synthesis of [^{11}C]methyl iodide

[^{11}C]Methyl iodide can be obtained either starting from [^{11}C]carbon dioxide or from [^{11}C]methane. The most frequently used method is the reduction of [^{11}C]carbon dioxide with lithium aluminium hydride. The formed [^{11}C]methanol is reacted with hydroiodic acid. Alternatively [^{11}C]methane, either obtained directly in the target or by on-line processes from [^{11}C]carbon dioxide, is reacted with iodine.

Synthesis of [^{11}C]methyl triflate

[^{11}C]methyl triflate can be prepared from [^{11}C]methyl iodide using a silver triflate-impregnated solid support such as graphitised carbon.

Synthesis of l-[*methyl*-^{11}C]methionine

The most widely used method to obtain L-[*methyl*-^{11}C]methionine is the alkylation of the sulfide anion, generated from L-homocysteine thiolactone, with [^{11}C]methyl iodide or [^{11}C]methyl triflate in alkaline conditions in a solvent such as acetone. The L-[*methyl*-^{11}C]methionine obtained can be purified by semi-preparative liquid chromatography. For example, a column packed with octadecylsilyl silica gel for chromatography eluted with a 9 g/L solution of sodium chloride is suitable.

l-Homocysteine thiolactone hydrochloride

Specific optical rotation (2.2.7): + 20.5 to + 21.5, determined on a 10 g/L solution at 25 °C.

Infrared absorption spectrophotometry (2.2.24).

Comparison Ph. Eur. reference spectrum of L-homocysteine thiolactone hydrochloride.

CHARACTERS

Appearance

Clear, colourless solution.

Half-life and nature of radiation of carbon-11

See general chapter 5.7. *Table of physical characteristics of radionuclides*.

IDENTIFICATION

A. Gamma-ray spectrometry.

Results The only gamma photons have an energy of 0.511 MeV and, depending on the measurement geometry, a sum peak of 1.022 MeV may be observed.

B. Radionuclidic purity (see Tests).

C. Examine the chromatograms obtained in the test for radiochemical purity.

Results The principal peak in the radiochromatogram obtained with the test solution is similar in retention time to the principal peak in the chromatogram obtained with reference solution (b).

TESTS

pH (2.2.3)

4.5 to 8.5.

Sterility

It complies with the test for sterility prescribed in the monograph on *Radiopharmaceutical preparations (0125)*. The injection may be released for use before completion of the test.

Bacterial endotoxins (2.6.14)

Less than 175/V IU/mL, V being the maximum recommended dose in millilitres. The injection may be released for use before completion of the test.

CHEMICAL PURITY

Impurity A, impurity B and methionine

Liquid chromatography (2.2.29).

Test solution The preparation to be examined.

Reference solution (a) Dissolve 0.6 mg of L-homocysteine thiolactone hydrochloride R, 2 mg of DL-homocysteine R and 2 mg of DL-methionine R in *water R* and dilute to V, V being the maximum recommended dose in millilitres.

Reference solution (b) Dissolve 2 mg of L-methionine R in the same solvent as used in the test solution and dilute to 10 mL with the same solvent.

Column:
— size: l = 0.25 m, Ø = 4.6 mm,
— stationary phase: spherical *octadecylsilyl silica gel for chromatography R* (5 μm) with a specific surface of 220 m^2/g, a pore size of 8 nm and a carbon loading of 6.2 per cent,
— temperature: 25 °C.

Mobile phase 1.4 g/L solution of *potassium dihydrogen phosphate R*.

Flow rate 1 mL/min.

Detection Spectrophotometer at 225 nm and radioactivity detector connected in series.

Injection Loop injector.

Run time 10 min.

Relative retention With reference to methionine (retention time = about 2.6 min): impurity B = about 0.8, impurity A = about 2.7.

System suitability Reference solution (a):
— resolution: minimum of 2.5 between the peaks due to methionine and impurity B.

Limits Examine the chromatogram obtained with the spectrophotometer:
— *impurity A*: not more than the area of the corresponding peak in the chromatogram obtained with reference solution (a) (0.6 mg/V),
— *impurity B*: not more than the area of the corresponding peak in the chromatogram obtained with reference solution (a) (2 mg/V),
— *methionine*: not more than the area of the corresponding peak in the chromatogram obtained with reference solution (a) (2 mg/V).

Residual solvents (2.4.24)

Maximum 50 mg/V for the concentration of acetone, V being the maximum recommended dose in millilitres.
The preparation may be released for use before completion of the test.

RADIONUCLIDIC PURITY

Carbon-11

Minimum 99 per cent of the total radioactivity.

A. Gamma-ray spectroscopy.

Comparison Standardised fluorine-18 solution, or by using an instrument calibrated with the aid of such a solution. Standardised fluorine-18 solutions and/or standardisation services are available from the competent authority.

Results The spectrum obtained with the solution to be examined does not differ significantly from that obtained with a standardised fluorine-18 solution.

B. Half-life: 19.9 min to 20.9 min.

The preparation may be released for use before completion of the test.

RADIOCHEMICAL PURITY

l-[Methyl-^{11}C]methionine and impurity E

Liquid chromatography (2.2.29) as described in the test for impurity A, impurity B and methionine.

Injection Test solution and reference solution (b).

Limits Examine the chromatogram obtained with the radioactivity detector:
— *total of L-[methyl-^{11}C]methionine and impurity E*: minimum of 95 per cent of the total radioactivity,

— other peaks in the chromatogram may be due to impurity C, impurity D and impurity F.

ENANTIOMERIC PURITY

Impurity E

Thin-layer chromatography (2.2.27).

Test solution   The preparation to be examined.

Reference solution (a)   Dissolve 2 mg of L-*methionine R* in *water R* and dilute to 10 mL with the same solvent.

Reference solution (b)   Dissolve 4 mg of DL-*methionine R* in *water R* and dilute to 10 mL with the same solvent.

Plate   TLC octadecylsilyl silica gel plate for chiral separations R.

Mobile phase   methanol R, water R (50:50 V/V).

Application   2-10 μL.

Development   Over a path of 8 cm.

Drying   In air for 5 min.

Detection   Spray with a 2 g/L solution of *ninhydrin R* in *ethanol R* and heat at 60 °C for 10 min. Determine the distribution of radioactivity using a suitable detector.

Retardation factors   L-[methyl-^{11}C]methionine = about 0.58; impurity E = about 0.51.

System suitability   The chromatogram obtained with reference solution (b) shows 2 clearly separated spots.

Limits:
— *total of* L-[methyl-^{11}C]methionine *and impurity E:* minimum 95 per cent of the total radioactivity,
— *impurity E:* maximum 10 per cent of the total radioactivity.

The preparation may be released for use before completion of the test.

RADIOACTIVITY

Measure the radioactivity using suitable equipment by comparison with a standardised fluorine-18 solution or by measurement in an instrument calibrated with the aid of such a solution.

LABELLING

The accompanying information specifies the maximum recommended dose in millilitres.

IMPURITIES

A. (3S)-3-aminodihydrothiophen-2(3H)-one (L-homocysteine thiolactone),

B. (2S)-2-amino-4-sulfanylbutanoic acid (L-homocysteine),

C. (2RS)-2-amino-4-(^{11}C]methylsulfonyl)butanoic acid (DL-[methyl-^{11}C]methionine S,S-dioxide),

D. (2RS)-2-amino-4-(^{11}C]methylsulfinyl)butanoic acid (DL-[methyl-^{11}C]methionine S-oxide),

E. (2R)-2-amino-4-(^{11}C]methylsulfanyl)butanoic acid (D-[methyl-^{11}C]methionine),

$$[^{11}C]H_3\text{-}OH$$

F. [11]C]methanol

_____ *Ph Eur*

Oxygen (^{15}O)

(*Ph Eur monograph 1620*)

Ph Eur _____

DEFINITION

Mixture of ^{15}O]oxygen in the gaseous phase and a suitable vehicle such as *Medicinal air (1238)*, for diagnostic use.

Purity:
— minimum 99 per cent of the total radioactivity corresponds to oxygen-15,
— minimum 97 per cent of the total radioactivity corresponds to oxygen-15 in the form of oxygen (O_2).

PRODUCTION

RADIONUCLIDIC PRODUCTION

Oxygen-15 is a radioactive isotope of oxygen which may be produced by various nuclear reactions such as proton irradiation of nitrogen-15 or deuteron irradiation of nitrogen-14.

RADIOCHEMICAL SYNTHESIS

In order to recover oxygen-15 as molecular oxygen from the nitrogen target gas, carrier oxygen is added at concentrations generally ranging from 0.2 per cent V/V to 1.0 per cent V/V. After irradiation, the target gas is usually passed through activated charcoal and a carbon dioxide scavenger, such as soda lime, before mixing with the vehicle.

CHARACTERS

Appearance

Colourless gas.

Half-life and nature of radiation of oxygen-15

See general chapter 5.7. *Table of physical characteristics of radionuclides.*

IDENTIFICATION

A. Gamma spectrometry.

Results   The only gamma photons have an energy of 0.511 MeV and, depending on the measurement geometry, a sum peak of 1.022 MeV may be observed.

B. Radionuclidic purity (see Tests).

C. Examine the chromatograms obtained in the test for radiochemical purity.

Results   The retention times of the principal peaks in the chromatogram obtained with the test gas using the radioactivity detector are similar to those of the principal peaks corresponding to oxygen in the chromatogram obtained with the reference gas using the thermal conductivity detector.

TESTS

The following tests are performed on [^{15}O]oxygen as described under radiochemical synthesis before mixing with the vehicle.

RADIONUCLIDIC PURITY

Oxygen-15

Minimum 99 per cent of the total radioactivity.

A. Gamma spectrometry.

Comparison Standardised fluorine-18 solution, or by using an instrument calibrated with the aid of such a solution. Standardised fluorine-18 solutions and/or standardisation services are available from the competent authority.

Results The spectrum obtained with the solution to be examined does not differ significantly from that obtained with a standardised fluorine-18 solution.

B. Half-life: 1.9 min to 2.2 min.

The preparation may be released for use before completion of the test.

RADIOCHEMICAL PURITY

Oxygen-15 in the form of O$_2$

Gas chromatography (*2.2.28*): use the normalisation procedure.

Test sample [^{15}O]oxygen as described under radiochemical synthesis.

Reference gas Nitrogen gas mixture R.

Column:
— *size:* l = 1.8 m, Ø1 = 6.3 mm and Ø2 = 3.2 mm,
— *stationary phase:* GC concentrical column R.

Carrier gas Helium for chromatography R.

Flow rate 65 mL/min.

Temperature:
— *column:* 40 °C,
— *injection port:* 40 °C,
— *thermal conductivity detector:* 70 °C.

Detection Thermal conductivity detector and radioactivity detector connected in series.

Injection Loop injector.

Run time 10 min.

Retention times Oxygen, nitrogen and carbon monoxide eluting from the inner column = about 0.4 min; carbon dioxide eluting from the inner column = about 0.8 min; oxygen eluting from the outer column = about 2.1 min; nitrogen eluting from the outer column = about 3.1 min; carbon monoxide eluting from the outer column = about 6.2 min.

System suitability Reference gas:
— 5 clearly separated principal peaks are observed in the chromatogram obtained using the thermal conductivity detector,
— *resolution:* minimum of 1.5 between the peaks due to carbon dioxide eluting from the inner column and oxygen eluting from the outer column, in the chromatogram obtained using the thermal conductivity detector.

Limits Examine the chromatogram obtained with the radioactivity detector and calculate the percentage content of oxygen-15 substances from the peak areas.
— *oxygen-15 gas in the form of O$_2$:* minimum 97 per cent of the total radioactivity,

— disregard the first peak corresponding to components co-eluting from the inner column.

RADIOACTIVITY

The radioactive concentration is determined before administration.

Measure the radioactivity using suitable equipment by comparison with a standardised fluorine-18 solution or by measurement in an instrument calibrated with the aid of such a solution.

—————————————————————— Ph Eur

Raclopride ([^{11}C]Methoxy) Injection

(Ph Eur monograph 1924)

Ph Eur ——————————————————————

DEFINITION

Sterile solution of 3,5-dichloro-*N*-[[(2*S*)-1-ethylpyrrolidin-2-yl]methyl]-2-hydroxy-6-([^{11}C]methoxy)benzamide.

Content

90 per cent to 110 per cent of the declared carbon-11 radioactivity at the date and time stated on the label.

Purity:
— minimum of 99 per cent of the total radioactivity corresponds to carbon-11,
— minimum of 95 per cent of the total radioactivity corresponds to carbon-11 in the form of [*methoxy*-^{11}C]raclopride.

Content of raclopride

Maximum of 10 µg per maximum recommended dose in millilitres.

PRODUCTION

RADIONUCLIDE PRODUCTION

Carbon-11 is a radioactive isotope of carbon most commonly produced by proton irradiation of nitrogen. Depending on the addition of either trace amounts of oxygen or small amounts of hydrogen, the radioactivity is obtained as [^{11}C]carbon dioxide or [^{11}C]methane, respectively.

RADIOCHEMICAL SYNTHESIS

[*Methoxy*-^{11}C]raclopride may be prepared by *O*-alkylation of the corresponding phenolate anion (*S*)-3,5-dichloro-2,6-dihydroxy-*N*-[(1-ethylpyrrolidin-2-yl)methyl]benzamide with iodo[^{11}C]methane or [^{11}C]methyl trifluoromethanesulfonate.

Synthesis of iodo[^{11}C]methane

Iodo[^{11}C]methane may be produced from [^{11}C]carbon dioxide or from [^{11}C]methane. The most frequently used method is reduction of [^{11}C]carbon dioxide with lithium aluminium hydride. The lithium aluminium [^{11}C]methanolate formed is reacted with hydroiodic acid to iodo[^{11}C]methane via [^{11}C]methanol. Alternatively [^{11}C]methane, either obtained directly in the target or by on-line processes from [^{11}C]carbon dioxide, is reacted with iodine.

Synthesis of [^{11}C]methyl trifluoromethanesulfonate

[^{11}C]Methyl trifluoromethanesulfonate may be prepared from iodo[^{11}C]methane using a solid support such as graphitised carbon impregnated with silver trifluoromethanesulfonate.

Synthesis of [*methoxy*-^{11}C]raclopride

Methylation with iodo[^{11}C]methane is performed under alkaline conditions in a solvent such as dimethyl sulfoxide. The methylation with [^{11}C]methyl trifluoromethanesulfonate is performed in a solvent such as dimethylformamide or acetone. The resulting [*methoxy*-^{11}C]raclopride may be purified by semi-preparative liquid chromatography using, for example, a column packed with octadecylsilyl silica gel for chromatography eluted with a mixture of 25 volumes of acetonitrile and 75 volumes of 0.01 M phosphoric acid.

PRECURSOR FOR SYNTHESIS

(*S*)-3,5-Dichloro-2,6-dihydroxy-*N*-[(1-ethylpyrrolidin-2-yl)methyl]benzamide hydrobromide

Melting point (*2.2.14*): 211 °C to 213 °C.

Specific optical rotation (*2.2.7*): + 11.3 to + 11.5, determined on a 15.0 g/L solution in *ethanol R* at 22 °C.

CHARACTERS

Appearance

Clear, colourless solution.

Half-life and nature of radiation of carbon-11

See general chapter *5.7*. *Table of physical characteristics of radionuclides*.

IDENTIFICATION

A. Gamma-ray spectrometry.

Results The only gamma photons have an energy of 0.511 MeV and, depending on the measurement geometry, a sum peak of 1.022 MeV may be observed.

B. It complies with test B for radionuclidic purity (see Tests).

C. Examine the chromatograms obtained in the test for radiochemical purity.

Results The principal peak in the radiochromatogram obtained with the test solution is similar in retention time to the principal peak in the chromatogram obtained with reference solution (d).

TESTS

pH (*2.2.3*)

4.5 to 8.5.

Sterility

It complies with the test for sterility prescribed in the monograph on *Radiopharmaceutical preparations (0125)*. The injection may be released for use before completion of the test.

Bacterial endotoxins (*2.6.14*)

Less than 175/*V* IU/mL, *V* being the maximum recommended dose in millilitres. The injection may be released for use before completion of the test.

CHEMICAL PURITY

Raclopride and impurity A

Liquid chromatography (*2.2.29*).

Test solution The preparation to be examined.

Reference solution (a) Dissolve 7.2 mg of *raclopride tartrate R* in *water R* and dilute to 50 mL with the same solvent.

Reference solution (b) Dissolve 1.2 mg of *(S)-3,5-dichloro-2,6-dihydroxy-N-[(1-ethylpyrrolidin-2-yl)methyl]benzamide hydrobromide R* in *methanol R* and dilute to 100 mL with the same solvent.

Reference solution (c) To 0.1 mL of reference solution (a) add 0.1 mL of reference solution (b) and dilute to *V* with *water R*, *V* being the maximum recommended dose in millilitres.

Reference solution (d) Dilute 1.0 mL of reference solution (a) to 10.0 mL with *water R*.

Column:
— *size*: *l* = 0.05 m, Ø = 4.6 mm,
— *stationary phase*: spherical end-capped octadecylsilyl silica gel for chromatography R (3.5 μm) with a specific surface area of 175 m^2/g, a pore size of 12.5 nm, a pore volume of 0.7 cm^3/g and a carbon loading of 15 per cent,
— *temperature*: 30 °C.

Mobile phase Dissolve 2 g of *sodium heptanesulfonate R* in 700 mL of *water R*, adjust to pH 3.9 with *phosphoric acid R* and dilute to 1000 mL with *acetonitrile R*.

Flow rate 1 mL/min.

Detection Spectrophotometer at 220 nm and radioactivity detector connected in series.

Injection Loop injector; inject the test solution and reference solutions (b) and (c).

Run time 10 min.

Relative retention With reference to raclopride: impurity A = about 0.46.

System suitability Reference solution (c):
— *resolution*: minimum of 5 between the peaks due to raclopride and to impurity A.

Limits Examine the chromatogram obtained with the spectrophotometer:
— *raclopride*: not more than the area of the corresponding peak in the chromatogram obtained with reference solution (c) (10 μg/*V*),
— *impurity A*: not more than the area of the corresponding peak in the chromatogram obtained with reference solution (c) (1 μg/*V*).

Residual solvents

Are limited according to the principles defined in the general chapter (*5.4*), using the general method (*2.4.24*).

The preparation may be released for use before completion of the test.

RADIONUCLIDIC PURITY

Carbon-11

Minimum 99 per cent of the total radioactivity.

The preparation may be released for use before completion of the test.

A. Gamma-ray spectrometry.

Comparison Standardised fluorine-18 solution, or by using a calibrated instrument. Standardised fluorine-18 solutions and/or standardisation services are available from the competent authority.

Results The spectrum obtained with the solution to be examined does not differ significantly from that obtained with a standardised fluorine-18 solution.

B. Half-life. 19.9 min to 20.9 min.

RADIOCHEMICAL PURITY

Liquid chromatography (*2.2.29*) as described in the test for raclopride and impurity A with the following modifications.

Injection Test solution and reference solution (d).

Limits Examine the chromatogram obtained with the radioactivity detector:
— [*Methoxy*-^{11}C] raclopride: minimum of 95 per cent of the total radioactivity.

RADIOACTIVITY

Mesure the radioactivity using suitable equipment by comparison with a standardised fluorine-18 solution or by using a calibrated instrument.

LABELLING

The accompanying information specifies the maximum recommended dose in millilitres.

IMPURITIES

A. 3,5-dichloro-N-[[(2S)-1-ethylpyrrolidin-2-yl]methyl]-2,6-dihydroxybenzamide.

_____ *Ph Eur*

Sodium Acetate ([1-^{11}C]) Injection

(Ph Eur monograph 1920)

CH$_3$^{11}COONa

Ph Eur _____

DEFINITION

Sterile solution of sodium [1-^{11}C]acetate, in equilibrium with [1-^{11}C]acetic acid.

Content

90 per cent to 110 per cent of the declared carbon-11 radioactivity at the date and time stated on the label.

PRODUCTION

RADIONUCLIDE PRODUCTION

Carbon-11 is a radioactive isotope of carbon which is most commonly produced by proton irradiation of nitrogen. By the addition of trace amounts of oxygen, the radioactivity is obtained as [^{11}C]carbon dioxide.

RADIOCHEMICAL SYNTHESIS

[^{11}C]Carbon dioxide may be separated from the target gas mixture by cryogenic trapping or by trapping on a molecular sieve at room temperature. [^{11}C]Carbon dioxide is then released from the trap using an inert gas such as nitrogen at a temperature higher than the trapping temperature.

[1-^{11}C]Acetate is usually prepared by reaction of [^{11}C]carbon dioxide with methylmagnesium bromide in organic solvents such as ether or tetrahydrofuran.

Hydrolysis of the product yields [1-^{11}C]acetic acid. It is purified by chromatographic procedures. The eluate is diluted with sodium chloride solution.

PRECURSOR FOR SYNTHESIS

Methylmagnesium bromide

The reactivity of methylmagnesium bromide is tested by decomposition of a defined amount with water. The amount of methane released during this reaction is not less than 90 per cent of the theoretical value.

CHARACTERS

Appearance

Clear, colourless solution.

Half-life and nature of radiation of carbon-11

See general chapter *5.7. Table of physical characteristics of radionuclides.*

IDENTIFICATION

A. Gamma-ray spectrometry.

Results The only gamma photons have an energy of 0.511 MeV and, depending on the measurement geometry, a sum peak of 1.022 MeV may be observed.

B. It complies with test B for radionuclidic purity (see Tests).

C. Examine the chromatograms obtained in the test for radiochemical purity.

Results The principal peak in the radiochromatogram obtained with the test solution is similar in retention time to the principal peak in the chromatogram obtained with the reference solution.

TESTS

pH *(2.2.3)*

4.5 to 8.5.

Sterility

It complies with the test for sterility prescribed in the monograph on *Radiopharmaceutical preparations (0125)*. The injection may be released for use before completion of the test.

Bacterial endotoxins *(2.6.14)*

Less than 175/*V* IU/mL, *V* being the maximum recommended dose in millilitres. The injection may be released for use before completion of the test.

CHEMICAL PURITY

Acetate

Liquid chromatography *(2.2.29)*.

Test solution The preparation to be examined.

Reference solution Dissolve 28 mg of sodium *acetate R* in *water R* and dilute to *V*, *V* being the maximum recommended dose in millilitres.

Column:
— *size*: $l = $ 0.25 m, Ø $= $ 4.0 mm;
— *stationary phase*: *strongly basic anion exchange resin for chromatography R* (10 µm);
— *temperature*: 25 °C.

Mobile phase *0.1 M sodium hydroxide* protected from atmospheric carbon dioxide.

Flow rate 1 mL/min.

Detection Spectrophotometer at 220 nm and radioactivity detector connected in series.

Injection Loop injector.

Run time 10 min.

System suitability Reference solution:
— *resolution*: minimum 4.0 between the peaks due to hold-up volume and acetate.

Limit Examine the chromatograms obtained with the spectrophotometer:
— *acetate*: not more than the area of the corresponding peak in the chromatogram obtained with the reference solution (20 mg per *V*).

Residual solvents

Are limited according to the principles defined in the general chapter *(5.4)*, using the general method *(2.4.24)*.

The preparation may be released for use before completion of the test.

RADIONUCLIDIC PURITY

Carbon-11

Minimum 99 per cent of the total radioactivity.

The preparation may be released for use before completion of the tests.

A. Gamma-ray spectrometry.

Comparison Standardised fluorine-18 solution, or by using a calibrated instrument. Standardised fluorine-18 solutions and/or standardisation services are available from laboratories recognised by the competent authority.

Results The spectrum obtained with the solution to be examined does not differ significantly from that obtained with a standardised fluorine-18 solution.

B. Half-life: 19.9 min to 20.9 min.

RADIOCHEMICAL PURITY

[1-^{11}C]Acetate

Liquid chromatography (*2.2.29*) as described in the test for acetate.

Limit Examine the chromatograms obtained with the spectrophotometer and the radioactivity detector:
— total of [1-^{11}C]acetate: minimum 95 per cent of the total radioactivity.

RADIOACTIVITY

Measure the radioactivity using suitable equipment by comparison with a standardised fluorine-18 solution or by measurement with a calibrated instrument.

LABELLING

The accompanying information specifies the maximum recommended dose in millilitres.

_____ *Ph Eur*

Sodium Chromate (^{51}Cr) Sterile Solution

(*Ph Eur monograph 0279*)

Ph Eur _____

DEFINITION

Sterile solution of sodium [^{51}Cr]chromate made isotonic by the addition of sodium chloride.

Chromium-51

90 per cent to 110 per cent of the declared chromium-51 radioactivity at the date and time stated on the label.

Specific radioactivity

Minimum 370 MBq of chromium-51 per milligram of chromate ion.

CHARACTERS

Appearance

Clear, colourless or slightly yellow solution.

Half-life and nature of radiation of chromium-51

See general chapter *5.7. Table of physical characteristics of radionuclides*.

IDENTIFICATION

A. Gamma-ray spectrometry.

Result The only gamma photon of chromium-51 has an energy of 0.320 MeV.

B. Examine the chromatogram obtained in the test for radiochemical purity (see Tests).

Result The retardation factor of the principal peak in the radiochromatogram obtained with the test solution is about 0.9.

TESTS

pH (*2.2.3*)

6.0 to 8.5.

Total chromate

Maximum 2.7 µg of chromate ion (CrO_4^{2-}) per MBq.

Test solution The preparation to be examined.

Reference solution 1.7 mg/L solution of *potassium chromate R*.

Measure the absorbance of the solutions (*2.2.25*) at the absorption maximum at 370 nm. If necessary, adjust the test solution and the reference solution to pH 8.0 by adding *sodium hydrogen carbonate solution R*. Calculate the content of chromate in the preparation to be examined using the measured absorbances.

Sterility

It complies with the test for sterility prescribed in the monograph *Radiopharmaceutical preparations (0125)*.

The preparation may be released for use before completion of the test.

RADIONUCLIDIC PURITY

Chromium-51

Gamma-ray spectrometry.

Result The spectrum obtained with the preparation to be examined does not differ significantly from that obtained with a standardised chromium-51 solution.

RADIOCHEMICAL PURITY

[^{51}Cr]Chromate ion

Ascending paper chromatography (*2.2.26*).

Test solution The preparation to be examined.

Paper *paper for chromatography R*.

Mobile phase *ammonia R*, *ethanol (96 per cent) R*, *water R* (25:50:125 *V/V/V*).

Application A volume of the solution sufficient for the detection method.

Development Immediately, for 2.5 h.

Detection Suitable detector to determine the distribution of the radioactivity.

Retardation factor Impurity A = 0.0 to 0.1; chromate ion = about 0.9.

Limit:
— *[^{51}Cr]chromate ion*: minimum 90 per cent of the total radioactivity due to chromium-51.

RADIOACTIVITY

Determine the radioactivity using a calibrated instrument.

IMPURITIES

A. [^{51}Cr]chromium(III) ion.

_____ *Ph Eur*

Sodium Fluoride (¹⁸F) Injection

(Ph Eur monograph 2100)

Ph Eur

DEFINITION

Sterile solution containing fluorine-18 in the form of sodium fluoride. It may contain carrier fluoride and a suitable buffer.

Content:

— *fluorine-18*: 90 per cent to 110 per cent of the declared fluorine-18 radioactivity at the date and hour stated on the label,

— *fluoride*: maximum 4.52 mg per maximum recommended dose in millilitres.

PRODUCTION

The radionuclide fluorine-18 is most commonly produced by proton irradiation of water enriched in oxygen-18. Fluorine-18 in the form of fluoride is recovered from the target water, generally by adsorption and desorption from anion-exchange resins or electrochemical deposition and redissolution.

CHARACTERS

Appearance

Clear, colourless solution.

Half-life and nature of radiation of fluorine-18

See general chapter 5.7. *Table of physical characteristics of radionuclides.*

IDENTIFICATION

A. Gamma-ray spectrometry.

Results The only gamma photons have an energy of 0.511 MeV and, depending on the measurement geometry, a sum peak of 1.022 MeV may be observed.

B. It complies with test B for radionuclidic purity (see Tests).

C. Examine the chromatograms obtained in the test for radiochemical purity (see Tests).

Results The principal peak in the radiochromatogram obtained with the test solution is similar in retention time to the principal peak in the chromatogram obtained with the reference solution. In the chromatogram obtained with the reference solution, the peak due to fluoride is negative.

TESTS

pH *(2.2.3)*

5.0 to 8.5.

Fluoride

Liquid chromatography *(2.2.29)*.

Test solution The preparation to be examined.

Reference solution Dissolve 10 mg of *sodium fluoride R* in *water R* and dilute to V with the same solvent, V being the maximum recommended dose in millilitres.

Column:

— *size: l = 0.25 m, Ø = 4 mm,*

— *stationary phase: strongly basic anion-exchange resin for chromatography R* (10 μm),

— *temperature:* constant, between 20 °C and 30 °C.

Mobile phase 4 g/L solution of *sodium hydroxide R*, protected from atmospheric carbon dioxide.

Flow rate 1 mL/min.

Detection Spectrophotometer at 220 nm and a radioactivity detector connected in series.

Injection 20 μL.

Run time 15 min.

System suitability Examine the chromatogram obtained with the reference solution using the spectrophotometer:

— *signal-to-noise ratio*: minimum 10 for the principal peak,

— *retention time of fluoride*: minimum 3 times the hold-up time.

Limit Examine the chromatogram obtained with the spectrophotometer:

— *fluoride*: not more than the area of the corresponding peak in the chromatogram obtained with the reference solution (4.52 mg/V).

Sterility

It complies with the test for sterility prescribed in the monograph on *Radiopharmaceutical preparations (0125)*. The injection may be released for use before completion of the test.

Bacterial endotoxins *(2.6.14)*

Less than 175/V IU/mL, V being the maximum recommended dose in millilitres. The injection may be released for use before completion of the test.

RADIONUCLIDIC PURITY

Fluorine-18

Minimum 99.9 per cent of the total radioactivity.

The preparation may be released for use before completion of the tests.

A. Gamma-ray spectrometry.

Determine the amount of fluorine-18 and radionuclidic impurities with a half-life longer than 2 h. For the detection and quantification of impurities, retain the preparation to be examined for a sufficient time to allow the fluorine-18 to decay to a level which permits the detection of impurities.

Results The spectrum obtained with the preparation to be examined does not differ significantly from that of a background spectrum.

B. Half-life: 105 min to 115 min.

RADIOCHEMICAL PURITY

[¹⁸F]fluoride

Liquid chromatography *(2.2.29)* as described in the test for fluoride. If necessary, dilute the test solution with water R to obtain a radioactivity concentration suitable for the radioactivity detector.

Limit Examine the chromatogram obtained with the radioactivity detector:

— *[¹⁸F]fluoride*: minimum 98.5 per cent of the total radioactivity.

RADIOACTIVITY

Determine the radioactivity using a calibrated instrument.

LABELLING

The label states the maximum recommended dose in millilitres.

_____ *Ph Eur*

Sodium Iodide (¹²³I) Injection

(Ph Eur monograph 0563)

Ph Eur ___

DEFINITION

Sterile solution containing iodine-123 in the form of sodium iodide; it may contain sodium thiosulfate or some other suitable reducing agent and a suitable buffer.

Content

90 per cent to 110 per cent of the declared iodine-123 radioactivity at the date and hour stated on the label.

PRODUCTION

Iodine-123 is obtained by proton irradiation of xenon enriched in xenon-124 (minimum 98 per cent) followed by the decay of xenon-123 which is formed directly and by the decay of caesium-123. No carrier iodide is added.

CHARACTERS

Appearance

Clear, colourless solution.

Half-life and nature of radiation of iodine-123

See general chapter 5.7. *Table of physical characteristics of radionuclides.*

IDENTIFICATION

A. Gamma-ray spectrometry.

Results The spectrum obtained with the preparation to be examined does not differ significantly from that of a standardised iodine-123 solution. The most prominent gamma photon has an energy of 0.159 MeV and is accompanied by the principal X-ray of 0.027 MeV.

B. Examine the chromatograms obtained in the test for radiochemical purity.

Results The principal peak in the radiochromatogram obtained with the test solution is similar in retention time to the principal peak in the chromatogram obtained with reference solution (a).

TESTS

pH (*2.2.3*)

7.0 to 10.0.

Sterility

It complies with the test for sterility prescribed in the monograph on *Radiopharmaceutical preparations (0125)*. The preparation may be released for use before completion of the test.

RADIONUCLIDIC PURITY

Iodine-123

Minimum 99.65 per cent of the total radioactivity.

Gamma-ray spectrometry.

Determine the relative amounts of iodine-123, iodine-125, tellurium-121 and other radionuclidic impurities present. For the detection of tellurium-121 and iodine-125, retain the preparation to be examined for a sufficient time to allow iodine-123 to decay to a level which permits the detection of radionuclidic impurities. No radionuclides with a half-life longer than that of iodine-125 are detected.

The preparation may be released for use before completion of the test.

RADIOCHEMICAL PURITY

[¹²³I]iodide

Liquid chromatography (*2.2.29*).

Test solution Dilute the preparation to be examined with a 2 g/L solution of *sodium hydroxide R* to a radioactive concentration suitable for the detector. Add an equal volume of a solution containing 1 g/L of *potassium iodide R*, 2 g/L of *potassium iodate R* and 10 g/L of *sodium hydrogen carbonate R* and mix.

Reference solution (a) Dilute 1 mL of a 26.2 mg/L solution of *potassium iodide R* to 10 mL with *water R*.

Reference solution (b) Dilute 1 mL of a 24.5 mg/L solution of *potassium iodate R* to 10 mL with *water R*. Mix equal volumes of this solution and reference solution (a).

Column:
— *size: l* = 0.25 m, Ø = 4.0 mm,
— *stationary phase: octadecylsilyl silica gel for chromatography R* (5 μm),
— *temperature*: constant between 20 °C and 30 °C.

Mobile phase Dissolve 5.85 g of *sodium chloride R* in 1000 mL of *water R*, add 0.65 mL of *octylamine R* and adjust to pH 7.0 with *dilute phosphoric acid R*; add 50 mL of *acetonitrile R* and mix.

Flow rate 1.5 mL/min.

Detection Spectrophotometer at 220 nm and a radioactivity detector connected in series.

Injection 20 μL.

Run time 12 min.

Relative retention With reference to iodide (retention time = about 5 min): iodate = 0.2 to 0.3.

System suitability Reference solution (b):
— *resolution*: minimum 2 between the peaks due to iodide and iodate in the chromatogram recorded with the spectrophotometer.

Limit Examine the chromatogram obtained with the test solution using the radioactivity detector and locate the peak due to iodide by comparison with the chromatogram obtained with reference solution (a) using the spectrophotometer:
— *[¹²³I]iodide*: minimum 95 per cent of the total radioactivity.

RADIOACTIVITY

Determine the radioactivity using a calibrated instrument.

LABELLING

The label states the name of any excipient.

IMPURITIES

A. [¹²³I]iodate ion.

___ *Ph Eur*

Sodium Iodide (¹²³I) Solution for Radiolabelling

(Ph Eur monograph 2314)

Ph Eur ___

DEFINITION

Strongly alkaline solution containing iodine-123 in the form of sodium iodide.

Content

90 per cent to 110 per cent of the declared iodine-123 radioactivity at the date and hour stated on the label.

PRODUCTION

Iodine-123 is obtained by proton irradiation of xenon highly enriched in xenon-124 followed by the decay of directly formed xenon-123 and by the decay of caesium-123. No carrier iodide or reducing agents are added.

CHARACTERS

Appearance

Clear, colourless solution.

Half-life and nature of radiation of iodine-123

See general *chapter 5.7. Table of physical characteristics of radionuclides.*

IDENTIFICATION

A. Gamma-ray spectrometry.

Results The most prominent gamma photon of iodine-123 has an energy of 0.159 MeV and is accompanied by the principal X-ray of 0.027 MeV.

B. Examine the chromatograms obtained in the test for radiochemical purity (see Tests).

Results The principal peak in the radiochromatogram obtained with the test solution is similar in retention time to the principal peak in the chromatogram obtained with reference solution (a).

TESTS

Alkalinity *(2.2.4)*

The solution is strongly alkaline.

RADIONUCLIDIC PURITY

Iodine-123

Minimum 99.7 per cent of the total radioactivity.

Gamma-ray spectrometry.

Determine the relative amounts of iodine-123, iodine-125, tellurium-121 and other radionuclidic impurities present. For the detection of tellurium-121 and iodine-125, retain the solution to be examined for a sufficient time to allow iodine-123 to decay to a level which permits the detection of radionuclidic impurities. No radionuclides with a half-life longer than that of iodine-125 are detected.

The solution may be released for use before completion of the test.

RADIOCHEMICAL PURITY

[^{123}I]iodide

Liquid chromatography *(2.2.29).*

Test solution Dilute the solution to be examined with an equal volume of a solution containing 1 g/L of *potassium iodide R*, 2 g/L of *potassium iodate R* and 10 g/L of *sodium hydrogen carbonate R* and mix. If necessary, first dilute the solution to be examined with a 2 g/L solution of *sodium hydroxide R* to ensure that the final mixture has a radioactivity concentration suitable for the radioactivity detector.

Reference solution (a) Dissolve 10 mg of *potassium iodide R* in *water R* and dilute to 10 mL with the same solvent.

Reference solution (b) Dissolve 20 mg of *potassium iodate R* in *water R* and dilute to 10 mL with the same solvent. Mix equal volumes of this solution and reference solution (a).

Column:
— *size: l* = 0.25 m, Ø = 4.0 mm;
— *stationary phase: octadecylsilyl silica gel for chromatography R* (5 µm);
— *temperature*: constant, between 20 °C and 30 °C.

Use stainless steel tubing.

Mobile phase Dissolve 5.85 g of *sodium chloride R* in 1000 mL of *water R*, add 0.65 mL of *octylamine R* and adjust to pH 7.0 with *dilute phosphoric acid R*; add 50 mL of *acetonitrile R* and mix.

Flow rate 1.5 mL/min.

Detection Spectrophotometer at 220 nm and a radioactivity detector connected in series.

Injection 20 µL.

Run time 12 min.

Relative retention With reference to iodide (retention time = about 5 min): iodate = 0.2 to 0.3.

System suitability Reference solution (b):
— *resolution*: minimum 2 between the peaks due to iodide and iodate in the chromatogram recorded with the spectrophotometer.

Examine the chromatogram obtained with the test solution using the radioactivity detector and locate the peak due to iodide by comparison with the chromatogram obtained with reference solution (a) using the spectrophotometer.

Limit:
— [^{123}I]iodide: minimum 95 per cent of the total radioactivity.

RADIOACTIVITY

Determine the radioactivity using a calibrated instrument.

LABELLING

The label states:
— the name of any excipient;
— that the solution is not for direct administration to humans.

IMPURITIES

A. iodine-125,

B. tellurium-121,

C. [^{123}I]iodate ion.

_____ *Ph Eur*

Sodium Iodide (^{131}I) Capsules for Diagnostic Use

(Ph Eur monograph 0938)

Ph Eur _____

DEFINITION

Capsules for diagnostic use containing iodine-131 in the form of sodium iodide on a solid support; they may contain sodium thiosulfate or some other suitable reducing agents and a suitable buffering substance. A package contains 1 or more capsules.

Content:
— iodine-131: maximum 37 MBq per capsule; the average radioactivity determined in the test for uniformity of content is 90 per cent to 110 per cent of the declared iodine-131 radioactivity at the date and hour stated on the label;
— iodide: maximum 20 µg per capsule.

PRODUCTION

Iodine-131 is obtained by neutron irradiation of tellurium or by extraction from uranium fission products. No carrier iodide is added.

CHARACTERS

Half-life and nature of radiation of iodine-131

See general chapter *5.7. Table of physical characteristics of radionuclides.*

IDENTIFICATION

A. Gamma-ray spectrometry.

Results The spectrum obtained with the preparation to be examined does not differ significantly from that of a standardised iodine-131 solution. The most prominent gamma photon has an energy of 0.365 MeV.

B. Examine the chromatograms obtained in the test for radiochemical purity.

Results The principal peak in the radiochromatogram obtained with test solution (b) is similar in retention time to the principal peak in the chromatogram obtained with reference solution (a).

TESTS

Disintegration

The contents of the capsule dissolve completely within 15 min.

In a water-bath at 37 °C, warm in a small beaker about 20 mL of a 2.0 g/L solution of *potassium iodide R*. Add a capsule to be examined. Stir magnetically at 20 r/min.

Uniformity of content

Determine the radioactivity of each of not fewer than 10 capsules. Calculate the average radioactivity per capsule. The radioactivity of no capsule differs by more than 10 per cent from the average, the relative standard deviation is not greater than 3.5 per cent.

Iodide

Liquid chromatography (*2.2.29*).

Test solution (a) Dissolve a capsule to be examined in 10 mL of *water R*. Filter through a 0.2 μm filter.

Test solution (b) Dissolve a capsule to be examined in *water R*. Filter through a 0.2 μm filter and dilute the filtrate with a 2 g/L solution of *sodium hydroxide R* to a radioactive concentration suitable for the detector. Add an equal volume of a solution containing 1 g/L of *potassium iodide R*, 2 g/L of *potassium iodate R* and 10 g/L of *sodium hydrogen carbonate R* and mix.

Reference solution (a) Dilute 1 mL of a 26.2 mg/L solution of *potassium iodide R* to 10 mL with *water R*.

Reference solution (b) Dilute 1 mL of a 24.5 mg/L solution of *potassium iodate R* to 10 mL with *water R*. Mix equal volumes of this solution and reference solution (a).

Blank solution Prepare a solution containing 2 mg/mL of each constituent stated on the label, apart from iodide.

Column:
— *size: l* = 0.25 m, Ø = 4.0 mm,
— *stationary phase: octadecylsilyl silica gel for chromatography R* (5 μm),
— *temperature*: constant between 20 °C and 30 °C.

Mobile phase Dissolve 5.85 g of *sodium chloride R* in 1000 mL of *water R*, add 0.65 mL of *octylamine R* and adjust to pH 7.0 with *dilute phosphoric acid R*; add 50 mL of *acetonitrile R* and mix.

Flow rate 1.5 mL/min.

Detection Spectrophotometer at 220 nm and radioactivity detector connected in series.

Injection 20 μL of test solution (a), reference solutions (a) and (b) and the blank solution.

Run time 12 min.

Relative retention With reference to iodide (retention time = about 5 min): iodate = 0.2 to 0.3.

System suitability:
— in the chromatogram obtained with the blank solution, none of the peaks has a retention time similar to that of the peak due to iodide,
— *resolution*: minimum 2 between the peaks due to iodide and iodate in the chromatogram obtained with reference solution (b) recorded with the spectrophotometer.

Limit Examine the chromatograms obtained with the spectrophotometer:
— *iodide*: not more than the area of the corresponding peak in the chromatogram obtained with reference solution (a) (20 μg/capsule).

RADIONUCLIDIC PURITY

Iodine-131

Minimum 99.9 per cent of the total radioactivity.

Gamma-ray spectrometry.

Determine the relative amounts of iodine-131, iodine-133, iodine-135 and other radionuclidic impurities present.

RADIOCHEMICAL PURITY

[^{131}I]iodide

Liquid chromatography (*2.2.29*) as described in the test for iodide with the following modifications.

Injection 20 μL of test solution (b) and reference solution (a).

Limit Examine the chromatogram obtained with the test solution using the radioactivity detector and locate the peak due to iodide by comparison with the chromatogram obtained with reference solution (a) using the spectrophotometer:
— [^{131}I]iodide: minimum 95 per cent of the total radioactivity.

RADIOACTIVITY

Determine the radioactivity of the package using a calibrated instrument.

LABELLING

The label states the name of any excipient and the number of capsules in the package.

IMPURITIES

A. [^{131}I]iodate ion.

                                         Ph Eur

Sodium Iodide (^{131}I) Capsules for Therapeutic Use

(*Ph Eur monograph 2116*)

Ph Eur ⎯⎯⎯⎯⎯⎯⎯⎯⎯⎯⎯⎯⎯⎯⎯⎯⎯⎯⎯

DEFINITION

Capsules for therapeutic use containing iodine-131 in the form of sodium iodide on a solid support; they contain sodium thiosulfate or some other suitable reducing agents and a suitable buffering substance.

Content:
— iodine-131: 90 per cent to 110 per cent of the declared radioactivity at the date and hour stated on the label,
— iodide: maximum 20 μg per capsule.

PRODUCTION

Iodine-131 is obtained by neutron irradiation of tellurium or by extraction from uranium fission products. No carrier iodide is added.

CHARACTERS

Half-life and nature of radiation of iodine-131

See general chapter *5.7. Table of physical characteristics of radionuclides.*

IDENTIFICATION

A. Gamma-ray spectrometry.

Results The spectrum obtained with the preparation to be examined does not differ significantly from that of a standardised iodine-131 solution. The most prominent gamma photon of iodine-131 has an energy of 0.365 MeV.

B. Examine the chromatograms obtained in the test for radiochemical purity.

Results The principal peak in the radiochromatogram obtained with test solution (b) is similar in retention time to the principal peak in the chromatogram obtained with reference solution (a).

TESTS

Disintegration

The contents of the capsule dissolve completely within 15 min.

In a water-bath at 37 °C, warm in a small beaker about 20 mL of a 2.0 g/L solution of *potassium iodide R*. Add a capsule to be examined. Stir magnetically at a rotation rate of 20 r/min.

Iodide

Liquid chromatography (*2.2.29*).

Test solution (a) Dissolve a capsule to be examined in 10 mL of *water R*. Filter through a 0.2 µm filter.

Test solution (b) Dissolve a capsule to be examined in *water R*. Filter through a 0.2 µm filter and dilute the filtrate with an equal volume of a solution containing 1 g/L of *potassium iodide R*, 2 g/L of *potassium iodate R* and 10 g/L of *sodium hydrogen carbonate R*. If necessary, first dilute the filtrate with a 2 g/L solution of *sodium hydroxide R* to ensure that the final mixture has a radioactivity concentration suitable for the radioactivity detector.

Reference solution (a) Dilute 1.0 mL of a 26.2 mg/L solution of *potassium iodide R* to 10.0 mL with *water R*.

Reference solution (b) Dilute 1 mL of a 24.5 mg/L solution of *potassium iodate R* to 10 mL with *water R*. Mix equal volumes of this solution with reference solution (a).

Blank solution Prepare a solution containing 2 mg/mL of each excipient stated on the label, apart from iodide.

Column:
— *size: l* = 0.25 m, Ø = 4.0 mm,
— *stationary phase:* octadecylsilyl silica gel for chromatography R (5 µm),
— *temperature:* constant, between 20 °C and 30 °C.

Use stainless steel tubing.

Mobile phase Dissolve 5.85 g of *sodium chloride R* in 1000 mL of *water R*, add 0.65 mL of *octylamine R* and adjust to pH 7.0 with *dilute phosphoric acid R*; add 50 mL of *acetonitrile R* and mix.

Flow rate 1.5 mL/min.

Detection Spectrophotometer at 220 nm and radioactivity detector connected in series.

Injection 20 µL of test solution (a), reference solutions (a) and (b) and the blank solution.

Run time 12 min.

Relative retention With reference to iodide (retention time = about 5 min): iodate = 0.2 to 0.3.

System suitability:
— in the chromatogram obtained with the blank solution, none of the peaks has a retention time similar to that of the peak due to iodide;
— *resolution:* minimum 2 between the peaks due to iodide and iodate in the chromatogram obtained with reference solution (b) using the spectrophotometer.

Limits Examine the chromatograms obtained with the spectrophotometer; locate the peak due to iodide by comparison with the chromatogram obtained with reference solution (a):
— *iodide:* not more than the area of the corresponding peak in the chromatogram obtained with reference solution (a) (20 µg/capsule).

RADIONUCLIDIC PURITY

Iodine-131

Minimum 99.9 per cent of the total radioactivity.

Gamma-ray spectrometry.

Determine the relative amounts of iodine-130, iodine-131, iodine-133, iodine-135 and other radionuclidic impurities present.

RADIOCHEMICAL PURITY

[131I]iodide

Liquid chromatography (*2.2.29*) as described in the test for iodide with the following modifications.

Injection 20 µL of test solution (b) and reference solution (a).

Limits Examine the chromatogram obtained with test solution (b) using the radioactivity detector and locate the peak due to iodide by comparison with the chromatogram obtained with reference solution (a) using the spectrophotometer:
— *[131I]iodide:* minimum 95 per cent of the total radioactivity.

RADIOACTIVITY

Determine the radioactivity of each capsule using a calibrated instrument.

LABELLING

The label states the name of any excipient.

IMPURITIES

A. [131I]iodate ion,

B. iodine-130,

C. iodine-133,

D. iodine-135.

Ph Eur

Sodium Iodide (131I) Solution

(*Ph Eur monograph 0281*)

Ph Eur

DEFINITION

Solution containing iodine-131 in the form of sodium iodide and also sodium thiosulfate or some other suitable reducing agent. It may contain a suitable buffer.

Content:
— *iodine-131:* 90 per cent to 110 per cent of the declared radioactivity at the date and hour stated on the label,
— *iodide:* maximum 20 µg in the maximum recommended dose in millilitres.

PRODUCTION

Iodine-131 is a radioactive isotope of iodine and may be obtained by neutron irradiation of tellurium or by extraction from uranium fission products. No carrier iodide is added.

CHARACTERS

Appearance

Clear, colourless solution.

Half-life and nature of radiation of iodine-131

See general chapter 5.7. *Table of physical characteristics of radionuclides.*

IDENTIFICATION

A. Gamma-ray spectrometry.

Results The spectrum obtained with the preparation to be examined does not differ significantly from that of a standardised iodine-131 solution. The most prominent gamma photon has an energy of 0.365 MeV.

B. Examine the chromatograms obtained in the test for iodide.

Results The principal peak in the radiochromatogram obtained with test solution (a) is similar in retention time to the principal peak in the chromatogram obtained with reference solution (a).

TESTS

pH (2.2.3)

7.0 to 10.0.

Sterility

If intended for parenteral administration, it complies with the test for sterility prescribed in the monograph on *Radiopharmaceutical preparations (0125)*. The solution may be released for use before completion of the test.

Iodide

Liquid chromatography (2.2.29).

Test solution (a) The preparation to be examined.

Test solution (b) Dilute the preparation to be examined with 0.05 M sodium hydroxide until the radioactivity is equivalent to about 74 MBq/mL. Add an equal volume of a solution containing 1 g/L of *potassium iodide R*, 2 g/L of *potassium iodate R* and 10 g/L of *sodium hydrogen carbonate R* and mix.

Reference solution (a) Dilute 1 mL of a 26.2 mg/L solution of *potassium iodide R* to V with *water R*, V being the maximum recommended dose in millilitres.

Reference solution (b) Dilute 1 mL of a 24.5 mg/L solution of *potassium iodate R* to V with *water R*, V being the maximum recommended dose in millilitres. Mix equal volumes of this solution and of reference solution (a).

Blank solution Prepare a solution containing 2 mg/mL of each of the components stated on the label, apart from iodide.

Column:
— *size:* l = 0.25 m, Ø = 4.0 mm,
— *stationary phase:* octadecylsilyl silica gel for chromatography R (5 μm),
— *temperature:* maintain at a constant temperature between 20 °C and 30 °C.

Use stainless steel tubing.

Mobile phase Dissolve 5.844 g of *sodium chloride R* in 1000 mL of *water R*, add 650 μL of *octylamine R* and adjust to pH 7.0 with *phosphoric acid R*; add 50 mL of *acetonitrile R* and mix.

Flow rate 1.5 mL/min.

Detection Spectrophotometer at 220 nm and radioactivity detector connected in series.

Injection 25 μL; inject test solution (a), the blank solution and reference solutions (a) and (b).

Run time 12 min.

Relative retention With reference to iodide (retention time = about 5 min): iodate = 0.2 to 0.3.

System suitability:
— in the chromatogram obtained with the blank solution, none of the peaks shows a retention time similar to that of the peak due to iodide,
— *resolution:* minimum 2 between the peaks due to iodide and iodate in the chromatogram obtained with reference solution (b) recorded with the spectrophotometer.

Limit Examine the chromatogram obtained with the spectrophotometer; locate the peak due to iodide by comparison with the chromatogram obtained with reference solution (a):
— *iodide:* not more than the area of the corresponding peak in the chromatogram obtained with reference solution (a).

RADIONUCLIDIC PURITY

Iodine-131

Minimum 99.9 per cent of the total radioactivity.

Gamma-ray spectrometry.

Determine the relative amounts of iodine-131, iodine-133, iodine-135 and other radionuclidic impurities present.

RADIOCHEMICAL PURITY

[^{131}I]Iodide

Liquid chromatography (2.2.29) as described in the test for iodide with the following modification.

Injection Test solution (b).

Limit Examine the chromatogram obtained with the radioactivity detector:
— *[^{131}I]iodide:* minimum 95 per cent of the total radioactivity.

RADIOACTIVITY

Measure the radioactivity using suitable equipment by comparison with a standardised iodine-131 solution or by using a calibrated instrument.

LABELLING

The label states:
— the name of any excipient,
— the maximum recommended dose, in millilitres,
— where applicable, that the preparation is suitable for use in the manufacture of parenteral preparations.

IMPURITIES

A. [^{131}I]iodate ion.

_____ *Ph Eur*

Sodium Iodide (^{131}I) Solution For Radiolabelling

(*Ph Eur monograph 2121*)

Ph Eur _____

DEFINITION

Strongly alkaline solution containing iodine-131 in the form of sodium iodide. It does not contain a reducing agent.

Content

90 per cent to 110 per cent of the declared iodine-131 radioactivity at the date and hour stated on the label.

PRODUCTION

Iodine-131 may be obtained by neutron irradiation of tellurium or by extraction from uranium fission products. No carrier iodide is added.

CHARACTERS

Appearance

Clear, colourless solution.

Half-life and nature of radiation of iodine-131

See general chapter 5.7. *Table of physical characteristics of radionuclides.*

IDENTIFICATION

A. Gamma-ray spectrometry.

Results The spectrum obtained with the preparation to be examined does not differ significantly from that of a standardised iodine-131 solution. The most prominent gamma photon of iodine-131 has an energy of 0.365 MeV.

B. Examine the chromatograms obtained in the test for radiochemical purity (see Tests).

Results The principal peak in the radiochromatogram obtained with the test solution is similar in retention time to the principal peak in the chromatogram obtained with reference solution (a).

TESTS

Alkalinity (2.2.4)

The preparation is strongly alkaline.

RADIONUCLIDIC PURITY

Iodine-131

Minimum 99.9 per cent of the total radioactivity.

Gamma-ray spectrometry.

Determine the relative amounts of iodine-130, iodine-131, iodine-133, iodine-135 and other radionuclidic impurities present.

RADIOCHEMICAL PURITY

[^{131}I]iodide

Liquid chromatography (2.2.29).

Test solution Dilute the preparation to be examined with an equal volume of a solution containing 1 g/L of *potassium iodide R*, 2 g/L of *potassium iodate R* and 10 g/L of *sodium hydrogen carbonate R* and mix. If necessary, first dilute the preparation to be examined with a 2 g/L solution of *sodium hydroxide R* to ensure that the final mixture has a radioactivity concentration suitable for the radioactivity detector.

Reference solution (a) Dissolve 10 mg of *potassium iodide R* in *water R* and dilute to 10 mL with the same solvent.

Reference solution (b) Dissolve 20 mg of *potassium iodate R* in *water R* and dilute to 10 mL with the same solvent. Mix equal volumes of this solution and reference solution (a).

Column:
— *size:* l = 0.25 m, Ø = 4.0 mm,
— *stationary phase:* octadecylsilyl silica gel for chromatography R (5 μm),
— *temperature:* constant, between 20 °C and 30 °C.

Use stainless steel tubing.

Mobile phase Dissolve 5.85 g of *sodium chloride R* in 1000 mL of *water R*, add 0.65 mL of *octylamine R* and adjust to pH 7.0 with *dilute phosphoric acid R*; add 50 mL of *acetonitrile R* and mix.

Flow rate 1.5 mL/min.

Detection Spectrophotometer at 220 nm and a radioactivity detector connected in series.

Injection 20 μL.

Run time 12 min.

Relative retention With reference to iodide (retention time = about 5 min): iodate = 0.2 to 0.3.

System suitability Reference solution (b):
— *resolution:* minimum 2 between the peaks due to iodide and iodate in the chromatogram recorded with the spectrophotometer.

Limit Examine the chromatogram obtained with the radioactivity detector:
— [^{131}I]iodide: minimum 95 per cent of the total radioactivity.

RADIOACTIVITY

Determine the radioactivity using a calibrated instrument.

LABELLING

The label states:
— the method of production of iodine-131,
— the name of any excipient,
— that the preparation is not for direct human use.

IMPURITIES

A. [^{131}I]iodate ion.

Ph Eur

Sodium Iodohippurate (^{123}I) Injection

(Ph Eur monograph 0564)

Ph Eur

DEFINITION

Sterile solution of sodium (2-[^{123}I]iodobenzamido)acetate. It may contain a suitable buffer and a suitable antimicrobial preservative such as benzyl alcohol.

Iodine-123

90 per cent to 110 per cent of the declared iodine-123 radioactivity at the date and time stated on the label.

Specific radioactivity

0.74 GBq to 10.0 GBq of iodine-123 per gram of sodium 2-iodohippurate.

CHARACTERS

Appearance

Clear, colourless solution.

Half-life and nature of radiation of iodine-123

See general chapter 5.7. *Table of physical characteristics of radionuclides.*

IDENTIFICATION

A. Gamma-ray and X-ray spectrometry.

Results The most prominent gamma photon has an energy of 0.159 MeV and is accompanied by an X-ray of 0.027 MeV.

B. Examine the chromatograms obtained in the test for radiochemical purity (see Tests).

Result The principal spot in the radiochromatogram obtained with the test solution is similar in retardation factor to the spot corresponding to 2-iodohippuric acid in the chromatogram obtained with the reference solution.

TESTS

pH (*2.2.3*)

3.5 to 8.5.

Sterility

It complies with the test for sterility prescribed in the monograph *Radiopharmaceutical preparations (0125)*. The preparation may be released for use before completion of the test.

RADIONUCLIDIC PURITY

The preparation may be released for use before completion of the test.

Radionuclides other than iodine-123

Maximum 0.35 per cent of the total radioactivity.

Gamma-ray and X-ray spectrometry.

Determine the relative amounts of iodine-125, tellurium-121 and other radionuclidic impurities present. For their detection, retain the preparation to be examined for a sufficient time to allow iodine-123 to decay to a level which permits the detection of radionuclidic impurities. Record the gamma-ray spectrum and X-ray spectrum of the decayed material. No radionuclides with a half-life longer than that of iodine-125 are detected.

RADIOCHEMICAL PURITY

2-[^{123}I]Iodohippuric acid

Thin-layer chromatography (*2.2.27*).

Test solution   Dissolve 1 g of *potassium iodide R* in 10 mL of *water R*, add 1 volume of this solution to 10 volumes of the preparation to be examined and use within 10 min of mixing. If necessary, dilute with the reference solution (carrier) to give a radioactive concentration sufficient for the detection method, for example 3.7 MBq per millilitre.

Reference solution (carrier)   Dissolve 40 mg of *2-iodobenzoic acid R* and 40 mg of *2-iodohippuric acid R* in 4 mL of a 4 g/L solution of *sodium hydroxide R*, add 10 mg of *potassium iodide R* and dilute to 10 mL with *water R*.

Plate   TLC silica gel GF$_{254}$ plate R.

Mobile phase   water R, glacial acetic acid R, butanol R, toluene R (1:4:20:80 *V/V/V/V*).

Application   10 µL.

Development   Over a path of 12 cm in about 75 min.

Drying   In air.

Detection   Examine in ultraviolet light at 254 nm and determine the distribution of radioactivity using a suitable detector.

Identification of spots   The chromatogram obtained with the reference solution shows a spot corresponding to 2-iodohippuric acid and nearer to the solvent front a spot corresponding to impurity D; impurity C remains near the point of application.

Limits:

— *2-[^{123}I]iodohippuric acid*: minimum 96 per cent of the total radioactivity due to iodine-123;

— *impurity C*: maximum 2 per cent of the total radioactivity due to iodine-123;

— *impurity D*: maximum 2 per cent of the total radioactivity due to iodine-123.

RADIOACTIVITY

Determine the radioactivity using a calibrated instrument.

STORAGE

Protected from light.

LABELLING

The label states whether or not the preparation is suitable for renal plasma-flow studies.

IMPURITIES

A. iodine-125,

B. tellurium-121,

C. [^{123}I]iodide,

D. 2-[^{123}I]iodobenzoic acid.

_____ *Ph Eur*

Sodium Iodohippurate (^{131}I) Injection

(*Ph Eur monograph 0282*)

Ph Eur _____

DEFINITION

Sterile solution of sodium 2-(2-[^{131}I]iodobenzamido)acetate. It may contain a suitable buffer and a suitable antimicrobial preservative such as benzyl alcohol.

Iodine-131

90 per cent to 110 per cent of the declared iodine-131 radioactivity at the date and time stated on the label.

Specific radioactivity

0.74 GBq to 7.4 GBq of iodine-131 per gram of sodium 2-iodohippurate.

CHARACTERS

Appearance

Clear, colourless solution.

Half-life and nature of radiation of iodine-131

See general chapter 5.7. *Table of physical characteristics of radionuclides*.

IDENTIFICATION

A. Gamma-ray spectrometry.

Result   The most prominent gamma photon of iodine-131 has an energy of 0.365 MeV.

B. Examine the chromatograms obtained in the test for radiochemical purity (see Tests).

Result   The principal peak in the radiochromatogram obtained with the test solution has a similar retardation factor as the spot corresponding to 2-iodohippuric acid in the chromatogram obtained with the reference solution.

TESTS

pH (*2.2.3*)

6.0 to 8.5.

Sterility

It complies with the test for sterility prescribed in the monograph *Radiopharmaceutical preparations (0125)*. The preparation may be released for use before completion of the test.

RADIONUCLIDIC PURITY

Iodine-131

Minimum 99.9 per cent of the total radioactivity.

Gamma-ray spectrometry.

Determine the relative amounts of iodine-131, iodine-133, iodine-135 and other radionuclidic impurities present.

RADIOCHEMICAL PURITY

2-[^{131}I]Iodohippuric acid

Thin-layer chromatography (*2.2.27*).

Test solution Dissolve 1 g of *potassium iodide R* in 10 mL of *water R*, add 1 volume of this solution to 10 volumes of the preparation to be examined and use within 10 min of mixing. If necessary dilute with the reference solution (carrier) to give a radioactive concentration sufficient for the detection method, for example 3.7 MBq/mL.

Reference solution (carrier) Dissolve 40 mg of *2-iodobenzoic acid R* and 40 mg of *2-iodohippuric acid R* in 4 mL of a 4 g/L solution of *sodium hydroxide R*, add 10 mg of *potassium iodide R* and dilute to 10 mL with *water R*.

Plate TLC silica gel GF_{254} *plate R*.

Mobile phase *water R*, *glacial acetic acid R*, *butanol R*, *toluene R* (1:4:20:80 *V/V/V/V*).

Application 10 μL.

Development Over a path of 12 cm in about 75 min.

Drying In air.

Detection In ultraviolet light at 254 nm and with a suitable detector to determine the distribution of radioactivity.

Identification of spots The chromatogram obtained with the reference solution shows a spot corresponding to 2-iodohippuric acid and nearer to the solvent front a spot corresponding to impurity C; impurity D remains near the point of application.

Limits:
— 2-[^{131}I]iodohippuric acid: minimum 96 per cent of the total radioactivity due to iodine-131;
— *impurity C*: maximum 2 per cent of the total radioactivity due to iodine-131;
— *impurity D*: maximum 2 per cent of the total radioactivity due to iodine-131.

RADIOACTIVITY

Determine the radioactivity using a calibrated instrument.

STORAGE

Protected from light.

LABELLING

The label states that the preparation is not necessarily suitable for renal plasma-flow studies.

IMPURITIES

A. iodine-133,

B. iodine-135,

C. 2-[^{131}I]iodobenzoic acid,

D. [^{131}I]iodide.

Ph Eur

Sodium Molybdate (^{99}Mo) Solution (Fission)

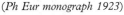

(Ph Eur monograph 1923)

Ph Eur _____

DEFINITION

Alkaline solution of sodium [^{99}Mo]molybdate obtained by extraction of fission products of uranium-235. It may contain stabilisers.

Content

90 per cent to 110 per cent of the declared molybdenum-99 radioactivity at the date and time stated on the label.

PRODUCTION

Molybdenum-99 is usually produced by fission of uranium enriched in uranium-235, which is caused by the absorption of a thermal neutron, resulting in high-specific-activity molybdenum-99. By the fission of uranium after neutron capture, more than 200 different radionuclides are produced. In approximately 6 per cent of the fissions, molybdenum-99 is formed after decay of a number of short-lived parent radionuclides. After dissolution of the target, the molybdenum-99 is separated from the mixture of nuclides and purified by using chromatographic processes in order to obtain molybdenum-99 with a high level of radionuclidic purity.

CHARACTERS

Appearance

Clear, colourless or almost colourless solution.

Half-life and nature of radiation of molybdenum-99

See general chapter 5.7. *Table of physical characteristics of radionuclides.*

IDENTIFICATION

A. Gamma-ray spectrometry.

Results The most prominent gamma photon of molybdenum-99 has an energy of 0.740 MeV; a peak with an energy of 0.141 MeV, due to technetium-99-m is also visible.

B. Examine the chromatograms obtained in the test for radiochemical purity (see Tests).

Results The principal peak in the radiochromatogram obtained with the test solution has a similar retardation factor to the principal spot in the chromatogram obtained with the reference solution.

TESTS

Solution S

Dilute the preparation to be examined to a radioactivity concentration of approximately 370 MBq/mL with a 2.42 g/L solution of *sodium molybdate R*.

Alkalinity

The preparation is alkaline (*2.2.4*).

RADIONUCLIDIC PURITY

Iodine-131, ruthenium-103 and tellurium-132:
— *iodine-131*: maximum 5×10^{-3} per cent of the total radioactivity;
— *ruthenium-103*: maximum 5×10^{-3} per cent of the total radioactivity;
— *tellurium-132*: maximum 5×10^{-3} per cent of the total radioactivity.

The following method has been found to be suitable; other validated methods, approved by the competent authority, may be used.

Gamma-ray spectrometry.

Condition a column with an internal volume of approximately 1.5 mL of *strongly basic anion exchange resin R* with a mixture of equal volumes of *glacial acetic acid R* and *water R*. All elutions of the column are made at a flow rate not exceeding 1 mL/min.

Test solution In a test-tube, successively add, with mixing, 1 mL of a 24.2 g/L solution of *sodium molybdate R*, 0.5 mL of *strong hydrogen peroxide solution R*, 2.5 mL of *glacial acetic acid R*, 1.0 mL of *iodine-123 and ruthenium-106 spiking solution R* and 1.0 mL of solution S. Allow to stand for 30 min at room temperature.

Reference solution Mix 1.0 mL of *iodine-123 and ruthenium-106 spiking solution R* and 4.0 mL of *water R*.

Apply the test solution to the column and elute. Just before the disappearance of the liquid from the top of the column, add 6 mL of a mixture of equal volumes of *glacial acetic acid R* and *water R* and elute. Transfer 5.0 mL of the

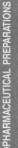

combined eluates to a counting tube. Determine the radioactivity of iodine-123, iodine-131, ruthenium-103, ruthenium-106 and iodine-132 at the gamma-ray energies of 0.159 MeV for iodine-123, 0.365 MeV for iodine-131, 0.497 MeV for ruthenium-103, 0.512 MeV for ruthenium-106 and 0.668 MeV for iodine-132. Determine in the same way the radioactivity of iodine-123 and ruthenium-106 in the reference solution and calculate the recovery of iodine-123 and ruthenium-106 in the combined eluates.

Calculate the radioactivity of iodine-131, iodine-132 and ruthenium-103 in the combined eluates, taking into account the recovery, the fraction of eluate used, the counting efficiency and the radioactive decay. From the radioactivity of iodine-132 (daughter radionuclide of tellurium-132), calculate the radioactivity of tellurium-132, taking into account the time of the test and the time of separation of molybdenum-99.

Total radioactivity due to strontium-89 and strontium-90

Maximum 6×10^{-5} per cent of the total radioactivity.

The following method has been found to be suitable; other validated methods, approved by the competent authority, may be used.

Liquid scintillation spectrometry.

Connect 2 columns, each with an internal volume of approximately 1.5 mL of *strongly basic anion exchange resin R*, in series and condition the columns with 10 mL of a 4 g/L solution of *sodium hydroxide R*. All elutions of the columns are made at a flow rate not exceeding 1 mL/min.

Test solution   In a test-tube, successively add, with mixing, 1.0 mL of solution S, 50 μL of *strontium-85 spiking solution R* and 0.05 mL of *strong sodium hypochlorite solution R*. Allow to stand for 10 min at room temperature.

Reference solution   Mix 50 μL of *strontium-85 spiking solution R* with 5.0 mL of a 9.5 g/L solution of *nitric acid R* in a vial for liquid scintillation counting and add 10 mL of *liquid scintillation cocktail R*.

Apply the test solution to the upper of the 2 columns and elute. Just before the disappearance of the liquid from the top of the upper column, add 3 mL of a 4 g/L solution of *sodium hydroxide R* and elute until the columns are dry. Combine the eluates and add 4 mL of a 947 g/L solution of *nitric acid R* (molybdenum-poor eluate). Determine the radioactivity due to molybdenum-99 using gamma-ray spectrometry. If the radioactivity due to molybdenum-99 is higher than 6×10^{-7} per cent of the radioactivity due to molybdenum-99 in 1 mL of solution S, repeat the above procedure using 2 new columns.

Condition a column with an internal volume of approximately 2 mL of *strontium selective extraction resin R* with 5 mL of a 473 g/L solution of *nitric acid R* and dry the column. All elutions of the column are made at a flow rate not exceeding 1 mL/min. Apply to the column the molybdenum-poor eluate and elute. Just before the disappearance of the liquid from the top of the column, add 20 mL of a 473 g/L solution of *nitric acid R* and elute until the column is dry. Rinse the column with 2 mL of a 9.5 g/L solution of *nitric acid R*, dry the column and discard the eluate. Elute the column with 8.0 mL of a 9.5 g/L solution of *nitric acid R* until the column is dry. Transfer 5.0 mL of the eluate into a vial for liquid scintillation counting and add 10 mL of *liquid scintillation cocktail R*.

Determine the total radioactivity due to strontium-89 and strontium-90 in this solution by liquid scintillation

spectrometry, and the radioactivity due to strontium-85 by gamma-ray spectrometry. Determine the radioactivity due to strontium-85 in the reference solution by gamma-ray spectrometry. Calculate the recovery of strontium-85 in the eluate. Calculate the measured total radioactivity of strontium-89 and strontium-90 in the eluate, taking into account the recovery of strontium and the fraction of eluate used.

Total radioactivity due to alpha-particle-emitting impurities

Maximum 1×10^{-7} per cent of the total radioactivity.

The following method has been found to be suitable; other validated methods, approved by the competent authority, may be used.

Alpha-ray spectrometry.

Test solution   To 0.2 mL of the preparation to be examined add 1.0 mL of *plutonium-242 spiking solution R*, 1.0 mL of *americium-243 spiking solution R* and 9.0 mL of a 927 g/L solution of *hydrochloric acid R*. Evaporate the sample to dryness. Dissolve the residue in 2 mL of a 927 g/L solution of *hydrochloric acid R*. Evaporate again to dryness. Dissolve the residue in 2 mL of a 10.3 g/L solution of *hydrochloric acid R*.

Apply the test solution to a column containing 0.7 g of *anion exchange resin R1*. Collect the eluate and wash the column with 1 mL of a 10.3 g/L solution of *hydrochloric acid R*. Evaporate the combined eluates to dryness and dissolve the residue in 2 mL of a 10.3 g/L solution of *hydrochloric acid R*. Apply this solution to a 2nd column containing 0.7 g of *anion exchange resin R1*. Collect the eluate and wash the column with 1 mL of a 10.3 g/L solution of *hydrochloric acid R*. Evaporate the combined eluates to dryness and dissolve the residue in 1 mL of *nitric acid R*. Evaporate to dryness. Dissolve the residue again in 1 mL of *nitric acid R*.

Add 1 mL of a 42.6 g/L solution of *anhydrous sodium sulfate R* and evaporate to dryness. Add 0.3 mL of *sulfuric acid R*. Warm until the residue is dissolved. Add 4 mL of *distilled water R* and 0.01 mL of *thymol blue solution R*. Add *concentrated ammonia R* dropwise until the colour changes from red to yellow.

Prepare an electrodeposition cell as follows.
An electropolished stainless steel planchet is fitted in the cap of a 20 mL polyethylene scintillation vial. The bottom of the vial has been cut off and a hole has been drilled through the centre of the cap for electrical connection to the planchet cathode. The planchet, 20 mm in diameter and 0.5 mm thick, is rinsed with *acetone R* and *water R* prior to use. The anode, a platinum spiral, is introduced through the bottom of the vial and fitted 5 mm from the cathode.

Pour the solution prepared as described above into the electrodeposition cell and rinse the container with a total of 5 mL of a 10 g/L solution of *sulfuric acid R* (the solution becomes slightly pink). Adjust to pH 2.1-2.4. with *concentrated ammonia R* or with a 200 g/L solution of *sulfuric acid R*. Electrolyse at 1.2 A for 75 min without stirring.

Add 1 mL of *concentrated ammonia R* about 1 min prior to switching off the current. Rinse the planchet with a 57 g/L solution of *ammonia R*. Rinse the planchet with *acetone R* and remove any residual solvent by patting the planchet with absorbent paper. Heat the planchet on a hot plate at 180 °C for 10 min.

Determine the radioactivity of alpha emitters by alpha-ray spectrometry, taking into account the recovery of the alpha-particle-emitting radionuclides (measured using the plutonium-242 and americium-243 spiking solutions).

Total of gamma-ray-emitting radionuclides other than molybdenum-99, technetium-99m, iodine-131, ruthenium-103 and tellurium-132

Maximum 1×10^{-2} per cent of the total radioactivity.

The following method has been found to be suitable; other validated methods, approved by the competent authority, may be used.

Gamma-ray spectrometry.

Allow the preparation to decay for 4-6 weeks. Examine the gamma-ray spectrum for the presence of other gamma-ray-emitting impurities. Identify and quantify other gamma-ray-emitting impurities. The preparation may be released for use before completion of the test.

RADIOCHEMICAL PURITY

[⁹⁹Mo]Molybdate

The following method has been found to be suitable; other validated methods, approved by the competent authority, may be used.

Thin-layer chromatography (2.2.27).

Test solution   Dilute the preparation to be examined with a 4.0 g/L solution of *sodium hydroxide R* to a radioactivity concentration suitable for the detector.

Reference solution   50 g/L solution of *sodium molybdate R* in a 4.0 g/L solution of *sodium hydroxide R*.

Plate   *TLC silica gel plate R.*

Mobile phase   10.6 g/L solution of *anhydrous sodium carbonate R*.

Application   5 μL of the test solution and 2 μL of the reference solution.

Development   Over 2/3 of the plate.

Drying   In a current of warm air.

Detection   Determine the distribution of radioactivity using a suitable detector and spray with a 2 g/L solution of *phenylhydrazine R* in *glacial acetic acid R*; heat at 100-105 °C for 5 min.

Retardation factor   Molybdate and pertechnetate = about 0.9.

Limit:
— sum of *[⁹⁹Mo]molybdate and [99mTc]pertechnetate*: minimum 95 per cent of the total radioactivity.

RADIOACTIVITY

Determine the radioactivity using a calibrated instrument.

LABELLING

The label states that the preparation is only suitable for the preparation of technetium-99m generators.

IMPURITIES

A. iodine-131,

B. ruthenium-103,

C. tellurium-132,

D. strontium-89,

E. strontium-90.

_____ *Ph Eur*

Sodium Pertechnetate (⁹⁹ᵐTc) Injection (Fission)

(Ph Eur monograph 0124)

Ph Eur _____

This monograph applies to sodium pertechnetate (⁹⁹ᵐTc) injection obtained from molybdenum-99 extracted from fission products of uranium. Sodium pertechnetate (⁹⁹ᵐTc) injection obtained from molybdenum-99 produced by neutron irradiation of molybdenum is described in the monograph Sodium pertechnetate (⁹⁹ᵐTc) injection (non-fission) (0283).

DEFINITION

Sterile solution containing technetium-99m in the form of pertechnetate ion and made isotonic by the addition of sodium chloride. The injection may be prepared from a sterile preparation of molybdenum-99 under aseptic conditions.

Technetium-99m

90 per cent to 110 per cent of the declared technetium-99m radioactivity at the date and time stated on the label.

CHARACTERS

Appearance

Clear, colourless solution.

Half-life and nature of radiation of technetium-99m

See general chapter 5.7. *Table of physical characteristics of radionuclides.*

IDENTIFICATION

Gamma-ray spectrometry.

Result: the most prominent gamma photon of technetium-99m has an energy of 0.141 MeV.

TESTS

pH (2.2.3)

4.0 to 8.0.

Aluminium

Maximum 5 ppm.

Test solution   In a test tube about 12 mm in internal diameter, mix 1 mL of *acetate buffer solution pH 4.6 R* and 2 mL of a 1 in 2.5 dilution of the preparation to be examined in *water R*. Add 0.05 mL of a 10 g/L solution of *chromazurol S R*.

Reference solution   Prepare at the same time and in the same manner as the test solution and using 2 mL of *aluminium standard solution (2 ppm Al) R*.

After 3 min, the colour of the test solution is not more intense than that of the reference solution.

Sterility

It complies with the test for sterility prescribed in the monograph *Radiopharmaceutical preparations (0125)*.

The preparation may be released for use before completion of the test.

RADIONUCLIDIC PURITY

Preliminary test   To obtain an approximate estimate before use of the preparation, take a volume equivalent to 37 MBq and determine the gamma-ray spectrum using a sodium iodide detector with a shield of lead, of thickness 6 mm, interposed between the sample and the detector.

The response in the region corresponding to the 0.740 MeV photon of molybdenum-99 does not exceed that obtained using 37 kBq of a standardised molybdenum-99 solution measured under the same conditions, when all measurements are expressed with reference to the date and time of administration.

Definitive test   Retain a sample of the preparation to be examined for a sufficient time to allow the technetium-99m radioactivity to decay to a sufficiently low level to permit the detection of radionuclidic impurities. All measurements of radioactivity are expressed with reference to the date and time of administration.
— *Impurity A*: Maximum 5×10^{-3} per cent of the total radioactivity.

Gamma-ray spectrometry. *Record the spectrum of the decayed material.*

Comparison   Suitable instrument calibrated with the aid of a standardised iodine-131 solution.

Results   The most prominent photon has an energy of 0.365 MeV; iodine-131 has a half-life of 8.04 days.
— *Impurity B*: maximum 0.1 per cent of the total radioactivity.

Gamma-ray spectrometry. *Record the spectrum of the decayed material.*

Comparison   Suitable instrument calibrated with the aid of a standardised molybdenum-99 solution.

Results   The most prominent photons have energies of 0.181 MeV, 0.740 MeV and 0.778 MeV; molybdenum-99 has a half-life of 66.0 h.
— *Impurity C*: maximum 5×10^{-3} per cent of the total radioactivity.

Gamma-ray spectrometry. *Record the spectrum of the decayed material.*

Comparison   Suitable instrument calibrated using a standardised ruthenium-103 solution.

Results   The most prominent photon has an energy of 0.497 MeV; ruthenium-103 has a half-life of 39.3 days.
— *Impurity D*: maximum 6×10^{-5} per cent of the total radioactivity.

Determine the presence of strontium-89 in the decayed material with an instrument suitable for the detection of beta rays. It is usually necessary first to carry out chemical separation of the strontium so that the standard and the sample may be compared in the same physical and chemical form.

Comparison   Standardised strontium-89 solution.

Results   Strontium-89 decays with a beta emission of 1.492 MeV maximum energy and has a half-life of 50.5 days.
— *Impurity E*: maximum 6×10^{-6} per cent of the total radioactivity.

Determine the presence of strontium-90 in the decayed material with an instrument suitable for the detection of beta rays. To distinguish strontium-90 from strontium-89, compare the radioactivity of yttrium-90, the daughter nuclide of strontium-90, with an yttrium-90 standard after the chemical separation of the yttrium. If prior chemical separation of the strontium is necessary, the conditions of radioactive equilibrium must be ensured. The yttrium-90 standard and the sample must be compared in the same physical and chemical form.

Results   Strontium-90 and yttrium-90 decay with respective beta emissions of 0.546 MeV and 2.284 MeV maximum energy and half-lives of 29.1 years and 64.0 h.
— *Other gamma-emitting impurities*: maximum 0.01 per cent of the total radioactivity.

Gamma-ray spectrometry.

Examine the spectrum of the decayed material for the presence of other radionuclidic impurities, which should, where possible, be identified and quantified.

— *Alpha-emitting impurities*: maximum 1×10^{-7} per cent of the total radioactivity.

Measure the alpha radioactivity of the decayed material to detect any alpha-emitting radionuclidic impurities, which should, where possible, be identified and quantified.

RADIOCHEMICAL PURITY
[⁹⁹ᵐTc]Pertechnetate ion
Descending paper chromatography (*2.2.26*).

Test solution   Dilute the preparation to be examined with *water R* to a suitable radioactive concentration.

Paper   *paper for chromatography R.*

Mobile phase   *water R, methanol R* (20:80 *V/V*).

Application   5 μL.

Development   For 2 h.

Drying   In air.

Detection   Suitable detector to determine the distribution of radioactivity.

Retardation factor   [⁹⁹ᵐTc]pertechnetate ion = about 0.6.
Limit:
— *[⁹⁹ᵐTc]pertechnetate ion*: minimum 95 per cent of the total radioactivity due to technetium-99m.

RADIOACTIVITY
Determine the radioactivity using a calibrated instrument.

IMPURITIES
A. iodine-131,

B. molybdenum-99,

C. ruthenium-103,

D. strontium-89,

E. strontium-90.

_____ *Ph Eur*

Sodium Pertechnetate (⁹⁹ᵐTc) Injection (Non-fission)

(*Ph Eur monograph 0283*)

Ph Eur _____

This monograph applies to sodium pertechnetate (⁹⁹ᵐTc) injection obtained from molybdenum-99 produced by neutron irradiation of molybdenum. Sodium pertechnetate (⁹⁹ᵐTc) injection obtained from molybdenum-99 extracted from fission products of uranium is described in the monograph Sodium pertechnetate (⁹⁹ᵐTc) injection (fission) (0124).

DEFINITION
Sterile solution containing technetium-99m in the form of pertechnetate ion and made isotonic by the addition of sodium chloride.

Technetium-99m
90 per cent to 110 per cent of the declared technetium-99m radioactivity at the date and time stated on the label.

CHARACTERS
Appearance
Clear, colourless solution.

Half-life and nature of radiation of technetium-99m
See general chapter *5.7. Table of physical characteristics of radionuclides.*

IDENTIFICATION
A. Gamma-ray spectrometry.

Result The most prominent gamma photon of technetium-99m has an energy of 0.141 MeV.

B. Examine the chromatogram obtained in the test for radiochemical purity (see Tests).

Result The retardation factor of the principal peak in the radiochromatogram obtained with the test solution is about 0.6.

TESTS

pH *(2.2.3)*

4.0 to 8.0.

Aluminium

Maximum 5 ppm.

Test solution In a test tube about 12 mm in internal diameter, mix 1 mL of *acetate buffer solution pH 4.6 R* and 2 mL of a 1 in 2.5 dilution of the preparation to be examined in *water R*. Add 0.05 mL of a 10 g/L solution of *chromazurol S R*.

Reference solution Prepare at the same time and in the same manner as the test solution and using 2 mL of *aluminium standard solution (2 ppm Al) R*.

After 3 min, the colour of the test solution is not more intense than that of the reference solution.

Sterility

It complies with the test for sterility prescribed in the monograph *Radiopharmaceutical preparations (0125)*. The preparation may be released for use before completion of the test.

RADIONUCLIDIC PURITY

Preliminary test To obtain an approximate estimate before use of the preparation, take a volume equivalent to 37 MBq and record the gamma-ray spectrum using a sodium iodide detector with a shield of lead, 6 mm thick, interposed between the sample and the detector. The response in the region corresponding to the 0.740 MeV photon of molybdenum-99 does not exceed that obtained using 37 kBq of a standardised molybdenum-99 solution measured under the same conditions, when all measurements are expressed with reference to the date and time of administration.

Definitive test Retain a sample of the preparation to be examined for a sufficient time to allow the technetium-99m radioactivity to decay to a sufficiently low level to permit the detection of radionuclidic impurities. All measurements of radioactivity are expressed with reference to the date and time of administration.

— *Impurity A*: maximum 0.1 per cent of the total radioactivity.

Gamma-ray spectrometry. Record the gamma-ray spectrum of the decayed material.

Comparison Standardised molybdenum-99 solution.

Results The most prominent gamma photons have energies of 0.181 MeV, 0.740 MeV and 0.778 MeV; molybdenum-99 has a half-life of 66.0 h.

— *Other gamma-emitting impurities*: maximum 0.01 per cent of the total radioactivity.

Gamma-ray spectrometry. Examine the gamma-ray spectrum of the decayed material for the presence of other radionuclidic impurities, which should, where possible, be identified and quantified.

RADIOCHEMICAL PURITY

[⁹⁹mTc]Pertechnetate ion

Descending paper chromatography *(2.2.26)*.

Test solution Dilute the preparation to be examined with *water R* to a suitable radioactive concentration.

Paper paper for chromatography R.

Mobile phase water R, methanol R (20:80 *V/V*).

Application 5 μL.

Development For 2 h.

Drying In air.

Detection Suitable detector to determine the distribution of radioactivity.

Retardation factor [⁹⁹mTc]pertechnetate ion = about 0.6.

Limit:

— *[⁹⁹mTc]pertechnetate ion*: minimum 95 per cent of the total radioactivity due to technetium-99m.

RADIOACTIVITY

Determine the radioactivity using a calibrated instrument.

IMPURITIES

A. molybdenum-99.

Ph Eur

Sodium Phosphate (³²P) Injection

(Ph Eur monograph 0284)

Ph Eur

DEFINITION

Sterile solution of disodium and monosodium (³²P) orthophosphates made isotonic by the addition of sodium chloride.

Phosphorus-32

90 per cent to 110 per cent of the declared phosphorus-32 radioactivity at the date and time stated on the label.

Specific radioactivity

Minimum 11.1 MBq of phosphorus-32 per milligram of orthophosphate ion.

CHARACTERS

Appearance

Clear, colourless solution.

Half-life and nature of radiation of phosphorus-32

See general chapter 5.7. *Table of physical characteristics of radionuclides.*

IDENTIFICATION

A. Beta-ray spectrometry.

Result The maximum energy of the beta radiation is 1.71 MeV.

B. Examine the chromatogram obtained in the test for radiochemical purity (see Tests).

Result The principal peak in the radiochromatogram obtained with the test solution is similar in retardation factor to the principal peak in the chromatogram obtained with the reference solution.

TESTS

pH *(2.2.3)*

6.0 to 8.0.

Phosphates

Maximum 89 μg/MBq.

Test solution Dilute the preparation to be examined with *water R* to give a radioactive concentration of 370 kBq of phosphorus-32 per millilitre. Mix in a volumetric flask, with shaking, 1.0 mL of this solution with a mixture of 0.5 mL of *ammonium molybdate solution R*, 0.5 mL of a 2.5 g/L solution of *ammonium vanadate R* and 1 mL of *perchloric acid R*, and dilute to 5.0 mL with *water R*.

Reference solution   Prepare at the same time and in the same manner as the test solution, using 1.0 mL of a solution containing 33 mg of orthophosphate ion per litre.

After 30 min, the test solution is not more intensely coloured than the reference solution.

Sterility
It complies with the test for sterility prescribed in the monograph *Radiopharmaceutical preparations (0125)*.
The preparation may be released for use before completion of the test.

RADIONUCLIDIC PURITY
Beta-ray spectrometry.

Result   The spectrum obtained with the preparation to be examined does not differ significantly from that obtained under the same conditions with a standardised phosphorus-32 solution.

RADIOCHEMICAL PURITY
[^{32}P]Phosphate
Ascending paper chromatography (*2.2.26*).

Test solution   Dilute the preparation to be examined with *water R* until the radioactivity is equivalent to 10 000-20 000 counts per minute per 10 μL.

Reference solution   A solution of *phosphoric acid R* containing 2 mg of phosphorus per millilitre.

Paper   Paper for chromatography *R*; use a strip of paper 25 mm wide and about 300 mm long.

Mobile phase   Mixture of 0.3 mL of *ammonia R*, 5 g of *trichloroacetic acid R*, 25 mL of *water R* and 75 mL of *2-propanol R*.

Application   10 μL of the reference solution, then apply to the same point of application 10 μL of the test solution.

Development   For 16 h.

Drying   In air.

Detection   Determine the position of the non-radioactive phosphoric acid by spraying with a 50 g/L solution of *perchloric acid R* and then with a 10 g/L solution of *ammonium molybdate R*. Expose the paper to *hydrogen sulfide R*. A blue colour develops. Determine the distribution of radioactivity using a suitable detector.

Limit:
— *[^{32}P]phosphate*: minimum 95 per cent of the total radioactivity due to phosphorus-32.

RADIOACTIVITY
Determine the radioactivity using a calibrated instrument.

Ph Eur

Strontium (^{89}Sr) Chloride Injection

(*Ph Eur monograph 1475*)

Ph Eur

DEFINITION
Sterile solution of [^{89}Sr]strontium chloride.

Strontium-89
90 per cent to 110 per cent of the declared strontium-89 radioactivity at the date stated on the label.

Specific radioactivity
Minimum 1.8 MBq of strontium-89 per milligram of strontium.

Strontium
6.0 mg/mL to 12.5 mg/mL.

CHARACTERS
Appearance
Clear, colourless solution.

Half-life and nature of radiation of strontium-89
See general chapter *5.7. Table of physical characteristics of radionuclides*.

IDENTIFICATION
A. Gamma-ray and X-ray spectrometry.

Result   The gamma photon detected has an energy of 0.909 MeV and is due to the short-lived daughter product, yttrium-89m (formed in 0.01 per cent of the disintegrations), in equilibrium with the strontium-89.

B. To 0.1 mL of the preparation to be examined, add 1 mL of a freshly prepared 1 g/L solution of *sodium rhodizonate R*. Mix and allow to stand for 1 min. A reddish-brown precipitate is formed.

C. To 0.1 mL of *silver nitrate solution R2* add 50 μL of the preparation to be examined. A white precipitate is formed.

TESTS
pH (*2.2.3*)
4.0 to 7.5.

Note: the following tests for aluminium, iron and lead may be carried out simultaneously with the test for strontium. If this is not the case, the reference solutions are prepared such that they contain strontium at approximately the same concentration as in the test solution.

Aluminium
Maximum 2 μg/mL.

Atomic emission spectrometry (plasma or arc method) (*2.2.22, Method I*).

Test solution   Dilute 0.2 mL of the preparation to be examined to a suitable volume with *dilute nitric acid R*.

Reference solutions   Prepare the reference solutions using *aluminium standard solution (10 ppm Al) R* diluted as necessary with *dilute nitric acid R*.

Iron
Maximum 5 μg/mL.

Atomic emission spectrometry (plasma or arc method) (*2.2.22, Method I*).

Test solution   Dilute 0.2 mL of the preparation to be examined to a suitable volume with *dilute nitric acid R*.

Reference solutions   Prepare the reference solutions using *iron standard solution (20 ppm Fe) R* diluted as necessary with *dilute nitric acid R*.

Lead
Maximum 5 μg/mL.

Atomic emission spectrometry (plasma or arc method) (*2.2.22, Method I*).

Test solution   Dilute 0.2 mL of the preparation to be examined to a suitable volume with *dilute nitric acid R*.

Reference solutions   Prepare the reference solutions using *lead standard solution (10 ppm Pb) R* diluted as necessary with *dilute nitric acid R*.

Strontium
6.0 mg/mL to 12.5 mg/mL.

Atomic emission spectrometry (*2.2.22, Method I*).

Test solution   Dilute 0.2 mL of the preparation to be examined to a suitable volume with *dilute nitric acid R*.

Reference solutions Prepare the reference solutions using *strontium standard solution (1.0 per cent Sr) R* diluted as necessary with *dilute nitric acid R*.

Sterility

It complies with the test for sterility prescribed in the monograph *Radiopharmaceutical preparations (0125)*.

RADIONUCLIDIC PURITY

The total radioactivity due to radionuclides other than strontium-89 is not more than 0.6 per cent.

Gamma emitters other than yttrium-89m

Maximum 0.4 per cent of the total radioactivity.

Gamma-ray and X-ray spectrometry.

Beta emitters

Evaporate to dryness 100 µL of the preparation to be examined under a radiant heat source. Dissolve the residue in 2 mL of *47 per cent hydrobromic acid R*, evaporate to dryness under the radiant heat source and dissolve the residue in 2 mL of *dilute hydrobromic acid R1*. Transfer the solution to the top of a column, 5-6 mm in diameter, packed with approximately 2 mL of *cation exchange resin R1* (100-250 µm), previously conditioned with *dilute hydrobromic acid R1* and elute the column with the same solvent until 10 mL of eluate has been collected into a container containing 50 µL of a 15 g/L solution of *anhydrous sodium sulfate R* in *1 M hydrochloric acid*.

To a liquid scintillation cocktail vial add an appropriate volume of *liquid scintillation cocktail R* followed by 1 mL of *water R*, 0.1 mL of a 15 g/L solution of *anhydrous sodium sulfate R* in *1 M hydrochloric acid* and 100 µL of eluate. Shake to obtain a clear solution. Using suitable counting equipment determine the radioactivity due to impurities A and B in the sample.

Taking into account the recovery efficiency of the separation, counting efficiency and radioactive decay, determine the radioactive concentration of impurities A and B in the sample and hence the percentage of total beta emitting impurities in the injection to be examined.

Result:
— *impurities A and B:* maximum 0.2 per cent of the total radioactivity.

RADIOACTIVITY

Determine the radioactivity using a calibrated instrument.

IMPURITIES

A. sulfur-35,

B. phosphorus-32.

Ph Eur

Technetium (⁹⁹ᵐTc) Albumin Injection

(Technetium (⁹⁹ᵐTc) Human Albumin Injection, Ph Eur monograph 0640)

Ph Eur

DEFINITION

Sterile, apyrogenic solution of human albumin labelled with technetium-99m. It is prepared using *Sodium pertechnetate (⁹⁹ᵐTc) injection (fission) (0124)* or *Sodium pertechnetate (⁹⁹ᵐTc) injection (non fission) (0283)*. It contains a reducing substance, such as a tin salt in an amount not exceeding 1 mg of Sn per millilitre. Although, at present, no definite value for a maximum limit of tin can be fixed, available evidence tends to suggest the importance of keeping the ratio

of tin to albumin as low as possible. It may contain a suitable buffer and an antimicrobial preservative. The human albumin used complies with the requirements of the monograph *Human albumin solution (0255)*.

Technetium-99m

90 per cent to 110 per cent of the declared technetium-99m radioactivity at the date and time stated on the label.

Albumin

90.0 per cent to 110.0 per cent of the quantity of albumin stated on the label.

CHARACTERS

Appearance

Clear, colourless or pale yellow solution.

Half-life and nature of radiation of technetium-99m

See general chapter 5.7. *Table of physical characteristics of radionuclides.*

IDENTIFICATION

A. Gamma-ray spectrometry.

Result The most prominent gamma photon of technetium-99m has an energy of 0.141 MeV.

B. Using a suitable range of species-specific antisera, carry out precipitation tests on the preparation to be examined. The test is to be carried out using antisera specific to the plasma proteins of each species of domestic animal currently used in the preparation of materials of biological origin in the country concerned. The preparation is shown to contain proteins of human origin and gives negative results with antisera specific to plasma proteins of other species.

C. Examine by a suitable immunoelectrophoresis technique. Using antiserum to normal human serum, compare normal human serum and the preparation to be examined, both diluted if necessary. The main component of the preparation to be examined corresponds to the main component of the normal human serum. The diluted preparation may show the presence of small quantities of other plasma proteins.

TESTS

pH *(2.2.3)*

2.0 to 6.5.

Albumin

Test solution The preparation to be examined.

Reference solution Dilute *human albumin solution R* with a 9 g/L solution of *sodium chloride R* to a concentration of 5 mg of albumin per millilitre.

To 1.0 mL of the test solution and to 1.0 mL of the reference solution add 4.0 mL of *biuret reagent R* and mix. After exactly 30 min, measure the absorbance *(2.2.25)* of each solution at 540 nm, using as the compensation liquid a 9 g/L solution of *sodium chloride R* treated in the same manner. From the absorbances measured, calculate the content of albumin in the preparation to be examined in milligrams per millilitre.

Tin

Maximum 1 mg/mL.

Test solution To 1.0 mL of the preparation to be examined add 1.0 mL of a 206 g/L solution of *hydrochloric acid R*. Heat in a water-bath at 100 °C for 30 min. Cool and centrifuge at 300 g for 10 min. Dilute 1.0 mL of the supernatant liquid to 10 mL with a 103 g/L solution of *hydrochloric acid R*.

Reference solution Dissolve 95 mg of *stannous chloride R* in a 103 g/L solution of *hydrochloric acid R* and dilute to 1000.0 mL with the same acid.

To 1.0 mL of each solution add 0.05 mL of *thioglycollic acid R*, 0.1 mL of *dithiol reagent R*, 0.4 mL of a 20 g/L solution of *sodium laurilsulfate R* and 3.0 mL of a 21 g/L solution of *hydrochloric acid R*. Mix. Measure the absorbance (*2.2.25*) of each solution at 540 nm, using a 21 g/L solution of *hydrochloric acid R* as the compensation liquid.
The absorbance of the test solution is not greater than that of the reference solution.

Physiological distribution
Inject a volume not greater than 0.5 mL and containing not more than 1.0 mg of albumin into a suitable vein such as a caudal vein or a saphenous vein of each of 3 male rats, each weighing 150-250 g. Measure the radioactivity in the syringe before and after the injection. Euthanise the rats 30 min after the injection. Take 1 ml of blood by a suitable method and remove the liver and, if a caudal vein has been used for the injection, the tail. Using a suitable instrument determine the radioactivity in these organs and blood. Determine the percentage of radioactivity in the liver and in 1 mL of blood with respect to the total radioactivity calculated as the difference between both measurements made on the syringe minus the activity in the tail (if a caudal vein has been used for the injection). Correct the blood radioactivity by multiplying by a factor of $m/200$ where m is the body mass of the rat in grams. In not fewer than 2 of the 3 rats used, the radioactivity in the liver is not more than 15 per cent and that in blood, after correction, is not less than 3.5 per cent.

Sterility
It complies with the test for sterility prescribed in the monograph *Radiopharmaceutical preparations (0125)*.
The preparation may be released for use before completion of the test.

Bacterial endotoxins (*2.6.14*)
Less than $175/V$ IU/mL, V being the maximum recommended dose in millilitres.

RADIOCHEMICAL PURITY

Impurity A
Thin-layer chromatography (*2.2.27*).

Test solution   The preparation to be examined.

Plate   TLC silica gel plate R; use silica gel as the coating substance on a glass-fibre sheet, heated at 110 °C for 10 min.

Mobile phase   methyl ethyl ketone R.

Application   5-10 µL and allow to dry.

Development   Over a path of 10-15 cm in about 10 min.

Drying   In air.

Detection   Suitable detector to determine the distribution of radioactivity.

Retardation factors   [^{99m}Tc]technetium human albumin = 0.0 to 0.1; impurity A = 0.9 to 1.0.

Limit:
— *impurity A*: maximum 5.0 per cent of the total radioactivity due to technetium-99m.

[^{99m}Tc]Technetium albumin fractions II to V
Size-exclusion chromatography (*2.2.30*).

Mobile phase (concentrated)   Dissolve 1.124 g of *potassium dihydrogen phosphate R*, 4.210 g of *disodium hydrogen phosphate R*, 1.17 g of *sodium chloride R* and 0.10 g of *sodium azide R* in *water R* and dilute to 100 mL with the same solvent.

Test solution   Mix 0.25 mL of the preparation to be examined with 0.25 mL of the mobile phase (concentrated). *Use immediately after dilution.*

Column:
— *size: l* = 0.6 m, Ø = 7.5 mm;
— *stationary phase: silica gel for size-exclusion chromatography R.*

Mobile phase   mobile phase (concentrated), *water R* (50:50 *V/V*).

Flow rate   0.6 mL/min.

Detection   Radioactivity detector set for technetium-99m.

Injection   200 µL.

Run time   At least 10 min after background level is reached.

Retention times of eluted peaks:

I	High molecular mass compound	19-20 min
II	Poly III-albumin	23-24 min
III	Poly II-albumin	25-27 min
IV	Poly I-albumin	28-29 min
V	Human serum albumin	32-33 min
VI	Tin colloid	40-47 min
VII	Pertechnetate	48 min

Limit:
— *[^{99m}Tc]technetium albumin fractions II to V*: minimum 80 per cent of the radioactivity due to technetium-99m applied to the column.

RADIOACTIVITY
Determine the radioactivity using a calibrated instrument.

LABELLING
The label states:
— the amount of albumin;
— the amount of tin, if any.

IMPURITIES
A. [^{99m}Tc]pertechnetate ion.

—————————— Ph Eur

Technetium (^{99m}Tc) Bicisate Injection

(*Ph Eur monograph 2123*)

Ph Eur ——————————————————————

DEFINITION
Sterile solution of a complex of technetium-99m with diethyl N,N′-ethylenedi-L-cysteinate. It may contain stabilisers and inert additives such as *Mannitol (0559)* and *Disodium edetate (0232)*.

Content
90 per cent to 110 per cent of the declared technetium-99m radioactivity at the date and hour stated on the label.

PRODUCTION
It is prepared from N,N′-(1,2-ethylenediyl)bis[(2R)-2-amino-3-sulfanylpropanoic acid] diethyl ester and *Sodium pertechnetate (^{99m}Tc) injection (fission) (0124)* or *Sodium pertechnetate (^{99m}Tc) injection (non-fission) (0283)* in the presence of reducing agents such as a stannous salt.

CHARACTERS

Appearance

Clear, colourless solution.

Half-life and nature of radiation of technetium-99m

See general chapter 5.7. *Table of physical characteristics of radionuclides.*

IDENTIFICATION

A. Gamma-ray spectrometry.

Results The most prominent gamma photon of technetium-99m has an energy of 0.141 MeV.

B. Examine the chromatograms obtained in the test for radiochemical purity (see Tests).

Results The principal peak in the chromatogram obtained with the test solution is similar in retardation factor to the principal peak in the chromatogram obtained with reference solution (a).

TESTS

pH *(2.2.3)*

6.5 to 7.5.

Sterility

It complies with the test for sterility prescribed in the monograph on *Radiopharmaceutical preparations (0125)*. The injection may be released for use before completion of the test.

RADIOCHEMICAL PURITY

Impurities A, B, C, D, E, F

Thin-layer chromatography *(2.2.27)*.

Test solution The preparation to be examined.

Reference solution (a) To vial B of *bicisate labelling kit CRS* in lead shielding add 2 mL of sodium pertechnetate (⁹⁹ᵐTc) injection (fission or non-fission) containing 400-800 MBq. Dissolve the contents of vial A of *bicisate labelling kit CRS* in 3 mL of a 9 g/L solution of *sodium chloride R*. Immediately transfer 1.0 mL of the solution contained in vial A to vial B. Mix and allow to stand for 30 min at room temperature.

Reference solution (b) Sodium pertechnetate (⁹⁹ᵐTc) injection (fission or non fission).

Plate TLC silica gel plate R.

Mobile phase ethyl acetate R.

Application 5 µL, allow the spots to dry for 5-10 min.

Development Over 4/5 of the plate.

Drying In air.

Detection Determine the distribution of radioactivity using a suitable detector.

Retardation factors technetium-99m bicisate = more than 0.4; impurities A, B, C, D, E and F = less than 0.2.

System suitability The retardation factor of the principal peak in the chromatogram obtained with reference solution (a) is clearly different from the retardation factor of the peak in the chromatogram obtained with reference solution (b).

Limit:

— sum of impurities A, B, C, D, E and F: not more than 6 per cent of the total radioactivity.

RADIOACTIVITY

Determine the radioactivity using a calibrated instrument.

IMPURITIES

A. technetium-99m in colloidal form,

B. [⁹⁹ᵐTc]pertechnetate ion,

C. complex of technetium-99m with ethyl hydrogen *N,N′*-ethylenedi-L-cysteinate,

D. complex of technetium-99m with *N,N′*-ethylenedi-L-cysteine,

E. complex of technetium-99m with mannitol,

F. complex of technetium-99m with disodium edetate.

Ph Eur

Technetium (⁹⁹ᵐTc) Colloidal Rhenium Sulfide Injection

Technetium (⁹⁹ᵐTc) Colloidal Rhenium Sulphide Injection

(Ph Eur monograph 0126)

Ph Eur

DEFINITION

Sterile colloidal dispersion of rhenium sulfide, the micelles of which are labelled with technetium-99m. It is prepared using *Sodium pertechnetate (⁹⁹ᵐTc) injection (fission) (0124)* or *Sodium pertechnetate (⁹⁹ᵐTc) injection (non fission) (0283)*. It is stabilised with gelatin. The pH of the injection may be adjusted by the addition of a suitable buffer such as citrate buffer.

Technetium-99m

90 per cent to 110 per cent of the declared technetium-99m radioactivity at the date and time stated on the label.

Rhenium

Maximum 0.22 mg/mL.

CHARACTERS

Appearance

Light brown liquid.

Half-life and nature of radiation of technetium-99m

See general chapter 5.7. *Table of physical characteristics of radionuclides.*

IDENTIFICATION

A. Gamma-ray spectrometry.

Result The most prominent gamma photon of technetium-99m has an energy of 0.141 MeV.

B. Examine the chromatogram obtained in the test for radiochemical purity (see Tests).

Result The retardation factor of the principal peak in the radiochromatogram obtained with the test solution is 0.0 to 0.1.

C. To 1 mL add 1 mL of a 200 g/L solution of *stannous chloride R* in hydrochloric acid R, 5 mL of *hydrochloric acid R* and 5 mL of a 50 g/L solution of *thiourea R*. A yellow colour develops.

TESTS

pH *(2.2.3)*

4.0 to 7.0.

Rhenium

Maximum 0.22 mg/mL.

Test solution   The preparation to be examined.

Reference solutions   Using a solution containing 100 μg of *potassium perrhenate R* (equivalent to 60 ppm of Re) and 240 μg of *sodium thiosulfate R* per millilitre, prepare a range of solutions and dilute to the same final volume with *water R*.

To 1 mL of the test solution and to 1 mL of each of the reference solutions add 1 mL of a 200 g/L solution of *stannous chloride R* in *hydrochloric acid R*, 5 mL of *hydrochloric acid R* and 5 mL of a 50 g/L solution of *thiourea R* and dilute to 25.0 mL with *water R*. Allow to stand for 40 min and measure the absorbance *(2.2.25)* of each solution at 400 nm, using a reagent blank as the compensation liquid. Using the absorbances obtained with the reference solutions, draw a calibration curve and calculate the concentration of rhenium in the preparation to be examined.

Physiological distribution

Inject a volume not greater than 0.2 mL into a caudal vein of each of 3 mice each weighing 20-25 g. Euthanise the mice 20 min after the injection, remove the liver, spleen and lungs and measure the radioactivity in the organs using a suitable instrument. Measure the radioactivity in the rest of the body after having removed the tail. Determine the percentage of radioactivity in the liver, the spleen and the lungs using the following expression:

$$\frac{A}{B} \times 100$$

A = radioactivity of the organ concerned,

B = total radioactivity in the liver, the spleen, the lungs and the rest of the body.

In each of the 3 mice at least 80 per cent of the radioactivity is found in the liver and spleen and not more than 5 per cent in the lungs. If the distribution of radioactivity in 1 of the 3 mice does not correspond to the prescribed proportions, repeat the test on a further 3 mice. The preparation complies with the test if the prescribed distribution of radioactivity is found in 5 of the 6 mice used. The preparation may be released for use before completion of the test.

Sterility

It complies with the test for sterility prescribed in the monograph *Radiopharmaceutical preparations (0125)*. The preparation may be released for use before completion of the test.

Bacterial endotoxins *(2.6.14)*

Less than 175/V IU/mL, V being the maximum recommended dose in millilitres.

RADIOCHEMICAL PURITY

[^{99m}Tc]Technetium in colloidal form

Ascending paper chromatography *(2.2.26)*.

Test solution   The preparation to be examined.

Paper   *paper for chromatography R.*

Mobile phase   9 g/L solution of *sodium chloride R*.

Application   10 μL.

Development   Immediately over a path of 10-15 cm.

Drying   In air.

Detection   Suitable detector to determine the distribution of radioactivity.

Retardation factors   [^{99m}Tc]technetium in colloidal form = 0.0 to 0.1; impurity A = about 0.6; other impurities = 0.8 to 0.9.

Limit:

— *[^{99m}Tc]technetium in colloidal form*: minimum 92 per cent of the total radioactivity due to technetium-99m.

RADIOACTIVITY

Determine the radioactivity using a calibrated instrument.

LABELLING

The label states the concentration of rhenium expressed in milligrams per millilitre.

IMPURITIES

A. [^{99m}Tc]pertechnetate ion.

Ph Eur

Technetium (^{99m}Tc) Colloidal Sulfur Injection

Technetium (^{99m}Tc) Colloidal Sulphur Injection

(Ph Eur monograph 0131)

Ph Eur

DEFINITION

Sterile, apyrogenic colloidal dispersion of sulfur, the micelles of which are labelled with technetium-99m. It is prepared using *Sodium pertechnetate (^{99m}Tc) injection (fission) (0124)* or *Sodium pertechnetate (^{99m}Tc) injection (non fission) (0283)*. It may be stabilised with a colloid-protecting substance based on gelatin. The pH of the injection may be adjusted by the addition of a suitable buffer, such as an acetate, citrate or phosphate buffer solution. The injection contains a variable amount of colloidal sulfur, according to the method of preparation.

Technetium-99m

90 per cent to 110 per cent of the declared technetium-99m radioactivity at the date and time stated on the label.

CHARACTERS

Appearance

Clear or opalescent, colourless or yellowish liquid.

Half-life and nature of radiation of technetium-99 m

See general chapter *5.7. Table of physical characteristics of radionuclides.*

IDENTIFICATION

A. Gamma-ray spectrometry.

Result   The most prominent gamma photon of technetium-99m has an energy of 0.141 MeV.

B. Examine the chromatogram obtained in the test for radiochemical purity (see Tests).

Result   The retardation factor of the principal peak in the radiochromatogram obtained with the test solution is 0.0 to 0.1.

C. In a test-tube 100 mm long and 16 mm in internal diameter, evaporate 0.2 mL of the preparation to be examined to dryness. Dissolve the sulfur by shaking the residue with 0.2 mL of *pyridine R* and add about 20 mg of *benzoin R*. Cover the open end of the tube with a filter paper moistened with *lead acetate solution R*. Heat the test-tube in a bath containing glycerol at 150 °C. The paper slowly becomes brown.

TESTS
pH (*2.2.3*)
4.0 to 7.0.

Physiological distribution
Inject a volume not greater than 0.2 mL into the caudal vein of each of 3 mice, each weighing 20-25 g. Euthanise the mice 20 min after the injection, remove the liver, spleen and lungs and measure the radioactivity in these organs using a suitable instrument. Measure the radioactivity in the rest of the body of each animal after having removed the tail. Determine the percentage of radioactivity in the liver, the spleen and the lungs using the following expression:

$$\frac{A}{B} \times 100$$

A = radioactivity of the organ concerned;
B = total radioactivity in the liver, the spleen, the lungs and the rest of the body.

In each of the 3 mice at least 80 per cent of the radioactivity is found in the liver and spleen and not more than 5 per cent in the lungs. If the distribution of radioactivity in 1 of the 3 mice does not correspond to the prescribed proportions, repeat the test on a further 3 mice. The preparation to be examined complies with the test if the prescribed distribution of radioactivity is found in 5 of the 6 mice used.
The preparation may be released for use before completion of the test.

Sterility
It complies with the test for sterility prescribed in the monograph *Radiopharmaceutical preparations (0125)*.
The preparation may be released for use before completion of the test.

Pyrogens
It complies with the test for pyrogens prescribed in the monograph *Radiopharmaceutical preparations (0125)*. Inject, per kilogram of the rabbit's mass, not less than 0.1 mL.
The preparation may be released for use before completion of the test.

RADIOCHEMICAL PURITY

[⁹⁹ᵐTc]Technetium in colloidal form
Ascending paper chromatography (*2.2.26*).

Test solution   The preparation to be examined.

Paper   *paper for chromatography R.*

Mobile phase   9 g/L solution of *sodium chloride R.*

Application   10 µL.

Development   Immediately, over a path of 10-15 cm.

Drying   In air.

Detection   Suitable detector to determine the distribution of radioactivity.

Retardation factors   [⁹⁹ᵐTc]technetium in colloidal form = 0.0 to 0.1; impurity A = about 0.6; other impurities = 0.8 to 0.9.

Limit:
— *[⁹⁹ᵐTc]technetium in colloidal form*: minimum 92 per cent of the total radioactivity due to technetium-99m.

RADIOACTIVITY
Determine the radioactivity using a calibrated instrument.

IMPURITIES
A. [⁹⁹ᵐTc]pertechnetate ion.

Technetium (⁹⁹ᵐTc) Colloidal Tin Injection

(*Ph Eur monograph 0689*)

Ph Eur

DEFINITION
Sterile, colloidal dispersion of tin labelled with technetium-99m. It is prepared using *Sodium pertechnetate (⁹⁹ᵐTc) injection (fission) (0124)* or *Sodium pertechnetate (⁹⁹ᵐTc) injection (non fission) (0283)*. The injection contains a variable quantity of tin not exceeding 1 mg of Sn per millilitre; it contains fluoride ions, it may be stabilised with a suitable, apyrogenic colloid-protecting substance and it may contain a suitable buffer.

Technetium-99m
90 per cent to 110 per cent of the declared technetium-99m radioactivity at the date and time stated on the label.

Tin
Maximum 1 mg/mL.

CHARACTERS
Appearance
Clear or opalescent, colourless solution.

Half-life and nature of radiation of technetium-99m
See general chapter 5.7. *Table of physical characteristics of radionuclides.*

IDENTIFICATION
A. Gamma-ray spectrometry.

Result   The most prominent gamma photon of technetium-99m has an energy of 0.141 MeV.

B. Mix 0.05 mL of *zirconyl nitrate solution R* with 0.05 mL of *alizarin S solution R*. Add 0.05 mL of the preparation to be examined. A yellow colour is produced.

TESTS
pH (*2.2.3*)
4.0 to 7.0.

Tin
Maximum 1 mg/mL.

Test solution   Dilute 3.0 mL of the preparation to be examined to 50.0 mL with a 103 g/L solution of *hydrochloric acid R.*

Reference solution   Dissolve 0.115 g of *stannous chloride R* in a 103 g/L solution of *hydrochloric acid R* and dilute to 1000.0 mL with the same acid.

To 1.0 mL of each solution add 0.05 mL of *thioglycollic acid R*, 0.1 mL of *dithiol reagent R*, 0.4 mL of a 20 g/L solution of *sodium laurilsulfate R* and 3.0 mL of a 21 g/L solution of *hydrochloric acid R*. Mix. Measure the absorbance (*2.2.25*) of each solution at 540 nm, using a 21 g/L solution of *hydrochloric acid R* as the compensation liquid.
The absorbance of the test solution is not greater than that of the reference solution.

Physiological distribution
Inject not more than 0.2 mL into a caudal vein of each of 3 mice, each weighing 20-25 g. Euthanise the mice 20 min after the injection and remove the liver, spleen and lungs. Measure the radioactivity in the organs using a suitable instrument. Measure the radioactivity in the rest of the body of each animal, after having removed the tail. Determine the percentage of radioactivity in the liver, the spleen and the lungs with respect to the total radioactivity of all organs and the rest of the body excluding the tail.

In each of the 3 mice at least 80 per cent of the radioactivity is found in the liver and spleen and not more than 5 per cent in the lungs. If the distribution of radioactivity in 1 of the 3 mice does not correspond to the prescribed proportions, repeat the test on a further 3 mice. The preparation to be examined complies with the test if the prescribed distribution of radioactivity is found in 5 of the 6 mice used.

Sterility

It complies with the test for sterility prescribed in the monograph *Radiopharmaceutical preparations (0125)*. The preparation may be released for use before completion of the test.

RADIOCHEMICAL PURITY

[^{99m}Tc]Technetium in colloidal form

Thin-layer chromatography (2.2.27).

Test solution   The preparation to be examined.

Plate   TLC silica gel plate R; use silica gel as the coating substance on a glass-fibre sheet heated at 110 °C for 10 min.

Mobile phase   9 g/L solution of *sodium chloride R* purged with *nitrogen R*.

Application   5-10 µL.

Development   Over a path of 10-15 cm in about 10 min.

Drying   In air.

Detection   Suitable detector to determine the distribution of radioactivity.

Retardation factors   [^{99m}Tc]technetium in colloidal form = 0.0 to 0.1; impurity A = 0.9 to 1.0.

Limit:
— *[^{99m}Tc]technetium in colloidal form*: minimum 95 per cent of the radioactivity due to technetium-99m.

RADIOACTIVITY

Determine the radioactivity using a calibrated instrument.

IMPURITIES

A. [^{99m}Tc]pertechnetate ion.

_____ *Ph Eur*

Technetium (^{99m}Tc) Etifenin Injection

(*Ph Eur monograph 0585*)

Ph Eur _____

DEFINITION

Technetium (^{99m}Tc) etifenin injection is a sterile solution which may be prepared by mixing sodium pertechnetate (^{99m}Tc) injection (fission or non-fission) with solutions of etifenin [[(2,6-diethylphenyl)carbamoylmethylimino]di-acetic acid; $C_{16}H_{22}N_2O_5$] and stannous chloride. The injection contains a variable quantity of tin (Sn) not exceeding 0.2 mg/mL. The injection contains not less than 90.0 per cent and not more than 110.0 per cent of the declared technetium-99m radioactivity at the date and hour stated on the label. Not less than 95.0 per cent of the radioactivity corresponds to technetium-99m complexed with etifenin.

It is prepared from sodium pertechnetate (^{99m}Tc) injection (fission or non-fission) using suitable, sterile ingredients and calculating the ratio of radionuclidic impurities with reference to the date and hour of administration.

CHARACTERS

A clear, colourless solution.

Technetium-99m has a half-life of 6.02 h and emits gamma radiation.

IDENTIFICATION

A. Record the gamma-ray spectrum using a suitable instrument. The spectrum does not differ significantly from that of a standardised technetium-99m solution either by direct comparison or by using an instrument calibrated with the aid of such a solution. Standardised technetium-99m and molybdenum-99 solutions are available from laboratories recognised by the competent authority. The most prominent gamma photon of technetium-99m has an energy of 0.140 MeV.

B. Examine by liquid chromatography (2.2.29).

Test solution   Dilute the injection to be examined with *methanol R* to obtain a solution containing about 1 mg of etifenin per millilitre.

Reference solution   Dissolve 5.0 mg of *etifenin CRS* in *methanol R* and dilute to 5.0 mL with the same solvent.

The chromatographic procedure may be carried out using:
— a column 0.25 m long and 4.6 mm in internal diameter packed with *octadecylsilyl silica gel for chromatography R* (5 µm to 10 µm),
— as mobile phase at a flow rate of 1 mL/min a mixture of 20 volumes of *methanol R* and 80 volumes of a 14 g/L solution of *potassium dihydrogen phosphate R* adjusted to pH 2.5 by the addition of *phosphoric acid R*,
— a spectrophotometer set at 230 nm.

Inject 20 µL of each solution. The principal peak in the chromatogram obtained with the test solution has a similar retention time to the principal peak in the chromatogram obtained with the reference solution.

TESTS

pH (2.2.3)
The pH of the injection is 4.0 to 6.0.

Physiological distribution

Inject 0.1 mL (equivalent to about 3.7 MBq) into a caudal vein of each of three mice, each weighing 20 g to 25 g. Euthanise the mice 1 h after the injection. Remove the liver, gall-bladder, small intestine, large intestine and kidneys, collecting excreted urine. Measure the radioactivity in the organs using a suitable instrument. Measure the radioactivity of the rest of the body, after having removed the tail. Determine the percentage of radioactivity in each organ from the expression:

$$\frac{A}{B} \times 100$$

A = radioactivity of the organ concerned,
B = radioactivity of all organs and the rest of the body, excluding the tail.

In not fewer than two mice the sum of the percentages of radioactivity in the gall-bladder and small and large intestine is not less than 80 per cent. Not more than 3 per cent of the radioactivity is present in the liver, and not more than 2 per cent in the kidneys.

Tin

Test solution   Dilute 1.0 mL of the injection to be examined to 5.0 mL with *1 M hydrochloric acid*.

Reference solution Prepare a reference solution containing 0.075 mg of *stannous chloride R* per millilitre in *1 M hydrochloric acid*.

To 1.0 mL of each solution add 0.4 mL of a 20 g/L solution of *sodium laurilsulfate R*, 0.05 mL of *thioglycollic acid R*, 0.1 mL of *dithiol reagent R* and 3.0 mL of *0.2 M hydrochloric acid*. Mix. Measure the absorbance (*2.2.25*) of each solution at 540 nm, using *0.2 M hydrochloric acid* as the compensation liquid. The absorbance of the test solution is not greater than that of the reference solution (0.2 mg of Sn per millilitre).

Sterility

It complies with the test for sterility prescribed in the monograph *on Radiopharmaceutical preparations (0125)*. The injection may be released for use before completion of the test.

RADIOCHEMICAL PURITY

Examine by thin-layer chromatography (*2.2.27*) using silicic acid as the coating substance on a glass-fibre sheet. Heat the plate at 110 °C for l0 min. The plate used should be such that during development the mobile phase moves over a distance of 10 cm to 15 cm in about 15 min.

Apply to the plate 5 µL to 10 µL of the injection to be examined. Develop immediately over a path of 10 cm to 15 cm using a 9 g/L solution of *sodium chloride R*. Allow the plate to dry. Determine the distribution of radioactivity using a suitable detector. Technetium-99m complexed with etifenin migrates almost to the middle of the chromatogram and pertechnetate ion migrates with the solvent front. Impurities in colloidal form remain at the point of application. The radioactivity corresponding to technetium-99m complexed with etifenin represents not less than 95.0 per cent of the total radioactivity of the chromatogram.

RADIOACTIVITY

Measure the radioactivity using suitable counting equipment by comparison with a standardised technetium-99m solution or by measurement in an instrument calibrated with the aid of such a solution.

Ph Eur

Technetium (⁹⁹ᵐTc) Exametazime Injection

(*Ph Eur monograph 1925*)

and enantiomer

Ph Eur

DEFINITION

Sterile solution of lipophilic technetium-99m exametazime which may be prepared by dissolving a racemic mixture of (3RS,9RS)-4,8-diaza-3,6,6,9-tetramethylundecane-2,10-dione bisoxime in the presence of a stannous salt in *Sodium pertechnetate (⁹⁹ᵐTc) injection (fission) (0124)* or *Sodium pertechnetate (⁹⁹ᵐTc) injection (non-fission) (0283)*. It may contain stabilisers and inert additives.

Content

90 per cent to 110 per cent of the declared technetium-99m radioactivity at the date and time stated on the label.

Purity

Minimum of 80 per cent of the total radioactivity corresponds to lipophilic technetium-99m exametazime and its *meso* isomer.

CHARACTERS

Appearance

Clear solution.

Half-life and nature of radiation of technetium-99m

see general chapter *5.7*. *Table of physical characteristics of radionuclides*.

IDENTIFICATION

A. Gamma-ray spectrometry.

Comparison Standardised technetium-99m solution, or by using a calibrated instrument. Standardised technetium-99m solutions and/or standardisation services are available from the competent authority.

Results The spectrum obtained with the solution to be examined does not differ significantly from that obtained with a standardised technetium-99m solution. The most prominent gamma photon has an energy of 0.141 MeV.

B. Examine the chromatograms obtained in the test Impurity A under Radiochemical purity.

Results The principal peak in the chromatogram obtained with the test solution is similar in retention time to the peak due to lipophilic technetium-99m exametazime in the chromatogram obtained with the reference solution.

TESTS

pH (*2.2.3*)
5.0 to 10.0.

Sterility

It complies with the test for sterility prescribed in the monograph on *Radiopharmaceutical preparations (0125)*. The injection may be released for use before completion of the test.

RADIOCHEMICAL PURITY

Impurity C

Thin-layer chromatography (*2.2.27*).

Test solution The preparation to be examined.

Plate TLC silica gel plate *R*; use a glass-fibre plate.

Mobile phase 9 g/L solution of *sodium chloride R*.

Application About 5 µL.

Development Immediate, over 2/3 of the plate.

Drying In air.

Detection Determine the distribution of radioactivity using a suitable detector.

Retardation factors impurity C = 0.8 to 1.0; lipophilic technetium-99m exametazime and impurities A, B, D and E do not migrate.

Limits:
— *impurity C*: maximum 10 per cent of the total radioactivity.

Total of lipophilic technetium-99m exametazime and impurity A

Thin-layer chromatography (*2.2.27*).

Test solution The preparation to be examined.

Plate TLC silica gel plate *R*; use a glass-fibre plate.

Mobile phase methyl ethyl ketone *R*.

Application   About 5 µL.

Development   Immediate, over 2/3 of the plate.

Drying   In air.

Detection   Determine the distribution of radioactivity using a suitable detector.

Retardation factors   lipophilic technetium-99m exametazime = 0.8 to 1.0, impurity A = 0.8 to 1.0, impurity C = 0.8 to 1.0; impurities B, D and E do not migrate.

Limits   Calculate the percentage of radioactivity due to impurities B, D and E from test B (*B*) and the percentage of the radioactivity due to impurity C from test A (*A*). Calculate the total percentage of lipophilic technetium-99m exametazime and impurity A from the expression:

$$100 - A - B$$

— *total of lipophilic technetium-99m exametazime and impurity A*: minimum 80 per cent of the total radioactivity.

Impurity A

Liquid chromatography (*2.2.29*).

Test solution   The preparation to be examined.

Reference solution   Dissolve the contents of a vial of *meso-rich exametazime CRS* in 0.5 mL of a 9 g/L solution of *sodium chloride R* and transfer to a lead-shielded, nitrogen-filled vial. Add 6 µL of a freshly prepared 1 g/L solution of *stannous chloride R* in *0.05 M hydrochloric acid* and 2.5 mL of sodium pertechnetate (⁹⁹ᵐTc) injection (fission or non-fission) containing 370-740 MBq. Mix carefully and use within 30 min of preparation.

Column:
— *size: l* = 0.25 m, Ø = 4.6 mm,
— *stationary phase*: *spherical base-deactivated end-capped octadecylsilyl silica gel for chromatography R* (5 µm) with a pore size of 13 nm and a carbon loading of 11 per cent.

Mobile phase   Mix 33 volumes of *acetonitrile R* and 67 volumes of *0.1 M phosphate buffer solution pH 3.0 R*.

Flow rate   1.5 mL/min.

Detection   Radioactivity detector.

Injection   Loop injector.

Run time   20 min.

Relative retention   With reference to lipophilic technetium-99m exametazime: impurity A = about 1.2.

System suitability   Reference solution:
— chromatogram similar to the chromatogram provided with *meso-rich exametazime CRS*,
— *resolution*: minimum of 2 between the peaks due to lipophilic technetium-99m exametazime and to impurity A.

Limits:
— *impurity A*: maximum 5 per cent of the radioactivity due to lipophilic technetium-99m exametazime and impurity A.

RADIOACTIVITY

Measure the radioactivity using suitable equipment by comparison with a standardised technetium-99m solution or by using a calibrated instrument.

IMPURITIES

A. *meso* isomer of lipophilic technetium-99m exametazime,

B. technetium-99m in colloidal form,

C. [⁹⁹ᵐTc]pertechnetate ion,

D. non lipophilic technetium-99m exametazime complex,

E. *meso* isomer of non lipophilic technetium-99m exametazime complex.

_____ Ph Eur

Technetium (⁹⁹ᵐTc) Gluconate Injection

(*Ph Eur monograph 1047*)

Ph Eur _____

DEFINITION

Sterile solution of a complex of technetium-99m with calcium gluconate. It is prepared using *Sodium pertechnetate (⁹⁹ᵐTc) injection fission (0124)* or *Sodium pertechnetate (⁹⁹ᵐTc) injection non fission (0283)*.

Technetium-99m

90 per cent to 110 per cent of the declared technetium-99m radioactivity at the date and time stated on the label.

CHARACTERS

Appearance

Slightly opalescent solution.

Half-life and nature of radiation of technetium-99m

See general chapter 5.7. *Table of characteristics of radionuclides.*

IDENTIFICATION

A. Gamma-ray spectrometry.

Result   The most prominent gamma photon of technetium-99m has an energy of 0.141 MeV.

B. 5 µL of the preparation to be examined complies with identification A prescribed in the monograph *Calcium gluconate (0172)*.

C. Examine the chromatograms obtained in tests A and B for radiochemical purity (see Tests).

Results:
— the retardation factor of the principal peak in the radiochromatogram obtained with the test solution in test A is 0.9 to 1.0;
— the retardation factor of the principal peak in the radiochromatogram obtained with the test solution in test B is 0.0 to 0.1.

TESTS

pH (*2.2.3*)

6.0 to 8.5.

Physiological distribution

Inject a volume not greater than 0.2 mL into the caudal vein of each of 3 rats weighing 150-250 g. Measure the radioactivity of the syringe before and after injection.

Euthanise the rats 30 min after the injection. Remove at least 1 g of blood by a suitable method and remove the kidneys, the liver, the bladder plus voided urine and the tail. Weigh the sample of blood.

Determine the radioactivity in the organs, the blood sample and the tail using a suitable instrument. Calculate the percentage of radioactivity in each organ and in 1 g of blood with respect to the total radioactivity calculated as the difference between the 2 measurements made on the syringe minus the activity in the tail. Correct the blood concentration by multiplying by a factor of $m/200$ where m is the body mass of the rat in grams.

In not fewer than 2 of the 3 rats used, the radioactivity is:
— *in the kidneys*: minimum 15 per cent,
— *in the bladder plus voided urine*: minimum 20 per cent,
— *in the liver*: maximum 5 per cent.
— *in the blood*, after correction: maximum 0.50 per cent.

Sterility

It complies with the test for sterility prescribed in the monograph *Radiopharmaceutical preparations (0125)*. The preparation may be released for use before completion of the test.

RADIOCHEMICAL PURITY

A. Impurity A. Thin-layer chromatography (*2.2.27*).

Test solution   The preparation to be examined.

Plate   *TLC silica gel plate R*; use silica gel as the coating substance on a glass-fibre sheet heated at 110 °C for 10 min.

Mobile phase   9 g/L solution of *sodium chloride R*.

Application   5-10 µL.

Development   Immediately over a path of 10-15 cm in about 10 min.

Drying   In air.

Detection   Suitable detector to determine the distribution of radioactivity.

Retardation factors   impurity A = 0.0 to 0.1; [^{99m}Tc]technetium gluconate and impurity B = 0.9 to 1.0.

B. Impurity B. Thin-layer chromatography (*2.2.27*).

Test solution   The preparation to be examined.

Plate   *TLC silica gel plate R*; use silica gel as the coating substance on a glass-fibre sheet heated at 110 °C for 10 min.

Mobile phase   methyl ethyl ketone R.

Application   5-10 µL and allow to dry.

Development   Over a path of 10-15 cm in about 10 min.

Drying   In a current of warm air.

Detection   Suitable detector to determine the distribution of radioactivity.

Retardation factors   [^{99m}Tc]technetium gluconate and impurity A = 0.0 to 0.1; impurity B = 0.9 to 1.0.

Limit:
— *sum of impurities A and B*: maximum 10 per cent of the radioactivity due to technetium-99m in the chromatograms obtained in tests A and B.

RADIOACTIVITY

Determine the radioactivity using a calibrated instrument.

IMPURITIES

A. [^{99m}Tc]technetium in colloidal form,

B. [^{99m}Tc]pertechnetate ion.

Technetium (^{99m}Tc) Macrosalb Injection

(*Ph Eur monograph 0296*)

Ph Eur

DEFINITION

Sterile suspension of human albumin in the form of irregular insoluble aggregates obtained by denaturing human albumin in aqueous solution. It is prepared using *Sodium pertechnetate (^{99m}Tc) injection (fission) (0124)* or *Sodium pertechnetate (^{99m}Tc) injection (non fission) (0283)*. The particles are labelled with technetium-99m and have a typical diameter between 10 µm and 100 µm. The injection contains reducing substances, such as tin salts; it may contain a suitable buffer such as acetate, citrate or phosphate buffer and also non-denatured human albumin and an antimicrobial preservative such as benzyl alcohol.

The human albumin employed complies with the requirements prescribed in the monograph *Human albumin solution (0255)*.

Technetium-99m   90 per cent to 110 per cent of the declared technetium-99m radioactivity at the date and time stated on the label.

Specific radioactivity   Minimum 37 MBq of technetium-99m per milligram of aggregated albumin at the date and time of administration.

CHARACTERS

Appearance

White suspension which may separate on standing.

Half-life and nature of radiation of technetium-99m   See general chapter 5.7. *Table of physical characteristics of radionuclides*.

IDENTIFICATION

A. Gamma-ray spectrometry.

Result   The most prominent gamma photon of technetium-99m has an energy of 0.141 MeV.

B. The tests for non-filterable radioactivity and particle size contribute to the identification of the preparation (see Tests).

C. Transfer 1 mL of the preparation to be examined to a centrifuge tube and centrifuge at 2500 *g* for 5-10 min. Decant the supernatant liquid. To the residue add 5 mL of *cupri-tartaric solution R2*, mix and allow to stand for 10 min. If necessary, heat to dissolve the particles and allow to cool. Add rapidly 0.5 mL of *dilute phosphomolybdotungstic reagent R*, mixing immediately. A blue colour develops.

TESTS

pH (*2.2.3*)

3.8 to 7.5.

Non-filterable radioactivity

Minimum 90 per cent of the total radioactivity.

Use a polycarbonate membrane filter 13-25 mm in diameter, 10 µm thick and with circular pores 3 µm in diameter. Fit the membrane into a suitable holder. Place 0.2 mL of the preparation to be examined on the membrane and filter, adding 20 mL of a 9 g/L solution of *sodium chloride R* during the filtration. Determine the radioactivity remaining on the membrane.

Particle size

not more than 10 particles have a maximum dimension greater than 100 µm and no particle having a maximum dimension greater than 150 µm is present.

Examine using a microscope. Dilute the preparation to be examined if necessary so that the number of particles is just low enough for individual particles to be distinguished. Using a syringe fitted with a needle having a calibre not less than 0.35 mm, place a suitable volume in a suitable counting chamber such as a haemocytometer cell, taking care not to overfill the chamber. Allow the preparation to be examined to settle for 1 min and, carefully add a cover slide without squeezing the sample. Scan an area corresponding to at least 5000 particles.

Aggregated albumin

Test solution   Transfer a volume of the preparation to be examined containing about 1 mg of aggregated albumin to a centrifuge tube and centrifuge at about 2500 *g* for 5-10 min. Decant the supernatant liquid. Resuspend the residue in 2.0 mL of a 9 g/L solution of *sodium chloride R*. Centrifuge at 2500 *g* for 5-10 min. Decant the supernatant liquid. Resuspend the residue in 5.0 mL of *sodium carbonate solution R1*. Heat in a water-bath at 80-90 °C to dissolve the aggregated albumin. Allow to cool, transfer to a volumetric flask and dilute to 10.0 mL with *sodium carbonate solution R1*.

Reference solutions   Prepare a range of solutions containing 0.05-0.2 mg of human albumin per millilitre by diluting *human albumin solution R* with *sodium carbonate solution R1*.

Introduce 3.0 mL of each solution separately into 25 mL flasks. To each flask add 15.0 mL of *cupri-tartaric solution R2*, mix and allow to stand for 10 min. Add rapidly 1.5 mL of *dilute phosphomolybdotungstic reagent R* and mix immediately. Allow to stand for 30 min and measure the absorbance (*2.2.25*) of each solution at 750 nm using *sodium carbonate solution R1* as the compensation liquid. Using the absorbances obtained with the reference solutions, draw a calibration curve and calculate the content of aggregated albumin in the preparation to be examined.

Tin

Maximum 3 mg/mL.

Test solution   To 1.0 mL of the preparation to be examined, add 1.0 mL of a 206 g/L solution of *hydrochloric acid R*. Heat in a water-bath for 30 min. Cool and centrifuge for 10 min at 300 *g*. Dilute 1.0 mL of the supernatant liquid to 25.0 mL with a 103 g/L solution of *hydrochloric acid R*.

Reference solution   Dissolve 0.115 g of *stannous chloride R* in a 103 g/L solution of *hydrochloric acid R* and dilute to 1000.0 mL with the same acid.

To 1.0 mL of each solution, add 0.05 mL of *thioglycollic acid R*, 0.1 mL of *dithiol reagent R*, 0.4 mL of a 20 g/L solution of *sodium laurilsulfate R* and 3.0 mL of a 21 g/L solution of *hydrochloric acid R*. Mix. Measure the absorbance (*2.2.25*) of each solution at 540 nm, using a 21 g/L solution of *hydrochloric acid R* as the compensation liquid. The absorbance of the test solution is not greater than that of the reference solution.

Physiological distribution

Inject a volume not greater than 0.2 mL into a caudal vein of each of 3 rats weighing 150-250 g. Euthanise the rats 15 min after the injection, remove the liver, the spleen and the lungs and measure the radioactivity in the organs using a suitable instrument. Measure the radioactivity in the rest of the body, including the blood, after having removed the tail. Determine the percentage of radioactivity in the lungs, the liver and the spleen from the following expression:

$$\frac{A}{B} \times 100$$

A =   radioactivity of the organ concerned;

B =   total radioactivity in the liver, the spleen, the lungs and the rest of the body.

In not fewer than 2 of the 3 rats used, at least 80 per cent of the radioactivity is found in the lungs and not more than a total of 5 per cent in the liver and spleen. The preparation may be released for use before completion of the test.

Sterility

It complies with the test for sterility prescribed in the monograph *Radiopharmaceutical preparations (0125)*.
The preparation may be released for use before completion of the test.

Bacterial endotoxins (*2.6.14*)

Less than 175/*V* IU/mL, *V* being the maximum recommended dose in millilitres.

RADIOACTIVITY

Determine the radioactivity using a calibrated instrument.

LABELLING

The label states:
— the concentration of tin expressed in milligrams per millilitre, if any;
— that the preparation is to be shaken before use;
— that the preparation is not to be used if after shaking, the suspension does not appear homogeneous.

Ph Eur

Technetium (⁹⁹ᵐTc) Mebrofenin Injection

(*Ph Eur monograph 2393*)

Ph Eur

DEFINITION

Sterile solution of a complex of technetium-99m with mebrofenin. It may contain stabilisers and inert additives.

Content

90 per cent to 110 per cent of the declared technetium-99m radioactivity at the date and time stated on the label.

PRODUCTION

It is prepared by dissolving [[[(3-bromo-2,4,6-trimethylphenyl)carbamoyl]methyl]imino]diacetic acid (mebrofenin) in the presence of a reducing agent such as a stannous salt in *Sodium pertechnetate (⁹⁹ᵐTc) injection (fission) (0124)* or *Sodium pertechnetate (⁹⁹ᵐTc) injection (non-fission) (0283)*.

CHARACTERS

Appearance

Clear, colourless solution.

Half-life and nature of radiation of technetium-99m

See general chapter *5.7. Table of physical characteristics of radionuclides*.

IDENTIFICATION

A. Gamma-ray spectrometry.

Results The most prominent gamma photon of technetium-99m has an energy of 0.141 MeV.

B. Examine the chromatogram obtained in the test for other radiochemical impurities (see Tests).

Results The principal peak in the chromatogram obtained with the test solution is similar in retention time to the peak due to technetium-99m mebrofenin in the chromatogram obtained with the reference solution.

TESTS

pH *(2.2.3)*
4.0 to 7.5.

Sterility

It complies with the test for sterility prescribed in the monograph on *Radiopharmaceutical preparations (0125)*. The injection may be released for use before completion of the test.

Bacterial endotoxins *(2.6.14)*

Less than 175/*V* IU/mL, *V* being the maximum recommended dose in millilitres.

RADIOCHEMICAL PURITY

Impurity A

Thin-layer chromatography *(2.2.27)*.

Test solution The preparation to be examined.

Reference solution (a) To 1 mL of a 1 g/L solution of *stannous chloride R* in *0.05 M hydrochloric acid* in a closed vial, add 2 mL of sodium pertechnetate (^{99m}Tc) injection (fission or non-fission). Use within 30 min after preparation.

Reference solution (b) Dissolve 40 mg of *mebrofenin CRS* in 2 mL of *water R* and adjust to pH 6.5 with a 40 g/L solution of *sodium hydroxide R*. To this solution add 25 µL of a 20 mg/mL solution of *stannous chloride R* in *0.05 M hydrochloric acid* and 400 MBq of sodium pertechnetate (^{99}Tc) injection (fission or non-fission) in a volume of 2 mL. Allow to stand for 15 min.

Plate TLC silica gel plate R; use a glass-fibre plate.

Mobile phase water R, acetonitrile R (40:60 *V/V*).

Application About 5 µL.

Development Immediately, over 4/5 of the plate.

Drying In air.

Detection Determine the distribution of radioactivity using a suitable detector.

Retardation factor impurity A = 0-0.1.

System suitability The retardation factor of the principal peak in the chromatogram obtained with reference solution (a) is not more than 0.1. The retardation factor of the principal peak in the chromatogram obtained with reference solution (b) is more than 0.7.

Other radiochemical impurities

Liquid chromatography *(2.2.29)*.

Test solution The preparation to be examined.

Reference solution Use reference solution (b) of the test for impurity A.

Column:
— *size: l* = 0.25 m, Ø = 4.0 mm;
— *stationary phase:* end-capped octadecylsilyl silica gel for chromatography with polar incorporated groups R (5 µm).

Mobile phase A 3.85 g/L solution of *ammonium acetate R*.

Mobile phase B acetonitrile R.

Time (min)	Mobile phase A (per cent *V/V*)	Mobile phase B (per cent *V/V*)
0 - 20	70	30
20 - 25	70 → 0	30 → 100
25 - 30	0	100

Flow rate 1.0 mL/min.

Detection Radioactivity detector.

Injection 20 µL.

Relative retention With reference to technetium-99m mebrofenin (retention time = about 20 min): impurity B = about 0.17.

Limits:
— *technetium-99m mebrofenin*: minimum 94 per cent of the total radioactivity.

Calculate the percentage of radioactivity due to technetium-99m mebrofenin using the following expression:

$$(100 - A) \times T$$

A = percentage of radioactivity due to impurity A determined in the test for impurity A under radiochemical purity;

T = proportion of the radioactivity in the peak due to technetium-99m mebrofenin relative to the total eluted radioactivity in the chromatogram obtained with the test solution.

RADIOACTIVITY

Determine the radioactivity using a calibrated instrument.

IMPURITIES

A. technetium-99m in colloidal form,

B. [^{99m}Tc]pertechnetate ion.

_____ *Ph Eur*

Technetium (^{99m}Tc) Medronate Injection

(Ph Eur monograph 0641)

Ph Eur _____

DEFINITION

Sterile solution of a complex of technetium-99m with sodium medronate. It is prepared using *Sodium pertechnetate (^{99m}Tc) injection (fission) (0124)* or *Sodium pertechnetate (^{99m}Tc) injection (non fission) (0283)*. The injection may contain antimicrobial preservatives, antioxidants, stabilisers and buffers.

Technetium-99m

90 per cent to 110 per cent of the declared technetium-99m radioactivity at the date and time stated on the label.

CHARACTERS

Appearance

Clear, colourless solution.

Half-life and nature of radiation of technetium-99m

See general chapter 5.7. *Table of physical characteristics of radionuclides.*

IDENTIFICATION

A. Gamma-ray spectrometry.

Result   The most prominent gamma photon of technetium-99m has an energy of 0.141 MeV.

B. Examine the chromatograms obtained in tests A and B for radiochemical purity (see Tests).

Results:
— the retardation factor of the principal peak in the radiochromatogram obtained with the test solution in test A is 0.9 to 1.0;
— the retardation factor of the principal peak in the radiochromatogram obtained with the test solution in test B is 0.0 to 0.1.

C. Thin-layer chromatography (*2.2.27*).

Test solution   Dilute the preparation to be examined with *water R* to obtain a solution containing about 0.1-0.5 mg/mL of sodium medronate.

Reference solution   Dissolve a suitable quantity (1-5 mg) of *medronic acid CRS* in a suitable mixture of a 9.0 g/L solution of *sodium chloride R* and *water R* and dilute to 10 mL with the same solvent mixture so as to obtain a solution similar to the test solution with regard to sodium medronate and sodium chloride concentrations.

Plate   *Cellulose for chromatography R* as the coating substance.

Mobile phase   *2-propanol R*, *1 M hydrochloric acid*, *methyl ethyl ketone R* (20:30:60 *V/V/V*).

Application   10 μL.

Development   Over a path of 12-14 cm in about 4 h.

Drying   In air.

Detection   Spray with *ammonium molybdate solution R4*, then expose to ultraviolet light at 254 nm for about 10 min.

Results   The principal spot in the chromatogram obtained with the test solution is similar in position and colour to the spot in the chromatogram obtained with the reference solution.

TESTS

pH (*2.2.3*)
3.5 to 7.5.

Tin
Maximum 3 mg/mL.

Test solution   Dilute 1.0 mL of the preparation to be examined to 50.0 mL with a 103 g/L solution of *hydrochloric acid R*.

Reference solution   Dissolve 0.115 g of *stannous chloride R* in a 103 g/L solution of *hydrochloric acid R* and dilute to 1000.0 mL with the same acid.

To 1.0 mL of each solution add 0.05 mL of *thioglycollic acid R*, 0.1 mL of *dithiol reagent R*, 0.4 mL of a 20 g/L solution of *sodium laurilsulfate R* and 3.0 mL of a 21 g/L solution of *hydrochloric acid R*. Mix. Measure the absorbance (*2.2.25*) of each solution at 540 nm, using a 21 g/L solution of *hydrochloric acid R* as compensation liquid. The absorbance of the test solution is not greater than that of the reference solution.

Physiological distribution
Inject a volume not greater than 0.2 mL, equivalent to not more than 0.05 mg of sodium medronate, into a suitable vein such as a caudal vein or the saphenous vein of each of 3 rats, each weighing 150-250 g. Measure the radioactivity in the syringe before and after injection. Euthanise the rats 2 h after the injection. Remove 1 femur, the liver, and some blood. Weigh the blood. Remove the tail if a caudal vein has been used for the injection. Using a suitable instrument measure the radioactivity in the femur, liver and blood, and in the tail

if a caudal vein has been used for the injection. Determine the percentage of radioactivity in each sample using the following expression:

$$\frac{A}{B} \times 100$$

A = radioactivity of the sample concerned;
B = total radioactivity, which is equal to the difference between the two measurements made on the syringe minus the radioactivity in the tail if a caudal vein has been used for the injection.

Calculate the radioactivity per unit mass in the blood. Correct the blood concentration by multiplying by a factor $m/200$ where m is the body mass of the rat in grams.

In not fewer than 2 of the 3 rats used, the radioactivity is:
— *in the liver*: maximum 1.0 per cent;
— *in the femur*: minimum 1.5 per cent;
— *in the blood after correction*: maximum 0.05 per cent per gram.

Sterility
It complies with the test for sterility prescribed in the monograph *Radiopharmaceutical preparations (0125)*.
The preparation may be released for use before completion of the test.

RADIOCHEMICAL PURITY
A. Impurity A. Thin-layer chromatography (*2.2.27*).

Test solution   The preparation to be examined.

Plate   *TLC silica gel plate R*; use silica gel as the coating substance on a glass-fibre sheet.

Mobile phase   136 g/L solution of *sodium acetate R*.

Application   5-10 μL.

Development   Immediately, over a path of 10-15 cm in about 10 min.

Drying   In air.

Detection   Suitable detector to determine the distribution of radioactivity.

Retardation factors   impurity A = 0.0 to 0.1; [^{99m}Tc]technetium medronate and impurity B = 0.9 to 1.0.

B. Impurity B. Thin-layer chromatography (*2.2.27*).

Test solution   The preparation to be examined.

Plate   *TLC silica gel plate R*; use silica gel as the coating substance on a glass-fibre sheet.

Mobile phase   methyl ethyl ketone R.

Application   5-10 μL; dry quickly.

Development   Over a path of 10-15 cm in about 10 min.

Drying   In air.

Detection   Suitable detector to determine the distribution of radioactivity.

Retardation factors   [^{99m}Tc]technetium medronate and impurity A = 0.0 to 0.1; impurity B = 0.9 to 1.0.

Limits:
— *impurity B*: maximum 2.0 per cent of the radioactivity due to technetium-99m in the chromatogram obtained in test B;
— *sum of impurities A and B*: maximum 5.0 per cent of the radioactivity due to technetium-99m in the chromatograms obtained in tests A and B.

RADIOACTIVITY
Determine the radioactivity using a calibrated instrument.

IMPURITIES

A. [^{99m}Tc]technetium in colloidal form;

B. [^{99m}Tc]pertechnetate ion.

Ph Eur

Technetium (^{99m}Tc) Mertiatide Injection

(*Ph Eur monograph 1372*)

Ph Eur

DEFINITION

Sterile solution of disodium oxo[*N*-[*N*-[*N*-(sulfanylacetyl)glycyl]glycyl]glycynato(5-)-κ^4*N*,*N'*,*N''*,*S*][^{99m}Tc]technetate(V). It may be prepared by either heating a mixture containing *S*-benzoylmercaptoacetyltriglycine (betiatide), a weak chelating agent such as tartrate, a stannous salt and *Sodium pertechnetate (^{99m}Tc) injection fission (0124)* or *Sodium pertechnetate (^{99m}Tc) injection non-fission (0283)*, or by mixing solutions of mercaptoacetyltriglycine (mertiatide), a stannous salt and *Sodium pertechnetate (^{99m}Tc) injection fission (0124)* or *Sodium pertechnetate (^{99m}Tc) injection non-fission (0283)* at alkaline pH. It may contain stabilisers and a buffer.

Technetium-99m

90 per cent to 110 per cent of the declared technetium-99m radioactivity at the date and time stated on the label.

CHARACTERS

Appearance

Clear, colourless solution.

Half-life and nature of radiation of technetium-99m

See general chapter 5.7. *Table of physical characteristics of radionuclides*.

IDENTIFICATION

A. Gamma-ray spectrometry.

Result The most prominent gamma photon of technetium-99m has an energy of 0.141 MeV.

B. Examine the chromatograms obtained in the test of other radiochemical impurities in the section Radiochemical purity (see Tests).

Result The principal peak in the radiochromatogram obtained with the test solution is similar in retention time to the principal peak in the chromatogram obtained with the reference solution.

TESTS

pH (*2.2.3*)

5.0 to 7.5.

Sterility

It complies with the test for sterility prescribed in the monograph *Radiopharmaceutical preparations (0125)*.

The preparation may be released for use before completion of the test.

RADIOCHEMICAL PURITY

Impurity A

Ascending paper chromatography (*2.2.26*).

Test solution The preparation to be examined.

Paper paper for chromatography R.

Mobile phase water R, acetonitrile R (40:60 *V/V*).

Application 2 μL.

Development Over a path of 15 cm.

Drying In air.

Detection Suitable detector to determine the distribution of radioactivity.

Retardation factor impurity A = 0.0-0.1.

Limit:

— *impurity A*: maximum 2.0 per cent of the total radioactivity.

Other radiochemical impurities

Liquid chromatography (*2.2.29*).

Test solution The preparation to be examined.

Reference solution Dissolve with heating on a water-bath 5 mg of *S-benzylmercaptoacetyltriglycine CRS* in 5 mL of *water R*. To 1 mL of this solution in a closed vial filled with *nitrogen R*, add 0.5 mL of a 40 g/L solution of *sodium potassium tartrate R*, 25 μL of a 4 g/L solution of *stannous chloride R* in a 5 g/L solution of *hydrochloric acid R* and 370-740 MBq of sodium pertechnetate (^{99m}Tc) injection (fission or non-fission) in a volume not exceeding 3 mL. Heat the mixture on a water-bath for 10 min and allow to cool to room temperature.

Column:

— *size: l* = 0.25 m, Ø = 4.0 mm;

— *stationary phase: octadecylsilyl silica gel for chromatography R* (5 μm).

Mobile phase A Mix 7 volumes of *anhydrous ethanol R* with 93 volumes of a 1.36 g/L solution of *potassium dihydrogen phosphate R*, adjusted to pH 6.0 with a 4 g/L solution of *sodium hydroxide R*.

Mobile phase B water R, methanol R (10:90 *V/V*).

Time (min)	Mobile phase A (per cent *V/V*)	Mobile phase B (per cent *V/V*)
0 - 10	100	0
10 - 25	0	100

Flow rate 1.0 mL/min.

Detection Suitable detector to determine the distribution of radioactivity.

Equilibration With mobile phase A for 20 min.

Injection 20 μL.

Limits:

— *sum of the areas preceding the principal peak (corresponding to hydrophilic impurities, including impurity B)*: maximum 3.0 per cent of the sum of the areas of all peaks in the chromatogram obtained with the test solution;

— *sum of the peaks following the principal peak (corresponding to lipophilic impurities)*: maximum 4.0 per cent of the sum of the area of all peaks in the chromatogram obtained with the test solution;

— *[^{99m}Tc]technetium mertiatide*: minimum 94 per cent of the radioactivity due to technetium-99m.

RADIOACTIVITY

Determine the radioactivity using a calibrated instrument.

IMPURITIES

A. [^{99m}Tc]technetium in colloidal form,

B. [^{99m}Tc]pertechnetate ion.

_____ *Ph Eur*

Technetium (^{99m}Tc) Microspheres Injection

(Ph Eur monograph 0570)

Ph Eur _____

DEFINITION

Sterile suspension of human albumin which has been denatured to form spherical insoluble particles. The particles are labelled with technetium-99m and have a typical diameter of 10-50 μm. It is prepared using *Sodium pertechnetate (^{99m}Tc) injection (fission) (0124)* or *Sodium pertechnetate (^{99m}Tc) injection (non fission) (0283)*.

The injection contains reducing substances, such as tin salts. It may contain a suitable buffer such as acetate, citrate or phosphate and additives such as wetting agents.

The human albumin used complies with the requirements of the monograph *Human albumin solution (0255)*.

Technetium-99m

90 per cent to 110 per cent of the declared technetium-99m radioactivity at the date and time stated on the label.

Radioactivity

Minimum 185 MBq of technetium-99m per million particles at the date and time of administration.

CHARACTERS

Appearance

Suspension of white, yellow or artificially coloured particles which may separate on standing.

Half-life and nature of radiation of technetium-99m

See general chapter 5.7. *Table of physical characteristics of radionuclides.*

IDENTIFICATION

A. Gamma-ray spectrometry.

Result   The most prominent gamma photon of technetium-99m has an energy of 0.141 MeV.

B. The tests for non-filterable radioactivity and particle size (see Tests) contribute to the identification of the preparation.

C. Transfer 1 mL of the preparation to be examined to a centrifuge tube and centrifuge at 2500 g for 5-10 min. Decant the supernatant liquid. To the residue add 5 mL of *cupri-tartaric solution R2*, mix and allow to stand for 10 min. If necessary, heat to dissolve the particles and allow to cool. Add rapidly 0.5 mL of *dilute phosphomolybdotungstic reagent R*, mix immediately. A blue colour develops.

TESTS

pH *(2.2.3)*

4.0 to 9.0.

Non-filterable radioactivity

Minimum 95 per cent of the total radioactivity.

Use a polycarbonate membrane filter 13-25 mm in diameter, 10 μm thick and with circular pores 3 μm in diameter. Fit the membrane into a suitable holder. Place 0.2 mL of the preparation to be examined on the membrane and filter, adding 20 mL of a 9 g/L solution of *sodium chloride R* during the filtration. Determine the radioactivity remaining on the membrane.

Particle size

Maximum 10 particles have a maximum dimension greater than 75 μm but no particle have a maximum dimension greater than 100 μm.

Examine using a microscope. Dilute the preparation if necessary so that the number of particles is just low enough for individual particles to be distinguished. Using a syringe fitted with a needle having a calibre not less than 0.35 mm, place a suitable volume in a suitable counting chamber such as a haemocytometer cell, taking care not to overfill the chamber. Allow the suspension to settle for 1 min and carefully add a cover slide without squeezing the sample. Scan an area corresponding to at least 5000 particles. The particles have a uniform spherical appearance.

Number of particles

Examine using a microscope. Fill a suitable counting chamber such as a haemocytometer cell with a suitable dilution of the preparation taking care that particles do not separate during the transfer. Count the number of particles in the chamber. Repeat this procedure twice and calculate the number of particles per millilitre of the preparation to be examined.

Tin

Maximum 3 mg/mL.

Test solution   To 1.0 mL of the preparation to be examined add 0.5 mL of *sulfuric acid R* and 1.5 mL of *nitric acid R*. Heat and evaporate to approximately 1 mL. Add 2 mL of *water R* and evaporate again to approximately 1 mL. Repeat this procedure twice, cool and dilute to 25.0 mL with a 103 g/L solution of *hydrochloric acid R*.

Reference solution   Dissolve 0.115 g of *stannous chloride R* in a 103 g/L solution of *hydrochloric acid R* and dilute to 1000.0 mL with the same acid.

To 1.0 mL of each solution add 0.4 mL of a 20 g/L solution of *sodium laurilsulfate R*, 0.05 mL of *thioglycollic acid R*, 0.1 mL of *dithiol reagent R* and 3.0 mL of a 21 g/L solution of *hydrochloric acid R*. Mix. Measure the absorbance *(2.2.25)* of each solution at 540 nm, using a 21 g/L solution of *hydrochloric acid R* as the compensation liquid.

The absorbance of the test solution is not greater than that of the reference solution.

Physiological distribution

Inject a volume not greater than 0.2 mL into a caudal vein of each of 3 rats weighing 150-250 g. Euthanise the rats 15 min after the injection, remove the liver, the spleen and the lungs and measure the radioactivity in these organs using a suitable instrument. Measure the radioactivity in the rest of the body, including the blood and voided urine, after having removed the tail. Determine the percentage of radioactivity in the liver, the spleen and the lungs, using the following expression:

$$\frac{A}{B} \times 100$$

A = radioactivity of the organ concerned,

B = total radioactivity in the liver, the spleen, the lungs and the rest of the body, including voided urine.

In not fewer than 2 of the 3 rats used, not less than 80 per cent of the radioactivity is found in the lungs and not more than a total of 5 per cent in the liver and spleen.

The preparation may be released for use before completion of the test.

Sterility

It complies with the test for sterility prescribed in the monograph *Radiopharmaceutical preparations (0125)*. The preparation may be released for use before completion of the test.

Bacterial endotoxins (2.6.14)

Less than $175/V$ IU/mL, V being the maximum recommended dose in millilitres.

RADIOACTIVITY

Determine the radioactivity using a calibrated instrument.

LABELLING

The label states:
— the concentration of tin expressed in milligrams per millilitre, if any,
— that the preparation is to be shaken before use.

———————————————————— Ph Eur

Technetium (^{99m}Tc) Pentetate Injection

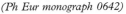

(Ph Eur monograph 0642)

Ph Eur _____

DEFINITION

Sterile solution of a complex of technetium-99m with sodium pentetate or calcium trisodium pentetate. It is prepared using *Sodium pertechnetate (^{99m}Tc) injection (fission) (0124)* or *Sodium pertechnetate (^{99m}Tc) injection (non fission) (0283)*. It may contain suitable antimicrobial preservatives, antioxidants, stabilisers and buffers.

Technetium-99m

90 per cent to 110 per cent of the declared technetium-99m radioactivity at the date and time stated on the label.

CHARACTERS

Appearance

Clear, colourless or slightly yellow solution.

Half-life and nature of radiation of technetium-99m

See general chapter 5.7. *Table of physical characteristics of radionuclides*.

IDENTIFICATION

A. Gamma-ray spectrometry.

Result The most prominent gamma photon of technetium-99m has an energy of 0.141 MeV.

B. Examine the chromatograms obtained in tests A and B for radiochemical purity (see Tests).

Results:
— the retardation factor of the principal peak in the radiochromatogram obtained with the test solution in test A is 0.9 to 1.0;
— the retardation factor of the principal peak in the radiochromatogram obtained with the test solution in test B is 0.0 to 0.1.

C. *Test solution.* In a clean, dry, 10 mL glass tube, place a volume of the preparation to be examined containing 2 mg of pentetate. Dilute, if necessary, to 1 mL with *water R*.

Reference solution In a clean, dry, 10 mL glass tube, place 1 mL of *water R*.

To each tube add 0.1 mL of a 1 g/L solution of *nickel sulfate R*, 0.5 mL of a 50 per cent *V/V* solution of *glacial acetic acid R* and 0.75 mL of a 50 g/L solution of *sodium hydroxide R*. Mix and check that the pH is not above 5. To each tube add 0.1 mL of a 10 g/L solution of *dimethylglyoxime R* in *ethanol (96 per cent) R*. Mix and allow to stand for 2 min. Adjust the pH in each tube to not less than 12 by adding a 100 g/L solution of *sodium hydroxide R*. Mix and check that the pH is not below 12. Allow to stand for 2 min. Heat the tubes gently on a water-bath for 2 min.

Results:
— the test solution remains clear and colourless throughout;
— the reference solution becomes red on addition of dimethylglyoxime solution and a red precipitate is formed when the tube is heated on the water-bath.

TESTS

pH (2.2.3)

4.0 to 7.5.

Tin

Maximum 1 mg/mL.

Test solution Dilute 1.5 mL of the preparation to be examined to 25.0 mL with a 103 g/L solution of *hydrochloric acid R*.

Reference solution Dissolve 0.115 g of *stannous chloride R* in a 103 g/L solution of *hydrochloric acid R* and dilute to 1000.0 mL with the same acid.

To 1.0 mL of each solution add 0.05 mL of *thioglycollic acid R*, 0.1 mL of *dithiol reagent R*, 0.4 mL of a 20 g/L solution of *sodium laurilsulfate R* and 3.0 mL of a 21 g/L solution of *hydrochloric acid R*. Mix. Measure the absorbance (2.2.25) of each solution at 540 nm, using a 21 g/L solution of *hydrochloric acid R* as the compensation liquid.

The absorbance of the test solution is not greater than that of the reference solution.

Sterility

It complies with the test for sterility prescribed in the monograph *Radiopharmaceutical preparations (0125)*. The preparation may be released for use before completion of the test.

RADIOCHEMICAL PURITY

A.

Impurity A

Thin-layer chromatography (2.2.27).

Test solution The preparation to be examined.

Plate TLC silica gel plate R; use silica gel as the coating substance on a glass-fibre sheet, previously heated at 110 °C for 10 min.

Mobile phase 9 g/L solution of *sodium chloride R*.

Application 5-10 µL.

Development Immediately, over a path of 10-15 cm in about 10 min.

Drying In air.

Detection Suitable detector to determine the distribution of radioactivity.

Retardation factors impurity A = 0.0 to 0.1; [^{99m}Tc]technetium pentetate and impurity B = 0.9 to 1.0.

B.

Impurity B

Thin-layer chromatography (2.2.27).

Test solution The preparation to be examined.

Plate TLC silica gel plate R; use silica gel as the coating substance on a glass-fibre sheet, previously heated at 110 °C for 10 min.

Mobile phase methyl ethyl ketone R.

Application 5-10 µL; allow to dry.

Development Over a path of 10-15 cm in about 10 min.

Drying In air.

Detection Suitable detector to determine the distribution of radioactivity.

Retardation factors [⁹⁹ᵐTc]technetium pentetate and impurity A = 0.0 to 0.1; impurity B = 0.9 to 1.0.

Limit:

— sum of impurities A and B: maximum 5.0 per cent of the radioactivity due to technetium-99m in the chromatograms obtained in tests A and B.

RADIOACTIVITY

Determine the radioactivity using a calibrated instrument.

IMPURITIES

A. [⁹⁹ᵐTc]technetium in colloidal form,

B. [⁹⁹ᵐTc]pertechnetate ion.

_____ *Ph Eur*

Technetium (⁹⁹ᵐTc) Sestamibi Injection

(Ph Eur monograph 1926)

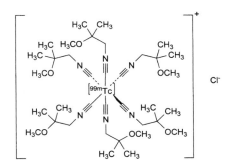

Ph Eur _____

DEFINITION

Sterile solution of (OC-6-11)-hexakis[1-(isocyano-κC)-2-methoxy-2-methylpropane][⁹⁹ᵐTc]technetium(I) chloride, which may be prepared by heating a mixture containing [tetrakis(2-methoxy-2-methylpropyl-1-isocyanide)copper (1+)] tetrafluoroborate, a weak chelating agent, a stannous salt and *Sodium pertechnetate (⁹⁹ᵐTc) injection (fission) (0124)* or *Sodium pertechnetate (⁹⁹ᵐTc) injection (non-fission) (0283)*.

Content

90 per cent to 110 per cent of the declared technetium-99m radioactivity at the date and hour stated on the label.

CHARACTERS

Appearance

Clear, colourless solution.

Half-life and nature of radiation of technetium-99m

See general chapter 5.7. *Table of physical characteristics of radionuclides*.

IDENTIFICATION

A. Gamma-ray spectrometry.

Results The spectrum obtained with the solution to be examined does not differ significantly from that of a standardised technetium-99m solution. The most prominent gamma photon has an energy of 0.141 MeV.

B. Examine the chromatograms obtained in the test for impurity C under Radiochemical purity.

Results The principal peak in the radiochromatogram obtained with the test solution is similar in retention time to the principal peak in the radiochromatogram obtained with the reference solution.

TESTS

pH *(2.2.3)*

5.0 to 6.0.

Sterility

It complies with the test for sterility prescribed in the monograph on *Radiopharmaceutical preparations (0125)*. The injection may be released for use before completion of the test.

RADIOCHEMICAL PURITY

Impurity A and other polar impurities

Thin-layer chromatography *(2.2.27)*.

Test solution The preparation to be examined.

Plate TLC octadecylsilyl silica gel plate R.

Mobile phase Mix 10 volumes of *tetrahydrofuran R*, 20 volumes of a 38.5 g/L solution of *ammonium acetate R*, 30 volumes of *methanol R* and 40 volumes of *acetonitrile R*.

Application About 5 µL.

Development Immediately over a path of 6 cm.

Drying In air.

Detection Determine the distribution of radioactivity using a radioactivity detector.

Retardation factors impurity B and apolar impurities = 0 to 0.1; impurity C and technetium-99m sestamibi = 0.3 to 0.6; impurity A and other polar impurities = 0.9 to 1.0.

Limit See test for impurity B.

Impurity B

Paper chromatography *(2.2.26)*. *If no activity is found at retardation factor 0 to 0.1 in the test for impurity A and other polar impurities, impurity B is absent and the test for impurity B may be omitted.*

Test solution The preparation to be examined.

Paper paper for chromatography R.

Mobile phase Mix equal volumes of *acetonitrile R, 0.5 M acetic acid* and a 20 g/L solution of *sodium chloride R*.

Application About 5 µL.

Development Over a path of 10 cm.

Drying In air.

Detection Determine the distribution of radioactivity using a radioactivity detector.

Retardation factors impurity B = 0 to 0.1; impurity A, impurity C and technetium-99m sestamibi = 0.8 to 1.0.

Limit:

— sum of impurity A and other polar impurities, and impurity B: maximum 5 per cent of the total radioactivity.

Impurity C

Liquid chromatography *(2.2.29)*.

Test solution The preparation to be examined.

Reference solution To a vial of *sestamibi labelling kit CRS* add 3 mL of a 9 g/L solution of *sodium chloride R* containing 700 MBq to 900 MBq of sodium pertechnetate (⁹⁹ᵐTc)

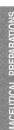

injection (fission or non-fission). Heat the mixture in a water-bath for 10 min and allow to cool to room temperature.

Column:
— *size:* $l = 0.25$ m, Ø = 4.6 mm,
— *stationary phase:* spherical *base-deactivated end-capped octadecylsilyl silica gel for chromatography R* (5 µm).

Mobile phase Mix 20 volumes of *acetonitrile R*, 35 volumes of a 6.6 g/L solution of *ammonium sulfate R* and 45 volumes of *methanol R*.

Flow rate 1.5 mL/min.

Detection Radioactivity detector.

Injection 25 µL.

Run time 25 min.

Relative retention With reference to technetium-99m sestamibi: impurity C = about 1.3.

System suitability Reference solution:
— the chromatogram is similar to the chromatogram provided with *sestamibi labelling kit CRS*,
— *relative retention* with reference to technetium-99m sestamibi: impurity C = minimum 1.2.

Limits:
— *impurity C*: not more than 3 per cent of the total radioactivity,
— *technetium-99m sestamibi*: minimum 94 per cent of the total radioactivity.

Calculate the percentage of radioactivity due to technetium-99m sestamibi from the expression:

$$\frac{(100 - B) \times T}{100}$$

B = percentage of radioactivity due to impurity B determined in the test for impurity B under Radiochemical purity,

T = area of the peak due to technetium-99m sestamibi in the chromatogram obtained with the test solution.

RADIOACTIVITY
Determine the radioactivity using a calibrated instrument.

IMPURITIES
A. $[^{99m}Tc]O_4^-$: (^{99m}Tc)pertechnetate ion,

B. technetium-99m in colloidal form,

C. (*OC*-6-22)-pentakis[1-(isocyano-κ*C*)-2-methoxy-2-methylpropane][1-(isocyano-κ*C*)-2-methylprop-1-ene][^{99m}Tc]technetium (1+).

Ph Eur

Technetium (^{99m}Tc) Succimer Injection

(*Ph Eur monograph 0643*)

Ph Eur

DEFINITION
Sterile solution of a complex of technetium-99m with meso-2,3-dimercaptosuccinic acid. It is prepared using *Sodium pertechnetate (^{99m}Tc) injection (fission) (0124)* or *Sodium pertechnetate (^{99m}Tc) injection (non fission) (0283)*. It contains a reducing substance, such as tin salt and may contain stabilisers, antioxidants such as ascorbic acid, and inert additives.

Technetium-99m
90 per cent to 110 per cent of the declared technetium-99m radioactivity at the date and time stated on the label.

CHARACTERS
Appearance
Clear, colourless solution.

Half-life and nature of radiation of technetium-99m
See general chapter 5.7. *Table of physical characteristics of radionuclides.*

IDENTIFICATION
A. Gamma-ray spectrometry.

Result The most prominent gamma photon of technetium-99m has an energy of 0.141 MeV.

B. Examine the chromatogram obtained in the test for radiochemical purity (see Tests).

Result The retardation factor of the principal peak in the radiochromatogram obtained with the test solution is 0.0 to 0.1.

C. Place 1 mL of the preparation to be examined in a test-tube and add 0.1 mL of *glacial acetic acid R* and 1 mL of a 20 g/L solution of *sodium nitroprusside R*. Mix. Carefully place a layer of *concentrated ammonia R* at the top of the solution. A violet ring develops between the layers.

TESTS
pH (*2.2.3*)
2.3 to 3.5.

Tin
Maximum 1 mg/mL.

Test solution Dilute 1.5 mL of the preparation to be examined to 25.0 mL with a 103 g/L solution of *hydrochloric acid R*.

Reference solution Dissolve 0.115 g of *stannous chloride R* in a 103 g/L solution of *hydrochloric acid R* and dilute to 1000.0 mL with the same solution.

To 1.0 mL of each solution add 0.05 mL of *thioglycollic acid R*, 0.1 mL of *dithiol reagent R*, 0.4 mL of a 20 g/L solution of *sodium laurilsulfate R* and 3.0 mL of a 21 g/L solution of *hydrochloric acid R*. Mix. Allow to stand for 60 min. Measure the absorbance (*2.2.25*) of each solution at 540 nm, using a 21 g/L solution of *hydrochloric acid R* as the compensation liquid. The absorbance of the test solution is not greater than that of the reference solution.

Physiological distribution
Inject a volume not greater than 0.2 mL and containing not more than 0.1 mg of dimercaptosuccinic acid into a suitable vein, such as a caudal vein or a saphenous vein, of each of 3 rats each weighing 150-250 g. Measure the radioactivity in the syringe before and after the injection. Euthanise the rats

1 h after the injection. Remove the kidneys, the liver, the stomach, the lungs and, if a caudal vein has been used for the injection, the tail. Using a suitable instrument determine the radioactivity in these organs. Determine the percentage of radioactivity in each organ with respect to the total radioactivity calculated as the difference between the 2 measurements made on the syringe minus the activity in the tail (if a caudal vein has been used for the injection).

In not fewer than 2 of the 3 rats used, the radioactivity is:
— in the kidneys: minimum 40 per cent;
— in the liver: maximum 10.0 per cent;
— in the lungs: maximum 5.0 per cent;
— in the stomach: maximum 2.0 per cent.

Sterility

It complies with the test for sterility prescribed in the monograph *Radiopharmaceutical preparations (0125)*. The preparation may be released for use before completion of the test.

RADIOCHEMICAL PURITY

Impurity A

Thin-layer chromatography (*2.2.27*).

Test solution   The preparation to be examined.

Plate   *TLC silica gel plate R*; use silica gel plate as the coating substance on a glass-fibre sheet, heated at 110 °C for 10 min.

Mobile phase   methyl ethyl ketone *R*.

Application   5-10 µL.

Development   Immediately, over a path of 10-15 cm in about 10 min.

Drying   In air.

Detection   Suitable detector to determine the distribution of radioactivity.

Retardation factors   [^{99m}Tc]technetium succimer = 0.0 to 0.1; impurity A = 0.9 to 1.0.

Limits:
— *[^{99m}Tc]technetium succimer*: minimum 95.0 per cent of the total radioactivity due to technetium-99m;
— *impurity A*: maximum 2.0 per cent of the total radioactivity due to technetium-99m.

RADIOACTIVITY

Determine the radioactivity using a calibrated instrument.

STORAGE

Protected from light.

IMPURITIES

A. [^{99m}Tc]pertechnetate ion.

———————————————————————— *Ph Eur*

Technetium (^{99m}Tc) Tin Pyrophosphate Injection

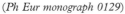

(*Ph Eur monograph 0129*)

Ph Eur ————————————————————————

DEFINITION

Sterile solution which may be prepared by mixing solutions of sodium pyrophosphate and stannous chloride with *Sodium pertechnetate (^{99m}Tc) injection (fission) (0124)* or *Sodium pertechnetate (^{99m}Tc) injection (non fission) (0283)*.

Technetium-99m

90 per cent to 110 per cent of the declared technetium-99m radioactivity at the date and time stated on the label.

Sodium pyrophosphate (Na$_4$P$_2$O$_7$,10H$_2$O)

1 mg/mL to 50 mg/mL.

Tin

Maximum 3.0 mg/mL.

CHARACTERS

Appearance

Clear, colourless solution.

Half-life and nature of radiation of technetium-99m

See general chapter *5.7. Table of physical characteristics of radionuclides.*

IDENTIFICATION

A. Gamma-ray spectrometry.

Result   The most prominent gamma photon of technetium-99m has an energy of 0.141 MeV.

B. Examine the chromatograms obtained in the tests A and B for radiochemical purity (see Tests).

Results:
— the retardation factor of the principal peak in the radiochromatogram obtained with the test solution in the test A is 0.9 to 1.0,
— the retardation factor of the principal peak in the radiochromatogram obtained with the test solution in the test B is 0.0 to 0.1.

C. To 1 mL add 1 mL of *acetic acid R*. Heat on a water-bath for 1 h. After cooling, add 10 mL of *nitro-molybdovanadic reagent R* and allow to stand for 30 min. A yellow colour develops.

D. To 1 mL add 0.05 mL of *thioglycollic acid R*, 0.1 mL of *dithiol reagent R*, 0.4 mL of a 20 g/L solution of *sodium laurilsulfate R*, 1 mL of *hydrochloric acid R*, 2 mL of a 30 per cent *V/V* solution of *sulfuric acid R* and allow to stand for 30 min. A pink colour develops.

TESTS

pH (*2.2.3*)

6.0 to 7.0.

Sodium pyrophosphate

1 mg/mL to 50 mg/mL.

Test solution   Use 1 mL of the preparation to be examined or a suitable dilution of it.

Reference solutions   Using a solution containing *sodium pyrophosphate R* and *stannous chloride R* in the same proportions as in the test solution, prepare a range of solutions and dilute to the same final volume with *water R*.

To the test solution and to 1 mL of each of the reference solutions add successively 10 mL of a 1 g/L solution of *disodium hydrogen phosphate R*, 10 mL of *iron standard solution (8 ppm Fe) R*, 5 mL of *glacial acetic acid R* and 5 mL of a 1 g/L solution of *hydroxylamine hydrochloride R*. Dilute each solution to 40 mL with *water R* and heat in a water-bath at 40 °C for 1 h. To each solution, add 4 mL of a 1 g/L solution of *phenanthroline hydrochloride R* and dilute to 50.0 mL with *water R*. Measure the absorbance (*2.2.25*) of each solution at 515 nm using as the compensation liquid a reagent blank containing hydrochloric acid (1.1 g/L HCl) instead of the *iron standard solution (8 ppm Fe) R*. Using the absorbances obtained with each of the reference solutions, draw a calibration curve and calculate the concentration of sodium pyrophosphate in the preparation to be examined.

Tin

Maximum 3.0 mg/mL.

Test solution   Use 1 mL of the preparation to be examined or a suitable dilution of it.

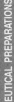

Reference solutions Using a solution in hydrochloric acid (6.2 g/L HCl) containing *sodium pyrophosphate R* and *stannous chloride R* in the same proportions as in the test solution, prepare a range of solutions and dilute to the same final volume with hydrochloric acid (6.2 g/L HCl).

To the test solution and to 1 mL of each of the reference solutions add 0.05 mL of *thioglycollic acid R*, 0.1 mL of *dithiol reagent R*, 0.4 mL of a 20 g/L solution of *sodium laurilsulfate R*, 1 mL of *hydrochloric acid R* and 2 mL of a 300 g/L solution of *sulfuric acid R*, and dilute to 15 mL with hydrochloric acid (6.2 g/L HCl). Allow the solutions to stand for 30 min and measure the absorbance (*2.2.25*) of each solution at 530 nm, using as the compensation liquid a reagent blank containing the same quantity of *sodium pyrophosphate R* as the test solution. Using the absorbances obtained with each of the reference solutions, draw a calibration curve and calculate the concentration of tin in the preparation to be examined.

Sterility

It complies with the test for sterility prescribed in the monograph *Radiopharmaceutical preparations (0125)*. The preparation may be released for use before completion of the test.

Bacterial endotoxins (*2.6.14*)
Less than $175/V$ IU/mL, V being the maximum recommended dose in millilitres.

RADIOCHEMICAL PURITY

A.

Impurity A.

Thin-layer chromatography (*2.2.27*).

Test solution The preparation to be examined.

Plate TLC silica gel plate R; use silica gel plate as the coating substance on a glass-fibre sheet heated at 110 °C for 10 min.

Mobile phase 136 g/L solution of *sodium acetate R*.

Application 5-10 μL.

Development Immediately, over a path of 10-15 cm in about 10 min.

Drying In air.

Detection Suitable detector to determine the distribution of radioactivity.

Retardation factors Impurity A = 0.0 to 0.1; [^{99m}Tc]technetium tin pyrophosphate and impurity B = 0.9 to 1.0.

B.

Impurity B

Thin-layer chromatography (*2.2.27*).

Test solution The preparation to be examined.

Plate TLC silica gel plate R; use silica gel plate as the coating substance on a glass-fibre sheet heated at 110 °C for 10 min.

Mobile phase methyl ethyl ketone R through which nitrogen has been bubbled in the chromatographic tank for 10 min immediately before the chromatography.

Application 5-10 μL and dry in a steam of nitrogen.

Development Over a path of 10-15 cm in about 10 min.

Drying In air.

Detection Suitable detector to determine the distribution of radioactivity.

Retardation factors [^{99m}Tc]technetium tin pyrophosphate = 0.0 to 0.1; impurity B = 0.95 to 1.0.

Limit:
— *sum of impurities A and B*: maximum 10 per cent of the total radioactivity due to technetium-99m in the chromatograms obtained in tests A and B.

RADIOACTIVITY
Determine the radioactivity using a calibrated instrument.

LABELLING
The label states:
— the concentration of sodium pyrophosphate expressed in milligrams per millilitre;
— the concentration of tin expressed in milligrams per millilitre.

IMPURITIES
A. [^{99m}Tc]technetium in colloidal form,
B. [^{99m}Tc]pertechnetate ion.

Ph Eur

Thallous (^{201}Tl) Chloride Injection

(*Ph Eur monograph 0571*)

Ph Eur

DEFINITION

Sterile solution of thallium-201 in the form of thallous chloride. It may be made isotonic by the addition of *Sodium chloride (0193)* and may contain a suitable antimicrobial preservative such as *Benzyl alcohol (0256)*.

Thallium-201
90 per cent to 110 per cent of the declared thallium-201 radioactivity, at the date and time stated on the label.

Specific radioactivity
Minimum 3.7 GBq per milligram of thallium.

CHARACTERS
Appearance
Clear, colourless solution.

Half-life and nature of radiation of thallium-201
See general chapter *5.7. Table of physical characteristics of radionuclides*.

IDENTIFICATION
A. Gamma-ray and X-ray spectrometry.

Results The most prominent gamma photons of thallium-201 have energies of 0.135 MeV, 0.166 MeV and 0.167 MeV; the X-rays have energies of 0.069 MeV to 0.083 MeV.

B. Examine the electropherogram obtained in the test for radiochemical purity (see Tests). The distribution of radioactivity contributes to the identification of the preparation.

TESTS
pH (*2.2.3*)
4.0 to 7.0.

Thallium

Test solution To 0.5 mL of the preparation to be examined add 0.5 mL of hydrochloric acid (220 g/L HCl) and 0.05 mL of *bromine water R*, and mix. Add 0.1 mL of a 30 g/L solution of *sulfosalicylic acid R*. After decolorisation add 1.0 mL of a 1 g/L solution of *rhodamine B R*. Add 4 mL of *toluene R* and shake for 60 s. Separate the toluene layer.

Reference solution Prepare at the same time and in the same manner as the test solution, using 0.5 mL of *thallium standard solution (10 ppm Tl) R*.

The toluene layer of the test solution is not more intensely coloured than the toluene layer of the reference solution.

Sterility

It complies with the test for sterility prescribed in the monograph *Radiopharmaceutical preparations (0125)*. The preparation may be released for use before completion of the test.

RADIONUCLIDIC PURITY

Thallium-201

Minimum 97.0 per cent of the total radioactivity.

Gamma-ray and X-ray spectrometry.

Determine the relative amounts of thallium-200, thallium-201, thallium-202, lead-201, lead-203 and other radionuclidic impurities present.

Result   The total radioactivity due to thallium-202 is not more than 2.0 per cent.

RADIOCHEMICAL PURITY

[²⁰¹Tl]Thallous ions

Zone electrophoresis *(2.2.31)*.

Use a suitable cellulose acetate strip as the supporting medium and a 18.6 g/L solution of *sodium edetate R* as the electrolyte solution. Soak the strip in the electrolyte solution for 45-60 min. Remove the strip with forceps taking care to handle the outer edges only. Place the strip between 2 absorbent pads and blot to remove excess solution.

Test solution   Mix equal volumes of the preparation to be examined and the electrolyte solution.

Apply not less than 5 µL of the test solution to the centre of the strip and mark the point of application. Apply an electric field of 17 V/cm for at least 10 min. Allow the strip to dry in air. Determine the distribution of radioactivity using suitable detector.

Result   Minimum 95.0 per cent of the radioactivity migrates towards the cathode.

RADIOACTIVITY

Determine the radioactivity using a calibrated instrument.

IMPURITIES

A. lead-201,

B. lead-203,

C. thallium-200,

D. thallium-202,

E. [²⁰¹Tl]thallic(III) ion.

_____ *Ph Eur*

Tritiated (³H) Water Injection

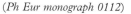

(Ph Eur monograph 0112)

Ph Eur _____

DEFINITION

Water for injections in which some of the water molecules contain tritium atoms in place of protium atoms. It may be made isotonic by the addition of sodium chloride.

Tritium

90 per cent to 110 per cent of the declared tritium radioactivity at the date stated on the label.

CHARACTERS

Appearance

Clear, colourless solution.

Half-life and nature of radiation of tritium

See general chapter *5.7. Table of physical characteristics of radionuclides*.

IDENTIFICATION

Beta-ray spectrometry as described in test A for radionuclidic purity (see Tests).

Result   The maximum energy of the beta radiation is 0.019 MeV.

TESTS

pH *(2.2.3)*

4.5 to 7.0.

Sterility

It complies with the test for sterility prescribed in the monograph *Radiopharmaceutical preparations (0125)*.

RADIONUCLIDIC PURITY

A. *Test solution*. Mix 100 µL of a suitable dilution of the preparation to be examined with 10 mL of *liquid scintillation cocktail R1*.

Reference solution   A standardised tritiated (³H) water having approximately the same radioactivity as the test solution.

Measure the radioactivity of the test solution in a liquid scintillation counter fitted with a discriminator. The count should be about 5000 impulses per second at the lowest setting of the discriminator. Record the count at different discriminator settings. For each measurement, count at least 10 000 impulses over a period of at least 1 min. Immediately determine in the same conditions the count for the reference solution.

Plot the counts at each discriminator setting, correcting for background activity, on semi-logarithmic paper, the discriminator settings being in arbitrary units as the abscissae. The vertical distance between the 2 curves obtained is constant. They obey the following mathematical relationship:

$$\frac{\dfrac{A_1}{B_1} - \dfrac{A_2}{B_2}}{\dfrac{A_1}{B_1}} \times 100 < 20$$

A_1 = radioactivity recorded for the reference solution at the lowest discriminator setting,

B_1 = radioactivity recorded for the test solution to be examined at the lowest discriminator setting,

A_2 = radioactivity recorded for the reference solution at the discriminator setting such that,

$$A_2 \approx A_1 \times 10^{-3}$$

B_2 = radioactivity recorded for the test solution to be examined at the latter discriminator setting.

B. Gamma-ray spectrometry. The instrument registers only background activity.

RADIOCHEMICAL PURITY

Place a quantity of the preparation to be examined equivalent to about 74 kBq, diluted to 50 mL with *water R*, in an all-glass distillation apparatus of the type used for the determination of distillation range *(2.2.11)*. Determine the radioactive concentration. Distil until about 25 mL of distillate has been collected. Precautions must be taken to avoid contamination of the air. If the test is carried out in a fume cupboard, the equipment must be protected from draughts. Determine the radioactive concentration of the distillate and of the liquid remaining in the distillation flask.

Neither of the radioactive concentrations determined after distillation differs by more than 5 per cent from the value determined before distillation.

RADIOACTIVITY

Determine the radioactivity using a liquid scintillation counter.

_____ Ph Eur

Water (^{15}O) Injection

(*Ph Eur monograph 1582*)

Ph Eur _____

DEFINITION

Sterile solution of [^{15}O]water for diagnostic use.

Oxygen-15

90 per cent to 110 per cent of the declared oxygen-15 radioactivity at the date and time stated on the label.

CHARACTERS

Appearance

Clear, colourless liquid.

Half-life and nature of radiation of oxygen-15

See general chapter 5.7. *Table of physical characteristics of radionuclides.*

IDENTIFICATION

A. Gamma-ray spectrometry.

Results The only gamma photons of [^{15}O]water have an energy of 0.511 MeV and, depending on the measurement geometry, a sum peak of 1.022 MeV may be observed.

B. Radionuclidic purity (see Tests).

C. Examine the chromatogram obtained in the test for radiochemical purity (see Tests). The retention time of the 2nd peak is due to the radioactivity eluting in the void volume.

TESTS

pH (*2.2.3*)

5.5 to 8.5.

Ammonium (*2.4.1*)

Maximum 10 ppm, determined on 1 mL. The preparation may be released for use before completion of the test.

Nitrates

Maximum 10 ppm. The preparation may be released for use before completion of the test.

Test solution To 1 mL add 49 mL of *nitrate-free water R*. Place 5 mL of this solution in a test-tube immersed in iced water, add 0.4 mL of a 100 g/L solution of *potassium chloride R*, 0.1 mL of *diphenylamine solution R* and, dropwise with shaking, 5 mL of *sulfuric acid R*. Transfer the tube to a water-bath at 50 °C.

Reference solution Prepare at the same time in the same manner as the test solution, using a mixture of 4.5 mL of *nitrate-free water R* and 0.5 mL of *nitrate standard solution (2 ppm NO$_3$) R*.

After 15 min, any blue colour in the test solution is not more intense than that in the reference solution.

Sterility

It complies with the test for sterility prescribed in the monograph *Radiopharmaceutical preparations (0125)*. The preparation may be released for use before completion of the test.

Bacterial endotoxins (*2.6.14*)

Less than 175/V IU/mL, V being the maximum recommended dose in millilitres. The preparation may be released for use before completion of the test.

RADIONUCLIDIC PURITY

The preparation may be released for use before completion of the test.

Oxygen-15

Minimum 99 per cent of total radioactivity.

Gamma-ray spectrometry.

Results:
— the spectrum obtained with the preparation to be examined does not differ significantly from that obtained with a standardised fluorine-18 solution;
— the half-life is between 1.9 min and 2.2 min.

RADIOCHEMICAL PURITY

The preparation may be released for use before completion of the test.

[^{15}O]Water

Liquid chromatography (*2.2.29*).

Test solution The preparation to be examined.

Column:
— size: l = 0.25 m, Ø = 4.0 mm;
— stationary phase: *aminopropylsilyl silica gel for chromatography R* (10 µm);
— temperature: constant, at 20-30 °C.

Mobile phase 10 g/L solution of *potassium dihydrogen phosphate R* adjusted to pH 3 with *phosphoric acid R*.

Flow rate 1 mL/min.

Detection Suitable detector to determine the distribution of radioactivity and internal recovery detection system, consisting of a loop of the chromatographic tubing between the injector and the column through the radioactivity detector, which has been calibrated for count recovery.

Run time 10 min.

Identification of peaks In the chromatogram obtained with the test solution, the 1st peak corresponds to the injected radioactivity of the test solution, the 2nd peak corresponds to the amount of radioactivity as [^{15}O]water.

Limit:
— [^{15}O]water: minimum 99 per cent of the total radioactivity due to oxygen-15.

RADIOACTIVITY

Determine the radioactivity using a calibrated instrument.

_____ Ph Eur

Xenon (^{133}Xe) Injection

(*Ph Eur monograph 0133*)

Ph Eur _____

DEFINITION

Sterile solution of xenon-133 that may be made isotonic by the addition of sodium chloride.

Xenon-133

80 per cent to 130 per cent of the declared xenon-133 radioactivity at the date and time stated on the label.

The injection is presented in a container that allows the contents to be removed without introducing air bubbles. The container is filled as completely as possible and any gas bubble present does not occupy more than 1 per cent of the volume of the injection as judged by visual comparison with a suitable standard.

CHARACTERS

Appearance
Clear, colourless solution.

Half-life and nature of radiation of xenon-133
See general chapter 5.7. *Table of physical characteristics of radionuclides.*

IDENTIFICATION
Gamma-ray and X-ray spectrometry.

Comparison   Standardised xenon-133 solution in a 9 g/L solution of *sodium chloride R.*

Results   The most prominent gamma photon of xenon-133 has an energy of 0.081 MeV and there is an X-ray (resulting from internal conversion) of 0.030 MeV to 0.035 MeV.

TESTS

pH (2.2.3)
5.0 to 8.0.

Sterility
It complies with the test for sterility prescribed in the monograph *Radiopharmaceutical preparations (0125)*.
The preparation may be released for use before completion of the test.

RADIONUCLIDIC PURITY
A. Gamma-ray and X-ray spectrometry.

Comparison   Standardised xenon-133 solution in a 9 g/L solution of *sodium chloride R.*

Result   The spectrum obtained with the preparation to be examined does not differ significantly from that obtained with a standardised xenon-133 solution in a 9 g/L solution of *sodium chloride R,* apart from any differences attributable to the presence of xenon-131m and xenon-133m.

B. Transfer 2 mL of the preparation to be examined to an open flask and pass a current of air through the solution for 30 min, taking suitable precautions concerning the dispersion of radioactivity. Measure the residual beta and gamma activity of the solution. The activity does not differ significantly from the background activity detected by the instrument.

RADIOACTIVITY
Weigh the container with its contents. Determine its total radioactivity using suitable counting equipment by comparison with a standardised xenon-133 solution or by measurement in an instrument calibrated with the aid of such a solution, operating in strictly identical conditions. If an ionisation chamber is used its inner wall should be such that the radiation is not seriously attenuated. Remove at least half the contents and re-weigh the container. Measure the total residual radioactivity of the container and the remaining contents as described above. From the measurements, calculate the radioactive concentration of xenon-133 in the preparation to be examined.

CAUTION
Significant amounts of xenon-133 may be present in the closures and on the walls of the container. This must be taken into account in applying the rules concerning the transport and storage of radioactive substances and in disposing of used containers

IMPURITIES
A. xenon-131m.

_____ *Ph Eur*

Monographs

Surgical Materials

Absorbent Cotton

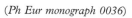

(Ph Eur monograph 0036)

Ph Eur _____

DEFINITION

Absorbent cotton consists of new fibres or good quality combers obtained from the seed-coat of various species of the genus *Gossypium* L., cleaned, purified, bleached and carefully carded. It may not contain any compensatory colouring matter.

CHARACTERS

It is white or almost white and is composed of fibres of average length not less than 10 mm, determined by a suitable method, and contains not more than traces of leaf residue, pericarp, seed-coat or other impurities. It offers appreciable resistance when pulled. It does not shed any appreciable quantity of dust when gently shaken.

IDENTIFICATION

A. Examined under a microscope, each fibre is seen to consist of a single cell, up to about 4 cm long and up to 40 μm wide, in the form of a flattened tube with thick and rounded walls and often twisted.

B. When treated with *iodinated zinc chloride solution R*, the fibres become violet.

C. To 0.1 g add 10 mL of *zinc chloride-formic acid solution R*. Heat to 40 °C and allow to stand for 2 h 30 min, shaking occasionally. It does not dissolve.

TESTS

Solution S

Place 15.0 g in a suitable vessel, add 150 mL of *water R*, close the vessel and allow to macerate for 2 h. Decant the solution, squeeze the residual liquid carefully from the sample with a glass rod and mix. Reserve 10 mL of the solution for the test for surface-active substances and filter the remainder.

Acidity or alkalinity

To 25 mL of solution S add 0.1 mL of *phenolphthalein solution R* and to another 25 mL add 0.05 mL of *methyl orange solution R*. Neither solution is pink.

Foreign fibres

Examined under a microscope, it is seen to consist exclusively of typical cotton fibres, except that occasionally a few isolated foreign fibres may be present.

Fluorescence

Examine a layer about 5 mm in thickness under ultraviolet light at 365 nm. It displays only a slight brownish-violet fluorescence and a few yellow particles. It shows no intense blue fluorescence, apart from that which may be shown by a few isolated fibres.

Neps

Spread about 1 g evenly between 2 colourless transparent plates each 10 cm square. Examine for neps by transmitted light and compare with *Cotton wool standard for neps CRS*. The product to be examined is not more neppy than the standard.

Absorbency

Apparatus A dry cylindrical copper wire basket 8.0 cm high and 5.0 cm in diameter. The wire of which the basket is constructed is about 0.4 mm in diameter, the mesh is 1.5 cm to 2.0 cm wide and the mass of the basket is 2.7 ± 0.3 g.

Sinking time Not more than 10 s. Weigh the basket to the nearest centigram (m_1). Take a total of 5.00 g in approximately equal quantities from 5 different places in the product to be examined, place loosely in the basket and weigh the filled basket to the nearest centigram (m_2). Fill a beaker 11 cm to 12 cm in diameter to a depth of 10 cm with water at about 20 °C. Hold the basket horizontally and drop it from a height of about 10 mm into the water. Measure with a stopwatch the time taken for the basket to sink below the surface of the water. Calculate the result as the average of 3 tests.

Water-holding capacity Not less than 23.0 g of water per gram. After the sinking time has been measured, remove the basket from the water, allow it to drain for exactly 30 s suspended in a horizontal position over the beaker, transfer it to a tared beaker (m_3) and weigh to the nearest centigram (m_4). Calculate the water-holding capacity per gram of absorbent cotton using the following expression:

$$\frac{m_4 - (m_2 + m_3)}{m_2 - m_1}$$

Calculate the result as the average of 3 tests.

Ether-soluble substances

Not more than 0.50 per cent. In an extraction apparatus, extract 5.00 g with *ether R* for 4 h at a rate of at least 4 extractions per hour. Evaporate the ether extract and dry the residue to constant mass at 100 °C to 105 °C.

Extractable colouring matter

In a narrow percolator, slowly extract 10.0 g with *alcohol R* until 50 mL of extract is obtained. The liquid obtained is not more intensely coloured (*2.2.2, Method II*) than reference solution Y_5, GY_6 or a reference solution prepared as follows: to 3.0 mL of blue primary solution add 7.0 mL of hydrochloric acid (10 g/L HCl). Dilute 0.5 mL of this solution to 10.0 mL with hydrochloric acid (10 g/L HCl).

Surface-active substances

Introduce the 10 mL portion of solution S reserved before filtration into a 25 mL graduated ground-glass-stoppered cylinder with an external diameter of 20 mm and a wall thickness of not greater than 1.5 mm, previously rinsed 3 times with *sulfuric acid R* and then with *water R*. Shake vigorously 30 times in 10 s, allow to stand for 1 min and repeat the shaking. After 5 min, any foam present must not cover the entire surface of the liquid.

Water-soluble substances

Not more than 0.50 per cent. Boil 5.000 g in 500 mL of *water R* for 30 min, stirring frequently. Replace the water lost by evaporation. Decant the liquid, squeeze the residual liquid carefully from the sample with a glass rod and mix. Filter the liquid whilst hot. Evaporate 400 mL of the filtrate (corresponding to 4/5 of the mass of the sample taken) and dry the residue to constant mass at 100 °C to 105 °C.

Loss on drying (*2.2.32*)

Not more than 8.0 per cent, determined on 5.000 g by drying in an oven at 105 °C.

Sulfated ash (*2.4.14*)

Not more than 0.40 per cent. Introduce 5.00 g into a previously heated and cooled, tared crucible. Heat cautiously over a naked flame and then carefully to dull redness at 600 °C. Allow to cool, add a few drops of *dilute sulfuric acid R*, then heat and incinerate until all the black particles have disappeared. Allow to cool. Add a few drops of *ammonium carbonate solution R*. Evaporate and incinerate carefully, allow to cool and weigh again. Repeat the incineration for periods of 5 min to constant mass.

STORAGE

Store in a dust-proof package in a dry place.

_____ *Ph Eur*

Absorbent Viscose Wadding

(*Ph Eur monograph 0034*)

Ph Eur _____

DEFINITION

Absorbent viscose wadding consists of bleached, carefully carded, new fibres of regenerated cellulose obtained by the viscose process, with or without the addition of titanium dioxide, of linear density 1.0 dtex to 8.9 dtex (dtex = mass of 10 000 m of fibre, expressed in grams) and cut to a suitable staple length. It does not contain any compensatory colouring matter.

CHARACTERS

It is white or very slightly yellow, has a lustrous or matt appearance, and is soft to the touch.

IDENTIFICATION

A. Viscose rayon fibres may be solid or hollow; hollow fibres may have a continuous lumen or be compartmented.

The fibres have an average length of 25 mm to 80 mm and when examined under a microscope in the dry state, or when mounted in *alcohol R* and *water R*, the following characters are observed. They are usually of a more or less uniform width, with many longitudinal parallel lines distributed unequally over the width. The ends are cut more or less straight. Matt fibres contain numerous granular particles of approximately 1 µm average diameter.

Solid fibres   In longitudinal view, the surface of the fibres may be uneven or crenate. Fibres having an approximately circular or elliptical cross section have a diameter of about 10 µm to 20 µm and those that are flattened and twisted ribbons vary in width from 15 µm to 20 µm as the twisting of the filament reveals first the major axis and then the minor axis. They are about 4 µm in thickness. Other solid cross sections are Y-shaped and have protruding limbs with the major axis 5 µm to 25 µm in length and the minor axis 2 µm to 8 µm wide.

Hollow fibres   Fibres with a continuous, hollow lumen have a diameter of up to about 30 µm; they are thin-walled, with a wall thickness of about 5 µm. When mounted in *alcohol R* and *water R*, the lumen is clearly indicated in many fibres by the presence of many entrapped air bubbles.

Compartmented fibres   These fibres may have a diameter of up to about 80 µm; they are hollow, having a central lumen which is divided up into several compartments. Individual compartments vary in size but typically may be up to about 60 µm in length and there may be more than one compartment across the width of each fibre. Some compartments show entrapped air bubbles when the fibres are mounted in *alcohol R* and *water R*.

B. When treated with *iodinated zinc chloride solution R*, the fibres become violet.

C. To 0.1 g add 10 mL of *zinc chloride-formic acid solution R*. Heat to 40 °C and allow to stand for 2 h 30 min, shaking occasionally. It dissolves completely except for the matt variety where titanium dioxide particles remain.

D. Dissolve the residue obtained in the test for sulfated ash by warming gently with 5 mL of *sulfuric acid R*. Allow to cool and add 0.2 mL of *dilute hydrogen peroxide solution R*. The solution obtained from the lustrous variety undergoes no change in colour; that from the matt variety shows an orange-yellow colour, the intensity of which depends on the quantity of titanium dioxide present.

TESTS

Solution S

Place 15.0 g in a suitable vessel, add 150 mL of *water R*, close the vessel and allow to macerate for 2 h. Decant the solution, squeeze the residual liquid carefully from the sample with a glass rod and mix. Reserve 10 mL of the solution for the test for surface-active substances and filter the remainder.

Acidity or alkalinity

To 25 mL of solution S add 0.1 mL of *phenolphthalein solution R* and to another 25 mL add 0.05 mL of *methyl orange solution R*. Neither solution is pink.

Foreign fibres

Examined under a microscope, it is seen to consist exclusively of viscose fibres, except that occasionally a few isolated foreign fibres may be present.

Fluorescence

Examine a layer about 5 mm in thickness under ultraviolet light at 365 nm. It displays only a slight brownish-violet fluorescence. It shows no intense blue fluorescence, apart from that which may be shown by a few isolated fibres.

Absorbency

Apparatus   A dry cylindrical copper-wire basket 8.0 cm high and 5.0 cm in diameter. The wire of which the basket is constructed is about 0.4 mm in diameter, the mesh is 1.5 cm to 2.0 cm wide and the mass of the basket is 2.7 ± 0.3 g.

Sinking time   Not more than 10 s. Weigh the basket to the nearest centigram (m_1). Take a total of 5.00 g in approximately equal quantities from 5 different places in the product to be examined, place loosely in the basket and weigh the filled basket to the nearest centigram (m_2). Fill a beaker 11 cm to 12 cm in diameter to a depth of 10 cm with water at about 20 °C. Hold the basket horizontally and drop it from a height of about 10 mm into the water. Measure with a stopwatch the time taken for the basket to sink below the surface of the water. Calculate the result as the average of 3 tests.

Water-holding capacity   Not less than 18.0 g of water per gram. After the sinking time has been measured, remove the basket from the water, allow it to drain for exactly 30 s suspended in a horizontal position over the beaker, transfer it to a tared beaker (m_3) and weigh to the nearest centigram (m_4). Calculate the water-holding capacity per gram of absorbent viscose wadding using the following expression:

$$\frac{m_4 - (m_2 + m_3)}{m_2 - m_1}$$

Calculate the result as the average of 3 tests.

Ether-soluble substances

Not more than 0.30 per cent. In an extraction apparatus, extract 5.00 g with *ether R* for 4 h at a rate of at least 4 extractions per hour. Evaporate the ether extract and dry the residue to constant mass at 100 °C to 105 °C.

Extractable colouring matter

In a narrow percolator, slowly extract 10.0 g with *alcohol R* until 50 mL of extract is obtained. The liquid obtained is not more intensely coloured (*2.2.2, Method II*) than reference solution Y_5, GY_6 or a reference solution prepared as follows: to 3.0 mL of blue primary solution add 7.0 mL of hydrochloric acid (10 g/L HCl) and dilute 0.5 mL of this solution to 10.0 mL with hydrochloric acid (10 g/L HCl).

Surface-active substances

Introduce the 10 mL portion of solution S reserved before filtration into a 25 mL graduated ground-glass-stoppered cylinder with an external diameter of 20 mm and a wall thickness of not greater than 1.5 mm, previously rinsed 3 times with *sulfuric acid R* and then with *water R*. Shake vigorously 30 times in 10 s, allow to stand for 1 min and repeat the shaking. After 5 min, any foam present does not cover the entire surface of the liquid.

Water-soluble substances

Not more than 0.70 per cent. Boil 5.00 g in 500 mL of *water R* for 30 min, stirring frequently. Replace the water lost by evaporation. Decant the liquid, squeeze the residual liquid carefully from the sample with a glass rod and mix. Filter the liquid whilst hot. Evaporate 400 mL of the filtrate (corresponding to 4/5 of the mass of the sample taken) and dry the residue to constant mass at 100 °C to 105 °C.

Hydrogen sulfide

To 10 mL of solution S add 1.9 mL of *water R*, 0.15 mL of *dilute acetic acid R* and 1 mL of *lead acetate solution R*. After 2 min, the solution is not more intensely coloured than a reference solution prepared at the same time using 0.15 mL of *dilute acetic acid R*, 1.2 mL of *thioacetamide reagent R*, 1.7 mL of *lead standard solution (10 ppm Pb) R* and 10 mL of solution S.

Loss on drying (*2.2.32*)

Not more than 13.0 per cent, determined on 5.000 g by drying in an oven at 105 °C.

Sulfated ash (*2.4.14*)

Not more than 0.45 per cent for the lustrous variety and not more than 1.7 per cent for the matt variety. Introduce 5.00 g into a previously heated and cooled, tared crucible. Heat cautiously over a naked flame and then carefully to dull redness at 600 °C. Allow to cool, add a few drops of *dilute sulfuric acid R*, then heat and incinerate until all the black particles have disappeared. Allow to cool. Add a few drops of *ammonium carbonate solution R*. Evaporate and incinerate carefully, allow to cool and weigh again. Repeat the incineration for periods of 5 min to constant mass.

STORAGE

Store in a dust-proof package in a dry place.

———————————————————————— *Ph Eur*

SUTURES

(*Ph Eur monograph 90004*)

Ph Eur ————————————————————————

INTRODUCTION

The following monographs apply to sutures for human use: Catgut, sterile (0317), Sutures, sterile non-absorbable (0324), Sutures, sterile synthetic absorbable braided (0667) and Sutures, sterile synthetic absorbable monofilament (0666). They cover performance characteristics of sutures and may include methods of identification. Sutures are medical devices as defined in Directive 93/42/EEC.

These monographs can be applied to show compliance with essential requirements as defined in Article 3 of Directive 93/42/EEC covering the following:

Physical performance characteristics: diameter, breaking load, needle attachment, packaging, sterility, information supplied by the manufacturer (see Section 13 of Annex 1 of Directive 93/42/EEC), labelling.

To show compliance with other essential requirements, the application of appropriate harmonised standards as defined in Article 5 of Directive 93/42/EEC may be considered.

———————————————————————— *Ph Eur*

Sterile Catgut

(*Ph Eur monograph 0317*)

Ph Eur ————————————————————————

DEFINITION

Sterile catgut consists of sutures prepared from collagen taken from the intestinal membranes of mammals. After cleaning, the membranes are split longitudinally into strips of varying width, which, when assembled in small numbers, according to the diameter required, are twisted under tension, dried, polished, selected and sterilised. The sutures may be treated with chemical substances such as chromium salts to prolong absorption and glycerol to make them supple, provided such substances do not reduce tissue acceptability.

Appropriate harmonised standards may be considered when assessing compliance with respect to origin and processing of raw materials and with respect to biocompatibility.

Sterile catgut is a surgical wound-closure device. Being an absorbable suture it serves to approximate tissue during the healing period and is subsequently metabolised by proteolytic activity.

PRODUCTION

Production complies with relevant regulations on the use of animal tissues in medical devices notably concerning the risk of transmission of animal spongiform encephalopathy agents.

Appropriate harmonised standards may apply with respect to appropriate validated methods of sterilisation, environmental control during manufacturing, labelling and packaging.

It is essential for the effectiveness and the performance characteristics during use and during the functional lifetime of catgut that the following physical properties are specified: consistent diameter, sufficient initial strength and firm needle attachment.

The requirements outlined below have been established, taking into account stresses which occur during normal conditions of use. These requirements can be used to demonstrate that individual production batches of sterile catgut are suitable for wound closure according to usual surgical techniques.

TESTS

If stored in a preserving liquid, remove the sutures from the sachet and measure promptly and in succession the length, diameter and breaking load. If stored in the dry state, immerse the sutures in alcohol R or a 90 per cent V/V solution of 2-propanol R for 24 h and proceed with the measurements as indicated below.

Length

Measure the length without applying to the suture more tension than is necessary to keep it straight. The length of each suture is not less than 90 per cent of the length stated on the label and does not exceed 350 cm.

Diameter

Carry out the test on 5 sutures. Use a suitable instrument capable of measuring with an accuracy of at least 0.002 mm and having a circular pressor foot 10 mm to 15 mm in diameter. The pressor foot and the moving parts attached to it are weighted so as to apply a total load of 100 ± 10 g to the suture being tested. When making the measurement, lower the pressor foot slowly to avoid crushing the suture. Measure the diameter at intervals of 30 cm over the whole length of the suture. For a suture less than 90 cm in length, measure at 3 points approximately evenly spaced along the suture. The suture is not subjected to more tension than is necessary to keep it straight during measurement.

The average of the measurements carried out on the sutures being tested and not less than two-thirds of the measurements taken on each suture are within the limits given in the columns under A in Table 0317.-1 for the gauge number concerned. None of the measurements is outside the limits given in the columns under B in Table 0317.-1 for the gauge number concerned.

Table 0317.-1.– *Diameters and Breaking Loads*

| Gauge number | Diameter (millimetres) | | | | Breaking load (newtons) | |
| | A | | B | | C | D |
	min.	max.	min.	max.		
0.1	0.010	0.019	0.005	0.025	-	-
0.2	0.020	0.029	0.015	0.035	-	-
0.3	0.030	0.039	0.025	0.045	0.20	0.05
0.4	0.040	0.049	0.035	0.060	0.30	0.10
0.5	0.050	0.069	0.045	0.085	0.40	0.20
0.7	0.070	0.099	0.060	0.125	0.70	0.30
1	0.100	0.149	0.085	0.175	1.8	0.40
1.5	0.150	0.199	0.125	0.225	3.8	0.70
2	0.200	0.249	0.175	0.275	7.5	1.8
2.5	0.250	0.299	0.225	0.325	10	3.8
3	0.300	0.349	0.275	0.375	12.5	7.5
3.5	0.350	0.399	0.325	0.450	20	10
4	0.400	0.499	0.375	0.550	27.5	12.5
5	0.500	0.599	0.450	0.650	38.0	20.0
6	0.600	0.699	0.550	0.750	45.0	27.5
7	0.700	0.799	0.650	0.850	60.0	38.0
8	0.800	0.899	0.750	0.950	70.0	45.0

Minimum breaking load

The minimum breaking load is determined over a simple knot formed by placing one end of a suture held in the right hand over the other end held in the left hand, passing one end over the suture and through the loop so formed (see Figure 0317.-1) and pulling the knot tight. Carry out the test on 5 sutures. Submit sutures of length greater than 75 cm to 2 measurements and shorter sutures to one measurement. Determine the breaking load using a suitable tensilometer. The apparatus has 2 clamps for holding the suture, one of which is mobile and is driven at a constant rate of 30 cm/min. The clamps are designed so that the suture being tested can be attached without any possibility of slipping. At the beginning of the test the length of suture between the clamps is 12.5 cm to 20 cm and the knot is midway between the clamps. Set the mobile clamp in motion and note the force required to break the suture. If the suture breaks in a clamp or within 1 cm of it, the result is discarded and the test repeated on another suture. The average of all the results, excluding those legitimately discarded, is equal to or greater than the value given in column C in Table 0317.-1

and no individual result is less than that given in column D for the gauge number concerned.

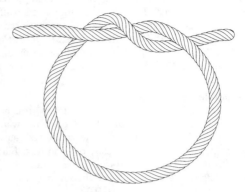

Figure 0317.-1. – *Simple knot*

Soluble chromium compounds

Place 0.25 g in a conical flask containing 1 mL of *water R* per 10 mg of catgut. Stopper the flask, allow to stand at 37 ± 0.5 °C for 24 h, cool and decant the liquid. Transfer 5 mL to a small test tube and add 2 mL of a 10 g/L solution of *diphenylcarbazide R* in *alcohol R* and 2 mL of *dilute sulfuric acid R*. The solution is not more intensely coloured than a standard prepared at the same time using 5 mL of a solution containing 2.83 µg of *potassium dichromate R* per millilitre, 2 mL of *dilute sulfuric acid R* and 2 mL of a 10 g/L solution of *diphenylcarbazide R* in *alcohol R* (1 ppm of Cr).

Needle attachment

If the catgut is supplied with an eyeless needle attached that is not stated to be detachable, it complies with the test for needle attachment. Carry out the test on 5 sutures. Use a suitable tensilometer, such as that described for the determination of the minimum breaking load. Fix the needle and suture (without knot) in the clamps of the apparatus in such a way that the swaged part of the needle is completely free of the clamp and in line with the direction of pull on the suture. Set the mobile clamp in motion and note the force required to break the suture or to detach it from the needle. The average of the 5 determinations and all individual values are not less than the respective values given in Table 0317.-2 for the gauge number concerned. If not more than one individual value fails to meet the individual requirement, repeat the test on an additional 10 sutures. The catgut complies with the test if none of these 10 values is less than the individual value in Table 0317.-2 for the gauge number concerned.

Table 0317.-2. – *Minimum Strengths of Needle Attachment*

Gauge number	Mean value (newtons)	Individual values (newtons)
0.5	0.50	0.25
0.7	0.80	0.40
1	1.7	0.80
1.5	2.3	1.1
2	4.5	2.3
2.5	5.6	2.8
3	6.8	3.4
3.5	11.0	4.5
4	15.0	4.5
5	18.0	6.0

STORAGE (PACKAGING)

Sterile catgut sutures are presented in individual sachets that maintain sterility and allow the withdrawal and use of the sutures in aseptic conditions. Sterile catgut may be stored dry or in a preserving liquid to which an antimicrobial agent but not an antibiotic may be added.

Sutures in their individual sachets (primary packaging) are kept in a protective cover (box) which maintains the physical and mechanical properties until the time of use.

The application of appropriate harmonised standards for packaging of medical devices shall be considered.

LABELLING

Reference may be made to the appropriate harmonised standards for labelling of medical devices.

The details strictly necessary for the user to identify the product properly are indicated on or in each sachet (primary packaging) and on the protective cover (box) and include at least:
— gauge number,
— length in centimetres or metres,
— if appropriate, that the needle is detachable,
— name of the product,
— intended use (surgical suture, absorbable).

Ph Eur

Sterile Synthetic Absorbable Braided Sutures

(*Ph Eur monograph 0667*)

Ph Eur

DEFINITION

Sterile synthetic absorbable braided sutures consist of sutures prepared from a synthetic polymer, polymers or copolymers which, when introduced into a living organism, are absorbed by that organism and cause no undue tissue irritation. They consist of completely polymerised material. They occur as multifilament sutures consisting of elementary fibres which are assembled by braiding. The sutures may be treated to facilitate handling and they may be coloured.

Appropriate harmonised standards may be considered when assessing compliance with respect to origin and processing of raw materials and with respect to biocompatibility.

Sterile synthetic absorbable braided sutures are wound-closure devices. Being absorbable they serve to approximate tissue during the healing period and subsequently lose tensile strength by hydrolysis.

PRODUCTION

Appropriate harmonised standards may apply with respect to appropriate validated methods of sterilisation, environmental control during manufacturing, labelling and packaging.

It is essential for the effectiveness and the performance characteristics during use and during the functional lifetime of these sutures that the following physical properties are specified: consistent diameter, sufficient initial strength and firm needle attachment.

The requirements below have been established, taking into account stresses which occur during normal conditions of use. These requirements can be used to demonstrate that individual production batches of these sutures are suitable for wound closure according to usual surgical techniques.

TESTS

Carry out the following tests on the sutures in the state in which they are removed from the sachet.

Length

Measure the length of the suture without applying more tension than is necessary to keep it straight. The length of each suture is not less than 95 per cent of the length stated on the label and does not exceed 400 cm.

Diameter

Unless otherwise prescribed, measure the diameter by the following method, using five sutures in the condition in which they are presented. Use a suitable instrument capable of measuring with an accuracy of at least 0.002 mm and having a circular pressor foot 10 mm to 15 mm in diameter. The pressor foot and the moving parts attached to it are weighted so as to apply a total load of 100 ± 10 g to the suture being tested. When making the measurements, lower the pressor foot slowly to avoid crushing the suture. Measure the diameter at intervals of 30 cm over the whole length of the suture. For a suture less than 90 cm in length, measure at three points approximately evenly spaced along the suture. During the measurement, submit the sutures to a tension not greater than one-fifth of the minimum breaking load shown in column C of Table 0667.-1 appropriate to the gauge number and type of material or 10 N whichever is less. For sutures of gauge number above 1.5 make two measurements at each point, the second measurement being made after rotating the suture through 90°. The diameter of that point is the average of the two measurements.

The average of the measurements carried out on the sutures being tested and not less than two-thirds of the measurements taken on each suture are within the limits given in the columns under A in Table 0667.-1 for the gauge number concerned. None of the measurements is outside the limits given in the columns under B in Table 0667.-1 for the gauge number concerned.

Minimum breaking load

The minimum breaking load is determined over a simple knot formed by placing one end of a suture held in the right hand over the other end held in the left hand, passing one end over the suture and through the loop so formed (see Figure 0667.-1) and pulling the knot tight.

Carry out the test on five sutures. Submit sutures of length greater than 75 cm to two measurements and shorter sutures to one measurement. Determine the breaking load using a suitable tensilometer. The apparatus has two clamps for holding the suture, one of which is mobile and is driven at a constant rate of 25 cm to 30 cm per minute. The clamps are designed so that the suture being tested can be attached without any possibility of slipping. At the beginning of the test the length of suture between the clamps is 12.5 cm to 20 cm and the knot is midway between the clamps. Set the mobile clamp in motion and note the force required to break the suture. If the suture breaks in a clamp or within 1 cm of it, the result is discarded and the test repeated on another suture. The average of all the results excluding those legitimately discarded is equal to or greater than the value given in column C in Table 0667.-1 and no individual result is less than that given in column D for the gauge number concerned.

Table 0667.-1. – *Diameters and breaking loads*

Gauge number	Diameter (millimetres)				Breaking load (newtons)	
	A		B		C	D
	min.	max.	min.	max.		
0.01	0.001	0.004	0.0008	0.005	-	-
0.05	0.005	0.009	0.003	0.012	-	-
0.1	0.010	0.019	0.005	0.025	-	-
0.2	0.020	0.029	0.015	0.035	-	-
0.3	0.030	0.039	0.025	0.045	0.45	0.23
0.4	0.040	0.049	0.035	0.060	0.70	0.35
0.5	0.050	0.069	0.045	0.085	1.4	0.7
0.7	0.070	0.099	0.060	0.125	2.5	1.3
1	0.100	0.149	0.085	0.175	6.8	3.4
1.5	0.150	0.199	0.125	0.225	9.5	4.8
2	0.200	0.249	0.175	0.275	17.7	8.9
2.5	0.250	0.299	0.225	0.325	21.0	10.5
3	0.300	0.349	0.275	0.375	26.8	13.4
3.5	0.350	0.399	0.325	0.450	39.0	18.5
4	0.400	0.499	0.375	0.550	50.8	25.4
5	0.500	0.599	0.450	0.650	63.5	31.8
6	0.600	0.699	0.550	0.750	-	-
7	0.700	0.799	0.650	0.850	-	-

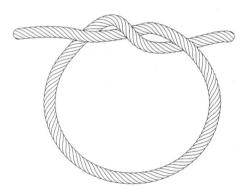

Figure 0667.-1. – *Simple knot*

Needle attachment

If the suture is supplied with an eyeless needle attached that is not stated to be detachable the attachment, it complies with the test for needle attachment. Carry out the test on five sutures. Use a suitable tensilometer, such as that described for the determination of the minimum breaking load. Fix the needle and suture (without knot) in the clamps of the apparatus in such a way that the swaged part of the needle is completely free of the clamp and in line with the direction of pull on the suture. Set the mobile clamp in motion and note the force required to break the suture or to detach it from the needle. The average of the five deter-minations and all individual values are not less than the respective values given in Table 0667.-2 for the gauge number concerned. If not more than one individual value fails to meet the individual requirement, repeat the test on an additional ten sutures. The attachment complies with the test if none of the ten

values is less than the individual value in Table 0667.-2 for the gauge number concerned.

Table 0667.-2. – *Minimum strengths of needle attachment*

Gauge number	Mean value (newtons)	Individual value (newtons)
0.4	0.50	0.25
0.5	0.80	0.40
0.7	1.7	0.80
1	2.3	1.1
1.5	4.5	2.3
2	6.8	3.4
2.5	9.0	4.5
3	11.0	4.5
3.5	15.0	4.5
4	18.0	6.0
5	18.0	7.0

STORAGE (PACKAGING)

Sterile synthetic absorbable braided sutures are presented in a suitable sachet that maintains sterility and allows the withdrawal and use of the sutures in aseptic conditions. The sutures must be stored dry.

They are intended to be used only on the occasion when the sachet is first opened.

Sutures in their individual sachets (primary packaging) are kept in a protective cover (box) which maintains the physical and mechanical properties until the time of use.

The application of appropriate harmonised standards for packaging of medical devices may be considered in addition.

LABELLING

Reference may be made to the appropriate harmonised standards for the labelling of medical devices.

The details strictly necessary for the user to identify the product properly are indicated on or in each sachet (primary packaging) and on the protective cover (box) and include at least:
— gauge number,
— length in centimetres or metres,
— if appropriate, that the needle is detachable,
— name of the product,
— intended use (surgical absorbable suture),
— if appropriate, that the suture is coloured,
— the structure (braided).

Ph Eur

Sterile Synthetic Absorbable Monofilament Sutures

(*Ph Eur monograph 0666*)

Ph Eur

DEFINITION

Sterile synthetic absorbable monofilament sutures consist of sutures prepared from a synthetic polymer, polymers or copolymers which, when introduced into a living organism, are absorbed by that organism and cause no undue tissue irritation. They consist of completely polymerised material.

They occur as monofilament sutures. The sutures may be treated to facilitate handling and they may be coloured.

Appropriate harmonised standards may be considered when assessing compliance with respect to origin and processing of raw materials and with respect to biocompatibility.

Sterile synthetic absorbable monofilament sutures are wound-closure devices. Being absorbable they serve to approximate tissue during the healing period and subsequently lose tensile strength by hydrolysis.

PRODUCTION

The appropriate harmonised standards may apply with respect to appropriate validated methods of sterilisation, environmental control during manufacturing, labelling and packaging.

It is essential for the effectiveness and the performance characteristics during use and during the functional lifetime of these sutures that the following physical properties are specified: consistent diameter, sufficient initial strength and firm needle attachment.

The requirements below have been established, taking into account stresses which occur during normal conditions of use. These requirements can be used to demonstrate that individual production batches of these sutures are suitable for wound closure according to usual surgical techniques.

TESTS

Carry out the following tests on the sutures in the state in which they are removed from the sachet.

Length

Measure the length of the suture without applying more tension than is necessary to keep it straight. The length of each suture is not less than 95 per cent of the length stated on the label and does not exceed 400 cm.

Diameter

Unless otherwise prescribed, measure the diameter by the following method, using five sutures in the condition in which they are presented. Use a suitable instrument cap-able of measuring with an accuracy of at least 0.002 mm and having a circular pressor foot 10 mm to 15 mm in diameter. The pressor foot and the moving parts attached to it are weighted so as to apply a total load of 100 ± 10 g to the suture being tested. When making the measurements, lower the pressor foot slowly to avoid crushing the suture. Measure the diameter at intervals of 30 cm over the whole length of the suture. For a suture less than 90 cm in length, measure at three points approximately evenly spaced along the suture. During the measurement, submit the sutures to a tension not greater than that required to keep them straight. The average of the measurements carried out on the sutures being tested and not less than two-thirds of the measurements taken on each suture are within the limits given in the columns under A in Table 0666.-1 for the gauge number concerned. None of the measurements is outside the limits given in the columns under B in Table 0666.-1 for the gauge number concerned.

Minimum breaking load

The minimum breaking load is determined over a simple knot formed by placing one end of a suture held in the right hand over the other end held in the left hand, passing one end over the suture and through the loop so formed (see Figure 0666.-1) and pulling the knot tight.

Table 0666.-1. – *Diameters and breaking loads*

Gauge number	Diameter (millimetres)				Breaking load (newtons)	
	A		B		C	D
	min.	max.	min.	max.		
0.5	0.050	0.094	0.045	0.125	1.4	0.7
0.7	0.095	0.149	0.075	0.175	2.5	1.3
1	0.150	0.199	0.125	0.225	6.8	3.4
1.5	0.200	0.249	0.175	0.275	9.5	4.7
2	0.250	0.339	0.225	0.375	17.5	8.9
3	0.340	0.399	0.325	0.450	26.8	13.4
3.5	0.400	0.499	0.375	0.550	39.0	18.5
4	0.500	0.570	0.450	0.600	50.8	25.4
5	0.571	0.610	0.500	0.700	63.5	31.8

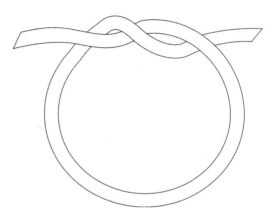

Figure 0666.-1. – *Simple knot*

Carry out the test on five sutures. Submit sutures of length greater than 75 cm to two measurements and shorter sutures to one measurement. Determine the breaking load using a suitable tensilometer. The apparatus has two clamps for holding the suture, one of which is mobile and is driven at a constant rate of 25 cm to 30 cm per minute. The clamps are designed so that the suture being tested can be attached without any possibility of slipping. At the beginning of the test the length of suture between the clamps is 12.5 cm to 20 cm and the knot is midway between the clamps. Set the mobile clamp in motion and note the force required to break the suture. If the suture breaks in a clamp or within 1 cm of it, the result is discarded and the test repeated on another suture. The average of all the results excluding those legitimately discarded is equal to or greater than the value given in column C in Table 0666.-1 and no individual result is less than that given in column D for the gauge number concerned.

Needle attachment

If the suture is supplied with an eyeless needle attached that is not stated to be detachable, the attachment complies with the test for needle attachment. Carry out the test on five sutures. Use a suitable tensilometer, such as that described for the determination of the minimum breaking load. Fix the needle and suture (without knot) in the clamps of the apparatus in such a way that the swaged part of the needle is completely free of the clamp and in line with the direction of pull on the suture. Set the mobile clamp in motion and note the force required to break the suture or to detach it from the needle. The average of the five determinations and all individual values are not less than the respective values given in Table 0666.-2 for the gauge number concerned. If not more than one individual value fails to meet the individual requirement, repeat the test on an additional ten sutures. The attachment complies with the test if none of the ten values is less than the individual value in Table 0666.-2 for the gauge number concerned.

Table 0666.-2. – *Minimum strengths of needle attachment*

Gauge number	Mean value (newtons)	Individual value (newtons)
0.5	0.80	0.40
0.7	1.7	0.80
1	2.3	1.1
1.5	4.5	2.3
2	6.8	3.4
2.5	9.0	4.5
3	11.0	4.5
3.5	15.0	4.5
4	18.0	6.0
5	18.0	7.0

STORAGE (PACKAGING)

Sterile synthetic absorbable monofilament sutures are presented in a suitable sachet that maintains sterility and allows the withdrawal and use of the sutures in aseptic conditions. The sutures must be stored dry.

They are intended to be used only on the occasion when the sachet is first opened.

Sutures in their individual sachets (primary packaging) are kept in a protective cover (box) which maintains the physical and mechanical properties until the time of use.

The application of appropriate harmonised standards for packaging of medical devices may be considered in addition.

LABELLING

Reference may be made to appropriate harmonised standards for the labelling of medical devices.

The details strictly necessary for the user to identify the product properly are indicated on or in each sachet (primary packaging) and on the protective cover (box) and include at least:

— gauge number,
— length in centimetres or metres,
— if appropriate, that the needle is detachable,
— name of the product,
— intended use (surgical absorbable suture),
— if appropriate, that the suture is coloured,
— the structure (monofilament).

———————————————————————————— Ph Eur

Sterile Non-absorbable Sutures

Sterile Non-absorbable Ligatures

(Ph Eur monograph 0324)

NOTE: *The name Nylon 6 as a synonym for Polyamide 6 and Nylon 6/6 as a synonym for Polyamide 6/6 may be used freely in many countries, including the United Kingdom, but exclusive proprietary rights in this name are claimed in certain other countries.*

Ph Eur ———————————————————————————————

DEFINITION

Sterile non-absorbable sutures are sutures which, when introduced into a living organism, are not metabolised by that organism. Sterile non-absorbable sutures vary in origin, which may be animal, vegetable, metallic or synthetic. They occur as cylindrical monofilaments or as multifilament sutures consisting of elementary fibres which are assembled by twisting, cabling or braiding; they may be sheathed; they may be treated to render them non-capillary, and they may be coloured.

Appropriate harmonised standards may be considered when assessing compliance with respect to origin and processing of raw materials and with respect to biocompatibility.

Sterile non-absorbable surgical sutures serve to approximate tissue during the healing period and provide continuing wound support.

Commonly used materials include the following:

Silk

Sterile braided silk suture is obtained by braiding a number of threads, according to the diameter required, of degummed silk obtained from the cocoons of the silkworm *Bombyx mori* L.

Linen

Sterile linen thread consists of the pericyclic fibres of the stem of *Linum usitatissimum* L. The elementary fibres, 2.5 cm to 5 cm long, are assembled in bundles 30 cm to 80 cm long and spun into continuous lengths of suitable diameter.

Poly(ethylene terephthalate)

Sterile poly(ethylene terephthalate) suture is obtained by drawing poly(ethylene terephthalate) through a suitable die. The suture is prepared by braiding very fine filaments in suitable numbers, depending on the gauge required.

Polyamide-6

Sterile polyamide-6 suture is obtained by drawing through a suitable die a synthetic plastic material formed by the polymerisation of ε-caprolactam. It consists of smooth, cylindrical monofilaments or braided filaments, or lightly twisted sutures sheathed with the same material.

Polyamide-6/6

Sterile polyamide-6/6 suture is obtained by drawing through a suitable die a synthetic plastic material formed by the polycondensation of hexamethylenediamine and adipic acid. It consists of smooth, cylindrical monofilaments or braided filaments, or lightly twisted sutures sheathed with the same material.

Polypropylene

Polypropylene suture is obtained by drawing polypropylene through a suitable die. It consists of smooth cylindrical mono-filaments.

Monofilament and multifilament stainless steel

Sterile stainless steel sutures have a chemical composition as specified in ISO 5832-1 - Metallic Materials for surgical implants - Part 1: Specification for wrought stainless steel and comply with ISO 10334 - Implants for surgery - Malleable wires for use as sutures and other surgical applications.

Stainless steel sutures consist of smooth, cylindrical monofilaments or twisted filaments or braided filaments.

Poly(vinylidene difluoride) (PVDF)

Sterile PVDF suture is obtained by drawing through a suitable die a synthetic plastic material which is formed by polymerisation of 1,1-difluorethylene. It consists of smooth cylindrical monofilaments.

IDENTIFICATION

Non-absorbable sutures may be identified by chemical tests. Materials from natural origin may also be identified by microscopic examination of the morphology of these fibres. For synthetic materials, identification by infrared spectrophotometry (*2.2.24*) or by differential scanning calorimetry may be applied.

Identification of silk

A. Dissect the end of a suture, using a needle or fine tweezers, to isolate a few individual fibres. The fibres are sometimes marked with very fine longitudinal striations parallel to the axis of the suture. Examined under a microscope, a cross-section is more or less triangular to semi-circular, with rounded edges and without a lumen.

B. Impregnate isolated fibres with *iodinated potassium iodide solution R*. The fibres are coloured pale yellow.

Identification of linen

A. Dissect the end of a suture, using a needle or fine tweezers, to isolate a few individual fibres. Examined under a microscope, the fibres are seen to be 12 μm to 31 μm wide and, along the greater part of their length, have thick walls, sometimes marked with fine longitudinal striations, and a narrow lumen. The fibres gradually narrow to a long, fine point. Sometimes there are unilateral swellings with transverse lines.

B. Impregnate isolated fibres with *iodinated zinc chloride solution R*. The fibres are coloured violet-blue.

Identification of poly(ethyleneterephthalate)

It is practically insoluble in most of the usual organic solvents, but is attacked by strong alkaline solutions. It is incompatible with phenols.

A. 50 mg dissolves with difficulty when heated in 50 mL of *dimethylformamide R*.

B. To about 50 mg add 10 mL of *hydrochloric acid R1*. The material remains intact even after immersion for 6 h.

Identification of polyamide-6

It is practically insoluble in the usual organic solvents; it is not attacked by dilute alkaline solutions (for example a 100 g/L solution of *sodium hydroxide R*) but is attacked by dilute mineral acids (for example a 20 g/L solution of *sulfuric acid R*), by hot *glacial acetic acid R* and by a 70 per cent *m/m* solution of *anhydrous formic acid R*.

A. Heat about 50 mg with 0.5 mL of *hydrochloric acid R1* in a sealed glass tube at 110 °C for 18 h and allow to stand for 6 h. No crystals appear.

B. 50 mg dissolves in 20 mL of a 70 per cent *m/m* solution of *anhydrous formic acid R*.

Identification of polyamide-6/6

It is practically insoluble in the usual organic solvents; it is not attacked by dilute alkaline solutions (for example a 100 g/L solution of *sodium hydroxide R*) but is attacked by dilute mineral acids (for example a 20 g/L solution of *sulfuric acid R*), by *hot glacial acetic acid R* and by an 80 per cent *m/m* solution of *anhydrous formic acid R*.

A. In contact with a flame it melts and burns, forming a hard globule of residue and gives off a characteristic odour resembling that of celery.

B. Place about 50 mg in an ignition tube held vertically and heat gently until thick fumes are evolved. When the fumes fill the tube, withdraw it from the flame and insert a strip of *nitrobenzaldehyde paper R*. A violet-brown colour slowly appears on the paper and fades slowly in air; it disappears almost immediately on washing with *dilute sulfuric acid R*.

C. To about 50 mg add 10 mL of *hydrochloride acid R1*. The material disintegrates in the cold and dissolves within a few minutes.

D. 50 mg does not dissolve in 20 mL of a 70 per cent *m/m* solution of *anhydrous formic acid R* but dissolves in 20 mL of an 80 per cent *m/m* solution of *anhydrous formic acid R*.

Identification of polypropylene

Polypropylene is soluble in decahydronaphthalene, 1-chloronaphthalene and trichloroethylene. It is not soluble in alcohol, in ether and in cyclohexanone.

A. It softens at temperatures between 160 °C and 170 °C. It burns with a blue flame giving off an odour of burning paraffin wax and of octyl alcohol.

B. To 0.25 g add 10 mL of *toluene R* and boil under a reflux condenser for about 15 min. Place a few drops of the solution on a disc of *sodium chloride R* slide and evaporate the solvent in an oven at 80 °C. Examine by infrared absorption spectrophotometry (*2.2.24*), comparing with the spectrum obtained with *polypropylene CRS*.

C. To 2 g add 100 mL of *water R* and boil under a reflux condenser for 2 h. Allow to cool. The relative density (*2.2.5*) of the material is 0.89 g/mL to 0.91 g/mL, determined using a hydrostatic balance.

Identification of stainless steel

Stainless steel sutures are identified by confirming that the composition is in accordance with ISO 5832 Part 1.

Identification of poly(vinylidene difluoride)

It is soluble in warm dimethylformamide. It is insoluble in ethanol, hot and cold isopropyl alcohol, ethyl acetate, tetrachlorethylene.

A. The strand melts between 170 °C and 180 °C. It melts in a flame and does not burn after removal of the flame. Place a small piece of suture on an annealed copper wire or sheet. Heat in an oxidising flame. No green colour is produced.

B. Dissolve 0.25 g of the suture in 10 mL of *dimethylformamide R* and boil under a reflux condenser for about 15 min. Place a few drops of the solution on a *sodium chloride R* slide and evaporate the solvent in an oven at 80 °C (1 h). Examine by infrared absorption spectrophotometry (*2.2.24*). The spectrum shows absorption maxima at the following wave-numbers: 838.3 ± 0.5 cm^{-1}, 873.3 ± 1 cm^{-1}, 1070.0 ± 2 cm^{-1}, 1165.0 ± 10 cm^{-1}, 1275 ± 0.5 cm^{-1}, 1399 ± 5 cm^{-1}.

C. To 2 g of suture add 100 mL of *water R* and boil under a reflux condenser for 2 h. Allow to cool. The relative density (*2.2.5*) of the material is 1.71 to 1.78.

PRODUCTION

The appropriate harmonised standards may apply with respect to appropriate validated methods of sterilisation, environmental control during manufacturing, labelling and packaging.

It is essential for the effectiveness and the performance characteristics during use and during the functional lifetime of these sutures that the following physical properties are specified: consistent diameter, sufficient initial strength and firm needle attachment.

The requirements below have been established, taking into account stresses which occur during normal conditions of use. These requirements can be used to demonstrate that individual production batches of these sutures are suitable for wound closure in accordance with usual surgical techniques.

TESTS

Remove the sutures from the sachet and measure promptly and in succession the length, diameter and minimum load.

If linen is tested the sutures are conditioned as follows: if stored in the dry state, expose to an atmosphere with a relative humidity of 65 ± 5 per cent at 20 ± 2 °C for 4 h immediately before measuring the diameter and for the determination of minimum breaking load immerse in *water R* at room temperature for 30 min immediately before carrying out the test.

Length

Measure the length without applying more tension than is necessary to keep them straight. The length of the suture is not less than 95 per cent of the length stated on the label and does not exceed 400 cm.

Diameter

Unless otherwise prescribed, measure the diameter by the following method using 5 sutures. Use a suitable mechanical instrument capable of measuring with an accuracy of at least 0.002 mm and having a circular pressor foot 10-15 mm in diameter. The pressor foot and the moving parts attached to it are weighted so as to apply a total load of 100 ± 10 g to the suture being tested. When making the measurements, lower the pressor foot slowly to avoid crushing the suture. Measure the diameter at intervals of 30 cm over the whole length of the suture. For a suture less than 90 cm in length, measure at 3 points approximately evenly spaced along the suture. During the measurement submit monofilament sutures to a tension not greater than that required to keep them straight. Submit multifilament sutures to a tension not greater than one-fifth of the minimum breaking load shown in column C of Table 0324.-1 appropriate to the gauge number and type of material concerned or 10 N whichever is less. Stainless steel sutures do not require tension to be applied during the measurement of diameter.

For multifilament sutures of gauge number above 1.5 make 2 measurements at each point, the second measurement being made after rotating the suture through 90°. The diameter of that point is the average of the 2 measurements. The average of the measurements carried out on the sutures being tested and not less than two-thirds of the measurements taken on each suture are within the limits given in the column under A in Table 0324.-1 for the gauge number concerned. None

Table 0324.-1. – *Diameters and minimum breaking loads*

| Gauge number | Diameter (millimetres) | | | | Minimum breaking load (newtons) | | | | | |
| | A | | B | | Linen thread | | All other non-absorbable strands | | Stainless steel | |
	min.	max.	min.	max.	C	D	C	D	C	D
0.05	0.005	0.009	0.003	0.012	-	-	0.01	-		
0.1	0.010	0.019	0.005	0.025	-	-	0.03	-		
0.15	0.015	0.019	0.012	0.025	-	-	0.06	0.01		
0.2	0.020	0.029	0.015	0.035	-	-	0.1	-		
0.3	0.030	0.039	0.025	0.045	-	-	0.35	0.06		
0.4	0.040	0.049	0.035	0.060	-	-	0.60	0.15	1.1	
0.5	0.050	0.069	0.045	0.085	-	-	1.0	0.35	1.6	
0.7	0.070	0.099	0.060	0.125	1.0	0.3	1.5	0.60	2.7	
1	0.100	0.149	0.085	0.175	2.5	0.6	3.0	1.0	5.3	4.0
1.5	0.150	0.199	0.125	0.225	5.0	1.0	5.0	1.5	8.0	6.0
2	0.200	0.249	0.175	0.275	8.0	2.5	9.0	3.0	13.3	10.0
2.5	0.250	0.299	0.225	0.325	9.0	5.0	13.0	5.0	15.5	11.6
3	0.300	0.349	0.275	0.375	11.0	8.0	15.0	9.0	17.7	13.3
3.5	0.350	0.399	0.325	0.450	15.0	9.0	22.0	13.0	33.4	25.0
4	0.400	0.499	0.375	0.550	18,0	11.0	27.0	15.0	46.7	35.0
5	0.500	0.599	0.450	0.650	26.0	15.0	35.0	22.0	57.9	43.4
6	0.600	0.699	0,.550	0.750	37.0	18.0	50.0	27.0	89.4	67.0
7	0.700	0.799	0.650	0.850	50.0	26.0	62.0	35.0	111.8	83.9
8	0.800	0.899	0.750	0.950	65.0	37.0	73.0	50.0	133.4	100.1
9	0.900	0.999	0.850	1.050					156.0	117.0
10	1.000	1.099	0.950	1.150					178.5	133.9

of the measurements are outside the limits given in the columns under B in Table 0324.-1 for the gauge number concerned.

Minimum breaking load

Unless otherwise prescribed, determine the minimum breaking load by the following method using sutures in the condition in which they are presented. The minimum breaking load is determined over a simple knot formed by placing one end of a suture held in the right hand over the other end held in the left hand, passing one end over the suture and through the loop so formed (see Figure 0324.-1) and pulling the knot tight. For stainless steel sutures gauges 3.5 and above, the minimum breaking load is determined on a straight pull. Carry out the test on 5 sutures. Submit sutures of length greater than 75 cm to 2 measurements and shorter sutures to 1 measurement. Determine the breaking load using a suitable tensilometer. The apparatus has 2 clamps for holding the suture, 1 of which is mobile and is driven at a constant rate of 30 cm/min. The clamps are designed so that the suture being tested can be attached without any possibility of slipping. At the beginning of the test the length of suture between the clamps is 12.5 cm to 20 cm and the knot is midway between the clamps. Set the mobile clamp in motion and note the force required to break the suture. If the suture breaks in a clamp or within 1 cm of it, the result is discarded and the test repeated on another suture. The average of all the results, excluding those legitimately discarded, is equal to or greater than the value given in column C in Table 0324.-1 and no value is less than that given in column D for the gauge number and type of material concerned.

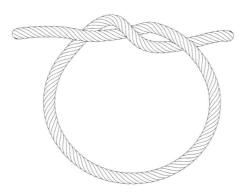

Figure 0324.-1. – *Simple knot*

Needle attachment

If the sutures are supplied with an eyeless needle attached that is not stated to be detachable, they comply with the test for needle attachment. Carry out the test on 5 sutures. Use a suitable tensilometer, such as that described for the determination of the minimum breaking load. Fix the needle and suture (without knot) in the clamps of the apparatus in such a way that the swaged part of the needle is completely free of the clamp and in line with the direction of pull on the suture. Set the mobile clamp in motion and note the force required to break the suture or to detach it from the needle. The average of the 5 determinations and all individual values are not less than the respective values given in Table 0324.-2 for the gauge number concerned. If not more than 1 individual value fails to meet the individual requirement, repeat the test on an additional 10 sutures. The attachment complies with the test if none of these 10 values is less than

the individual value in Table 0324.-2 for the gauge number concerned.

Table 0324.-2. – *Minimum strengths of needle attachment*

Gauge number	Mean value (newtons)	Individual value (newtons)
0.4	0.50	0.25
0.5	0.80	0.40
0.7	1.7	0.80
1	2.3	1.1
1.5	4.5	2.3
2	6.8	3.4
2.5	9.0	4.5
3	11.0	4.5
3.5	15.0	4.5
4	18.0	6.0
5	18.0	7.0
6	25.0	12.5
7	25.0	12.5
8	50.0	25
9	50.0	25
10	75.0	37.5

Extractable colour

Sutures that are dyed and intended to remain so during use comply with the test for extractable colour. Place 0.25 g of the suture to be examined in a conical flask, add 25.0 mL of *water R* and cover the mouth of the flask with a short-stemmed funnel. Boil for 15 min, cool and adjust to the original volume with *water R*. Depending on the colour of the suture, prepare the appropriate reference solution as described in Table 0324.-3 using the primary colour solutions (*2.2.2*).

The test solution is not more intensely coloured than the appropriate reference solution.

Table 0324.-3. – *Colour reference solutions*

Colour of strand	Composition of reference solution (parts by volume)			
	Red primary solution	Yellow primary solution	Blue primary solution	*Water R*
Yellow-brown	0.2	1.2	-	8.6
Pink-red	1.0	-	-	9.0
Green-blue	-	-	2.0	8.0
Violet	1.6	-	8.4	-

Monomer and oligomers

Polyamide-6 suture additionally complies with the following test for monomer and oligomers. In a continuous-extraction apparatus, treat 1.00 g with 30 mL of *methanol R* at a rate of at least 3 extractions per hour for 7 h. Evaporate the extract to dryness, dry the residue at 110 °C for 10 min, allow to cool in a desiccator and weigh. The residue weighs not more than 20 mg (2 per cent).

STORAGE (PACKAGING)

Sterile non-absorbable sutures are presented in a suitable sachet that maintains sterility and allows the withdrawal and use of a suture in aseptic conditions. They may be stored dry or in a preserving liquid to which an antimicrobial agent but no antibiotic may be added.

Sterile non-absorbable sutures are intended to be used only on the occasion when the sachet is first opened.

Sutures in their individual sachets (primary packaging) are kept in a protective cover (box) which maintains the physical and mechanical properties until the time of use.

The application of appropriate harmonised standards for packaging of medical devices shall be considered in addition.

LABELLING

Reference may be made to the appropriate harmonised standards for the labelling of medical devices.

The details strictly necessary for the user to identify the product properly are indicated on or in each sachet (primary packaging) and on the protective cover (box) and include at least:
— gauge number,
— length, in centimetres or metres,
— if appropriate, that the needle is detachable,
— name of the product,
— intended use (surgical suture, non-absorbable),
— if appropriate, that the suture is coloured,
— if appropriate, the structure (braided, monofilament, sheathed).

_____ *Ph Eur*